Grossm
Baim's

Handbook of Cardiac Catheterization, Angiography, and Intervention

MAURO MOSCUCCI | MD, MBA, MPH

Adjunct Professor of Medicine
University of Michigan
Ann Arbor, Michigan

ASSOCIATE EDITOR
MARC D. FELDMAN, MD

Adjunct and Emeritus Professor
University of Texas Health
San Antonio, Texas

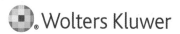. Wolters Kluwer

Philadelphia • Baltimore • New York • London
Buenos Aires • Hong Kong • Sydney • Tokyo

Senior Acquisitions Editor: James Sherman
Senior Development Editor: Ashley Fischer
Editorial Coordinator: Sunmerrilika Baskar
Marketing Manager: Kirsten Watrud
Production Project Manager: Nancy Devaux
Manager, Graphic Arts & Design: Stephen Druding
Manufacturing Coordinator: Bernard Tomboc
Prepress Vendor: TNQ Technologies

First edition

Library of Congress Cataloging-in-Publication Data

ISBN-13: 978-1-4963-9928-1

Cataloging in Publication data available on request from publisher.

This work is provided "as is," and the publisher disclaims any and all warranties, express or implied, including any warranties as to accuracy, comprehensiveness, or currency of the content of this work.

This work is no substitute for individual patient assessment based upon healthcare professionals' examination of each patient and consideration of, among other things, age, weight, gender, current or prior medical conditions, medication history, laboratory data and other factors unique to the patient. The publisher does not provide medical advice or guidance and this work is merely a reference tool. Healthcare professionals, and not the publisher, are solely responsible for the use of this work including all medical judgments and for any resulting diagnosis and treatments.

Given continuous, rapid advances in medical science and health information, independent professional verification of medical diagnoses, indications, appropriate pharmaceutical selections and dosages, and treatment options should be made and healthcare professionals should consult a variety of sources. When prescribing medication, healthcare professionals are advised to consult the product information sheet (the manufacturer's package insert) accompanying each drug to verify, among other things, conditions of use, warnings and side effects and identify any changes in dosage schedule or contraindications, particularly if the medication to be administered is new, infrequently used or has a narrow therapeutic range. To the maximum extent permitted under applicable law, no responsibility is assumed by the publisher for any injury and/or damage to persons or property, as a matter of products liability, negligence law or otherwise, or from any reference to or use by any person of this work.

QUADM0923

To my mentors and colleagues—Bill Grossman and Donald Baim—recognizing their charismatic vision and persistence in creating and sustaining the original textbook and in training and mentoring multiple generations of cardiologists.

And to my wife Adriana and to my children, Alessandra and Matteo, for their love and unwavering support over the many years of my journey in cardiology.

Preface

Since the first coronary angiogram performed by Marvin Sones in 1958 and the first percutaneous transluminal coronary angioplasty performed by Andreas Grundzig in 1977, the use of diagnostic and therapeutic cardiovascular interventions has continued to grow exponentially. New applications include the recent expansion to other vascular beds beyond the coronary artery system and more recently further expansion to the management of structural heart disease. This tremendous expansion has led to the new concept of the heart team, which brings together the expertise of multiple subspecialties including nurses, cardiovascular technicians, interventional cardiologists, cardiac surgeons, vascular surgeons, interventional radiologists, anesthesiologists, and cardiac imaging specialists.

In 2010, I was honored to be asked by Wolters Kluwer to take over as the new editor of *Grossman and Baim's Cardiac Catheterization, Angiography, and Intervention*. Given the tremendous growth of cardiac catheterization, preparing the eighth edition of the textbook was a major effort. The total number of chapters was increased from 34 to 46 and every chapter from the prior edition was updated and expanded with further emphasis on hemodynamic data, hemodynamic tracings, interventions, and images. As the field of interventional cardiology continued to expand, the ninth edition then followed. The "Grossman and Baim's" textbook remains my key reference when I want to review in detail any aspect of cardiac catheterization and intervention. Yet, I often thought about the potential utility of having a concise version, quickly accessible and easy to carry around. Following further discussion with the Wolters Kluwer team, the idea for this handbook was developed.

The purpose of this handbook is to provide a comprehensive, yet easily accessible reference to the entire cardiac team including cardiovascular technologists, nurses, physicians, and fellows in training. The handbook follows the general layout of the Grossman and Baim's textbook, and it includes a total of seven sections. The first section is on general principles and it addresses issues surrounding the imaging chain, radiation safety, complications, adjunctive pharmacotherapy, and legal considerations as well as issues specifically related to cardiovascular technologists and nursing care. Section two, three, and four cover basic techniques, hemodynamic principles, and angiographic techniques. Section five addresses the evaluation of cardiac function, whereas section six and seven are dedicated respectively to special catheter techniques and interventional procedures. Throughout the handbook, a major effort has been made to retain the content of the chapters from the ninth edition of the Grossman and Baim's textbook, and to provide the material in an easily readable, concise format, with an emphasis on figures and tables.

This handbook would not have been possible without the outstanding work of my associate editor, Dr Marc Feldman, who provided enthusiastic support through the project.

I hope that the information provided will be helpful as a quick reference to the entire cardiac team, and eventually it will be beneficial to our patients.

Mauro Moscucci, MD, MBA, MPH
Adjunct Professor of Medicine
University of Michigan
Ann Arbor, Michigan

Acknowledgments

First and foremost, I would like to thank Dr. William Grossman and Dr. Donald Baim for their charismatic mentorship and guidance during my 2 years of training in the early 1990s and for their continued friendship during the following decades. I would also like to thank the entire Wolters Kluwer team, with whom I have been working since 2008. Fran DeStefano, as the Acquisitions Editor of prior editions, had a critical role while I was shaping and planning the eighth edition. Following Fran's retirement, Julie Goolsby, as Acquisitions Editor, and Leanne Vandetty, as Product Manager, provided outstanding assistance for the eighth edition. Sharon Zinner, in her role of Executive Editor, was instrumental in providing support for the ninth edition of the textbook, and for the initial development of this handbook. In addition, I would like to thank Ashley Fischer, for her outstanding assistance and patience as Senior Development Editor through my many projects with Wolters Kluwer, including this handbook, and James Sherman, who as Senior Content Editor for Wolters Kluwer took over the oversight of this project. The incredible support (and patience) of the Wolters Kluwer team is what has made this handbook become true. Finally, I am extremely grateful to all the authors who contributed to the ninth edition of the Grossman and Baim's textbook, as portions of their chapters were retained in the handbook, and to Dr. Paolo Angelini, as the image in the cover was reproduced with permission from his classic textbook on coronary artery anomalies (Angelini P. Coronary Artery Anomalies: A Comprehensive Approach. Philadelphia, PA: Lippincott Williams & Wilkins; 1999).

Contents

SECTION I
General Principles

1

Cardiac Catheterization History and Current Practice Standards[1]

As Andre Cournand remarked in his Nobel lecture of December 11, 1956, "the cardiac catheter was ... the key in the lock." By turning this key, Cournand and his colleagues led us into a new era in the understanding of normal and disordered cardiac function in humans.

According to Cournand, cardiac catheterization was first performed (and so named) by Claude Bernard in 1844. The subject was a horse, and both the right and left ventricles were entered by a retrograde approach from the jugular vein and carotid artery. However, it is Reverend Stephen Hales who perhaps can be credited with the first invasive hemodynamic assessment, as he measured the blood pressure of a horse by inserting a brass rod in the femoral artery and observing the column of blood rising in a 9-foot glass tube connected to the brass rod. In further experiments, which he published in 1733, he proceeded toward identifying how much blood goes through the heart in 1 minute and determining the capacity of the left ventricle.

Following the initial studies by Claude Bernard, in 1861 Chaveau and Marey published their work on the measurement of intracardiac pressure. They performed the first simultaneous measurement of left ventricular (LV) and central aortic pressures, and they determined that ventricular systole and apical beat are simultaneous.

Werner Forssmann is credited with performing the first cardiac catheterization of a living person—himself. At the age of 25 years, while receiving clinical training in surgery in Germany, he passed a 65-cm catheter through one of his left antecubital veins, guiding it by fluoroscopy until it entered his right atrium. He then walked to the radiology department (which was on a different level, where the catheter position was documented by a chest roentgenogram; **Figure 1.1**). During the next 2 years, Forssmann continued to perform catheterization experiments. Bitter criticism, based on an unsubstantiated belief in the danger of his experiments, caused Forssmann to eventually pursue a different career as a urologist. Nevertheless, for his contribution and foresight, he shared the Nobel Prize in Medicine with Andre Cournand and Dickinson Richards in 1956.

Others appreciated the potential of using Forssmann's technique as a diagnostic tool. The next four decades were characterized by major advances in our understanding of cardiac physiology and heart disease through the application of cardiac catheterization (**Table 1.1**).

The introduction by Andreas Gruntzig in 1977 of percutaneous transluminal coronary angioplasty (PTCA) and the more recent development of new techniques for the treatment of structural heart disease have further expanded the use of cardiac catheterization to therapeutic interventions and spearheaded its exponential growth.

---

[1]We gratefully acknowledge the Grossman & Baim's *Cardiac Catheterization, Angiography, and Intervention*, 9th edition contributions of Dr. Mauro Moscucci, as portions of the chapter, Cardiac Catheterization History and Current Practice Standard, were retained in this text.

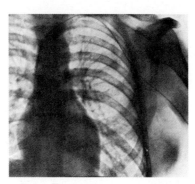

Figure 1.1 The first documented cardiac catheterization. At the age of 25 y, while receiving clinical instruction in surgery at Eberswalde, Werner Forssmann passed a catheter 65 cm through one of his left antecubital veins until its tip entered the right atrium. He then walked to the radiology department where this roentgenogram was taken. (From Forssmann W. Die Sondierung des Rechten Herzens. *Klin Wochenschr.* 1929;8:2085.)

INDICATIONS FOR CARDIAC CATHETERIZATION

As performed today, cardiac catheterization is a combined hemodynamic and angiographic procedure undertaken for diagnostic and therapeutic purposes. Indications for the use of catheterization and coronary intervention in the management of stable angina, unstable angina, and ST-elevation myocardial infarction (MI) have been developed by the American College of Cardiology (ACC) and the American Heart Association (AHA) and are available online at https://www.acc.org/Guidelines (accessed May 13, 2023).

The basic principle is that cardiac catheterization is recommended to confirm the presence of a clinically suspected condition, define its anatomic and physiologic severity, and determine the presence or absence of associated conditions when a therapeutic intervention is planned in a symptomatic patient. The most common indication for cardiac catheterization today thus consists of patients with an acute coronary ischemic syndrome (unstable angina or acute MI) and patients with structural heart disease in whom an invasive therapeutic percutaneous or surgical intervention is contemplated. Whether *all* patients being considered for heart surgery should undergo preoperative cardiac catheterization and coronary angiography has been the topic of debate. The introduction of computed tomography coronary angiography has provided a less invasive approach to the evaluation of low-risk patients undergoing valve surgery. According to the ACC/AHA 2020 Guideline for the Management of Patients with Valvular Heart Disease, "In selected patients with a low to intermediate pretest probability of CAD, contrast-enhanced coronary CT angiography is reasonable to exclude the presence of significant obstructive CAD (Class of Recommendation 2a; Level of Evidence B)." However, current guidelines still recommend cardiac catheterization in patients who might be at higher risk of coronary artery disease independent of age, or in patients for whom additional information might be required.

Catheterization data can also inform other nonsurgical therapeutic considerations. For example, although a clinical diagnosis of primary pulmonary hypertension can often be made by echocardiography, cardiac catheterization is usually required (1) to confirm the diagnosis and (2) to assess potential responsiveness to pharmacologic agents.

Table 1.1 Cardiac Catheterization: Historic Milestones

1733—Stephen Hales. Measurement of blood pressure of a horse.

1844—Claude Bernard. Right and left retrograde cardiac catheterization. It was described in 2 volumes, the first *Chaleur animal*" and the second *Physiologie animal* published in 1876.

1861—Chaveau and Marey. Measurement of intracardiac pressure. Determination that ventricular systole and apical beat are simultaneous. First simultaneous measurement of LV and central aortic pressures

1929—Werner Forssmann. Right heart catheterization in human heart

1931—Werner Forssmann. Injection of contrast material in the human heart

1930—Klein. Measurement of cardiac output in man according to the Fick principle

1932—Padillo. Right heart catheterization and measurement of cardiac output in 2 subjects

1941—1950s—Cournand and Richards. Cardiac catheterization in many clinical conditions including hypertension, circulatory shock and chronic lung disease

1947—Dexter. Studies on congenital heart disease. Catheter passed to the distal pulmonary artery. Oxygen saturation and pulmonary wedge position.

1950—Zimmerman and others; Limon-Lason and Bouchard. Retrograde left heart catheterization.

1953—Seldinger. Development of the percutaneous (rather than cutdown) technique.

1958—Mason Sones. First coronary angiography

1959—Ross and Cope. Transseptal catheterization

1962—Ricketts and Abrams. Coronary angiography modification for a percutaneous approach.

1967—Judkins. Transfemoral percutaneous coronary angiography.

1970—Swan and Ganz. Balloon-tipped, flow-guided catheter techniques

1977—Gruntzig. **P**ercutaneous **t**ransluminal **c**oronary **a**ngioplasty (PTCA)

Research

On occasion, cardiac catheterization is performed primarily as a research proce-dure. Research often relates to the evaluation of new therapeutic devices in patients who would be undergoing diagnostic and therapeutic catheterization in any event. All such studies require prior approval of the U.S. Food and Drug Administration (FDA) in the form of an Investigational Device Exemption, of the local Committee on Human Research at the institution (Institutional Review Board, or IRB), and attain-ment of informed consent after the details of the risks and potential benefits of the procedure and its alternatives have been thoroughly explained. Doing such research requires meticulous attention to protocol details, inclusion/exclusion criteria, data collection, and prompt reporting of any complications.

Catheterization can also be performed solely for the purpose of a research investigation (as a 6-month follow-up angiogram or intravascular coronary ultrasound imaging after a new stent might be). Such studies should be carried out only by an experienced investigator who is expert in cardiac catheterization, using a protocol that has been carefully scrutinized and approved by the IRB at the investigator's institution.

Contraindications

Over the years, the concepts of contraindications have been modified by the fact that patients with acute MI, cardiogenic shock, intractable ventricular tachycardia, and other extreme conditions now tolerate cardiac catheterization and coronary angiography surprisingly well.

At present, the only *absolute* contraindication to cardiac catheterization is the refusal of a mentally competent patient to consent to the procedure. Relative contraindications to cardiac catheterization are listed in **Table 1.2**. For example, hypertension increases predisposition to ischemia, pulmonary edema, or bleeding and should be controlled before and during catheterization. Other conditions that should be controlled before elective catheterization include intercurrent febrile illness, decompensated left heart failure, active bleeding, digitalis toxicity, and hypokalemia. Unexplained worsening renal function is a strong indication to postpone cardiac catheterization, given the associated high risk of acute renal failure following administration of radiographic contrast in this context. Allergy to radiographic contrast agent is a relative contraindication to cardiac angiography, but proper premedication and use of low-osmolar contrast agents can substantially reduce the risks of a major adverse reaction, as discussed in Chapters 2 and 4.

Anticoagulant therapy is more controversial as a contraindication. The view regarding oral anticoagulants (eg, warfarin) that it is best to reverse the prolonged prothrombin time to an international normalized ratio of <2 (and in most labs to <1.5) before cardiac catheterization represents a complex problem. This is best done by withholding warfarin for 3 to 5 days before the procedure, potentially switching to subcutaneous low-molecular-weight heparin or intravenous heparin for a strong anticoagulant indication (eg, atrial fibrillation, a mechanical heart valve). If more rapid reversal of oral anticoagulation is required, fresh frozen plasma (FFP) is commonly used. We reserve its use only for clinical conditions where urgent reversal is indicated, as administration of FFP requires a high-volume load and it is associated with a low, though not insignificant, risk of infections and of transfusion-related acute lung injury (TRALI). Prothrombin complex concentrates (PCCs) have been introduced as a new option to reverse anticoagulation in patients receiving warfarin. They have the advantage of rapid reversal, have no association with TRALI, and require administration of a significantly lower volume when compared with FFP. However, the major drawback with PCCs has been the risk of thrombotic complications. Their use in reversing oral anticoagulation prior to cardiac catheterization has not been assessed.

Factors Influencing the Choice of Approach

Certain approaches to cardiac catheterization have only historical interest (transbronchial approach, posterior transthoracic left atrial puncture, suprasternal puncture of the left atrium).

The great vessels and all cardiac chambers can be entered in nearly all cases by percutaneous approach from various sites including femoral or radial arteries, femoral or internal jugular veins, transseptal catheterization of the left heart, and apical puncture of the left ventricular apex. The choice depends on patient issues (aortic occlusion,

Table 1.2 **Relative Contraindications to Cardiac Catheterization and Angiography**

Condition	Increased Risk
Hyperkalemia, hypokalemia, or digitalis toxicity	Arrhythmias
Uncontrolled hypertension	Bleeding, hemorrhagic stroke following anticoagulation, heart failure, and myocardial ischemia during angiography
Febrile illness	Infection
Ongoing anticoagulation with warfarin (INR >1.5 commonly used as a cutoff)	Bleeding
Severe thrombocytopenia. The general consensus is that a platelet count of 40,000/mL to 50,000/mL is sufficient to perform major invasive procedures with safety, in the absence of associated coagulation abnormalities.[a]	Bleeding
History of severe allergy to contrast media	Life-threatening anaphylactoid reactions
Decompensated heart failure	Pulmonary edema following contrast administration. Inability to lay flat during the procedure
Severe renal insufficiency and or anuria, unless dialysis is planned to remove fluid and as renal replacement therapy	Volume overload and pulmonary edema, nephropathy requiring dialysis
Worsening renal function: unexplained or following radiocontrast administration	Acute renal failure requiring dialysis
Active bleeding including gastrointestinal bleeding	Major bleeding secondary to administration of antiplatelets and antithrombotic agents

INR, international normalized ratio.
[a]Schiffer A, Anderson KC, Bennett CL, et al. Platelet transfusion for patients with cancer: clinical practice guidelines of the american society of clinical oncology. *J Clin Oncol*. 2001;19:1519-1538.

morbid obesity), procedural issues (need for use of larger bore catheters), and patient/operator preference. Ideally, the physician performing cardiac catheterization should be well versed in several of these methods. More recently, the radial artery approach has become the preferred approach of many operators (Chapter 7). It appears to have a lower complication rate when compared to femoral artery access and allows early ambulation. In general, the radial artery is the preferred approach in any setting that might increase the risk of bleeding, including, among others, morbid obesity or the need to resume anticoagulation following a diagnostic or therapeutic procedure.

DESIGN OF THE CATHETERIZATION PROTOCOL
Every cardiac catheterization should have a protocol, that is, a carefully reasoned sequential plan designed specifically for the individual patient.

Certain general principles should be considered in the design of a protocol if it includes hemodynamic measurements. First, hemodynamic measurements should generally precede angiographic studies, so that crucial pressure and flow measurements may be made as close as possible to the basal state. Second, pressures and selected oxygen saturations should be measured and recorded in each chamber "on the way in," that is, immediately after the catheter enters and before it is directed toward the next chamber. If a problem should develop during the later stages of a catheterization procedure (atrial fibrillation or other arrhythmia, pyrogen reaction, hypotension, or reaction to contrast material), it will be beneficial to have the pressures and saturations already measured in advance, rather than waiting until the time of catheter pullback. Third, measurements of pressure and cardiac output (using true Fick, Fick with estimated oxygen consumption, or thermodilution) should be made as simultaneously as possible.

Beyond these general guidelines, the protocol will reflect differences from patient to patient and factor in changes when unexpected findings are encountered (eg, finding an unexpected marked elevation of LV end diastolic pressure may cause addition of a right heart catheterization to the protocol).

In a patient with an elevated creatinine in whom coronary intervention is anticipated, the LV angiogram should be replaced by a noninvasive evaluation of ventricular function and even the number of baseline coronary injections should be limited. With regard to angiography, it is important to limit contrast injections to the most important diagnostic considerations in a given patient.

The Checklist

Checklists are commonly used (and are often a necessity) in several industries and professions. They allow a detailed breakdown of the process in each individual component and prevent skipping key steps, which could result in an adverse outcome. The field of interventional cardiology, with its evolution toward the execution of more complex procedures requiring the expertise and interaction of multiple subspecialties, is an ideal area for an effective use of checklists. **Figure 1.2** illustrates a simple checklist for patients referred for invasive procedures.

Preparation and Premedication of the Patient

Current guidelines by the American Society of Anesthesiologists recommend a minimum of 2 hours fasting period after clear liquids, and 6 hours after a light meal. Complete vital signs should be recorded before the patient leaves the floor (for inpatients), or shortly after arriving at the ambulatory center (for outpatients).

Once the question of indications and contraindications has been dealt with and the patient's consent obtained, attention can be directed toward the matter of premedications. Antibiotic prophylaxis can be considered if there have been any breaks in sterile technique, in immunocompromised patients, or if a vascular closure device is being used in a patient with diabetes mellitus. Antibiotic prophylaxis is also commonly used prior to implantation of certain devices, such as atrial septal or ventricular septal defect occluders, percutaneous aortic valves, and electrophysiology devices. A single dose of a cephalosporin administered 30 to 60 minutes prior to the procedure is adequate in providing suitable tissue concentrations for several hours. As an alternative, vancomycin can be used although the recommendation is that it should be given 120 minutes prior to the procedure.

Various sedatives have been used for premedication. Patient's state of alertness and need for sedation is assessed once they are on the catheterization table. Per conscious sedation guidelines, small, repeated doses of midazolam (Versed) 0.5 to

Patient name	MRN	Procedure date	
Planned Procedure: (circle all that apply)	Diagnostic Cardiac Catheterization (L, R, simultaneous) Coronary angiography Left ventriculography Intravascular Imaging/Hemodynamic Assessment (IVUS, OCT, FFR) Possible PCI Planned PCI Other		
History and Physical Examination:			
Elective Outpatient Procedures: H&P documented with in 30 days?		Yes	No
Inpatient Procedures: H&P documented within 24 hours of admission?		Yes	No
History of prior PCI or CABG: Yes No If yes, report/s obtained?		Yes	No
Stress test/LVSF assessment: Yes No If yes, report/s obtained?		Yes	No
Candidacy for DES:			
1. Major surgery in the past month or next year?		Yes	No
2. Is there any clinically overt or suspected bleeding?		Yes	No
3. Is patient on chronic anticoagulation (e.g., warfarin, TSOAC)?		Yes	No
4. Is there history of/anticipated medication non-adherence?		Yes	No
Allergies:			
1. Contrast: Yes No If yes, was the patient pretreated?		Yes	No
2. Aspirin: Yes No If yes, was the patient desensitized?		Yes	No
3. Heparin (HIT) Yes No If yes, consider alternative anti-thrombotic agents (DTI)			
4. Latex Yes No If yes, remove all latex products from procedural use			
Medications:			
1. Did patient take aspirin within the past 24 h?		Yes	No
2. Did patient take clopidogrel, prasugrel, or ticagrelor within the past 24 h?		Yes	No
3. Did patient take metformin within the past 24 h?		Yes	No
4. Did patient take sildenafil (or other PDE5 inhibitor) within the past 24 h?		Yes	No
5. Did patient receive LMWH within the past 12 h?		Yes	No
If yes for LMWH, time of last dose _____			
6. Did patient take anticoagulants		Yes	No
If yes, which agent _____ and when was last dose _____			
Informed Consent:			
Was informed consent obtained within 30 days?		Yes	No
Is there a healthcare proxy?		Yes	No
Is the patient DNR or DNI?		Yes	No
If Yes, was it revoked for procedure?		Yes	No
Sedation, Anesthesia and Analgesia:			
Are ASA and Mallampati Class documented?		Yes	No
Is there any contraindication to sedation present?		Yes	No
Risk scores applied?		Yes	No
Bleeding		Yes	No
CIN		Yes	No
Mortality		Yes	No
Laboratories and Studies:			
CBC and renal profile within 30 days (outpatient) or 24 h (inpatient)?		Yes	No
Hgb _____			
eGFR _____			
Was ECG performed within 24 h?		Yes	No
PT/INR performed within 24 h (for patients on warfarin)?		Yes	No
INR ≤ 1.8?		Yes	No
Urine/serum hcg in woman of childbearing age?		Yes	No
Does the patient require preprocedure hydration?		Yes	No
Preferred vascular access:		R L TR TF	
Same Day Discharge candidate?		Yes	No

Figure 1.2 Example of a simple nursing checklist for patients referred for cardiac catheterization or any other invasive procedure. The checklist can be easily included in the workflow when using either paper charts or a full electronic medical record. ASA, American Society of Anesthesiologists; CABG, coronary artery bypass graft; CBC, complete blood count; CIN, contrast-induced nephropathy;

Figure 1.2 Continued

DES, drug-eluting stents; DNI, Do Not Intubate; DNR, Do Not Resuscitate; DTI, direct thrombin inhibitor; ECG, electrocardiogram; eGFR, estimated glomerular filtration rate; FFR, fractional flow reserve; H&P, history and physical; hcg, human chorionic gonadotropin; Hgb, hemoglobin; HIT, heparin-induced thrombocytopenia; INR, international normalized ratio; IVUS, intravascular ultrasound; L, left; LMWH, low-molecular-weight heparin; LVSF, left ventricular systolic function; MRN, medical record number; OCT, optical coherence tomography; PCI, percutaneous coronary intervention; PDE5, phosphodiesterase 5; PT, prothrombin; R, right; TF, trans femoral; TR= trans radial; TSOAC, target-specific oral anticoagulant. (Reproduced with permission from Naidu SS, Aronow HD, Box LC, et al. SCAI expert consensus statement: 2016 best practices in the cardiac catheterization laboratory – (Endorsed by the Cardiological Society of India, and sociedad Latino Americana de Cardiologia intervencionista; Affirmation of value by the Canadian Association of Interventional Cardiology - Association canadienne de cardiologie d'intervention). *Catheter Cardiovasc Interv.* 2016;88:407-423.)

1.0 mg intravenously and/or fentanyl 25 to 50 mg intravenously are administered to maintain a comfortable but arousable state. Premedication of patients with prior history of allergic reactions to contrast media is listed in Chapter 4.

Universal Protocol and Time-Out

In 2002, the Joint Commission established the National Patient Safety Goals program aimed toward addressing specific areas of concern related to patient safety. The "Universal Protocol" is focused on preventing "wrong-site/wrong-surgery" through implementation of a standardized protocol. The Universal Protocol includes the time-out, which involves communication among the immediate members of the procedure team before the beginning of the procedure: the individual performing the procedure, anesthesia providers, circulating nurse, operating room technician, and other active participants who will be participating in the procedure from the beginning. A fire risk assessment should also be included in the Universal Protocol and time-out, as fire risk can be an issue with hybrid procedures performed in the modern cardiac catheterization suite. Details of the time-out are listed in **Table** 1.3.

THE CARDIAC CATHETERIZATION FACILITY

The modern cardiac catheterization laboratory has been evolving toward the new concept of the "hybrid suite" and today requires an area ranging from 850 to 1500 square feet, within which will be housed a conglomeration of highly sophisticated electronic and radiographic equipment (**Figure** 1.3). Reports of the Inter-Society Commission for Heart Disease Resources on optimal resources for cardiac catheterization facilities have been published and updated from 1971 through 2018.

A recent Society for Coronary Angiography & Interventions statement on best practices in the cardiac catheterization laboratory has further expanded the focus on the optimal catheterization laboratory team and periprocedural best practices (see *Suggested Readings*).

Location Within a Hospital vs Freestanding

The issue of whether cardiac catheterization laboratories should be hospital based, freestanding, or mobile has been the subject of much debate. In agreement with the observed reduction in the risk of adverse outcomes that has been observed over the past 2 decades, the Centers for Medicare & Medicaid Services (CMS) January 2019 Update of the Ambulatory Surgical Center (ASC) Payment System has included 11 cardiac catheterization procedures, "which are not expected to pose a significant risk to beneficiary safety when performed in an ASC, and would not be expected to require

Table 1.3 **Time-Out (The Joint Commission Hospital National Patient Safety Goals Effective January 1, 2020—Elements of Performance for UP.01.03.01)**

1	Conduct a time-out immediately before starting the invasive procedure or making the incision.	
2	The time-out has the following characteristics:	• It is standardized, as defined by the hospital. • It is initiated by a designated member of the team. • It involves the immediate members of the procedure team, including the individual performing the procedure, the anesthesia providers, the circulating nurse, the operating room technician, and other active participants who will be participating in the procedure from the beginning.
3	When two or more procedures are being performed on the same patient, and the person performing the procedure changes, perform a time-out before each procedure is initiated.	
4	During the time-out, the team members agree, at a minimum, on the following:	• Correct patient identity • The correct site • The procedure to be done
5	Document the completion of the time-out.	*Note: The hospital determines the amount and type of documentation.*

UP, Universal Protocol.
Based on National Patient Safety Goals Effective January 2020. *The Joint Commission website.* https://www.jointcommission.org/-/media/tjc/documents/standards/national-patient-safety-goals/2020/npsg_chapter_ahc_jan2020.pdf

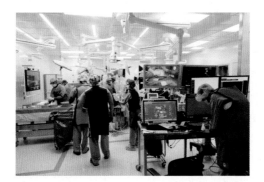

Figure 1.3 Modern cardiac catheterization suite. Multimodality imaging hybrid room that can be transformed into an operating room and used for procedures requiring an open access approach such as the transapical approach for transcatheter aortic valve implantation.

active medical monitoring and care of the beneficiary at midnight following the pro-cedure." The list can be accessed at https://www.cms.gov/Outreach-and-Education/Medicare-Learning-Network-MLN/MLNMattersArticles/downloads/MM11108.pdf (accessed May 13, 2023).

Immediately available cardiac surgical backup can be critical for laboratories that perform diagnostic catheterization on unstable or high-risk patients, as well as for those that perform coronary angioplasty, endomyocardial biopsy, or transseptal catheterization. As of today, several states allow performance of acute MI and even elective coronary intervention in hospitals without on-site cardiac surgery and in ambulatory surgery centers, as long as it is performed by operators active at other sites and with a formal plan for transfer within 1 hour to a facility with cardiac sur-gery on-site (eg, an ambulance standing by, and an agreement with a nearby surgical facility to provide timely backup if needed).

Outpatient Cardiac Catheterization

Outpatient cardiac catheterization has been demonstrated by a variety of groups to be safe, practical, and highly cost-efficient and is now widely practiced throughout the world. Outpatient catheterization can be accomplished by the radial, brachial, or femoral approaches, which allow the patient to be ambulatory within minutes of the completion of the catheterization study. For femoral procedures, hemostasis can be obtained by manual compression for 10 minutes over the femoral artery, followed by bed rest for 2 to 4 hours, or use of a femoral closure device (see Chapter 6) with 1 to 2 hours of bed rest before discharge. More recently, several studies have shown that outpatient percutaneous coronary intervention (PCI) with same day discharge is safe and feasible in selected patients. As a result, in November 2019, the CMS issued its final rule on PCI and approved the addition of 6 PCI CPT (Current Procedural Terminology) codes to the ASC-covered procedures list.

TRAINING STANDARDS

Training in the performance and interpretation of hemodynamic and angiographic data derived from cardiac catheterization is an important part of fellowship training in cardiovascular disease. The most recent Core Cardiology Training Statement in cardiac catheterization (COCATS 4) calls for a minimum of 4 months of diagnos-tic catheterization experience (100 cases, level 1), with an additional 8 months of catheterization experience (200 additional cases, level 2) for individuals wishing to perform *diagnostic catheterization* in practice, within the basic 3-year cardiovascular disease fellowship. Level 3 advanced training in interventional cardiac catheteriza-tion requires 12 months of additional training and the performance of 250 PCI as primary operator.

In 1999, the Accreditation Council for Graduate Medical Education (ACGME) established the structural, content, and faculty requirements for creating an accred-ited fellowship in interventional cardiology, requiring an additional 12 months beyond the 3-year general cardiovascular training period, during which at least 250 interventional procedures should be performed.

In parallel, the American Board of Internal Medicine (ABIM) recognized the body of knowledge subsumed by interventional cardiology by offering a voluntary 1-day proctored examination to individuals who met certain eligibility requirements—documented prior performance of 500 coronary interventions (the practice path-way, no longer open after 2003), or completion of an ACGME-approved inter-ventional fellowship (the fellowship pathway). Candidates able to pass this examination receive Board Certification via a Certificate of Additional Qualification in interventional cardiology (**Table 1.4**). Several thousand individuals continue to

Table 1.4 Medical Content, Sample Topics, and Relative Percentage Included in the Interventional Cardiology Board Exam

Medical Content	Topics	Relative Percentage
Case selection and management	Chronic ischemic heart disease and acute coronary syndromes (clinical characteristics [demographics and comorbidities], laboratory abnormalities and cardiac catheterization [hematology, coagulation, and chemistry], renal insufficiency and cardiac catheterization, noninvasive testing before diagnostic catheterization, selection of treatment modality, interventional therapy, surgical therapy, medical therapy, preoperative cardiac evaluation for noncardiac surgery, preoperative revascularization before noncardiac surgery), unstable angina and non–ST-segment elevation myocardial infarction (UA and NSTEMI) (evaluation and risk stratification of the UA and NSTEMI patient, UA/NSTEMI—pharmacologic management, UA/NSTEMI—timing of cardiac catheterization, UA/NSTEMI—percutaneous coronary intervention [PCI]), ST-segment elevation myocardial infarction (STEMI) (STEMI systems of care, primary PCI—procedure, primary PCI—stents, primary PCI—thrombectomy, primary PCI—outcomes, right ventricular infarction, multivessel PCI, primary PCI following cardiopulmonary arrest, STEMI—differential diagnosis, acute aortic dissection, therapeutic hypothermia, fibrinolytic therapy, transfer for PCI, rescue PCI, surgical therapy in STEMI, medical management after STEMI), STEMI complications (shock, electrophysiologic complications, emergency pacing, acute respiratory distress, mechanical complications [mitral regurgitation (MR), ventricular septal defect (VSD), rupture, pseudoaneurysm], advanced cardiovascular life support [ACLS]).	20%
Procedural techniques	Planning and execution of interventional procedures (general decision-making for access-site selection, radial access, femoral access, other access sites [ulnar, brachial], vascular access closure devices, pericardiocentesis, right heart catheterization, right ventricular biopsy), lesion subsets (ostial, bifurcation, long, tortuous, calcified, restenosis, complex, single-vessel disease, multivessel disease, saphenous vein graft disease, coronary artery bridge, PCI in the anomalous coronary, left main, chronic total occlusion), selection and use of equipment (guiding catheters, guidewires, balloon catheters, bare metal stents, drug-eluting stents rotational atherectomy, embolic protection devices, intra-aortic balloon pump counterpulsation, Impella, TandemHeart PTVA, extracorporeal membrane oxygenation [ECMO]), PCI technical troubleshooting and problem-solving (failure to engage guide catheter, to cross lesion with guidewire, to cross lesion with device, to dilate lesion).	20%

(Continued)

Table 1.4 Medical Content, Sample Topics, and Relative Percentage Included in the Interventional Cardiology Board Exam (Continued)

Medical Content	Topics	Relative Percentage
Complications of coronary intervention	Cardiac (coronary dissection, abrupt closure of coronary artery, stent thrombosis, coronary thromboembolism, air embolism, no reflow, periprocedural myocardial infarction, perforation, tamponade), noncardiac (systemic thromboembolism, cerebrovascular complications, bleeding and hemorrhage, vascular access and major vessel dissection, aortic dissection [due to PC]), acute limb ischemia).	8%
Catheter-based management of noncoronary disease	Hemodynamics (arterial pressure evaluation, right heart catheterization, valvular stenosis, valvular regurgitation, shunt quantification), evaluation and case selection in structural and valvular heart disease (structural heart disease, mitral valve, aortic valve, pulmonic valve, tricuspid valve, hypertrophic cardiomyopathy, patent foramen ovale atrial septal defect, coarctation, ventricular septal defect), evaluation and case selection in noncardiac vascular disease (carotid disease, subclavian disease, aortic disease, chronic aortic dissection, renal artery stenosis, iliac and femoral arterial disease, peripheral interventional therapy, ankle-brachial index).	13%
Basic science	Vascular biology (normal vascular biology, atherosclerosis, atherosclerotic plaque, vascular injury, vasoreactivity, reperfusion injury, effects of diabetes mellitus, restenosis after balloon percutaneous transluminal coronary angioplasty [PTCA], restenosis after stent PCI, vascular remodeling, microvascular dysfunction), physiology (clotting cascade, platelet function, thrombosis and thrombolysis, lipid metabolism, and lipid abnormalities).	6%
Anatomy, anatomic variants, anatomic pathology	Cardiac (normal coronary anatomy, dominance, anomalous left circumflex, anomalous left coronary, anomalous right coronary, indications for surgery for coronary anomalies, collateral vessels, coronary fistulae, coronary ectasia and aneurysm, other anatomic abnormalities, angiographic assessment of coronary flow [Thrombolysis In Myocardial Infarction (TIMI) Trial flow grade, TIMI frame count], angiographic assessment of microcirculation [TIMI myocardial perfusion grade], flow and perfusion effects of arterial spasm or microembolization, left ventriculography, left ventricular dysfunction—stunning and hibernation, takotsubo syndrome, surgical shunts and baffles), extracardiac (aortic arch anatomy and variants, arterial anatomy of the cerebral vessels, arterial anatomy of the upper extremities and variants, arterial anatomy of the abdominal vessels, arterial anatomy of the lower extremities and variants, superior vena cava [SVC] and inferior vena cava [IVC] anatomy and variants).	6%

Table 1.4 **Medical Content, Sample Topics, and Relative Percentage Included in the Interventional Cardiology Board Exam (Continued)**

Medical Content	Topics	Relative Percentage
Pharmacology	General (vasopressors, inotropes, vasodilators, moderate sedation, reversal agents, local anesthetic agents, drug-eluting stent [DES] compounds, fibrinolytic agents, antiarrhythmic agents, antianginal agents, antilipid agents), intravenous antiplatelet agents, (abciximab, eptifibatide, tirofiban, cangrelor), oral antiplatelet agents (aspirin, clopidogrel, prasugrel, ticagrelor, cilostazol, vorapaxar), platelet function testing (genotype and phenotype), intravenous anticoagulants (unfractionated heparin, low-molecular-weight heparins, bivalirudin), oral anticoagulants (warfarin, novel oral anticoagulants), contrast agents (contrast physics, osmolality and other properties, contrast-induced nephropathy, contrast allergy, and anaphylactoid reactions).	12%
Cardiac imaging and assessment	General tests (stress testing, stress test imaging, transthoracic echocardiography, transesophageal echocardiography, intracardiac echocardiography, magnetic resonance imaging, computed tomography angiography [CTA], structural cardiac imaging), diagnostic coronary imaging (catheter shapes and sizes, angiographic views and techniques, coronary lesion morphology [plaque, stenosis, thrombus], fractional flow reserve [FFR], instantaneous wave-free ratio [IFR], volumetric flow rate [VFR] and coronary flow reserve [CFR], intravascular ultrasonography [IVUS], optical coherence tomography [OCT], vulnerable plaque imaging), x-ray radiography (radiation physics and safety, radiographic imaging chain, radiation exposure parameters, risks, injury, and methods of control, equipment operation, and imaging techniques).	9%
Miscellaneous	Ethical and legal issues and risks (patient consent, patient safety, ethics and professionalism, documentation requirements for operative and invasive procedures), procedure-related data (statistics and literature interpretation, epidemiology, cost, cost-effectiveness, and quality of life), quality of care and appropriateness (clinical quality measurement and performance improvement, appropriate use criteria [AUC], adverse event reporting, and device surveillance).	6%

Adapted from American Board of Internal Medicine. *Interventional Cardiology Certification Examination Blue Print*. ABIM website. Accessed October 11, 2021. https://www.abim.org/Media/gaendtbx/interventional-cardiology.pdf

perform interventional procedures without the benefit of such certification or do not recertify after expiration of the initial certification. However, many hospitals today require active certification for renewal of privileges.

As the field of interventional cardiology expands, it is increasingly recognized that knowledge and skill in coronary intervention do not necessarily confer the ability to safely perform *peripheral* vascular intervention. Some content relating to peripheral vascular procedures is tested in the interventional exam, but individuals interested in performing complex lower extremity or carotid intervention are increasingly undertaking an additional training period after their interventional fellowship to gain the necessary skills and experience. This training should occur under the proctorship of a formally trained vascular interventionalist and includes some degree of training in vascular medicine and noninvasive testing for peripheral vascular disease. Certifications by a general examination in vascular medicine and an endovascular specialty examination are available through the American Board of Vascular Medicine. Details on eligibility criteria and the examinations can be found at https://www.vascularboard.org/cert_reqs.cfm (accessed May 13, 2023).

Physician and Laboratory Caseload

Use levels and optimal physician caseload are important issues in invasive cardiology. It is generally accepted that high-volume laboratories and operators tend to have better outcomes. In addition, low-volume laboratories might be associated with the risk of inadequate equipment and staffing due to financial limitations. At the same time, a cardiologist should not have such an excessive caseload that interferes with proper precatheterization evaluation of the patient and adequate postcatheterization interpretation of the data, report preparation, patient follow-up, and continuing medical education.

For interventional cardiology, the guidelines have recommended for the laboratory to perform a minimum of 200 procedures (more than 400 being ideal), and each operator to perform a minimum of 75 cases per year, to remain proficient. In actuality, these numbers are generally not enforced except at the level of hospital privileging (compliance with minimal volumes is required in some states, however), and a segment of the interventional community still performs as few as 25 to 50 interventions per year. Outcome data suggest that higher-volume operators working in higher-volume interventional centers do have greater procedural success and fewer adverse complications. However, other data suggest that while the trend between operator and outcomes continues to exist with contemporary PCI, some lower-volume operators can still practice safely, particularly if they work side by side with more-experienced operators in high-volume centers and if they limit the complexity of the procedures they attempt. With the current very low rate of major complications associated with interventional procedures and the difficulties in accurately adjusting outcomes for differences in case complexity, it would be very difficult to draw statistically valid conclusions about this issue. All that said, as in other areas of procedural medicine, there is a compelling truth to the adage that "practice makes perfect." It should be noted that well-defined volume standards have been recently set by the CMS in the National Coverage Determination (NCD) for transcatheter aortic valve replacement (TAVR) and transcatheter mitral valve repair. These standards clearly state the lifetime and annual or biannual volumes for members of the cardiac team performing the procedure and for the hospital. For further details, the reader is referred to the NCD.

The Catheterization Laboratory Director and Quality Assurance

The director should have at least 5 years of postfellowship experience in procedural performance and should be board-certified in both cardiology and interventional cardiology (ie, the Certificate of Additional Qualification as described in the previous section). Important roles of the director include selection and upkeep scheduling of all equipment, oversight of device ordering systems and procedural policies, training supervision of ancillary personnel (nurses, cardiovascular technicians, and radiographic technicians), and development of an equitable case scheduling methodology. The director usually also has fiduciary responsibilities to the hospital for the safe and efficient use of catheterization lab time, personnel, and supplies, as well as oversight of the hospital billing activity for catheterization procedures. In exchange, the director often receives partial salary support from the hospital to cover time taken away from remunerative clinical practice.

One of the most important roles of the catheterization laboratory director is the systematic collection of outcomes data and a fair assessment of the quality of care provided by individual operators. In addition to clinical outcomes, data collection should include comorbidities and procedure variables. This can be achieved by participation in a regional or national registry. Participation in a regional registry (Northern New England, Michigan BMC2, New York State, Massachusetts, Washington State, and other regional registries) and in the national ACC CathPCI Registry provides the added value of comparative risk-adjusted data that can be used for benchmarking and for quality improvement.

The director should organize a clinical conference where data are presented to identify laboratory-wide solutions to certain problems, didactic conferences for the fellows and faculty and periodic "cath conferences" in which interesting cases, complications, and cases performed with new technologies are presented. In addition, an assessment of the appropriateness of procedure performed according to available guidelines should be included in the quality assurance program. In short, the director is responsible for overseeing the safe, effective, and up-to-date operation of the laboratory, with the commitment to provide the best and most appropriate patient care.

PERFORMING THE PROCEDURE

In individual cardiac catheterization procedures, the choice of procedure components draws selectively on the techniques that are described throughout this handbook. The methods described in this handbook have been found to be safe, successful, and practical. That said, *readers should also note that the techniques described throughout this text are not proposed as the only correct approaches to cardiac catheterization (many laboratories and operators take different approaches, and still obtain excellent results),* and that personal practice will continue to evolve based on new clinical trial data and individual preference.

SUGGESTED READINGS

1. 2019 ESC guidelines for the diagnosis and management of chronic coronary syndromes: the task force for the diagnosis and management of chronic coronary syndromes of the European Society of Cardiology (ESC). *Eur Heart J.* 2019;41(3):407-477.
2. Accessed May 13, 2023. https://intersocietal.org/programs/cardiovascular-catheterization/standards/
3. American Society of Anesthesiologists Task Force on Sedation and Analgesia by Non-Anesthesiologists. Practice guidelines for sedation and analgesia by non-anesthesiologists. *Anesthesiology.* 2002;96(4):1004-1017.
4. Amsterdam EA, Wenger NK, Brindis RG, et al; ACC/AHA Task Force Members. 2014 AHA/ACC guideline for the management of patients with non-ST-elevation acute coronary syndromes: a report of the American College of Cardiology/American Heart Association Task Force on Practice Guidelines. *Circulation.* 2014;130(25):e344-e426.
5. Anderson KO, Masur FT. Psychologic preparation for cardiac catheterization. *Heart Lung.* 1989;18(2):154-163.
6. Anderson JL, Adams CD, Antman EM, et al. 2011 ACCF/AHA focused update incorporated into the ACC/AHA 2007 guidelines for the management of patients with unstable angina/non-ST-elevation myocardial infarction: a report of the American College of Cardiology Foundation/American Heart Association Task Force on practice guidelines. *Circulation.* 2011;123(18):e426-e579.
7. Bashore TM, Bates ER, Berger PB, et al. American College of cardiology/society for cardiac angiography and interventions clinical expert consensus document on cardiac catheterization laboratory standards. A report of the American College of cardiology task force on clinical expert consensus documents. *J Am Coll Cardiol.* 2001;37(8):2170-2214.

8. Bashore TM, Balter S, Barac A, et al. 2012 American College of cardiology Foundation/society for cardiovascular angiography and interventions expert consensus document on cardiac catheterization laboratory standards update: a report of the American College of cardiology Foundation task force on expert consensus documents developed in collaboration with the society of thoracic surgeons and society for vascular medicine. *J Am Coll Cardiol.* 2012;59(24):2221-2305.

9. Boothman RC, Blackwell AC. Legal considerations: informed consent and disclosure practices. In: Moscucci M, ed. *Complications of Cardiovascular Procedures: Risk Factors, Management and Bailout Techniques.* Wolter Kluwer/Lippincott Williams & Wilkins; 2011:37-52.

10. Chambers CE, Eisenhauer MD, McNicol LB, et al. Infection control guidelines for the cardiac catheterization laboratory: society guidelines revisited. *Catheter Cardiovasc Interv.* 2006;67(1):78-86.

11. Conti CR. Presidents' page: cardiac catheterization laboratories – hospital-based, free-standing or mobile? *J Am Coll Cardiol.* 1990;15(3):748-750.

12. Cope C. Technique for transseptal catheterization of the left atrium: preliminary report. *J Thorac Surg.* 1959;37(4):482-486.

13. Cournand AF, Ranges HS. Catheterization of the right auricle in man. *Proc Soc Exp Biol Med.* 1941;46:462.

14. Cournand AF, Riley RL, Breed ES, et al. Measurement of cardiac output in man using the technique of catheterization of the right auricle or ventricle. *J Clin Invest.* 1945;24:106.

15. Cournand AF. Nobel lecture, December 11, 1956. In: *Nobel Lectures, Physiology and Medicine 1942-1962*: Elsevier; 1964:529.

16. Cournand A. Cardiac catheterization. Development of the technique, its contributions to experimental medicine, and its initial application in man. *Acta Med Scand Suppl.* 1975;579:1-32.

17. Creager MA, Gornik HL, Gray BH, et al. COCATS 4 task force 9: training in vascular medicine. *J Am Coll Cardiol.* 2015;65(17):1832-1843.

18. Creager MA, Hamburg NM, Calligaro KD, et al. 2021 ACC/AHA/SVM/ACP advanced training statement on vascular medicine (Revision of the 2004 ACC/ACP/SCAI/SVMB/SVS clinical competence statement on vascular medicine and catheter-based peripheral vascular interventions). *Circ Cardiovasc Interv.* 2021;14(2):e000079.

19. Decision Memo for Transcatheter Mitral Valve Repair (TMVR) (CAG-00438N). Accessed August 5, 2020. https://www.cms.gov/medicare-coverage-database/details/nca-decision-memo.aspx?NCAId=273

20. Forssmann W. *Experiments on Myself; Memoirs of a Surgeon in Germany*. St. Martin's Press; 1974.

21. Freeman RV, O'Donnell M, Share D, et al. For the Blue Cross Blue Shield of Michigan Cardiovascular Consortium (BMC2). Nephropathy requiring dialysis after percutaneous coronary interventions: incidence, risk factors and the critical role of an adjusted contrast dose. *Am J Cardiol.* 2002;90(10):1068-1073.

22. Gruntzig A, Myler R, Hanna R, Turina M. Coronary transluminal angioplasty. *Circulation.* 1977;56(II):319.

23. Grüntzig AR, Senning A, Siegenthaler WE. Nonoperative dilatation of coronary-artery stenosis: percutaneous transluminal coronary angioplasty. *N Engl J Med.* 1979;301(2):61-68.

24. Gurm HS, Dixon SR, Smith DE, et al. Renal function-based contrast dosing to define safe limits of radiographic contrast media in patients undergoing percutaneous coronary interventions. *J Am Coll Cardiol.* 2011;58(9):907-914.

25. Hales S. Statical Essays: Containing Haemastatics – or, an Account of Some Hydraulic and Hydrostatical Experiments Made on the Blood and Blood-Vessels of Animals. To Which Is Added, an Appendix, with an index to Both vs Vol II. 3rd ed. v 2 of 2-. (Reproduction of original writings available through: Gale Eighteenth Century Collection Online Print Editions).

26. Haynes AB, Weiser TG, Berry WR, et al. A surgical safety checklist to reduce morbidity and mortality in a global population. *N Engl J Med.* 2009;360(5):491-499.

27. Judkins MP. Selective coronary arteriography: a percutaneous transfemoral technique. *Radiology.* 1967;89(5):815-824.

28. Kaplan AV, Baim DS, Smith JJ, et al. Medical device development: from prototype to regulatory approval. *Circulation.* 2004;109(25):3068-3072.

29. King SB III, Babb JD, Bates ER, et al. COCATS 4 Task Force 10: training in cardiac catheterization. *J Am Coll Cardiol.* 2015;65(17):1844-1853.

30. King SB III. The development of interventional cardiology. *J Am Coll Cardiol.* 1998;31(4 suppl B):64B-88B.

31. Levine GN, Bates ER, Blankenship JC, et al. 2011 ACCF/AHA/SCAI guideline for percutaneous coronary intervention: a report of the American College of cardiology Foundation/American heart association task force on practice guidelines and the society for cardiovascular angiography and interventions. *Circulation.* 2011;124(23):e574-e651.
32. Moscucci M, Rogers EK, Montoye C, et al. Association of a continuous quality improvement initiative with practice and outcome variations of contemporary percutaneous coronary interventions. *Circulation.* 2006;113(6):814-822.
33. Mueller RL, Sanborn TA. The history of interventional cardiology: cardiac catheterization, angioplasty, and related interventions. *Am Heart J.* 1995;129(1):146-172.
34. Naidu SS, Aronow HD, Box LC, et al. SCAI expert consensus statement: 2016 best practices in the cardiac catheterization laboratory – (Endorsed by the Cardiological Society of India, and sociedad Latino Americana de Cardiologia intervencionista; Affirmation of value by the Canadian Association of Interventional Cardiology – association canadienne de cardiologie d'intervention). *Catheter Cardiovasc Interv.* 2016;88(3):407-423.
35. O'Gara PT, Kushner FG, Ascheim DD, et al. 2013 ACCF/AHA guideline for the management of ST-elevation myocardial infarction: a report of the American College of cardiology Foundation/American heart association task force on practice guidelines. *J Am Coll Cardiol.* 2013;61(4):e78-e140.
36. Otto CM, Nishimura RA, Bonow RO, et al. 2020 ACC/AHA guideline for the management of patients with valvular heart disease: a report of the American College of Cardiology/American Heart Association Joint Committee on Clinical Practice guidelines. *Circulation.* 2021;143(5):e72-e227.
37. Ross J Jr.. Transeptal left heart catheterization: a new method of left atrial puncture. *Ann Surg.* 1959;149(3):395-401.
38. Sones FM Jr., Shirey EK, Prondfit WL, Westcott RN. Cinecoronary arteriography. *Circulation.* 1959;20:773.
39. Sorensen B, Spahn DR, Innerhofer P, Spannagl M, Rossaint R. Clinical review: prothrombin complex concentrates – evaluation of safety and thrombogenicity. *Crit Care.* 2011;15(1):201.
40. Swan HJ, Ganz W, Forrester J, Marcus H, Diamond G, Chonette D. Catheterization of the heart in man with use of a flow directed balloon-tipped catheter. *N Engl J Med.* 1970;283(9):447-451.
41. Tait AR, Voepel-Lewis T, Moscucci M, Brennan-Martinez CM, Levine R. Patient comprehension of an interactive, computer-based information program for cardiac catheterization: a comparison with standard information. *Arch Intern Med.* 2009;169(20):1907-1914.
42. WHO's patient-safety checklist for surgery. *Lancet.* 2008;372:1.

2 Cineangiographic Imaging, Radiation Safety, and Contrast Agents[1]

Working knowledge of radiation safety and the technology of fluoroscopic equipment is part of core competencies of interventional cardiologists and allied health care providers. Most importantly, patient safety is a continuing concern because fluoroscopic radiation injuries ranging from inconsequential to devastating continue to occur.

BASIC X-RAY PHYSICS

X-rays are a form of electromagnetic radiation similar to visible light and radio waves. The x-ray beam is often described as a stream of photons (ie, discrete packets of electromagnetic radiation, each containing a defined amount of energy). Each x-ray photon contains thousands of times the energy of a photon of visible light. This explains why different and more potent biologic effects occur when an x-ray photon is absorbed by or scattered from living tissue.

X-rays are predominantly produced when high-energy electrons are decelerated by interaction with a metallic target (in our case tungsten). This is called *bremsstrahlung* (breaking radiation). The resulting x-ray beam contains a spectrum of photon energies ranging from approximately 20 keV up to the maximum voltage applied to the x-ray tube. Characteristic x-rays are also produced when the incoming electrons interact with the orbital electrons of the target's atoms. The x-ray spectrum emitted toward the patient is modified by filters placed between the x-ray tube and the patient. The shape of the x-ray spectrum strongly affects both image contrast and patient dose. Too "soft" a spectrum needlessly increases patient dose; too hard a spectrum decreases image contrast.

Radiation quantities and units needed to describe the use of x-rays in the interventional laboratory are summarized in **Table 2.1**.

CLINICAL MEASUREMENT OF PATIENT IRRADIATION

Radiation can be measured in many ways and at many locations (**Figure 2.1**). Of these, the image-receptor entrance point is best for assessing image noise and the patient entrance point is best for assessing the risk of skin injury. If dose maps are not available on a given system, reference point air kerma ($K_{a,r}$) is a reasonable surrogate for predicting tissue reactions such as skin injuries. Cancer risk is related to the dose received by each of the organs in the body and its radiosensitivity. Organ dose is not directly measurable. However, kerma-area product (P_{KA}) can be used to estimate cancer risk. Fluoroscopy time is not a useful indicator of either risk. Because of this, potentially high radiation dose procedures should not be done using equipment that can only display fluoroscopic time.

Measuring and tracking radiation during a fluoroscopic procedure provides critical safety information to the operator. Interventional fluoroscopes conforming to the International Electrotechnical Commission 60601-2-43 standard incorporate mandatory instrumentation to monitor $K_{a,r}$, P_{KA}, and fluoro time.

[1]We gratefully acknowledge the Grossman & Baim's *Cardiac Catheterization, Angiography, and Intervention*, 9th edition contributions of Drs. Stephen Balter and Mauro Moscucci, as portions of their chapter, Cineangiographic Imaging, Radiation Safety, and Contrast Agents, were retained in this text.

Table 2.1 Clinically Important Dosimetric Definitions

Quantity	Description	SI Unit	Related Units
Exposure, $K_{a,r}$	The radiation present at a point in space. It is currently described as air kerma (kinetic energy released in matter) in units of gray. At fluoroscopic energies, air kerma is the dose delivered to air. By itself, exposure gives no information regarding how much radiation energy is delivered to tissue or the biologic effects that irradiation might have.	Gray (Gy) In air	Roentgen (R) 100 R = 0.87 Gy (air)
Dose, $D_{material}$	The local concentration of energy absorbed by a small volume of a specified material (eg, air) or specified tissue (eg, myocardium) from the x-ray beam. Tissue dose is usually stated in units of gray (1 Gy = 1 J/kg) or milligray (mGy). The dose delivered to different portions of a patient from an initially uniform x-ray beam is always nonuniform because of x-ray beam size limits, x-ray absorption, and x-ray scatter. It is incorrect to describe the physical dose distribution in a patient or staff member using a single number. 1 Gy (specific substance) = 1 J (absorbed)/kg (specific substance).	Gray (Gy) In soft tissue or another specified material	RAD 100 RAD = 1 Gy
Peak skin dose **(PSD)**	The highest dose received by any portion of the patient's skin from a procedure. Presently, there is no commercially available technology to map skin dose distribution while a procedure is in progress. However, real-time skin mapping is anticipated in the near future. Several film-based technologies are available to produce a skin dose map after the patient has been removed from the table.	Gray (Gy) Includes backscatter from patient	
Effective dose **(E)**	A calculated quantity that was introduced by the ICRP for managing stochastic radiation risks experienced by large populations. This usage has also been adopted by the NCRP. The calculation includes a complex convolution of radiation type and organ sensitivity in a hypothetical standard person. Effective dose is not intended to characterize the radiation risk experienced by any individual. Its use for such purposes is specifically rejected by both the ICRP and NCRP. Effective dose is a useful metric for generally comparing different types of procedures or different protocols. ED (Sv) = $\sum$ [Dose to a volume of tissue (Gy)] × Radiosensitivity of that tissue	Sievert (Sv)	100 REM = 1 Sv

(Continued)

Table 2.1 Clinically Important Dosimetric Definitions (Continued)			
Quantity	**Description**	**SI Unit**	**Related Units**
Air kerma–area product (**KAP,** P_{KA})	A measure of the total x-ray energy in a beam. In simple terms, it is the product of the dose measured at a point in the center of the beam and the cross-sectional area of the beam at that point. Following this definition, dose-area product (DAP) is usually stated in units of Gy cm². P_{KA} has the same value anywhere between the x-ray tube and the patient's entrance surface. DAP and anatomical information can be combined to estimate effective dose using conversion factors derived from Monte-Carlo simulations. P_{KA} is the best dose metric for estimating patient stochastic risk and the amount of scatter in the procedure room.	Gy cm²	See **Figure 2.1**
Reference point air kerma ($K_{a,r}$)	The total air kerma accumulated at an internationally defined reference point during a procedure. For an isocentric fluoroscope, the reference point is located 15 cm from the isocenter along a line from the isocenter to the x-ray tube's focal spot. This point approximates the skin location for a nonmoving beam. $K_{a,r}$ is the best currently available dose metric for managing the possibility of skin injury.	Gy	See **Figure 2.1**
Fluoroscopic time	This is not a useful dose metric because fluoroscopic time does not reflect patient size, beam orientation, or the use of cine. The use of fluoroscopic time as a dose metric or equipment that can only display fluoroscopic time for interventional procedures is strongly discouraged.	Minutes	See **Figure 2.1**

ED, equivalent dose; ICRP, International Commission on Radiological Protection; NCRP, National Council on Radiation Protection and Measurements.

IMAGE FORMATION
Image Contrast

Images are formed when different structures in the body absorb different amounts of radiation from the beam. The beam is modulated by different absorption, and it is detected and converted into a useful image by an image receptor. A structure in the patient can only be seen if its detected signal is sufficiently different from the surrounding structures. The visibility of the primary signal is degraded by scattered radiation and obscured by image noise.

The primary signal is produced by differences in x-ray absorption attributable to differences in thickness, physical density (gm/cc), or atomic number (Z) between

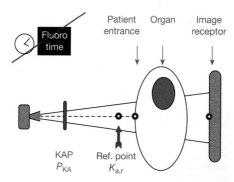

Figure 2.1 Important radiation measurement points. The best estimates of radiogenic risk can be made when the tissue dose distribution on the patient's skin and the dose delivered to each internal organ are known. Present technology provides measurement and in-lab display of the total dose at a defined reference point ($K_{a,r}$ as well as the total kerma-area product [P_{KA}] from the procedure). $K_{a,r}$ and P_{KA} are practical real-time measurements for assessing skin injury and late cancer risk, respectively. Fluoroscopy time does not provide an accurate assessment of either. Although fluoro time is widely available, it has an uncertainty of at least a factor of 10 when used to estimate either $K_{a,r}$ or P_{KA}. KAP, kerma-area product.

the target and its surrounds. Natural differences between structures are enhanced by the use of a contrast agent. The contrast agents used in the catheterization laboratory (cath lab) usually contain iodine (atomic number 53). Iodine is a strong absorber of x-ray photons in the range from 31 to 70 keV. This property allows visualization of small vessels when the iodinated contrast agent displaces blood during angiography.

X-ray production is automatically controlled by most fluoroscopes by changing factors including the voltage applied across the x-ray tube and beam filtration. For long tissue paths (due to patient size and/or beam angulation), the x-ray spectrum is displaced above the photon energy range that produces optimum visibility of iodine or steel (eg, stents or guidewires). This produces less beam modulation and is one of the reasons why the visibility of contrast media and devices vary from view to view and from patient to patient.

Image Noise

The radiographic image of a totally uniform object has random variations in brightness from point to point and over time due to both x-ray quantum effects and other sources. These random fluctuations are called *image noise*. Noise reduces the ability to detect low-contrast structures. Image noise includes an avoidable component attributable to the imaging system itself (structural noise) and a second component unavoidably attributable to the physics of the x-ray beam (quantum mottle). Quantum mottle is caused by the statistical photon nature of the x-ray beam. Fewer detected x-ray photons result in a noisier image (**Figure 2.2**).

Image Sharpness

The primary sharpness of an object in a fluoro image is affected by interactions between (1) the size of the x-ray tube's focal spot; (2) the position of the object between the x-ray tube and the image receptor; (3) the object's motion; and (4) the spatial resolution properties of the image receptor.

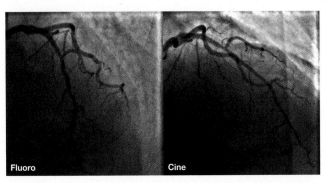

Figure 2.2 Image receptor dose per frame and system settings affect image appearance. The image on the left is a frame from a stored fluoroscopic run. The image on the right is a cine frame. These images were acquired a few seconds apart. The increased noise in the last-image hold results from less dose used in its production. The increased contrast seen in the cine image results from system programming to a lower kVp, different beam filtration, and different image processing parameters.

The x-ray tube focal spot is the area of the anode surface which receives the beam of electrons from the cathode. Larger focal spots are needed for high-power imaging, with the limitation of greater loss of sharpness in the x-ray image from large focal spots at high geometric magnification.

Scattered Radiation

Scattered radiation is produced when the x-ray beam interacts with the patient or other objects and is redirected rather than completely absorbed. Scattered radiation reduces contrast, it is the principal source of exposure of the patient's body parts outside of the direct beam, and it is the primary source of exposure of laboratory staff. The amount of scatter is proportional to the intensity of the x-ray beam and the size of the x-ray field (ie, proportional to P).

Optimizing Patient Exposure and Image Quality

Producing an x-ray image involves balancing many factors including image contrast (needed to detect an object), spatial and temporal sharpness (needed to characterize the object), image noise, and patient exposure.

Most modern fluoroscopes contain a large set of preprogrammed techniques intended to provide an optimal balance between patient size, image quality, patient exposure for a wide variety of different imaging tasks, and include image-processing and display parameters that further affect image appearance.

THE CINEFLUOROGRAPHIC SYSTEM

The purpose of an x-ray cinefluorographic system is to produce fluoroscopic and fluorographic optimized images of relevant anatomy at minimum patient exposure. The technical means to do this include the production of a collimated x-ray beam of appropriate quality and intensity, projection of that beam through the patient at the required angle, detection of the modulated x-ray beam after it passes through the patient, processing and storing the resultant images, and, last but not least, displaying these images to the operator. The principal components needed for these tasks are illustrated in **Figure 2.3**.

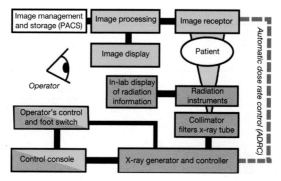

Figure 2.3 Block diagram of a medical fluoroscope. Fluoroscopic systems consist of components needed to produce x-rays, detect the modulated beam passing through the patient, process and display images to the operator, and store images for later use. The automatic dose rate control (ADRC) system stabilizes the image-receptor signal against changes in path length in the patient. The operator can profoundly influence both patient irradiation and image appearance by changing examination sets or irradiation mode. PACS, picture archiving and communication system.

Radiation Production and Control

The cinefluorographic x-ray generator delivers controlled amounts of electrical power to the x-ray tube. One circuit selects the appropriate x-ray tube filament and heats that filament to produce an electron beam at a current ranging between 1 and 1000 milliamperes (mA). A second circuit supplies a voltage ranging from 50 to 125 kilovolts peak (kVp) to accelerate the electrons toward the anode of the x-ray tube. X-rays are usually produced as a series of pulses. This is accomplished by electrically switching the electron beam on and off to produce the pulses.

X-Ray Tubes

The x-ray tube is a device that converts electrical energy into x-rays (**Figure 2.4**). It consists of an evacuated glass or metal housing. Its key components are 1 or more tungsten filaments (housed in a focusing cup) and an anode disk (tungsten alloy, 100-200 mm in diameter), which rotates at more than 10,000 rpm (**Figure 2.4**). Electrons are emitted from the selected filament by thermionic emission. These electrons are accelerated toward the anode by the electric field (50-125 kV) supplied by the generator. X-rays are produced when the electrons hit the anode.

For sharpest imaging, the point of impact of the electron beam on the anode should be as small as possible so that x-ray emission appears to come from a single "point" focal spot. The actual size of the focal spot represents a balance between the requirements for sharp imaging and the need to avoid melting the target. X-ray tubes have 2 filaments and hence 2 focal spots. The smaller focal spot (typically 0.3-0.5 mm) is used for fluoroscopy. The larger focal spot (typically 0.81 mm) accommodates the higher power requirements of adult cine.

Spatial and Spectral Shaping of the X-Ray Beam

The x-ray beam contains a spectrum of photon energies. These range from the maximum determined by the peak voltage supplied by the generator (kVp) to a lower energy determined by the filters in the beam. Images are mainly formed by photons of intermediate energies. Higher energy photons strongly penetrate both tissue and iodine; this

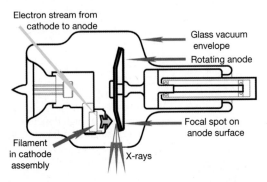

Electron stream from cathode to anode

Glass vacuum envelope

Rotating anode

Focal spot on anode surface

Filament in cathode assembly

X-rays

Figure 2.4 Medium-power rotating anode x-ray tube. See text for discussion.

reduces contrast. Low-energy x-ray photons are easily absorbed by the patient's tissues; they contribute to risk but not to image formation.

The size of the x-ray beam can always be reduced by the use of the collimator control. Actively confining the beam to the smallest area of immediate clinical interest as a procedure progresses reduces both patient and staff irradiation while simultaneously improving image contrast (by limiting scatter).

Many systems also have movable semitransparent copper shutters (also called wedge filters) that can be positioned over the lung fields up to the heart border in each projection. These improve the visibility of vessels and devices as well as overall image quality by reducing excessive image brightness in the lung fields.

Imaging Modes

Dedicated cardiac fluoroscopes have two principal modes of operation: fluoroscopy (fluoro) and cinefluorographic acquisition (cine). Multipurpose units have an additional digital subtraction angiography (DSA) mode. A single cine frame delivers about as much dose to the patient as 10 fluoro frames; a single DSA frame delivers as much as 10 cine frames (100 fluoro frames). **Figure 2.2** illustrates the differences in image appearance between fluoro and cine.

Fluoroscopy

Fluoroscopy provides a real-time x-ray image with adequate quality for observing motion and guiding device manipulations.

At present, the most common frame rates for adult coronary angiography are 7.5 or 15 frames per second. Decreasing frame rate saves dose at the expense of visual smoothness of the transition between frames. The required dose rate scales against the square root of the frame rate for equal visual perception of noise. This scaling law is used by some (but not all) types of interventional fluoroscopes.

Acquisition (Cine)

Cine requires images of sufficient quality for single-frame viewing. Higher x-ray input dose rates are therefore needed to reduce noise and optimize clinical visualization. It is therefore worthwhile to remember that a minute of cine is essentially equivalent to 10 minutes of fluoroscopy.

Many current systems also provide a choice of cine dose rates. Low dose–rate cine should be used whenever it does not reduce the clinical value of the images.

Digital Subtraction Angiography

The digital subtraction angiography (DSA) process begins with the acquisition of a series of images of the same anatomical area. Typically, contrast media is injected during this acquisition. The first image in the series is usually used as a mask. The mask is digitally subtracted from the remaining images in the series. The remainder shows the difference between the mask and the target image (usually a faint image of contrast plus artifacts due to motion). Display contrast is increased to improve visibility. Quantum noise is not removed by the subtraction process because it is random. Thus, all of the images in the original series must be acquired at high dose to reduce their noise content. As noted above, the dose needed for a single DSA frame is approximately 10 times higher than that needed for a cine frame. Because of the high dose per frame, DSA images should be acquired at the lowest clinically usable frame rate and for the shortest possible time.

Automatic Dose Rate Control

Fluoroscopic systems use automatic dose rate control (ADRC) to monitor the dose at the image receptor and automatically adjust x-ray production to produce the requisite receptor level. The normal function of this circuit has a profound influence on patient skin dose. X-ray intensity is increased if the detector measures too dim a signal and decreased if it measures too bright a signal. This means that the patient's entrance port skin dose increases substantially for heavy patients and when compound projection angles are used. Increasing the tissue path length from 10 to 40 cm will increase patient's skin dose rate by more than a factor of 10 for fluoroscopy and more than a factor of 100 for cine (**Figure 2.5**).

ADRC's primary goal is to maintain the programmed image receptor dose rate irrespective of patient size. Competing goals include optimizing the visibility of iodinated contrast as well as minimizing patient irradiation.

In most fluoroscopes, responding to increased tissue path length requires an increase in the kVp. This moves the x-ray spectrum away from the region of maximum iodine absorption. The primary x-ray contrast is further reduced because the

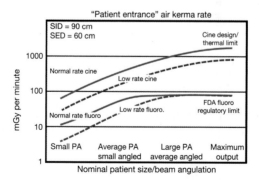

Figure 2.5 Automatic dose rate control (ADRC). Illustration of the range of patient entrance air kerma rates a function of path length in the patient. Angled beams in small patients can have a path length exceeding the PA (posterior-anterior) dimension of average or large patients. This example is of a system with two fluoroscopic and two cine dose rate modes. Fluoroscopy is limited by the FDA and state regulations. Maximum cine rates are limited by engineering design considerations. In this example, the two fluoro modes reach the limit for different size patients. The two cine modes always differ by a factor of 2. FDA, U.S. Food and Drug Administration; SED, source-to-entry skin distance; SID, source-to-image receptor distance.

same opaque vessel produces less modulation against a long tissue path than in a short path. In addition, more scattered radiation is generated in long-path situations. Some of this scatter reaches the image receptor and further degrades the visibility of vessels and devices by reducing both net beam modulation and the signal-to-noise ratio of the entire image.

CLINICAL PROGRAMS AND PROGRAMMING

Most if not all interventional fluoroscopes are configured to perform any specific type of procedure (eg, coronary angiography; EP mapping) by selecting a preprogrammed examination set from a menu on the control desk. Each set transforms the fluoroscope into a highly specialized imaging tool by configuring its x-ray acquisition and image display properties. *Operators should personally verify that the correct set has been selected as part of each preprocedure time-out.*

IMAGE DETECTION, PROCESSING, AND RECORDING

The x-ray image formed by the interaction of the x-ray beam and the patient must be detected and transformed into a usable format. The fluoroscopic screen was the original x-ray detector used by Roentgen. The image intensifier was introduced in the 1950s and it was the enabling technology for coronary angiography because it provided enough light to expose cine film. In the last two decades, the image intensifier itself has been substantially replaced by solid-state detectors (commonly called flat-panel detectors [FPDs]).

IMAGE INTENSIFIER

The structure of a single-mode image intensifier is shown in **Figure 2.6**. The modulated x-ray beam emerging from the patient enters the image intensifier and is detected and converted to visible light by a cesium iodide (CsI) fluorescent layer. This visible light image is converted into an electron image by a photocathode. Focusing electrodes in the tube accelerate and minify the electrons onto a small output screen. The output screen converts the electron image back into a smaller and brighter visible light image.

Image intensifiers usually offer several magnification modes. When a specific magnification is selected, the electronics focuses a larger or smaller portion of the input screen onto the fixed-size output screen. Smaller fields of view (FOVs) require higher input dose rates than do larger FOVs. Vascular image intensifiers remain available with FOVs exceeding 40 cm. These devices require substantially higher dose

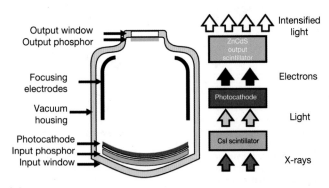

Figure 2.6 X-ray image intensifier. See text for discussion.

rates than cardiac image intensifiers when they are used at the typical 17 cm cardiac FOV. In addition, the larger bulk of vascular tubes limits beam angulation. Moving the image intensifier away from the patient to obtain the necessary angles further increases patient dose rate.

The resolution of an image intensifier tube is limited by the characteristics of its output screen. In most cases, decreasing FOV (increasing zoom) increases the spatial resolution of the image intensifier tube. The downside is the additional radiation needed for small FOVs. Patient dose can be minimized by working at the largest FOV consistent with seeing clinically relevant structures. Visibility can sometimes be improved in heavy patients by increasing the FOV and collimating the beam to the region of interest.

FLAT-PANEL X-RAY DETECTORS

Over the past 2 decades, the image intensifier and its video camera have been replaced by integrated image receptors, commonly called flat-panel detectors (FPDs).

Figure 2.7 schematically illustrates the structure of FPDs.

The FPD by itself will not appreciably affect patient dose. However, in newer systems, better dose-management algorithms, spectral shaping, and reduced frame rates for both fluoro and cine have combined to substantially reduce the overall dose required to perform procedures.

The imaging behavior of a flat-panel system differs from an image-intensifier system in two important respects:

1. The optical diaphragm between the image intensifier and the video camera delivers the same light level to the camera for both fluoro and cine. Thus, the camera noise is the same for both modes. Because there is no diaphragm inside the flat panel, the electronics must use a greater degree of amplification during fluoro relative to cine.

2. Flat panels require a slightly higher fluoroscopic entrance dose rate to overcome the additional electronic noise resulting from the additional amplification. However, because of control programming differences, fluoroscopic patient entrance dose rates are not primarily affected by image receptor type.

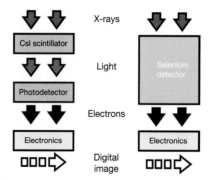

Figure 2.7 Indirect and direct flat-panel image receptors. The indirect (left) detector uses a CsI scintillator, virtually identical to that in an image intensifier, to convert the x-ray signal into light. A photodetector converts the light into an electron signal. This signal is then digitized. The direct detector (right) uses a selenium layer to directly convert the x-ray signal into an electrical charge distribution. This signal is then digitized.

IMAGE PROCESSING AND DISPLAY

Digital images are always highly processed before they are displayed. Processing techniques include:

1. Grayscale transformations (change overall contrast level and the relative contrast of objects of different brightness);
2. Edge enhancement (improves the visibility of small high-contrast structures such as stents at the expense of increasing the visibility of noise);
3. Smoothing (reduces the effect of noise in a single frame at the expense of edge sharpness);
4. Temporal averaging. This last function provides a time-weighted average of several image frames and it reduces noise by averaging while maintaining the sharpness of nonmoving structures.

Many systems offer the ability to store the current fluoroscopy loop as if it were a cine run. When clinically possible (eg, documenting a balloon inflation), the use of retrospectively stored fluoroscopy instead of cine is an excellent dose reduction technique.

DIGITAL IMAGING AND COMMUNICATION IN MEDICINE AND PICTURE ARCHIVING AND COMMUNICATION SYSTEM

Within the fluoroscopic system, displayed digital cardiac images are usually formatted to a nominal 1024 × 1024 pixel matrix. The internal bit depth of each pixel is usually 10 to 12 bits (1024-4096 potential shades of gray). These images are usually stored in the fluoroscope and displayed at full resolution in the laboratory. Cardiac studies are usually downsampled and archived to PACS (picture archiving and communication system) in a 512 × 512 × 8 bit image format. This format was specified in the 1995 DICOM (Digital Imaging and Communication in Medicine) standard so that most studies would fit onto a single CD-ROM disk.

THE ANGIOGRAPHIC ROOM

The angiographic room must have sufficient space to house the fluoroscope, an increasing array of ancillary equipment (eg, intravascular ultrasound, intra-aortic balloon pump), and work and storage areas. Larger rooms can increase working efficiency while providing staff space away from tableside.

The control room should be large enough to accommodate working staff, physiological monitors, and an increasing number of computer workstations. The scattered radiation field around the fluoroscope is complex and changes with beam angles (**Figure** 2.8). Whenever possible, staff required to be in the procedure room should work at a distance from the x-ray table and be positioned behind fixed or mobile x-ray shielding, unless delivering direct services to the patient.

The centerpiece of the cardiac cath lab is the gantry that holds the x-ray tube and image receptor in correct alignment while providing a full range of two-dimensional rotation (left to right anterior oblique) and skew (cranial to caudal) of the direction with which the x-ray beam passes through the patient. The 2 axes of rotation meet at a single point called the isocenter. An object, such as the patient's heart, placed at isocenter will remain centered on the screen as the beam direction is changed. The patient is supported on an adjustable-height flat-top table. The tabletop can be panned in the left-right or head-foot direction to move the patient relative to the x-ray beam. Ceiling-suspended gantries can be moved as well if additional panning range is needed. Some tables feature a tilt capability to put the patient into Trendelenburg or reverse Trendelenburg positions.

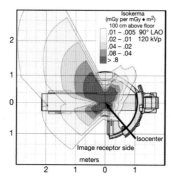

Figure 2.8 Scatter isodose curves around an interventional fluoroscope. This figure illustrates the radiation scatter levels 1 m above the floor for a full lateral beam. Isokerma lines are in units of Gy per Gy m² of kerma-area product. The asymmetry is caused by backscatter from the patient coupled with attenuation by the patient and equipment. Such curves are found in the operator's manual. LAO, left anterior oblique. (Illustration by courtesy of Koninklijke Philips N.V.)

IMAGING EQUIPMENT QUALITY ASSURANCE

Any new room requires both a radiation safety survey and an equipment acceptance test to assure compliance with regulatory requirements and conformance to the manufacturer's specifications. Testing needs to be done after installation and before first clinical use, after major repairs (eg, replacement of an x-ray tube or image receptor), and on a periodic basis.

In addition, safety and quality testing of the fluoroscope, along with an audit of its configuration, should be done by a qualified medical physicist (this is a regulatory requirement in some states).

BIOLOGICAL EFFECTS OF RADIATION

Radiation injuries are induced by 1 of 2 mechanisms. The *stochastic* mechanism of action is triggered by unrepaired radiation damage to the DNA of even a single viable cell. In contrast, *tissue reactions* are caused by radiation killing large numbers of cells (*deterministic* mechanism). Radiation management differs for these 2 mechanisms.

Stochastic Effects

The word *stochastic* implies chance or probability. Stochastic effects are presumably induced when a single photon causes unrepaired injury to the DNA of a single viable cell.

Radiogenic cancer is the principal stochastic risk in the interventional laboratory. Because clinical disease requires cellular proliferation, radiogenic cancer will take years to decades before it becomes clinically apparent.

Every person is irradiated by a variety of natural and human-made sources. In the United States, the typical annual effective dose from natural background is around 3 to 4 mSv/y. The actual amount of natural background varies depending on where individuals live, housing construction, and other factors. The natural background rate in Denver is about 1 mSv/y higher than in New York City.

Almost all human-made exposure (approximately 3 mSv/y in the United States) comes from medical exposure. Presuming that each imaging procedure is clinically justified and technically optimized, the expected clinical benefits of using radiation almost always outweigh the radiogenic risks of the procedure. This is not true for unnecessary procedures and may not be true for procedures performed using too much radiation. The goal is to use no more radiation than is necessary to safely meet the needs of each patient. This meets the radiation-protection concept of "As Low As Reasonably Achievable" or ALARA.

Radiogenic Cancer

Most dose-risk models used for radiation protection purposes predict an increase in cancer with increased procedural and lifetime dose.

Low-dose risks are *estimated* by extrapolating from the effects high-level irradiations (ie, atomic bomb survivors) back to the low dose region. The commonly used linear no threshold (LNT) model is an example of such an extrapolation. Other models, such as the linear-quadratic, are possible and are used to model specific cancers.

Effective dose can be used to estimate the order of magnitude of radiogenic risk. For example, a typical adult diagnostic coronary angiogram yields a calculated E in the range of a few mSv. The resultant cancer risk is likely to be in the order of magnitude of 0.1%. By way of comparison, a 60-year-old cancer-free male with no special risk factors has a 16% probability of being diagnosed with cancer in the next 10 years of his life. One can conclude that the stochastic risk of neoplasm from an adult diagnostic coronary angiogram is small in comparison with the natural incidence of cancer in the typical patient population receiving this procedure.

Radiation risk management in children is different from that for adults. Radiogenic neoplasm is related to age at exposure and is gender dependent. Females are more susceptible than males because of greater breast sensitivity. Additionally, because of a smaller body, a greater portion of a child's radiosensitive tissues is in close proximity to the x-ray beam during cardiologic procedures. Fortunately, because of small body size, pediatric dose rates and total doses are relatively low.

The Pregnant Patient

At low fetal dose, the principal risk is radiation-induced cancer. The lifetime radiogenic risks induced by an in utero exposure are likely to be similar to the newborn's radiogenic risk. The specific risks are determined by actual fetal dose and gestation age. Fetal doses >50 mGy place the child at risk for tissue reactions such as central nervous system damage, growth retardation, malformation, or miscarriage. Fetal doses in this range seldom happen unless the uterus is heavily irradiated.

Procedures that involve structures above the diaphragm are unlikely to induce fetal tissue reactions if direct irradiation of the fetus is minimized. However, the fetus will still receive scattered radiation from the irradiated area. The carcinogenic risk to the child is the principal concern, and this risk must be weighed in relation to the anticipated clinical benefits to the mother. Minimizing the total use of radiation, applying good collimation, and avoiding unnecessary direct irradiation of the uterus during pregnancy contribute to minimizing fetal injury. Protective measures including avoiding extreme cranial angulations and using a radial approach reduce fetal radiation risk. A consultation with a medical physicist regarding fetal dose management prior to the procedure can be very helpful.

Radiation-Induced Heritable Effects

Genetic risk is applicable only to individuals who become future parents. Thus, the main concerns for radiation-induced genetic damage should be focused on pediatric patients and younger adults. Patient risk can be managed by reducing total patient dose, and minimizing gonadal irradiation, while staff risk can be reduced by applying actions to reduce staff dose.

Tissue Reactions

Tissue reactions occur when a significant number of existing cells are sufficiently damaged so as to cause observable injury. Acute injury occurs when there is massive immediate cell killing (extremely uncommon under fluoroscopic conditions) or there is a physiological response to dose levels that may produce serious injury in the subsequent months. Skin and subcutaneous tissue injuries appear when damaged cells die off and are not adequately replaced. Such injuries manifest a few weeks after irradiation and may take a year or more to fully mature. The time and dose thresholds for injury and recovery are shown in **Table 2.2**. At higher doses, microvasculature is denuded and subcutaneous necrosis can occur. Biopsies of such injuries frequently result in nonhealing tracks resulting in an increased risk of infection.

The patient's state of health may modify the normal response of skin or other organs to radiation, with collagen vascular disease, diabetes mellitus, and hyperthyroidism making the patient more susceptible to injury.

Radiation-induced skin injury is the most common tissue reaction occurring after fluoroscopically guided cardiac procedures. A severe skin injury is illustrated in **Figure 2.9**. The common thread in most of cases of debilitating injuries from cardiac procedures is that the operators were seldom aware that their use of radiation caused the injuries.

Table 2.2 presumes that the entire irradiation occurred in less than a day and that the skin was not previously irradiated. Tissue will tolerate a higher total dose if the irradiation is divided over several sessions with enough time between sessions for DNA repair. In general, skin will require at least 1 month for the affected cells to die and at least 2 months for tissue regeneration. At higher doses, subcutaneous microvasculature is damaged, and regeneration is incomplete.

If the beam angles are not changed during prolonged portions of the procedure, the lesion will be a well-demarcated square or rectangle of several centimeters on a side. Major injuries extend into subcutaneous tissues to a depth of several centimeters and may result in radionecrosis of an underlying rib.

Patient Radiation Management

The amount of radiation used in a simple diagnostic study performed on a moderately large adult cardiac patient is highly unlikely to cause either a tissue reaction or a late cancer. Radiation use increases with increasing patient size and clinical complexity. The population of pediatric patients is at increased stochastic risk relative to an adult population who received the same nominal effective dose because of the increased radio-carcinogenic sensitivity of children.

Operators are not legally restricted to a maximum patient radiation dose. They are expected to reduce the amount of fluoroscopy and cine to the clinically required minimum. Equipment features, preprogrammed examination sets, and user selections provide the operator with a great deal of control over x-ray dose rates and beam sizes.

Imaging geometry matters. This includes both gantry configuration and placement of the gantry relative to the patient. For example, when the heart is placed in the fluoroscopy unit's isocenter, it appears to rotate without moving as the gantry is rotated and skewed. This minimizes the need to reposition the patient when the x-ray projection angle is changed.

The best general advice is to position the table height to a level comfortable for the primary operator. This should help reduce overall patient (and staff) dose by facilitating efficiency. However, when clinically possible, it is prudent to increase the x-ray tube to patient-skin distance when the beam port has already been highly irradiated. This step helps reduce patient entrance dose rate in this small area.

Table 2.2 Skin Injury: Local Skin Dose and Time of Onset

Band	Single-Site Acute Skin-Dose Range (Gy)[a]	NCI Skin Reaction Grade	Approximate Time of Onset of Effects			
			Prompt	**Early**	**Midterm**	**Long Term**
A1	0-2	NA	No observable effects expected	No observable effects expected	No observable effects expected	No observable effects expected
A1	2-5	1	Transient erythema	Epilation	Recovery from hair loss	No observable results expected
B	5-10	1-2	Transient erythema	Erythema, epilation	Recovery; at higher doses, prolonged erythema, permanent partial epilation	Recovery; at higher doses, dermal atrophy or induration
C	10-15	2-3	Transient erythema	Erythema, epilation; possible dry or moist desquamation; recovery from desquamation	Prolonged erythema; permanent epilation	Telangiectasia[b]; dermal atrophy or induration; skin likely to be weak
D	>15	3-4	Transient erythema; after very high doses, edema and acute ulceration; long-term surgical intervention likely to be required	Erythema, epilation; moist desquamation	Dermal atrophy; secondary ulceration due to failure of moist desquamation to heal; surgical intervention likely to be required; at higher doses, dermal necrosis, surgical intervention likely to be required	Telangiectasia[b]; dermal atrophy or induration; possible late skin breakdown; wound might be persistent and progress into a deeper lesion; surgical intervention likely to be required

NA, not applicable; NCI, National Cancer Institute.
Tissue reactions from single-delivery radiation dose to skin of the neck, torso, pelvis, buttocks, or arms.
Note: Applicable to normal range of patient radiosensitivities in the absence of mitigating or aggravating physical or clinical factors. Data do not apply to the skin of the scalp. Dose and time bands are not rigid boundaries. Signs and symptoms are expected to appear earlier as skin dose increases. Prompt is <2 wk; early, 2-8 wk; midterm, 6-52 wk; long term, >40 wk.
Data from Balter S, Hopewell JW, Miller DL, Wagner LK, Zelefsky MJ. Fluoroscopically guided interventional procedures: a review of radiation effects on patients' skin and hair. *Radiology*. 2010;254:326-341.
[a]Skin doses refer to actual skin dose (including backscatter). This quantity is not the reference point air kerma described by the U.S. Food and Drug Administration (21 CFR § 1020.32 [2008]) or International Electrotechnical Commission. Skin dosimetry is unlikely to be more accurate than ±50%.
[b]Refers to radiation-induced telangiectasia. Telangiectasia associated with area of initial moist desquamation or healing of ulceration may be present earlier.

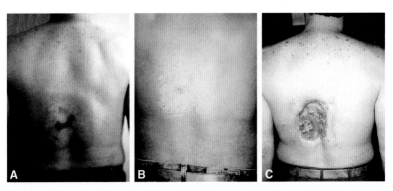

Figure 2.9 Timeline of a major radiation injury. Early erythema and blistering at approximately 8 weeks is seen in **(A)**. This has resolved by approximately 20 weeks **(B)**; however, the tissue is necrotic. The tissue has broken down by 20 months **(C)**. Details of this case were reported by Shope. (Data from Shope TB. Radiation-induced skin injuries from fluoroscopy. *Radiographics.* 1996;16(5):1195-1199.)

Minimizing the gap between the patient and the image receptor will reduce patient irradiation and scatter in the laboratory. This should be checked and done every time the gantry or table is moved.

Collimating the x-ray beam within the working FOV is an important radiation management tool that is often neglected by interventionalists. Collimation decreases the total radiation load on the patient and facilitates beam motion without field overlap. In addition, less scatter is produced in a collimated beam in comparison to an uncollimated beam (**Figure 2.10**).

At a minimum, all systems should be set up by the equipment's service provider to have a small unirradiated margin on all sides of the "fully opened beam" for all FOVs and source-to-image receptor distances (SIDs). This assures that all of the radiation reaching the patient produces clinically useful information. Collimator shifts, visible during routine clinical procedures, should be promptly corrected.

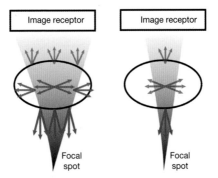

Figure 2.10 Collimation reduces scatter in the lab. Collimation reduces the volume of irradiated tissue. This reduces the production of scattered radiation and results in better image contrast plus less staff irradiation.

Moving the beam should be considered when clinically practicable, especially if $K_{a,r}$ > 3000 mGy. Changing beam angulation during the procedure reduces peak skin dose provided the beam ports do not overlap. Smaller input field sizes at the patient's entrance skin require smaller minimum changes in beam angle to be effective. Larger changes provide a margin of safety.

Clinical Dose Monitoring

Any form of radiation used inside or outside the cath lab must be justified. To do so, documentation of clinical appropriateness and quantitative radiological data is required. Tracking radiation use while a procedure is in progress is the operator's responsibility. This is of increasing importance at dose levels where skin injuries are possible.

For other systems, reference point air kerma ($K_{a,r}$) is the best available metric for managing skin injury, while P_{KA} is the metric for estimating late cancer risk.

For interventional fluoroscopes, $K_{a,r}$ is defined at a point on the beam axis 15 cm from isocenter toward the x-ray tube. Depending on table height and patient size, this point is seldom exactly on the patient's skin and may be either inside or outside the patient. Furthermore, the reference point moves with the gantry as the beam is rotated or skewed. For these reasons, $K_{a,r}$ is not a precise measurement of skin dose. It tracks well enough for clinical use in laboratories without real-time dose maps. The laboratory's medical physicist should be consulted for further information on this topic.

Unfortunately, many laboratories continue to rely on fluoroscopic time as a primary dose measure. Fluoro time is a poor predictor of radiogenic risk because it does not account for the effects of patient size and beam orientation, cine usage, and other factors. As shown in **Figure 2.11**, there is an order of magnitude range of $K_{a,r}$ at almost any fluoro time. Similar noncoronary plots have an almost 2 orders of magnitude span due to both the wide range in tissue thicknesses in different procedures and the relative use of fluoroscopy versus acquisition in such procedures.

Postprocedural documentation of radiation should be a universal requirement as is documentation of drug and contrast medium use.

Including radiation reviews in the laboratory's continuous quality improvement program is important for patient safety as well as increasingly becoming accreditation or regulatory requirements. These should include individual reviews of patients with suspected or actual radiation injuries, examination of high-dose procedures, and periodic statistical reviews of the entire laboratory's experience.

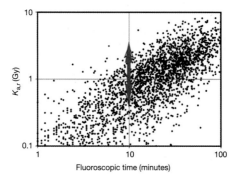

Figure 2.11 Fluoroscopic time is a poor predictor of dose. The plot illustrates the relationship between fluoro time and clinical dose. For most fluoro times, there is an order of magnitude range of different clinical doses (arrow).

Staged and Multiple Procedures

Staging a procedure allows time for DNA repair and tissue regeneration. A few months are required for skin and subcutaneous tissue regeneration to be as complete as biologically possible at skin doses above a few Gy. The required time interval increases with increasing skin dose. In addition, increasing skin dose results in losses of the local microvasculature and other forms of incomplete repair.

Patients who have previously undergone fluoroscopically guided procedures or radiation therapy may have a lower threshold for radiation injury in subsequent procedures. Extreme caution is needed when reirradiating a known radiogenic skin injury. By definition, repair is incomplete in an active injury. Substantial reirradiation of such regions can be catastrophic.

The skin of patients with a history of irradiation should be examined before starting a new procedure. Injured areas can be outlined with radio-opaque markers before the procedure. Operators should stay outside of the marked areas whenever clinically possible.

Radiogenic cancer may also be a consideration: decreases in radiosensitivity with age and the years to decades between irradiation and clinical cancer can be important. In addition, the LNT model states that an individual's radiogenic cancer risk depends on the total effective dose (E) accumulated over a lifetime. However, according to the LNT model, the carcinogenic risk of a procedure is independent of the patient's past radiation history. Thus, the anticipated radiation use in a planned procedure is the quantity of importance for use for preprocedure benefit-risk assessment.

Patient Education, Consent, and Follow-Up

The possibility of late radiogenic cancer or skin injury should be appropriately included in the informed consent process. Informed consent details should be enhanced for a patient who is at increased risk for 1 or more reasons. Radiogenic cancer is the primary risk for small (<50 kg) pediatric patients. Skin injury is a risk for patients who are expected to undergo a particularly long and complex procedure, have had multiple recent procedures, have received or are scheduled to receive radiotherapy to the chest, or who are extremely obese (>150 kg).

Appropriate postprocedure patient education and a follow-up plan are necessary for all patients where a substantial amount of radiation was used. The basics are informing the patient that radiation was used and to have his or her back examined by a family member approximately 2 and 4 weeks after the procedure. The laboratory is to be called if a red area "the size of a hand" is seen. Any reported reaction should be presumed to be radiogenic until proven otherwise. The patient should be instructed to avoid abrading or otherwise damaging the affected skin. They should also tell other health care providers that the lesion is of possible radiogenic etiology. The operator is responsible for follow-up for a year after the procedure. Patients with suspected radiation injuries should be seen in the operator's clinic for evaluation and referral if necessary.

Staff Radiation Safety

Staff radiation safety differs from patient radiation safety. Irradiation of staff is one of the risks of the job. Providers have a social obligation to provide care even if there is some risk. Nevertheless, available protective measures can reduce all forms of radiogenic risks to low levels.

Staff Tissue Reaction

Staff tissue reactions should never happen in an interventional setting. Nevertheless, there are reports of hair loss on the legs of interventional cardiologists (below the lead apron) after many years of practice. There are also reports of chronic skin changes and basal cell carcinoma in practitioners. Unnecessary hand irradiation is often seen in the interventional cardiology laboratory.

There has been a great deal of evidence collected in the past few years documenting radiation-induced opacities in the eyes of interventionalists and support staff. Based on this evidence, the National Council on Radiation Protection and Measurements (NCRP) and International Commission on Radiological Protection (ICRP) have recommended reducing the dose limit for the eyes to 50 mSv/y (NCRP) or 20 mSv/y (ICRP). The new recommended limit can be exceeded by a busy interventionalist who does not use supplemental eye protection.

Staff Cancer Risk

Cancer induction is a topic of real concern to staff members. Multiple studies of physician fluoroscopic users including interventional cardiologists, over the last 30 years, have produced only anecdotal reports with no confirmed evidence of increased cancer mortality in these populations. Nevertheless, interventional staff members are clearly exposed to radiation in the course of their duties, and the LNT model predicts a small increased risk.

Staff stochastic risk can be estimated using radiation monitors worn by a staff member. This should be an appropriately calculated value and not simply the raw reading from a monitor worn outside the lead apron. Radiation monitoring of interventionalists is currently tending toward a single badge worn at the collar outside all radiation personal protective equipment (RPPE). This provides a good estimate of eye dose and is used to estimate total body irradiation. An additional under-lead monitor may be of interest to some. The most highly irradiated operators in a properly functioning interventional laboratory probably receive an effective dose of a few mSv/y. Most laboratory staff receive <1 mSv/y. By way of comparison, the natural background radiation level in Denver exceeds that in New York City by about 1 mSv/y.

Basic Principles of Reducing Staff Radiation Exposure

Operators can use several methods to reduce their exposure to radiation. One important factor under the operator's control is reducing patient dose—the ultimate source of exposure of the operator and staff. Procedure strategies aimed at reducing exposure to radiation are summarized in **Table 2.3**.

Staff Radiation Monitoring

Radiation monitors are individually assigned and are to be worn whenever that individual is in a radiation environment. Always using the correct badge in its assigned position is critical to interpretation of the results. The primary badge should be worn at collar level above all radioprotective garments (RPPE). This badge monitors eye dose and provides an estimate of stochastic risk. Some facilities require a second badge worn at chest level under RPPE. Its reading is used to refine the stochastic risk assessment. The second monitor also assesses the performance of RPPE. If the reading of the "inside dosimeter" is high, additional RPPE is needed. If it is low, lighter weight RPPE might be enough to provide appropriate radiation protection to the wearer with reduced risk of orthopedic injury (from the weight of the RPPE).

Female workers in 2-badge facilities who are or might become pregnant should wear the inside badge at waist level to provide a better estimate of potential fetal dose. An additional "fetal dose" monitor is supplied in most facilities to monitor fetal dose once pregnancy is declared.

Table 2.3 Strategies to Reduce Exposure to Radiation

- Reduce fluoro and cine time
- Increase distance from the x-ray beam
- Use of appropriate radiation shielding
- Use of tableside protective drapes, pull-down eye shields, and roll-around shields
- Use of radioprotective garments. Wraparound one-piece or two-piece styles are preferred in the cath lab. Attenuation is usually stated in terms of lead equivalence with 0.35 mm being typical in the United States. High-lead–equivalent garments are heavy and often impose hazardous muscular-skeletal loads.
- Concerns regarding radiogenic cataract is reflected by the NCRP and ICRP reductions of the annual dose limit to the eye. Interventionalists will exceed this level without proper eye protection. Ideally, shielding includes a combination of pull-down shields and radioprotective eyewear. Monitoring of one's eye dose with a collar badge is essential.
- Situational awareness of when radiation is being produced.
- Beam angulation influences the scatter field near the operator. For example, in the lateral position, there is an order of magnitude more scatter on the x-ray tube side of the patient relative to the image receptor side.

ICRP, International Commission on Radiological Protection; NCRP, National Council on Radiation Protection and Measurements.

There is no substitute for having each individual in the laboratory always monitor his or her own exposure using "radiation badges." In addition to this being a legal requirement, routine monitoring is an indispensable tool for managing and minimizing operators' risk.

INTRAVASCULAR CONTRAST AGENTS

The development of iodinated contrast agents has led to the major advancements in x-ray-based imaging that have characterized the past century.

Iodinated Contrast Agents

Modern contrast agents are based on *iodine,* which by virtue of its high atomic number and chemical versatility has proved to be an excellent agent for intravascular opacification. Inorganic iodine (sodium iodide), however, causes marked toxic reactions. Experiments in 1929 thus explored an organic iodide preparation (Selectan) that contained 1 iodine atom per benzoic acid ring. In the 1950s, a series of substituted *triiodobenzoic acid* derivatives were developed, which contain 3 iodine atoms per ring. These agents differ from each other in terms of the specific side chains used in positions 1, 3, and, influencing both solubility and toxicity.

Ratio-1.5 ionic compounds are substituted ionic triiodobenzoic acid derivatives that contain 3 atoms of iodine for every 2 ions (that is, the substituted benzoic acid ring and the accompanying cation). Included in this family of *high-osmolar* contrast agents are agents such as Renografin (Bracco), Hypaque (Nycomed), and Angiovist (Berlex), which are mixtures of the meglumine and sodium salts of diatrizoic acid. Functionally similar agents are based on iothalamic acid (Conray [Mallinckrodt]) or metrizoic acid (Isopaque). These agents have a sodium concentration roughly equal to blood, pH titrated between 6.0 and 7.0, and a low concentration (0.1-0.2 mg/mL) of calcium disodium ethylenediaminetetraacetic acid. Higher or lower sodium concentrations may contribute to ventricular arrhythmias during coronary injection, and calcium binding by sodium citrate may cause greater myocardial depression. To have an iodine concentration of 320 to 370 mg I/mL, as is required for left ventricular and coronary contrast injection, solutions of these agents are markedly hypertonic (with an osmolality >1500 mOsm/kg, roughly 6 times that of blood).

In the mid-1980s, the first *ratio-3* lower-osmolality contrast materials were introduced. Although it is still ionic (as a mixture of meglumine and sodium salts), ioxaglate (Hexabrix [Mallinckrodt]) is a ratio-3 agent by virtue of its unique dimeric structure that includes 6 molecules of iodine on the dimeric ring (three atoms of iodine for every ion). To achieve an iodine concentration of 320 mg I/mL, ioxaglate has an osmolality roughly twice that of blood and contributes to a lower incidence of undesirable side effects related to hypertonicity.

A more significant modification in the late 1980s, however, was the introduction of true *nonionic ratio-3* contrast agents. These low-osmolality contrast agents are water soluble in a noncharged form, without an associated cation. Examples include iopamidol (Isovue [Bracco]), iohexol (Omnipaque [Nycomed]), metrizamide (Amipaque [Winthrop]), ioversol (Optiray [Mallinckrodt]), and ioxilan (Oxilan [Cook]), each containing three atoms of iodine for every molecule. Their viscosity (which influences ease of injection through small-lumen catheters) is roughly 6 to 10 times that of water.

In the late 1990s, a *ratio-6* nonionic dimeric compound (iodixanol, Visipaque [Nycomed]) was released as an *iso-osmolar* contrast agent.

In summary, available contrast media can be classified as high osmolar (1500-2000 mOsm/kg), low osmolar (600-1000 mOsm/kg), and iso-osmolar (290 mOsm/kg). There is extensive evidence that low-osmolar and iso-osmolar contrast media produce fewer episodes of bradycardia and hypotension, precipitate less angina, and cause less nausea and sensation of heat than traditional high-osmolar contrast agents. There is also evidence that the nonionic ratio-3 and ratio-6 agents produce fewer allergic side effects and are less nephrotoxic in human studies. For all of these reasons, coronary and vascular angiography is now routinely performed with low-osmolar contrast agents.

Most studies have been unable to demonstrate a clear advantage of the iso-osmolar agent iodixanol over low-osmolar contrast agents with regard to contrast-induced nephropathy (CIN). It should also be noted that randomized clinical trials and meta-analysis have shown a benefit of the iso-osmolar agent iodixanol when compared with iohexol and ioxaglate, but no benefit when compared with iopamidol, ioversol, or iopromide. It has been suggested that in addition to the osmolarity, the viscosity of the contrast agent might play a role in the development of CIN, with a higher viscosity associated with a higher risk.

Gadolinium

Gadolinium is a rare earth metal that has paramagnetic properties. In its salt form, gadolinium is very toxic. However, through a process of chelation by which large molecules create a complex surrounding gadolinium ions, less toxic gadolinium compounds have been developed and are currently used for magnetic resonance imaging.

Due to the risk of CIN with the use of iodinated contrast agents in patients with chronic renal failure, there was initial enthusiasm in the development of gadolinium-enhanced coronary angiography. However, more recent studies have shown that gadolinium does not seem to provide added benefit when compared to iodinated contrast agents in the prevention of CIN in high-risk patients. In addition, there have been several reports on the development of a rare systemic fibrosing disease, nephrogenic systemic fibrosis, in patients with chronic renal failure receiving gadolinium contrast agents. Therefore, the current recommendation is to avoid the use of gadolinium in patients with advanced renal failure (glomerular filtration rate <30 mL/min/1.73 m^2), in patients on dialysis, and in patients with hepatorenal syndrome.

Carbon Dioxide

Carbon dioxide (CO_2) gas was initially used in the 1950s as a contrast agent for the diagnosis of pericardial effusions. The development of DSA has expanded the use of CO_2 and as of today CO_2 angiography has emerged as an alternative approach that provides the advantage of virtually no risk of allergic reactions or renal toxicity. Familiarity with the technique is critical to minimize the risk of air contamination, or the accumulation of CO_2 bubbles that can lead to embolism or occlusion of small vessels. Given an association of CO_2 angiography with a risk of cerebral, coronary, and spinal artery embolization, its use has been limited to vascular beds below the diaphragm.

SUGGESTED READINGS

1. Accessed February 21, 2021. https://www.dicomstandard.org/current/
2. American College of Radiology. *Manual on Contrast Media—Version 10.3.* 2018.
3. Aspelin P, Aubry P, Fransson SG, Strasser R, Willenbrock R, Berg KJ; Nephrotoxicity in High-Risk Patients Study of Iso-Osmolar and Low-Osmolar Non-Ionic Contrast Media Study Investigators. Nephrotoxic effects in high-risk patients undergoing angiography. *N Engl J Med.* 2003;348(6):491-499.
4. Balter S, Hopewell JW, Miller DL, Wagner LK, Zelefsky MJ. Fluoroscopically guided interventional procedures: a review of radiation effects on patients' skin and hair. *Radiology.* 2010;254(2):326-341.
5. Balter S. Fundamental properties of digital images. *Radiographics.* 1993;13(1):129-141.
6. Balter S. Digital images. *Catheter Cardiovasc Interv.* 1999;46(4):487-496.
7. Balter S. Prognostic value of the flat fluoroscopic detector. *Catheter Cardiovasc Interv.* 2004;63(3):331.
8. Bertrand ME, Esplugas E, Piessens J, Rasch W. Influence of a nonionic, iso-osmolar contrast medium (iodixanol) versus an ionic, low-osmolar contrast medium (ioxaglate) on major adverse cardiac events in patients undergoing percutaneous transluminal coronary angioplasty: a multicenter, randomized, double-blind study. Visipaque in Percutaneous Transluminal Coronary Angioplasty [VIP] Trial Investigators. *Circulation.* 2000;101(2):131-136.
9. Cantone MC, Ginjaume M, Miljanic S, et al. Report of IRPA task group on the impact of the eye lens dose limits. *J Radiol Prot.* 2017;37(2):527-550.
10. Cousins C, Miller DL, Bernardi G, et al. ICRP publication 120: radiological protection in cardiology. *Ann ICRP.* 2013;42:1-125.
11. Eagan JT Jr., Jones CT. Cutaneous cancers in an interventional cardiologist: a cautionary tale. *J Interv Cardiol.* 2011;24(1):49-55.
12. FDA. Federal performance standard for diagnostic x-ray systems and their major components—FDA. Final rule. *Fed Regist.* 2005;70:33998-34042.
13. Hawkins IF, Caridi JG. Carbon dioxide (CO2) digital subtraction angiography: 26-year experience at the University of Florida. *Eur Radiol.* 1998;8(3):391-402.
14. Heinz-Peer G, Neruda A, Watschinger B, et al. Prevalence of NSF following intravenous gadolinium-contrast media administration in dialysis patients with endstage renal disease. *Eur J Radiol.* 2010;76(1):129-134.
15. Hirshfeld JW Jr., Ferrari VA, Bengel FM, et al. 2018 ACC/HRS/NASCI/SCAI/SCCT expert consensus document on optimal use of ionizing radiation in cardiovascular imaging-best practices for safety and effectiveness, part 1. Radiation physics and radiation biology: a report of the American College of Cardiology Task Force on expert consensus decision pathways. *J Am Coll Cardiol.* 2018;71(24):2811-2828.
16. Hirshfeld JW Jr., Ferrari VA, Bengel FM, et al. 2018 ACC/HRS/NASCI/SCAI/SCCT expert consensus document on optimal use of ionizing radiation in cardiovascular imaging-best practices for safety and effectiveness, part 2. Radiological equipment operation, dose sparing methodologies, patient and medical personnel protection: a report of the American College of Cardiology Task Force on expert consensus decision pathways. *J Am Coll Cardiol.* 2018;71(24):2829-2855.
17. IAE Agency. *Dosimetry in Diagnostic Radiology: An International Code of Practice.* International Atomic Energy Agency; 2007.
18. IEC 60601. *Medical Electrical Equipment—Part 2-43 2nd Edition: Particular Requirements for the Safety of X-ray Equipment for Interventional Procedures.* 2010.
19. Justinvil GN, Leidholdt EM Jr., Balter S, et al. Preventing harm from fluoroscopically guided interventional procedures with a risk-based analysis approach. *J Am Coll Radiol.* 2019;16(9 pt A):1144-1152.
20. Lopez PO, Dauer LT, Loose R, et al. ICRP publication 139: occupational radiological protection in interventional procedures. *Ann ICRP.* 2018;47(2):1-118.

21. Measurements NCoRPa Report 115. *Risk Estimates for Radiation Protection.* NCRP; 1993.
22. Measurements NCoRPa Report 168. *Radiation Dose Management for Fluoroscopically Guided Interventional Medical Procedures*; 2010.
23. Measurements NCoRPa. *Composite Glossary 1991-2 006. NCRP Report.* NCRP; 2006.
24. Mettler FA Jr., Huda W, Yoshizumi TT, Mahesh M. Effective doses in radiology and diagnostic nuclear medicine: a catalog. *Radiology.* 2008;248(1):254-263.
25. Miller DL, Vano E, Bartal G, et al. Occupational radiation protection in interventional radiology: a joint guideline of the Cardiovascular and Interventional Radiology Society of Europe and the Society of interventional radiology. *J Vasc Interv Radiol.* 2010;21(5):607-615.
26. Nickoloff EL. AAPM/RSNA physics tutorial for residents: physics of flat-panel fluoroscopy systems—survey of modern fluoroscopy imaging—flat-panel detectors versus image intensifiers and more. *Radiographics.* 2011;31(2):591-602.
27. Rajaraman P, Doody MM, Yu CL, et al. Cancer risks in U.S. radiologic technologists working with fluoroscopically guided interventional procedures, 1994-2008. *AJR Am J Roentgenol.* 2016;206(5):1101-1108. quiz 1109.
28. Reed M, Meier P, Tamhane UU, Welch KB, Moscucci M, Gurm HS. The relative renal safety of iodixanol compared with low-osmolar contrast media: a meta-analysis of randomized controlled trials. *JACC Cardiovasc Interv.* 2009;2(7):645-654.
29. Schwab SJ, Hlatky MA, Pieper KS, et al. Contrast nephrotoxicity: a randomized controlled trial of a nonionic and an ionic radiographic contrast agent. *N Engl J Med.* 1989;320(3):149-153.
30. Seals KF, Lee EW, Cagnon CH, Al-Hakim RA, Kee ST. Radiation-induced cataractogenesis: a critical literature review for the interventional radiologist. *Cardiovasc Intervent Radiol.* 2016;39(2):151-160.
31. Spinosa DJ, Angle JF, Hartwell GD, Hagspiel KD, Leung DA, Matsumoto AH. Gadolinium-based contrast agents in angiography and interventional radiology. *Radiol Clin North Am.* 2002;40(4):693-710.

3 Integrated Imaging Modalities in the Cardiac Catheterization Lab[1]

The emergence of a multitude of new therapeutic cardiac interventions has been allowed by the development of 2 critical technologies. The first type of technology includes therapeutic devices, often accompanied by novel delivery systems. The second type is medical imaging, which allows the therapeutic device to be used. The subject of this chapter is the new cardiac catheterization–based imaging paradigm, which includes new imaging modalities and their integration into the cardiac catheterization laboratory.

LIMITATIONS OF TRADITIONAL IMAGING SYSTEMS

Fluoroscopy is a real-time imaging modality; the proceduralist activates the x-ray system with the foot pedal and can immediately see the instantaneous movement of catheters, assuming they are manufactured with materials that are radiopaque. One of the limitations of fluoroscopic imaging includes the format of the resultant image; the image is abstract and not inherently a complete anatomic image. This flat 2-dimensional (2D) projection image is analogous to a "shadow image" but with a broader range of gray scales proportional to the variable penetration of x-rays. Years of experience and technology refinements, including the development of storage and replay of image acquisitions and road-mapping using angiographic images to facilitate equipment navigation, have made fluoroscopy the workhorse modality of the cardiac catheterization laboratory.

Diagnostic and therapeutic procedures, such as percutaneous coronary intervention, extensively use a system for catheter advancement called the "over-the-wire" technique. This technique is used as an alternative to the difficulty and potential danger associated with the unassisted advancement of catheters in the 3-dimensional (3D) branching vascular beds, both leading to the heart and also within the coronary tree. The "over-the-wire" technique converts this 3D pathway to the target into a 2D-like linear rail needed to complete the intervention using the simplicity, familiarity, and other virtues of only traditional fluoroscopy. Furthermore, relatively small amounts of contrast can be intermittently injected to visualize the small tubular vascular structures during the final placement of therapeutic devices such as coronary stents.

Most recently, the development of new interventions targeting dynamic soft-tissue structures and requiring new navigation in large cardiac chambers has led to the realization that the imaging needs to guide cardiovascular therapies are often different from the imaging needs of diagnostic procedures. These differences are important to understand when considering new imaging modalities (**Table 3.1**).

EVOLUTION OF IMAGING NEEDS IN THE CARDIAC CATHETERIZATION SUITE

The purpose of medical imaging during a therapeutic cardiac catheterization is to enable the efficient, safe, and effective performance of the sequential tasks needed for the specific intervention. The choice of imaging is dictated by the task to be performed.

[1]We gratefully acknowledge the Grossman & Baim's *Cardiac Catheterization, Angiography, and Intervention*, 9th edition contributions of Drs. Robert A Quaife and John D Carroll as portions of their chapter, Integrated Imaging Modalities in the Cardiac Catheterization Lab, were retained in this text.

Table 3.1	Major Differences Between Cardiac Imaging for Dedicated Diagnostic Purposes Versus Image Guidance of Therapeutic Procedures
Dedicated Diagnostic Medical Imaging	**Image Guidance of Therapeutic Procedures**
Comprehensive with image sets for visualization and other derived parameters needed to assess structures and function	Focused with images to visualize equipment and targets to guide task completion and to assess immediate pre/postresults and potential complications
Standardized protocols for image acquisition with predetermined list of views with minor ad hoc changes in imaging views	Flexible protocols for image guidance that are optimized ad hoc to complete specific tasks such as (1) optimize hand-eye coordination of interventionalist; (2) 3D alignment of a device and target anatomy
Image acquisition and interpretation often completed separately	Real-time acquisition with immediate use and concurrent interpretation in dynamic environment
Outcome: A report with diagnostic value	Outcome: Successful and uncomplicated intervention
Assessment of value of diagnostic imaging modality: Evaluation using hierarchical fashion and leading to appropriateness criteria	Assessment of value of image guidance modality: Evaluation more technical and incorporation in interventional guidelines (problematic)
Imaging modality used determined by diagnostic and patient considerations	Imaging modality used determined by type of intervention
Physician skill set related to modality and experience in its diagnostic use	Physician skill set related to modality and experience in both diagnostic and therapeutic guidance use

Each imaging modality has unique features, and the same modality might have different versions. The performance of tasks as part of an intervention requires real-time imaging, of which there are only 2 types: fluoroscopy and ultrasound. **Table 3.2** provides a comparison of these 2 modalities as an additional overview to understand the emergence of new approaches in the cardiac catheterization laboratory.

As seen with the evolution of intravascular ultrasound or intracoronary imaging, a key to the efficient use of new technology is its integration into the cardiac catheterization laboratory infrastructure. There are multiple levels of integration, including image acquisition, processing, display, and archiving; the commercially available products that incorporate these needs for integration are rapidly evolving. Display of targeted key structures uses either a focused or wide field of view (FOV) to enable cardiac procedures. Inherent to each modality chosen (ie, CT angiography [CTA], cardiac MR, cardiac 2D or 3D echocardiography, or intrachamber echocardiography) are the characteristics to display fine versus gross or still versus moving structures.

The imaging workstation, often with table-side controls, is one addition to the cardiac catheterization facility required by multimodality imaging. Processing of fluoroscopic and angiographic images has become part of the internal workings of

Table 3.2	**Overview of Real-Time Imaging Modalities to Guide the Performance of Diagnostic and Interventional Tasks in Cardiac Catheterization Laboratory**	
Modality	**Fluoroscopy**	**Ultrasound**
Field of view (FOV)	Variable and includes large field that can include whole heart, surrounding structures, and entire thorax or abdomen	Variable but upper limit of multiple cardiac chambers
System for acquisition	Limited to gantry. Either with 1 or 2 gantries (ie, single vs biplane)	Transducer based. Diversity of probes including external application to skin, transesophageal, and intracardiac
Operator	Interventionalist	Sometimes interventionalist but transesophageal echocardiography requires echocardiographers (both physician and sonographer)
Experience with guidance of interventions	Extensive and well established over decades	Growing over last decade
Integration of technology in cardiac catheterization laboratory	Complete	Incomplete
Safety	Radiation-related risks	Probe-related risks
Strengths and weaknesses in visualization: 1. Current generation of intravascular equipment and devices 2. Navigation in vascular pathway to heart 3. Navigation in cardiac chamber 4. Navigation and interaction with soft-tissue targets such as native valves and chamber defects 5. Navigation and interaction with coronary target 6. Navigation and interaction with other vascular targets	1. Excellent 2. Excellent 3. Excellent for simple tasks but fair to good even with contrast injection for complex tasks 4. Poor and limited to intermittent contrast visualization 5. Excellent with contrast injection 6. Excellent with contrast injection	1. Limited 2. Limited to access point 3. Excellent 4. Excellent with caveat that high level of expertise required 5. Poor and nonexistent for active guidance 6. Limited
Real-time 3D visualization and create views of target/anatomy that are independent of location of image acquisition system	No	Yes
Future adaptability to robotic guidance systems and holographic display	Limited without fusion with 3D images from another modality	Yes

modern x-ray systems, but image processing involving 3D volumetric image formats, segmentation, and multimodality image fusion with registration requires the imaging workstation. Direct digital links to the CTA and magnetic resonance angiography (MRA) hospital archival system are needed to enable the intraprocedure use of previously acquired images in patients now undergoing an intervention.

The emergence of multimodality imaging has changed the requirements standards of display systems. Monitors must be able to show not only gray scales but also the color used to represent "depth" in 3D ultrasound images. The potential of displaying medical images in a holographic format is a new exciting development that may be initially tested in the cardiac catheterization environment and studied for its impact on the performance of interventions optimally performed with 3D visualization. With this transformation in image display, the 3D image is displayed in 3D space, and the operator uses the human visual system's ability to perceive depth rather than the color-coding and shading necessary to represent 3D aspects of the image on a traditional 2D monitor.

The skill sets of the proceduralist, as well as the nature of the team performing these new procedures, are evolving as rapidly as the technology. Specifically, the interventional cardiologist in the past was proficient predominantly in using fluoroscopy and performing angiography. The interventional cardiologist of today and of the future must be proficient not only in these older techniques but also in CTA, MR, different forms of cardiac ultrasound, OCT (optical coherence tomography) technology, and in their use for preplanning and for the actual performance of interventions. Examples of different imaging guidance strategies are listed in **Table 3.3**. This evolution has also led to an expansion of the team of physicians and staff. With complex structural heart disease interventions (SHDIs), it has become essential that a colleague expert in ultrasound, including 3D transesophageal echocardiography (TEE), be part of the interventional team.

Table 3.3   Examples of Study Designs to Determine Relative Merits of Different Image Guidance Strategies

Procedure	Image Guidance Modality Comparison	Outcome Metrics
Coronary angiography	Rotational vs conventional angiography (multiple fixed gantry positions)	Radiation exposure, contrast volume, time to completion, image content
Transcatheter atrial septal defect and PFO closure	Intracardiac echocardiography vs transesophageal echocardiography	Successful closure, complications, fluoroscopy time, procedure time, costs, need for general anesthesia, patient satisfaction
Atrial flutter ablation	Fluoroscopy alone vs fluoroscopy with real-time 3D transesophageal echocardiography	Rate of complete bidirectional block, number of radiofrequency applications to achieve block, complications, procedural time, radiation exposure

PFO, patent foramen ovale.

Value Assessment

Table 3.4 summarizes factors that are felt important in the evaluation of an image guidance modality. Technical performance is routinely evaluated. Single-center studies are sometimes conducted measuring ease of use and intermediate markers of clinical outcomes. Occasional randomized trials are conducted comparing different imaging approaches. Yet, new technologies are difficult to evaluate due to several factors. First, they must be studied on a procedure-specific basis to assess outcomes. Second, the number of patients studied may need to be large in order to show an impact on infrequent events such as major complications. Third, the relative contribution of the imaging modality on clinical outcomes may be difficult to differentiate from the relative contribution of other determinants. Finally, the approval process for new image guidance technology by governmental regulatory agencies is often based on technical performance and general safety issues rather than on improved patient outcomes. Thus, pivotal randomized trials measuring clinical endpoints are generally not performed. This does limit the claims of what benefit a product may bring by imaging companies and often precludes imaging technologies from being incorporated into professional society clinical management guidelines that use level of evidence from clinical trials to determine necessity and value.

NEW IMAGING MODALITIES

Current methods such as x-ray fluoroscopy, 2D echocardiography, 3D echocardiography (3DE), cardiac MR, and cardiac CT have developed independently and merged into important adjuncts that enable the execution of complex structural interventions. **Figure 3.1** demonstrates the concepts of preplanning, orientation, sizing, and then fused image guidance of left atrial appendage closure exemplifying SHDIs.

Echocardiography

Ultrasound image generation is dependent upon either transmission or reflection of propagated sound waves and the return frequencies characteristically produced

Table 3.4 Assessment of Image Guidance Technology

Technological assessment: accuracy, image quality, reliability, graphic user interface, integration into cardiac catheterization laboratory, integration into image archiving system

Scope of use: General or niche applications: specific diagnostic and therapeutic procedures for which technology is appropriate (proven or expected)

Competency and training needed: relevance to board certification or hospital credentialing, learning curve of users, additional personnel needed and with what specific skill sets

Impact on procedure performance (relevant to image guidance technology): duration, specific task performance metrics, radiation exposure, contrast volume, rate of successful procedure completion, rate of complications, confidence of operator during performance of procedure.

Impact on patient outcomes (relevant to image guidance technology): mortality, frequency and outcomes of complications, successful vs unsuccessful procedures

System, cost, and reimbursement issues: infrastructure and other support availability for new modality, direct costs, capital costs, other infrastructural issues, personnel time

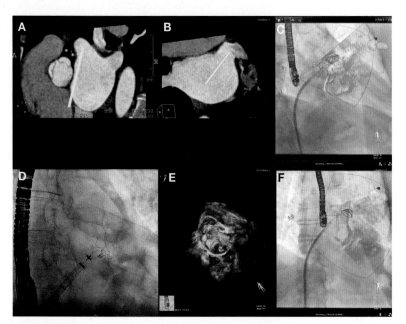

Figure 3.1 Steps of planning left atrial appendage (LAA) occlusion shown in the panels. Panels A and B are transseptal puncture location and LAA os measurement. 3D image guidance fused echocardiography and fluoroscopy (Panel C) and fluoroscopy with catheter and device alone (Panel D) and then 3D-TEE image from left atrial view with catheter and device (Panel E) and then fused catheter device; models all displayed in a single format for procedural guidance (Panel F).

by different tissues. The frequencies used in medical imaging are tuned to both the target tissues and the depth needing to be imaged. These ultrasound images provide the anatomic landscape for interventional procedures. However, the interaction of highly reflective devices such as a "J" wire causes reverberation or signal dropout that must be mentally integrated with tissue effects when attempting to understand the anatomic landscape. Conversely, some catheters or wires, such as a "Glidewire," demonstrate very little ultrasound signature, thus making visibility almost impossible. The quality of the ultrasound image of a structure is dependent on the volume and characteristics of the tissue between the transducer and the target of image acquisition. Finally, for visualization of catheters and wires, ultrasound image quality is best when the target is laid out perpendicular to the ultrasound waves and, conversely, may be "invisible" when parallel to the ultrasound waves. Therefore, greater flexibility in where the transducer system(s) is located is important and is an advantage of catheter-based ultrasound systems that can be moved to locations to optimize visualization.

2D-TEE is capable of measuring structural defects, guiding navigation of catheters, and monitoring the delivery of devices. The safety and effectiveness of 2D-TEE are well established in ASD/VSD (atrial septal defect/ventricular septal defect) device sizing, equipment navigation, device deployment, and assessment of postprocedural complications such as thrombus formation. However, the incorporation of 3D technologies has suggested greater precision sizing of aortic annular diameter and likely translates to other anatomical targets such as septal defects and the entire mitral and tricuspid valve complexes incompletely visualized by standard 2D methods. Complementary use of echocardiography with x-ray imaging results in reduced radiation exposure when ultrasound guidance for navigation is performed in combination with an effort to reduce fluoroscopy. The advantage of enhanced guidance is balanced by the risk of long interventions that require general anesthesia.

Real-time 3D transthoracic echocardiography (RT3D-TTE) has been clinically implemented to improve endomyocardial biopsy accuracy and off-pump mitral valve (MV) edge-to-edge repair in a pig model. This was expanded to successful percutaneous pediatric ASD closure. The development of RT3D imaging with both 3D-TTE and 3D-TEE integrates moving structures with the definition of tissue structure and depth in wide FOVs, providing superior structure resolution. This allows the definition of cardiac defects, chambers, and valves while directly and simultaneously monitoring the movements of interventional devices.

Volume rendering and perspective are accomplished through color shading of the volume, thereby creating a sense of depth, but precise distances are not well validated within RT3D acquisitions. Complete volume data-gated acquisition takes advantage of the RT3D-TEE's wide FOV by scanning and integrating a volumetric echosector, thereby displaying moving cardiac structures. This is a summation of 4 adjacent wedge-shaped volumetric data sets that are acquired sequentially over 4 cardiac cycles, with subsequent fusion into a single large echosector (**Figure 3.2C**). The data set may be viewed online or offline in operator-defined cropped planes in any axis and orientation, offering several visual vantage points ideal for preprocedural planning.

RT3D images may be acquired via 2 modes: (1) larger FOV with focused thickness (**Figure 3.2B**) volume that segments heart valves, complex defects, masses, and might allow visualization of the right ventricle; (2) high magnification mode, which acquires images using an obtuse view angle and a limited sector region of interest with less depth (**Figure 3.2A**). The wider FOV and greater perspective make it ideal for navigating catheters and interventional devices, while the thin sector 3D is better for determining edges of ASDs or leaflet insertion in valve clip procedure. Both volumetric data sets may be rotated or tilted to define desired structures and can be viewed in cropped planes of any axis and orientation. However, a systematic approach to the movement of the volume is critical to avoid anatomic confusion. Thus, one could first tilt the image to gain a top view from which rotation like a clock can occur and then move toward key structures like the aortic valve positioned at 12 o'clock to provide standard perspectives such as the "surgeon's view" of the left atrium. These methods provide the advantage of online manipulation of the data set, performed from different viewing angles or perspectives without probe repositioning or causing associated workflow interruptions for a proceduralist.

While individual procedures emphasize specific elements of the process of executing structural interventions, common elements include preprocedural planning, targeting, detection/positioning/tracking, mechanical biofeedback/eye-hand coordination, precise repositioning, alignment, navigation, 3D localization, deployment surveillance, and postprocedure inspection (**Figure 3.3**).

Rotational Angiography

The planar nature of x-ray imaging visualizes insufficiently soft tissue and requires operators to mentally reconstruct cardiac structures. The development of flat-panel detectors has blurred the difference between true x-ray imaging and tomographic technologies. Full 3D data such as coronary vascular trees are extracted from the entire volume to evaluate angulation, foreshortening, and motion from a single cor-

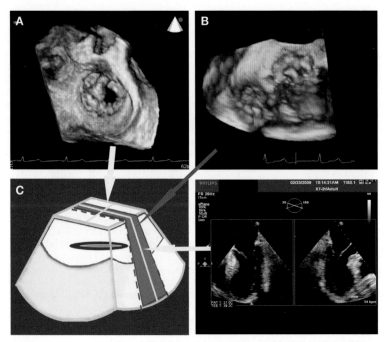

Figure 3.2 Graphic display of the volume images is shown by the 3 different 3D echocardio-graphic methods. Real-time (RT)3D-TEE focused method is shown in Panel A, which is at a focused depth that magnified 3D data set (creme color). Shown in Panel B is the narrow sector RT3D "live" method (blue color); note the larger field of view but with less depth or thickness. Lastly, Panel C the steerable biplane technique shows the orthogonal nature of the planes (yellow lines).

onary tree acquisition. A modality called C-arm CT uses rotation with segmented or continuous acquisition and simulates CT imaging. Using advanced gated 180° circular flat-panel rotation in combination with contrast injection, whole-heart CT-like image can be obtained. This provides large anatomic structure and muscle volume rendering adequate for the execution of complex congenital and structural heart disease interventions.

Intracardiac Echocardiography

Intracardiac echocardiography (ICE) provides superior image quality due to its close proximity to the structures from the right atrial position and other locations. It obviates the need for general anesthesia and is capable of guiding the navigation of catheters and devices, visualizing adjacent structures, and sizing defects. Currently, the evidence supports ICE as the modality of choice in percutaneous patent foramen ovale and ASD closure. However, ICE has fewer imaging planes than 2D-TEE and may interfere with guiding procedures performed from the right side of the heart. To date, ICE has limited 3D imaging capabilities for the guidance of complex procedures.

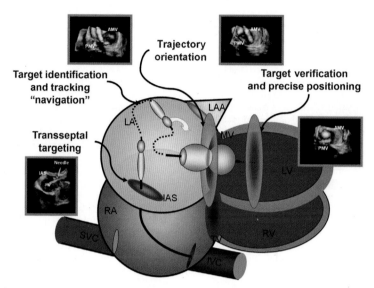

Figure 3.3 Steps for image guidance are shown. Using a mitral valve balloon valvuloplasty as an example, each key stage is shown: first, transseptal puncture; second, identification of the target; positioning and definition of trajectory; and target verification and precision adjustment. Each step is important for preplanning and procedural guidance. AMV, anterior mitral valve leaflet; IAS, interatrial septum; IVC, inferior vena cava; LA, left atrium; LAA, left atrial appendage; LV, left ventricle; MV, mitral valve; PMV, posterior mitral valve leaflet; PW, posterior wall; RA, right atrium; RV, right ventricle; SVC, superior vena cava.

Computed Tomography Angiography

Fine resolution of cardiac structures requires 2 key factors: (1) absolute resolution of the imaging system and (2) the ability to effectively stop cardiac motion. CT is a 360° map of x-ray attenuation. This map is then converted into intensity values ranging from −300 air to −100 fat; 0 fluid and +300 calcium. Injection of contrast materials high in iodine content in combination with CT allows visualization of chambers and vessels. The advent of faster gantry rotation speeds, increased numbers of detectors, and dual sources have improved both spatial and temporal resolution, thereby allowing the application of multislice CT scanners in SHD.

Implementation of both multiphase contrast injectors and high-concentration contrast agents (Isovue 370 mg/mL) has dramatically improved the image quality, a necessary requirement for delineation of fine structures (ie, atrial baffles, perivalvular leaks, valve leaflet morphology, and origin of the great vessels). Imaging of delicate structures present in SHDIs requires, at a minimum, a 64-row detector system. Cardiac structure visualization may be enhanced with new 256- or 320-detector row CT systems that allow "whole heart" data acquisition within 1 to 4 heartbeats. CTA image resolution is still based on lowering heart rate (approximately 60 BPM) to obtain the greatest image quality and simultaneously allow the lowest radiation exposure. Dual detector (2 head/tube) systems expand the heart rate range while maintaining high-quality images. Cardiac motion is least prominent during end-systole and mid- to late-diastole, making electrocardiographic gating a requirement of any cardiac CT exam. The use of oral or intravenous beta-blockers slows the heart rate, thereby limiting cardiac motion and subsequently improving image quality.

High flow rate and multiphase contrast injections allow high-quality images by minimizing contrast artifacts and providing high-contrast differential chamber delineations. Creating a contrast concentration gradient between structures or chambers is important for the accurate evaluation of anatomic targets, whether this is an ASD or a perivalvular leak. In a typical cardiac exam using a 64-slice scanner, approximately 75 mL of iodinated contrast (iopamidol [Isovue]; 370 mg/mL) is injected in the right antecubital vein at 5 mL/s followed by a 30 to 50 mL saline chase also delivered at 3 to 4 mL/s. These methods provide differential chamber contrast concentration necessary for the identification of the shunts (**Figure 3.4**), delineation of fine structures, orthogonal planes, and 3D special relationships often required for preprocedural planning in SHD.

Information regarding the potential right-to-left direction of ASD shunting can be determined by performing a dynamic contrast-enhanced cardiac exam. The orientation of a contrast jet on dynamic contrasted cardiac CT can be helpful in the differentiation of Secundum ASD from patent foramen and in shunt visualization of ischemic VSDs, left atrial appendage occlusion, perivalvular leak, or other complex congenital heart diseases (**Figures 3.4** and **3.5**).

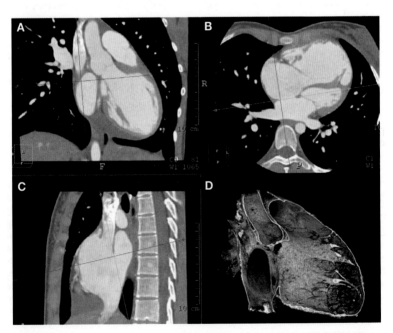

Figure 3.4 A large secundum atrial septal defect (ASD) is shown employing CT angiography. Orthogonal views (Panels A-C) define the size of the ASD with volumetric 3D display in the lower right image (Panel D). Note the lack of inferior rim, a finding that defines a likely unsuccessful percutaneous closure of the ASD.

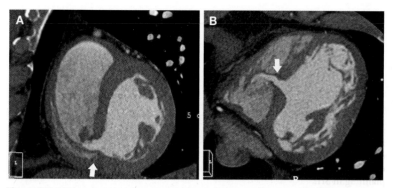

Figure 3.5 CTA images of an inferoseptal ventricular septal defect are shown (white arrow). Note the contrast gradient between the right and left ventricles shown in short-axis (Panel A) and horizontal long-axis (Panel B) projection.

Optimal acquisition protocols are critical for SHD evaluations. Reducing radiation exposure with the CT component is critical, especially when planning complex interventional procedures which have their own dose costs. ECG phase dose modulation or prospectively gated "step and shoot" sequential axial imaging technologies provide standard dose reduction strategies. Consideration of patient size is also required to properly tailor tube current and voltage to deliver the minimum radiation dose to the patient that answers the important question.

Successful percutaneous correction of SHD requires a thorough clinical evaluation and comprehensive preprocedure imaging, detailing the structural abnormality.

As shown in **Figure 3.6**, advanced cardiac imaging provides a valuable resource of heart- and vessel-specific information to evaluate exclusion characteristics, preprocedure sizing of devices, procedural risk assessment, and possible subsequent complications.

Magnetic Resonance Imaging and Angiography

Cardiac MRI (CMR) imaging is a valuable technique employed to evaluate patients with SHD. The key characteristic of CMR is the stimulation of tissue protons that in turn, provides radiofrequency energy specific to different tissue types, thus creating independent tissue signatures, which do not require contrast administration. Using these characteristics, cardiac structure, tissue signature, and flow can be determined by this technique. CMR routinely includes 4 major pulse sequence types used in the routine assessment of cardiovascular patients. They can be categorized as bright-blood cine sequence; dark blood T2-weighted sequence; phase-contrast sequence, and MRA. Cardiac gating is generally necessary to stop cardiac motion and reduce imaging blurring. Usually, CMR acquisition also employs breath-holding to remove respiratory motion.

Cardiac function and quantification of volumes and ejection fraction are performed using a bright-blood cine steady-state free precession sequence that produces a series of images, which are played as a composite movie loop averaged over multiple cardiac cycles (cinematic display). Cine images are acquired in standard cardiac axes allowing the determination of structural anatomy and physiologic motion.

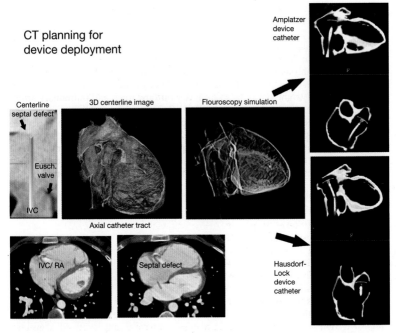

Figure 3.6 Diagrammatic processing of an atrial septal defect (ASD) is shown. The CTA preplanning is shown with centerline defining a potential pathway from the inferior vena cava through the defect into the left atrium. 3D images are shown in the center with a rapid prototype model testing different ASD closure delivery catheters on the right. IVC, inferior vena cava; RA, right atrium.

Dark blood sequence, on the other hand, produces images only at a single cardiac phase with bright soft-tissue structures (myocardium and vessel walls), but dark blood signals inside ventricles and vessel lumen again employing a breath-hold technique. Dark blood images are used to evaluate morphology, tissue characteristic, and connections of the cardiovascular structures. Adding a third inversion pulse provides enhanced proton signal that helps distinguish fluid or edema from fat or tissue.

Phase-contrast sequences generate quantitative velocity mapping similar to Doppler echocardiography. This method is useful for quantifying regurgitant volumes and Q_p/Q_s calculations present in perivalvular leaks and shunt pathology lesions. Phase-contrast sequences for coronary artery disease are used to quantify flow and pressure gradient estimated from velocity by the Bernoulli equation. Total flow is calculated by summing velocity across the luminal cross-section with a known slice thickness providing absolute flow and volume. Therefore, cardiac output, shunt ratio, and valvular regurgitation can be quantified.

MRA can be divided into contrast-enhanced technique and non–contrast-enhanced technique. Contrast-enhanced MRA produces high-resolution images, but due to the inherent noncubical (nonisotropic voxels) resolution, this technique is slightly more limited in evaluating thin structures often present in SHD. MRA is a volumetric technique that allows multiplanar reformatting of the bright, contrast-filled blood vessel, 3D data. Typically, this technique is not cardiac-gated and is used for evaluating noncardiac structures, such as the aorta and the pulmonary arteries. Administration of a gadolinium-based contrast agent is required at a concentration of between 0.1 and 0.2 mmol/kg for this technique.

MRA images can be postprocessed similarly to those of CTA. Multiplanar reformats and maximum intensity projections image orientation and display are the hallmark of image analysis for SHD. Selection of the timed segments of the dynamic gadolinium contrast injection is most critical to identify cardiac structures such as RA (right atrium), RV (right ventricle), pulmonary outflow tract, and pulmonary artery versus pulmonary veins, LA (left atrium), LV (left ventricle), and aorta. Once the segment is selected, MR vendors often have preset image "galleries" or color-coded volumetric 3D display packages to render the 2D image into a 3D format. Since CMR has less signal-to-noise ratio than CTA, these presets are often too stringent for these images and require individual manipulation. Despite this minor limitation of MRA images, similar image quality is provided to that of CTA once adjusted correctly.

IMAGE AND MODALITY COREGISTRATION

Medical diagnoses commonly rely on the assessment of both the functional status and the anatomic condition of the patient. The emergence of multidetector CT and MRI of anatomic structures changes the paradigm. The volumetric 3D nature of these images can potentially be used for both planning and execution of invasive procedures that typically involve a therapeutic intervention. Such volumetric data sets are imported into the angiographic suite and displayed either adjacent to the fluoroscopic images or as a true image overlay coregistered with the x-ray image.

Before the tracking process is initiated, the 3D multimodality-based data set needs to be registered with the patient's location and orientation on the table during the intervention. Navigation systems linked to interventions must have accurate, perfectly registered data sets that compensate for cardiac and respiratory motion to correlate with the patient's physical condition. The 3D CT or MR volumetric overlay provides tissue characterization of major structures coupled to catheter or guidewire manipulation and guidance, which tract C-arm rotation and movement. As part of the preprocedural planning, centerlines can be imported as well-defining pathways for the successful completion of the SHDI (**Figure 3.7**). While only a single cardiac phase depiction, the model sheds light on the size, orientation, and adjacencies around the target point. The addition of cinematic motion to these images often allows significantly improved visualization of such abnormal structures, but currently is technically challenging. The use of these preprocedural imaging methods hopefully improves safety and possibly shortens the time of SHDIs.

RT3D-TEE imaging is the technical leader in advanced guidance of complex interventional procedures. Target structures are usually centered within biplane orthogonal image before proceeding to the zoom mode. The perception of depth is created by portraying light surface color and deep structure as dark colors. Crisp 2D-TEE images are required to start with minimum gain necessary to define a homogeneous target structure. Next, appropriate standardized display of common structures allows orientation of the operator. Perspective is a key element that requires identification of the target and a view that provides clear visualization of motion. The advantage of RT3D-TEE is 3D imaging during cardiac contraction and structural motion. The direct visualization of catheter or device movement that is coupled with the manipulation of these devices allows enhanced eye-hand coordination to guide tasks.

MODALITY SELECTION

Advanced cardiac imaging techniques are usually performed after a screening echocardiogram. Selection of the appropriate imaging modality is probably related most to the type of SHD problem to be addressed, but may also be determined by availa-

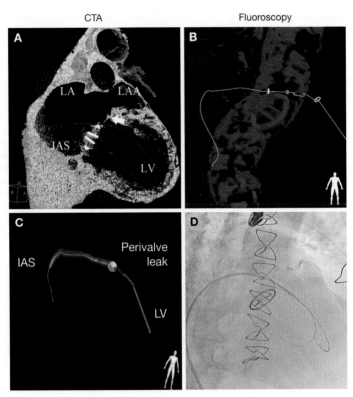

CTA

Fluoroscopy

Figure 3.7 Preprocedural planning is shown for a perivalvular leak. The centerline is drawn planning the pathway from the inferior vena cava through the interatrial septum to the lateral mitral perivalvular leak (Panel A). Note the overlay of the centerline into the fluoroscopic image with aortic calcification shown in red (Panel B). The guidewire through the orifice is shown by fluoroscopy and follows the previously planned route and trajectory (Panels C and D). IAS, interatrial septum; LA, left atrium; LAA, left atrial appendage; LV, left ventricle.

bility and local expertise. The decision for selection of the optimal imaging modality should be based on consideration of the absolute spatial resolution, temporal resolution, FOV, and characterization of different tissue types. Either CT or CMR provides extended FOV compared to echocardiography. This characteristic is important for pathway planning in the preprocedural evaluation process. CTA possesses inherently greater absolute resolution between 0.4 and 0.6 mm but is at the cost of lower temporal resolution even when large doses of beta-blockers are used to lower the heart rate and improve nonmotion imaging. CMR, in general, can be performed at most physiologic heart rates without heart rate-lowering medications and provides similar angiographic imaging but without ionizing radiation dose. These are usually only 1 cardiac phase and acquired at separate times, thus limiting the real-time use for active procedural guidance. 3D-TEE clearly provides the best real-time imaging methodology for SHD guidance. Given its excellent spatial and temporal resolution, it is currently the most useful technique for navigating the delivery of interventional devices.

VISUALIZATION: 2-DIMENSIONAL TO 3-DIMENSIONAL
3-Dimensional Fluoroscopy and Coregistration of Computed Tomography Imaging

Cardiovascular CT imaging in the preprocedural planning of complex SHDIs has the potential to streamline the intervention, reducing extensive diagnostic angiography and its concomitant radiation and contrast risks. Combined CT and fluoroscopy coregistered data can be used to directly guide SHDIs for pulmonary vascular complex problems. Cardiac phases that most clearly depict the pulmonary artery are used to segment cardiac chambers and cardiac vessels. Centerline segmentation algorithms are used to project and identify the expected trajectory through the interventional target in the pulmonary artery. 3D centerline simulated trajectories can be imported into the catheterization lab and coregistered to fluoroscopic images from a single cardiac phase CT image data set. CT image data are projected into similar fluoroscopic views to define optimal viewing projections. The same viewing plane as in catheterization lab C-arm and overlaid onto live fluoroscopy can be used to identify positions of initiation and procedure guidance. Target reorientation or dilation followed by device deployment can be determined on the fly when superimposed onto contrast angiographic images (**Figure 3.7**). Importantly, planning of orientation and identification of best angiographic views can be performed well in advance of the interventional procedure (**Figure 3.8**).

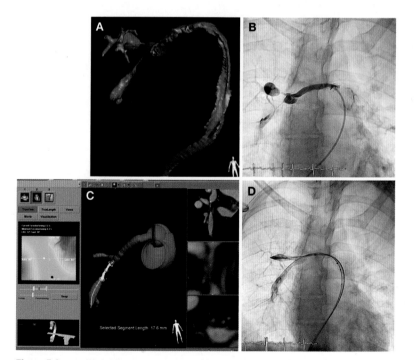

Figure 3.8 CT overlay with CTA is shown displayed in the interventional suite. Centerline with fluoroscopy shows the pathway for a pulmonary artery intervention and stenting. The best "TrueView" image is shown to determine the best angulation by fluoroscopy to perform the procedure (Panels A and C). Shown on the right panels are pulmonary artery angiogram before (Panels B and D) and after angioplasty and stenting.

Real-Time Echocardiographic 3-Dimensional

Spatially orienting and localizing targets for interventions is enhanced with RT3D-TEE.

Targeted volumetric imaging can center defects and simultaneously monitor catheters and guidewires. Orientation of these catheters in 3D space is difficult to predict and constantly changes during repositioning when using 2D echocardiographic views. RT3D-TEE, however, allows changing perspective on the fly while providing visual biofeedback. Visual feedback enables the operator to be reoriented to the external inputs corresponding to moving the delivery system.

New imaging technologies are being developed to synchronize the x-ray and RT3D-TEE images and to allow the interventionalist to define the perspective best suited for the SHDI. An integrated echocardiographic and fluoroscopic imaging system for interventional use has recently been developed that registers the TEE probe with the x-ray C-arm integrated 3D-TEE and fluoroscopic images (**Figure 3.9**). The technology provides images in multiple 3D views simultaneously with table-side control by the interventionalist.

Preprocedural virtual planning and device selection

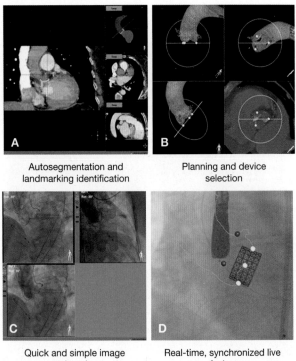

Autosegmentation and landmarking identification	Planning and device selection
Quick and simple image registration	Real-time, synchronized live fusion

Figure 3.9 Shown are steps of planning, device selection, and image registration for rotational CT "road-mapping" to define correct aortic annular plane and optimal view for displaying aortic cusps (Panels A and B). Angiographic display with cusps marked (Panel C) and with device in place (Panel D).

New technologies have increased the usable FOV in 3D (X8-2t probe Phillips Healthcare, Andover, MA) and also increased frequency sampling to approximately 15 Hz when acquiring both zoomed 3D and color flow data sets. The specific impact of novel features such as x-ray-echo registration, multiple 3D perspectives, and the proceduralist's control of TEE-derived images is evolving. This includes projected models segmented from the 3D-TEE data sets that provide a real-time understanding of structures and relationships, and boundaries important for new, more complex SHDIs.

NEW FRONTIERS

Seamless integration of imaging technologies into hybrid interventional spaces and expansion of intervention for SHD are driving the use of combined modality imaging to simultaneously visualize cardiac boundaries, adjacent structures, specific tissue targets, and pathways (**Figures 3.10** and **3.11**). Incorporation of rapid prototyping with either using 3D-printed models or advanced modeling software will determine patient-specific device fit and sizing.

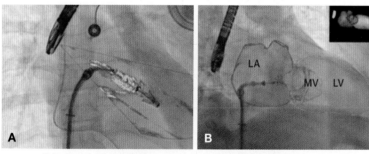

Color Doppler fluoro overlay   3D TEE Heart model fluoro overlay

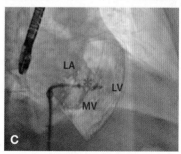

3D TEE fluoro overlay

Figure 3.10 Real-time 3D-TEE fluoro overlay use of color flow jet as a target during procedural guidance (Panel A). Derived models from 3D-TEE provide orientation and direction of clip manipulation during mitral valve (MV) intervention (Panel B). Volume fusion of tissue with color flow and "ghosted" volumes to provide the entire volume during an MV intervention (Panel C). LA, left atrium; LV, left ventricle. (From Jone PN, Haak A, Petri N, et al. Echocardiography-fluoroscopy fusion imaging for guidance of congenital and structural heart disease interventions. *JACC Cardiovasc Imaging.* 2019;12:1279-1282.)

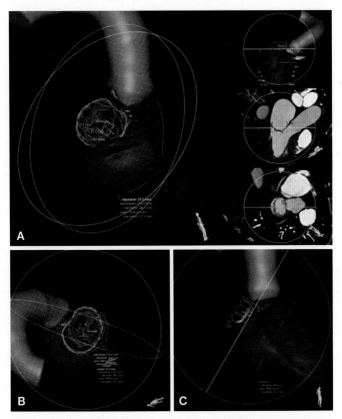

Figure 3.11 Virtual planning for transcatheter mitral valve interventions. (Panel A) Model of the mitral prosthesis (red stent lattice) positioned in the native mitral annulus (blue ring) (main window); 3-dimensional reconstruction (right panel); visualization in oblique planes (middle and bottom windows). (Panels B and C) Review of the virtual prosthesis from different angles. Yellow circle is the plane of the mitral annulus and the green circle represents a perpendicular plane. (Panel C) In this view, the mitral annular plane shown as the straight line, representing the best C-arm position for the valve deployment. The appropriate depth of prosthesis implantation can be determined. (Reproduced with permission from Jelnin V, Kliger C, Zucchetta F, Ruiz CE. Use of computed tomography to guide mitral interventions. *Intervent Cardiol Clin.* 2016;5:33-43.)

It is also expected that, eventually, separate modalities will merge as already tested in interventional MR systems to provide intervention-based navigation, using emitter units located at the tip of a catheter.

The future paradigm shift will be the high-resolution acquisition and characterization of cardiovascular tissues with the structural abnormalities within which the interventionalist navigates to achieve the target objective.

SUGGESTED READINGS

1. Alkhouli et al., 2016 Alkhouli M, Rihal CS, Holmes DR. Transseptal techniques for emerging structural heart interventions. *JACC Cardiovasc Interv.* 2016;9(24):2465-2480.
2. Amitai ME, Schnittger I, Popp RL, Chow J, Brown P, Liang DH. Comparison of three-dimensional echocardiography to twodimensional echocardiography and fluoroscopy for monitoring of endomyocardial biopsy. *Am J Cardiol.* 2007;99(6):864-866.
3. Anwar S, Singh GK, Miller J, et al. 3D printing is a transformative technology in congenital heart disease. *JACC Basic Transl Sci.* 2018;3(2):294-312.
4. Bartel T, Konorza T, Arjumand J, et al. Intracardiac echocardiography is superior to conventional monitoring for guiding device closure of interatrial communications. *Circulation.* 2003;107(6):795-797.
5. Bashir F, Quaife R, Carroll JD. Percutaneous closure of ascending aortic pseudoaneurysm using Amplatzer septal occluder device: the first clinical case report and literature review. *Catheter Cardiovasc Interv.* 2005;65(4):547-551.
6. Becerra JM, Almeria C, de Isla LP, Zamorano J. Usefulness of 3D transoesophageal echocardiography for guiding wires and closure devices in mitral perivalvular leaks. *Eur J Echocardiogr.* 2009;10(8):979-981.
7. Biaggi P, Fernandez-Golfin C, Hahn R, Corti R. Hybrid imaging during transcatheter structural heart interventions. *Curr Cardiovasc Imaging Rep.* 2015;8(9):33.
8. Bruckheimer E, Rotschild C, Dagan T, et al. Computer-generated real-time digital holography: first-time use in clinical medical imaging. *Eur Heart J Cardiovasc Imaging.* 2016;17(8):845-849.
9. Campbell-Washburn AE, Tavallaei MA, Pop M, et al. Real-time MRI guidance of cardiac interventions. *J Magn Reson Imaging.* 2017;46(4):935-950.
10. Carroll JD, Mack M. Facilities: the SHD interventional lab and the hybrid operating room. In: Carroll JD, Webb J, eds. *Manual of Structural Heart Disease Interventions.* Lippincott, Williams & Wilkins; 2011.
11. Carroll JD. The future of image guidance of cardiac interventions. *Catheter Cardiovasc Interv.* 2007;70(6):783.
12. Cavalcante JL, Wang DD. Structural heart interventional imagers – the new face of cardiac imaging. *Arq Bras Cardiol.* 2018;111(5):645-647.
13. Chan FP. MR and CT imaging of the pediatric patient with structural heart disease. *Semin Thorac Cardiovasc Surg Pediatr Card Surg Annu.* 2009;12:99-105.
14. Eng MH, Salcedo EE, Quaife RA, Carroll JD. Implementation of real time three-dimensional transesophageal echocardiography in percutaneous mitral balloon valvuloplasty and structural heart disease interventions. *Echocardiography.* 2009;26(8):958-966.
15. Fagan TE, Truong UT, Jone PN, et al. Multimodality 3-dimensional image integration for congenital cardiac catheterization. *Methodist Debakey Cardiovasc J.* 2014;10(2):68-76.
16. Funabashi N, Asano M, Sekine T, Nakayama T, Komuro I. Direction, location, and size of shunt flow in congenital heart disease evaluated by ECG-gated multislice computed tomography. *Int J Cardiol.* 2006;112(3):399-404.
17. Garcia J, Eng MH, Chen SY, Carroll JD. Image guidance of percutaneous coronary and structural heart disease interventions using a computed tomography and fluoroscopic integration. *Vasc Dis Manag.* 2007;4(3):89-87.
18. Garcia JA, Agostoni P, Green NE, et al. Rotational vs. standard coronary angiography: an image content analysis. *Catheter Cardiovasc Interv.* 2009;73(6):753-761.
19. Garcia JA, Bhakta S, Kay J, et al. On-line multislice computed tomography interactive overlay with conventional X-ray: a new and advanced imaging fusion concept. *Int J Cardiol.* 2009;133(3):e101-e105.
20. Gatehouse PD, Keegan J, Crowe LA, et al. Applications of phasecontrast flow and velocity imaging in cardiovascular MRI. *Eur Radiol.* 2005;15(10):2172-2184.
21. Gill EA, Liang DH. Interventional three-dimensional echocardiography: using real-time three-dimensional echocardiography to guide and evaluate intracardiac therapies. *Cardiol Clin.* 2007;25(2):335-340.
22. Green NE, Hansgen AR, Carroll JD. Initial clinical experience with intracardiac echocardiography in guiding balloon mitral valvuloplasty: technique, safety, utility, and limitations. *Catheter Cardiovasc Interv.* 2004;63(3):385-394.
23. Gutierrez FR, Ho ML, Siegel MJ. Practical applications of magnetic resonance in congenital heart disease. *Magn Reson Imaging Clin N Am.* 2008;16(3):403-435, v.
24. Hahn RT. Transcathether valve replacement and valve repair: review of procedures and intraprocedural echocardiographic imaging. *Circ Res.* 2016;119(2):341-356.
25. Holmes DR, Jr., Lakkireddy DR, Whitlock RP, Waksman R, Mack MJ. Left atrial appendage occlusion: opportunities and challenges. *J Am Coll Cardiol.* 2014;63(4):291-298.

26. Huang X, Shen J, Huang Y, et al. En face view of atrial septal defect by two-dimensional transthoracic echocardiography: comparison to real-time three-dimensional transesophageal echocardiography. *J Am Soc Echocardiogr.* 2010;23(7):714-721.

27. Hudson PA, Eng MH, Kim MS, Quaife RA, Salcedo EE, Carroll JD. A comparison of echocardiographic modalities to guide structural heart disease interventions. *J Interv Cardiol.* 2008;21(6):535-546.

28. Jelnin V, Dudiy Y, Einhorn BN, Kronzon I, Cohen HA, Ruiz CE. Clinical experience with percutaneous left ventricular transapical access for intervention in structural heart disease defects: a safe access and secure exit. *JACC Cardiovasc Interv.* 2011;4(8):868-874.

29. Jelnin V, Kliger C, Zucchetta F, Ruiz CE. Use of computed tomography to guide mitral interventions. *Interv Cardiol Clin.* 2016;5(1):33-43.

30. Jone PN, Haak A, Petri N, et al. Echocardiography-fluoroscopy fusion imaging for guidance of congenital and structural heart disease interventions. *JACC Cardiovasc Imaging.* 2019;12(7 pt 1):1279-1282.

31. Kilger C, Eiros R, Isasti G, et al. Review of surgical prosthetic para-valvular leak: diagnosis and catheter-based closure. *Eur Heart J.* 2013;34:638-649.

32. Kim MS, Hansgen AR, Wink O, Quaife RA, Carroll JD. Rapid prototyping – a new tool in understanding and treating structural heart disease. *Circulation.* 2008;117(18):2388-2394.

33. Kim SS, Hijazi ZM, Lang RM, Knight BP. The use of intracardiac echocardiography and other intracardiac imaging tools to guide noncoronary cardiac interventions. *J Am Coll Cardiol.* 2009;53(23):2117-2128.

34. Kliger C, Jelnin V, Sharma S, et al. CT angiography-fluoroscopy fusion imaging for percutaneous transapical access. *JACC Cardiovasc Imaging.* 2014;7(2):169-177.

35. Lange A, Palka P, Burstow DJ, Godman MJ. Three-dimensional echocardiography: historical development and current applications. *J Am Soc Echocardiogr.* 2001;14(5):403-412.

36. Quaife RA, Carroll JD. CT evaluation of the interatrial septum in atrial septal defects? In: Hijazi ZM, Feldman T, Abdullah Al-Qbandi MH, Sievert H, eds. *Transcatheter Closure of Atrial Septal Defects & Patent Foramen Ovale: A Comprehensive Assessment.* Cardiotext; 2010:125-138.

37. Quaife RA, Carroll JD. Cardiac CT and MRI in patient assessment and procedural guidance in structural heart disease interventions. In: Carroll JD, Webb J, eds. *Manual of Structural Heart Disease Interventions.* Lippincott, Williams & Wilkins; 2011.

38. Quaife RA, Chen MY, Kim M, et al. Pre-procedural planning for percutaneous atrial septal defect closure: transesophageal echocardiography compared with cardiac computed tomographic angiography. *J Cardiovasc Comput Tomogr.* 2010;4(5):330-338.

39. Quaife RA, Salcedo EE, Carroll JD. Procedural guidance using advance imaging techniques for percutaneous edge-to-edge mitral valve repair. *Curr Cardiol Rep.* 2014;16(2):452.

40. Salcedo EE, Carroll JD. Echocardiography in patient assessment and procedural guidance in structural heart disease interventions. In: Carroll JD, Webb J, eds. *Manual of Structural Heart Disease Interventions.* Lippincott, Williams & Wilkins; 2011.

41. Salcedo EE, Carroll JD. Echocardiographic guidance of structural heart disease interventions. In: Otto CM, ed. *The Practice of Clinical Echocardiography.* 4th ed. Elsevier; 2012.

42. Schwartz JG, Neubauer AM, Fagan TE, Noordhoek NJ, Grass M, Carroll JD. Potential role of three-dimensional rotational angiography and C-arm CT for valvular repair and implantation. *Int J Cardiovasc Imaging.* 2011;27(8):1205-1222.

43. Suematsu Y, Marx GR, Stoll JA, et al. Three-dimensional echocardiography – guided beating-heart surgery without cardiopulmonary bypass: a feasibility study. *J Thorac Cardiovasc Surg.* 2004;128(4):579-587.

44. Valente AM, Powell AJ. Clinical applications of cardiovascular magnetic resonance in congenital heart disease. *Cardiol Clin.* 2007;25(1):97-110.

45. Zamorano JL, Badano LP, Bruce C, et al. EAE/ASE recommendations for the use of echocardiography in new transcatheter interventions for valvular heart disease. *J Am Soc Echocardiogr.* 2011;24(9):937-965.

4

Complications[1]

INTRODUCTION

The determinants of the risk for sustaining a complication during an invasive procedure include the clinical characteristics of the patient, the procedure type, equipment limitations, and operator experience.

Familiarity with the risks of complications can be of immeasurable value in (1) taking extra precautions to avoid them (eg, implementation of a hydration protocol to reduce the risk of contrast nephropathy in patients with baseline chronic kidney disease), (2) promptly recognizing complications when they occur (eg, perforation of the right atrium during a transseptal puncture), and (3) taking corrective and potentially lifesaving action (eg, pericardiocentesis for perforation-induced tamponade).

DEATH

Death as a Complication of Diagnostic Catheterization

Death as a complication of diagnostic catheterization has declined progressively over the last 30 years. A 1% mortality was seen with diagnostic catheterization in the 1960s, whereas an analysis of the registry of the Society for Cardiac Angiography and Interventions including 58,332 patients studied in 1990 has shown an overall mortality of 0.08%, with a 1.5% incidence of any major complication. A number of baseline variables (including New York Heart Association class, multivessel disease, congestive heart failure, and renal insufficiency) were identified, whose presence was associated with up to 8-fold increase in major complication rates, from 0.3% in patients with none of these factors to 2.5%.

Left Main Disease

Although there has been a progressive reduction in the overall mortality of diagnostic cardiac catheterization over the last 25 years, patients with severe left main coronary disease remain at increased risk. Because roughly 7% of patients undergoing coronary angiography have significant left main disease, the protocol used for coronary angiography should always begin with careful catheter entry into the left coronary ostium to facilitate early recognition of ostial left main disease through catheter pressure damping or performance of a test "puff" immediately after engagement. Even without these early warnings of left main disease, we routinely perform the first left coronary injection in the right anterior oblique (RAO) projection with caudal angulation to screen for mid- and distal left main disease and get the maximal anatomic information on the first injection. If ostial left main stenosis is suspected, a straight anterior (anteroposterior) injection may be performed. If severe left main disease is present, the only other left coronary injection needed is an RAO projection with cranial angulation (to see the left anterior descending and its diagonal branches). Performing superfluous contrast injections in a patient with critical left main disease offers little more in the way of important anatomical information and increases the risk of triggering the vicious cycle of ischemia/hypotension/more ischemia that may lead to irreversible collapse.

---

[1]We gratefully acknowledge the Grossman & Baim's *Cardiac Catheterization, Angiography, and Intervention*, 9th edition contribution of Dr. Mauro Moscucci, as portions of his chapter, Complications, were retained in this text.

Left Ventricular Dysfunction

Patients with cardiogenic shock in the setting of acute myocardial infarction or severe chronic left ventricular dysfunction (ejection fraction <30%) have a severalfold increased risk of procedural morbidity and mortality.

Although right-sided heart catheterization is no longer routine, it should be performed before angiography in a patient with poor left ventricular ejection fraction because it provides valuable data about baseline hemodynamic status and allows ongoing monitoring of pulmonary artery pressure as an early warning about hemodynamic decompensation before frank pulmonary edema ensues. If the baseline pulmonary capillary wedge pressure is >30 mmHg, every effort should be made to improve hemodynamic status before angiography is attempted.

Valvular Heart Disease

Despite the preponderance of coronary artery disease as the indication for diagnostic cardiac catheterization, patients with severe valvular heart disease are also at increased risk for dying during cardiac catheterization. With current noninvasive methods for assessing the severity of valvular lesions, there has been debate about whether it is necessary to cross severely stenotic valves during preoperative cardiac catheterization.

Prior Coronary Artery Bypass Graft Surgery

Patients who have previously undergone coronary bypass surgery make up a growing subgroup of diagnostic and interventional catheterizations. They are typically 5 years older, have more diffuse coronary and generalized atherosclerosis, have worse left ventricular function, and require a lengthier and more complex procedure to image both native coronary arteries and all grafts. Despite these adverse risk factors, the Post CABG Trial looked at 2635 diagnostic angiograms performed in stable patients and found 0% mortality, with major complications in 0.7% (myocardial infarction 0.08%, stroke 0.19%, vascular trauma requiring transfusion or surgery 0.4%).

Pediatric Patients

Pediatric patients may be at higher risk. One review of 4952 patients (median age 2.9 years) performed at the Hospital for Sick Children in Toronto found a mortality of 1.2% confined to patients younger than 5 years (half in critically ill neonates <30 days of age). Although the risk was lower for diagnostic than for electrophysiologic or interventional procedures, there were 3 deaths (0.1%) among the 3149 diagnostic procedures.

Death in the Course of an Interventional Procedure

With the introduction of coronary stents, the overall mortality for elective coronary intervention has fallen, but the extension of intervention to other high-risk subsets, including patients with acute myocardial infarction undergoing primary percutaneous coronary intervention (PCI), has kept overall mortality close to 1%—roughly 10-fold higher than purely diagnostic catheterization. Several multivariable models that predict procedural mortality have been developed based on age, ejection fraction, treatment for acute myocardial infarction/shock, urgent/emergent priority, and so on. In general, there is a wide variation in risk of death in the course of coronary intervention—based on patient comorbidities, clinical indication, and procedure type.

MYOCARDIAL INFARCTION

Although transient myocardial ischemia is relatively common during diagnostic catheterization and occurs routinely during coronary intervention, myocardial infarction is an uncommon but important complication of diagnostic cardiac catheterization.

Interventional Procedures

Coronary interventions may produce myocardial infarction by a variety of mechanisms that include dissection, abrupt vessel closure, "snowplow" occlusion of side branches, spasm of the epicardial or arteriolar vessels (no reflow), thrombosis, or distal embolization.

The official definition of periprocedural myocardial infarction has been broadened to include non-Q-wave infarctions (more properly called non-ST-elevation myocardial infarctions) detected by elevation of cardiac biomarkers above the 99th percentile of the upper limit of normal. According to the updated fourth universal definition of myocardial infarction, PCI-related myocardial infarction (type 4a) is defined as an elevation of cardiac troponin to values >5 times the 99th percentile of the upper reference limit (URL) in patients with normal baseline values and in association with evidence of new myocardial ischemia. The evidence of myocardial ischemia might be based on electrocardiogram (ECG) changes, or on procedure-related complications resulting in impairment of coronary blood flow including coronary dissection, occlusion of a major epicardial artery or a side branch, disruption of collateral flow, slow flow or no reflow, or distal embolization. Patients with these low-level enzyme elevations are more likely to have some degree of chest discomfort due to occlusion of small side branches or distal microembolization (**Figure 4.1**), but this finding is common also in patients without enzyme elevation, where it presumably represents stimulation of adventitial pain receptors by local stretching at the treatment site. In the absence of evidence of myocardial ischemia, "myocardial injury" is defined as any increases of troponin values >99th percentile of the URL in patients with normal

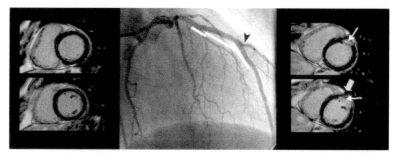

Figure 4.1 Two basal short-axis images (left) in a patient before left anterior descending coronary artery (LAD) percutaneous coronary intervention (PCI) showing no delayed hyperenhancement. Contrast-enhanced images in the same image plane after PCI (right) reveal new anterolateral wall hyperenhancement (long arrows) adjacent to LAD stent (block arrow). Middle panel shows post-PCI angiogram with position of 3 stents highlighted and good flow in LAD and second diagonal branch (likely affected territory; black arrowhead). (Reproduced with permission from Selvanayagam JB, Porto I, Channon K, et al. Troponin elevation after percutaneous coronary intervention directly represents the extent of irreversible myocardial injury: insights from cardiovascular magnetic resonance imaging. *Circulation.* 2005;111(8):1027-1032.)

baseline values or a rise of troponin values >20% of the baseline value when the baseline troponin is already elevated or falling (**Table 4.1**).

Several studies have evaluated the relationship between elevations of creatine kinase myocardial band (CK-MB) and long-term mortality. Although elevation above 5 or 8 times normal corresponds to a significant amount of myocardial necrosis and carries the same adverse impact on long-term prognosis as a Q-wave infarction, long-term follow-up of patients from several multicenter trials has shown that patients with even low-level (1-3 times normal) elevation of postprocedural CK after PCI

Table 4.1	Definitions of Periprocedural Myocardial Injury and Myocardial Infarction
Myocardial injury[a]	Cardiac procedural myocardial injury is arbitrarily defined by increases of cTn values (>99th percentile URL) in patients with normal baseline values (<99th percentile URL) or a rise of cTn values >20% of the baseline value when it is above the 99th percentile URL but it is stable or falling.
Type 4a myocardial infarction (MI)[a]	Coronary intervention-related MI is arbitrarily defined by an elevation of cTn values more than 5 times the 99th percentile URL in patients with normal baseline values. In patients with elevated preprocedural cTn in whom the cTn levels are stable (<20% variation) or falling, the postprocedural cTn must rise by >20%. However, the absolute postprocedural value must still be at least 5 times the 99th percentile URL. In addition, one of the following elements is required:
	• New ischemic ECG changes. • Development of new pathological Q-waves. • Imaging evidence of new loss of viable myocardium or new regional wall motion abnormality in a pattern consistent with an ischemic etiology. • Angiographic findings consistent with a procedural flow-limiting complication such as coronary dissection, occlusion of a major epicardial artery or a side branch occlusion/thrombus, disruption of collateral flow, or distal embolization.
Type 4b myocardial infarction[a]	Stent/scaffold thrombosis, as documented by angiography or autopsy using the same criteria utilized for type 1 MI.
Type 4c myocardial infarction[a]	Restenosis-associated MI using the same criteria utilized for type 1 MI.
Society of Coronary Angiography and Interventions (SCAI) definition[b]	In patients with normal baseline values, elevation of CK-MB values >10 times URL or TnT values >70 times URL, or elevation of CK-MB values >5 times URL or TnT values >35 times URL, and new pathological Q-waves in 2 contiguous leads or new persistent LBB in ECG. In patients with elevated baseline values but stable or falling values, increment rise of CK-MB >10 times URL or TnT values >70 times URL. In patients with elevated baseline CK-MB (or cTn) in whom the biomarker levels have not been stable or falling, increment rise of CK-MB (or cTn) plus new ST-segment elevation or expression, and signs consistent with a clinically relevant MI.

CK-MB, creatine kinase myocardial band; cTn, cardiac troponin; LBB, left bundle block; URL, upper reference limits.
[a]Adapted from Thygesen K, Alpert JS, Jaffe AS, et al. Fourth universal definition of myocardial infarction (2018). *Circulation*. 2018;138:e618-e651.
[b]From Moussa ID, Klein LW, Shah B, et al. Consideration of a new definition of clinically relevant myocardial infarction after coronary revascularization: an expert consensus document from the Society for Cardiovascular Angiography and Interventions (SCAI). *J Am Coll Cardiol*. 2013;62:1563-1570.

have a greater incidence of late adverse outcomes. Similar results have been shown by analysis evaluating the relationship between troponin elevations and long-term mortality. Whether any such relationship is cause and effect or simply an association of both periprocedural cardiac biomarker elevation and late events with a common confounding variable (such as the diffuse underlying atherosclerosis) remains to be determined. It has also been suggested that, due to the higher sensitivity of troponin, a larger percentage of patients will meet the definition of 4a myocardial infarction when troponin is used when compared with the same patients when CK-MB is used. Some of these patients will not have any evidence of myocardial necrosis even when a very sensitive imaging modality such as contrast-enhanced cardiac magnetic resonance is used.

CEREBROVASCULAR COMPLICATIONS

Cerebrovascular accidents (strokes) are uncommon but potentially devastating complications of diagnostic cardiac catheterization, with a reported incidence of 0.07% in the Society for Cardiac Angiography registries.

The risk of stroke is somewhat higher with coronary intervention, as expected based on the use of guiding catheters, multiple equipment exchanges in the aortic root, aggressive anticoagulation, and longer procedure times. Although cerebral hemorrhage must always be excluded, the main cause of catheterization-related strokes seems to be embolic. There is some evidence that many such emboli are dislodged from unsuspected aortic plaque or diffuse atherosclerosis, given the observation that atherosclerotic debris is liberated from the wall of the aorta in 40% to 60% of cases during advancement of large-lumen guiding catheters over a 0.035-in guidewire. Most neuro-ophthalmologic complications (ie, retinal artery embolization) and the syndrome of diffuse cholesterol embolization also appear to be caused by emboli released by disruption of unrecognized plaques on the walls of the aorta, liberating cholesterol crystals, calcified material, or platelet-fibrin thrombus into the aortic root.

Embolic material may also originate in the cardiac chambers, in thrombotic coronary arteries, or on the surface of cardiac valves. In addition, there can be no excuse for contributory technical malfeasance such as sloppy catheter flushing, introduction of air bubbles during contrast injection, inadvertent placement of wires and catheters into the arch vessels, prolonged (>3 minutes) wire dwell times during attempts to cross a stenotic aortic valve, or failure to carefully wipe and immerse guidewires in heparinized saline before their reintroduction during left-sided heart catheterization. The question of embolic risk also invariably comes up when it is necessary to perform catheterization on patients with endocarditis of left-sided (aortic and mitral) heart valves. With current noninvasive techniques for assessing the left ventricle and mitral valve, it is not necessary to enter the left ventricle in a patient with left-sided endocarditis.

LOCAL VASCULAR COMPLICATIONS

Local complications at the catheter introduction site are among the most common problems seen after cardiac catheterization procedures and probably are the single greatest source of procedure-related morbidity. Specific problems include vessel thrombosis, distal embolization, dissection, poorly controlled bleeding at the puncture site, the development of pseudoaneurysm, arteriovenous fistula, retroperitoneal hematoma (RPH), and the development of femoral neuropathy.

With the femoral approach, poorly controlled bleeding may present as free hemorrhage, femoral or retroperitoneal hematoma, pseudoaneurysm, or arteriovenous fistula. Although frank hemorrhage and hematoma are generally evident within 12 hours of the procedure, the diagnosis of pseudoaneurysm may not be evident for days or even weeks after the procedure. Brachial complications tend to be thrombotic, whereas femoral complications tend to be hemorrhagic, but exceptions to this general rule can and do occur.

Femoral Artery Thrombosis

Femoral artery thrombosis can occur in patients with a small common femoral artery lumen (peripheral vascular disease, diabetes, female gender), in whom a large-diameter catheter or sheath (eg, an intra-aortic balloon pump) has been placed, particularly when the catheter dwell time is long or when prolonged postprocedural compression is applied. Such patients have a white painful leg with impaired distal sensory and motor function, as well as absent distal pulses. If this develops during the catheterization procedure and is not corrected promptly by sheath removal, a flow-obstructing dissection or thrombus at the femoral artery puncture site or a distal arterial embolus should be suspected. This requires urgent attention via vascular surgery consultation. Alternatively, operators skilled in peripheral intervention may be able to puncture the contralateral femoral artery and address a common femoral occlusion percutaneously (**Figure 4.2**). Either way, failure to restore limb flow within 2 to 6 hours may result in extension of thrombosis or muscle necrosis requiring fasciotomy or even amputation and predisposes to the development of renal failure.

Femoral Vein Thrombosis

Femoral venous thrombosis and pulmonary embolism are rare complications of diagnostic femoral catheterization. A small number of clinical cases have been reported, however, particularly in the setting of venous compression by a large arterial hematoma, sustained mechanical compression, or prolonged procedures with multiple venous lines (eg, electrophysiologic studies).

Hemorrhagic Complications

Although thrombotic complications do occur, poorly controlled bleeding from the arterial puncture site is a more common problem after cardiac catheterization by the femoral approach. Uncontrollable free bleeding around the sheath suggests laceration of the femoral artery. Anticoagulation may be reversed, and an attempt is made to remove the sheath and control bleeding with prolonged (30- to 60-minute) compression or to place a femoral closure device.

Formation of a hematoma—a collection of blood within the soft tissues of the upper thigh—is more common than free bleeding. It tends to cause a tender mass, the size of a baseball or softball. If ongoing bleeding stops with manual compression, the hematoma will usually resolve over 1 to 2 weeks as the blood gradually spreads and is reabsorbed from the soft tissues. Larger hematomas may require transfusion, but surgical repair of a hematoma is generally not required. The level of anticoagulation and antiplatelet therapy as well as increased sheath size, female gender, and advanced age all increase the risk of hemorrhagic complications.

Retroperitoneal Bleeding

Retroperitoneal bleeding or hematoma is a relatively rare complication that is associated with high morbidity and mortality. In an analysis of 112,340 consecutive patients undergoing PCI in a large, multicenter registry, RPH occurred in 482 patients (0.4%). In that study, female sex, body surface area <1.8 m², emergency procedure, history of chronic obstructive pulmonary disease, cardiogenic shock, use of preprocedural intravenous (IV) heparin, use of preprocedural glycoprotein IIb/IIIa inhibitors, adoption of sheath size >8F, and use of vascular closure devices emerged as independent predictors of RPH, whereas the use of bivalirudin was associated with a lower risk. When

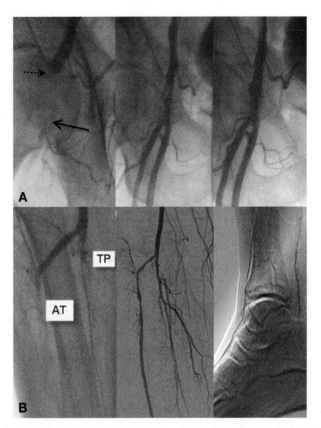

Figure 4.2 Femoral artery thrombosis. In the morning after AngioSeal closure of the right femoral artery, this patient experienced sharp pain and swelling at the site, managed by 30 minutes of compression. After that, he reported severe pain and loss of sensation in a white limb. Upper left. Crossover from the contralateral side showed occlusion of the common femoral with reconstitution (arrows). Upper center. After balloon dilation, there was a prominent filling defect consistent with thrombus. Upper right. After AngioJet thrombectomy, the filling defect has decreased in size. Lower left. Distal injection, however, showed thrombotic occlusion of both the anterior tibial (AT) and the tibioperoneal (TP) trunk. Lower center. After catheter suction, patency of these vessels was restored. Lower right. Distal angiogram shows filling of both the dorsalis pedis and posterior tibial vessels. (Case courtesy of Dr. Andrew Eisenhauer, Brigham and Women's Hospital.)

compared with patients who did not develop RPH, the development of RPH was associated with a higher frequency of postprocedural myocardial infarction (5.81% vs 1.67%, $P < .0001$), infection and/or sepsis (17.43% vs 3.00%, $P < .0001$), and heart failure (8.00% vs 1.63%, $P < .0001$). The overall mortality rate in patients who developed RPH was 6.6%. RPH may occur if the front or back wall of the femoral artery is punctured above the inguinal ligament, allowing the resulting hematoma to extend into the retroperitoneal space. Trauma or perforation of the inferior epigastric artery and, in rare instances, bleeding from a common femoral artery entry site can also lead

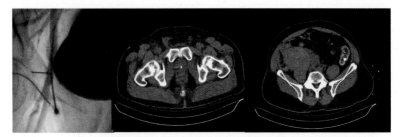

Figure 4.3 Retroperitoneal bleeding. A 67-year-old man underwent coronary intervention. Left. The sheath injection shows a relatively high puncture entering the common femoral artery at the top (rather than the middle) of the femoral head (arrow). On the day after AngioSeal closure, he felt a pop and pain in his groin and became hypotensive, responding only briefly to atropine and fluids, with a fall in hematocrit from 42% to 35%. Center. A computed tomography (CT) scan at the level of the femoral neck shows the common femoral artery bilaterally. Right. A CT scan slice in the lower abdomen shows a large right retroperitoneal bleed obliterating the psoas muscle. With continued fall in his hematocrit, he was taken to the operating room, where active bleeding was found from the anterior wall of the external iliac artery, from which the closure device had dislocated. He was discharged on day 9 after a total of 15 units of packed red cells.

to the development of RPH. Such bleeding should be considered whenever a patient develops unexplained hypotension (particularly, if it responds only briefly to aggressive volume loading), fall in hematocrit, or ipsilateral flank pain following a femoral catheterization procedure. The diagnosis may be confirmed by computed tomography scanning or abdominal ultrasound (**Figure 4.3**). More recently, effective catheter-based interventions have emerged as alternatives to conservative management with IV fluids, transfusion, and bed rest for the management of RPH. They include an ipsilateral (or contralateral if the problem is low in the iliac) approach for localization and tamponade of the retroperitoneal bleeding site, using a peripheral angioplasty balloon followed by placement of a covered stent, as possible alternatives. **Figure 4.4** illustrates a proposed algorithm for the management of patients with suspected RPH.

Femoral Neuropathy

Femoral neuropathy is another rare complication of femoral artery access. It can occur from direct trauma to the femoral nerve, from compression by a hematoma, or from direct prolonged compression during achievement of hemostasis. Two different clinical syndromes have been recognized. The first (and most concerning) syndrome is associated with large RPHs resulting in a lumbar plexopathy involving the femoral, obturator, or lateral femoral cutaneous nerves. In these patients, sensory neuropathy and motor deficit might persist. In the second syndrome, a groin hematoma or false aneurysm can result in paresthesias involving the medial and intermediate cutaneous branches of the femoral nerve.

Pseudoaneurysm and Arteriovenous Fistula

A pseudoaneurysm may develop if a hematoma remains in continuity with the arterial lumen (**Figure 4.5**). Blood flowing in and out of the arterial puncture expands the hematoma cavity during systole and allows it to decompress back into the arterial lumen in diastole. Since the hematoma cavity contains no normal arterial wall structures (ie, media or adventitia), this condition is referred to as false or pseudoaneurysm. It can often be distinguished from a simple hematoma on

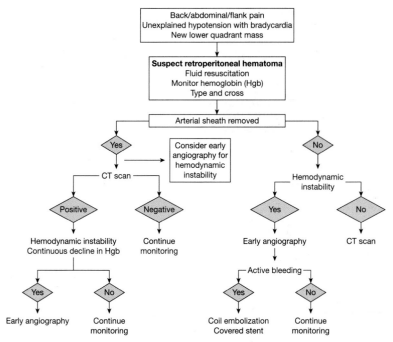

Figure 4.4 Suggested algorithm for the management of patients with suspected retroperitoneal hematoma. CT, computed tomography. (Reproduced with permission from Chetcuti SJ, Cohen GC, Moscucci M. Local arterial and venous vascular access site complication. In: Moscucci M, ed. *Complications of Cardiovascular Procedures: Incidence, Risk Factors and Bailout Techniques.* Lippincott Williams & Wilkins; 2011.)

physical examination by the presence of pulsation and an audible bruit over the site, but Duplex ultrasound scanning is confirmatory. Since all but the smallest (<2-cm diameter) false aneurysms tend to enlarge and ultimately rupture, we usually have them managed by ultrasound compression, and if ultrasound compression fails, by surgical repair. Ultrasound-guided compression of the narrow neck through which blood exits the femoral artery for 30 to 60 minutes, injection of the false aneurysm cavity with procoagulant solutions, or embolization coils during ultrasound, or contralaterally inserted balloon occlusion of the aneurysm neck are usually effective.

The key steps to avoiding pseudoaneurysm formation are accurate puncture of the common femoral artery and effective initial control of bleeding after sheath removal.

An arteriovenous fistula results from ongoing bleeding from the femoral arterial puncture site that decompresses into an adjacent venous puncture site (see **Figure 4.5**). This can be recognized by a to-and-fro continuous bruit over the puncture site and may not be clinically evident until days after a femoral catheterization procedure. These fistulae may enlarge with time, but at least one-third close spontaneously within 1 year, after which surgical repair should be entertained. The most common findings at surgery are a low puncture (ie, of the superficial femoral or profunda, transecting a small venous branch), emphasizing the importance of careful puncture technique in avoiding this femoral vascular complication.

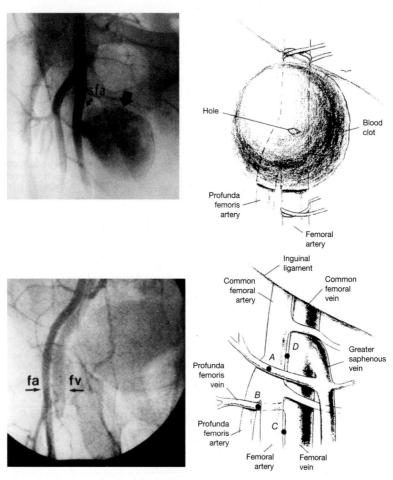

Figure 4.5 Common significant femoral vascular complications. Upper left. Angiographic appearance of a false aneurysm of right femoral artery (arrow) that developed 4 to 5 d following percutaneous retrograde femoral arterial catheterization complicated by a significant local hematoma after groin compression. Note that the arterial puncture had been made in the superficial (rather than common) femoral artery. Upper right. Schematic diagram showing the surgical approach to the false aneurysm cavity and the underlying puncture. Lower left. Angiographic appearance of an arteriovenous fistula with simultaneous filling of the femoral artery (left) and vein (right). Lower right. Diagram showing the potential anatomic situations (overlying arterial and venous branches) that may underlie fistula formation after femoral puncture. (From Fukumoto Y, Tsutsui H, Tsuchihashi M, Masumoto A, Takeshita A. The incidence and risk factors of cholesterol embolization syndrome, a complication of cardiac catheterization: a prospective study. *J Am Coll Cardiol.* 2003;42(2):211-226, with permission.)

ARRHYTHMIAS OR CONDUCTION DISTURBANCE

Various cardiac arrhythmias (tachycardia or bradycardia) or conduction disturbance may occur during the course of diagnostic or therapeutic cardiac catheterization. Most, like ventricular premature beats during catheter entry into the right or left ventricle, are devoid of clinical consequence. Others, like asystole or ventricular fibrillation, pose immediate risk. Some rhythm disturbances (like atrial fibrillation) are well tolerated in most patients but may trigger profound hemodynamic decompensation in patients with severe coronary disease, aortic stenosis, or hypertrophic cardiomyopathy by excessively increasing heart rate or eliminating the atrial "kick" needed to maintain diastolic filling of a stiff left ventricle.

The ability to promptly recognize and reverse major rhythm disturbances can avoid progression to full cardiopulmonary arrest that would require the institution of cardiopulmonary resuscitation. All operators and cardiac catheterization support staff should be current in their basic and advanced cardiac life support (ACLS) certification and prepared to institute ventilatory and circulatory support without delay, when necessary.

Ventricular Fibrillation

Although ventricular tachycardia and ventricular fibrillation may result from catheter manipulation, the most common cause is intracoronary injection into the right coronary artery, particularly when the catheter is subselectively engaged in the right coronary artery conus branch. The incidence of ventricular fibrillation may be somewhat higher, in patients with baseline prolongation of the QT interval.

Some of the most refractory ventricular ectopy is seen in the setting of profound transmural ischemia or early myocardial infarction. Ventricular fibrillation or unstable ventricular tachycardia should be treated with prompt countershock, whereas lower-grade ventricular ectopy may respond to loading with intravenous amiodarone (150 mg over 10 minutes, with additional boluses of 150 mg over 10 minutes for breakthrough ectopy, followed by an infusion of 1 mg/min for 6 hours, and then 0.5 mg/min). Magnesium sulfate (1-2 g intravenously over 2 minutes) may be given for suspected hypomagnesemia or torsades de pointes). However, it is rare for witnessed and promptly treated ventricular fibrillation as occurs in the catheterization laboratory to result in a prolonged arrest. In that case, however, the full ACLS protocol should be initiated. Of course, precordial compression and bag/mask ventilation should be begun as arrangements for endotracheal intubation are made, in the case of ventricular fibrillation that does not respond immediately to countershock.

Atrial Arrhythmias

Atrial extrasystoles are common during catheter advancement from the right atrium to the superior vena cava or during looping of the catheter in the right atrium to facilitate passage in a patient with enlargement of the right-sided heart chambers. These extrasystoles usually subside once the catheter is repositioned, although they may progress to atrial flutter or fibrillation in sensitive patients. Both rhythms tend to revert spontaneously over a period of minutes to hours but may require additional therapy if they produce ischemia or hemodynamic instability. Atrial flutter can be treated by a brief (15-second) but rapid (300-400 beats/min) burst of right atrial pacing, following which reversion to sinus rhythm or onset of atrial fibrillation (with a more controlled ventricular response) can be expected. Care must be taken, however, to ensure a stable atrial pacing location, since catheter migration into the ventricle during burst pacing may trigger ventricular fibrillation.

Atrial flutter or atrial fibrillation is generally benign during catheterization but may cause clinical sequelae if the ventricular response is rapid (>100); if the loss of the atrial kick causes hypotension in a patient with mitral stenosis, hypertrophic cardiomyopathy, or diastolic left ventricular dysfunction; or if the duration of atrial fibrillation is prolonged, thus leading to an increased risk of embolic stroke. Thus, if it does not convert spontaneously to normal sinus rhythm, atrial fibrillation or flutter may require synchronized DC cardioversion.

Bradyarrhythmias

Transient slowing of the heart rate used to occur commonly during coronary angiography, particularly at the end of a right coronary artery injection performed using a high-osmolar ionic contrast agent. Since forceful coughing helps to clear contrast from the coronaries, support aortic pressure and cerebral perfusion during asystole, and restore normal cardiac rhythm, patients should be warned at the beginning of the procedure that they may be asked to cough forcefully and that they must do so without hesitation when asked. This problem is no longer an issue with the widespread use of low-osmolar agents (see Chapter 2).

Vasovagal reactions, in which bradycardia is associated with hypotension, nausea, yawning, and sweating, should be suspected when bradycardia is more prolonged. This is a common complication (with a roughly 3% incidence) seen in the cardiac catheterization laboratory, triggered by pain and anxiety, particularly in the setting of hypovolemia. Some elderly patients may exhibit the hypotensive findings of a vasovagal reaction without the hallmark finding of bradycardia. In a study by Landau et al, more than 80% of such reactions occurred as vascular access was being obtained, with 16% occurring during sheath removal. This highlights the importance of adequate preprocedural sedation and adequate administration of local anesthetic before catheter insertion is attempted. The treatment of vasovagal reaction consists of the following: (1) cessation of the painful stimulus; (2) rapid volume administration (elevation of the legs on a linen pack and hand pumping of saline through the sidearm of the venous sheath or peripheral intravenous line); and (3) atropine (0.6-1.0 mg intravenously). If hypotension persists, additional pressor support (norepinephrine or Neo-Synephrine) may be needed. When the vasovagal constellation occurs during catheter manipulation (instead of sheath insertion or removal), it should still be treated as outlined above, but the operator should be aware that vagal stimulation is one of the earliest findings in cardiac perforation (see below) as the pericardium is irritated by blood or in the setting of an RPH.

Conduction disturbances (bundle branch block or complete atrioventricular block) are an uncommon but potentially serious cause of bradycardia during cardiac catheterization. They may be precipitated when the catheter impacts the area of the right bundle during right-sided heart catheterization. With right bundle branch block superimposed on preexisting left bundle branch block, asystole and cardiovascular collapse may ensue unless an adequate escape rhythm (ie, a junctional escape) takes over. The same scenario may be seen when left bundle branch block is produced as the aortic valve is crossed in a patient with preexisting right bundle branch block.

When complete heart block develops, atropine is rarely helpful in the setting of inadequate junctional escape and hemodynamic deterioration but should be given anyway, since it has few adverse effects. Coughing may help support the circulation and maintain consciousness as a temporary pacing catheter is inserted. Isoproterenol hydrochloride can be helpful but is rarely indicated in the cardiac catheterization laboratory where temporary pacing can be rapidly initiated. At one time, temporary pacing catheters were placed prophylactically in patients with bundle branch block or planned right coronary intervention, but this has been abandoned because frank asystole is rare and there is generally adequate time for insertion of a pacing catheter. The only procedures for which we currently place prophylactic right-sided pacing catheters are rotational atherectomy, rheolytic thrombectomy (particularly in the right and circumflex coronary arteries), alcohol ablation for hypertrophic cardiomyopathy, and transcatheter aortic valve replacement.

PERFORATION OF THE HEART OR GREAT VESSELS

Perforation of the cardiac chambers, coronary arteries, or the intrathoracic great vessels is fortunately a rare event in diagnostic catheterization.

When cardiac perforation does occur, it is usually heralded by bradycardia and hypotension owing to vagal stimulation (see vasovagal reaction, above). As blood accumulates in the pericardium, the cardiac silhouette may enlarge and the normal pulsation of the heart borders on fluoroscopy will become blunted. Hemodynamic findings of tamponade may develop in the form of pulsus paradox and elevation of the right atrial pressure with loss of the "y" descent. If the patient is hemodynamically stable, a transthoracic echocardiogram can document the presence of blood in the pericardial space, but if hemodynamic compromise is severe or progressive, immediate pericardiocentesis should be performed via the subxiphoid approach. Once pericardiocentesis has stabilized the situation, the operator must decide whether or not emergency surgery will be needed to close the site of perforation. Most perforations will seal so that surgery is unnecessary.

With the use of hydrophilic-coated guidewire, and more aggressive atherectomy technologies, the incidence of coronary perforation may be as high as 1%. A classification of coronary artery perforation is listed in **Table 4.2**. Some perforations, particularly those limited to deep injury to the vessel wall with localized perivascular contrast staining, can simply be observed (type I perforation). In contrast, free perforations (type III) may lead to the development of frank tamponade within seconds to minutes (**Figure 4.6**). The first countermeasure is to seal the site of leakage by inflation of a balloon catheter that spans the perforated segment. Once this is done, anticoagulation should generally be reversed (ie, giving protamine).

Table 4.2 Ellis Classification of Coronary Artery Perforation

	Morphology	Clinical Sequelae
Type I	Extraluminal crater without extravasation	Almost always benign; treated effectively with stent placement
Type II	Pericardial or myocardial blush without contrast jet extravasation and without a ≥1-mm exit hole	Can result in late presentation of tamponade; requires close observation
Type III	Extravasation through a frank perforation with a ≥1-mm exit hole	High risk of tamponade; requires reversal of anticoagulation and immediate treatment
Type III—Cavity spilling	Perforation into an anatomic chamber, such as coronary sinus, atria, or ventricles	Can often have a benign course; may result in fistulae formation; large perforation requires repair to avoid coronary steal

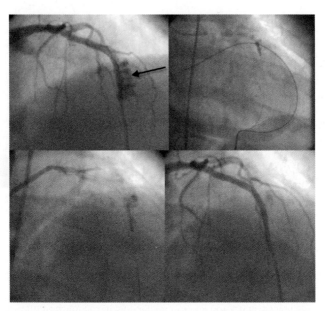

Figure 4.6 Coronary perforation and management. Upper left. Immediately after 18 atm post-dilation of a mid-left anterior descending coronary artery stent through a 6F catheter, coronary perforation with free extravasation of contrast was noted (arrow). Upper right. The patient became hypotensive within minutes, and the angioplasty balloon was reinflated within the area of perforation to seal the leak as pericardiocentesis was performed via the subxiphoid route. Lower left. Via the contralateral groin, an 8F guiding catheter was engaged in the left coronary ostium, and a wire and Jomed covered stent were advanced to the point of perforation. Lower right. After this stent was deployed, there was no further extravasation, and the heparin was not reversed as the platelet glycoprotein IIb/IIIa receptor blocker was continued to protect the patency of the stents that had been placed in the right and proximal left anterior descending coronary arteries.

Pericardiocentesis may also be necessary if hemodynamic embarrassment is present. Although many localized coronary perforations will seal with just prolonged balloon inflation and reversal of anticoagulation, ongoing bleeding is the rule for free perforations. Nonsurgical options then include coil embolization if the bleeding site is in a small distal branch or placement of a covered stent to seal the perforation site in a larger proximal vessel. A free perforation with ongoing leakage, however, is a strong indication for emergent surgical repair.

Perforation of the great vessels (aorta or pulmonary artery) is extremely rare. Aortic puncture may occur, however, during attempted transseptal puncture with too anterior a needle orientation. Ascending aortic dissection can also result from vigorous use of a guiding catheter or extension from a proximal coronary dissection (**Figure 4.7**).

Rupture of the pulmonary artery is also rare, but care must be taken not to use stiff-tip guidewires in these thinner-walled vessels. Perforation of the branch pulmonary arteries has been reported when balloon flotation catheters are inflated while positioned in a distal branch (rather than in the left or right main pulmonary artery). Patients typically develop massive hemoptysis of bright red blood and respiratory distress. This requires tamponade of the proximal pulmonary artery, embolization of

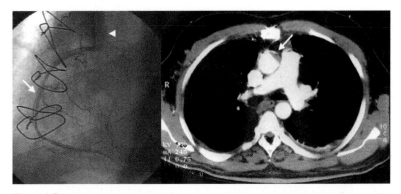

Figure 4.7 Guiding catheter dissection of right coronary artery extending into the aortic root. Left. During attempted angioplasty of the right coronary artery, an extensive coronary dissection was produced (arrow) with contrast extending into the wall of the aortic root (arrowhead). Right. Computed tomography (CT) angiogram showed a localized hematoma in the right side of the aorta (arrow), which was managed expectantly and resolved on follow-up CT studies. (Reprinted with permission from Goldstein JA, Casserly IP, Katsiyiannis WT, Lasala JM, Taniuchi M. Aortocoronary dissection complicating a percutaneous coronary intervention. *J Invasive Cardiol.* 2003;15:89-92.)

the bleeding branch, and placement of a double-lumen endotracheal tube to protect the uninjured lung (or even emergency lobectomy or pneumonectomy). To avoid this serious complication, a balloon-tip catheter should never be inflated in a distal position without a clear pulmonary artery trace, and then only in a slow gradual fashion just until the waveform changes shape (ie, from pulmonary artery to pulmonary capillary wedge).

INFECTIONS AND PYROGEN REACTIONS

Because cardiac catheterization is an inherently sterile procedure, infection is extremely unusual. Recommended technique includes shaving and cleaning the catheter introduction site with chlorhexidine gluconate, use of a nonporous drape, and adequate operator clothing (including a scrub suit, gown, and sterile gloves). Endocarditis prophylaxis is not recommended when cardiac catheterization is performed with standard sterile precautions, but bacteremia has been reported after long or complex PCI interventions. Administration of a single dose of cephalosporin 30 to 60 minutes prior to the procedure can be considered when a delayed intervention is performed by exchanging sheaths placed in an earlier diagnostic procedure, in a patient at high risk (prosthetic valve) undergoing a complex procedure, or when any break in sterile technique is suspected. Special care should also be taken when performing catheterization through a femoral graft since such grafts appear more prone to infection with potentially disastrous consequences and when implanting a foreign body (eg, a femoral closure device).

ALLERGIC AND ANAPHYLACTOID REACTIONS

Cardiac catheterization may precipitate allergic or anaphylactoid reactions to 3 materials: (1) local anesthetic, (2) iodinated contrast agent, or (3) protamine sulfate. True allergies to local anesthetic do occur but are more common with older ester agents (eg, procaine) than with newer amide agents (lidocaine, bupivacaine). Some purported allergic reactions to these agents are actually vasovagal episodes or reactions to preservatives. For patients who claim this history, preservative-free anesthetic (bupivacaine or mepivacaine) or the use of other class (amide vs ester) are practical alternatives to performing the procedure without local anesthetic.

The most common allergic reactions (<1% of procedures) are triggered by iodinated contrast agents. In contrast to true anaphylactic reactions (which are mediated by IgE), reactions to contrast appear to involve degranulation of circulating basophils and tissue mast cells by direct complement activation (ie, anaphylactoid reactions). Release of histamine and other agents causes the clinical manifestations (sneezing, urticaria, angioedema of lips and eyelids, bronchospasm, or, in extreme cases, shock with warm extremities owing to profound systemic vasodilation), which can be classified as mild, moderate, or severe (**Table 4.3**). Risk of such reactions is increased in patients on beta-blockers and in patients with other atopic disorders, allergy to penicillin, or allergy to food products and may be as high as 15% to 35% in patients who have had a prior reaction to contrast. Premedication is recommended for patients with a strong history of atopic reactions and with prior history of reactions to contrast administration. It should be noted that there are currently no data linking allergies to shellfish and allergic reactions to contrast media. Thus, premedication is currently not recommended for patients allergic to shellfish or seafood. A widely used premedication protocol includes (1) prednisone 50 mg by mouth 13 hours, 7 hours, and 1 hour before contrast administration; (2) diphenhydramine (Benadryl) 50 mg intravenously, intramuscularly, or by mouth 1 hour before contrast injection; and (3) + H_2 blockers. The addition of antihistamines can reduce the incidence of adverse reactions and particularly of cutaneous reactions. In addition, it is currently recommended to hold beta-blockers in patients with prior history of adverse reactions. The availability of newer low- and iso-osmolar nonionic contrast agents adds a further margin of safety, since the rate of severe cross reactions in patients with prior reaction to an ionic contrast agent is also <1%. For this indication, the true nonionic agents are preferable to ionic low-osmolar agents. In patients with a severe prior allergic reaction to contrast,

Table 4.3 Classification of Hypersensitivity Reactions

	Classification #1	Classification #2
Mild	Single episode of emesis, nausea, sneezing, or vertigo	Cough, erythema, hives, nasal congestion, pruritus, scratchy throat, sneezing
Moderate	Hives, erythema, emesis more than once, or fever or chills (or both)	Bradycardia, bronchospasm, chest pain, dyspnea, facial edema, hypertension, transient hypotension, mild hypoxemia, tachycardia, diffuse urticaria
Severe	Shock, bronchospasm, laryngospasm or laryngeal edema, loss of consciousness, convulsions, fall or rise in blood pressure, cardiac arrhythmia, angina, angioedema, or pulmonary edema	Cardiopulmonary arrest, refractory hypotension, moderate or severe hypoxemia, laryngeal edema

Reprinted with permission from Moscucci M. Complications of contrast media: contrast induced nephropathy, allergic reactions, and other idiosyncratic reactions. In: Moscucci M, ed. *Complications of Cardiovascular Procedures: Incidence, Risk Factors and Bailout Techniques.* Williams & Wilkins; 2011.

use of a nonionic contrast agent is combined with steroid and antihistamine premedication, although even then breakthrough allergic reactions may occur.

When a patient with a well-documented prior severe contrast reaction needs to undergo repeat catheterization, aortic pressure should be recorded before the catheter is cleared with contrast, since even this small amount of contrast can cause significant histamine release. Coronaries angiography should be performed first, since a severe contrast reaction to the left ventriculogram may preclude further angiography.

Although reactions to contrast are the most common allergic reaction in the cardiac catheterization laboratory, reactions to protamine sulfate, a biologic product derived from salmon eggs, can also occur. These reactions seem to be more common in insulin-dependent diabetic patients who have received NPH insulin (which contains protamine). **Table 4.4** summarizes the guidelines for the management of individual reactions.

Another allergic reaction that should be considered—even though it is rarely seen in the cardiac catheterization laboratory itself—is heparin-induced thrombocytopenia (HIT). Up to 10% of patients will have a fall in platelet count to <50,000 after 4 days of heparin exposure owing to a direct nonimmune mechanism (so called HIT-1). But a much smaller number (<1%) will exhibit a more profound fall in platelets combined with arterial and venous thrombosis owing to an antibody that binds to the complex of heparin with platelet factor 4 and causes platelet activation (HIT-2 or HITT [heparin-induced thrombocytopenia and thrombosis]). This usually does not develop until day 5, unless there has been prior sensitization to heparin, and can be diagnosed by blood testing, which should be done in any postprocedure patient who develops thrombocytopenia. If positive, an alternative nonheparin anticoagulant agent should be used. If thrombocytopenia develops after a coronary interventional procedure, the assay for heparin antibodies is particularly important to distinguish it from the thrombocytopenia that develops in 1% to 3% of patients treated with a IIb/IIIa receptor blocker.

Table 4.4	**Recommended Management of Adverse Reactions**
Urticaria and skin itching	1. No treatment. 2. Diphenhydramine 25-50 mg IV. ***Unresponsive:*** 3. Epinephrine 0.3 mL of 1:1000 solution sub-Q q 15 min up to 1 mL. 4. Cimetidine 300 mg or ranitidine 50 mg in 20 mL NS IV over 15 min
Broncho-spasm	1. (a) O$_2$ by mask; (b) oximetry. 2. ***Mild:*** Albuterol inhaler 2 puffs. ***Moderate:*** Epinephrine 0.3 mL of 1:1000 solution sub-Q **q** 15 min up to 1 mL. ***Severe:*** Epinephrine IV as a bolus(es) of 10 µg/min and then an infusion of 1-4 µg/min; observe for desired effect with blood pressure (BP) and ECG monitoring. 3. Diphenhydramine 50 mg IV. 4. Hydrocortisone 200-400 mg IV. 5. Optional: H$_2$ blocker as outlined. ***Preparation of epinephrine IV:*** Bolus dose: 0.1 mL of 1:1000 solution or 1 mL of 1:10,000 diluted to 10 mL (10 µg/mL). Infusion dose: 1 mL of 1:1000 or 10 mL of 1:10,000 in 250 mL **NS** (4 µg/mL).

(Continued)

Table 4.4	**Recommended Management of Adverse Reactions (Continued)**
Facial edema and laryngeal edema	**Call anesthesia Assess airway:** a. O$_2$ by mask. b. Intubation. c. Tracheostomy tray. **Mild:** Epinephrine 0.3 mL of 1:1000 solution sub-Q **q** 15 min up to 1 mL. **Moderate/severe:** 1. Epinephrine IV as outlined. 2. Diphenhydramine 50 mg IV. 3. Oximetry/arterial blood gas (ABG). 4. Optional: H$_2$ blocker as outlined.
Hypotension/shock	**Call anesthesia Assess airway:** a. O$_2$ by mask. b. Oximetry/ABG. c. Intubation. d. Tracheostomy tray. Simultaneous administration: a. Epinephrine IV—bolus(es) 10 µg/min IV until desired BP response obtained, then infuse 1-4 µg/min to maintain desired BP. Preparation of solution as outlined above. b. Large volumes of 0.9% NS (1-3 L in first hour). 1. Diphenhydramine 50-100 mg IV. 2. Hydrocortisone 400 mg IV. 3. CVP/Swan-Ganz. ***Unresponsive:*** 1. H2 blocker as outlined. 2. Dopamine 2-15 µg/kg/min IV. 3. Advanced cardiac life support.

CVP, central venous pressure; NS, normal saline.
From Moscucci M. Complications of contrast media: contrast induced nephropathy, allergic reactions, and other idiosyncratic reactions. In: Moscucci M, ed. *Complications of Cardiovascular Procedures: Incidence, Risk Factors and Bailout Techniques*. Williams & Wilkins; 2011. Adapted from Goss JE, Chambers CE, Heupler FA Jr. Systemic anaphylactoid reactions to iodinated contrast media during cardiac catheterization procedures: guidelines for prevention, diagnosis, and treatment. Laboratory Performance Standards Committee of the Society for Cardiac Angiography and Interventions. *Cathet Cardiovasc Diagn*. 1995;34(2):99-104.

CONTRAST-INDUCED NEPHROPATHY/ACUTE KIDNEY INJURY

Temporary or permanent renal dysfunction is a serious potential complication of cardiac angiography. The potential mechanisms of contrast-induced nephropathy (CIN) include vasomotor instability, increased glomerular permeability to protein, direct tubular injury, or tubular obstruction. At least 5% of patients experience a transient rise in serum creatinine (>0.5 mg/dL or a relative increase of 25%) following cardiac angiography, making CIN the third most common cause of hospital-acquired renal failure. It may occur in 15% of the general catheterized population or <50% of patients who have risk factors including diabetes, preexisting renal dysfunction, multiple myeloma, volume depletion, or other drug therapy (eg, gentamicin, angiotensin-converting enzyme inhibitors, nonsteroidal anti-inflammatory drugs). Most such creatinine elevations are nonoliguric, peak within 1 to 2 days, and then return to baseline by 7 days, but may rarely go on to require chronic dialysis. The occurrence of CIN increases the length of hospital stay and is associated with up to 5-fold increase of in-hospital mortality. If dialysis is required, there is a further increase in mortality (from 1.1% to 7.1% with CIN to 35.7% with CIN plus dialysis). Several investigators have developed risk prediction rules for the development of CIN.

The main defense against CIN is limitation of total contrast volume. In patients with reduced renal function and especially with diabetes, extra attention must be paid to limiting unnecessary angiographic views and multiple contrast puffs during interventional wire and device placement. As described in Chapter 2, available contrast agents can be classified as high osmolar, low osmolar, and iso-osmolar. There is now evidence that low-osmolar contrast agents are associated with a lower incidence of CIN in patients with renal insufficiency when compared with high-osmolar contrast agents. The role of iso-osmolar, nonionic contrast media (iodixanol) in further reducing the incidence of CIN when compared with low-osmolar contrast media is controversial.

Several studies and meta-analyses have suggested that iodixanol is associated with a lower incidence of CIN when compared with iohexol and ioxaglate but not when compared with iopamidol, ioversol, or iopamidate. Adequate prehydration is also critically important in any patient with impaired baseline renal function. In a classic study, 26% of patients with a mean baseline serum creatinine of 2.1 mL/dL had a rise in serum creatinine by >0.5 mg/dL. Hydration with 1/2 normal saline for 12 hours before and after the contrast procedure provided the best protection against creatinine rise (which then occurred in 11%), but 26% to 28% of patients who received hydration in combination with either furosemide or mannitol had such a rise. Another landmark study has shown that hydration with 0.9% normal saline appears to be superior when compared with 0.45% normal saline. Promising results were also shown with the use of sodium bicarbonate (154 mEq/L). Postprocedural hemofiltration in the intensive care unit has also been reported to reduce the incidence of CIN in a study. However, its overall benefit remains unclear and its routine use in high-risk patients is not recommended.

The free-radical scavenger N-acetylcysteine (600 mg orally before and twice a day after contrast exposure) has shown some benefit in a small clinical trial. However, following a more recent negative randomized clinical trial and registry analysis, the use of N-acetylcysteine is no longer recommended. Finally, when available, the use of biplane coronary angiography, by allowing obtaining 2 orthogonal angiographic views with a single contrast injection, will help in reducing the total amount of contrast dose.

A strategic approach toward the prevention of CIN, including hydration protocols, is summarized in **Table 4.5**.

Another cause of renal failure following cardiac catheterization is systemic cholesterol embolization. This clinical syndrome is seen in 0.15% of catheterizations, but cholesterol emboli can be identified pathologically in many more patients. Patients at greatest risk are those with diffuse atherosclerosis or abdominal aortic aneurysm, in whom insertion of a guiding catheter will frequently produce a shower of glistening particles on the table drape. The hallmarks of cholesterol embolization are evidence of peripheral embolization (including livedo reticularis, abdominal or foot pain, and purple toes). Renal failure due to cholesterol embolization tends to develop slowly (over weeks to months, rather than over 1-2 days as is seen with CIN). Half of the patients with this syndrome progress to frank renal failure. Renal biopsy can confirm the presence of cholesterol clefts but is seldom necessary for diagnosis. Treatment is purely supportive.

Table 4.5 Practical Approach to Prevention of Contrast-Induced Nephropathy

Patients at Risk and Procedure Strategy—Minimize Contrast Amount

All patients receiving intravenous or intra-arterial contrast media should undergo assessment of baseline renal function and clinical assessment for the identification of additional risk factors for the development of contrast-induced nephropathy (CIN).

Several studies have shown increasing risk of CIN with increasing contrast doses, and the additional importance of a contrast dose threshold, including either <125 mL or a weight- and creatinine-adjusted contrast dose calculated using the formula (5 mL of contrast/serum creatinine in mg/dL × body weight in kg).

Minimize total amount of contrast media by avoiding unnecessary views or unnecessary tests, eg, left ventriculography when ejection fraction is already available from noninvasive tests, and by using biplane angiography if available.

Use of smaller catheter might be associated with a lower amount of contrast per case. Use of biplane angiography can help in minimizing the amount of contrast used for visualization of coronary artery segments.

Hydration Protocols

Isotonic 0.9% normal saline is superior to 0.45% saline.

0.9% NS 1 mL/kg/h starting 12 h before the procedure and continued for 12 h after the procedure. (This approach might be applied to inpatients, while more aggressive hydration protocols are more suitable for outpatient settings.)

A 3-mL/kg bolus infusion of 154 mEq/L of sodium bicarbonate 1 h before contrast administration, followed by an infusion of 1.5 mL/kg/h during the procedure and for 4 h thereafter is an alternative to 0.9% NS, but on the basis of most recent data, it does not appear to provide any advantage.

A 3-mL/kg bolus infusion of 154 mEq/L of NaCl (0.9% NS) 1 h before contrast administration, followed by an infusion of 1.5 mL/kg/h during the procedure and for 4 h thereafter.

Role of Contrast Media and of Pharmacological Interventions

Among the characteristics of contrast media, a higher viscosity and higher osmolarity appear to be associated with an increased risk of CIN. Thus, low-osmolar contrast media should be used.

It remains to be determined whether the use of iso-osmolar (280-290 mOsm/kg) contrast media is associated with additional benefits.

Of the many pharmacological interventions tested in the prevention of CIN, N-acetylcysteine is no longer recommended.

Preprocedural statin use has been found to be associated with a lower incidence of CIN and other complications of PCI, and therefore it is generally recommended.

Modified from Moscucci M. Complications of contrast media: contrast induced nephropathy, allergic reactions, and other idiosyncratic reactions. In: Moscucci M, ed. *Complications of Cardiovascular Procedures: Incidence, Risk Factors and Bailout Techniques.* Williams & Wilkins; 2011.

OTHER COMPLICATIONS
Hypotension
Reduction in arterial blood pressure is one of the most common problems seen during catheterization. This reduction represents the final common manifestation of a variety of conditions including the following: (1) hypovolemia, owing to inadequate prehydration, blood loss, or excessive contrast-induced diuresis; (2) reduction in cardiac output, owing to ischemia, tamponade, arrhythmia, or valvular regurgitation; or (3) inappropriate systemic arteriolar vasodilation, owing to vasovagal, excessive nitrate administration, or a vasodilator response to contrast or mixed inotrope-vasodilator drugs such as dopamine or dobutamine.

Low filling pressures mandate rapid volume administration through the peripheral intravenous line and consideration of potential sites of blood loss (expanding thigh hematoma, retroperitoneal bleeding).

In addition, the potential for coexisting sepsis or massive pulmonary embolism should be considered when the severity of coronary anatomy does not match the severity of hemodynamic instability.

Volume Overload
Patients in the cardiac catheterization laboratory are prone to volume overload owing to the administration of hypertonic contrast agents, myocardial depression or ischemia induced by contrast, poor baseline left ventricular function, as well as their supine position and attempts to volume load patients at risk for contrast-induced renal dysfunction. The best treatments are prevention by optimizing volume status before or early during the procedure. Once pulmonary edema develops, aggressive treatment is warranted. Allowing the patient to sit up partially while morphine and nitroprusside are administered to bring filling pressures down may be necessary. If respiratory failure seems imminent, anesthesia support should be requested early enough to allow intubation before a full arrest develops.

Anxiety/Pain
Cardiac catheterization procedures should be well tolerated with oral sedative pretreatment (midazolam [Versed] 1-2 mg and fentanyl 25-50 µg) and liberal use of local anesthetics at the catheter insertion site. However, the amount of discomfort, level of anxiety, and tolerance for either vary widely from patient to patient. Guidelines for monitoring conscious sedation require monitoring of blood pressure, respiratory rate, and pulse oximetry after such medications are administered. The antagonist drugs—naloxone (Narcan) for opiates and flumazenil (Mazicon) for benzodiazepines—should also be stocked wherever the agonist drugs are used for conscious sedation.

Respiratory Insufficiency
Problems with adequate ventilation or oxygenation are not uncommon in the cardiac catheterization laboratory; they may result from pulmonary edema, baseline lung disease, allergic reaction, obstructive sleep apnea, or oversedation. Patients are monitored throughout the procedure with a finger pulse oximeter to detect progressive desaturation.

Retained Equipment
Although diagnostic and therapeutic cardiac catheters have a high degree of reliability, failures can occur whereby devices knot, become entrapped, or leave fragments in the circulation. Operators should be familiar with the use of vascular snares, bioptomes, baskets, and other devices and techniques that can be used to recover the errant fragments when devices do fail (**Figure 4.8**).

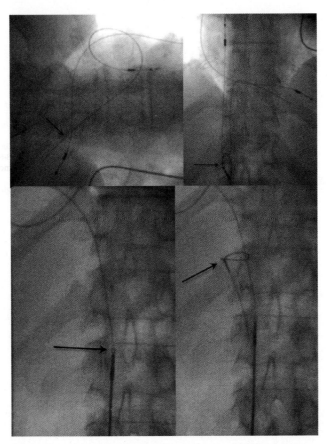

Figure 4.8 Retrieval of a fractured pacemaker lead. When this biventricular pacemaker ceased to pace the atrium, the fractured end of the lead was found free in the right ventricle (upper left, arrow), the loop of this lead was grasped with a deflectable mapping catheter (upper right, arrow), and the free end was pulled down into the inferior vena cava. The free end was grasped with a bioptome (lower left, arrow), and a goose-neck snare was advanced over the lead to allow it to be removed through a 12F femoral venous sheath (lower right). (Case provided courtesy of Dr. Laurence Epstein, Brigham and Women's Hospital.)

CONCLUSION

Advances in technology and in adjunctive pharmacotherapy have resulted in a marked increase in the safety of cardiac catheterization and of cardiovascular interventional procedures. However, complications will occur. Therefore, it is critical that operators performing cardiac catheterization are familiar with factors associated with an increased risk of complications, with their recognition, and with bailout techniques.

SUGGESTED READINGS

1. ACT Investigators. Acetylcysteine for prevention of renal outcomes in patients undergoing coronary and peripheral vascular angiography: main results from the randomized acetylcysteine for contrast-induced nephropathy trial (ACT). *Circulation.* 2011;124(11):1250-1259.

2. Blanco VR, Moris C, Barriales V, Gonzalez C. Retinal cholesterol emboli during diagnostic cardiac catheterization. *Cathet Cardiovasc Interv.* 2000;51(3):323-325.
3. Boehrer JD, Lange RA, Willard JE, Hillis LD. Markedly increased periprocedure mortality of cardiac catheterization in patients with severe narrowing of the left main coronary artery. *Am J Cardiol.* 1992;70(18):1388-1390.
4. Brar SS, Shen AY, Jorgensen MB, et al. Sodium bicarbonate vs sodium chloride for the prevention of contrast medium-induced nephropathy in patients undergoing coronary angiography: a randomized trial. *J Am Med Assoc.* 2008;300(9):1038-1046.
5. Brieger DB, Mak KH, Kottke-Marchant K, Topol EJ. Heparin-induced thrombocytopenia. *J Am Coll Cardiol.* 1998;31(7):1449-1459.
6. HIV and Occupational Exposure. Accessed June 1, 2023. https://www.cdc.gov/hiv/workplace/healthcareworkers.html
7. Chambers CE, Eisenhauer MD, McNicol LB, et al. Infection control guidelines for the cardiac catheterization laboratory: society guidelines revisited. *Cathet Cardiovasc Interv.* 2006;67(1):78-86.
8. Ellis SG, Ajluni S, Arnold AZ, et al. Increased coronary perforation in the new device era. Incidence, classification, management, and outcome. *Circulation.* 1994;90(6):2725-2730.
9. Folland ED, Oprian C, Giacomini J, et al. Complications of cardiac catheterization and angiography in patients with valvular heart disease. VA Cooperative Study on Valvular Heart Disease. *Cathet Cardiovasc Diagn.* 1989;17(1):15-21.
10. Friedrich SP, Berman AD, Baim DS, Diver DJ. Myocardial perforation in the cardiac catheterization laboratory: incidence, presentation, diagnosis, and management. *Cathet Cardiovasc Diagn.* 1994;32(2):99-107.
11. Fuchs S, Stabile E, Kinnaird TD, et al. Stroke complicating percutaneous coronary interventions: incidence, predictors, and prognostic implications. *Circulation.* 2002;106(1):86-91.
12. Fukumoto Y, Tsutsui H, Tsuchihashi M, Masumoto A, Takeshita A; Cholesterol Embolism StudyCHEST Investigators. The incidence and risk factors of cholesterol embolization syndrome, a complication of cardiac catheterization: a prospective study. *J Am Coll Cardiol.* 2003;42(2):211-216.
13. Gobel FL, Stewart WJ, Campeau L, et al. Safety of coronary arteriography in clinically stable patients following coronary bypass surgery. Post CABG Clinical Trial Investigators. *Cathet Cardiovasc Diagn.* 1998;45(4):376-381.
14. Goss JE, Chambers CE, Heupler FA Jr.. Systemic anaphylactoid reactions to iodinated contrast media during cardiac catheterization procedures: guidelines for prevention, diagnosis, and treatment. Laboratory Performance Standards Committee of the Society for Cardiac Angiography and Interventions. *Cathet Cardiovasc Diagn.* 1995;34(2):99-104; discussion 105.
15. Johnson LW, Lozner EC, Johnson S, et al. Coronary arteriography 1984-1987: a report of the registry of the society for cardiac angiography and interventions. I–results and complications. *Cathet Cardiovasc Diagn.* 1989;17(1):5-10.
16. Kelm M, Perings SM, Jax T, et al. Incidence and clinical outcome of iatrogenic femoral arteriovenous fistulas: implications for risk stratification and treatment. *J Am Coll Cardiol.* 2002;40(2):291-297.
17. Kent KC, Moscucci M, Gallagher SG, DiMattia ST, Skillman JJ. Neuropathy after cardiac catheterization: incidence, clinical patterns, and long-term outcome. *J Vasc Surg.* 1994;19(6):1008-1013; discussion 1013-1004.
18. Kim D, Orron DE, Skillman JJ, et al. Role of superficial femoral artery puncture in the development of pseudoaneurysm and arteriovenous fistula complicating percutaneous transfemoral cardiac catheterization. *Cathet Cardiovasc Diagn.* 1992;25(2):91-97.
19. Koreny M, Riedmuller E, Nikfardjam M, Siostrzonek P, Mullner M. Arterial puncture closing devices compared with standard manual compression after cardiac catheterization: systematic review and meta-analysis. *J Am Med Assoc.* 2004;291(3):350-357.
20. Landau C, Lange RA, Glamann DB, Willard JE, Hillis LD. Vasovagal reactions in the cardiac catheterization laboratory. *Am J Cardiol.* 1994;73(1):95-97.
21. Laskey W, Boyle J, Johnson LW. Multivariable model for prediction of risk of significant complication during diagnostic cardiac catheterization. The Registry Committee of the Society for Cardiac Angiography & Interventions. *Cathet Cardiovasc Diagn.* 1993;30(3):185-190.
22. Mak GY, Daly B, Chan W, Tse KK, Chung HK, Woo KS. Percutaneous treatment of post catheterization massive retroperitoneal hemorrhage. *Cathet Cardiovasc Diagn.* 1993;29(1):40-43.
23. Marenzi G, Marana I, Lauri G, et al. The prevention of radiocontrastagent-induced nephropathy by hemofiltration. *N Engl J Med.* 2003;349(14):1333-1340.
24. Mehran R, Aymong ED, Nikolsky E, et al. A simple risk score for prediction of contrast-induced nephropathy after percutaneous coronary intervention: development and initial validation. *J Am Coll Cardiol.* 2004;44(7):1393-1399.

25. Moscucci M, Mansour KA, Kent KC, et al. Peripheral vascular complications of directional coronary atherectomy and stenting: predictors, management, and outcome. *Am J Cardiol.* 1994;74(5):448-453.
26. Moscucci M, Kline-Rogers E, Share D, et al. Simple bedside additive tool for prediction of in-hospital mortality after percutaneous coronary interventions. *Circulation.* 2001;104(3):263-268.
27. Moscucci M, Rogers EK, Montoye C, et al. Association of a continuous quality improvement initiative with practice and outcome variations of contemporary percutaneous coronary interventions. *Circulation.* 2006;113(6):814-822.
28. Moscucci M, ed. *Complications of Cardiovascular Procedures: Incidence, Risk Factors and Bailout Techniques.* Lippincott & Wilkins; 2011.
29. Moussa ID, Klein LW, Shah B, et al. Consideration of a new definition of clinically relevant myocardial infarction after coronary revascularization: an expert consensus document from the Society for Cardiovascular Angiography and Interventions (SCAI). *J Am Coll Cardiol.* 2013;62(17):1563-1570.
30. Mueller C, Buerkle G, Buettner HJ, et al. Prevention of contrast media-associated nephropathy: randomized comparison of 2 hydration regimens in 1620 patients undergoing coronary angioplasty. *Arch Intern Med.* 2002;162(3):329-336.
31. Noto TJ Jr., Johnson LW, Krone R, et al. Cardiac catheterization 1990: a report of the registry of the society for cardiac angiography and interventions (SCA&I). *Cathet Cardiovasc Diagn.* 1991;24(2):75-83.
32. Peterson ED, Dai D, DeLong ER, et al. Contemporary mortality risk prediction for percutaneous coronary intervention: results from 588,398 procedures in the National Cardiovascular Data Registry. *J Am Coll Cardiol.* 2010;55(18):1923-1932.
33. Ramsdale DR, Aziz S, Newall N, Palmer N, Jackson M. Bacteremia following complex percutaneous coronary intervention. *J Invasive Cardiol.* 2004;16(11):632-634.
34. Reed M, Meier P, Tamhane UU, Welch KB, Moscucci M, Gurm HS. The relative renal safety of iodixanol compared with low-osmolar contrast media: a meta-analysis of randomized controlled trials. *JACC Cardiovasc Interv.* 2009;2(7):645-654.
35. Ricciardi MJ, Wu E, Davidson CJ, et al. Visualization of discrete microinfarction after percutaneous coronary intervention associated with mild creatine kinase-MB elevation. *Circulation.* 2001;103(23):2780-2783.
36. Samal AK, White CJ, Collins TJ, Ramee SR, Jenkins JS. Treatment of femoral artery pseudoaneurysm with percutaneous thrombin injection. *Cathet Cardiovasc Interv.* 2001;53(2):259-263.
37. Sandoval AE, Laufer N. Thromboembolic stroke complicating coronary intervention: acute evaluation and management in the cardiac catheterization laboratory. *Cathet Cardiovasc Diagn.* 1998;44(4):412-414.
38. Shammas RL, Reeves WC, Mehta PM. Deep venous thrombosis and pulmonary embolism following cardiac catheterization. *Cathet Cardiovasc Diagn.* 1993;30(3):223-226.
39. Solomon R, Werner C, Mann D, D'Elia J, Silva P. Effects of saline, mannitol, and furosemide on acute decreases in renal function induced by radiocontrast agents. *N Engl J Med.* 1994;331(21):1416-1420.
40. Thygesen K, Alpert JS, Jaffe AS, et al; Executive Group on behalf of the Joint European Society of Cardiology ESC/American College of Cardiology ACC/American Heart Association AHA/World Heart Federation WHF Task Force for the Universal Definition of Myocardial Infarction, American College of Cardiology, American Heart Association, World Heart Federation Task Force for the Universal Definition of Myocardial I. Fourth universal definition of myocardial infarction (2018). *Circulation.* 2018;138(20):e618-e651.
41. Trimarchi S, Smith DE, Share D, et al. Retroperitoneal hematoma after percutaneous coronary intervention: prevalence, risk factors, management, outcomes, and predictors of mortality—a report from the BMC2 (Blue Cross Blue Shield of Michigan Cardiovascular Consortium) registry. *JACC Cardiovasc Interv.* 2010;3(8):845-850.
42. Tsang TS, Freeman WK, Barnes ME, Reeder GS, Packer DL, Seward JB. Rescue echocardiographically guided pericardiocentesis for cardiac perforation complicating catheter-based procedures. The Mayo Clinic experience. *J Am Coll Cardiol.* 1998;32(5):1345-1350.
43. Vitiello R, McCrindle BW, Nykanen D, Freedom RM, Benson LN. Complications associated with pediatric cardiac catheterization. *J Am Coll Cardiol.* 1998;32(5):1433-1440.

5 Adjunctive Pharmacology for Cardiac Catheterization[1]

There is little doubt that refinements in antiplatelet and anticoagulant adjunctive pharmacology have contributed significantly to the improvements in percutaneous coronary intervention (PCI) success, safety, and durability over the last decade. This chapter focuses on evidence-based recommendations for antithrombotic therapy during PCI, highlighting the guidelines.

ANTIPLATELET AGENTS

The 3 classes of antiplatelet agents that are approved for use in patients undergoing PCI include cyclooxygenase inhibitors (aspirin), platelet $P2Y_{12}$ ADP receptor antagonists (ticlopidine, clopidogrel, prasugrel, ticagrelor), and glycoprotein (GP) IIb/IIIa inhibitors. In general, the use of GP IIb/IIIa inhibitors has declined significantly in the past decade and is reserved for excessive clot formation. In addition, current guidelines recommend dual antiplatelet therapy (DAPT) with aspirin and an ADP receptor antagonist for all patients undergoing PCI based on reduction of ischemic events and stent thrombosis following coronary intervention.

Aspirin

Mechanism of Action and Pharmacokinetics

Aspirin (acetylsalicylic acid) exerts its antiplatelet effect primarily by interfering with the biosynthesis of cyclic prostanoids (eg, thromboxane A2 [TXA2]). Aspirin irreversibly inhibits the cyclooxygenase activity of prostaglandin H synthase 1 (Cox-1) and prostaglandin H synthase 2 (Cox-2), which produce intermediate compounds that are used to generate several prostanoids including arachidonic acid-derived TXA2, which promotes platelet aggregation. Aspirin irreversibly acetylates key serine residues on Cox-1 and Cox-2 and prevents conversion of arachidonic acid to prostanoid precursors. The platelet-activating prostanoid TXA is mainly produced by Cox-1, while the vasodilator and platelet inhibitor prostacyclin (PGI_2) is primarily produced by Cox-2. Higher aspirin doses are required to inhibit Cox-2 compared with Cox-1, which is the reason why aspirin exerts antiplatelet effects at half the dose that is required for analgesia (80-100 vs 325 mg). Aspirin is rapidly absorbed in the upper gastrointestinal tract (GI), and plasma levels peak in <40 minutes after administration. Aspirin-mediated platelet inhibition is seen within 40 to 60 minutes of ingestion, and Cox is irreversibly inhibited for the life of the platelet (7-10 days).

Dosing for Percutaneous Coronary Intervention

The optimal aspirin dose for PCI is not firmly established, but randomized trials have shown inhibition of Cox-1 at doses ranging between 50 and 100 mg/d. Clinical studies have demonstrated that aspirin doses of 75 to 150 mg are as effective as higher doses for the prevention of cardiovascular events. When given in combination with warfarin or the ADP receptor antagonist class of antiplatelet agents, the aspirin dose should probably be lowered to 80 to 100 mg based on a post hoc analysis of data from the Clopidogrel in Unstable Angina to Prevent Recurrent Events (CURE) study in

[1]We gratefully acknowledge the Grossman & Baim's Cardiac *Catheterization, Angiography, and Intervention*, 9th edition contributions of Drs Kevin Croce, Mehdi H. Shishehbor, and Daniel I. Simon as portions of their chapter, Adjunctive Pharmacology for Cardiac Catheterization, were retained in this text.

which similar efficacy, but less major bleeding, was seen in the low-dose (<100 mg) aspirin group.

In the CURRENT/OASIS-7 (Clopidogrel Optimal Loading Dose Usage to Reduce Recurrent Events/Organization to Assess Strategies in Ischemic Syndromes) trial, patients undergoing coronary angiography for acute coronary syndromes (ACS) were randomized in a 2 × 2 factorial manner to open-label low-dose (75-100 mg daily) versus high-dose (300-325 mg daily) aspirin and to standard-dose (300 mg loading dose followed by 75 mg daily thereafter) or high-dose (600 mg loading dose followed by 150 mg daily for 7 days and then 75 mg daily thereafter) clopidogrel for 1 month. The results of the trial did not show significant differences in efficacy between low- and high-dose aspirin.

Evidence for Use in Patients Undergoing Percutaneous Coronary Intervention

Aspirin is a cornerstone treatment of coronary artery disease (CAD) because 4 randomized trials have demonstrated that aspirin therapy results in approximately 50% reduction in the risk of death or myocardial infarction (MI) in patients with unstable angina (UA) and non-ST-segment elevation myocardial infarction (NSTEMI).

Adverse Reactions

Because of its antiplatelet effects, aspirin increases the risk of bleeding. Meta-analysis studies have demonstrated a 60% increase in the risk of a major extracranial bleed with aspirin therapy, although aspirin does not appear to increase the risk of fatal bleeding. Aspirin sensitivity includes anaphylactoid reactions, respiratory sensitivity, and cutaneous sensitivity (urticaria and/or angioedema). Aspirin-allergic patients who require aspirin therapy for PCI and stenting can be desensitized so that they can tolerate DAPT following stent implantation.

Adenosine Diphosphate Receptor Antagonists
Mechanism of Action and Pharmacokinetics

ADP receptor antagonists attenuate platelet activation by selectively and irreversibly (clopidogrel, prasugrel, ticlopidine) or reversibly (ticagrelor) binding and inhibiting the platelet $P2Y_{12}$ ADP receptor, which plays a critical role in orchestrating platelet activation and aggregation. When given in combination with aspirin, ADP receptor antagonists inhibit platelet aggregation to a greater extent than either agent alone.

Ticlopidine

Ticlopidine is the first-generation ADP receptor antagonist that was approved for use as an antiplatelet agent in 1991. Ticlopidine is a thienopyridine class ADP receptor antagonist, which is an inactive prodrug that requires conversion by hepatic cytochrome P450-3A4 enzymes to produce active metabolites. The inhibition of platelet aggregation by ticlopidine is concentration dependent, and ticlopidine metabolites bind irreversibly to the $P2Y_{12}$ receptor, resulting in inhibition for the life of the platelet. However, due to high rates of neutropenia, ticlopidine has been largely replaced by clopidogrel (a second-generation thienopyridine) because of its better safety profile.

Clopidogrel

The second-generation thienopyridine clopidogrel differs structurally from ticlopidine by the addition of a carboxymethyl group. Clopidogrel is also a prodrug that requires hepatic cytochrome P450-3A4 conversion to produce active metabolites. The activation processes involved in clopidogrel metabolism lead to a delay in peak antiplatelet effect that varies from 6 to 9 hours depending on the loading dose.

Clopidogrel is 6 times more potent than ticlopidine, and these 2 drugs do not share common metabolites. The inhibition of platelet aggregation by clopidogrel is concentration dependent and irreversible. Following cessation of clopidogrel therapy, platelet function recovers in 5 to 7 days due to the synthesis of new platelets.

The degree of platelet inhibition achieved with clopidogrel is affected by several clinical factors, such as compliance, age, ethnicity, body weight, diabetes, dyslipidemia, renal function, MI presentation, congestive heart failure, and interaction with drugs that alter prodrug conversion. In addition, specific polymorphisms that reduce the activity of hepatic CYP2C19 enzymes (eg, CYP2C19*2 and CYP2C19*3) decrease hepatic conversion of clopidogrel, and carriers of these reduced-function CYP2C19 alleles have significantly lower levels of active metabolite, diminished platelet inhibition, and higher rates of adverse cardiovascular events and stent thrombosis following PCI. The prevalence of CYP2C19 polymorphisms is significant and varies from 30% to 60%, particularly in Asians. Polymorphisms in genes that influence GI absorption, such as ABCB1, also influence platelet inhibition.

Medications that inhibit CYP activity such as certain proton pump inhibitors appear to decrease clopidogrel efficacy by diminishing clopidogrel conversion to the active metabolite. The clinical importance of ABCB1 polymorphisms and clopidogrel drug-drug interactions (eg, atorvastatin and omeprazole) remains uncertain with regard to their effect on cardiovascular outcomes in patients undergoing PCI.

Prasugrel

Compared with ticlopidine and clopidogrel, the third-generation irreversible thienopyridine ADP receptor antagonist prasugrel has more rapid onset of action (1-2 hours), achieves a greater degree of platelet inhibition, has fewer drug-drug interactions, and has less interindividual response variability (**Figure 5.1**). Prasugrel is also a prodrug; however, compared with clopidogrel, prasugrel conversion occurs via more efficient hepatic oxidation pathways that result in rapid metabolite production and peak platelet inhibition 30 to 60 minutes after loading dose administration. Prasugrel activity is not altered by genetic polymorphisms in hepatic CYP2C19 enzymes.

Ticagrelor

The third-generation nonthienopyridine ADP receptor antagonist ticagrelor is a reversibly binding, direct acting, noncompetitive agent. Ticagrelor and prasugrel are similar in the timing of their onset of action (<60 minutes), and both of these newer agents provide a greater degree of platelet inhibition with less interindividual variability compared with clopidogrel. Ticagrelor is not a prodrug and thus does not require hepatic conversion to an active metabolite. In addition, because ticagrelor is a reversible inhibitor, platelet function normalizes within 3 to 5 days following the last dose.

Cangrelor

Cangrelor is an intravenous reversible active ADP receptor antagonist with very short half-life (3-6 minutes) and immediate onset of effect. In general, cessation of drug allows normal platelet activity within 1 hour. Because of its short half-life and rapid onset of action, it has been evaluated as a pharmacologic bridge in patients undergoing coronary artery bypass grafting (CABG) surgery requiring $P2Y_{12}$ inhibition.

Dosing for Percutaneous Coronary Intervention

The recommended loading dose of clopidogrel is 600 mg in the setting of PCI, which is followed by 75 mg daily. In patients undergoing PCI, the clopidogrel loading dose should be given as early as possible. Higher clopidogrel dosing (600-900 mg) has been

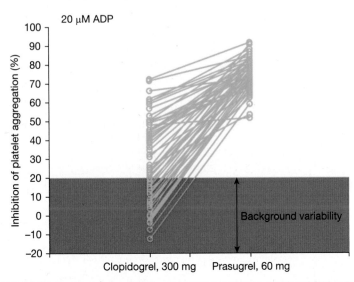

Figure 5.1 Relationship between inhibition of platelet activation by clopidogrel (300 mg) versus prasugrel (60 mg) in response to 20 pmol/L adenosine diphosphate (ADP) 24 hours after loading. Subjects were administered both clopidogrel and prasugrel in a crossover fashion. These data illustrate the point that clopidogrel has significant interindividual variability compared with prasugrel. (Reprinted from Brandt JT, Payne CD, Wiviott SD, et al. A comparison of prasugrel and clopidogrel loading doses on platelet function: magnitude of platelet inhibition is related to active metabolite formation. *Am Heart J.* 2007;153:66. Copyright © 2007 Elsevier. With permission.)

shown to shorten the onset of action, reduce interindividual variability, and improve early outcomes without increasing bleeding. Despite the ability of high-maintenance-dose clopidogrel to increase platelet inhibition, high maintenance dosing strategies have not consistently improved cardiovascular outcomes when patients with poor clopidogrel response are prospectively identified with platelet function testing.

In the setting of PCI, prasugrel is administered with a 60 mg loading dose followed by 10 mg daily. Because of the rapid onset of action, prasugrel preloading was not routinely done prior to diagnostic angiography in clinical studies.

Ticagrelor dosing for PCI is accomplished with a 180-mg load followed by 90 mg twice daily. When prescribing ticagrelor, aspirin should be used at low doses, 81 to 100 mg, because ticagrelor had reduced clinical efficacy in clinical trials when coadministered with high-dose aspirin.

Cangrelor should be administered via the intravenous (IV) route with a 30-pg/kg single-dose bolus followed immediately by 4-pg/kg/min continuous IV infusion. The bolus should be administered prior to PCI, and infusion should be continued for at least 2 hours or for the duration of PCI, whichever is longer. An oral $P2Y_{12}$ platelet inhibitor (eg, ticagrelor, prasugrel, or clopidogrel) should be administered to maintain platelet inhibition. Prasugrel 60 mg orally (PO) or clopidogrel 600 mg PO may be administered after discontinuation of the cangrelor infusion. Prasugrel or clopidogrel should not be administered prior to discontinuation of cangrelor. However, ticagrelor 180 mg PO may be administered at any time during or immediately after discontinuation of cangrelor infusion.

Evidence for Use in Patients Undergoing Percutaneous Coronary Intervention

When aspirin is used in combination with a thienopyridine, several studies have demonstrated up to 5-fold reductions in acute and subacute stent thrombosis compared with aspirin alone, warfarin, heparin, or long-term low-molecular-weight heparin (LMWH) (**Figure 5.2**).

The CURE study randomized 12,362 patients who presented within 24 hours of symptoms to receive clopidogrel 300-mg load, followed by 75 mg daily and aspirin versus aspirin and placebo. There was a significant reduction (9.3% vs 11.4%, relative risk reduction 20%, *P* < .001) in the primary endpoint (death from cardiovascular cause, nonfatal MI, or stroke) in the group receiving clopidogrel. The benefit with clopidogrel was noted early and was observed in all patients with ACSs regardless of their level of risk.

The Clopidogrel to Reduce Events During Observation (CREDO) trial demonstrated the benefit of clopidogrel pretreatment and long-term therapy in a relatively stable CAD population undergoing stenting. Patients loaded with clopidogrel were continued on active drug from day 28 through 12 months, and those patients in the control group received placebo. There was a significant 27% (*P* = .02) reduction in death, MI, or stroke in patients receiving clopidogrel, suggesting that clopidogrel therapy in addition to aspirin should be continued for a minimum of 9 months post PCI.

Prasugrel was compared head-to-head with clopidogrel in TRITON TIMI 38, which tested the hypothesis that a newer antiplatelet agent with greater potency and less variable response would reduce ischemic events compared with standard-dose clopidogrel. The study randomized 13,608 patients with moderate- to high-risk ACS undergoing PCI to prasugrel or clopidogrel for a median duration 14 months. The primary efficacy endpoint was death from cardiovascular causes, nonfatal MI, or nonfatal stroke, and the primary safety endpoint was non-CABG TIMI major bleeding. The primary efficacy endpoint occurred in 9.9% of patients receiving prasugrel and 12.1% of patients receiving clopidogrel (confidence interval [CI], 0.73-0.90; *P* < .001). There were significant reductions in the prasugrel group in the rates of MI (prasugrel, 7.4% vs clopidogrel, 9.7%; *P* < .001), urgent target-vessel revascularization (prasugrel, 2.5% vs clopidogrel, 3.7%; *P* < .001), and stent thrombosis (prasugrel, 1.1% vs clopidogrel, 2.4%; *P* < .001).

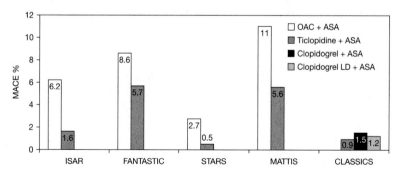

Figure 5.2 Comparison of major adverse clinical events (MACE) after bare-metal stenting in the CLASSICS, ISAR, FANTASTIC, STARS, and MATTIS trials. These events largely reflect the incidence of subacute stent thrombosis. ASA, acetylsalicylic acid (aspirin); LD, loading dose; OAC, oral anticoagulant. (Reprinted with permission from Bertrand ME, Rupprecht HJ, Urban P, et al. Double-blind study of the safety of clopidogrel with and without a loading dose in combination with aspirin compared with ticlopidine in combination with aspirin after coronary stenting study (CLASSICS). *Circulation.* 2000;102:628.)

The reversible ADP receptor antagonist ticagrelor was also compared head-to-head against clopidogrel in the Platelet Inhibition and Patient Outcomes (PLATO) trial. The primary endpoint, a composite of death from vascular causes, MI, or stroke, occurred in 9.8% of patients receiving ticagrelor as compared with 11.7% of those receiving clopidogrel (CI, 0.77-0.92; $P < .001$). In secondary endpoint analyses, ticagrelor reduced the rate of MI (5.8% in the ticagrelor group vs 6.9% in the clopidogrel group, $P = .005$) and death from vascular causes (4.0% vs 5.1%, $P = .001$).

Cangrelor was evaluated in CHAMPION PCI (Cangrelor Versus Standard Therapy to Achieve Optimal Management of Platelet Inhibition-PCI) and CHAMPION PLATFORM in patients undergoing PCI. CHAMPION PCI randomly assigned 8716 patients to receive either a bolus and infusion of cangrelor followed by 600 mg clopidogrel or only clopidogrel 600 mg loading dose within 30 minutes of the start of PCI. Patients with UA, NSTEMI, and ST-segment elevation myocardial infarction (STEMI) were included. The infusion began within 30 minutes before PCI and continued for at least 2 hours or until the conclusion of the procedure. Similarly, in CHAMPION PLATFORM, 5362 patients with NSTEMI and naive to $P2Y_{12}$ inhibitors were randomized to IV bolus and infusion of cangrelor followed by 600 mg of clopidogrel or received 600 mg loading dose of clopidogrel. Cangrelor was not superior to clopidogrel in either of the 2 trials with respect to the primary endpoint of death from any cause, MI, or ischemia-driven revascularization at 48 hours, and both trials were terminated prematurely by the Data and Safety Monitoring Board for futility. In CHAMPION PHOENIX, a total of 11,145 patients who were undergoing urgent or elective PCI were randomized to IV cangrelor versus a loading dose of clopidogrel. The study met its primary endpoint of 4.7% in cangrelor and 5.9% in clopidogrel group ($P = .005$) without an increase in bleeding rates. However, the trial has been criticized given second-generation $P2Y_{12}$ inhibitors were not tested.

Adverse Reactions

All of the ADP receptor antagonists increase the risk of bleeding. In CURE, clopidogrel use with aspirin was associated with an increase in bleeding compared with placebo with aspirin (3.7% vs 2.7%; relative risk, 1.38; $P = .001$), and in the Clopidogrel Aspirin Stent International Cooperative Study (CLASSICS), major bleeding complications were similar between clopidogrel (1.3%) and ticlopidine (1.2%).Compared with clopidogrel, the more potent agents prasugrel and ticagrelor do increase bleeding in patients undergoing PCI. In TRITON TIMI 38, prasugrel use was associated with increased life-threatening bleeding (prasugrel, 1.4% vs clopidogrel, 0.9%; $P = .01$), Similarly, in PLATO ticagrelor caused a higher rate of major bleeding not related to CABG (ticagrelor, 4.5% vs clopidogrel, 3.8%, $P = .03$)

Post hoc subgroup analysis of TRITON TIMI 38 identified less clinical efficacy and greater bleeding in patients with prior history of stroke or transient ischemic attack, in elderly patients (age > 75 years), in patients with low body weight (<60 kg), and in patients undergoing urgent CABG. Increased risk of bleeding in these subgroups resulted in an US Food and Drug Administration black box warning stating that prasugrel should not be prescribed to these patient subgroups. The 2 most common nonhemorrhagic side effects seen with ticagrelor are dyspnea (ticagrelor, 13.8% vs clopidogrel 7.8%) and bradycardia/ventricular pauses (ticagrelor 6.0% vs clopidogrel 3.5%).

Guideline Recommendations

The 2021 ACCF/AHA/SCAI Guidelines for Percutaneous Coronary Intervention specifically address oral ADP receptor antagonists for patients undergoing PCI. The recommendations are as follows:

A loading dose of a $P2Y_{12}$ receptor inhibitor should be given to patients undergoing PCI with stenting (class 1, level of evidence: B). Options include:

Clopidogrel 600 mg (ACS and non-ACS patients)
Prasugrel 60 mg (ACS patients)
Ticagrelor 180 mg (ACS patients)

The duration of $P2Y_{12}$ inhibitor therapy after stent implantation should generally be as follows:

In patients receiving a stent (bare-metal stent [BMS] or drug-eluting stent [DES]) during PCI for ACS, $P2Y_{12}$ inhibitor therapy should be given for at least 12 months. Options include clopidogrel 75 mg daily, prasugrel 10 mg daily, and ticagrelor 90 mg twice daily. In patients receiving DES for a non-ACS indication, clopidogrel 75 mg daily should be given for at least 12 months if patients are not at high risk of bleeding. In patients receiving BMS for a non-ACS indication, clopidogrel should be given for a minimum of 1 month and ideally up to 12 months (unless the patient is at increased risk of bleeding; then it should be given for a minimum of 2 weeks).

Intravenous Glycoprotein IIb/IIIa Inhibitors
Mechanism of Action and Pharmacokinetics
Platelet GP IIb/IIIa receptors mediate the "final common pathway" of platelet aggregation by binding fibrinogen and other adhesive proteins that bridge adjacent platelets and have thus served as a primary focus of pharmacologic antiplatelet strategies. Two parental GP IIb/IIIa receptor antagonists, eptifibatide and tirofiban, are currently available for clinical use.

Eptifibatide
The cyclic heptapeptide eptifibatide is based on a 73-amino-acid peptide isolated from the venom of the Southeastern pygmy rattlesnake. With the recommended bolus (180 µg/kg followed by second 180 µg/kg bolus) and infusion (2 µg/kg/min) regimen, peak plasma levels are established shortly after the bolus dose, and slightly lower concentration is subsequently maintained throughout the infusion period. Plasma concentrations decrease rapidly after the infusion is discontinued, and eptifibatide has an elimination half-life of 2.5 hours, with the majority of the drug eliminated through renal mechanisms. A lower infusion dose (1 µg/kg/min) of eptifibatide is recommended in patients with creatinine clearance less than 50 mL/min.

Tirofiban
Tirofiban is a peptidomimetic inhibitor that occupies the binding pocket on GP IIb/IIIa and thereby competitively inhibits platelet aggregation mediated by fibrinogen or von Willebrand factor. The stoichiometry of both eptifibatide and tirofiban needed to achieve full platelet inhibition is >100 molecules of drug per GP IIb/IIIa receptor. This compares with a stoichiometry of 1.5 molecules of abciximab for each receptor. Like eptifibatide, substantial recovery of platelet aggregation is apparent within 4 hours of stopping the infusion.

Evidence for Use in Patients Undergoing Percutaneous Coronary Intervention
Although GP IIb/IIIa inhibitors have demonstrated an ability to reduce adverse cardiovascular events (**Figure 5.3**), in the modern era of thienopyridine use and stenting, the clinical benefit of routine GP IIb/IIIa inhibitors has been inconsistent. The CADILLAC (Controlled Abciximab and Device Investigation to Lower Late Angioplasty Complications) trial demonstrated that patients with STEMI treated with stenting did not benefit

Table 5.1 Dosing of Parenteral Anticoagulants During PCI

Drug	Patient Has Received Previous Anticoagulant Therapy	Patient Has Not Received Previous Anticoagulant Therapy
UFH	Additional UFH as needed (eg, 2000-5000 U) to achieve an ACT of 250-300 s[a]	70-100 U/kg initial bolus to achieve target ACT of 250-300 s[a]
Enoxaparin	For previous treatment with enoxaparin, if the last SC dose was administered 8-12 h earlier or if only 1 SC dose of enoxaparin has been administered, an IV dose of 0.3 mg/kg of enoxaparin should be given If the last SC dose was administered within the previous 8 h, no additional enoxaparin should be given	0.5-0.75 mg/kg IV bolus
Bivalirudin	For patients who have received UFH, repeat ACT If ACT is not in therapeutic range, then give 0.75 mg/kg IV bolus, then 1.75 mg/kg/h IV infusion	0.75 mg/kg bolus, 1.75 mg/kg/h IV infusion
Argatroban	200 µg/kg IV bolus, then 15 µg/kg/min IV infusion	350 µg/kg, then 15 µg/kg/min IV infusion

ACS, acute coronary syndrome; ACT, activated clotting time; CTO, chronic total occlusion; PCI, percutaneous coronary intervention; UFH, unfractionated heparin.
[a]Target ACTs for UFH dosing shown for HemoTec (GmbH, Switzerland) or I-Stat (Abbott) device. For Hemochron ACT (Werfen) devices, ACT goals are 50 s higher. In the case of CTO or ACS, consider higher target ACT. If IV glycoprotein IIb/IIIa receptor inhibitor is planned, target ACT 200-250 s.
Reproduced with permission from Lawton JS, Tamis-Holland JE, Bangalore S, et al. 2021 ACC/AHA/SCAI guideline for coronary artery revascularization: a report of the American College of Cardiology/American Heart Association Joint Committee on Clinical Practice guidelines. *Circulation.* 2022;145:e18-e114.

as much as patients treated with balloon angioplasty. In low-risk elective patients undergoing PCI who were preloaded with 600 mg of clopidogrel, abciximab increased bleeding and did not improve ischemic outcomes. Although there is no benefit to routine GP IIb/IIIa inhibitor use in thienopyridine-treated low-risk elective PCI cohorts, data do justify targeted GP IIb/IIIa inhibitor use in high-risk patients. In the Intracoronary Stenting and Antithrombotic Regimen: Rapid Early Action for Coronary Treatment-2 (ISAR-REACT-2) study, abciximab reduced ischemic endpoints without increasing bleeding in high-risk patients with ACS.

A recent study performed in the thienopyridine and stenting era showed that, in patients with ACS undergoing invasive management, upstream GP IIb/IIIa inhibitor use increased bleeding to the same degree that it reduced ischemic events compared with a strategy of provisional GP IIb/IIIa inhibitor use at the time of PCI. Similarly, the Facilitated Intervention with Enhanced Reperfusion Speed to Stop Events(FINESSE) trial demonstrated that in patients with STEMI, early abciximab use increased bleeding without clinical benefit when compared with provisional use during PCI.

Adverse Reactions

As outlined above, when GP IIb/IIIa inhibitors are utilized with dose-adjusted heparin and early sheath removal, studies demonstrate a 0% to 1% absolute increase

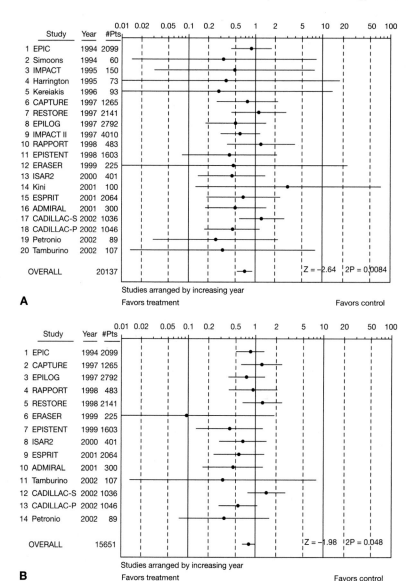

Figure 5.3 Meta-analysis of glycoprotein IIb/IIIa inhibitors and mortality reduction. Mortality at 30-day **(A)** and at 6-month **(B)** follow-up. P, PTCA; S, stenting. (From Karvourni E, Katritsis DG, Loannidis JPA. Intravenous glycoprotein IIb/IIIa receptor antagonists reduce mortality after percutaneous coronary interventions. *J Am Coll Cardiol.* 2003;41:30. Copyright © 2003 American College of Cardiology Foundation. With permission.)

in major bleeding at femoral access sites. In a meta-analysis of 8 clinical trials, abciximab increased the incidence of mild thrombocytopenia (>50,000 < 100,000) compared with placebo group (4.2% vs 2.0%, P < .001; odds ratio [OR] 2.13). Eptifibatide or tirofiban with heparin did not increase mild thrombocytopenia compared with placebo with heparin (OR 0.99). Patients receiving abciximab with heparin had more than twice the incidence of severe thrombocytopenia (defined as >20,000 and <50,000) than those receiving placebo with heparin (1.0% vs 0.4%, P = .01). While uncommon, severe and profound (<20,000) thrombocytopenia requires immediate cessation of GP IIb/IIIa therapy. HIT and pseudothrombocytopenia secondary to platelet clumping needs to be ruled out. Severe and profound thrombocytopenia from GP IIb/IIIa receptor inhibitors are infrequent and are more commonly associated with abciximab use. The mechanism(s) of thrombocytopenia is unknown. The platelet count falls within hours of GP IIb/IIIa administration while it takes days to occur with HITS. Readministration of abciximab, but not the small-molecule inhibitors (eptifibatide and tirofiban), is associated with a small increased risk of thrombocytopenia.

ANTITHROMBOTIC AGENTS

Adjunctive antithrombotic agents for PCI function by inhibiting protease activity of blood coagulation enzymes (**Figure** 5.4) resulting in decreased thrombin

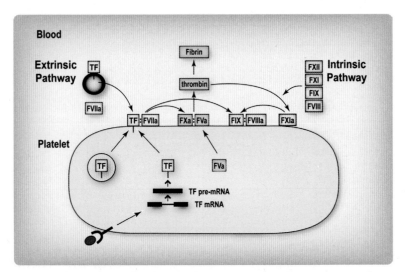

Figure 5.4 Potential role of platelets and the different coagulation pathways in the generation of thrombin and fibrin. Platelets have 3 sources of tissue factor (TF): cell-derived microparticles (MP) TF, TF stored in alpha-granules, and de novo synthesized TF. These different sources participate in the initiation and amplification of the clotting cascade. Assembly of the intrinsic pathway on the surface of the platelet also amplifies the clotting cascade. Finally, platelets bind plasma factor (F) Va, which is internalized, processed, and stored as FVa. This FVa is rapidly mobilized to the cell surface after platelet activation. (Reproduced with permission from Mackman N, Tilley RE, Key NS. Role of the extrinsic pathway of blood coagulation in hemostasis and thrombosis. *Arterioscler Thromb Vasc Biol.* 2007;27(8):1687-1693.)

production or activity and decreased fibrin formation. The main antithrombotic agents used during PCI include UFH, LMWHs (enoxaparin and dalteparin), factor Xa agents (fondaparinux), and direct thrombin inhibitors (DTIs; bivalirudin and argatroban).

Unfractionated Heparin

UFH is a commonly used anticoagulant during PCI. UFH is a heterogeneous mixture of polysaccharide molecules that range from 2000 to 30,000 Da. The anticoagulant mechanism of action of UFH is related to factor Xa inhibition by a specific pentasaccharide moiety and to thrombin inhibition by long-chain saccharide units. The long pentasaccharide chains (>18 units) bind to antithrombin, resulting in a 1000-fold increase in antithrombin inhibitory activity. The UFH:antithrombin complex inactivates multiple proteases including factors Xa, IXa, XIa, XIIa, and thrombin. The inhibitory activity of UFH is a ratio of 1 to 1 for factor Xa and thrombin. By inhibiting thrombin activation, UFH prevents fibrin formation and inhibits thrombin-induced platelet activation. UFH binds to a number of plasma proteins and cell surface proteins that attenuate its activity. This nonspecific protein binding results in variable anticoagulant activity and thus requires monitoring of the therapeutic effect via activated clotting time (ACT) measurements. The half-life of UFH is approximately 30 minutes following administration of an IV bolus of 25 U/kg.

Low-Molecular-Weight Heparin

LMWHs are produced by depolymerizing UFH polysaccharide chains. LMWHs range from 2000 to 10,000 Da, and although they contain the pentasaccharide sequence necessary to bind to antithrombin, LMWHs are too short to cross-link antithrombin and thrombin. Therefore, the primary effect of LMWHs is limited to anti-thrombin-dependent factor Xa inhibition. In comparison with UFH where the ratio of factor Xa:thrombin inhibition is 1:1, LMWHs preferentially inhibit factor Xa and have a factor Xa:thrombin inhibition ratio that varies from 2:1 to 4:1. The most commonly used LMWHs enoxaparin and dalteparin have respective anti-Xa:antithrombin ratios of 3.8:1 and 2.7:1. Compared with UFH, LMWHs bind less avidly to plasma and cell surface proteins and therefore have more predictable pharmacokinetics profiles. Laboratory monitoring of LMWH anticoagulant effect is not routinely required, although the therapeutic effect can be assessed by measuring anti-Xa levels. Following subcutaneous injection, LMWHs are 90% bioavailable and the measured anti-Xa effect peaks 3 to 5 hours after administration. LMWHs are cleared by kidney-dependent mechanisms, and the drug accumulates in a linear fashion in patients who have impaired renal function. In patients with normal renal function, the half-life of LMHWs is 3 to 6 hours after subcutaneous administration.

Factor Xa Inhibitors

Fondaparinux, which is a selective factor Xa inhibitor, is a synthetic 1728-Da LMWH that contains an antithrombin inhibitory pentasaccharide sequence, but because fondaparinux is not long enough to bridge antithrombin to thrombin, it has no thrombin-inhibitory activity. After subcutaneous injection, fondaparinux is 100% bioavailable. The half-life of fondaparinux is 17 hours, and because the primary mechanism of clearance is renal, fondaparinux is contraindicated in patients with severe renal dysfunction. Similar to LMWHs, the anticoagulant effect of fondaparinux can be assessed by measuring anti-factor Xa levels. However, due to the minimal nonspecific binding to plasma and cell surface proteins and the predictable anticoagulant effect, routine anticoagulation monitoring is not required.

Direct Thrombin Inhibitors

DTIs (lepirudin, argatroban, and bivalirudin) have been used during PCI in lieu of UFH. Of these agents, bivalirudin has been the most extensively studied. DTIs do not require antithrombin, and they exert their anticoagulant effect by directly binding to and inhibiting thrombin catalytic activity. In addition to inhibiting thrombin-dependent fibrin production, DTIs also reduce thrombin-mediated platelet activation and aggregation. Compared with other antithrombotic agents used for PCI, DTIs bind to and inhibit clot-bound thrombin in addition to circulating free thrombin, which provides a theoretical advantage.

The original DTI hirudin was isolated from the salivary gland of leeches. Lepirudin is a recombinant form of hirudin. Renal clearance is the primary mechanism of elimination, and dose reduction is required in patients with renal dysfunction. Lepirudin is mainly used as an anticoagulant in patients with HIT. Argatroban is a competitive small-molecule thrombin inhibitor that undergoes hepatic clearance. No dose adjustment is required for patients with renal dysfunction, although argatroban should be used cautiously in patients with liver dysfunction. Argatroban is primarily used as an anticoagulant in patients with HIT. Bivalirudin is the best validated and most commonly used DTI for PCI. Bivalirudin is a synthetic 20-amino-acid polypeptide derivative of hirudin. Bivalirudin interacts with thrombin in a 1:1 ratio. Bivalirudin undergoes hepatic metabolism with some dependence on renal excretion. Because of the partial renal excretion, bivalirudin is administered at reduced doses in patients with severe renal dysfunction. Clinical data support the use of bivalirudin in UA/NSTEMI prior to initiation of cardiac catheterization, instead of UFH plus GP IIb/IIIa inhibitor during primary PCI for STEMI, and for anticoagulation treatment of patients with HIT.

Dosing Percutaneous Coronary Intervention

Guideline–based dosing recommendations for common antithrombotic agents used during PCI are summarized in **Table 5.1**. UFH dosing is guided by ACT monitoring during PCI because the required level of anticoagulation is beyond the linear range of the partial thromboplastin time. Studies have retrospectively related ACT values to clinical outcomes after PCI. An analysis of data from 5216 patients receiving heparin during PCI suggested that ischemic complications at 7 days were 34% lower with an ACT in the range of 350 to 375 seconds than they were with an ACT between 171 and 295 seconds ($P = .001$). This was at the cost of progressively increased bleeding from 8.6% at ACT <350 seconds to 12.4% at ACT 350 to 375 seconds. Importantly, these studies were performed in patients given heparin without adjunctive GP IIb/IIIa inhibitors who require lower ACT targets.

Heparin is given in doses of 70 to 100 IU/kg to achieve a target ACT between 250 and 350 seconds in the absence of adjunctive GP IIb/IIIa inhibition. In contrast, the target ACT is 200 to 250 seconds when heparin (bolus dose of UFH 40-60 IU/kg) is given in conjunction with a GP IIb/IIIa inhibitor. Removal of the femoral sheath should be delayed until the ACT is between 150 and 180 seconds, unless a puncture closure device is used. Heparin is no longer used routinely after PCI because several randomized studies have shown that prolonged heparin infusion increases bleeding at catheter insertion sites and has no ischemic benefit.

Enoxaparin dosing during PCI is dependent on whether patients received a dose prior to initiation of the procedure, and in patients who received enoxaparin prior to the initiation of PCI, the administration of additional anticoagulation therapy is dependent on the timing of the last dose of enoxaparin (**Table 5.1**). Routine procedural anticoagulation monitoring is not recommended.

Lepirudin is typically administered intravenously as a 0.4-mg/kg bolus followed by a 0.15-mg/kg/h infusion, which is titrated to achieve an activated partial thromboplastin time (aPTT) that is 1.5 to 2.5 times control. Argatroban is given as a continuous intravenous infusion at a dose of 2 mg/kg/min with titration to achieve an aPTT 1.5 to 3 times control. Bivalirudin is administered intravenously for PCI procedures as a 0.75-mg/kg bolus followed by a 1.75-mg/kg/h infusion, which is continued for the duration of the PCI procedure. In patients with severe renal dysfunction, the half-life of bivalirudin may be increased, and sheath removal should be delayed for 2 hours, up to 8 hours for patients on dialysis. Bivalirudin increases the ACT in a nonlinear fashion, and routine monitoring of the anticoagulant effect is not required. However, it is still recommended to obtain an ACT after the intravenous bolus to confirm that it has been appropriately administered.

Evidence for Use in Patients Undergoing Percutaneous Coronary Intervention

Evidence for Unfractionated Heparin Use in Percutaneous Coronary Intervention
Guideline recommendations for UFH use in ACS are based on meta-analyses of placebo-controlled trials with UFH for treatment of UA/NSTEMI. In these studies, treatment with aspirin and UFH compared with aspirin alone resulted in a 54% reduction in death and MI, where ACT values were between 300 and 350. However, bleeding was increased in the heparin-treated group.

Evidence for Low-Molecular-Weight Heparin Use in Percutaneous Coronary Intervention
The use of the LMWH as an alternative anticoagulant to UFH in the PCI setting has been largely driven by trials showing superiority of enoxaparin compared with UFH in the medical treatment (ie, noninterventional) of patients with ACSs. The Efficacy and Safety of Subcutaneous Enoxaparin in Non-Q-Wave Coronary Events (ESSENCE) trial compared enoxaparin (1 mg/kg twice daily subcutaneous administration) with standard UFH (5000-U bolus), followed by an infusion titrated to an aPTT of 55 to 86 seconds. The composite outcome of death, MI, or recurrent angina was reduced by 16.2% at 14 days with enoxaparin (19.8% UFH vs 16.6% enoxaparin, $P = .019$) and by 19% at 30 days (23.3% vs 19.8%, $P = .017$). Similarly, the TIMI 11B trial randomized patients with UA/NSTEMI to enoxaparin (30-mg intravenous initial bolus immediately followed by subcutaneous injections of 1 mg/kg every 12 hours) or UFH (70-U/kg bolus followed by an infusion of 15 U/kg/h) titrated to a target aPTT 1.5 to 2.5 times control. The composite endpoint of death, MI, or need for an urgent revascularization was reduced at 8 days from 14.5% to 12.4% ($P = .048$) and at 43 days from 19.6% to 17.3% ($P = .048$). The risk of minor bleeding, however, was increased both in and out of hospital with enoxaparin.

Four randomized studies have compared the safety and efficacy of UFH with enoxaparin during PCI. In the Coronary Revascularization Using Integrilin and Single Bolus Enoxaparin (CRUISE) study, patients undergoing PCI were randomized to eptifibatide and enoxaparin or eptifibatide plus UFH. The primary endpoint of the study, the bleeding index (change in hemoglobin corrected for blood transfusions), was 0.8 in the patients randomized to enoxaparin and 1.1 in patients randomized to UFH ($P = .15$). The rate of vascular access site complications was 9.3% in the enoxaparin arm versus 9.8% in the UFH arm ($P = $ NS). There were no significant differences in the composite of death, MI, or urgent Target Vessel Revascularization (TVR) at 30 days (enoxaparin 8.5% vs UFH 7.6%, $P = $ NS). CRUISE demonstrated comparable safety and efficacy of enoxaparin to UFH during PCI in a randomized controlled study. The Integrilin and Enoxaparin Randomized Assessment of Acute Coronary Syndrome Treatment (INTERACT) study randomized 746 patients with high-risk ACS to receive eptifibatide plus either enoxaparin (1 mg/kg twice daily subcutaneously for 48 hours) or weight-adjusted UFH for 48 hours. Cardiac catheterization and coronary revascularization were performed at the discretion of the investigator (63% of patients underwent angiography, 28.5%

underwent PCI). The primary safety endpoint was the incidence of major non-CABG-related bleeding at 96 hours. Compared with UFH, enoxaparin significantly reduced the rate of non-CABG-related major bleeding: 3.8% versus 1.1% at 48 hours ($P = .014$) and 4.6% versus 1.8% at 96 hours ($P = .03$), respectively. The rate of the secondary endpoint, death or MI, was significantly lower in the enoxaparin group than in the UFH group (5% vs 9%, respectively; $P = .03$). Recurrent ischemia, determined by continuous electrocardiographic monitoring, was significantly lower in the enoxaparin group compared with the UFH group, both during the initial 48 hours (14.3% vs 25.4%; $P = .0002$) and from 48 to 96 hours following study entry (12.7% vs 25.9%; $P < .0001$).

The Aggrastat to Zocor (A to Z) study was designed to assess efficacy and safety of the combination of enoxaparin and tirofiban compared with UFH and tirofiban in patients with non-ST-elevation ACS. The primary endpoint of death, recurrent MI, or refractory ischemia occurred in 8.4% of patients randomized to enoxaparin compared with 9.4% of patients randomized to UFH (95% CI, 0.71-1.08). This met the prespecified criterion for noninferiority.

In the SYNERGY trial, 10,027 high-risk patients with ACS were randomized to enoxaparin (1 mg/kg twice daily subcutaneously) or UFH (60-U/kg bolus followed by 12-U/kg/h infusion) with a goal of early invasive therapy. The primary composite clinical endpoint of all-cause death or nonfatal MI during the first 30 days occurred in 14% of patients assigned to enoxaparin and 14.5% of patients assigned to UFH (CI, 0.86-1.06). No differences in ischemic events during PCI were observed between enoxaparin and UFH groups. More bleeding was observed with enoxaparin, with an increase in TIMI major bleeding (9.1% vs 7.6%, $P = .008$).

In summary, enoxaparin appears to be equally effective as UFH during PCI at preventing major adverse clinical events with modest excess of major bleeding.

Evidence for Direct Thrombin Inhibitor Use in Percutaneous Coronary Intervention

DTIs offer a number of theoretical advantages over UFH such as direct action, predictable pharmacokinetics, and inhibition of clot-bound thrombin and thrombin-mediated platelet activation. The Bivalirudin Angioplasty Trial (BAT) randomized 4098 high-risk patients with ACS undergoing PCI to high-dose heparin bolus or to bivalirudin. Bleeding complications were reduced with bivalirudin and ischemic complications were lower in the subset of patients with postinfarction angina. Reanalysis of these data using a contemporary combined endpoint of death, MI, or repeat revascularization showed a significant reduction in this endpoint with bivalirudin compared with UFH (6.2% vs 7.9%, $P = .039$, respectively).

The Randomized Evaluation in PCI Linking Angiomax to Reduced Clinical Events (REPLACE-2) trial assigned 6010 patients undergoing PCI to intravenous bivalirudin with provisional GP IIb/IIIa inhibition, or heparin with planned GP IIb/IIIa inhibition (abciximab or eptifibatide). The primary composite endpoint was 30-day incidence of death, MI, urgent repeat revascularization, or in-hospital major bleeding and occurred among 9.2% of patients in the bivalirudin group and 10.0% of patients in the heparin plus GP IIb/IIIa group (CI, 0.77-0.80; $P = .32$). The secondary composite endpoint of death, MI, or urgent revascularization occurred in 7.6% of patients in the bivalirudin group versus 7.1% of patients in the heparin plus GP IIb/IIIa group (0.90-1.32; $P = .40$). Bivalirudin with provisional GP IIb/IIIa blockade was thus statistically noninferior to heparin plus planned GP IIb/IIIa blockade and, by historical comparisons, statistically superior to heparin alone in suppressing acute ischemic endpoints with less associated bleeding. In-hospital major bleeding rates were significantly reduced by bivalirudin (2.4% vs 4.1%; $P < .001$). The use of bivalirudin may be particularly useful in patients with conditions associated with increased bleeding risk. It is now recognized that 5% of patients who received prolonged intravenous UFH develop HIT. Bivalirudin is now the anticoagulant of choice in patients with a history of HIT who are undergoing PCI.

In the Acute Catheterization and Urgent Intervention Triage Strategy (ACUITY) study, 13,189 patients with high-risk ACS were randomized to 1 of 3 treatment strategies that included (1) UFH or enoxaparin plus GP IIb/IIIa inhibitor, (2) bivalirudin plus GP IIb/IIIa inhibitor, or (3) bivalirudin alone. Although bivalirudin alone was noninferior with respect to the combined ischemic endpoint, it was superior with regard to bleeding outcomes compared with the other 2 strategies that incorporated GP IIb/IIIa inhibitors (3.0% vs 5.7% for UFH/enoxaparin plus GP IIb/IIIa, $P < .001$). The improved bleeding outcomes resulted in a superior net clinical benefit with bivalirudin alone (10.1% vs 11.7%, $P = .02$).

Bivalirudin use in STEMI was evaluated in the Harmonizing Outcomes with Revascularization and Stents in Acute Myocardial Infarctions (HORIZONS-AMI) trial. Patients with STEMI ($n = 3602$) were randomized to UFH plus GP IIb/IIIa inhibition or to treatment with bivalirudin alone during primary PCI. The bivalirudin-alone group demonstrated lower rates of death (2.1% vs 3.1%, $P = .047$) and major bleeding (4.9% vs 8.3%; $P < .001$) at 30 days compared with the heparin plus GP IIb/IIIa group. Reduced bleeding resulted in a significantly lower rate of the net adverse clinical event endpoint, which included death, ischemic, and bleeding events (9.2% bivalirudin vs 12.1% UFH/GP IIb/IIIa, $P = .005$). The bivalirudin group, however, had a 1% absolute increase in the rate of acute stent thrombosis. Bivalirudin treatment was associated with reduced 1-year rates of cardiac mortality (2.1% vs 3.8%, CI, 0.38-0.84, $P = < .005$) and all-cause mortality (3.5% vs 4.8%, CI, 0.51-0.98, $P = .037$), respectively. **Figure 5.5**

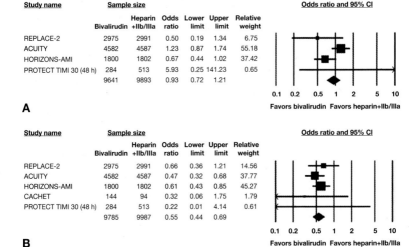

Figure 5.5 Meta-analysis of bivalirudin versus unfractionated heparin or enoxaparin plus glycoprotein IIb/IIIa inhibitors. The data demonstrate that anticoagulation with bivalirudin monotherapy results in similar ischemic adverse events **(A)** and a significant reduction in major bleeding **(B)**. (Reprinted from Lee MS, Liao H, Yang T, et al. Comparison of bivalirudin vs heparin plus glycoprotein IIb/IIIa inhibitors in patients undergoing an invasive strategy: a meta-analysis of randomized clinical trials. *Int J Cardiol.* 2011;152:369-374. Copyright © 2010 Elsevier Ireland Ltd.)

presents data from a meta-analysis evaluating the efficacy and safety of bivalirudin compared with UFH or enoxaparin plus GP IIb/IIIa inhibitors in patients undergoing PCI.

Adverse Reactions

In addition to causing bleeding, UFH can cause immune-mediated platelet activation or HIT. HIT mechanistically results from binding of heparin-dependent IgG antibodies to a platelet factor-4 and to Fc receptors on the platelet surface. This antibody binding results in platelet activation and increased platelet clearance and sets off a cascade of platelet-initiated events that create a markedly prothrombotic state and cause venous and arterial thrombosis.

The anticoagulant effect of enoxaparin can be partially reversed with protamine. Protamine attenuates the antithrombin effect of enoxaparin. It has a limited effect on enoxaparin inhibition of factor Xa. The reversal dose for patients treated with enoxaparin is 1 mg of protamine for each 1 mg of enoxaparin. Compared with UFH, enoxaparin is less likely to induce antiplatelet factor-4 antibodies and is less likely to induce HIT in patients with preformed antiplatelet factor-4 antibodies.

Duration of Antiplatelet Therapy

A number of studies have evaluated 3 to 6 months of therapy compared with the longer 12 months recommendation. Five randomized controlled trials (RCTs) have evaluated shorter 3-6 months DAPT compared with 12 months. The use of DAPT beyond 12 months has also been extensively studied in 6 RCTs. The 2016 focused update on duration of dual antiplatelet therapy recommends DAPT for at least 1 month for BMS and 6 months for those patients receiving DES and presenting with non-ACS. However, for those with NSTEMI or STEMI, 12 months of DAPT has been recommended. Second-generation $P2Y_{12}$ inhibitors have a class IIa recommendation over clopidogrel.

Use of antiplatelet therapy in patients treated with direct oral anticoagulants (OACs) has posed new challenges. Trials have evaluated the clinical equivalency of single antiplatelet therapy with an OAC (dual) therapy versus triple therapy. Overall, dual therapy is associated with lower bleeding risk and should be the default therapy for majority of patients on OAC requiring DAPT. Very little data are currently available for prasugrel or ticagrelor, and these agents should be avoided in conjunction with direct OACs.

SUGGESTED READINGS

1. Angiolillo DJ, Firstenberg MS, Price MJ, et al. Bridging antiplatelet therapy with cangrelor in patients undergoing cardiac surgery: a randomized controlled trial. *J Am Med Assoc.* 2012;307(3):265-274.
2. Bennett CL, Weinberg PD, Rozenberg-Ben-Dror K, Yarnold PR, Kwaan HC, Green D. Thrombotic thrombocytopenic purpura associated with ticlopidine. A review of 60 cases. *Ann Intern Med.* 1998;128(7):541-544.
3. Bittl JA, Strony J, Brinker JA, et al. Treatment with bivalirudin (Hirulog) as compared with heparin during coronary angioplasty for unstable or postinfarction angina. Hirulog Angioplasty Study Investigators. *N Engl J Med.* 1995;333(12):764-769.
4. Brener SJ, Barr LA, Burchenal JE, et al. Randomized, placebo-controlled trial of platelet glycoprotein IIb/IIIa blockade with primary angioplasty for acute myocardial infarction. ReoPro and Primary PTCA Organization and Randomized Trial (RAPPORT) Investigators. *Circulation.* 1998;98(8):734-741.
5. CAPTURE investigators. Randomised placebo-controlled trial of abciximab before and during coronary intervention in refractory UA: the CAPTURE Study. *Lancet.* 1997;349:1429-1435.
6. Chew D, Bhatt D, Lincoff A, et al. Defining the optimal activated clotting time during percutaneous coronary intervention: aggregate results from 6 randomized, controlled trials. *Circulation.* 2001;103(7):961-966.
7. Coller BS. Platelet GPIIb/IIIa antagonists: the first anti-integrin receptor therapeutics. *J Clin Invest.* 1997;100(11 suppl l):S57-S60.

8. Cuisset T, Frere C, Quilici J, et al. Benefit of a 600-mg loading dose of clopidogrel on platelet reactivity and clinical outcomes in patients with non-ST-segment elevation acute coronary syndrome undergoing coronary stenting. *J Am Coll Cardiol.* 2006;48(7):1339-1345.
9. EPISTENT Investigators. Randomised placebo-controlled and balloon-angioplasty-controlled trial to assess safety of coronary stenting with use of platelet glycoprotein-IIb/IIIa blockade. Evaluation of Platelet IIb/IIIa Inhibitor for Stenting. *Lancet.* 1998;352:87-92.
10. Erlinge D, Omerovic E, Frobert O, et al. Bivalirudin versus heparin monotherapy in myocardial infarction. *N Engl J Med.* 2017;377(12):1132-1142.
11. ESPRIT Investigators. Novel dosing regimen of eptifibatide in planned coronary stent implantation (ESPRIT): a randomised, placebo-controlled trial. *Lancet.* 2000;356:2037-2044.
12. FRagmin and Fast Revascularisation during InStability in Coronary Artery Disease Investigators. Invasive compared with non-invasive treatment in unstable coronary-artery disease: FRISC II prospective randomised multicentre study. *Lancet.* 1999;354:708-715.
13. Gilard M, Arnaud B, Cornily JC, et al. Influence of omeprazole on the antiplatelet action of clopidogrel associated with aspirin: the randomized, double-blind OCLA (Omeprazole CLopidogrel Aspirin) study. *J Am Coll Cardiol.* 2008;51(3):256-260.
14. Gurbel PA, Tantry US. Clopidogrel response variability and the advent of personalised antiplatelet therapy. A bench to bedside journey. *Thromb Haemost.* 2011;106(2):265-271.
15. Handeland GF, Abildgaard U, Holm HA, Arnesen KE. Dose adjusted heparin treatment of deep venous thrombosis: a comparison of unfractionated and low molecular weight heparin. *Eur J Clin Pharmacol.* 1990;39(2):107-112.
16. Kastrati A, Mehilli J, Schuhlen H, et al. A clinical trial of abciximab in elective percutaneous coronary intervention after pretreatment with clopidogrel. *N Engl J Med.* 2004;350(3):232-238.
17. Kuo KH, Kovacs MJ. Fondaparinux: a potential new therapy for HIT. *Hematology.* 2005;10(4):271-275.
18. Levine GN, Bates ER, Blankenship JC, et al. 2021 ACC/AHA/SCAI guidelines for coronary artery interventions: a report of the American College of Cardiology Foundation/American Heart Association task force on practice guidelines and the society for cardiovascular angiography and interventions. *Circulation.* 2011;124(23):e574-e651.
19. Levine GN, Bates ER, Bittl JA, et al. 2016 ACC/AHA guideline focused update on duration of dual antiplatelet therapy in patients with coronary artery disease: a report of the American College of Cardiology/American Heart Association task force on clinical practice guidelines. *J Am Coll Cardiol.* 2016;68(10):1082-1115.
20. Lewis B, Matthai W, Cohen M, Moses J, Hursting M, Leya F; ARG-216/310/311 Study Investigators. Argatroban anticoagulation during percutaneous coronary intervention in patients with heparin-induced thrombocytopenia. *Catheter Cardiovasc Interv.* 2002;57(2):177-184.
21. Lincoff AM, Bittl JA, Harrington RA, et al. Bivalirudin and provisional glycoprotein IIb/IIIa blockade compared with heparin and planned glycoprotein IIb/IIIa blockade during percutaneous coronary intervention: REPLACE-2 randomized trial. *J Am Med Assoc.* 2003;289(7):853-863.
22. Lokhandwala JO, Best PJ, Butterfield JH, et al. Frequency of allergic or hematologic adverse reactions to ticlopidine among patients with allergic or hematologic adverse reactions to clopidogrel. *Circ Cardiovasc Interv.* 2009;2(4):348-351.
23. Lopes RD, Heizer G, Aronson R, et al. Antithrombotic therapy after acute coronary syndrome or PCI in atrial fibrillation. *N Engl J Med.* 2019;380(16):1509-1524.
24. Mauri L, Kereiakes DJ, Yeh RW, et al. Twelve or 30 months of dual antiplatelet therapy after drug-eluting stents. *N Engl J Med.* 2014;371(23):2155-2166.
25. Mega JL, Close SL, Wiviott SD, et al. Cytochrome p-450 polymorphisms and response to clopidogrel. *N Engl J Med.* 2009;360(4):354-362.
26. Mehran R, Lansky AJ, Witzenbichler B, et al. Bivalirudin in patients undergoing primary angioplasty for acute myocardial infarction (HORIZONS-AMI): 1-year results of a randomised controlled trial. *Lancet.* 2009;374(9696):1149-1159.
27. Mehta SR, Yusuf S, Peters RJ, et al. Effects of pretreatment with clopidogrel and aspirin followed by long-term therapy in patients undergoing percutaneous coronary intervention: the PCI-CURE study. *Lancet.* 2001;358(9281):527-533.
28. Merlini PA, Rossi M, Menozzi A, et al. Thrombocytopenia caused by abciximab or tirofiban and its association with clinical outcome in patients undergoing coronary stenting. *Circulation.* 2004;109(18):2203-2206.
29. Montalescot G, Barragan P, Wittenberg O, et al. Platelet glycoprotein IIb/IIIa inhibition with coronary stenting for acute myocardial infarction. *N Engl J Med.* 2001;344(25):1895-1903.
30. O'Shea J, Hafley G, Greenberg S, et al. Platelet glycoprotein IIb/IIIa integrin blockade with eptifibatide in coronary stent intervention: the ESPRIT trial—a randomized controlled trial. *J Am Med Assoc.* 2001;285(19):2468-2473.
31. Patrono C, Garcia Rodriguez LA, Landolfi R, Baigent C. Low-dose aspirin for the prevention of atherothrombosis. *N Engl J Med.* 2005;353(22):2373-2383.

32. Price MJ, Endemann S, Gollapudi RR, et al. Prognostic significance of post-clopidogrel platelet reactivity assessed by a point-of-care assay on thrombotic events after drug-eluting stent implantation. *Eur Heart J.* 2008;29(8):992-1000.

33. (PRISM-PLUS) Study InvestigatorsPlatelet Receptor Inhibition in Ischemic Syndrome Management in Patients Limited by Unstable Signs and Symptoms (PRISM-PLUS) Study Investigators. Inhibition of the platelet glycoprotein IIb/IIIa receptor with tiro-fiban in UA and non-Q-wave myocardial infarction. *N Engl J Med.* 1998;338:1488-1497.

34. PURSUIT. Inhibition of platelet glycoprotein IIb/IIIa with eptifi-batide in patients with acute coronary syndromes. The PURSUIT trial investigators. Platelet glycoprotein IIb/IIIa in UA: receptor suppression using integrilin therapy. *N Engl J Med.* 1998;339:436-443.

35. Robson R, White H, Aylward P, Frampton C. Bivalirudin pharmacokinetics and pharmacodynamics: effect of renal function, dose, and gender. *Clin Pharmacol Ther.* 2002;71(6):433-439.

36. Rossini R, Angiolillo DJ, Musumeci G, et al. Aspirin desensitization in patients undergoing percutaneous coronary interventions with stent implantation. *Am J Cardiol.* 2008;101(6):786-789.

37. Stone GW, Grines CL, Cox DA, et al. Comparison of angioplasty with stenting, with or without abciximab, in acute myocardial infarction. *N Engl J Med.* 2002;346(13):957-966.

38. Stone GW, Witzenbichler B, Guagliumi G, et al. Bivalirudin during primary PCI in acute myocardial infarction. *N Engl J Med.* 2008;358(21):2218-2230.

39. Stone GW, Maehara A, Witzenbichler B, et al. Intracoronary abciximab and aspiration thrombectomy in patients with large anterior myocardial infarction: the INFUSE-AMI randomized trial. *J Am Med Assoc.* 2012;307(17):1817-1826. doi:10.1001/jama.2012.421

40. Topol EJ, Byzova TV, Plow EF. Platelet GPIIb-IIIa blockers. *Lancet.* 1999;353(9148):227-231.

41. Topol EJ, Moliterno DJ, Herrmann HC, et al. Comparison of two platelet glycoprotein IIb/IIIa inhibitors, tirofiban and abciximab, for the prevention of ischemic events with percutaneous coronary revascularization. *N Engl J Med.* 2001;344(25):1888-1894.

42. Wallentin L, Becker RC, Budaj A, et al. Ticagrelor versus clopidogrel in patients with acute coronary syndromes. *N Engl J Med.* 2009;361(11):1045-1057.

43. Warkentin TE, Levine MN, Hirsh J, et al. Heparin-induced thrombocytopenia in patients treated with low-molecular-weight heparin or unfractionated heparin. *N Engl J Med.* 1995;332(20):1330-1335.

44. Weitz JI. Low-molecular-weight heparins. *N Engl J Med.* 1997;337(10):688-698.

45. Wiviott SD, Braunwald E, McCabe CH, et al. Prasugrel versus clopidogrel in patients with acute coronary syndromes. *N Engl J Med.* 2007;357(20):2001-2015.

46. Yusuf S, Zhao F, Mehta SR, Chrolavicius S, Tognoni G, Fox KK; Clopidogrel in Unstable Angina to Prevent Recurrent Events Trial Investigators. Effects of clopidogrel in addition to aspirin in patients with acute coronary syndromes without ST-segment elevation. *N Engl J Med.* 2001;345(7):494-502.

6

Informed Consent and Legal Considerations[1]

INTRODUCTION

The risk of injury is inherent to nearly every aspect of a medical professional's work. When patients experience unplanned outcomes, some accept the complication and its ramifications to their lives without question, while other patients decide to seek legal advice and sue. Studies exploring reasons why some patients choose to sue their doctors yield common themes: (1) the need for an explanation; (2) a desire to ensure the safety of others; (3) sense of accountability; and (4) compensation. A common thread among this group is the element of surprise; being effectively forewarned diminishes the sense of surprise and softens the demand for answers. Physicians who understand the development of the duty to obtain informed consent will not only better comprehend how to satisfy this important legal requirement but will also appreciate its value as an effective risk management strategy.

THE ORIGINS OF THE DUTY TO OBTAIN INFORMED CONSENT

The legal requirement of informed consent derives from well-established legal and behavioral norms: we may only touch those who consent to be touched. Touching without consent is called battery, even where the battery does not cause physical injury.

One of the earliest known American cases clearly established the claim of battery in the context of medical care. In *Mohr v. Williams*, an opinion issued in 1905, the Supreme Court of Minnesota considered a case in which the patient complained of problems with her *right* ear and consented to surgery after a clinic examination revealed a large perforation of her tympanic membrane and the presence of a large polyp. After the patient was anesthetized, however, the surgeon undertook an examination of her *left* ear and concluded that it was more seriously diseased than the right: the eardrum was perforated and, in addition, it appeared that the bones of the middle ear were "diseased and dead." After consultation with the patient's primary care physician while the patient was still anesthetized, the surgeon elected to operate on the *left* ear, not the right as previously planned. Although the operation was deemed a success, the patient sued claiming that the surgery was, "wrongful and unlawful, constituting an assault and battery." The court disregarded that the surgery was deemed successful, rejected as disingenuous the suggestion that the surgery was performed under emergency circumstances, but considered whether the surgeon had "implied consent" to operate on the other ear. The court rejected the surgeon's arguments and characterized his actions bluntly: "It was a violent assault, not a mere pleasantry; and, even though no negligence is shown, it was wrongful and unlawful."

DOCUMENTING INFORMED CONSENT AND THE ROLE OF THE CONSENT FORM

Any basic discussion about the informed consent process must include the importance of documentation. Studies have established that patients' memories of the details of consent discussions are highly unreliable. Patients are influenced by subsequent events, human

[1]We gratefully acknowledge Richard C. Boothman, JD and Amy C. Blackwell JD contribution in Dr. Moscucci's "*Complications of Cardiovascular Procedures*" first edition, as portions of their chapter, Legal considerations: informed consent and disclosure practices, were retained in this text.

factors, the effects of anesthesia, and organic changes in short-term and long-term memory caused by the surgery or procedures themselves.

The following represents a list of most legal requirements and recommended practices:

- Informed consent is not simply securing a signature on a consent form. It is educating patients and providing sufficient information to make a knowing decision. This includes minimally a comprehensive discussion of the proposed treatment and the alternatives and the relative risks and benefits of each and culminates in an agreement obtained from an informed patient.
- The duty is generally considered a nondelegable one of the physician proposing the therapy. Ideally, clinical programs would be constructed so the physician performing the procedure would be the person obtaining the patient's informed consent. While surrogates like residents, fellows, PAs, and nurses are often expected to secure the patient's consent, the physician doing the procedure is bound by the adequacy of that conversation. In addition, any clinical workflow should allow a meaningful conversation between the person set to perform the procedure and the patient.
- The conversation in which the patient is informed and after which the patient makes a decision must happen before the procedure and under circumstances that are not coercive and when the patient is clear-headed.
- Programs and practitioners should construct practices and a workflow to accomplish the purpose of allowing most patients to make an intelligent choice.
- Practices must be flexible enough to recognize and respond to individual needs for departures from the usual in order to accomplish the purposes of informed consent. Marginally competent, illiterate, foreign, elderly, and hearing-impaired patients are examples of individuals who may present challenges, small and large, to the usual process.
- Ultimately, it is the nondelegable duty of the proceduralist to make sure reasonable efforts are made to effectively achieve informed consent given the specific needs of each patient.

There are two components to proper informed consent: content and documentation. The content is the substantive discussion that occurs with patients aimed at educating them about their condition, the proposed treatment and its accompanying risks, benefits, and alternatives.

According to the Joint Commission Standard RI.01.03.01, EP 2, "The informed consent process includes a discussion about the following:

1. The patient's proposed care, treatment, and services.
2. Potential benefits, risks, and side effects of the patient's proposed care, treatment, and services;
3. The likelihood of the patient achieving his or her goals; and any potential problems that might occur during recuperation.
4. Reasonable alternatives to the patient's proposed care, treatment, and services. The discussion encompasses risks, benefits, and side effects related to the alternatives and the risks related to not receiving the proposed care, treatment, and services."
5. The consent form should include the signature of the provider obtaining consent, date, and time.

Standardized consent forms are generally viewed as the "permit" allowing the physician to perform the proposed procedure. They are practical, simple, and require little time and effort on the part of the clinician. When used to their best advantage, they can ensure informed consent is documented in the patient's chart reliably. To be most useful, standardized consent forms should be concise and written in language patients will understand and have a hard time disavowing later.

A common misconception related to standardized consent forms is that "if the complication is listed, I should not be able to be sued for its occurrence." The simple response is: "Yes, but the patient never consented to a negligently performed procedure." Healthcare providers are not immune from a claim of negligence merely because the patient was told of the risk beforehand and still agreed to the procedure. For example, a standardized consent form for a cardiac catheterization might include retroperitoneal bleeding as a risk. This does not mean that a patient who suffers a retroperitoneal bleed as a result of a negligently performed catheterization cannot successfully sue. Conversely, if a patient sustains a complication that is not listed on the standardized consent form, it does not necessarily follow that this is proof the procedure was done negligently. Some complications may be unknown, unforeseen, and not discussed with the patient in advance. These exceedingly rare, unforeseen complications are not the type that should be itemized on a standardized consent form for a particular case.

Standardized consent forms have their limitations. They are often presented to the patient along with many other forms for signing. The patient may not take the time to read, understand, and digest what is written, let alone ask questions. The forms are typically written in technical, medical terms that are beyond the understanding of most patients. The forms can easily become outdated and do not encourage documentation or discussion of risks, benefits, and alternatives that may be unique to that particular patient. This is why a detailed, contemporaneous clinical note outlining the informed consent discussion is valuable.

A tailored clinical note in the patient's chart memorializing that the informed consent conversation occurred, identifying the participants to that conversation, the salient points made and the patient's agreement, coupled with a statement that all the patient's questions were answered resulting in the patient's agreement and request to proceed is a very valuable compliment to the usual operative or procedure consent and powerful evidence of the carefully obtained consent (**Table 6.1**).

THE OPPORTUNITY TO MANAGE RISK WITH INFORMED CONSENT

Practically speaking, most patients seek legal help after they were surprised by an outcome and explanations they could trust were not offered as they struggled to understand what happened to them. Solid risk management begins *before* a prob-

Table 6.1 **Example of Consent Documentation in a Clinical Note[a]**
This is a note to document the current plans of percutaneous coronary intervention for Robert L. Mr. L. is a 69-year-old man who was referred from outside hospital X following admission for non-ST segment elevation myocardial infarction. Coronary angiography reportedly showed a 90% stenosis of his right coronary artery. I have reviewed the cath lab films that were sent to me, and indeed these reveal a 90% stenosis in the mid right coronary artery. I think that percutaneous coronary intervention with drug-eluting stent placement as had been suggested by Dr. B., is indeed the best option. I discussed my assessment thoroughly with Mr. L., explained my recommendations, together with his other options and attendant risks of each, and he agrees to proceed. The procedure is scheduled for tomorrow morning, October 12, 2007. I encouraged Mr. L. to feel free to ask any other questions or concerns he might have in the interim.

[a]This is in addition to the consent form the patient signs.

lem develops. Obtaining informed consent remains the most underutilized opportunity to set reasonable expectations and sensitize the patient to the difficulties and potential adverse outcomes. Logically, a patient who is well informed before a problem occurs will more easily understand what happened if a problem develops later. Although they may need assistance to remember the consent discussion and process what happened to them, thoughtful informed consent will have prepared them better to embrace the idea that the complication alone does not mean that the practitioner was negligent.

The obligation to provide informed consent becomes for some an opportunity to create unrealistic expectations. Practitioners who find themselves saying things like, "you'll be up and running in no time," "you're in good hands – I've got the best complication rate in the state," and "you'll feel better as soon as you wake up" are really communicating: "It won't happen to you." Reciting remote statistical chances deceives patients into believing their personal risk is the same as the risk of a large study population. No individual patient experiences 0.3% death or complication. If the complication occurs to your patient, he or she experiences 100% of that complication. Statistics may have bearing in an informed consent discussion, but any recitation of a statistical risk should be placed in context and balanced with strong personal reminders that regardless of a population's risk, if a complication happens to a patient it could change the patient's life dramatically.

Informed Consent and Off-Label Medical Device Use

It has become relatively common for physicians, and interventionalists in particular, to use US Food and Drug Administration (FDA)-approved devices "off-label" (ie, for a use other than one specifically approved by the FDA). It is instructive to understand exactly how this happens. The FDA does not have the authority, and does not want the authority, to regulate the practice of medicine. The Federal Food, Drug, and Cosmetic Act specifically states that "nothing in this Act shall be construed to limit or interfere with the authority of a health care practitioner to prescribe or administer any legally marketed device to a patient for any condition or disease within a legitimate health care practitioner-patient relationship." The FDA has recognized that:

> "Good medical practice and the best interests of the patient require that physicians use legally available … devices according to their best knowledge and judgment. If physicians use a product for an indication not in the approved labeling, they have the responsibility to be well informed about the product, to base its use on firm scientific rationale and on sound medical evidence, and to maintain records of the product's use and effects. Use of a marketed product in this manner when the intent is the "practice of medicine" does not require the submission of an Investigational New Drug Application (IND), Investigational Device Exemption (IDE) or review by an Institutional Review Board (IRB). However, the institution at which the product will be used may, under its own authority, require IRB review or other institutional oversight."

Thus, it has become generally accepted that physicians may use devices off-label, provided the use is consistent with the "best interests of the patient" and based on "firm, scientific rationale and on sound medical evidence." The use should be recognized as within the standard of care for the specific specialist, which means in the case of an interventional cardiologist that "a reasonably prudent cardiologist of the same education, training and expertise would have used the device in that manner under the same or similar circumstances." It is the responsibility of the interventionalist to ensure the use is safe, effective, and supported by medical literature, scientific rationale, and patient need. Assuming the physician is well informed about the device and is basing its use on something founded in science and medical evidence, the question then becomes: when using approved devices off-label, what should patients be told about the regulatory status of the device as part of the informed consent process? Or, more to the point, how can advising the patient ahead of time avoid the kind of surprise and discovery afterward that would make the patient think something inappropriate or even illegal occurred in the procedure?

There is nothing in the Federal Food, Drug, and Cosmetic Act that requires that patients are advised of the regulatory status of a device, not surprising given the explicit exclusion in the Act of any pretense that it regulates the practice of medicine. But the absence in the FDA Act does not mean physicians are absolved of any preprocedure disclosure and certainly does not mean no preprocedure disclosure is a good idea. Importantly, nothing in the Act or regulations prohibits states or courts (via case law) from requiring disclosure of the regulatory status of a device in the informed consent process.

In general, the closer the off-label use is to the approved use, the lower the perceived need to make a special disclosure in the preprocedure visits. The less widespread the use nationally, the harder it will be to convince the patient after-the-fact that it was appropriate. The existence of robust controversy in the literature almost guarantees that absent full disclosure ahead of time and specific informed consent by the patient, the patient will both believe it was wrong and have no problem finding physicians to validate this belief as they offer their services as experts in the ensuing malpractice case. While off-label use of a device that is only incidental to the procedure may warrant no attention at all in the informed consent discussion, off-label use of a device for an essential purpose to the procedure takes on more importance in the preprocedure discussions, especially if there are less-controversial alternatives that will accomplish the same purpose. Whether to mention an intended off-label use or not in the conversation before the procedure at least should be considered against these and other considerations, but it is a choice ultimately left to the sound discretion of the physician, as informed by the standard of care.

That being said, if there is any question about the wisdom of doing so, cardiologists should err on the side of disclosure. Presumably, off-label use of the device is being considered because the patient's doctor has concluded that the patient will benefit from its use; if that is true, there should be no harm in sharing that judgment with the patient. Before the caregiver decides what form the disclosure should take and its content, they should consider a number of factors that would include the sophistication of the patient, the significance of the role the device will play, and the potential complications among them. The manner of the disclosure and education may range from making it a part of the informed consent discussion to use of special information sheets and a specific written consent form.

DISCLOSURE OF ADVERSE OUTCOMES

Study after study have demonstrated the same point: patients seek legal advice when they find they cannot get honest answers they can trust, when they sense the absence of accountability, and when no one is there to help them put the pieces together in a credible way. Answering questions directly leads to credibility and offers an opportunity to answer questions and clarify misconceptions. In one study, 24% of patients sued their doctors because they felt that their doctors were not being honest.

Disclosure of an unanticipated outcome is a process, not a single event. We do not recommend that any caregiver handle disclosure of a serious complication without first getting good advice. When adverse consequences happen as a result of well-intended medical care, caregivers experience a complex set of emotions and it is prudent to get an independent view of the situation and advice before undertaking a full disclosure. Committing to disclose once the facts are clear, but reserving a time frame to consult with resources like a risk management office or counsel and gather facts, not simply expressing assumptions and uninformed opinions, is always a good idea. The process of disclosure should begin as soon as the adverse outcome is appreciated, if only to promise full disclosure once the facts are in. As additional facts and information about the event are accumulated, further discussions with the patient and families need to occur. Well-executed and well-documented informed consent before the procedure sets the stage for these difficult conversations later, allowing the caregiver and the risk manager to build on what was established before the problem developed.

Practical Points

- The informed consent process should be viewed also as a tool to manage risk. It is an opportunity to set reasonable expectations for the patient to minimize surprise when complications occur.
- Informed consent is not completing a consent form. It is the agreement that arises from the conversation between physician and patient during which the patient is educated sufficiently to make an informed decision about medical treatment.
- In general, adequate informed consent discussions should include a description of the proposed procedure and alternatives, including material risks and benefits of each in language a layman can understand and in sufficient detail to create a reasonably educated patient.
- The person intending to perform the procedure should secure the consent in a noncoercive way when the patient is fully competent and with time to change their mind.
- Ideally, informed consent should be documented in both a well-written, up-to-date standardized consent form and a contemporary clinical note in the patient's chart.
- Whether to mention an off-label use of devices or medications in the informed consent conversation should be considered in every case. Disclosure of the off-label use is recommended if there is any question about whether to discuss the off-label use in advance.
- Well-executed and well-documented informed consent beforehand sets the stage for difficult disclosure conversations that may be required later. It allows the caregiver and risk manager to build on the discussion of potential risks and complications established before the problem occurred.
- Disclosure of adverse outcomes is the ethical thing to do for all involved, makes practical sense, is a necessary precursor to learning from mistakes, and makes sense from a claims management perspective but should never be done without help.
- Disclosure of an adverse outcome is a process, not a single event and should be handled in a way that is attentive to the patient and family's needs, and also in a way that is prudent and deliberate.

SUGGESTED READINGS

1. Boothman R, Blackwell A, Campbell D, Anderson S, Commiskey E. A better approach to medical malpractice claims? The university of Michigan approach. *J Health Life Sci Law.* 2009;2:125-159.
2. Canterbury v Spence, 464 F2d 772 (DC Cir 1972). Available at: https://casetext.com/case/canterbury-v-spence/case-summaries. (Accessed July 16, 2023).
3. Federal Food, Drug and Cosmetic Act, Sec. 906. [21 USC §396] Practice of Medicine. Page last visited February 7, 2009. http://www.fda.gov/ScienceResearch/SpecialTopics/RunningClinicalTrials/GuidancesInformationSheetsandNotices/ucm116355.htm

4. Hickson GB, Clayton EW, Githens PB, Sloan FA. Factors that prompted families to file medical malpractice claims following perinatal injuries. *JAMA*. 1992;267(10):1359-1363.

5. Mohr v Williams, 104 NW 12 (Minn. 1905). https://en.wikipedia.org/wiki/Mohr_v._Williams

6. National Quality Forum (NQF). *Safe Practices for Better Healthcare–2009 Update: A Consensus Report*. NQF; 2009. Safe Practice 5: Informed Consent.

7. Robinson G, Merav A. Informed consent: recall by patients tested postoperatively. *Ann Thorac Surg*. 1976;22(3):209-212.

8. Schloendorff v the Society of the New York Hospital, 211 NY 125, 105 NE 92, 93. 1914.

9. Southard v Temple University Hospital, 781 A2d 101, 107-08 (Pa. 2001); Earle v. Ratliff, 998 S.W.2d 882, 891-92 (Tex. 1999); Hansen v. Universal Health Services, 974 P.2d 1158, 1159-60 (Nev. 1999); Packard v. Razza, 927 So.2d 529, 534 (La. App. 2006); Sita v. Long Island Jewish-Hillside Medical Center, 803 N.Y.S.2d 112, 114 (A.D. 2005) Blazoski v. Cook, 346 256, 787 A.2d 910 (N.J. Super. A.D. 2002); Osburn v. Danek Medical, Inc., 520 S.E.2d 88, 92 (N.C. App. 1999), aff'd, 530 S.E.2d 54 (N.C. 2000); Alvarez v. Smith, 714 So. 2d 652, 654 (Fla. App. 1998); Klein v. Biscup, 109 3d 855, 673 N.E.2d 225, 231 (Ohio App. 1996); Balderston v. Medtronic Sofamor Danek, Inc., 285 F.3d 238, 239 n.2 (3d Cir. 2002) (applying Pennsylvania law); Bogle v. Sofamor Danek Group, Inc., 1999 WL 1132313, at *7 (S.D. Fla. Apr. 9, 1999); In re Orthopedic Bone Screw Products Liability Litigation, 1996 WL 107556, at *3-5 (E.D. Pa. Mar. 8, 1996), reconsideration denied, 1996 WL 900351 (E.D. Pa. May 21, 1996).

10. Vincent C, Young M, Phillips A. Why do people sue doctors? A study of patients and relatives taking legal action. *Lancet*. 1994;343(8913):1609-1613. doi:10.1016/s0140-6736(94)93062-7

7

Radial Artery Approach[1]

The development of evidence demonstrating the superiority of transradial access (TRA) when compared with transfemoral access (TFA) has led professional societies to endorse the TRA approach as a first choice for PCI. A recent scientific statement from the American Heart Association strongly supported a "radial-first" access strategy for patients with acute coronary syndromes (ACSs). In addition, the most recent Revascularization Guidelines from the European Society of Cardiology (ESC) and European Association for Cardio-Thoracic Surgery endorse TRA as a standard approach by experienced operators with a class I recommendation and level of evidence A to decrease bleeding and vascular complications in all patients undergoing PCI and mortality in patients undergoing PCI for ACS.

ANATOMICAL CONSIDERATIONS

The radial and ulnar arteries arise together from the bifurcation of the brachial artery just below the bend of the elbow. The radial artery has an average diameter of 2.8 mm in women and 3.1 mm in men. It passes along the lateral side of the forearm from the neck of the radius to the styloid process in the wrist. The distal portion of the artery in the forearm is superficial, covered by the integument and fascia, and lies between the tendons of the brachioradialis and flexor carpi radialis over the prominence of the radius. It then winds laterally around the lateral side of the carpus and crosses the floor of the anatomical snuffbox, between the tendons of the extensors pollicis longus and brevis muscles. Then it passes forward between the 2 heads of the first interosseous dorsalis muscle, into the palm of the hand, joining with the deep branch of the ulnar artery and forming the deep palmar arch. The artery is accompanied by a pair of venae comitantes throughout its whole course, which can be used to perform right-sided heart catheterization (RHC). For catheterization procedures, the radial artery can be accessed at the level of the wrist or more distally at the anatomic snuffbox.

The ulnar artery, with a similar diameter compared with the radial artery, courses between the tendons of the flexor digitorum superficialis and the flexor carpi ulnaris in the medial aspect of the wrist. Distally, it traverses to the hand through the Guyon canal along with the ulnar nerve, lateral to the pisiform bone. In contrast to the radial artery, the ulnar artery is mobile, deep lying, and adjacent to the ulnar nerve; its pulse is not easily palpable; and it lacks a bony compression surface. For these reasons, the ulnar artery is in general utilized as second-line access for coronary procedures, as an alternative to TRA to minimize crossover to TFA. Complication risks are comparable with TRA, with a trend toward higher risk of access site failure and local hematomas. Case series have reported that the use of the ulnar artery after failed radial access or in the presence of chronic ipsilateral radial occlusion is not associated with ischemic complications.

The operator should be aware of uncommon anatomic anomalies that may prevent the advancement of wires or catheters to the ascending aorta and result in pro-

---

[1]We gratefully acknowledge the Grossman & Baim's *Cardiac Catheterization, Angiography, and Intervention,* 9th edition contributions of Mauricio G Cohen, Tejas Patel, and Sunil V. Rao as portions of their chapter, Radial Artery Approach, were retained in this text.

Table 7.1 **Anatomical Variations of the Radial Artery**

Type of Radial Artery Variation	Frequency (%)
High radial artery origin at the level of the mid or upper arm.	7
Loop in the proximal radial artery.	2.3
Severe tortuosity.	2
Miscellaneous anomalies.	2.5
Bilateral anomalies.	8
Origin of the subclavian artery from distal segment of posterior aspect of aortic arch (arteria lusoria).	1

cedural failure. These anatomic variations are present in 15% to 20% of cases and include tortuous radial configurations, stenoses, hypoplasia, radioulnar loops, aberrant right subclavian artery (arteria lusoria), and abnormal origin of the radial artery (**Table 7.1**).

Figure 7.1 displays an algorithm for selecting access and crossover to TFA according to the type of procedure.

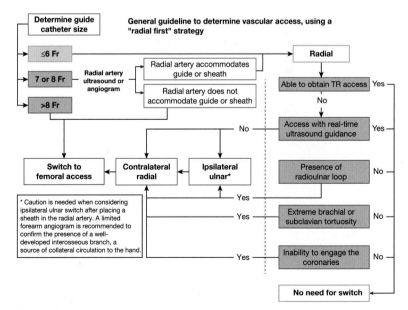

Figure 7.1 Algorithm for selecting radial access and crossing over to other vascular access.

TECHNICAL ASPECTS
Patient Preparation

All patients undergoing TRA procedures in the catheterization laboratory need to follow standard preparation guidelines as mandated by local policies. Depending on operators' preference, the groins can be prepped along with the wrists. Placement of intravenous lines in the vicinity of the wrist should be avoided. Sedation is strongly recommended to decrease catecholamine release that can potentially contribute to radial spasm.

Testing for dual circulation of the hand with pulse oximetry and plethysmography using the Barbeau test (modified Allen test) is not recommended as a tool to determine the feasibility of TRA. The Barbeau test has never been shown to predict ischemia or vascular complications of the hand. In addition to the radial and ulnar arteries, the interosseous branches along with a rich collateral system supply circulation to the hand. The RADAR study (Should Intervention Through RADial Approach be Denied to Patients With Negative Allen's Test Results?) examined the relationship between dual hand circulation using the Barbeau test and lactate levels in the thumb (a surrogate for hand ischemia), ulnar frame count (a surrogate for collateralization between the radial and ulnar arteries), and strength and discomfort of the hand after TRA. Among 203 patients undergoing TRA cardiac catheterization, the lactate levels were identical regardless of the Barbeau test result; even while an occlusive sheath was placed in the radial artery, lactate levels did not vary across Barbeau test results. Similar findings were observed for handgrip and hand discomfort with respect to the Barbeau test. Therefore, collateral flow testing is not a reliable predictor of hand ischemia after TRA procedures.

Patient Positioning—Right Versus Left Radial Access

TRA can be performed through the left or the right radial artery. Regardless of the side, a comfortable position for the patient and the operator is crucial for the successful performance of TRA procedures. For right-sided TRA, an arm board that provides transitional support between the wrist and the table for placement of interventional equipment (wires, catheters, etc.) is attached to the right side of the procedure table. Multiple arm boards in different shapes and designs are commercially available (**Figure 7.2**). The patient's right arm is placed on the board and abducted at a 30°

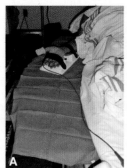 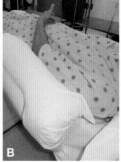

Figure 7.2 Positioning of the arm for right or left radial access. **A,** The right arm is placed on the board abducted at a 30° angle. **B,** The left arm rest on a large pillow placed on a regular arm board that guides the forearm toward the midsection of the patient's body, placing the left wrist on top of the left groin.

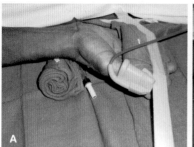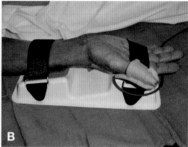

Figure 7.3 Positioning of the hand for transradial access. The hand is hyperextended with use of a rolled towel behind the wrist and tape holding the fingers **(A)**, or with use of a dedicated positioning splint **(B)**.

angle. The right wrist is placed in a hyperextended position using commercially available splints or a rolled towel behind the wrist with the fingers taped to the arm board (**Figure 7.3**). Both groins may be prepped as well, depending on the anticipated need for femoral access.

For left TRA, the patient setup varies widely across catheterization laboratories. As with right TRA, the operator stands at the right side of the patient to avoid disruption of the traditional laboratory setup. The patient is positioned supine on the table, the left wrist is propped using blankets or pillows, and the elbow is slightly flexed and pronated toward the midsection of the patient's body where the wrist can rest on the left thigh in proximity to the left groin. For enhanced patient and operator comfort, snuffbox access may be preferred for left TRA procedures, as the hand can be prepped with full pronation, resting on the patient's lower abdomen. There are a number of commercially available systems to arm positioning for left TRA (**Figure 7.2**). Coronary artery engagement from left TRA resembles TFA. Cannulation of left internal mammary artery (LIMA) bypass grafts is easier through left TRA. Left TRA is also more convenient for diagnostic and interventional procedures of infradiaphragmatic pathology in tall patients (height more than 170 cm) because there is no need to traverse the aortic arch from the left side, thereby saving almost 10 cm of catheter length. Moreover, entering the descending aorta is easier and straighter in most cases through left TRA. Even for addressing stenoses in left subclavian, left vertebral, and left internal mammary arteries, this is a convenient approach.

Sheath Selection

There are a number of TRA kits available in the market. In general, these kits include a micropuncture needle, a short 0.018- to 0.021-in wire, and a 10- to 13-cm hydrophilic-coated arterial sheath. Hydrophilic coating allows for easier sheath removal and is associated with less spasm and patient discomfort. Some operators recommend longer sheaths to avoid spasm and difficult catheter manipulation. However, a 2 × 2 factorial randomized study in 790 patients undergoing TRA PCI comparing shorter (13 cm) versus longer (23 cm) sheaths with or without hydrophilic coating showed that sheath length did not have any effect in the occurrence of spasm or patient discomfort. On the other hand, hydrophilic coating was associated with a significant reduction in radial spasm and patient discomfort. Operators should consider downsizing to smaller sheath size (5Fr) to decrease trauma to the radial artery and reduce the risk of radial artery occlusion (RAO). However, sheaths smaller than 6Fr cannot support the techniques or devices required for complex coronary interventions. To overcome the size limitations of TRA, slender thin-walled sheaths with an outer diameter close to that of a 5Fr sheath, but with an inner diameter compatible with 6Fr guiding catheters, have been developed and have gained popularity among radial operators because they minimize radial artery injury without compromising guiding catheter size. Slender sheaths are also available in outer/inner diameters of 4/5Fr and 6/7Fr. Of note, these thin-walled slender sheaths kink easily and should never be used in the femoral artery.

Radial Puncture Technique

TRA procedures can be successfully completed in more than 95% of cases. The radial artery has a high propensity to develop spasm due to its smaller-caliber, large muscular media, and higher receptor-mediated vasomotion in comparison with similar arteries (**Figure 7.4**).Spasm should be routinely prevented using a hydrophilic-coated sheath and vasodilators through the sidearm of the sheath immediately after obtaining access (**Figure 7.5**). Commonly used vasodilators in order of frequency include the combination of verapamil and nitroglycerin, verapamil or nitroglycerin alone, nicardipine, lidocaine, and papaverine. The radial artery is usually punctured 2 cm proximal to the radial styloid process, where the artery is most superficial. Approximately 2 to 3 mL of 1% lidocaine using a small syringe and a 25G needle is injected subcutaneously (**Figure 7.6**). Sedation is recommended to prevent radial artery spasm secondary to the release of catecholamines associated with the emotional stress and fear that patients experience before a procedure. The artery can be punctured with either a short 2.5-cm stainless steel 21G needle or a micropuncture intravenous (IV) catheter that consists of a fine metal needle and a 22G plastic cannula compatible with a 0.018- to 0.021-in guidewire. While feeling the pulse with the left hand, the operator advances the needle with the right hand, toward the radial artery at a 30° angle (**Figure 7.7**). Two puncture techniques have been described. With the single-wall technique, a stainless-steel needle is advanced through the front wall of the artery into the lumen, and once blood is noticed in the needle hub, the wire can be advanced (**Figure 7.8**). The operator should never force the wire because

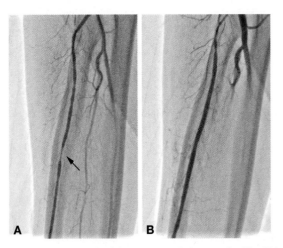

Figure 7.4 Angiographic evidence of radial artery spasm. **A,** An example of focal RA spasm (arrow). **B,** RA spasm was relieved after injection of vasodilator cocktail.

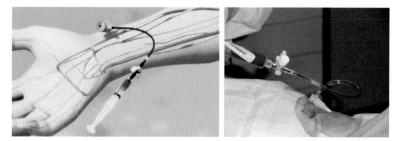

Figure 7.5 Transradial access technique—prevention of radial spasm. Once the sheath is in place, the spasmolytic cocktail is administered through the sidearm.

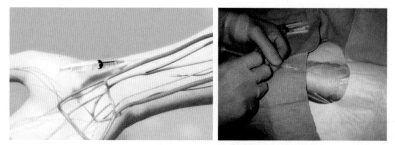

Figure 7.6 Transradial access technique (Step 1). After sterile preparation and draping, the wrist area is locally anesthetized with lidocaine using a 25G needle and a small 3-mL syringe.

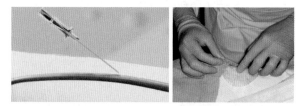

Figure 7.7 Transradial access technique—Front-wall technique (Step 2). With the front-wall technique, a short 2.5-cm 21G stainless steel needle is used to puncture the radial artery.

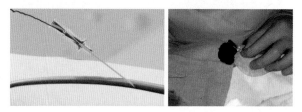

Figure 7.8 Transradial access technique—Front-wall technique (Step 3). The needle is advanced into the radial artery. The blood return indicates the intraluminal needle position. The blood return is rarely pulsatile or brisk.

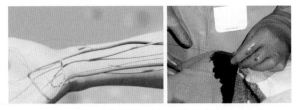

Figure 7.9 Transradial access technique—Front-wall technique (Step 4). A 0.018-in short guidewire is advanced without resistance through the needle into the proximal radial artery. Then the needle is exchanged for a hydrophilic-coated sheath.

of the risk of arterial dissection. The needle should be carefully rotated clockwise or counterclockwise until the wire can be easily advanced without resistance (**Figure 7.9**). With the dual-wall or back-wall technique, a micropuncture catheter is advanced through the front wall into the lumen of the artery until blood is noticed in the hub and then intentionally pushed through the back wall of the artery (**Figure 7.10**). The fine needle is removed, and the Teflon microcatheter is slowly withdrawn until the appearance of brisk pulsatile flow (**Figures 7.11** and **7.12**). Then the wire can be freely advanced and the microcatheter exchanged for the arterial sheath (**Figure 7.13**). The orifice in the back wall of the radial artery is sealed once the sheath is

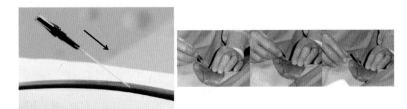

Figure 7.10 Transradial access technique—Back-wall technique (Step 2). The microcatheter and needle are advanced in a 30° angle through the skin into the radial artery. The presence of blood in the hub of the needle indicates that the artery has been punctured. The needle is advanced forward through the backwall of the radial artery.

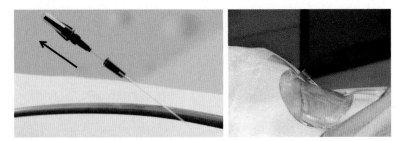

Figure 7.11 Transradial access technique—Back-wall technique (Step 3). Once the tip of the microcatheter and needle are advanced through the back wall of the radial artery, the needle is removed and the microcatheter left in place across the radial artery.

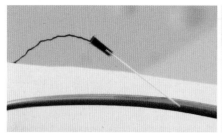
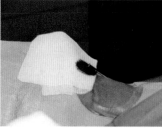

Figure 7.12 Transradial access technique—Back-wall technique (Step 4). The microcatheter is retrieved very slowly until the appearance of brisk pulsatile blood return that confirms that the distal tip is in the lumen of the radial artery.

in position, eliminating the risk of bleeding (**Figure 7.14**). The back-wall puncture technique is simpler, more reproducible, easier to teach, and facilitates advancement of the wire and the arterial pulsatile blood return is easier to recognize.

Real-time ultrasound guidance is strongly recommended to facilitate TRA, especially in patients with weak radial pulse, diminutive radial artery, or lack of pulsatility due to calcification (**Figure 7.15**). In addition, ultrasound scanning of the forearm prior to the procedure may be helpful for planning and identification of the largest vessel in the wrist (ulnar or radial) and identification of anomalies.

Distal Transradial Approach

Since its first publication in 2011, distal transradial approach is slowly becoming popular as an alternative route among transradial operators.

The distal radial artery is typically palpable at the junction of the base of the thumb and first finger over the bony structures of the snuffbox. The patient is positioned with the arm in a semiprone position (**Figure 7.16A**). Once the patient is prepared in sterile fashion, the planned site of puncture is anesthetized with approximately 1 to 5 mL of lidocaine, and the puncture is performed using a 21G needle with a plastic cannula (**Figure 7.16B and C**). The introducer sheath is placed in the usual fashion (**Figure 7.16D**). When the artery is not easily palpable, ultrasound is useful

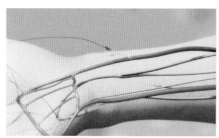
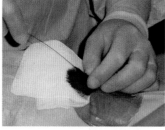

Figure 7.13 Transradial access technique—Back-wall technique (Step 5). A short 0.018-in wire, usually included in the micropuncture transradial access kit, is advanced without resistance through the microcatheter into the proximal radial artery. In case of resistance, a limited angiogram can be performed through the microcatheter to verify the intraluminal position and rule out the presence of vascular anomalies.

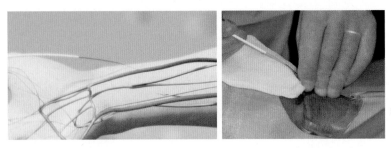

Figure 7.14 Transradial access technique (Step 6). The sheath, preferably hydrophilic coated, is advanced over the wire.

to guide the puncture and measure the arterial diameter to confirm adequate sizing for the planned procedure. After sheath placement, the arm is kept in a semiprone or prone position comfortable for the patient and operator. For left distal TRA, moving the left arm toward the operator no longer requires rotation of the wrist as the elbow is flexed to optimize the position, and the patient remains orthopedically comfortable, as the joints are not stressed.

Hemostasis is different after snuffbox radial access. The dorsal part of the hand is more mobile, and common hemostasis bands may loosen with hand movements. A

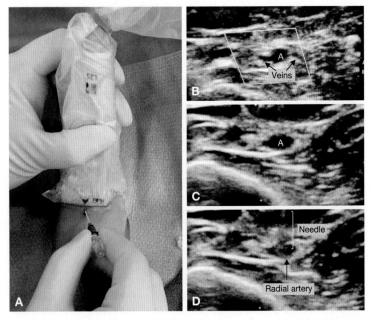

Figure 7.15 Ultrasound guidance for radial access. The ultrasound is positioned over the radial artery. The arrow on the probe marks the centerline and the place where the needle should enter the skin **(A)**. The radial artery is round and pulsatile, accompanied by 2 radial veins that are easily compressible **(B** and **C)**. The puncture needle is entering the radial artery **(D)**.

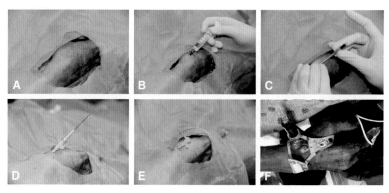

Figure 7.16 Distal radial artery puncture and hemostasis. **A,** The arm is kept in a semiprone position for distal transradial approach. **B,** The sterile puncture site is anesthetized using approximately 1 to 2 mL of 1% lidocaine in a small syringe. **C,** The arterial puncture is performed using a 21G needle with plastic cannula. **D,** The introducer sheath is placed in the usual fashion. **E,** The arm is kept in a semiprone position comfortable for the patient and operator. **F,** A commercial pneumatic compression device is placed for hemostasis.

useful solution is to place a rolled-up gauze at the arterial access site wrapped with a tight elastic bandage. Hemostatic systems specifically designed for snuffbox hemostasis are commercially available and appear to work well in practice (**Figure 7.16E**) (PreludeSYNC Distal, Merit Medical); however, there are no published systematic assessments on the efficacy of these bands.

Learning Curve

A steep learning curve for TRA procedures has been described. As operator experience increases, higher risk cases are selected for TRA. In a seminal study, Spaulding et al. documented an initial access failure rate greater than 10% that decreased dramatically to about 2% after the first 80 cases.

Figure 7.17 shows reasons for failure are different according to operator volume and experience.

Navigating the Upper Extremity Arterial System

Once arterial access is obtained, a 0.035-in guidewire and a catheter of choice are advanced into the ascending aorta traversing the upper extremity arterial system. A J-tipped wire may follow the path of larger vessels and may not selectively enter small radial or brachial branches. However, the tip of a regular J wire has a radius of 3 mm, which is larger than the diameter of the radial artery and may cause vasospasm. A small J tip wire ("Baby-J") with a radius of 1.5 mm is better suited to navigate the upper extremity vasculature. Angled-tip hydrophilic guidewires with stiff shafts are ideal for negotiating tortuous anatomy, especially in the subclavian artery and brachiocephalic trunk, but these wires need to be advanced under close fluoroscopic surveillance, as they may inadvertently enter into and perforate small branches of the radial or brachial arteries. As full anticoagulation is usually administered during transradial procedures, a small branch perforation can result in significant hematoma formation.

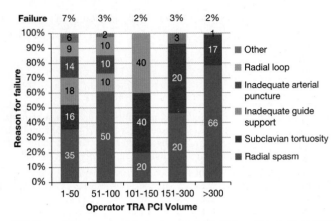

Figure 7.17 Transradial access experience and mechanisms of failure. (Adapted from Ball W, Ball WT, Sharieff W, et al. Characterization of operator learning curve for transradial coronary interventions. *Circ Cardiovasc Interv*. 2011;4:336-341.)

Failure

In a small proportion of cases, the transradial operator will encounter anatomic variations that may prevent the advancement of guidewires or catheters into the ascending aorta. Owing to the relatively small size of the upper extremity arterial system, the operator should never force any equipment against resistance because of the risk of vessel injury, dissection, or reactive spasm. Instead, a limited retrograde angiographic assessment should be performed to identify a vascular anomaly or unusual tortuosity, plan a strategy, and avoid complications. Techniques such as balloon-assisted tracking (BAT) and "Mother-in-Child" technique and familiarity with wires are important for effective navigation. BAT facilitates passage of catheters in vessels that are too narrow or tortuous (**Figure 7.18A and B**). An inflated coronary balloon is partially protruded through the distal end of a guide catheter or a diagnostic catheter and deployed at 3 or 6 atmos-

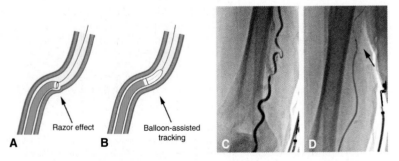

Figure 7.18 Schematic representation of "Razor" effect and "balloon-assisted tracking (BAT)." **A,** Guiding catheter edge leading to razor effect in tortuous segment.
B, Smooth tracking of guide catheter without razor effect in tortuous segment.
C, Severe RA tortuosity. **D,** Catheter is advanced using BAT (arrow).

pheres. For 5F catheters, a balloon diameter of 1.5 mm is recommended. For 6F guide catheters, a balloon diameter of 2.0 mm is recommended. A balloon length of 10 mm or 15 mm is sufficient. Once the balloon is partially protruded from the distal end of the catheter and deployed, the entire assembly is advanced over a soft-tipped 0.014-in coronary wire, thus allowing smooth and atraumatic advancement through difficult vascular anatomy (**Figure 7.18C and D**). Anatomical situations that may require BAT include a very small-caliber radial artery (diameter less than 1.5 mm), tortuous radial or brachial artery, severe and resistant radial spasm, atherosclerotic disease, complex loops, severe subclavian tortuosity, and subclavian stenosis. The Mother-in-Child technique consists of telescoping a long 75-cm 5Fr multipurpose or JR4 catheter through a 6- or 7-Fr guiding catheter to create a smooth transition between the wire and the guiding catheter eliminating a leading edge. It can be useful for navigating a guiding catheter through complex vascular anatomy without significant trauma or local pain.

Radioulnar loops and tortuosity in the radial or brachial arteries can be negotiated with the 0.014-in coronary wire of choice with the support of a 4F hydrophilic-coated Cobra or angled catheter compatible with a 0.035-in guidewire (**Figure 7.19A and B**). When the guidewire crosses the loop, its tip is parked as high as possible (ie, high brachial, axillary, or subclavian region). Then the catheter can be advanced. Usually, the loop opens up spontaneously during the passage of a catheter (**Figure 7.19C**). At times a catheter can be easily advanced over the wire across a loop without disturbing its shape (**Figure 7.19D**). If a catheter cannot be negotiated through a loop or the patient complains of significant pain, the operator may consider an alternative vascular access route.

Occasionally, in the presence of a radioulnar loop, the guidewire will advance through a small accessory communicating vessel between the loop and the proximal brachial artery without resistance (the so-called accessory radial artery). Under fluoroscopy, the wire will appear as it follows the expected trajectory, but upon advancement of the catheter the operator will encounter unusual resistance and the patient will experience severe pain due to spasm. Once this problem is identified, the operator may opt for downsizing the catheter size but should recognize that the accessory radial artery is often extremely small and advancement of catheters into this artery carries the risk of dissection or perforation. Instead, it is recommended that the operator negotiates the radioulnar loop in the forearm or go to the other radial artery to complete the procedure.

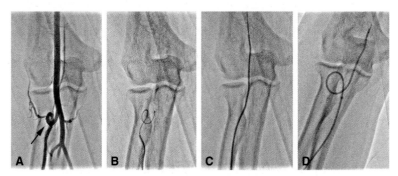

Figure 7.19 Negotiating a radial loop. **A,** A 360° loop with a very small diameter (arrow). **B,** A flexible J-tipped hydrophilic guidewire was used to cross the loop. **C,** The loop was straightened by pull-back of the entire assembly. **D,** A 5F guide catheter was successfully negotiated through a complex 360° loop using balloon-assisted tracking technique.

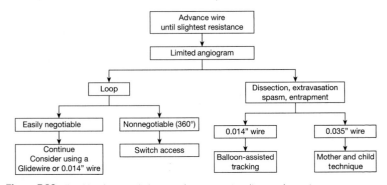

Figure 7.20 Algorithm for negotiating complex upper extremity vascular anatomy.

A high origin of the radial artery from the proximal segment of the brachial artery is a relatively common anomaly and may present additional challenges to the operator. In this case, diagnostic catheterization can be performed without much difficulty and minimal discomfort to the patient; however, when ad hoc PCI is planned, unusual resistance may be felt by the operator when the leading edge of the guiding catheter encounters the angulated origin of the anomalous radial artery. In these situations, the Mother-in-Child or BAT technique can be useful. **Figure 7.20** provides a simple algorithm for negotiating complex upper extremity vascular anatomy.

Resistance to the movement of a guidewire and/or a catheter in the subclavian region should prompt consideration of subclavian tortuosity (**Figure 7.21A-D**). Significant subclavian tortuosity can be negotiated by careful manipulation of the catheter and the use of a stiff shaft hydrophilic-coated guidewire. Deep inspiration elongates the subclavian artery and facilitates the entry of guidewire and catheter in the ascending aorta. The tortuous segment usually straightens as the stiff part of the wire passes through. Maintaining the wire in the catheter while attempting to cannulate the coronaries can facilitate catheter manipulation and cannulation. The guidewire can be removed once the catheter is in stable position. It should be emphasized that all catheter and wire manipulations to negotiate difficult anatomy must be performed under fluoroscopic guidance to prevent damage to carotid, vertebral, or internal mammary artery ostia. The less experienced operator may feel more comfortable using left TRA during the steep portion of the learning curve because the left subclavian artery is less tortuous with fewer areas of resistance compared with the right subclavian artery.

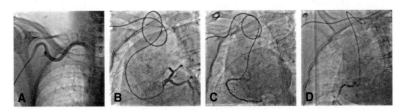

Figure 7.21 Negotiating subclavian tortuosity. **A,** An example of simple subclavian tortuosity. **B,** An example of left coronary artery cannulation through a complex subclavian tortuosity. **C,** An example of right coronary artery (RCA) cannulation through a complex subclavian tortuosity. **D,** Another example of RCA cannulation through a complex subclavian tortuosity.

CATHETER SELECTION

Diagnostic Angiography

Standard femoral catheter shapes, such as the Judkins family of catheters, perform well from the left or right radial approach. For the left coronary, it is recommended to downsize the curve of the JL catheter from 4.0 to 3.5, and for the right coronary to use either a JR4 or JR5. All catheter exchanges for TRA procedures should be performed over exchange length (260 cm) guidewires, especially in patients with tortuous radial or subclavian anatomy.

A single-catheter technique using the same catheter to engage both coronary arteries reduces the number of catheter exchanges, fluoroscopy time, and radiation exposure. Catheter shapes include the multipurpose, Kimny (Boston Scientific, Marlborough, MA, USA), Tiger, Jacky (Terumo, Tokyo, Japan), Ultimate (Merit Medical, South Jordan, Utah), DxTerity TRA (Medtronic, Minneapolis, Minnesota), and Ikari (Terumo, Tokyo, Japan) catheters. These universal catheters usually have a side hole just proximal to the tip to decompress a forceful contrast injection preventing coronary dissection when the tip of the catheter is not coaxial and directed against the vessel wall. Regardless of catheter selection, manipulation for diagnostic or interventional TRA cases should always be performed with small, finger-based, clock- and counterclockwise torquing movements and active catheter holding due to the multiple friction points in the subclavian artery and the aorta.

For patients with prior coronary artery bypass grafting, the left radial approach is preferred because it allows easy cannulation of the LIMA, usually with an IMA or a VB-1 catheter. For saphenous vein grafts, the left TRA is less challenging than the right TRA approach. The multipurpose or JR4 catheters can be used to cannulate right-sided grafts. Amplatz left catheters are well suited for grafts arising from the anterior or left walls of the aorta.

Percutaneous Coronary Intervention

Most TFA guide shapes are well suited for TRA, including the Judkins, Amplatz, and extra backup (EBU) catheters. As a rule, catheters should be coaxially aligned with the ostium to avoid traumatic iatrogenic dissections. Respiratory variation can cause a back-and-forth motion of the catheter, which can displace the coaxial positioning and lead to a lack of support or traumatic damage to the aorta, ostium, or proximal right coronary artery (RCA). EBU catheters provide the most support and are the most widely utilized for the left coronary artery PCI. The JR guide catheter is considered the workhorse catheter for the majority of RCA interventions. If greater support is needed, the JR4 can be advanced deeply into the mid-RCA by applying forward force and clockwise torque. This maneuver facilitates device delivery and increases backup support, and can also cause endothelial injury and vessel dissection. Amplatz left catheters are an excellent option for RCA interventions that require additional backup support (chronic total occlusion, tortuosity, heavy calcification) and arteries with shepherd's crook configuration.

Lack of backup support can be easily overcome by using a guide catheter extensions to deeply intubate the target vessel, such as GuideLiner (Teleflex, Morrisville, NC), Guidezilla II (Boston Scientific, Marlborough, MA), or Telescope (Medtronic PLC, Dublin, Ireland). Sheathless catheter insertion allows for larger guiding catheter diameters, overcoming the sizing limitations of TRA. There are 2 approaches to sheathless techniques. The first approach includes using a standard 7- to 8-Fr guiding catheter advanced over a 0.035-in wire and a long 75-cm 5-Fr diagnostic catheter that provides a "taper" and a smooth pass through the arteriotomy and skin. The second approach includes the use of dedicated hydrophilic-coated sheathless catheters with a long tapered central dilator with

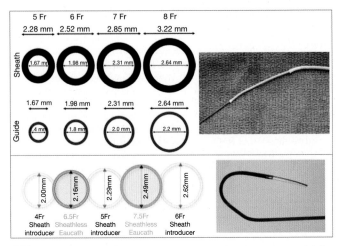

Figure 7.22 Sheathless transradial intervention using standard guide catheters and dedicated hydrophilic-coated sheathless catheters. (Modified from From AM, Gulati R, Prasad A, Rihal CS. Sheathless transradial intervention using standard guide catheters. *Catheter Cardiovasc Interv.* 2010;76:911-916.)

a seamless transition between wire, dilator, and guide catheter and atraumatic entry and passage through the skin into the radial artery (Asahi Intecc, Aichi, Japan). Sheathless catheters have an external diameter of 6.5Fr, which is actually smaller than that of a 5Fr sheath, or 7.5Fr, smaller than that of a 6Fr sheath. The hydrophilic coating on these catheters reduces frictional forces, discomfort, and radial artery spasm (**Figure 7.22**).

TRA for Peripheral Vascular Interventions

The rationale of TRA for peripheral vascular interventions is based on 2 important considerations. TRA is the preferred approach for renal artery stenting. The renal arteries generally have a varying degree of craniocaudal course after their origin from the abdominal aorta. Conventional coronary guide catheters (JR or multipurpose) offer better coaxial alignment and backup support using TRA. TRA for common and external iliac interventions is possible. It is also possible to address mesenteric, superficial femoral, and subclavian stenosis. Generally, for most infradiaphragmatic lesions, the left radial approach should be preferred, as it eliminates the extra length of the aortic arch, and using the available hardware, most lesions can be addressed. Complex cerebrovascular interventions are also possible using TRA.

RADIAL HEMOSTASIS-PREVENTION OF RADIAL ARTERY OCCLUSION

Multiple methods for radial hemostasis have been described. Gentle manual compression with 1 or 2 fingers at the arteriotomy site is an effective method. Alternatively, a rolled piece of gauze can be placed longitudinally at the arteriotomy site and wrapped with an elastic bandage or a hemoband around the wrist to maintain prolonged hemostatic pressure. The disadvantage of these methods is the complete interruption of arterial flow because of the inability to gauge the hemostatic pressure, increasing the risk of RAO. In contrast, balloon-based hemostatic devices that apply selective pressure to the radial artery allow fine adjustments of the hemostatic pressure and direct visualization of the arteriotomy site through the transparent balloon material. Elastic bandages and hemobands interrupt venous return resulting in congestion and edema of the hand and are not recommended.

RAO occurs in approximately 5% to 10% of transradial procedures, most likely due to vessel injury and thrombosis, and is usually manifested as asymptomatic loss of radial pulse due to the extensive collateral circulation in the hand from the ulnar and interosseous arteries that prevent ischemia. Approximately 25% to 50% of RAO cases recanalize spontaneously at 30 days. Assessment of radial artery patency should be performed in all patients before discharge. Palpation of the radial pulse is inaccurate and leads to underestimation of RAO. The Barbeau test using oximetry-plethysmography provides a simple and inexpensive method of indirect evaluation of radial artery patency. Procedural factors associated with RAO include lack of anticoagulation, larger-diameter sheaths, multiple procedures through the same radial artery, spasm, and prolonged occlusive hemostasis.

RAO can be prevented by using full anticoagulation during the procedure, usually with 50 to 70 IU/kg up to a maximum of 5000 IU of unfractionated heparin, and by applying minimum pressure for less than 2 hours during hemostasis. Maintaining flow in the radial artery during hemostasis minimizes RAO. The "patent" nonocclusive hemostasis technique consists of positioning a balloon-based device 2 to 3 mm proximal to the skin entry site and a pulse oximeter attached to the ipsilateral thumb. While the sheath is being removed, the balloon is fully inflated with 15 to 18 mL of air to completely occlude the radial artery. Air is removed from the device until some bleeding can be seen and reinflated just to maintain hemostasis. Radial patency is assessed with the reverse Barbeau test with manual pressure applied to the ulnar artery at the level the Guyon canal, lateral to the pisiform bone. Gradual deflation is performed until oximetry becomes positive and a plethysmographic waveform can be visualized. This technique assures the presence of antegrade flow in the radial artery during hemostasis. Two hours later, 5 mL of air can be released every 15 minutes, until the device is completely deflated and then removed. Using this technique, late occlusion rates can be reduced to approximately less than 5%. In case of early RAO, occurring on the same day of the procedure and/or before discharge, applying 1 hour of ulnar artery occlusive compression with a balloon-based hemostatic device can increase peak velocity flow into the radial artery with reestablishment of forward flow. With intense procedural anticoagulation, meticulous patent hemostasis, careful vigilance for early RAO managed with ulnar compression, and shorter hemostasis duration, the RAO incidence can be reduced to less than 1%.

Hand ischemia after TRA procedures is extremely rare and has been described in a handful of cases. In most of these, RAO was successfully treated with antegrade angioplasty. Amputation of the index finger secondary to gangrene in a patient with RAO was reported in one unfortunate case. In other series, RAO has been associated with forearm and access site pain without hand ischemia. Empiric short courses of 1 to 4 weeks of low-molecular-weight heparin led to late recanalization in the majority of patients.

Complications

Complications of TRA are relatively rare and can be classified as intraprocedural or postprocedural and bleeding or nonbleeding. **Table 7.2** displays the most common complications associated with TRA.

Radial Artery Spasm

Radial artery spasm is a common TRA complication and a reason for failure and crossover to TFA in up to 15% to 20% of cases. In the catheterization laboratory, radial

Table 7.2 Complications of Transradial Access

Intraprocedural		Postprocedural	
Bleeding	**Nonbleeding**	**Bleeding**	**Nonbleeding**
Radial artery perforation	Radial spasm	Forearm hematoma	Radial artery occlusion
	Catheter entrapment	Compartment syndrome	Pseudoaneurysm
	Radial dissection		Arteriovenous fistula
	Catheter kink		Regional pain syndrome
			Infection

Reprinted with permission from Sandoval Y, Bell MR, Gulati R. Transradial artery access complications. *Circ Cardiovasc Interv*. 2019;12:e007386.

spasm is manifested with severe forearm pain and unusually difficult manipulation of the catheters and the sheath. Independent predictors of radial spasm include the presence of radial artery anomalies, multiple puncture attempts, number of catheter exchanges, pain during radial cannulation, larger catheter diameter, and small radial artery caliber. In extreme cases, eversion radial endarterectomy has been reported after forceful removal of the radial sheath. When spasm occurs, additional doses of intra-arterial vasodilators, sedation, and downsizing to smaller 4- to 5-Fr catheters to complete the procedure are usually recommended. If after these measures the patient still complains of substantial pain and the catheters are difficult to manipulate, a limited upper extremity angiography is recommended. Anatomical variations particularly the anomalous origin of the radial artery from high brachial or axillary artery and radiobrachial loops are commonly misinterpreted as radial artery spasm. In case of catheter or sheath entrapment due to spasm, flow-mediated vasodilatation with a blood pressure cuff inflated to 30 mmHg above the average systolic blood pressure for approximately 3 minutes has been shown to cause reactive hyperemia and successfully relieve spasm. Other measures include warm wet compresses or heat applied over the skin of the upper extremity. In extreme cases, regional nerve block or general anesthesia may be required.

Hematoma and Bleeding

Forearm bleeding and hematoma formation should be suspected in the presence of significant pain and swelling during or after the procedure. Awareness and early detection in the catheterization laboratory or the recovery area are important to prevent compartment syndrome, one of the most feared TRA complications. Small hematomas are usually managed conservatively with ice, analgesics, arm elevation, and light compression, while large hematomas are managed with cessation/reversal of anticoagulants, circumferential compression of the forearm with an elastic bandage or blood pressure cuff, and aggressive blood pressure control. A pulse oximeter should be placed in the ipsilateral thumb to monitor for hand ischemia. In cases of large perforations, vascular ultrasound is recommended to rule out the presence of a pseudoaneurysm in the forearm. In extreme cases, compartment syndrome can develop with the need for surgical fasciotomy of the forearm (**Figure 7.23**).

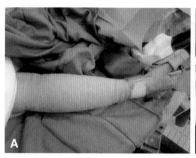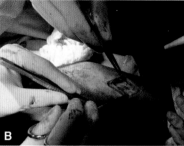

Figure 7.23 Prevention and treatment of compartment syndrome after forearm hematoma formation. After a vascular perforation in the forearm with early hematoma formation, the forearm can be wrapped with elastic bandage to prevent compartment syndrome, as depicted in **A**. Once compartment syndrome develops, it is treated with fasciotomy, as shown in **B**.

Radial Artery Perforation and Dissection

Radial artery perforation is a rare but serious complication of TRA with an incidence of <1%. Risk factors for vascular perforation include anatomic variations, such as radial artery tortuosity or looping, high radial-ulnar bifurcation, and short ascending aorta, as well as aggressive wire manipulation (hydrophilic wires in particular), female sex, short stature, hypertension, and excessive anticoagulation. In many instances, the leading edge of a guiding catheter sliding over a wire can create a "razor effect" that causes injury and perforation to tortuous or anomalous radial arteries.

If a perforation is suspected, the diagnosis should be confirmed with a limited radial angiogram. Perforations need to be recognized and managed immediately to avoid progression to hematoma or compartment syndrome. The recommended approach is to place a catheter across the perforation, with similar outer diameter to the radial lumen, to occlude the vessel and "tamponade" the perforation to prevent further blood extravasation. It usually takes 20 minutes for the perforation to be sealed. If the radial artery cannot be traversed with a catheter or continued extravasation is noted, external compression with elastic bandage or a blood pressure cuff for approximately 20 to 30 minutes is recommended. Vascular surgery can be consulted after all these maneuvers fail. The use of polytetrafluoroethylene-covered stent grafts to seal radial perforations has been reported.

Radial Artery Pseudoaneurysm

Radial artery pseudoaneurysm is an uncommon complication of TRA procedures. Pseudoaneurysms usually develop as a consequence of inadequate hemostasis with persistence of turbulent flow between the adventitia and the media, which over time creates a cavity surrounded by fibrous tissue connected to the arterial lumen through a neck. Clinically, a pseudoaneurysm can be recognized as a painful, tender, pulsatile mass days to weeks post procedure. Independent risk factors include systemic anticoagulation and elevated body mass index. Diagnosis is made by duplex ultrasound, and the treatment depends on the size of the pseudoaneurysm. Options include compression with a radial hemostasis device, ultrasound-guided compression, thrombin injection, or surgical repair.

TRANSRADIAL ACCESS AND RADIATION EXPOSURE

Most randomized trials have consistently shown that TRA is associated with a small but significant increase in fluoroscopy time for diagnostic and interventional procedures. A meta-analysis of 24 randomized clinical trials conducted between 1995 and 2014 including 19,328 patients demonstrated that TRA was associated with an incremental fluoroscopy duration of approximately 1 minute for diagnostic and interventional procedures. In addition, TRA was associated with a modest excess in radiation dose to the patient and operator. A metaregression examining secular trends in radiation exposure showed that the overall difference between TRA and TFA has substantially decreased over time by 75% from 2 minutes in 1996 to 30 seconds in 2014 ($P < .0001$).

In summary, the data consistently show slightly increased radiation exposure with TRA that is even apparent among high-volume experienced TRA operators; however, the increase in patient radiation exposure is well below the level at which deterministic effects (2 Gy) may be seen. Radiation exposure to the operator can be further reduced with the use of the approaches described in Chapter 2.

BRACHIAL VENOUS ACCESS FOR RIGHT-SIDED HEART CATHETERIZATION

RHC through the upper extremity is a simple procedure, and it can be easily performed concomitantly with TRA left-sided heart catheterization through one of the large veins located in the anticubital fossa, even in fully anticoagulated patients.

Venous access with an 18-gauge catheter, preferably in the medial antecubital vein, can be obtained by a nurse in the holding area in anticipation of the procedure. In the catheterization laboratory, the IV catheter is exchanged for a 5-Fr or 6-Fr sheath using a short 0.021-in wire. If a peripheral vein cannot be cannulated before the procedure, the brachial vein can be punctured with a 2-in-long 18-gauge stainless steel needle using ultrasound guidance in the catheterization laboratory (**Figure 7.24**). A tourniquet is placed in the upper arm to facilitate visualization of the vein with ultrasound. Usually, 2 brachial veins can be identified in close proximity to the brachial artery. The vein is usually elliptical and easily compressible in contrast to the artery, which is round and pulsatile. In comparison with arteries, veins are distensible and spasm is not a problem, but there is significant anatomic variability in the venous system with multiple collaterals and redundant passages.

Subsequently, a 5Fr or 6Fr 120-cm-long balloon-tipped catheter is advanced into the superior vena cava with or without the use of a 0.025-in guidewire. Once the tip

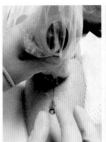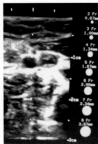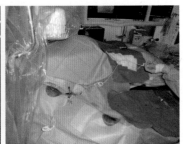

Figure 7.24 Ultrasound-guided access and setup for brachial venous transradial catheterization.

of the catheter is located in the chest, the balloon can be inflated and the catheter is flow-directed into the pulmonary artery. Passage of the catheter is usually straightforward and can be performed without fluoroscopy by observing the hemodynamic waveforms. In case of venous anatomical variation or tortuosity, a 0.014-in coronary guidewire can be used to facilitate catheter navigation. In patients with dilated right atria, the catheter tends to loop in the atrium. In these situations, forceful injection of 10 mL of saline can transiently straighten the catheter and facilitate passage into the RV. Hemostasis can be easily obtained with manual pressure after removing the sheath at the end of the procedure. Alternatively, the sheath can be exchanged for a 14-gauge angiocath that can be used as intravenous access, a useful measure for patients who need to return to hospital wards after the procedure.

TRANSRADIAL ACCESS AND OUTCOMES

Over the past decade, it has been recognized that bleeding after PCI has a significant unfavorable impact on short- and long-term adverse cardiovascular outcomes. As a consequence, the management focus has shifted from the prevention of ischemic complications to the prevention of bleeding. Widespread implementation of bleeding avoidance strategies has been associated with improved survival. Systematic adoption of TRA is considered an important bleeding avoidance strategy and has consistently demonstrated a reduction in bleeding and vascular complications in observational registries and randomized trials.

In aggregate, the available evidence indicates that TRA is superior to TFA among patients with ACS, supporting a radial-first strategy. The benefit appears to concentrate in sicker patients, such as those with ST-elevation myocardial infarction (STEMI), and cases performed by operators at high-volume centers. Of note, systematic TRA use for primary PCI results in a slightly longer door-to-balloon time, even with experienced operators, but it does not seem to affect the mortality benefit of TRA. The 2017 ESC STEMI guidelines endorse the use of TRA over TFA for primary PCI if performed by an experienced operator with a recommendation IA.

CONCLUSION

TRA has become the standard approach for cardiac catheterization and PCI in many parts of the world and is slowly gaining ground in the United States as newly trained operators go into practice. A radial-first approach for cardiovascular interventional procedures is currently endorsed by professional societies. TRA implementation requires a learning curve of approximately 50 to 100 cases and is associated with slightly increased fluoroscopy time and access crossover rates. However, once mastered and implemented as an institutional program, TRA is associated with less access-related bleeding, vascular injury, improved patient comfort, and significant cost savings for the healthcare system.

SUGGESTED READINGS

1. Abdelaal E, Rao SV, Gilchrist IC, et al. Same-day discharge compared with overnight hospitalization after uncomplicated percutaneous coronary intervention: a systematic review and metaanalysis. *JACC Cardiovasc Interv.* 2013;6(2):99-112.
2. Barbeau GR, Arsenault F, Dugas L, Simard S, Lariviere MM. Evaluation of the ulnopalmar arterial arches with pulse oximetry and plethysmography: comparison with the Allen's test in 1010 patients. *Am Heart J.* 2004;147(3):489-493.
3. Bernat I, Aminian A, Pancholy S, et al. Best practices for the prevention of radial artery occlusion after transradial diagnostic angiography and intervention: an international consensus paper. *JACC Cardiovasc Interv.* 2019;12(22):2235-2246.
4. Burzotta F, Trani C, Hamon M, Amoroso G, Kiemeneij F. Transradial approach for coronary angiography and interventions in patients with coronary bypass grafts: tips and tricks. *Catheter Cardiovasc Interv.* 2008;72(2):263-272.

 5. Burzotta F, Trani C, De Vita M, Crea F. A new operative classification of both anatomic vascular variants and physiopathologic conditions affecting transradial cardiovascular procedures. *Int J Cardiol.* 2010;145(1):120-122.
 6. Burzotta F, Trani C, Mazzari MA, et al. Vascular complications and access crossover in 10,676 transradial percutaneous coronary procedures. *Am Heart J.* 2012;163(2):230-238.
 7. Calvino-Santos RA, Vazquez-Rodriguez JM, Salgado-Fernandez J, et al. Management of iatrogenic radial artery perforation. *Catheter Cardiovasc Interv.* 2004;61(1):74-78.
 8. Campeau L. Percutaneous radial artery approach for coronary angiography. *Cathet Cardiovasc Diagn.* 1989;16(1):3-7.
 9. Caputo RP, Tremmel JA, Rao S, et al. Transradial arterial access for coronary and peripheral procedures: executive summary by the Transradial Committee of the SCAI. *Cathet Cardiovasc Interv.* 2011;78(6):823-839.
10. Collins N, Wainstein R, Ward M, Bhagwandeen R, Dzavik V. Pseudoaneurysm after transradial cardiac catheterization: case series and review of the literature. *Catheter Cardiovasc Interv.* 2012;80(2):283-287.
11. Corcos T. Distal radial access for coronary angiography and percutaneous coronary intervention: a state-of-the-art review. *Catheter Cardiovasc Interv.* 2019;93(4):639-644.
12. Dehghani P, Mohammad A, Bajaj R, et al. Mechanism and predictors of failed transradial approach for percutaneous coronary interventions. *JACC Cardiovasc Interv.* 2009;2(11):1057-1064.
13. Ferrante G, Rao SV, Juni P, et al. Radial versus femoral access for coronary interventions across the entire spectrum of patients with coronary artery disease: a meta-analysis of randomized trials. *JACC Cardiovasc Interv.* 2016;9(14):1419-1434.
14. Gilchrist IC, Kharabsheh S, Nickolaus MJ, Reddy R. Radial approach to right heart catheterization: early experience with a promising technique. *Catheter Cardiovasc Interv.* 2002;55(1):20-22.
15. Goldsmit A, Kiemeneij F, Gilchrist IC, et al. Radial artery spasm associated with transradial cardiovascular procedures: results from the RAS registry. *Catheter Cardiovasc Interv.* 2014;83(1):E32-E36.
16. Ibanez B, James S, Agewall S, et al. 2017 ESC Guidelines for the management of acute myocardial infarction in patients presenting with ST-segment elevation: the Task Force for the management of acute myocardial infarction in patients presenting with ST-segment elevation of the European Society of Cardiology (ESC). *Eur Heart J.* 2018;39(2):119-177.
17. Jolly SS, Yusuf S, Cairns J, et al. Radial versus femoral access for coronary angiography and intervention in patients with acute coronary syndromes (RIVAL): a randomised, parallel group, multicentre trial. *Lancet.* 2011;377(9775):1409-1420.
18. Jolly SS, Cairns J, Niemela K, et al. Effect of radial versus femoral access on radiation dose and the importance of procedural volume: a substudy of the multicenter randomized RIVAL trial. *JACC Cardiovasc Interv.* 2013;6(3):258-266.
19. Kedev S, Zafirovska B, Dharma S, Petkoska D. Safety and feasibility of transulnar catheterization when ipsilateral radial access is not available. *Catheter Cardiovasc Interv.* 2014;83(1):E51-E60.
20. Kiemeneij F, Laarman GJ. Percutaneous transradial artery approach for coronary stent implantation. *Cathet Cardiovasc Diagn.* 1993;30(2):173-178.
21. Kiemeneij F. Prevention and management of radial artery spasm. *J Invasive Cardiol.* 2006;18(4):159-160.
22. Kiemeneij F. Left distal transradial access in the anatomical snuffbox for coronary angiography (ldTRA) and interventions (ldTRI). *EuroIntervention.* 2017;13(7):851-857.
23. Klutstein MW, Westerhout CM, Armstrong PW, et al. Radial versus femoral access, bleeding and ischemic events in patients with non-ST-segment elevation acute coronary syndrome managed with an invasive strategy. *Am Heart J.* 2013;165(4):583-590.e1.
24. Kooiman J, Seth M, Dixon S, et al. Risk of acute kidney injury after percutaneous coronary interventions using radial versus femoral vascular access: insights from the Blue Cross Blue Shield of Michigan Cardiovascular Consortium. *Circ Cardiovasc Interv.* 2014;7(2):190-198.
25. Le May M, Wells G, So D, et al. Safety and efficacy of femoral access vs radial access in ST-segment elevation myocardial infarction: the SAFARI-STEMI randomized clinical trial. *JAMA Cardiol.* 2020;5(2):126-134.
26. Lo TS, Nolan J, Fountzopoulos E, et al. Radial artery anomaly and its influence on transradial coronary procedural outcome. *Heart.* 2009;95(5):410-415.
27. Mason PJ, Shah B, Tamis-Holland JE, et al. An update on radial artery access and best practices for transradial coronary angiography and intervention in acute coronary syndrome: a scientific statement from the American heart association. *Circ Cardiovasc Interv.* 2018;11(9):e000035.
28. Michael TT, Alomar M, Papayannis A, et al. A randomized comparison of the transradial and transfemoral approaches for coronary artery bypass graft angiography and intervention: the RADIAL-CABG Trial (RADIAL versus Femoral Access for Coronary Artery Bypass Graft Angiography and Intervention). *JACC Cardiovasc Interv.* 2013;6(11):1138-1144.

29. Mitchell MD, Hong JA, Lee BY, Umscheid CA, Bartsch SM, Don CW. Systematic review and cost-benefit analysis of radial artery access for coronary angiography and intervention. *Circ Cardiovasc Qual Outcomes.* 2012;5(4):454-462.
30. Neumann FJ, Sousa-Uva M, Ahlsson A, et al. 2018 ESC/EACTS Guidelines on myocardial revascularization. *Eur Heart J.* 2019;40(2):87-165.
31. Patel T, Shah S, Pancholy S, et al. Utility of transradial approach for peripheral vascular interventions. *J Invasive Cardiol.* 2015;27(6):277-282.
32. Plourde G, Pancholy SB, Nolan J, et al. Radiation exposure in relation to the arterial access site used for diagnostic coronary angiography and percutaneous coronary intervention: a systematic review and meta-analysis. *Lancet.* 2015;386(10009):2192-2203.
33. Plourde G, Abdelaal E, MacHaalany J, et al. Comparison of radiation exposure during transradial diagnostic coronary angiography with single- or multi-catheters approach. *Catheter Cardiovasc Interv.* 2017;90(2):243-248.
34. Rao SV, Ou FS, Wang TY, et al. Trends in the prevalence and outcomes of radial and femoral approaches to percutaneous coronary intervention: a report from the National Cardiovascular Data Registry. *JACC Cardiovasc Interv.* 2008;1(4):379-386.
35. Rao SV, Tremmel JA, Gilchrist IC, et al. Best practices for transradial angiography and intervention: a consensus statement from the society for cardiovascular angiography and intervention's transradial working group. *Catheter Cardiovasc Interv.* 2014;83(2):228-236.
36. Rashid M, Kwok CS, Pancholy S, et al. Radial artery occlusion after transradial interventions: a systematic review and meta-analysis. *J Am Heart Assoc.* 2016;5(1):e002686.
37. Rathore S, Stables RH, Pauriah M, et al. Impact of length and hydrophilic coating of the introducer sheath on radial artery spasm during transradial coronary intervention: a randomized study. *JACC Cardiovasc Interv.* 2010;3(5):475-483.
38. Safley DM, Amin AP, House JA, et al. Comparison of costs between transradial and transfemoral percutaneous coronary intervention: a cohort analysis from the Premier research database. *Am Heart J.* 2013;165(3):303-309.e2.
39. Sandoval Y, Bell MR, Gulati R. Transradial artery access complications. *Circ Cardiovasc Interv.* 2019;12(11):e007386.
40. Seto AH, Roberts JS, Abu-Fadel MS, et al. Real-time ultrasound guidance facilitates transradial access: RAUST (Radial Artery access with Ultrasound Trial). *JACC Cardiovasc Interv.* 2015;8(2):283-291.
41. Seto AH, Shroff A, Abu-Fadel M, et al. Length of stay following percutaneous coronary intervention: an expert consensus document update from the society for cardiovascular angiography and interventions. *Catheter Cardiovasc Interv.* 2018;92(4):717-731.
42. Shroff AR, Gulati R, Drachman DE, et al. SCAI expert consensus statement update on best practices for transradial angiography and intervention. *Catheter Cardiovasc Interv.* 2020;95(2):245-252.
43. Singh S, Singh M, Grewal N, Khosla S. The fluoroscopy time, door to balloon time, contrast volume use and prevalence of vascular access site failure with transradial versus transfemoral approach in ST segment elevation myocardial infarction: a systematic review & meta-analysis. *Cardiovasc Revasc Med.* 2015;16(8):491-497.
44. Spaulding C, Lefevre T, Funck F, et al. Left radial approach for coronary angiography: results of a prospective study. *Cathet Cardiovasc Diagn.* 1996;39(4):365-370.
45. Tizon-Marcos H, Barbeau GR. Incidence of compartment syndrome of the arm in a large series of transradial approach for coronary procedures. *J Interv Cardiol.* 2008;21(5):380-384.
46. Valgimigli M, Campo G, Penzo C, et al. Transradial coronary catheterization and intervention across the whole spectrum of Allen test results. *J Am Coll Cardiol.* 2014;63(18):1833-1841.
47. Valgimigli M, Gagnor A, Calabro P, et al. Radial versus femoral access in patients with acute coronary syndromes undergoing invasive management: a randomised multicentre trial. *Lancet.* 2015;385(9986):2465-2476.
48. van Leeuwen MAH, van der Heijden DJ, Hermie J, et al. The longterm effect of transradial coronary catheterisation on upper limb function. *EuroIntervention.* 2017;12(14):1766-1772.

8 Percutaneous Transfemoral, Transseptal, Transcaval, and Apical Approach[1]

Recent data have shown that utilization of the radial artery for vascular access has been rising because of improved outcomes and reduced vascular complications. However, despite the rise in the utilization of transradial access, adherence to best practices for femoral artery access still remains a critical component of current practice of interventional cardiology.

CATHETERIZATION VIA THE FEMORAL ARTERY AND VEIN
Patient Preparation

After palpation of the femoral arterial pulse within the inguinal area, a safety razor is used to shave an area approximately 10 cm in diameter surrounding this point. Although most catheterizations can be performed quickly and easily from a single groin, it is generally routine to have both groins prepared. In the past, the shaved areas were traditionally scrubbed with a povidone-iodine/detergent mixture. More recently, most laboratories have replaced povidone-iodine solution with chlorhexidine-alcohol-based antiseptic preparations, which have been shown to be more effective and less irritant.

Selection of Puncture Site

It is important to puncture the femoral artery at the correct level, that is, at the mid common femoral artery, above the arterial bifurcation into the profunda and superficial femoral artery, and 1 or 2 cm below the inguinal ligament (**Figure 8.1A and B**). The position of the skin crease itself is not a reliable marker for the puncture site, and it can instead be misleading in obese patients. The appropriate localization of the skin puncture should be first identified by fluoroscopic landmarks; a radiopaque marker (ie, mosquito forceps that routinely come within the sterile instrument package) should be placed on top of the inguinal area where the pulse appears stronger and adjusted by fluoroscopy in the anteroposterior view so that it is positioned overlying the inferior quadrant of the femoral head (**Figure 8.1A and D**). Making the skin nicks at this level increases the chance that needle puncture will take place in the common femoral segment (overlying the middle of the femoral head) rather than either too high (above the inguinal ligament) or too low (in the superficial femoral or profunda branches of the common femoral artery). The femoral artery should be easily palpable and the femoral vein will lie approximately 1 fingerbreadth medial to the artery along a parallel course. More recently, the use of intraprocedure vascular ultrasound guidance has emerged as an alternative method to identify each vessel and select the puncture site (**Figure 8.2A and B**). The femoral artery appears as a pulsatile circle, usually with thicker and brighter delineation of the walls and on occasion with atherosclerotic and calcific plaques. Upon gentle pressure with the vascular probe, the artery is not compressible, and the pulsations become more evident. A needle guide can be used to fix the angle of the needle and to intersect the ultrasound plane at the desired depth and avoid bifurcation. Medial to the femoral artery (or occasionally underneath) lies the

[1]We gratefully acknowledge the Grossman & Baim's *Cardiac Catheterization, Angiography, and Intervention*, 9th edition contributions of Drs Abdulla Damluji and Mauro Moscucci as portions of their chapter, Percutaneous Transfemoral, Transseptal, Transcaval, and Apical Approach, were retained in this text.

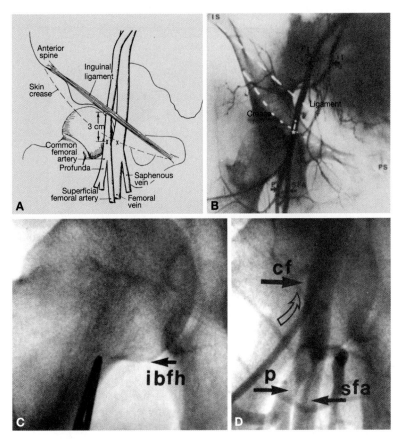

Figure 8.1 Regional anatomy relevant to percutaneous femoral arterial and venous catheterization. **A,** Schematic diagram showing the right femoral artery and vein coursing underneath the inguinal ligament, which runs from the anterior superior iliac spine to the pubic tubercle. The arterial skin nick (indicated by X) should be placed approximately 3 cm below the ligament and directly over the femoral arterial pulsation, and the venous skin nick should be placed at the same level but approximately 1 fingerbreadth more medial. **B,** Corresponding radiographic anatomy as seen during abdominal aortography. **C,** Fluoroscopic localization of skin nick (marked by clamp tip) to the inferior border of the femoral head (ibfh). **D,** Catheter (open arrow) inserted via this skin nick has entered the common femoral artery (cf), safely above its bifurcation into the superficial femoral (sfa) and profunda (p) branches. (For further details, see Kim D, Orron DE, Skillman JJ, et al. Role of superficial femoral artery puncture in the development of pseudoaneurysm and arteriovenous fistula complicating percutaneous transfemoral cardiac catheterization. *Cathet Cardiovasc Diagn*. 1992;25:91.)

femoral vein, which can be identified because of its thinner and smoother walls as well as the compressibility upon gentle pressure with the vascular probe.

A high puncture of the artery at or above the inferior epigastric artery or above the inguinal ligament predisposes to inadequate compression, hematoma formation, and/or retroperitoneal bleeding following catheter removal (see Chapter 4). A low

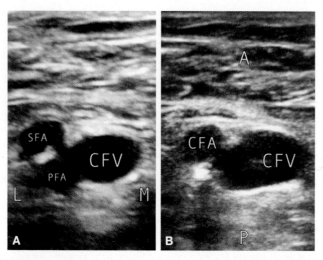

Figure 8.2 A, Still frame image from vascular ultrasound of right common femoral artery (CFA) and its bifurcation into superficial femoral artery (SFA) and profunda femoral artery (PFA). L, lateral; M, medial. After the CFA bifurcation, the common femoral vein (CFV) is visualized medially. **B,** Still frame image from vascular ultrasound of right CFA and CFV. A, anterior; P, posterior.

puncture of the artery (at or below the femoral bifurcation) increases the chance that the puncture will be at the bifurcation of the profunda and superficial femoral branches and will fail to enter the arterial lumen. Puncture of either one of the branches increases the risk of false aneurysm formation or thrombotic occlusion owing to smaller vessel caliber. Because the superficial femoral artery frequently overlies the femoral vein, low venous punctures may pass inadvertently through the superficial femoral artery, leading to excessive bleeding and possible arteriovenous (A-V) fistula formation (see Chapter 4).

Local Anesthesia

Once the appropriate entry site has been identified, the femoral artery is palpated along its course using the 3 middle fingers of the left hand. Without moving the left hand, a linear intradermal wheal of 1% or 2% lidocaine is raised slowly by tangential insertion of a 25- or 27-gauge needle along a course overlying both the femoral artery and vein at the desired level of entry. The smaller needle is then replaced by a 22-gauge 1.5-in needle, which is used to infiltrate the deeper tissues along the intended trajectory for arterial and venous entry. As this needle is advanced, small additional volumes of lidocaine are infiltrated by slow injection. Each incremental infiltration should be preceded by aspiration so that intravascular boluses can be avoided. The patient should be warned that they may experience some burning as the anesthetic is injected but that the medication should prevent any subsequent sharp sensations.

Femoral Vein Puncture

If right-sided heart catheterization is to be performed, the femoral venous puncture is usually performed prior to arterial puncture. With the left hand palpating the femoral artery along its course below the inguinal ligament, the needle is introduced through the more medial aspect.

Classically, an 18-gauge thin-walled Seldinger needle was used in the past; this needle consists of a blunt, tapered external cannula through which a sharp solid obturator project (**Figure 8.3**). The technique involved advancing the needle through the anterior and posterior wall of the vessel, and then slowly withdrawing the needle until back flow was obtained through a syringe connected to the needle.

However, nowadays the technique widely used is a modified Seldinger, where instead an 18- to 21-gauge single-wall puncture needle with a sharpened tip and without the inner obturator connected to a 10-mL syringe is used. Placement of a fluid-filled syringe on the needle's hub allows direct front-wall entry of the vein without the need to first exit the back wall and then pull back. With the left hand stabilizing the needle, the right hand is used to remove the syringe and to advance a 0.018- to 0.038-in J guidewire into the hub of the needle. The curved wire tip may be straightened by hyperextension of the wire shaft in the right hand or by leaving the tip of the wire within the plastic introducer supplied by the manufacturer. The wire should slide through the needle and 30 cm into the vessel with no perceptible resistance. Fluoroscopy should then show the tip of the guidewire just to the left (patient's right) of the spine.

If difficulty is encountered in advancing the guidewire, it should never be overcome by the application of force. Fluoroscopy may reveal that the tip of the wire has lodged in a small lumbar branch; it can be drawn back slightly and redirected or gently prolapsed up the iliac vein. When resistance to advancement is encountered at or just beyond the tip of the needle, however, even greater care is required. This resistance may be caused by apposition of the tip of the needle to the back wall of the vein, which can be corrected by further depression of the needle hub or slightly reorienting the hub to one side or the other, with or without slight withdrawal of the needle shaft. If this maneuver fails to allow free advancement of the wire, however, the wire should be removed and the syringe should be reattached to the needle hub to ensure that free flow of venous blood is still present before additional wire manipula-

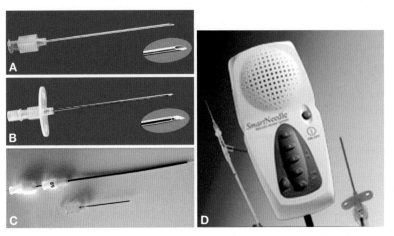

Figure 8.3 Percutaneous needles and guidewire. **A,** An 18-gauge thin-wall needle. **B,** Seldinger needle with its sharp solid obturator in place. **C,** Micropuncture Introducer Set (Cook, Inc, Bloomington, IN, USA): 21-gauge needle, 5F introducer and dilator, and 0.018-in nitinol wire. **D,** A Doppler-guided SmartNeedle. (**A-C,** Permission for use granted by Cook Medical, Bloomington, Indiana. **D,** Image courtesy of Teleflex Incorporated. ©2020 Teleflex Incorporated. All rights reserved.)

tion is attempted. If it is necessary to withdraw the wire, this should always be done gently, since it is possible for the wire to snag on the tip of the needle. To prevent this, the needle and wire should be removed as a unit. In some cases, puncturing the vein during a Valsalva maneuver or after giving a bolus of intravenous fluids may help by distending the femoral vein and making clean puncture more likely.

After the wire has freely entered the vein, the needle is removed, leaving the wire well within the vein, and secured at the skin entry site by the left hand. The protruding wire is wiped with a moistened gauze pad, and its free end is threaded into the lumen of a sheath and dilator combination adequate to accept the intended right-sided heart catheter. (Note: if a micropuncture kit is used, a 4F or 5F sheath and dilator are used over the 0.018-in wire in order to exchange for an 0.035- to 0.038-in wire, over which the intended sheath appropriate for the right-sided heart catheter is then inserted.) All current sheaths are equipped with a back-bleed valve and side-arm connector to control bleeding around the catheter shaft and to provide means of administering drugs or extra intravenous fluids during the right-sided heart catheterization. The operator must make sure that they have control of the proximal end of the guidewire and that it is held in a fixed position as the sheath and dilator are introduced through the skin. Insertion is eased if the sheath and dilator are rotated as a unit while they are advanced progressively through the soft tissues. If excessive resistance is encountered, it may be necessary to remove the dilator from the sheath and to introduce the dilator alone before attempting to introduce the combination. If inspection shows that initial attempts have created significant burring at the end of the sheath, a new sheath should be obtained. Care should be taken when advancing the introducer and sheath with the dilator in obese patients and those with significant soft tissue in the pelvic and abdominal space. In these patients, the use of a 150- to 180-cm-long 0.035- to 0.038-in wire can ensure that there is enough wire length within the intravascular space to avoid losing the wire in the soft tissue while advancing the sheath. In rare instances, the dilator and the sheath do not track well over the J-tipped 0.035- to 0.038- in wire, and the use of an Amplatz Super Stiff Guidewire might be needed to advance the dilator and the sheath. While these challenges are not common, the use of a long introducer sheath (23 or 45 cm) can ensure that the sheath remains in the intravascular space during the procedure and does not move with catheter(s) exchange or manipulation.

If needed, the sheath can be connected via a sterile length of intravenous extension tubing to provide a carrier for drug administration by the nurse.

Catheterizing the Right-Sided Heart From the Femoral Vein

Right-sided heart catheterization is no longer routinely done in patients with a primary diagnosis of coronary artery disease, unless they have symptoms of congestive heart failure, noninvasive evidence of depressed left ventricular (LV) function, associated valvular disease, or history of pulmonary hypertension.

While conventional woven Dacron catheters were commonly used in the past, as of today it is considerably safer to use 7F balloon flotation catheters, which provide the additional advantage to perform thermodilution measurements of cardiac output.

Deviation of the catheter tip from its paraspinous position during advancement from the leg suggests entry into a renal or hepatic vein, which can be corrected by slight withdrawal and rotation of the catheter. Once the catheter is above the diaphragm and within the right atrium, it is rotated counterclockwise to face the lateral wall of the right atrium. Additional counterclockwise rotation and gentle advancement allow passage of the catheter tip into the superior vena cava, which is contiguous with the posterolateral wall of the right atrium. In contrast, anterior orientation of the catheter tip at this point may result in its entrapment in the right atrial appendage and inability to reach the superior vena cava. If passage to the superior vena cava is difficult, the tip of the catheter can be withdrawn to the inferior vena cava, where a J guidewire can be introduced to traverse the straight-line path from the inferior to the superior vena cava along the back wall of the right atrium. Once in position, a baseline superior vena caval blood sample is obtained for measurement of oxygen saturation. The catheter is then flushed with heparinized saline solution and withdrawn to the right atrium for pressure measurement.

Figure 8.4 illustrates the different steps required to advance a catheter from the femoral vein to the pulmonary artery. Final advancement of the catheter from the right ventricular outflow tract to the pulmonary artery may be facilitated if performed as the patient takes a deep breath.

If the maneuvers described in **Figure 8.4A-F** fail to achieve access to the pulmonary artery owing to enlargement of the right atrial and ventricular chambers, the catheter may be withdrawn to the right atrium and formed into a large reverse loop, which allows the tip of the catheter to cross the tricuspid valve in an upward orientation (similar to that when right-sided heart catheterization is performed from above), which makes it more likely to enter the outflow tract (**Figure 8.4G and H**). If further difficulties are encountered in cases of severe pulmonary hypertension, the utilization of a 0.025-in J-tipped wire can be helpful when kept inside the catheter (ie, without advancing it outside the balloon-tipped catheter). This technique provides the catheter with additional stiffness while advancing it against high pulmonary pressures. If needed, after deflating the balloon, navigation from the outflow tract into the pulmonary artery can also be achieved by advancing the 0.025-in J-tipped wire to the pulmonary artery trunk. Once the wire is in the pulmonary trunk, the balloon-tipped catheter can be advanced over the wire, the wire is taken out, and the balloon is inflated again. Having the patient take a deep breath and cough during advancement often helps to achieve a wedge position. Alternatively, a small amount of air may be released from the balloon to decrease its size and facilitate wedging in a smaller, more distal branch of the pulmonary artery. Catheters advanced from the leg are more likely to seek the left pulmonary artery, whereas catheters advanced from above tend to seek the right pulmonary artery. If needed, either pulmonary artery can be catheterized by appropriate manipulation or careful introduction of a curved J guidewire, but extending a guidewire into the thin-walled pulmonary arteries should be avoided unless absolutely necessary.

Attempts to perform right-sided heart catheterization occasionally result in entry into other structures. A catheter advanced in the right atrium with a posteromedial orientation may cross a patent foramen ovale and enter the left atrium. This can be recognized by a change to a left atrial pressure waveform, position of the catheter tip across the spine and frequently out into the left lung field (ie, into a pulmonary vein, **Figure 8.5A and B**), and the ability to withdraw fully oxygenated blood from the catheter tip. A woven Dacron catheter can also enter the ostium of the coronary sinus, located inferiorly and posteriorly to the tricuspid orifice. There will be continued presence of a right atrial waveform, but blood sampling will disclose far lower oxygen saturation (20%-30%) than was present in the superior vena cava. In the right anterior oblique (RAO) projection, the catheter will be seen to remain in the atrioventricular groove rather than passing rightward into the ventricle. Anatomic abnormalities can also be suspected when the catheter takes an unusual position. **Figure 8.5C-E** depicts the appearance of the right-sided heart catheter course in 3 such congenital abnormalities.

In patients with elevated right-sided heart pressures or prior placement of an inferior vena caval filter or umbrella, those undergoing specialized procedures

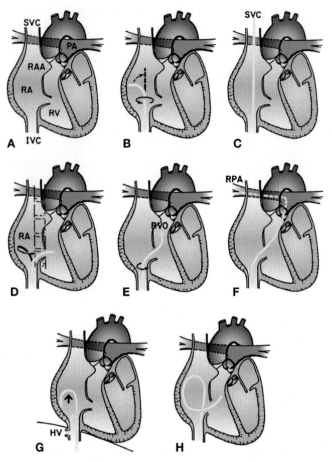

Figure 8.4 Right-sided heart catheterization from the femoral vein, shown in cartoon form. Top row. The right-sided heart catheter is initially placed in the right atrium (RA) aimed at the lateral atrial wall. Counterclockwise rotation aims the catheter posteriorly and allows advancement into the superior vena cava (SVC). Clockwise catheter rotation into an anterior orientation would lead to advancement into the right atrial appendage (RAA), precluding SVC catheterization. Center row. The catheter is then withdrawn back into the right atrium and aimed laterally. Clockwise rotation causes the catheter tip to sweep anteromedially and cross the tricuspid valve. Additional clockwise rotation causes the catheter to point straight up, allowing for advancement into the main pulmonary artery and from there into the right pulmonary artery (RPA). Bottom row. Two maneuvers useful in catheterization of dilated right side of the heart. A larger loop with a downward-directed tip may be required to reach the tricuspid valve and can be formed by catching the catheter tip in the hepatic vein (HV) and advancing the catheter quickly into the right atrium. The reverse loop technique (bottom right) gives the catheter tip an upward direction, aimed toward the outflow tract.

(endomyocardial biopsy, coronary sinus catheterization), or those in whom prolonged postprocedural monitoring with a balloon flotation catheter is desired, the right upper extremity (subclavian or median basilic vein, see Chapter 7) or the right internal jugular vein offers an excellent alternative to the femoral vein.

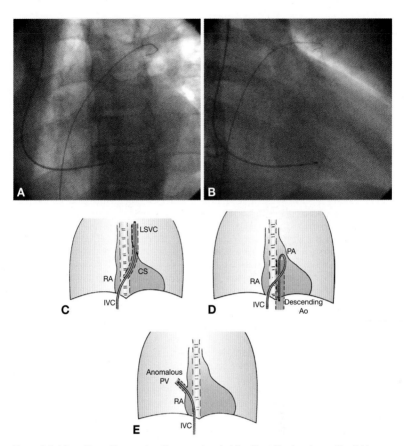

Figure 8.5 Alternative paths occasionally encountered while attempting to advance the right-sided heart catheter from right atrium to ventricle. **A** and **B,** A J-tipped guidewire has crossed a patent foramen ovale into the left atrium and left upper pulmonary vein; the right anterior oblique view confirms that the guidewire has remained on the atrial side of the atrioventricular plane and thus could not be in the pulmonary artery. **C,** The course of a catheter passed from the femoral vein to the inferior vena cava (IVC), right atrium (RA), coronary sinus (CS), and up into an anomalous left superior vena cava (LSVC). **D,** The catheter crossing from the pulmonary artery (PA) to the descending aorta (Ao) by way of a patent ductus arteriosus. **E,** The catheter entering an anomalous pulmonary vein that drains into the right atrium.

Femoral Artery Puncture

Once the fluoroscopic landmarks have been identified, vascular ultrasound can help visualize a single anterior wall stick above the bifurcation and in the common femoral artery as explained above. When the artery is accessed without ultrasound imaging guidance, the needle is inserted at approximately 45° along the axis of the femoral artery (depending on degree of obesity of patient) as palpated by the 3 middle fingers of the left hand. Occasionally, the "bounce" technique can be used. With this technique, the proximity to the artery can be confirmed based on the pulsation transmitted to the needle; if the needle is on top of the artery, the movement is north to south, while when the needle is lateral to the artery, the pulsation is transmitted laterally and the movement of the needle is from side to side. This technique is more obvious when using a 21-gauge needle.

The guidewire introduced through the needle should move freely up the aorta (located to the right [patient's left] side of the spine on fluoroscopy). When difficulty in advancing the guidewire is encountered at or just beyond the tip of the needle and is not corrected by slight depression or slight withdrawal of the needle, the guidewire should be withdrawn to ensure that brisk arterial flow is still present before any further wire manipulation is attempted. If flow is not brisk or if the wire still cannot be advanced, the needle should be removed and the groin should be compressed for 5 minutes.

If wire motion is initially free but resistance is encountered after several centimeters (particularly if the patient complains of any discomfort during wire advancement), extensive iliac disease and subintimal wire position are distinct possibilities. The wire should be pulled back slightly under fluoroscopic control, and the needle should be removed as the left hand is used to stabilize the wire and control arterial bleeding. After the wire is wiped with a moist gauze pad, a small (4F or 5F) dilator can be cautiously introduced to a point just below where wire movement became difficult. The wire is then withdrawn from the dilator, blood is aspirated to ensure free flow, and a small bolus of diluted low-osmolar contrast medium is then injected gently under fluoroscopic monitoring. This should disclose the anatomic reason for difficult wire advancement—generally iliac tortuosity, stenosis, or dissection. Problems advancing the wire above the aortic bifurcation may also suggest the presence of an abdominal aortic aneurysm. Either can usually be overcome by use of a floppy steerable (Wholey wire, Mallinckrodt, Hazelwood, MO) or hydrophilic (Glidewire, Terumo) guidewire, carefully reintroduced through the dilator in an attempt to reach the descending aorta, using extreme care to avoid perforation, dissection, or dislodgment of atherothrombotic debris.

In an aging population with diffuse atherosclerotic disease, the question of performing left-sided heart catheterization via a prosthetic (eg, aortobifemoral) graft arises frequently. While this is not an ideal approach, if needed, the graft should be identified as a separate structure from the adjacent native femoral artery and punctured using a front-wall approach, under vascular ultrasound. Even if the graft hood is punctured correctly, the guidewire may pass through the anastomosis and into the native femoral artery rather than proximally up the graft. In that event, contrast injections through a small dilator in an RAO projection (ipsilateral) will disclose the problem. Partial withdrawal of the dilator and the use of special steerable guidewires may then allow the wire to be redirected into the graft lumen and thereby reach the descending aorta (**Figure 8.9B**).

Serial dilators may be needed to facilitate sheath passage through the tough graft wall. Hydrophilic sheaths can also be used in order to facilitate sheath insertion. Some operators choose to administer prophylactic antibiotics (Kefzol 1 g every 8 hours for 24 hours) when achieving vascular access via a prosthetic graft.

Catheterizing the Left-Sided Heart From the Femoral Artery

Once the guidewire has been advanced to the level of the diaphragm and the needle has been removed, the operator's left hand is used to stabilize the wire and control arterial bleeding while the wire is wiped with a moistened gauze pad to remove any adherent blood. All left-sided heart catheterizations from the femoral approach are now performed using an appropriate-sized vascular sheath (eg, a 6F sheath for a 6F catheter) that is equipped with a back-bleed valve and side-arm tubing as described above. The 15-cm-long sheath is commonly used for diagnostic catheterization. In the presence of severe tortuosity or catheterization of obese patients, it may be preferable to use a 23-cm-long, or even a 45-cm-long, sheath, which is sufficiently long to enter the distal aorta above the bifurcation. This helps improve the torque responsiveness of diagnostic catheters under those circumstances.

After removal of the dilator, and following aspiration and flushing, the sheath can be connected to a pressurized flush system to avoid clot formation in the sheath. Alternatively, this side arm can be connected to a manifold for monitoring arterial pressure at a separate site (eg, during passage of a pigtail catheter across a stenotic aortic valve). This sheath should be flushed before insertion and after removal of each catheter.

In the classic approach as described above, the guidewire was removed once the sheath had been inserted. This required that the desired left-sided heart catheter be flushed and loaded with a 145-cm J guidewire before its nose was introduced into the back-bleed valve of the sheath. The soft end of the guidewire is then advanced carefully through the catheter to the level of the diaphragm before the catheter itself is advanced. One concern, however, is that readvancement of the guidewire out the end of the sheath can cause vascular injury in the presence of severe iliac tortuosity or disease. We therefore adopted a modified technique in which a short exchange length (175 cm) Newton J (Cook, Inc) is placed through the access needle, and its tip is left at the level of the diaphragm as the dilator is removed from the sheath, the sheath is flushed, and the left-sided heart catheter is inserted over the wire and through the sheath lumen. This obviates the need to renegotiate complex iliofemoral anatomy with the guidewire, and it allows exchanging catheters above the diaphragm.

Once the catheter has been advanced to the desired level (either above the diaphragm or into the ascending aorta), the guidewire is removed. The catheter is connected to the arterial manifold and double flushed (withdrawal and discarding of 10 mL of blood, followed by injection of heparinized saline solution).

A Word About Heparin

The use of systemic heparinization for simple diagnostic catheterizations is no longer indicated. However, systemic anticoagulation is appropriate for more prolonged or complex diagnostic catheterizations, during transseptal catheterization (after the transseptal puncture has been completed), during mitral or aortic valvuloplasty, and (absolutely) for all percutaneous coronary, structural, or peripheral interventions.

If systemic heparinization is used, its effects can be reversed at the termination of the left-sided heart catheterization and associated angiography by the administration of protamine (1 mL equals 10 mg of protamine for every 1000 IU of heparin). The operator should be watchful for potential adverse reactions to protamine, which are more common in insulin-dependent diabetic patients and patients with previous protamine exposure. With the increasing use of vascular closure devices, protamine is now rarely used to reverse heparin. When bivalirudin is used (not reversible), the sheaths are routinely removed 2 hours after discontinuation of the drip due to its short half-life.

Catheter Selection

The initial left-sided heart catheter in most cases is a pigtail catheter with end and multiple side holes (**Figure 8.6**). A straight dual-lumen catheter is commonly used when evaluating intraventricular or transvalvular gradients. In patients without known aortic valve disease, the traditional pigtail catheter can be pulled back for pressure recording from the left ventricle apex to the ascending aorta.

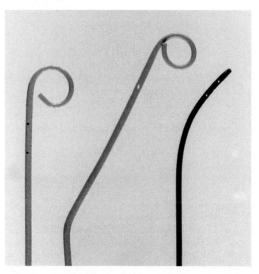

Figure 8.6 Left-sided heart catheters used from the femoral approach. Left to right. Pigtail, 145° angled pigtail, and Teflon Gensini catheter (no longer in common use). All 3 catheters have an end hole to allow placement over a guidewire and multiple side holes to minimize the tendency for catheter whipping or intramyocardial injection during power injection of contrast.

Crossing the Aortic Valve

After measurement of the ascending aortic pressure, the pigtail catheter is then advanced across the aortic valve and into the left ventricle. In most cases it may be necessary to advance the pigtail down into one of the sinuses of Valsalva to form a secondary loop (**Figure 8.7**). As the catheter is withdrawn slowly, this loop will open to span the full diameter of the aorta, at which point a very subtle further withdrawal will often cause the pigtail to fall across the valve.

If significant aortic stenosis is present, the pigtail must be advanced across the valve with the aid of a straight 0.038-in guidewire (**Figure 8.7**). A left Amplatz (AL1) catheter if the aortic root is normal or dilated, or a Judkins right coronary catheter if the aortic root is unusually narrow, can facilitate directing the straight wire and crossing the stenotic valve. As of today, the AL1 catheter is the preferred catheter by most operators to cross a stenotic aortic valve. In rare instances, the use of a straight glide hydrophilic-coated guidewire may be necessary, particularly in cases where critical aortic valve stenosis is encountered. In other instances, the guidewire can cross the aortic valve orifice, but the catheter may not be able to cross. In these rare events, the use of a hydrophilic-coated catheter may facilitate advancement into the left ventricle.

It is important to note that, when crossing the aortic valve with catheters other than the pigtail, a left anterior oblique (LAO) or anteroposterior view should be used in order to prevent inadvertent advancement of the straight wire in the coronary ostium. Once the tip of the wire has crossed the valve, the RAO view should be used to visualize the position of the wire in the ventricular cavity and prevent perforations. Once the catheter is in the left ventricle, the wire is immediately withdrawn and the catheter is aspirated vigorously, flushed, and hooked up for pressure monitoring, so that a gradient

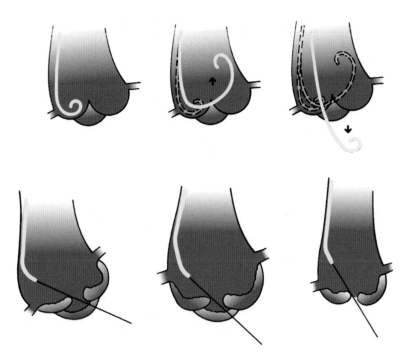

Figure 8.7 Crossing the aortic valve with a pigtail catheter. Top left. Although a correctly oriented pigtail catheter will frequently cross a normal aortic valve directly, it may also come to rest in the right or noncoronary sinus of Valsalva. Top center. Further advancement of the catheter enlarges the loop to span the aortic root and positions the catheter. Top right. Slow withdrawal causes the catheter to sweep across the aortic orifice and fall into the left ventricle. Bottom left. To cross a stenotic aortic valve, the pigtail catheter must be led by a segment of straight guidewire. Increasing the length of protruding guidewire straightens the catheter curve and causes the wire to point more toward the right coronary ostium; reducing the length of protruding wire restores the catheter curve and causes the wire to point more toward the left coronary ostium. Once the correct length of wire and the correct rotational orientation of the pigtail catheter have been found, repeated advancement and withdrawal of both the catheter and guidewire as a unit will allow the wire to cross the valve. Bottom center. In a dilated aortic root, an angled pigtail provides more favorable wire positions. Bottom right. In a small aortic root, a Judkins right coronary catheter may be preferable.

can be measured even if the catheter is rapidly ejected from the left ventricle or must be withdrawn because of arrhythmias. When using a left Amplatz catheter to cross a stenotic valve, however, we prefer to cross the valve with a full exchange length (260 cm) guidewire. Once the tip of this wire has entered the left ventricle, it is left in position as the Amplatz catheter is removed and a conventional dual-lumen pigtail catheter is substituted before an attempt is made to measure LV pressure.

Bioprosthetic and Mechanical Valves

The same approach applies to retrograde catheterization across a porcine aortic valve prosthesis, although it is more common to use a J-tipped guidewire to help avoid the area between the support struts and the aortic wall. Ball valves (Starr-Edwards) can be crossed retrograde with this approach, but use of a small (4F or 5F) catheter will minimize the amount of aortic regurgitation resulting from catheter interference with diastolic ball seating. Tilting-disk valves (Bjork-Shiley, St. Jude, Carbomedics), however, should not be crossed retrograde because of the potential for producing torrential aortic regurgitation, catheter entrapment, or even disk dislodgement if the catheter passes across the smaller (minor) orifice.

Control of the Puncture Site Following Sheath Removal

Originally, standard groin management required the effect of heparin to wear off or be reversed by protamine to an activated clotting time (ACT) <160 seconds before the arterial catheter and sheath were removed and manual pressure was applied. The manual pressure method is best applied using 3 fingers of the left hand that are positioned sequentially up the femoral artery beginning at the skin puncture. With the fingers in this position, there should be no ongoing bleeding into the soft tissues or through the skin puncture, and it should be possible to apply sufficient pressure to obliterate the pedal pulses and then release just enough pressure to allow them to barely return. Pressure is then gradually reduced over the next 10 to 15 minutes, at the end of which time pressure is removed completely. The venous sheath is usually removed 5 minutes after compression of the arterial puncture has begun, with gentle pressure applied over the venous puncture using the right hand. If relocation of the patient to a hospital bed is to be performed prior to sheath removal, it is important that the sheaths are secured in place (sutured) to prevent them from being pulled out during transport.

When procedures are performed using larger arterial sheaths or with thrombolytic agents or IIb/IIIa receptor blockers, more prolonged (30- to 45-min) compression is typically required. To avoid fatigue of the operator or other laboratory personnel performing compression, occasionally a mechanical device (Compressar [Applied Vascular Dynamics, Portland, OR], the Clamp Ease device [Semler Technologies, Inc. dba Advanced Vascular Dynamics, Milwaukie, OR], or FemoStop [Abbott Cardiovascular, Plymouth, MN]) can be used to apply similar local pressure. These devices can be equally or even more effective in prolonged holds but are uncomfortable for the patients. It should be emphasized that a trained person must be in attendance throughout the compression to ensure that the device is providing adequate control of puncture site bleeding and is not compromising distal perfusion.

After compression has been completed, the puncture site and surrounding area are inspected for hematoma formation and active oozing, and the quality of the distal pulse is assessed before application of a bandage. The patient is usually kept at bed rest with the leg straight for 4 to 6 hours following a diagnostic percutaneous femoral catheterization. The use of a sandbag over the puncture site has not been shown to decrease the incidence of hematoma formation and it is not indicated.

Elevation of the head and chest to 30° to 45° by the electrical or manual bed control, without muscular effort by the patient, will greatly increase the patient's comfort and will not increase the risk of local bleeding. Before ambulation and again before discharge, the puncture site should be reinspected for recurrent bleeding, hematoma formation, development of a bruit suggestive of pseudoaneurysm or A-V fistula formation, or loss of distal pulses.

Vascular Closure Devices

The potential for ongoing bleeding leading to additional complications, and a desire to promote early ambulation and improve patients' comfort, has prompted the development of a variety of devices that seek to provide more positive closure of the arterial puncture site (**Figure 8.8** and **Table 8.1**). These closure devices allow sheath removal in the catheterization laboratory in even a fully anticoagulated patient and shorten the time to hemostasis and ambulation.

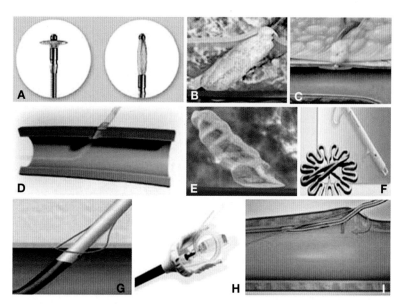

Figure 8.8 Schematic diagrams of various devices for the closure of femoral arterial punctures. **A,** Catalyst. **B,** Exoseal. **C,** Angio-Seal. **D,** FISH (Femoral Introducer Sheath and Haemostasis). **E,** Mynx. **F,** StarClose. **G,** Perclose ProGlide. **H,** Prostar. **I,** Axera. (See text for details.)

There are different types of vascular closure devices; *they can be grouped into passive or active,* depending on their mechanism. The simplest devices are the passive ones, which enhance hemostasis by providing prothrombotic material at the time of mechanical compression. The most common of this type are the hemostasis pads coated with procoagulant material: Chito-Seal (Abbott Vascular, Redwood City, California), Clo-Sur PAD (Scion Cardiovascular, Miami, Florida), SyvekPatch (Marine Polymer Technologies, Inc, Dankers, Massachusetts), Neptune Pad (Biotronik, Berlin, Germany), and D-Stat Dry (Teleflex Incorporated, Wayne, PA). Nevertheless, small randomized trials with patients undergoing diagnostic or interventional procedures have not demonstrated that the use of these pads shorten the time to ambulation, and the influence on hemostasis appears to be small; hence they are currently not considered true closure devices but tools to aid manual compression to obtain hemostasis.

The Cardiva Catalyst (II and III) (previously Boomerang; Cardiva Medical, Inc, Sunnyvale, California) is also a passive closure device that consists of a nitinol-braided mesh disk. The device is introduced through the arteriotomy sheath, and once the tip is within the arterial lumen, the disk is deployed and the sheath removed. The disk is gently pulled against the arterial wall where it is held in place by a tension clip in the skin to provide temporary intravascular tamponade, facilitating physiologic vessel contraction and thrombosis. After 15 minutes (120 minutes for interventional cases) the device is withdrawn and light manual compression can be applied. This device appears to reduce time for ambulation, and the Catalyst III can be used in patients who have received heparin.

The Exoseal (Cordis Corporation, Bridgewater, NJ) is also considered a passive closure device that consists of deployment of a polyglycolic acid plug (absorbed within 90 days) over the arteriotomy site for hemostasis, delivered through the

Table 8.1 Vascular Closure Devices

Closure Device	Mechanism	Indication	Sheath Size	Reaccess	Details
Catalyst III	Passive	Diagnostic/PCI	5-7F up to 25 cm	Immediate	Nitinol disk protamine coated (Catalyst III)
Exoseal	Passive	Diagnostic/PCI	5-7F up to 12 cm	>30 d	Polyglycolic acid plug over arteriotomy
Angio-Seal	Active/passive	Diagnostic/PCI	6-8F	>90 d (or 1 cm above)	Intra-arterial polymer and extravascular collagen plug
FISH	Active/passive	Diagnostic	5-8F	>30 d (or 2 cm above)	Intra-arterial porcine biomaterial as reabsorbable plug
Mynx	Passive	Diagnostic/PCI	5-7F	>30 d	Polyethylene glycol extravascular
StarClose	Active	Diagnostic/PCI	5-6F	Immediate	Nitinol clip
ProGlide	Active	Diagnostic/PCI	5-8F	Immediate	Suture-mediated closure
Prostar	Active	Diagnostic/PCI	8.5-10F	Immediate	Suture-mediated closure
Axera	Active	Diagnostic	5-6F	Immediate	Internal hemodynamic pressure to help close access
MANTA	Active	Large bore	12-25F	Immediate	Absorbable collagen and absorbable polymer anchor

FISH, Femoral Introducer Sheath and Haemostasis; PCI, percutaneous coronary intervention.

procedural sheath after diagnostic or interventional procedures. It should not be used in vessels of diameters <5 mm.

The MynxGrip device (Cordis Corporation, Bridgewater, NJ) consists of a polyethylene glycol matrix (degrades by hydrolysis in less than 30 days) that deploys outside the artery while a balloon occludes the arteriotomy site within the artery. This is introduced through the existing procedural sheath, and a small semi-compliant balloon is inflated within the artery and pulled back to the arterial wall, serving as an anchor to ensure proper placement. The sealant is delivered just outside the arterial wall where it expands to achieve hemostasis. The balloon is deflated and removed through the tract leaving the expanded sealant.

Active vascular closure devices range from simple to more complex mechanism of action.

The Angio-Seal closure device (Terumo Interventional Systems, Somerset, NJ) combines active and passive techniques. It consists of positioning a rectangular absorbable intra-arterial polymer anchor tethered by a polymer filament to an extravascular small collagen plug pushed against the outside of the artery, which provides a procoagulant state. The existing arterial sheath is exchanged for a specially designed 6F or 8F sheath with an arteriotomy locator. Once blood return confirms proper positioning within the arterial lumen, the sheath is held in place while the guidewire and arteriotomy locator are removed. The Angio-Seal device is inserted into the sheath until it snaps in place. The anchor is deployed and pulled back against the arterial wall. As the device is withdrawn further the collagen plug is exposed just outside the arterial wall and the remainder of the device is removed from the tissue track. Finally, the suture, which connects all the elements of the device, is cut below skin level leaving behind the anchor, collagen plug, and suture, all of which are absorbable by hydrolysis within 90 days.

The FISH (Femoral Introducer Sheath and Haemostasis) device (Morris Innovative, Bloomington, Indiana) is an active closure device that uses a combined procedural sheath and bioabsorbable extracellular matrix "patch" made from porcine small intestinal submucosa, which is inserted through the arteriotomy so that it straddles the arterial wall. After insertion, a wire is pulled to release the "patch" from the device, creating a reabsorbable plug in the artery wall.

The StarClose SE device (Abbott Vascular, Redwood City, California) is another active closure device that achieves hemostasis by deploying a 4-mm nitinol clip that approximates the edges of the arteriotomy. The device is inserted into the arterial lumen, and the clip is deployed just outside the arterial wall, grasping the edges of the arteriotomy and drawing them together for closure.

The Perclose ProGlide (Abbott Vascular, Redwood City, CA) consists of suture-mediated active closure. The device is inserted over a guidewire until blood return indicates positioning within the lumen. A lever is then pulled to deploy a "foot" within the arterial lumen. The device is pulled back positioning the foot against the anterior arterial wall. Two simultaneous needles are deployed through the anterior wall of the femoral artery engaging a nonbiodegradable polypropylene suture that is then pulled back through the arterial wall to form a suture loop. The device (containing the needles) is then removed, leaving behind the 2 suture tails. A knot is tied and pushed toward the arteriotomy to achieve hemostasis. This device has been shown to decrease time taken to achieve hemostasis and bed rest. Using the "preclosure" technique, the ProGlide can be used to close larger arteriotomies. In this case, after placing a 6F sheath and performing a femoral angiogram, the sheath is replaced with 2 subsequent ProGlide devices, the needles are deployed using perpendicular angles on the artery, and the ProGlide devices are removed leaving behind only the suture. A larger sheath can then be placed for the procedure, and at the conclusion of the procedure, the sutures are tied and pushed toward the arteriotomy for closure.

The Prostar XL (Abbott Vascular, Redwood City, CA) relies on the use of a sheath-like device to perform suture-mediated closure of the arterial puncture site. This device has undergone several design updates to improve the ease of delivery, and it relies on the passage of fine nitinol needles through the margins of the arterial puncture and out through the skin tunnel, where they can be tied to provide surgical hemostasis. It is currently mainly used for large sheaths.

The Axera device (Arstasis, Redwood City, CA) is an active closure device that does not leave any foreign material behind, and it is approved only for diagnostic cases with still limited data. It consists of creating an optimal predetermined shallow angle puncture allowing native hemodynamic pressure to close the access channel.

The percutaneous MANTA vascular closure device (Teleflex Incorporated, Wayne, PA) is a collagen-based device that was developed for large-bore vascular access. This technology includes an 8F puncture location dilator, a sheath, a closure unit (14F or 18F MANTA Closure Device), and a delivery system containing the implantable closure unit. This closure unit consists of an absorbable collagen hemostat and an absorbable polymer anchor (also known as toggle) that are connected by a suture. The device is utilized to facilitate hemostasis following the use of 10 to 20F devices or sheaths (ie, 12-25F outer diameter) for endovascular catheterization procedures. An anchor-arteriotomy-collage sandwich is achieved by mechanical compression resulting in hemostasis.

Randomized studies consistently have demonstrated that vascular closure devices shorten time to hemostasis and ambulation when compared with manual compression without any benefit in reducing vascular complications. Current recommendations are that it is reasonable to use closure devices after percutaneous interventions to improve comfort and reduce time to ambulation, but the use of closure devices is considered a class III indication for the reduction of vascular complications.

Contraindications to Femoral Approach to Left-Sided Heart Catheterization

As discussed in Chapter 1, the choice of catheterization approach is usually a function of operator, institution, and patient preference. Recognition of relative contraindications including peripheral vascular disease (femoral bruits or diminished lower extremity pulses), abdominal aortic aneurysm, marked iliac tortuosity, prior femoral arterial graft surgery, or gross obesity may favor the use of the percutaneous radial, brachial, or axillary approach rather than the transfemoral approach.

ALTERNATIVE SITES FOR LEFT-SIDED HEART CATHETERIZATION

The techniques described above for percutaneous insertion of a femoral catheter can also be used successfully from the axillary, brachial, or radial arteries, or even the lumbar aorta, with the use of an introducing sheath. In certain cases, access to the left side of the heart may be gained by transseptal puncture from the right atrium to the left atrium or even by direct percutaneous entry via the left ventricular apex.

Percutaneous Entry of the Axillary, Brachial, Radial Arteries, and Lumbar Aorta

For a review of axillary, brachial, and radial artery approaches, our readers are referred to Chapters 7 and 9. Percutaneous puncture of the lumbar aorta is a technique that had been used by radiologists to study patients with extensive peripheral vascular disease since the early 1980s and was then adapted to the performance of coronary angiography. The procedure must be done with the patient prone, thus limiting angiographic views and resuscitative efforts. Owing to the additional inability to apply direct pressure over the arterial entry site, this approach has not gained any popularity.

Percutaneous Transcaval Access

The transcaval access is a novel percutaneous vascular approach that has been introduced to allow large-bore access for patients who have unfavorable transfemoral, transaortic, and transapical anatomy. So far, it has been used successfully in numerous structural heart disease procedures (**Figure 8.9A-D**).

Transseptal Puncture

The development of catheter-based treatment of arrhythmias and of interventions for structural heart disease has led to a resurgence of transseptal cardiac catheterization,

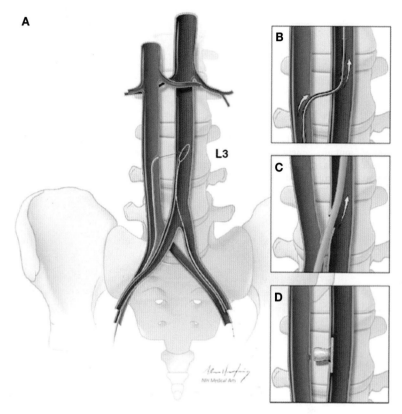

Figure 8.9 Transcaval access for transcatheter aortic valve replacement (TAVR). **A,** Transcaval access is obtained over an electrified guidewire directed from the inferior vena cava toward a snare in the abdominal aorta. **B,** After delivering a microcatheter to exchange for a stiff guidewire, **(C)** the transcatheter heart valve introducer sheath is advanced from the femoral vein into the abdominal aorta for conventional transfemoral retrograde TAVR. **D,** The aortocaval access site is closed with a nitinol cardiac occluder. (From Greenbaum AB, Babaliaros VC, Chen MY, et al. Transcaval access and closure for transcatheter aortic valve replacement: a prospective investigation. *J Am Coll Cardiol.* 2017;69:511-521.)

The goal of transseptal catheterization is to cross from the right atrium to the left atrium through the fossa ovalis. In approximately 10% of patients, this maneuver is performed inadvertently during right-sided heart catheterization because of the presence of a patent foramen ovale, but in the remainder, mechanical puncture of this area with a needle and catheter combination is required to enter the left atrium. The danger of the transseptal approach lies in the possibility that the needle and catheter will puncture an adjacent structure (ie, the posterior wall of the right atrium, the coronary sinus, or the aortic root). To minimize this risk, the operator must have a detailed familiarity with the regional anatomy of the atrial septum (**Figure 8.10**). The fossa ovalis is approximately 2 cm in diameter, it is bounded superiorly by a ridge—the limbus, and it is posterior and caudal to the aortic root

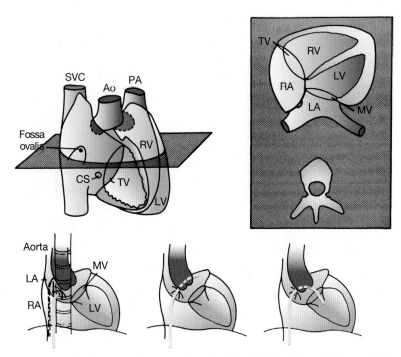

Figure 8.10 Regional anatomy for transseptal puncture. Top left. The position of the fossa ovalis is shown relative to the superior vena cava (SVC), aortic root (Ao), coronary sinus (CS), and tricuspid valve (TV). Top right. A cross section through the fossa (looking up from the feet) demonstrating the posteromedial direction of the interatrial septum (bold line) and the proximity of the lateral free wall of the right atrium. Bottom row. The appearance of the transseptal catheter as it is withdrawn from the SVC in a posteromedial orientation. As the catheter tip slides over the aortic root (bottom left, dotted position) it appears to move rightward onto the spine. Slight further withdrawal leads to more rightward movement into the fossa (solid position). Bottom center. Puncture of the fossa with advancement of the catheter into the left atrium. Bottom right. Advancement into the left ventricle with the aid of a curved tip occluder. (Redrawn from Ross J Jr. Considerations regarding the technique for trans-septal left heart catheterization. *Circulation.* 1966;34:391.)

and anterior to the free wall of the right atrium. It is located superiorly and posteriorly to the ostium of the coronary sinus and well posterior of the tricuspid annulus and right atrial appendage.

This anatomy can be distorted somewhat by the presence of aortic or mitral valve disease. In aortic stenosis, the plane of the septum becomes more vertical, and the fossa may be located slightly more anteriorly. In mitral stenosis, the intra-atrial septum becomes flatter with a more horizontal orientation and the fossa tends to lie lower. Intraprocedural transthoracic, transesophageal, or intracardiac ultrasound may aid in identifying the optimal location for puncture of the intra-atrial septum (**Figure 8.11**).

Classically, transseptal catheterization is performed from the right femoral vein, although the transjugular or left femoral vein approach is feasible but more complicated. A step-by-step approach to transseptal catheterization is illustrated in **Figure 8.12**).

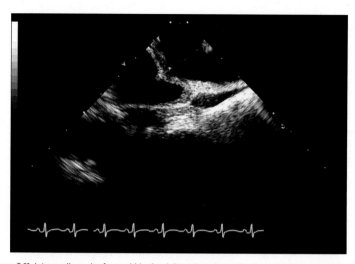

Figure 8.11 Intracardiac echo from within the right atrium shows the fossa ovalis and the left atrium clearly. Images during positioning of the transseptal needle show clear tenting of the foramen by the needle and reduce the uncertainty regarding correct puncture position. (Reproduced with permission from Moscucci M, Dairywala IT, Chetcuti S, et al. Balloon atrial septostomy in end-stage pulmonary hypertension guided by a novel intracardiac echocardiographic transducer. *Catheter Cardiovasc Interv.* 2001;52:530-534.)

The main risk during transseptal catheterization is inadvertent puncture of adjacent structures. As long as the patient is not anticoagulated and perforation is limited to the 21-gauge tip of the Brockenbrough needle, this is usually benign. However, if the 8F catheter itself is advanced into the pericardium or aortic root, potentially fatal complications may occur, underscoring the need for the operator to monitor closely the location of the transseptal apparatus by fluoroscopy, pressure, and oxygen saturation at each stage of the procedure. Damped pressure waveform may indicate puncture into the pericardium or simply incomplete penetration of a thickened interatrial septum. Injection of a small amount of contrast through the needle can be useful in this case by staining the atrial septum and allowing confirmation of an appropriate position in the LAO and RAO projection before more forceful needle advancement is attempted (**Figure 8.12**). If the initial attempt at transseptal puncture is unsuccessful, the operator may wish to repeat the catheter positioning procedure by removing the transseptal needle from the catheter, withdrawing the catheter slightly, and reinserting the 0.032-in guidewire into the superior vena cava. In general, one should never attempt to reposition the catheter-needle combination in the superior vena cava in any other way, since perforation of the right atrium or atrial appendage is a distinct possibility during such maneuvers.

Complications of transseptal catheterization for diagnostic purposes are generally infrequent (**Table 8.2**) in experienced hands.

Apical Left Ventricular Puncture

Historically, a variety of direct puncture techniques were used to enter the cardiac chambers before the introduction of percutaneous left- and right-sided heart catheterization. These techniques included transbronchial and transthoracic approaches

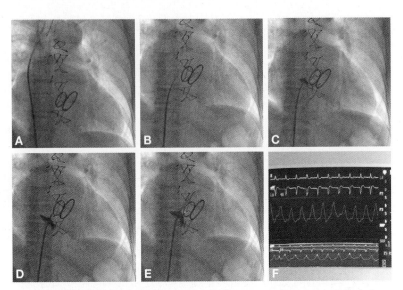

Figure 8.12 Steps of transseptal puncture as seen with fluoroscopy using common anatomical landmarks (spine, cardiac silhouette, left bronchus) and in this case prosthetic valves. **A,** Transseptal (TS) kit in the superior vena cava. **B,** Descent of the TS kit into the foramen ovale. The direction indicator of the needle is firmly controlled with the right hand and used to rotate the needle clockwise during this withdrawal from the superior vena cava until the arrow is oriented posteromedially (4 o'clock when looking from below). As the tip of the catheter enters the right atrium, it moves slightly toward the patient's left. As the catheter tip slips over the bulge of the ascending aorta, it again moves rightward to overlie the vertebrae in the anterior projection. Further slow withdrawal maintaining the 4-o'-clock orientation will be associated with a third rightward movement as the catheter tip "snaps" into the fossa ovalis. **C,** Staining of the interatrial septum. **D,** TS puncture and advancement into the left atrium (LA). **E,** Advancement of the TS sheath into the LA. **F,** Hemodynamic tracing of LA pressure. (Courtesy of Dr. Ruiz and Dr. Jelnin. Department of Interventional and Structural heart disease. Lenox Hill Institute of New York, and Reproduced with permission from Martinez C, Moscucci M. Complications of trans-septal cardiac catheterization. In: Moscucci M, ed. *Complications of Cardiovascular Procedures: Incidence, Risk Factors and Bailout Techniques.* Lippincott & Wilkins; 2011.)

to the left atrium, the suprasternal puncture technique of Radner, and apical LV puncture. Of these, only the last has survived and has gained popularity as the preferred approach to measure LV pressure in patients where retrograde and transseptal catheterization of the left ventricle are precluded by the presence of mechanical aortic and mitral prostheses, as well as for the treatment of specific structural heart disease conditions that do not have either an alternative access approach or a better anatomical access (ie, paravalvular leaks). A step-by-step approach to left ventricular apical puncture is summarized in **Table 8.3** (**Figure 8.13**).

Major complications (tamponade or pneumothorax) occur in roughly 3% of patients, although tamponade is very rare in postoperative patients (who have adhesive pericardium). Other complications of apical puncture can include hemothorax, intramyocardial injection, and ventricular fibrillation, as well as pleuritic chest discomfort (approximately 10%) and reflex hypotension owing to vagal stimulation (approximately 5%).

Table 8.2 Complications of Transseptal Puncture

Complications During Transseptal Puncture

Perforation:
- Roof of the LA
- Posterior LA wall
- LAA
- SVC or IVC
- Aorta
- Pulmonary vein perforation

Arrhythmias

Puncture or dissection of coronary sinus

Embolization
From:
- Layered thrombus in the LA wall
- LA myxoma
- Air
To:
- Brain
- Coronaries
- Systemic

Instrumental fracture due to breakage of the 21-gauge needle tip at its junction with the 18-gauge

Bezold-Jarisch-like vasovagal response: ST-segment elevation in the inferior leads without chest pain, associated with hypotension, bradycardia, and normal coronary arteries and reversed by atropine

Transient migraine

Thrombophlebitis and pulmonary embolism after complicated venous access

Pericarditis after injection of dye into the pericardium

Serious bleeding into posterior pericardial space

Inferior ST elevation

Residual atrial septal shunt

Hemothorax

Puncturing of the posterior RA creating a stitch phenomenon by reentering the LA

Atrial-aorto fistula

LA, left atrium; LAA, left atrial appendage; IVC, inferior vena cava; SVC, superior vena cava.
Reproduced with permission from Martinez C, Moscucci M. Complications of trans-septal cardiac catheterization. In: Moscucci M, ed. *Complications of Cardiovascular Procedures: Incidence, Risk Factors and Bailout Techniques.* Lippincott & Wilkins, 2011.

	Table 8.3 Step-by-Step Approach to Left Ventricular Apical Puncture
1	Preprocedure imaging with CT can help in identifying puncture site
2	Site of the apical impulse is located by palpation, confirmed by echocardiography, and marked. Confirmation by echocardiography is important, as in some patients the true apex might be located significantly more laterally than the palpated apical impulse in the setting of right ventricular enlargement.
3	After local anesthesia, a 21-gauge needle is introduced at the apex and directed along the long axis of the left ventricle. Contact with the LV wall can usually be felt as a very distinct impulse (and the onset of ventricular premature beats).
4	A 0.036-in 65-cm-long J guidewire is advanced through the needle into the left ventricle.
5	A 4F dilator followed by a 4F pigtail catheter to allow pressure measurement and/or LV angiography is then advanced over the guidewire.
6	Hemostasis at the end of the procedure is obtained depending on the size of the sheath inserted. Small sheaths can be manually pulled without major complications, and larger sheaths, up to 9F, have been removed by using off-label ventricular closure devices at the ventriculostomy site. When this fails, an open mini thoracotomy may be required to stitch close or to patch the puncture site.

CT, computed tomography.

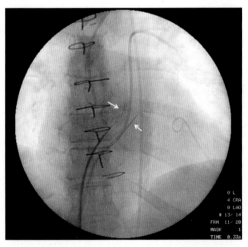

Figure 8.13 Direct apical puncture and transseptal puncture in a patient with St. Jude valves in aortic and mitral position. Cine frame in right anterior oblique view. There is a pigtail catheter inserted in the left ventricle through a transthoracic apical LV puncture, a second pigtail catheter positioned in the ascending aorta, a Mullins catheter advanced into the left atrium through the transseptal approach, and a Swan-Ganz catheter positioned in the pulmonary artery. The mitral and aortic St. Jude valve prostheses are visible on the left of the spine (arrows). (Reproduced with permission from Turgut T, Deeb M, Moscucci M. Left ventricular apical puncture: a procedure surviving well into the new millennium. *Catheter Cardiovasc Interv*. 2000;49:68-73.)

SUGGESTED READINGS

1. Ambrose JA, Lardizabal J, Mouanoutoua M, et al. Femoral micropuncture or routine introducer study (FEMORIS). *Cardiology*. 2014;129(1):39-43.
2. Applegate RJ, Turi Z, Sachdev N, et al. The angio-seal evolution registry: outcomes of a novel automated angio-seal vascular closure device. *J Invasive Cardiol*. 2010;22(9):420-426.
3. Bashore TM, Balter S, Barac A, et al. 2012 American College of Cardiology Foundation/Society for Cardiovascular Angiography and Interventions expert consensus document on cardiac catheterization laboratory standards update: a report of the American College of Cardiology Foundation Task Force on Expert Consensus documents developed in collaboration with the Society of Thoracic Surgeons and Society for Vascular Medicine. *J Am Coll Cardiol*. 2012;59(24):2221-2305.
4. Bhatt DL, Raymond RE, Feldman T, et al. Successful "pre-closure" of 7Fr and 8Fr femoral arteriotomies with a 6Fr suture-based device (the Multicenter Interventional Closer Registry). *Am J Cardiol*. 2002;89(6):777-779.
5. Castillo D, McEwen DS, Young L, Kirkpatrick J. Micropuncture needles combined with ultrasound guidance for unusual central venous cannulation: desperate times call for desperate measures—a new trick for old anesthesiologists. *Anesth Analg*. 2012;114(3):634-637.
6. Deuling JHH, Vermeulen RP, Anthonio RA, et al. Closure of the femoral artery after cardiac catheterization: a comparison of angio-seal, starclose, and manual compression. *Catheter Cardiovasc Interv*. 2008;71(4):518-523.
7. Greenbaum AB, Babaliaros VC, Chen MY, et al. Transcaval access and closure for transcatheter aortic valve replacement: a prospective investigation. *J Am Coll Cardiol*. 2017;69(5):511-521.
8. Harrison JK, Davidson CJ, Phillips HR, Harding MB, Kisslo KB, Bashore TM. A rapid, effective technique for retrograde crossing of valvular aortic stenosis using standard coronary catheters. *Catheter Cardiovasc Diagn*. 1990;21:51-54.
9. Jelnin V, Dudiy Y, Einhorn BN, Kronzon I, Cohen HA, Ruiz CE. Clinical experience with percutaneous left ventricular transapical access for interventions in structural heart defects a safe access and secure exit. *JACC Cardiovasc Interv*. 2011;4(8):868-874.
10. Kim D, Orron DE, Skillman JJ, et al. Role of superficial femoral artery puncture in the development of pseudoaneurysm and arteriovenous fistula complicating percutaneous transfemoral cardiac catheterization. *Cathet Cardiovasc Diagn*. 1992;25(2):91-97.
11. Koreny M, Riedmuller E, Nikfardjam M, Siostrzonek P, Mullner M. Arterial puncture closing devices compared with standard manual compression after cardiac catheterization: systematic review and meta-analysis. *J Am Med Assoc*. 2004;291(3):350-357.
12. Lesnefsky EJ, Carrea FP, Groves BM. Safety of cardiac catheterization via peripheral vascular grafts. *Cathet Cardiovasc Diagn*. 1993;29(2):113-116.
13. Martin JL, Pratsos A, Magargee E, et al. A randomized trial comparing compression, Perclose Proglide and Angio-Seal VIP for arterial closure following percutaneous coronary intervention: the CAP trial. *Catheter Cardiovasc Interv*. 2008;71:1-5.
14. Nguyen N, Hasan S, Caufield L, Ling FS, Narins CR. Randomized controlled trial of topical hemostasis pad use for achieving vascular hemostasis following percutaneous coronary intervention. *Catheter Cardiovasc Interv*. 2007;69(6):801-807.
15. Nishihara Y, Kajiura T, Yokota K, Kobayashi H, Okubo T. Evaluation with a focus on both the antimicrobial efficacy and cumulative skin irritation potential of chlorhexidine gluconate alcohol-containing preoperative skin preparations. *Am J Infect Control*. 2012;40(10):973-978.
16. Ren JF, Marchlinski FE. Training methodology for transseptal catheterization should incorporate difficult anatomic conditions and the use of intracardiac echocardiographic imaging. *J Am Coll Cardiol*. 2012;59(3):291-292; author reply 292.
17. Roelke M, Smith AJ, Palacios IF. The technique and safety of transseptal left heart catheterization: the Massachusetts general hospital experience with 1,279 procedures. *Cathet Cardiovasc Diagn*. 1994;32(4):332-339.
18. Scheinert D, Sievert H, Turco MA, et al. The safety and efficacy of an extravascular, water-soluble sealant for vascular closure: initial clinical results for Mynx. *Catheter Cardiovasc Interv*. 2007;70(5):627-633.
19. Seto AH, Abu-Fadel MS, Sparling JM, et al. Real-time ultrasound guidance facilitates femoral arterial access and reduces vascular complications: FAUST (Femoral Arterial Access with Ultrasound Trial). *JACC Cardiovasc Interv*. 2010;3(7):751-758.
20. Shroff A, Pinto D. *Vascular Access Management and Closure Best Practices*. The Society for Cardiovascular Angiography and Interventions (SCAI); 2019. Accessed December 3, 2019. http://www.scai.org/ebook-VAMC/
21. Wong SC, Bachinsky W, Cambier P, et al. A randomized comparison of a novel bioabsorbable vascular closure device versus manual compression in the achievement of hemostasis after percutaneous femoral procedures: the ECLIPSE (Ensure's Vascular Closure Device Speeds Hemostasis Trial). *JACC Cardiovasc Interv*. 2009;2(8):785-793.

9 Cutdown Approach: Brachial, Femoral, Axillary, Aortic, and Transapical[1]

Although the brachial cutdown (or Sones) approach was once the dominant technical approach to cardiac catheterization and angiography, it is now used in only a few (<1%) cardiac catheterization procedures, and the skills required for brachial arterial and venous cutdown and vascular repair are rapidly vanishing among the invasive cardiology community. Because this approach may still be of value in occasional patients, this chapter summarizes the technique as a guide for those learning to perform it, or as a refresher for those previously trained in the brachial approach who require the use of this technique in a particular patient. In addition, this chapter summarizes techniques for open femoral, axillary, aortic, and transapical access, which have become important alternatives for vascular access required for structural heart interventions.

INDICATIONS

The brachial approach may be indicated for patients with (1) severe peripheral vascular disease, (2) urgent or emergent cardiac catheterization with an increased risk for bleeding (owing to chronic oral anticoagulation or recent thrombolytic therapy), or (3) a need for early ambulation or mobility. Many of these situations can be addressed by percutaneous radial artery catheterization (see Chapter 7), but the brachial cutdown approach can provide the following additional advantages: (1) the ability to obtain upper extremity arterial access in patients without a patent radial artery or with a contraindication to radial artery access; (2) reliable venous access to perform concomitant right-sided heart catheterization; (3) assured arterial access for 7F or greater catheter sizes; (4) access to large veins to allow for foreign body retrieval (from the superior and inferior vena cava, right ventricle, or pulmonary artery).

Relative contraindications to brachial artery cutdown include absence of a brachial pulse, presence of an arteriovenous fistula, overlying soft-tissue infection, severe ipsilateral axillary or subclavian vascular disease, and inability to extend the arm at the elbow or supinate the hand.

PREPROCEDURAL EVALUATION

The general location for arterial cutdown will be approximated 2 to 3 cm above the antecubital skin folds, slightly superior to the level of the humeral epicondyles, and medial to the biceps tendon. A cutdown below this level is not recommended because the artery subsequently courses under the biceps tendons and bifurcates. A cutdown performed above this level is feasible but may be awkward owing to the medial course of the artery.

A diminished brachial pulse and/or bruits should lead the operator to anticipate proximal vascular occlusive disease and plan accordingly with consideration for a contralateral procedure, femoral access, or the use of soft and steerable guidewires.

---

[1]We gratefully acknowledge the Grossman & Baim's *Cardiac Catheterization, Angiography, and Intervention*, 9th edition contributions of Drs. Ronald P. Caputo, Charles J. Lutz, and William Grossman as portions of their chapter, Cutdown Approach: Brachial, Femoral, Axillary, Aortic, And Transapical, were retained in this text.

INCISION, ISOLATION OF VESSELS, AND CATHETER INSERTION

With the arm fully extended flat on the arm board and the hand supinated, the brachial artery (**Figure 9.1**) is identified by palpation and local anesthesia is induced in the overlying soft tissues using 1% to 2% lidocaine. If anesthesia is achieved properly, the catheter insertion site ought to be virtually painless throughout the procedure.

Prior to starting the procedure, the proper instruments shown in **Figure 9.2** should be on hand.

A transverse incision is made with a no. 15 surgical blade just proximal to (ie, approximately 2 cm above) the flexor crease. If right- and left-sided heart catheterization is contemplated, the incision is wide and made over the palpable brachial artery; if a right-sided heart study alone is planned, the incision is narrow and made directly over a previously identified medial vein. Even large veins of the lateral antecubital fossae usually drain into the cephalic system, through which it may be difficult to navigate the catheter into the right atrium, whereas the medial veins drain into either the basilic or brachial venous systems (which join the axillary vein by direct continuation) and thus provide the easiest routes to the superior vena cava (SVC) and right atrium (**Figure 9.3**).

The operator performs blunt dissection through the subcutaneous fat with a curved hemostat, simultaneously performing lateral retraction, while the assistant retracts medially. As the handheld retractors are applied to the lateral ends of the incision, the self-retaining retractor is applied superoinferiorly. This provides optimal exposure, particularly when substantial amounts of adipose tissue are present. After the fascia overlying the brachial artery is exposed, the artery is pal-

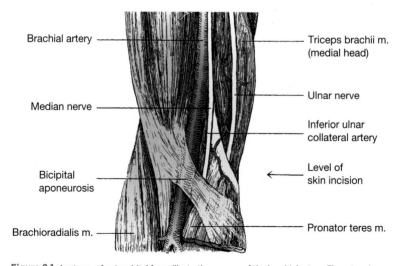

Figure 9.1 Anatomy of antecubital fossa illustrating course of the brachial artery. The artery is best sought at or slightly above the antecubital skin crease, medial to the bicipital aponeurosis. Care must be taken not to disturb the median nerve, which usually lies medial to the brachial artery. (Reprinted with permission from Clemente C. *Gray's Anatomy of the Human Body*. 30th American ed. Lea & Febiger; 1985.)

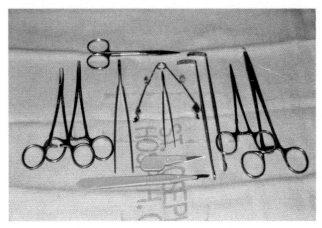

Figure 9.2 Instruments used for brachial cutdown: 2 Halstead curved 5-in mosquito hemo-stats, 1 Halstead straight mosquito 5-in hemostat, 1 thumb dressing 6-in forceps without teeth, 1 straight iris forceps without teeth, 1 short-handled scalpel (no. 11 blade), 1 long-handled scalpel (no. 15 blade), 1 Grieshaber wire self-retaining retractor, 2 Davis double-end soft-tissue retractors, 1 straight 4-inch iris scissors, and 1 Halsey 5-inch needle holder. All except scalpels are from Pilling Instruments, Washington, PA.

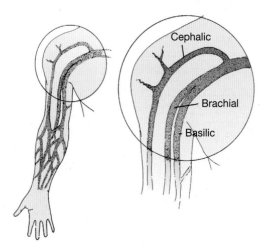

Figure 9.3 Venous anatomy of the arm. Brachial and basilic veins are medial to the cephalic vein within the antecubital fossa. Note that the brachial and basilic veins continue directly into the axillary and subclavian system, whereas the cephalic system frequently joins the subclavian vein at a right angle. Passage of a catheter from the cephalic system to the right atrium may thus be quite difficult; the medial veins provide the straightest pathway.

pated again and blunt dissection through the fascia is then performed immediately overlying or lateral to the artery. This further decreases the chance for median nerve injury.

At this point, the artery is easily recognized by its pulsation and characteristic silvery white color. Veins, in contrast, are nonpulsatile, much darker in color, and usually of smaller caliber.

The median nerve is yellowish with a slightly corrugated surface and should not be further manipulated. A few patients have an accessory brachial artery, which is smaller and usually not suitable for catheterization. This vessel has a more superficial course and generally is not surrounded by veins, but deeper palpation will often reveal the location of the true brachial artery. The tissues are separated by blunt dissection with a curved Kelly forceps, and an appropriate vein is brought to the surface, separated from adjacent nerves and fascia, and tagged proximally and distally with a loop of 3-0 or 4-0 silk suture material. The brachial artery is similarly brought to the surface with a curved Kelly forceps; isolated from adjacent nerves, veins, and fascia; and tagged proximally and distally with moistened umbilical tape or silicone-elastomer surgical tape (**Figure 9.4**).

The brachial artery is cleaned and positioned by applying gentle pressure on the hemostats or umbilical tapes using thumb and index fingers to stretch the artery longitudinally (**Figure 9.5**). This maneuver is critical because it allows for arterial positioning, stabilization, and (with adequate tension) excellent hemostatic control. Most operators incise it transversely by making a small (2-mm) nick in its anterior surface with a no. 11 surgical blade. Others favor a longitudinal arteriotomy with the no. 11 surgical blade held at a 30° angle to the artery and the sharp edge facing upward (toward the ceiling) to minimize risk of injury to the posterior wall. The longitudinal direction requires a more cautious repair to avoid narrowing the lumen.

An appropriately selected left-sided heart catheter (see the following section) is flushed. Tapered tip catheters, such as the Sones or multipurpose ones, can be inserted without a sheath (**Figure 9.6**), but a sheath may be preferable when multiple catheter exchanges are planned or when catheters with a nontapered tip, such as guiding catheters for percutaneous coronary interventions, are used.

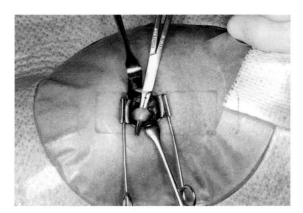

Figure 9.4 Isolation of the brachial artery. The incision is held open superoinferiorly by the self-retractor and laterally by the manual retractors while a curved hemostat is manipulated underneath the artery.

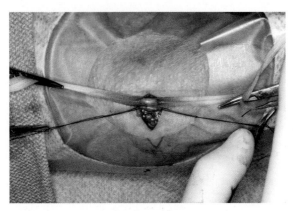

Figure 9.5 Isolating and securing the brachial artery and adjacent vein. The brachial artery is secured superiorly and inferiorly with moistened umbilical tapes fixed with curved hemostats. The isolated segment of vein is secured in similar fashion with 4-0 suture.

Many laboratories administer heparin solution (eg, 50 units/kg) to help prevent thromboembolic events to the hand. This can be given into the distal brachial artery, into the central aorta, or intravenously.

CATHETER SELECTION
Right-Sided Heart Catheters

Classic woven Dacron right-sided heart catheters (eg, Goodale-Lubin and Cournand, **Figure** 9.7) have now been replaced by flow-directed balloon flotation catheters. If right-sided angiography is planned, a closed-end catheter with multiple side-holes can be used.

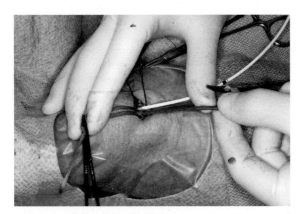

Figure 9.6 Insertion of an 8F Sones I catheter (Cordis Corp., Miami, FL) into the brachial artery during gentle retraction exerted by the thumb and index finger on umbilical tapes to control bleeding. A 7F balloon-tipped Swan-Ganz catheter has already been placed into the adjacent vein.

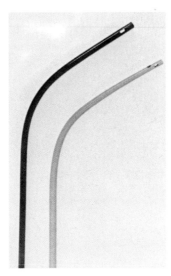

Figure 9.7 Useful traditional catheters for right- and left-sided heart catheterization. (Left) The Goodale-Lubin catheter has an end hole and 2 side holes and is ideal for right-sided heart catheterization, including measurement of pulmonary capillary wedge pressure. (Right) The polyurethane Sones catheter tapers to a 5F tip with an end hole and 4 side holes; it is useful for coronary angiography and for left ventriculography (at low flow rates).

Left-Sided Heart Catheters

The classic Sones B or a multipurpose catheter can be used for most coronary and left ventriculographic purposes, although they tend to recoil at injection rates greater than 8 mL/s and have to be positioned carefully within the left ventricle to avoid myocardial staining. Thus, from a safety perspective, it is preferable to use pigtail catheters for left ventriculography.

Coronary angiography can usually be completed with the Sones catheter or with multipurpose type I and type II catheters. Alternatively, Castillo or Amplatz 1, 2, or 3 type curves are available and are very useful for angiography of coronary artery bypass grafts, for coronary engagement in patients with large aortic roots, and in situations where more forceful torque must be applied. The Sones A type curve is also useful for patients with a high takeoff of the left coronary artery. From the right brachial approach, the femoral mammary catheter is adequate for angiography of the right internal mammary artery, whereas the brachial mammary catheter or a multistep approach (1) gaining access to the left subclavian artery with a Castillo or Amplatz catheter, (2) advancing an exchange wire into the axillary artery, and (3) exchanging for the femoral mammary catheter is required for angiography of the left internal mammary (see the section that follows).

ADVANCING THE RIGHT-SIDED HEART CATHETER

The right-sided heart catheter is advanced under fluoroscopic control to the SVC (**Figure 9.8**). If a balloon-tipped catheter is used, advancement is generally straightforward. However, if the cephalic vein is entered rather than the brachial vein, there may be resistance due to the angle of entry at the level of the subclavian vein. If there is difficulty entering the subclavian vein/SVC, it is sometimes helpful to try the following maneuvers:

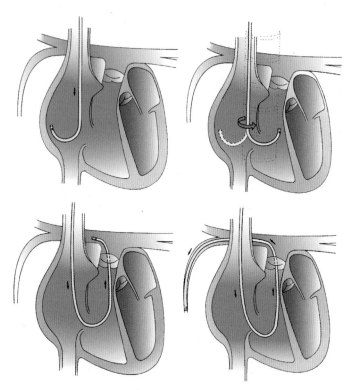

Figure 9.8 Advancing the right-sided heart catheter. In navigating from right atrium to pulmonary artery, the J loop technique should be tried first. (Top left) The catheter is advanced so that its tip catches on the lateral right atrial wall and forms the letter J. (Top right) It is then rotated counterclockwise so that the catheter tip sweeps the anterior right atrial wall (thus avoiding the coronary sinus) and jumps across the tricuspid valve into the right ventricle. (Bottom left) The catheter tip, pointing toward the right ventricular outflow tract, can be easily advanced into the pulmonary artery. (Bottom right) The patient takes a deep breath, and the catheter is advanced to the "wedge" position (see text).

have the patient take a deep breath; raise the right arm and shoulder toward the head (ask the patient to shrug their right shoulder); turn the patient's head to the extreme left; remove the patient's pillow. On occasion, a guidewire may be helpful in passing from the subclavian vein into the SVC. Arterial or venous spasm may develop and inhibit catheter movement. It may resolve if the catheter is withdrawn by a distance of 10 to 20 cm, and the same cocktail of intravenous nitroglycerine and verapamil or other calcium channel blockers may be administered as used in radial artery catheterization.

ADVANCING THE LEFT-SIDED HEART CATHETER

After the right-sided heart catheter has been advanced to the pulmonary artery or wedge position, an appropriately selected left-sided heart catheter is inserted into the brachial artery as described previously. This catheter is then advanced into the ascending aorta just above the aortic valve. Advancement over a J-tipped guidewire is the preferred approach. Passage may be aided by deep and held inspiration while lifting the chin and rotating the head leftward and over the left shoulder, but severe tortuosity may then impair catheter control once the aortic root has been reached.

Once the catheter is in the ascending aorta, central aortic pressure is measured and recorded. The catheter is then advanced across the aortic valve into the left ventricle by probing the valve with small to-and-fro excursions while gradually rotating the catheter through 360° so that the catheter tip moves up and down on the aortic valve over its entire plane. The soft-tipped Cordis polyurethane Sones catheter may be advanced directly (tip first) into the left ventricle, or it may be prolapsed across the aortic valve, loop first, as illustrated in **Figure 9.9**.

Internal Mammary Arteries

The mammary arteries usually originate from the subclavian arteries with inferior take-offs opposite to the origin of the vertebral arteries. Although the internal mammary artery is best engaged from an ipsilateral brachial approach using preformed femoral catheters, it is usually possible to engage the left mammary from the right brachial approach using 1 of 2 techniques. An Amplatz catheter (generally an AL 0.75, AL 1, or AL 2) is advanced into the descending aorta distal to the origin of the left subclavian artery. The catheter is manipulated into its natural configuration, and as it is slowly withdrawn using gentle rotation, the left subclavian artery is engaged. An exchange length wire is passed through this catheter into the axillary artery and used to exchange the Amplatz for a femoral mammary catheter. The second technique utilizes a preshaped brachial mammary catheter

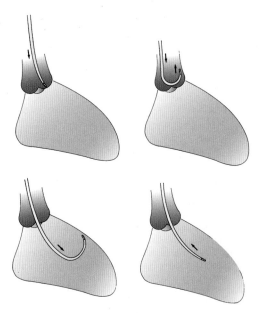

Figure 9.9 Technique for retrograde catheterization of the left ventricle using the Sones catheter. (Top left) The catheter is advanced to touch the aortic valve. (Top right) Further advancement usually produces a loop in the ascending aorta, which prolapses readily (bottom left) into the left ventricle. (Bottom right) The catheter is then withdrawn to eliminate the loop and obtain a proper axial orientation for left ventriculography.

that is passed into the aortic root and secondary curve is banked off the aortic valve while the tip is advanced toward the subclavian artery. This is done with the support of a 0.35-in or 0.38-in wire. After the tip engages the subclavian artery, the catheter is advanced and rotated to engage the mammary artery.

SPECIAL TECHNIQUES
Coronary Bypass Grafts

Aortocoronary vein grafts have a high takeoff compared with coronary arteries; therefore, a longer-curve Sones or multipurpose catheter (such as a Sones A or MP 2) should be used. However, preshaped catheters such as the Castillo or Amplatz type 1 (vein grafts to the right coronary), 2 (vein grafts to the left coronary arteries), or 3 curves (widened aortic root) are generally preferable.

Anomalous Coronary Takeoff

Preshaped catheters with Castillo or Amplatz curves are preferable for anomalous origins not easily reached with the Sones or multipurpose curves. Some catheter recommendations for specific situations include the following:

1. Right coronary artery with inferior takeoff or horizontal heart—AR 2, Castillo/AL 1
2. Right coronary artery with anterior takeoff—Castillo/AL 1 or 2
3. Left coronary artery with a high takeoff—Castillo/AL 3, Sones A, MP 1
4. Left circumflex coronary originating from the right coronary—Sones or MP 1 or 2 curves are optimal with the tip directed inferiorly; AR 2, Castillo/AL 1 if the Sones catheter overshoots the origin of the circumflex that is very proximal or is immediately adjacent to the right coronary ostium
5. Right coronary artery with anomalous takeoff from the left sinus of Valsalva or left coronary artery arising from the right sinus of Valsalva—Castillo/AL 2 or 3 to "scan" the aortic wall seeking the ostium. Kimny or JL 3.5 catheters can also be effective

REPAIR OF VESSELS AND AFTERCARE

Repair of the brachial arteriotomy may be done in many ways (purse-string, interrupted, continuous sutures). Prior to initiation of arterial repair, pressure on the proximal loop is released briefly to allow generous antegrade bleeding and flush out thrombi that may have formed around the catheter. The proximal bleeding is then controlled, and pressure on the distal umbilical tape is released to allow for retrograde (collateral-fed) bleeding to ensure patency of the distal artery. If there is brisk back-bleeding, no further maneuvers are indicated and arterial closure can commence. If no back-bleeding is present, the area overlying the radial and distal brachial artery should be manually "milked" or massaged in distal to proximal fashion to dislodge and remove any thromboemboli. If there is still no retrograde flow, a Sones or multipurpose catheter can be inserted distally through the arteriotomy, carefully advanced until resistance is met, and then slowly withdrawn while gentle suction is applied to its lumen with a syringe. If these maneuvers fail to restore back-bleeding, a Fogarty embolectomy procedure is then warranted.

A common approach to arteriotomy repair calls for stabilization of the vessel by applying pressure with the umbilical tapes or placing a large forceps transversely beneath the artery (**Figures 9.10** and **9.11**).

Minor bleeding around the sutures can often be controlled with gentle manual pressure and/or temporary application of a small Gelfoam pad. Once the assistant has confirmed the presence of an adequate radial pulse, the skin and subcutaneous

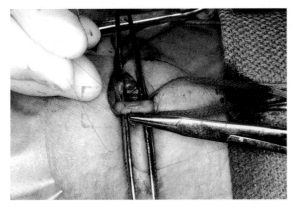

Figure 9.10 Suture repair of the brachial arteriotomy. The artery is stabilized by placing a large forceps underneath in transverse orientation. A stay suture has been placed above the superior margin of the longitudinal incision. Lockstitch running sutures will be placed beyond the inferior margin of the incision to close the arteriotomy.

tissues are closed using absorbable suture material and the subcutaneous technique. Two or three 0.25-in Steri-Strips are then applied in transverse fashion across the incision. A small Telfa pad coated with an antibacterial ointment is applied directly over the site and covered with a small stack of 4 × 4 gauze pads that are then wrapped in firm fashion with a 3-in-wide Ace bandage.

After repairing the arteriotomy successfully, the vein used in the right-sided heart catheterization may be tied off or repaired (a purse-string repair is usually adequate), followed by flushing the wound with copious quantities of fresh sterile saline solution followed by 10% povidone-iodine solution (Pharmadine, Sherwood Pharmaceutical, Mahwah, NJ). The skin is closed using a subcuticular stitch of an absorbable suture (4-0 Dexon Plus, Davis and Geck, Inc, Manati, Puerto Rico, on a cutting needle), thereby avoiding the need for suture removal. Antibiotic ointment is placed on

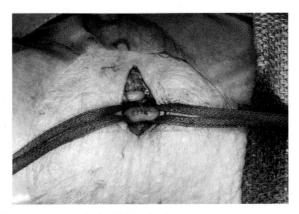

Figure 9.11 Completed repair of a brachial arteriotomy.

the suture line and covered with a firm dressing (although not so firm that it diminishes the radial pulse).

During the postprocedure period, blood pressure measurements should not be performed on the arm for 24 hours. Distal pulses, sensation, motor function, and local bleeding should be assessed without unwrapping the Ace bandage. The Ace bandage is first released 2 hours following the procedure to reassess the surgical site and then rewrapped firmly but comfortably for 48 hours. The incision should be kept dry for at least 3 days, with the Steri-Strips removed in 1 week.

TROUBLESHOOTING
Loss of Radial Pulse

The most frequent causes of an absent or diminished radial pulse following a brachial procedure are thrombosis at the arteriotomy site, embolization to the radial artery, dissection at the arteriotomy site, inappropriate suturing, and spasm. If arterial spasm was not a factor during catheter manipulation, it is unlikely to develop after arteriotomy repair and, therefore, should not be assumed to be responsible for a poor radial pulse.

Hand Numbness

Hand numbness may result from impaired circulation or median nerve compromise. If the brachial dressing is not overly tight and the radial pulse is palpable, the cause of numbness is unlikely to be circulatory. Severe median nerve injury during cutdown is usually apparent immediately as the patient experiences a striking and characteristic discomfort (electric shock sensation). The most common cause of later median nerve injury is compression induced by hematoma formation following skin closure. This usually develops gradually over the course of several hours post procedure and should be evacuated promptly to avoid potentially irreversible damage from long-standing median nerve compression.

FEMORAL, AXILLARY, AORTIC, AND TRANSAPICAL ACCESS

The success of procedures such as transcatheter aortic valve replacement exemplifies how multidisciplinary teams comprising interventional cardiologists and cardiac and vascular surgeons may achieve procedural excellence. Yet despite complementary skill sets, all team members should possess a fundamental technical knowledge of the exposure, cannulation, and closure of common sites of access to the central vasculature and the thorax.

Open Femoral Arterial Access

While the common femoral artery and its branches can be accessed using both general and local anesthesia, procedures of any significant duration would best be performed under general anesthesia. For simple exposure of the anterior wall of the common femoral artery, local anesthesia using 20 mL of 1% to 2% lidocaine produces sufficient analgesia.

Adequate access of the common femoral artery may be achieved through either a vertical or oblique skin incision. The vertical skin incision should be made using a no. 15 scalpel directly over the palpable femoral pulse from several centimeters above the groin crease inferiorly for another 5 to 7 cm (**Figure 9.12**). An oblique skin incision follows the course of the inguinal ligament just inferior to that structure and ideally measures 5 to 7 cm in length, centered on the palpable femoral pulse. If no femoral pulse is palpable, the vertical incision should be centered on the pubic escutcheon or located two-thirds of the way between the anterior superior iliac spine and symphysis pubis. The deep subcutaneous tissue overlying the femoral vessels

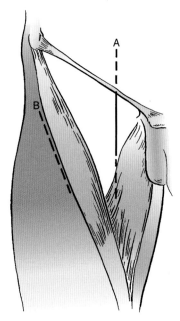

Figure 9.12 Illustration of the proximal thigh depicting a vertical incision A (dotted and solid lines) and oblique incision B (dotted lines). A is used in femoral bifurcation exposures; B is used in distal exposure of profunda femoral artery.

is dissected sharply or using electrocautery to expose the femoral sheath. Electrocautery is preferred for this dissection to seal the numerous lymphatic vessels and superficial veins encountered during the dissection. In general, limiting dissection to the anterior portion of the femoral artery and vein will minimize the risk of seroma formation. Sharp dissection in the periadventitial plane of Leriche using Metzenbaum scissors subsequently allows for safe exposure of the femoral artery and its branches. Self-retaining Weitlaner retractors provide excellent exposure to the depth of the common femoral artery. Superior retraction of the inguinal ligament by an assistant facilitates dissection of the external iliac artery when higher access is required. One must remain cautious not to inadvertently divide the circumflex iliac vein as it crosses the distal external iliac artery, as troublesome bleeding may occur.

Depending upon the diameter of the device being inserted into the common femoral artery, the lumen may be directly accessed either using the Seldinger technique or through an arteriotomy. The Seldinger technique requires a purse-string suture of 5-0 polypropylene to be placed in the anterior wall of the vessel and drawn into a tourniquet. A needle is then advanced into the lumen through the center of the purse-string suture followed by a wire. Catheters and cannulae up to 22F can be safely inserted into the common femoral artery following proper sequential dilatation in most vessels 7 mm or larger in diameter (Estech, Vascular Dilator Kit, San Ramon, CA). To facilitate passage of larger dilators, a no. 11 blade scalpel can be used to incise the anterior superior vessel wall inside the purse-string against a dilator once the dilator is in position in the vessel. Failure to advance a catheter or cannula or significant resistance should alert the operator to abandon the approach and consider alternative sites for surgical access.

Purse-string sutures aid hemostasis when using the Seldinger technique and are tied to close the arteriotomy following the procedure. Additional interrupted 5-0 polypropylene sutures placed vertically may be necessary to achieve hemostasis. A palpable pulse in the distal superficial femoral artery suggests adequate distal perfusion, but this should then be verified through palpation of the pedal pulses. Questionable distal perfusion mandates proximal and distal control of the common femoral artery, removal of the purse-string closure, and transverse closure of the arteriotomy using running or interrupted 5-0 polypropylene sutures.

Heavily diseased or calcified femoral vessels often require circumferential mobilization and proximal and distal control for intravascular access through open arteriotomy. Once the fascia overlying the femoral artery has been divided, dissection continues in the periadventitial plane medially and laterally from below the inguinal ligament superiorly to the bifurcation of the common femoral artery inferiorly (**Figure 9.13**). Small arterial branches of the common femoral artery can be either ligated with 3-0 silk suture or clipped with small titanium clips prior to sharp division. The femoral nerve and common femoral vein are nearby but protected within their own anatomic compartments. Silastic vessel loops should be passed twice around the common femoral artery superiorly and the branch vessels inferiorly for control. Prior to occlusion of the common femoral artery, heparin should be administered and anticoagulation confirmed by an activated clotting time (ACT) reading. Once the vessel loops are tightened or the vascular clamps applied, the common femoral artery may then be sharply opened transversely using a no. 11 or no. 15 scalpel and Potts scissors.

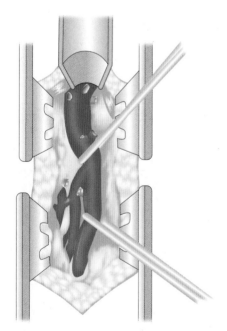

Figure 9.13 Silastic vessel loops placed around the inferior common femoral artery (superiorly) and the superficial femoral artery (inferiorly). The circumflex iliac vein has been divided to pass a silastic loop around the superior common femoral artery.

Guidewires and catheters may then be passed proximally into the central circulation by controlling the proximal silastic loop or partially releasing the common femoral arterial clamp. Serial dilators (Estech, Vascular Dilator Kit, San Ramon, CA) may be helpful in creating a larger proximal vessel even through an open arteriotomy. Introduction of larger vascular devices requires that the arteriotomy be performed midway between the inferior epigastric artery and the common femoral bifurcation. Closure of the transverse arteriotomy using running 5-0 or 6-0 polypropylene is much more reliable than purse-string closure to prevent vessel narrowing.

Meticulous technique of groin closure is the key to avoid complications. The wound itself and all 3 layers of closure should be copiously irrigated with antibiotic-containing saline solution. The deep soft tissue or fascia lata should be closed first using absorbable 2-0 polyglactin suture, taking bites of the femoral sheath to obliterate deeper dead space against the femoral vessels. The superficial subcutaneous tissue is then approximated again with 2-0 polyglactin suture. The skin may be closed using suture material or skin staples. A subcuticular absorbable 4-0 poliglecaprone suture provides a good cosmetic result and avoids the requirement to remove staples.

Common complications of femoral artery exposure include lymph fistulas and lymphocele or seroma formation. Other complications of femoral arterial access include bleeding, infection, femoral nerve injury, limb ischemia, and hematoma, pseudoaneurysm, or arteriovenous fistula formation. Secure arterial closure and vigilant assessment of distal perfusion provide the best defense here.

Axillary/Subclavian Artery Access

Patients with severe iliofemoral or distal aortic disease, severe femoral artery calcification, or small vessel diameter may require alternative access to the central circulation. In such cases, the axillary or subclavian artery provides sufficient arterial diameter and proximity to the aorta. In general, the left subclavian artery is preferred for access to the ascending aorta given its favorable trajectory along the curve of the aortic arch. Access to the subclavian or axillary artery is best performed under general anesthesia. The patient is positioned supine (semi-Fowler position) with the head rotated to the opposite side and the neck slightly hyperextended. The ipsilateral neck, chest, shoulder, and the entire clavicle should be included in the operative field.

A transverse or slightly oblique 3- to 5-cm skin incision is created using a no. 15 scalpel inferior to middle and lateral third of the clavicle. Beneath the subcutaneous tissue, the fascia overlying the pectoral muscles is identified and divided. The fibers of the pectoralis major are divided along their length and held apart by placing a self-retaining Weitlaner retractor. The underlying pectoralis minor tendon may require release laterally but often can be retracted to avoid division. In the fat pad deep to the pectoral muscles, there exist a number of venous tributaries to the subclavian vein. These veins should be divided using either clips or 3-0 silk ties to facilitate superior retraction of the subclavian vein to expose the deeper subclavian artery. The subclavian artery exists medial to the outer border of the first rib at which point it becomes the axillary artery. Regardless of this, this arterial structure has few branches at this location, having proximally given off the internal mammary artery, vertebral artery, and thyrocervical trunk.

At least 3 to 5 cm of the subclavian artery should be dissected free to obtain proximal and distal control with silastic or rubber vessel loops passed twice around the vessel (**Figure 9.14**). Caution should be exercised when passing vessel loops to avoid small posterior arterial branches and to recognize the thin-walled nature of this vessel and its sometimes tortuous course. With vessel loops safely in place, anticoagulation must then be administered.

A transverse arteriotomy created using a no. 11 scalpel and Potts scissors provides excellent exposure even when using the Seldinger technique for arterial access. Guidewires and dilators may be passed proximally directly through the skin incision

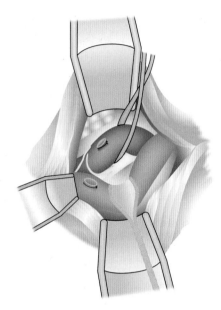

Figure 9.14 The distal subclavian and proximal axillary artery controlled with a silastic vessel loop under the divided pectoralis major and minor.

or may require a more laterally placed access incision if the angle through the skin incision is too acute. Alternatively, anastomosis of an 8-mm Dacron graft to the subclavian artery provides a route to more easily pass guidewires and catheters remote from the vessel itself. To place this Dacron graft, a longitudinal arteriotomy is created using a no. 11 scalpel. A 4.4-mm aortic punch typically used for coronary anastomoses can then be placed through the arteriotomy and fired several times to create an oval arteriotomy. The Dacron graft is then anastomosed to the subclavian artery in an end-to-side fashion using 5-0 or 6-0 polypropylene suture. To close the Dacron graft, place a small vascular clamp across the graft close to the subclavian vessel, divide, and oversew the graft end with 6-0 polypropylene. Closure of the incision requires 2-0 polyglactin for deeper tissues and 4-0 poligle-caprone or staples for skin closure. Although no drain is required, note that pneumothorax may complicate this access route given the adherence of the pleura to the deep wall of the subclavian artery. As always, the access procedure is not complete until distal perfusion has been assessed as adequate. Complications associated with axillary or subclavian access include stroke, arterial or aortic dissection, thrombus formation, and limb ischemia.

Direct Transthoracic Aortic Access

Upper ministernotomy and right anterior thoracotomy provide access to the ascending aortic and are common approaches used for open isolated aortic valve replacement by cardiac surgeons. Both approaches require general anesthesia. Ministernotomy requires a 6-cm vertical skin incision centered on the angle of Louis at the sternomanubrial junction. The sternum is divided from the manubrium to the level of the third intercostal space. A transverse division of the sternum into the third interspace bilaterally or unilaterally to the right provides visualization of the upper mediastinum including the ascending aorta. This approach generally avoids entry into either thorax, accessing the mediastinum directly. Once the thymic fat has been divided, the pericardium is divided vertically and tacked up to the skin using 2-0 silk sutures to create a "pericardial well" centered on the ascending aorta. Vascular access of the ascending aorta follows as routinely performed by cardiac surgeons to institute cardiopulmonary bypass. Two Teflon felt pledgeted purse-string 3-0 polypropylene sutures are placed in the ascending aorta through which vascular access may be obtained in either an antegrade or a retrograde fashion. Alternatively, a side-biting vascular clamp can be placed on the ascending aorta to permit the creation of an aortotomy using a no. 11 scalpel. The aortotomy is then enlarged using a 4.4-mm punch tool to create a defect large enough to allow for anastomosis of an 8-mm Dacron graft in an end-to-side fashion using 5-0 or 6-0 polypropylene. Vascular access can then occur remote from the aorta through the Dacron graft. The Dacron graft can be oversewn at the completion of the procedure using 5-0 polypropylene. Chest closure requires sternal wires and closed mediastinal drainage.

Right anterior thoracotomy provides aortic access similar to that of the upper ministernotomy but requires entry into the thorax. Patient positioning and preparation are identical to a ministernotomy. A 5- to 7-cm transverse skin incision is created over the right second intercostal space adjacent to the sternum. Dividing the pectus major and the underlying intercostal muscle above the third rib reveals the right side of the mediastinum. The right internal mammary artery and vein are typically divided between medium titanium hemoclips, although in some cases they can be spared. The upper pericardium is then divided vertically along the right side of the ascending aorta, and stay stitches (2-0 silk) are placed through the pericardium and skin to distract the upper mediastinum to the patient's right side. The ascending aorta lies at the base of the incision for access identical to that through the ministernotomy. Rib approximation may not be necessary for closure of a small thoracotomy, but chest tube placement is recommended.

One advantage to both ministernotomy and small right thoracotomy is that catastrophic complications of procedures performed through small chest incisions are more easily converted to open operations with institution of cardiopulmonary bypass if necessary.

Left Ventricular Apical Access

Access to the left ventricular apex is a surgical procedure that should be performed under general anesthesia using a double-lumen endotracheal tube or bronchial blocker to provide single (right) lung ventilation during the procedure. The patient is positioned supine and the entire chest, abdomen, and pelvis should be included in the operative field. The left ventricular apex is approached through a 5- to 7-cm transverse skin incision placed to the left of the sternum, roughly centered on the midclavicular line. The level of the skin incision should provide access to the fifth and sixth intercostal spaces. Preoperative computed tomography scanning is helpful in planning the location of the skin incision. In addition, transthoracic echocardiography using a sterile sleeve can assist in identifying the left ventricular apex. The left ventricular apex may also be palpable to guide incision location.

Dissection of the subcutaneous tissue and division of the fibers of the underlying pectus major reveals the underlying bony chest wall. Electrocautery is used to divide the intercostal muscle along the superior aspect of the chosen rib to provide entry to the thorax and to avoid the intercostal neurovascular bundle. If the apex is not apparent, either another interspace can be entered through the same skin incision or the rib can be notched with a rib shear. As a rule, it is better to be too low rather than too high when approaching the left ventricular apex because stay sutures of 2-0 polypropylene can be distracted downward into view. These stay sutures are passed through the longitudinally divided pericardium and then through the skin.

Two 2-0 polypropylene purse-string sutures on an MH needle with Teflon felt pledgets are placed ideally on the anterior left ventricular wall to include the apex. In this location,

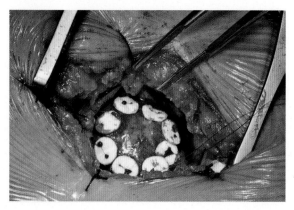

Figure 9.15 Transapical ventricular approach. The left ventricular apex has been exposed and prepared for transapical aortic valve replacement. Concentric purse-string sutures reinforced with pledgets have been placed at the left ventricular apex. (Courtesy of Alan W. Heldman, MD, University of Miami.)

there is less epicardial fat and a greater likelihood that sutures have achieved significant purchase of myocardium but without entering the left ventricular cavity. These sutures are then passed through tourniquets to control bleeding as catheters or devices are placed through the apex (**Figures 9.15** and **9.16**). Care should be taken to acknowledge the location of the left anterior descending coronary artery to avoid injury.

Closure of the left ventricular apex requires tying the purse-string sutures following the procedure (**Figure 9.17**) and is greatly facilitated by the use of a titanium knot fastener (Cor-knot, LSI Solutions, Victor, NY). Additional pledgeted 3-0 or 4-0 polypropylene sutures may be required to achieve hemostasis, and the thin left ventricular apex represents a true surgical challenge in this regard. The pericardium may be closed with interrupted 2-0 silk sutures or left open. A left pleural chest tube (28F or 32F) is required, although a small pericardial drain is preferred by some (19F).

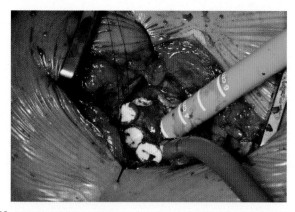

Figure 9.16 Transapical ventricular approach for aortic valve replacement. Insertion of the introducer sheath through the left ventricular apex. (Courtesy of Alan W. Heldman, MD, University of Miami.)

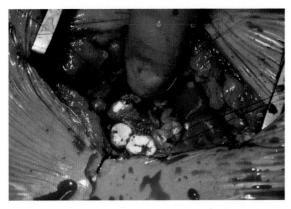

Figure 9.17 Transapical aortic valve replacement. The introducer sheath has been removed and the purse-string sutures have been tied to secure hemostasis. (Courtesy of Alan W. Heldman, MD, University of Miami.)

Pericostal sutures are required to approximate the interspace only if a rib was divided or notched (no.1 polyglactin). The pectoral fibers are then closed in a running fashion (0 polyglactin) as is the subcutaneous tissue (2-0 polyglactin). The skin should be closed with a running subcuticular stitch (4-0 poliglecaprone). The chest tubes are then placed to −20 cm water suction to complete the procedure. The potential complications of this vascular access route primarily include bleeding, coronary artery damage, false aneurysm formation, and respiratory complications.

SUGGESTED READINGS

1. Baker LD, Leshin SJ, Mathur VS, Messer JV. Routine Fogarty thrombectomy in arterial catheterization. *N Engl J Med.* 1968;279(22):1203-1205.
2. Bleiziffer S, Piazza N, Mazzitelli D, Opitz A, Bauernschmitt R, Lange R. Apical-access-related complications associated with trans-catheter aortic valve implantation. *Eur J Cardio Thorac Surg.* 2011;40(2):469-474.
3. Bruschi G, De Marco F, Fratto P, et al. Direct aortic access through right minithoracotomy for implantation of self-expanding aortic bioprosthetic valves. *J Thorac Cardiovasc Surg.* 2010;140(3):715-717.
4. Bruschi G, Fratto P, De Marco F, et al. The trans-subclavian retrograde approach for transcatheter aortic valve replacement: singlecenter experience. *J Thorac Cardiovasc Surg.* 2010;140(4):911-915, 915.e1-2.
5. Bruschi G, De Marco F, Botta L, et al. Direct transaortic corevalve implantation through right minithoracotomy in patients with patent coronary grafts. *Ann Thorac Surg.* 2012;93(4):1297-1299.
6. Caceres M, Braud R, Roselli EE. The axillary/subclavian artery access route for transcatheter aortic valve replacement: a systematic review of the literature. *Ann Thorac Surg.* 2012;93(3):1013-1018.
7. Etienne PY, Papadatos S, El Khoury E, Pieters D, Price J, Glineur D. Transaortic transcatheter aortic valve implantation with the Edwards Sapien valve: feasibility, technical considerations, and clinical advantages. *Ann Thorac Surg.* 2011;92(2):746-748.
8. Stoney RJ, Effeney DJ. *Comprehensive Vascular Exposures.* Lippincott-Raven; 1998.
9. Walther T, Dewey T, Borger MA, et al. Transapical aortic valve implantation: step by step. *Ann Thorac Surg.* 2009;87(1):276-283.
10. Willson A, Toggweiler S, Webb JG. Transfemoral aortic valve replacement with the SAPIEN XT valve: step-by-step. *Semin Thorac Cardiovasc Surg.* 2011;23(1):51-54.
11. Wong DR, Ye J, Cheung A, Webb JG, Carere RG, Lichtenstein SV. Technical considerations to avoid pitfalls during transapical aortic valve implantation. *J Thorac Cardiovasc Surg.* 2010;140(1):196-202.
12. Zierer A, Wimmer-Greinecker G, Martens S, Moritz A, Doss M. The transapical approach for aortic valve implantation. *J Thorac Cardiovasc Surg.* 2008;136(4):948-953.
13. Zierer A, Wimmer-Greinecker G, Martens S, Moritz A, Doss M. Is transapical aortic valve implantation really less invasive than minimally invasive aortic valve replacement? *J Thorac Cardiovasc Surg.* 2009;138(5):1067-1072.

10 Diagnostic Catheterization in Childhood and Adult Congenital Heart Disease[1]

As a growing population reaches adulthood after being treated during infancy for congenital heart disease, a significant proportion of patients undergoing cardiac catheterization for congenital cardiac abnormalities now is older than 18 years. The majority of surviving patients have increasingly complex anatomy and physiology, given that >60% of adult patients with congenital heart disease have had at least 1 surgery prior to their adult years, and approximately half of these patients have had a reoperation during adulthood. A complete review of every aspect of individual "natural" and prior operated history (**Table 10.1**) and anatomy (with particular attention to the specifics of each intervention) is required prior to embarking upon any catheter-based investigation (**Table 10.2**). This should be coupled with a full understanding of anatomic and physiologic variations and sequelae, as well as awareness and potential to perform intervention, as needed.

GENERAL PRINCIPLES IN THE CATHETERIZATION OF PATIENTS WITH CONGENITAL HEART DISEASE
Vascular Access/Vessel and Chamber Entry

Although femoral or jugular arterial and venous access can be used in larger children and adults, special access routes are usually required in neonates and infants.

Umbilical Vessels

Umbilical vessels have decreasing patency over the first 72 postnatal hours, but their use allows sparing of other vessels. Vascular access via the umbilical vein (5F umbilical catheter entry) directs catheter position posteriorly in the right atrium (RA), which assists balloon atrial septostomy but adds considerable difficulty to achieving stable right ventricle (RV) and pulmonary artery (PA) access. Given the nearly 180° turns involved in catheter passage (umbilical vein portal vein ductus venosus inferior vena cava [IVC] right atrium), concomitant angiographic delineation of course during entry is suggested. Hand-administered contrast injection to demonstrate ductus patency, combined with the use of either a tip-deflecting or a torque-controlled wire, permits posterior advancement of the catheter, avoidance of intubation of the liver, and successful passage of the umbilical vein catheter to the IVC, where it is exchanged for an access sheath after angiographic corroboration.

Direct Hepatic Vein

Direct hepatic vein entry can be considered when the femoral veins are impassable. A Chiba needle is passed between the mid and anterior axillary line, near the costal margin between the diaphragm and the inferior liver edge. The needle is typically advanced using ultrasound guidance, passing posteriorly and cephalad toward the intrahepatic IVC or just caudal to the IVC-RA junction, to within a few centimeters of the right border of the spine. Contrast injection confirms entry into a large central

[1]We gratefully acknowledge the Grossman & Baim's *Cardiac Catheterization, Angiography, and Intervention*, 9th edition contributions of Drs. Gabriele Egidy Assenza and Michael J Lndzberg as portions of their chapter, Diagnostic Catheterization in Childhood and Adult Congenital Heart Disease, were retained in this text.

Table 10.1 **Typical Categorization of Surgical Repairs**

Name	Typical Lesion Application	Surgical Connection	
Glenn (classic)	Single ventricle/TA	SVC to (right) pulmonary artery	End-to-end
(bidirectional)	Single ventricle/TA	SVC to R/MPA	End-to-side
Fontan (atriopulmonary)	Single ventricle/TA	Atrial appendage to RV or PA	
(cavopulmonary)		IVC-SVC intra- or extracardiac baffle to PAs	
Waterston	TOF/DORV/ pulmonary atresia	Ascending aorta to RPA	Side-to side
Potts	TOF/DORV/ pulmonary atresia	Descending aorta to LPA	Side-to-side
Blalock-Taussig (classic)	TOF/DORV/ pulmonary atresia	Subclavian artery to branch PA	End-to-side
(modified)	TOF/DORV/ pulmonary atresia	Conduit from subclavian artery to branch PA	Side-to-side
Mustard/Senning (atrial switch)	TGA	Baffle directing SVC-IVC flow to subpulmonary LV, pulmonary venous flow to subsystemic RV	End-to-end
Arterial switch	TGA	Translocation of more-posterior MPA to anterior supra-LV position, more-anterior aorta to posterior supra-PA position, coronary arterial reimplantation	
Rastelli	TGA/TOF	Conduit between subpulmonary ventricle and PA	
Norwood	HLHS	Translocation of proximal MPA to supra-LV position, end-to-side anastomosis of distal MPA to aorta, modified Blalock-Taussig shunt	
Double switch	TGA	Atrial switch + arterial switch	

DORV, double outlet right ventricle; HLHS, hypoplastic left heart syndrome; IVC, inferior vena cava; LPA, left pulmonary artery; LV, left ventricle; MPA, main pulmonary artery; PA, pulmonary artery; RPA, right pulmonary artery; RV, right ventricle; SVC, superior vena cava; TA, tricuspid atresia; TGA, transposition of the great arteries (L, left; D, right); TOF, tetralogy of Fallot.
All patients have variations mandating detailed review of operative reporting.

Table 10.2	Typical Indications for Diagnostic Catheterizations/Preferred Imaging Modalities/ Interventions		
Typical Lesion(s)	**Diagnostic Cath Typical Indications**	**Preferred Imaging Modalities**	**Cath Indication: Interventional**
ASD secundum	No: useful for PVR when PHT suspect → ASD test occlusion; PHT vasodilator testing; HD-based management of RV and LV dysfunction	TEE/ICE	ASD closure
PFO	No	TEE/ICE	PFO closure when indicated
ASD sinus venosus	Debated: higher incidence PHT: useful for PVR when PHT suspect; see above	MRI	
ASD primum	No	TEE	
AV canal defect	No: with increasing age, increased risk of PHT→ check PVR; see above	TEE	
TAPVR	Debated: PVR, PV anatomy, and rule out stenoses	Cath/MRI	
VSD, membranous	No: uncommon need to assess PVR	TTE/MRI	Investigational closure
VSD, multiple muscular	No: HD-based management of ventricular dysfunction, when indicated	TTE/MRI	VSD closure
AS/ regurgitation: subvalvular/ supravalvar	Debated: hemodynamic changes remain the standard for intervention in children and young adults with valvar AS Supravalvar AS: useful to define relationship to CA origins AR: demonstration of fistulous connections when indicated	TTE/TEE/MRI	AS: valve dilations
Aortic coarctation	No: hemodynamic changes remain the standard for intervention in children and adults	MRI	Dilation/stent
PDA	No: PA pressure when PHT suspect → PDA test occlusion	TTE/MRI	PDA closure
Valvar PS	No: HD-based management of RV failure when appropriate	TTE/MRI	Valve dilation
Peripheral PS	No: HD-based management of RV failure or PHT when appropriate	Nuclear scintigraphy/MRI	PA dilation/stent

Typical Lesion(s)	Diagnostic Cath Typical Indications	Preferred Imaging Modalities	Cath Indication: Interventional
TOF, preoperative	No: anatomy when CAs, VSDs, Ao-PA collaterals cannot be otherwise sufficiently imaged	TTE/MRI	Close muscular VSDs
TOF, postoperative	Assess for residual shunts; HD-based management of RV or LV dysfunction; PHT therapy	TTE/MRI	Close residual shunts/VSDs; PA or conduit dilation/stent
TOF, pulmonary atresia	Yes: define PA anatomy and hemodynamics	MRI	Close Ao-PA connections; dilate/stent stenoses
Pulmonary atresia/intact septum	In children, define coronary anatomy; in adults, define CA anatomy or HD-based management of ventricular dysfunction, as indicated		
TGA-D, preoperative	No	TTE	Atrial septostomy
TGA-D, postoperative atrial switch	Assessment of residual shunting; HD-based management of systemic ventricular dysfunction or PHT	MRI	Shunt closure
TGA-D VSD/PS; truncus; DORV postoperative	No; HD-based management of systemic ventricular dysfunction or PHT	MRI	Shunt closure; conduit dilation/stent
TGA-D, postoperative arterial switch	Assessment of PA stenoses, coronary arterial stenoses	MRI; IVUS	CA dilation/stent
TGA-L	HD-based management of systemic ventricular dysfunction	MRI	
Single ventricle, preoperative	Yes: hemodynamics/PVR	TTE/MRI	Close collaterals, PA dilation/stent
Single ventricle, post-Fontan	Yes: HD-based management of load and ventricular function	MRI	Conduit and PA dilation/stent; close collaterals

Table 10.2 **Typical Indications for Diagnostic Catheterizations/Preferred Imaging Modalities/Interventions (Continued)**

Ao, aorta; AR, aortic regurgitation; AS, aortic stenosis; ASD, atrial septal defect; AV, atrioventricular; CA, coronary artery; DORV, double outlet right ventricle; HD, hemodynamics; ICE, intracardiac echocardiography; IVUS, intravascular ultrasonography; LV, left ventricle; MRI, magnetic resonance imaging; PA, pulmonary artery; PFO, patent foramen ovale; PHT, pulmonary hypertension; PS, pulmonary stenosis; PV, pulmonary valve; PVR, pulmonary vascular resistance; RV, right ventricle; TAPVR, total anomalous pulmonary venous return; TEE, transesophageal echocardiography; TGA, transposition of the great arteries (L, left; D, right); TOF, tetralogy of Fallot; TTE, transthoracic echocardiography; VSD, ventricular septal defect.

hepatic vein, where a sheath and a dilator are advanced over a guidewire to the RA. Large sheath entry and transseptal passage can be performed without complication via this route. At the end of the procedure, a catheter 1F size smaller than the entry catheter is exchanged, and this sheath is withdrawn, with hand injection of contrast until the sheath is out of the vessel and within the liver parenchymal tract. This tract is then filled with either coils or Gelfoam.

Intracardiac Catheter Manipulation

Entry to the superior vena cava (SVC) is easiest via advancement of a straight wire or catheter from the IVC (soft catheters tend to advance anteriorly toward the atrial appendage, away from the SVC). A straight catheter may be gently advanced with a soft counterclockwise rolling to ensure freedom of the catheter tip.

On occasion, interruption of the IVC, with azygous continuation, may complicate catheter passage, markedly elongating the catheter course. Multiple curves along the catheter course make further posterior or transseptal passage extremely difficult from this access.

Entry of the RV can be facilitated either by advancement of a preformed catheter with curvature aimed toward the tricuspid valve (TV) or with a soft-tipped catheter into which the preformed bend on the stiff end of a wire or a tip-deflecting wire may be introduced, *always leaving the wire within the catheter rather than allowing it to protrude into the vasculature*. The guidewire-soft-catheter technique allows for adjustment of entry angle and length of curvature by balancing the distance of the guidewire tip from the catheter end, prior to catheter advancement over the guidewire. Particular care must be taken with this approach to ensure that the catheter tip is moving freely, prior to further manipulation or balloon tip inflation.

Intubation of a normally positioned RV outflow/main pulmonary artery (MPA) may be difficult when (1) the RV is particularly dilated or (2) the TV is regurgitant. Passage via an internal jugular or subclavian vein approach may increase stability and aid in anterior angulation to and through the RV outflow tract. A multipurpose or similarly precurved soft-tipped catheter can be turned gently in clockwise fashion, with either concomitant contrast injection or use of a torque-controlled wire. Similarly, a soft balloon end-hole catheter can be stiffened at its distal end either with a sharp S-shaped bend to the stiff end of a 0.035-in guidewire or with a tip-deflecting wire, to facilitate passage to the RV outflow tract. An alternative approach requires the creation of a controlled loop in the RA to enhance catheter stability to engage the RV outflow and MPA.

When the PAs are posteriorly directed (TGA [transposition of the great arteries]), entry via the subpulmonary left ventricle (LV) is generally performed with a soft-tipped, balloon end-hole catheter placed in the LV apex. After ensuring that the catheter tip is free, a tip-deflecting wire is placed within the catheter, proximal to its tip, and is deflected with sufficient traction to guide the catheter tip in a posterior direction, away from the ventricular apex, and toward the base of the heart. A slight retraction of both catheter and guidewire, as a unit, is typically performed, allowing alignment with the LV outflow. The guidewire is held firmly, acting as a fulcrum from which the catheter is extruded, away from the ventricular apex and into the LV outflow.

Left atrial entry via a transseptal approach can be accomplished on retraction from the SVC with gentle counterclockwise rotation of a leftward-facing catheter or with clockwise advancement from a similarly leftward-facing catheter positioned near the TV. Biplane fluoroscopic assessment facilitates safe transseptal passage. Typical antero-posterior (AP) location of the atrial septum is frequently just rightward of the center of the spine. Posterior, clockwise catheter rotation from this position will facilitate passage into the pulmonary veins, which may be probed with use of a torque-controlled guidewire. The position of the wire/catheter should be checked using a lateral projection to ensure that the wire/catheter takes a posterior course and is not located within the left atrial appendage, or anteriorly toward the aorta. Lower pulmonary vein entry is frequently facilitated by use of a tight, near-180°C-shaped compound curve to the stiff end of a guidewire placed within the entry catheter, directing it to the vessel orifice. Left pulmonary venous entry is typically routine on crossing the atrial septum, although it may be complicated by entry into the atrial appendage. Considerable catheter retraction and further posterior redirection outside of the appendage typically facilitates left pulmonary venous entry. The right-sided pulmonary veins typically require further posterior, clockwise rotation until the catheter tip appears on AP projection to be to the right of the spine, and then subsequent catheter advancement.

High-volume shunts (Waterston/Pott/alternative central aorta to PA) may be entered via transiently inflated, balloon-tipped flotation catheters, or with preformed individually adjusted catheters (eg, Judkins right coronary catheter modified by cutting its distal tip) directed manually or via tip-deflecting or torque-controlled wires. A preformed Cobra catheter or a modified pigtail (individually cut to approximately 180°) may facilitate torque-controlled wire passage from the subclavian artery through a Blalock-Taussig shunt.

The ductus arteriosus was one of the original congenital defects intubated during early catheterization attempts, although this is rarely present in adult congenital cardiac cases. The ductus, when present, can be intubated relatively easily from either an anterograde venous or retrograde arterial approach. From the descending aorta, a preshaped catheter (Cobra, right Judkins, or multipurpose in children; left Judkins in adults) directs a soft-tipped torque-controlled guidewire across the ductus. From a venous approach, stationing of a multipurpose catheter within the MPA angled slightly leftward to the MPA-LPA junction allows similar passage of a soft-tipped straight or torque-controlled guidewire across the ductus.

Pressure Measurements and Oximetry

Pressure and systolic or diastolic gradient measurements require stability of loading conditions and contractility, as well as precise localization of the catheter tip.

Oximetry remains the gold standard for shunt detection. Modern high-fidelity oximeters have an error range of approximately ±3%. This, combined with flow sampling and venous mixing errors, leads to a required oximetric saturation difference between 4% and 9% to be assured of the presence of left to right shunting. Commonly utilized formulas for shunt and resistance calculation and a box diagram for displaying hemodynamic and oximetric data are shown in **Table 10.3** and **Figure 10.1**.

Factors regarding congenital heart disease–related oximetry and measure of vascular flow and resistance that should be recognized include:

1. Shunt detection is enhanced in the presence of low systemic venous saturation.
2. Total pulmonary vascular resistance (PVR) is lowered by recruitment of any additional conduit for flow, regardless of resistance of that vessel (PVR is calculated in series).
3. PVR is typically flow dependent. Recruitment of additional zones of pulmonary blood flow at greater amounts of pulmonary blood flow allows for decrease in overall resistance. Hence, surgical elimination of shunt flow to the lungs may not, in fact, lead to decrease in pulmonary pressures (as would be estimated if pulmonary blood flow decreased with a constant PVR) but rather may allow for persistently elevated pulmonary pressures due to reduction in Qp and elevation in PVR.
4. When multiple sources of pulmonary blood flow with differing oxygen saturations (eg, Qp effective from a systemic venous shunt along with ineffective sys-

Table 10.3 Commonly Utilized Formulas for Shunt and Resistance Calculations

Parameter	Working Equation* Without Supplemental O_2	Working Equation* With Supplemental O_2
BSA Mosteller (m^2)	$\sqrt{[(Weight*Height)/3600]}$	
BSA Dubois (m^2)	$0.007184*(Height^{0.725})*(Weight^{0.425})$	
Qp (L/min)	$VO_2/(PVsat-PAsat)*(Hgb*1.36*10)$	$VO_2/[(PVsat)*(Hgb*1.36*10) + (PVpO_2*0.03)] - [(PAsat)*(Hgb*1.36*10)]$
Qpi (L/min/m^2)	$(VO_2/BSA)/(PVsat-PAsat)*(Hgb*1.36*10)$	$(VO_2/BSA)/[(PVsat)*(Hgb*1.36*10) + (PVpO_2*0.03)] - [(PAsat)*(Hgb*1.36*10)]$
Qs (L/min)	$VO_2/(Aosat-SVCsat)*(Hgb*1.36*10)$	$VO_2/[(Aosat)*(Hgb*1.36*10) + (AopO_2*0.03)] - [(MVsat)*(Hgb*1.36*10)]$
Qsi (L/min/m^2)	$(VO_2/BSA)/(Aosat-SVCsat)*(Hgb*1.36*10)$	$(VO_2/BSA)/[(Aosat)*(Hgb*1.36*10) + (AopO_2*0.03)] - [(MVsat)*(Hgb*1.36*10)]$
Qp/Qs	(Aosat-SVCsat)/(PVsat-PAsat)	
PVR (WU)	Mean PA pressure-PCW/Qp	
PVRi (WU*m^2)	Mean PA pressure-PCW/Qpi	
SVR (WU)	Mean Ao pressure-SVC/Qs	
SVRi (WU*m^2)	Mean Ao pressure-SVC/Qsi	
Effective Qp (Qs) (L/min)	$VO_2/(PVsat-SVCsat)(Hgb*1.36*10)$	$VO_2/[(PVsat)*(Hgb*1.36*10) + (PVpO_2*0.03)] - [(MVsat)*(Hgb*1.36*10)]$
Left-to-right shunt (L/min)	Qp-effective Qp	
Right-to-left shunt (L/min)	Qs-effective Qs	
% Left-to-right shunt (%)	(PAsat-SVCsat)/(PVsat-SVCsat)	
% Right-to-left shunt (%)	(PVsat-Aosat)/(PVsat-SVCsat)	
ΔO_2 (%)	$1.36*Hgb*(Aosat-SVCsat)$	$[(1.36*Hgb*10*Aosat) + (AopO_2*0.03)] - (1.36*Hgb*10*MVsat)$
VO_2 (male) (mL/min)	$BSA*[138.1 - (11.49*lnAge) + (0.378*HR)]$	
VO_2 (female) (mL/min)	$BSA*[138.1 - (17.04*lnAge) + (0.378*HR)]$	

Ao, aorta; Hgb, hemoglobin (gr/dL); MV, mixed venous; p, pulmonary; PA, pulmonary artery; PV, pulmonary vein; PVR, pulmonary vascular resistance; Q, flow; s, systemic; sat, saturation; SVC, superior vena cava; SVR, systemic vascular resistance; VO_2, oxygen consumption.

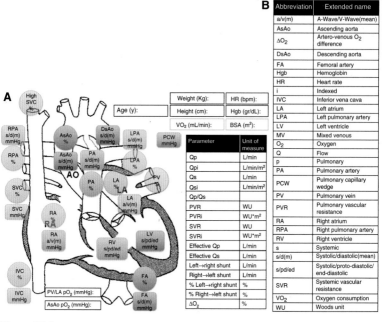

B Abbreviation	Extended name
a/v(m)	A-Wave/V-Wave(mean)
AsAo	Ascending aorta
ΔO₂	Artero-venous O₂ difference
DsAo	Descending aorta
FA	Femoral artery
Hgb	Hemoglobin
HR	Heart rate
i	Indexed
IVC	Inferior vena cava
LA	Left atrium
LPA	Left pulmonary artery
LV	Left ventricle
MV	Mixed venous
O₂	Oxygen
Q	Flow
p	Pulmonary
PA	Pulmonary artery
PCW	Pulmonary capillary wedge
PV	Pulmonary vein
PVR	Pulmonary vascular resistance
RA	Right atrium
RPA	Right pulmonary artery
RV	Right ventricle
s	Systemic
s/d(m)	Systolic/diastolic(mean)
s/pd/ed	Systolic/proto-diastolic/end-diastolic
SVR	Systemic vascular resistance
VO₂	Oxygen consumption
WU	Woods unit

Figure 10.1 Commonly used box diagram for displaying hemodynamic and oximetric data. *Open circles* surround oximetric percent at a given location, whereas pressures are recorded directly where they were measured. Full color box and circles denote standard location for pressure measurement and saturation sampling. Lighter color box and circles are often used in the presence of complex congenital defect with shunt and/or abnormal pulmonary vein drainage or connection.

temic arterial flow from an aortopulmonary shunt) exist in given lung segments or in the entire lung, segmental or total Qp cannot be directly measured. However, isolation of each source of flow, temporary occlusion of all but 1 source, and measure of pulmonary blood flow (mean PA and PV pressures, PA and PV saturations) from that single source to the lung segment(s) in question can allow calculation of PVR, albeit at a typically lower flow ("worst case scenario" of PVR).

5. Single ventricular (Fontan circulation) palliative physiology is particularly sensitive to increases of PVR or decreases in pulmonary vascular capacitance and, as such, challenges the ability of hemodynamic-driven parameters to accurately reflect the real burden of vascular impedance. In addition, Fontan circulation relies on very low hydraulic energy dissipation profile, as no ventricle supports the pulmonary circulation. Sophisticated approaches using computational fluid dynamic investigations and in vitro hydraulic measurements of hydraulic power loss have demonstrated that energy dissipation in Fontan is influenced by branch point configuration of the Fontan pathway, minimal lumen area, and flow distribution between LPA and RPA. The ability of catheter-based measurements to collect such important information is limited, thus affecting the role of diagnostic catheterization to detect subtle changes contributing to hemodynamic compromise and functional well-being in persons with Fontan circulation.

6. Measurement of vascular pressures and resistance may be affected by recent trauma (vascular intervention) or inflammation/infection, localized compression (eg, by adjacent structures, surrounding effusion, or atelectasis), contrast administration, or changes in systemic adrenergic state, local pH, pCO_2, or pO_2. Optimally, key aspects of hemodynamic assessment are performed prior to significant contrast exposure, perturbation of resting stable state, or intervention.

7. Cardiac output can be measured using thermodilution principle in subjects without intravascular shunting; in the presence of intracardiac or central intravascular shunting this will lead to under- or overestimation of pulmonary and/or systemic output. Accordingly, determination of pulmonary and systemic cardiac output using the oxygen-based Fick principle is of paramount importance in patients with congenital heart disease (**Table 10.3**).

Angiography

Viewing vessels, chambers, and their connections requires multiple (typically orthogonal) views that minimize overlap and foreshortening of critical areas (**Table 10.4**). Optimally, biplane or multiplane imagery is utilized to decrease radiation and contrast exposure. Recording of individualized angiographic angles and views utilized enhances accuracy of later comparisons.

Contrast administration is typically limited to a dose per injection that is tolerated by the involved ventricle (eg, segmental or subsegmental PA injections are preferable to larger branch or MPA injections in patients with elevated PVR or RV contractile dysfunction).

Given that total contrast administration is designed to optimally be <5 mL/kg/catheterization, complete angiographic planning should be performed before the procedure.

1. Specific angiographic views serve as reasonable starting points for imaging sites or lesions, with individualized adjustment (**Table 10.4**).

2. The best angiography may be performed with greatest fidelity and least contrast exposure when angiography is performed via a side-hole angiographic catheter or via injection through a large-bore, "guiding" sheath, at the site, upstream, or downstream of flow through the region of question in order to maximize anatomic imaging.

3. Retrograde imaging via wedge angiography may assist in delineation of otherwise unreachable vessels or chambers. Some patients, as a result of a congenital defect or prior cardiac surgery, have complete occlusion of a proximal PA (typically the left). Owing to bronchial arterial collateralization of the more distal portion of the occluded branch PA, this vessel may remain patent even decades later. A balloon-tipped end-hole catheter can be placed into the draining vessel (typically the corresponding PV) from which the image is desired (typically the occluded PA). With the balloon inflated, <0.3 mL/kg of nonionic contrast agent is injected and followed immediately by an equal volume of saline. The parenchymal vessels are usually well outlined by this method, with back-filling, if present, of the mediastinal segment. On occasion, the main and contralateral PA may also fill in, if they are in continuity. The use of biplane cineangiography can facilitate the accurate identification of the degree of proximal extension of the vessel relative to landmarks, such as the bronchus, on that side.

4. Rotational angiography has recently been introduced as a useful diagnostic tool for complex 3-dimensional anatomies. Images are acquired using a synchronized gantry rotation during continuous contrast injection into the target anatomy (**Figure 10.2**). In the event of high-flow structure (such as aorta,

Table 10.4 **Typical Angiographic Projections and Lesions Best Imaged**

Projection	Degrees	Vessel/Chamber Imaged	Lesion(s)
Long axial oblique	70° LAO, 30° cranial	LV	Membranous VSD, conotruncal VSD, LVOT obstruction
Hepatoclavicular	45° LAO, 45° cranial	LV	AV canal defect, mid-muscular VSD
		4 chambers	LV-RA connections
Lateral	90°	RV/branch PAs	PS/PPS/TGA/DORV
		Descending aorta	Coarctation/PDA
LAO	60°-70° LAO	Aorta	Coarctation/aortic valve disease
LAO-cranial	15° LAO, 30° cranial	MPA-branch origins	TOF/PA stenoses
Steep LAO-cranial	60° LAO, 15° cranial	Atrial septum	ASD, PFO
AP-cranial	0° LAO, 30° cranial	RV/conduits	TOF/PS/DORV
AP-caudal	0° LAO, 45° caudal	Ascending aorta/ coronary artery origins	TGA/DORV/anomalous CA origins
AP	0°	RV, peripheral PAs	TGA/DORV/peripheral PS
		Pulmonary veins	Pulmonary vein stenoses/ anomalies of origin/connection
RAO	30° RAO, with or without caudal angulation	LV, RVOT	Anterior VSD, mitral valve disease, failing RVOT

Ao, aorta; ASD, atrial septal defect; AV, atrioventricular; CA, coronary artery; DORV, double outlet right ventricle; LAO, left anterior oblique; LV, left ventricle; LVOT, left ventricular outflow tract; PA, pulmonary artery; PDA, patent ductus arteriosus; PFO, patent foramen ovale; (P)PS, (peripheral) pulmonary stenosis; RAO, right anterior oblique; RV, right ventricle; RVOT, right ventricular outflow tract; TGA, transposition of the great arteries (L, left; D, right); TOF, tetralogy of Fallot; VSD, ventricular septal defect.

pulmonary arteries), rapid ventricular pacing is required to transiently reduce stroke cardiac volume and allow for increasing structure delineation. To reduce contrast volume administration, a 60% saline dilution of contrast media is usually performed. Rotational angiography can provide full volume assessment of complex anatomy, resulting in a reduction of procedural time and improvement of interventional planning by allowing rapid roadmap guidance of complex interventions.

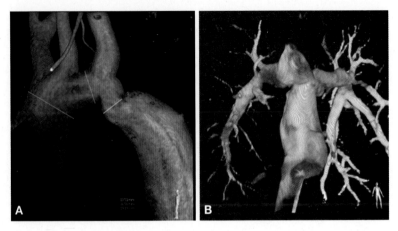

Figure 10.2 Three-dimensional reconstruction of 2 rotational angiographies in 2 patients with congenital heart disease. **A,** Coarctation of the aorta with moderate aortic arch hypoplasia. **B,** Lateral tunnel total cavopulmonary anastomosis with branch pulmonary arteries. In this last case, flow streaming does not allow perfect and balanced delineation of both pulmonary arteries as well as superior vena cava. Thoughtful positioning of angiographic catheter and appropriate use of injection-acquisition time delay is warranted to maximize image quality and diagnostic performance.

SPECIAL CIRCUMSTANCES

Certain circumstances lead to specific diagnostic considerations for individuals affected by congenital heart disease.

Pregnancy

Increased preload, heart rate, and cardiac output, coupled with varying ventricular contractile function, may exacerbate preexisting hemodynamic compromise. Catheterization is safe to mother and fetus when limited to those circumstances (usually mitral or ventricular outflow obstruction) where a combined cardiology and high-risk obstetrics team determines that catheter-based diagnostics or interventions are required despite adequate volume and heart rate control.

Choice in timing of catheterization may not be feasible, but the procedure should be timed to optimize maternal safety while minimizing fetal teratogenicity or mortality risk.

Overall uterine radiation exposure should be minimized (direct shielding with lead aprons may intensify rather than reduce exposure and should be avoided). Availability of fetal monitoring and urgent access to the delivery room should be determined by the obstetrical staff prior to catheterization.

Down Syndrome

The adult patient with Down syndrome frequently has increasing medical comorbidities (thyroid disease, upper and lower airway disease, gastrointestinal reflux, limited communication skills, and dementia). Despite restricted alimentation, the patient with Down syndrome should be considered to have a "full stomach" and to be at increased aspiration risk. Hemodynamic assessment of PVR should take into account alterations in ventilation and increased incidence of pulmonary vascular disease. Mechanical ventilation to ensure adequate assessment of PVR should be utilized as necessary.

Pulmonary Ventricular Failure and Pulmonary Vascular Disease

Elevation of subpulmonary ventricular systolic pressure is often seen in adult patients with repaired congenital heart disease. This may be related to fixed obstruction at the level of right ventricular outflow tract (such as in patients with dysfunctional RV-to-PA conduit or reconstructed outflow tract) or at the level of peripheral PA branches (such as in patients with complex cases of tetralogy of Fallot with or without pulmonary atresia or in patients who underwent unifocalization of aorta-to-PA collaterals). In a significant proportion of cases, the increase in subpulmonary ventricular afterload is due to progressive remodeling of pulmonary vascular bed, leading to elevation of PVR (pulmonary arterial hypertension, PAH).

The most recently accepted definition of PAH requires a mean pulmonary arterial pressure above 20 mmHg (at rest) with relatively preserved wedge pressure (<15 mmHg) and elevated PVR above 2 indexed Wood units (WU) (**Table 10.5**).

In some patients with open left-to-right shunt lesions (such as atrial septal defect [ASD]), the pulmonary arterial pressure and transpulmonary gradient can be elevated in the setting of high-flow circulation (given the very high Qp/Qs); in these cases, the measured PVR can fall within normal limits, although select patients may remain at risk over time for development of further changes in PVR.

Therapeutic advances for patients with acquired or congenital pulmonary vascular disease have markedly improved potential for improved quantity and quality of life. Historically, the assessment of pulmonary vascular reactivity as a marker for further surgical or medical therapy began in the congenital catheterization laboratories, and it has taken on an increasingly meaningful role in guiding care.

Extreme care should be taken to avoid acute confounding in-laboratory worsening of PVR by excessive sedation-induced hypoventilation, anesthetic-induced negative inotropy, pain, hemorrhage, acidemia, or severe alterations of loading conditions. Potential for in-laboratory support with intravenous (prostacyclin) or inhaled (nitric oxide, prostacyclin) pulmonary vasodilators or mechanical assist may be requisites for even basic hemodynamic assessments in such patients.

Acute vasodilator testing is recommended in every patient with PAH because it will improve risk stratification and guide therapeutic decision. **Table 10.6** summarizes route of administration and dose titration of the most common recommended regimens to perform acute vasodilator testing. The most recent and widely accepted definition of a positive response includes reduction of mean pulmonary arterial pressure of at least 10 mmHg to an actual value below 40 mmHg, with preserved cardiac output. Caution should be advised for those patients who present with very high capillary wedge pressure at rest (>25-30 mmHg) who may experience worsening pulmonary edema in the setting of acute vasodilator testing using inhaled NO. In patients with shunt lesion and evidence of prevalent left-to-right shunt but elevated PVR (see **Table 10.6**), controversies exist regarding potential for shunt closure and lesion repair. In this setting acute vasoreactivity testing has been proposed to guide closure recommendation. Although this approach did not receive universal acceptance, an acute reduction of PVRi below 6 WU and/or PVR/systemic vascular resistance ratio below 0.3 may be considered a reliable indicator for acute tolerance of shunt closure; however, concerns remain regarding postoperative, long-term development of PAH (see **Table 10.6**), which is characterized by an ominous clinical course.

A complete and patient-specific understanding of the PVR profile is required to guide transcatheter interventions in those patients with left-to-right shunt lesions that may be suitable for percutaneous closure. The concept of transcatheter tem-

Table 10.5 **Definition of Pulmonary Hypertension; Classification of Pulmonary Hypertension Associated With Congenital Heart Defect; Systemic-to-Pulmonary Shunt Lesion Recommendation for Closure**

Definition	Characteristics	Clinical Group
PH	mPAP > 20 mmHg	All
Precapillary PH	mPAP > 20 mmHg PCW < 15 mmHg PVR >2 WU	Pulmonary arterial hypertension PH due to lung disease Chronic thromboembolic disease PH with unclear and/or multifactorial mechanisms
Isolated postcapillary PH	mPAP > 20 mmHg PCW > 15 mmHg PVR < 2 WU	PH due to left-sided heart
Combined postcapillary PH	mPAP > 20 mmHg PAWP > 15 mmHg PVR > 2 WU	
Exercise PH	mPAP/CO slope between rest and exercise >3 mmHg/L/min	

PAH Associated With CHD	Definition	Comment
Eisenmenger syndrome	Includes all large intra- and extracardiac defects that begin as systemic-to-pulmonary shunts and progress with time to severe elevation of PVR and to reversal (pulmonary-to-systemic) or bidirectional shunting; cyanosis, secondary erythrocytosis, and multiple organ involvement are usually present. Closing the defects is contraindicated.	Cyanosis at rest
PAH associated with prevalent systemic-to-pulmonary shunts	• Correctable • Noncorrectable Includes moderate to large defects; PVR is mildly to moderately increased, systemic-to-pulmonary shunting is still prevalent, whereas cyanosis at rest is not a feature	See below for recommendation for closure
PAH with small/coincidental defects	Markedly elevated PVR in the presence of cardiac defects considered hemodynamically nonsignificant (usually ventricular septal defects <1 cm and atrial septal defects <2 cm of effective diameter assessed by echocardiography), which themselves do not account for the development of elevated PVR. The clinical picture is very similar to IPAH. Closing the defects is contraindicated.	NA

Table 10.5 Definition of Pulmonary Hypertension; Classification of Pulmonary Hypertension Associated With Congenital Heart Defect; Systemic-to-Pulmonary Shunt Lesion Recommendation for Closure (Continued)

Definition	Characteristics	Clinical Group
PAH after defect correction	Congenital heart disease is repaired, but PAH either persists immediately after correction or recurs/develops months or years after correction in the absence of significant postoperative hemodynamic lesions	

Recommendations	Class[a]	Level[b]
In patients with an ASD, VSD, or PDA and a PVR < 3 WU, shunt closure is recommended	I	C
In patients with an ASD, VSD, or PDA and a PVR of 3-5 WU, shunt closure should be considered	IIa	C
In patients with an ASD and a PVR > 5 WU that declines to <5 WU with PAH treatment, shunt closure may be considered	IIb	C
In patients with a VSD or PDA and a PVR >5 WU, shunt closure may be considered after careful evaluation in specialized centers	IIb	C
In patients with an ASD and a PVR >5 WU despite PAH treatment, shunt closure is not recommended	III	C

ASD, atrial septal defect; CHD, congenital heart defect; CO, cardiac output; IPAH, idiopathic pulmonary arterial hypertension; mPAP, mean pulmonary arterial pressure; NA, not applicable; PAH, pulmonary arterial hypertension; PAWP, pulmonary arterial wedge pressure; PCW, pulmonary capillary wedge; PDA, patent ductus arteriosus; PH, pulmonary hypertension; PVR, pulmonary vascular resistance; PVRi, indexed pulmonary vascular resistance; VSD, ventricular septal defect; WU, Woods unit.
Decisions on shunt closure should not be made on hemodynamic numbers alone; a multiparametric strategy should be followed.
(Adapted from: Humbert M , Kovacs G , Hoeper MM , et al. 2022 ESC/ERS Guidelines for the diagnosis and treatment of pulmonary hypertension. *Eur Heart J.* 2022;43:3618-3731.)
[a]Class of recommendation.
[b]Level of evidence.

Table 10.6	Agents for Acute Vasodilator Testing		
	Epoprostenol	**Adenosine**	**Nitric Oxide**
Route of administration	Intravenous infusion	Intravenous infusion	Inhaled
Dose titration	2 ng/kg/min every 10-15 min	50 µg/kg every 2 min	None
Dose range	2-10 ng/kg/min	50-250 µg/kg/min	10-80 ppm
Side effects	Headache, nausea, lightheadedness	Dyspnea, chest pain, atrioventricular block	Increased left-sided heart filling

porary balloon occlusion to mimic the acute physiologic change of defect closure was pioneered by pediatric cardiologists for the management of surgically placed fenestrations in Fontan baffles, establishing criteria to best estimate the long-term cardiopulmonary tolerance of a removal of a pop-off between circulatory systems. Extrapolation of these criteria to the older adult population with RV dysfunction and cyanosis is unsubstantiated but serves as a guide for at least acute testing of physiologic tolerance. Performance of temporary balloon defect occlusion with compliant large balloon catheters and subsequent measure of change in cardiac output and RA pressures is recommended in highest-risk patients contemplating catheter-based or surgical ASD closure. Care must be taken to avoid obstruction of associated flow (eg, pulmonary veins, mitral valve).

Right Ventricular Outflow Failure

Use of transannular patch repair, persistence or recurrence of right ventricular outflow obstruction, or elevation of distal PA pressure in patients with tetralogy of Fallot may contribute to increased incidence of right ventricular outflow and pulmonary arterial aneurysmal dilation.

Right ventricular to PA conduit placement is used to treat a variety of conotruncal malformations including (but not limited to) truncus arteriosus, double outlet RV, transposition of the great arteries with pulmonary stenosis, and pulmonary atresia with intact ventricular septum. Pulmonary homograft to restore RV to PA continuity is used in the Ross procedure to treat the spectrum of congenital left ventricular outflow tract obstruction in addition to native pulmonary autograft translocation.

Catheterization of such patients may be indicated to define hemodynamics and anatomy in the setting of changing exercise capacity, worsening arrhythmia, chest pain, or cyanosis and with either suspected encroachment of pulmonary venous drainage or pulmonary arterial dissection.

A variety of abnormal course and origin of coronary arteries is described in this group of diseases. To avoid coronary artery compression during percutaneous valve implantation, in selected cases, selective coronary angiography is simultaneously performed with balloon dilation of right ventricular outflow tract to assess for dynamic compression of origin or proximal segment of coronary arteries (**Figure 10.3**).

Cyanosis

Long-standing effects of hypoxia-mediated secondary erythrocytosis lessen the glomerular filtration rate and increase viscosity, raising the risk for contrast-induced acute tubular necrosis and vascular thrombosis. Catheterization should be planned

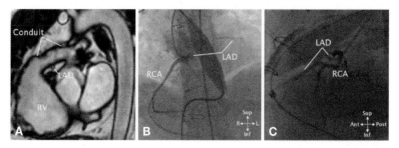

Figure 10.3 Right ventricular outflow tract transcatheter intervention and coronary artery anatomy. Cardiovascular magnetic resonance imaging **(A)** demonstrates findings in a patient with repaired tetralogy of Fallot. An anomalous left anterior descending (LAD) artery originating from the right coronary artery (RCA) runs behind a right ventricle (RV)-to-pulmonary artery conduit. **B** and **C**, show dynamic compression of proximal LAD during high-pressure balloon dilation within the conduit. No compression is noted on the proximal RCA. This scenario precluded transcatheter placement of pulmonary valve.

appropriately in such patients and may be accompanied by preprocedural organized reduction in red blood cell mass. Presence of right-to-left shunting at the level of systemic veins to pulmonary veins, atrial baffle leaks, patent foramen ovale, and PA to pulmonary veins should be explored and potentially treated in the catheterization laboratory. Similarly, pulmonary venous desaturation in the setting of pulmonary venous hypertension due to (1) systolic or diastolic subaortic ventricular failure, (2) AV valve regurgitation, (3) intravascular obstruction or extravascular compression by an enlarging RA or PA should be explored for potential medical, surgical, or transcatheter intervention.

Systemic Ventricular "Heart Failure"

The inability of the heart and lungs to meet the metabolic demands imposed by the patient with congenital heart disease may have unique anatomic and physiologic etiologies and widely differing therapies than those utilized for children or adults with acquired heart disease (Table 10.7). Use of tailored, hemodynamic-based changes in medical therapy, to date, has not been studied in patients with congenital heart disease.

Coronary Artery Disease

Patients may have abnormalities of coronary artery origin, passage (intramural or between the great arteries), and vessel characteristics (such as those seen in anomalous left coronary artery origin from the pulmonary artery, Kawasaki disease, or coronary reimplantation during arterial switch for TGA).

Vascular Anatomy Before Cardiac Surgery

Reoperation to treat residual defect, sequelae, or original repair failure is frequently performed in adults and adolescents with congenital heart disease, and it is associated with an increased risk for complications due to the additional challenges of multiple adhesions and unusual structural anatomy.

Fontan

Total cavopulmonary connection (TCPC) is a staged surgical palliation for patients with very complex congenital heart defect in which biventricular surgical repair can-

Table 10.7	Etiologies of "Heart Failure" in the Congenital Cardiac Patient
Afterload	
Vascular obstruction	
Abnormal arterial impedance	
Structural	
Neurohormonal	
Systemic right/single ventricle	
Preload	
Residual/acquired shunts	
Single ventricle	
Valvar/paravalvular regurgitation	
Renal/hepatic disease and volume retention	
Abnormal venous capacitance	
Atrial function/fluid conductance	
Fontan, single ventricle/tricuspid atresia, atrial switch: transposition of great arteries	
Loss of subpulmonary ventricle function (Fontan)	
Loss of native atrioventricular synchrony	
Atrial flutter → fibrillation	
Artificial pacing	
Ventricular ectopy	
Abnormal epicardial/intramural coronary artery flow/formation	
Anomalous left coronary artery origin from the pulmonary artery (ALCAPA)	
Transposition of the great arteries, s/p arterial switch	
Coronary artery between great arteries/intramural/single	

not be achieved (**Figure** 10.4). It does consist of direct routing of systemic venous return into the lung circulation without interposition of a supporting ventricle. Long-term failure of such palliation does occur in a high proportion of adult patients. The so-called Fontan failure, however, is a nonspecific term because the clinical picture of adults surviving after TCPC includes a heterogeneous cluster of signs and symptoms

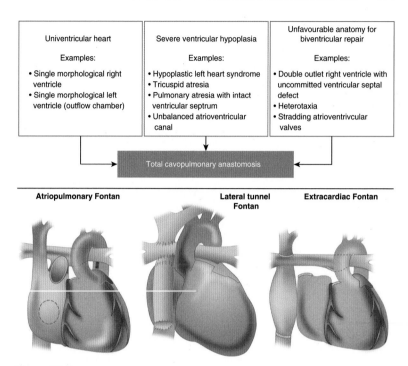

Univentricular heart	Severe ventricular hypoplasia	Unfavourable anatomy for biventricular repair
Examples:	Examples:	Examples:
• Single morphological right ventricle • Single morphological left ventricle (outflow chamber)	• Hypoplastic left heart syndrome • Tricuspid atresia • Pulmonary atresia with intact ventricular septum • Unbalanced atrioventricular canal	• Double outlet right ventricle with uncommitted ventricular septal defect • Heterotaxia • Stradding atrioventrivcular valves

Total cavopulmonary anastomosis

Atriopulmonary Fontan   Lateral tunnel Fontan   Extracardiac Fontan

Figure 10.4 Common congenital heart defect leading to staged surgical creation of total cavo-pulmonary anastomosis. In the bottom diagram, evolution of the surgical technique is demonstrated. Nowadays the lateral tunnel (intracardiac anastomosis) and conduit (extracardiac anastomosis) are usually performed. (Bottom illustrations from Garcia MJ. *Noninvasive Cardiovascular Imaging: A Multimodality Approach.* Wolters Kluwer; 2012.)

including refractory ascites, plastic bronchitis, protein-losing enteropathy, thromboembolic events, complex atrial and ventricular arrhythmias, systemic ventricular systolic/diastolic dysfunction, and cyanosis. Cardiac catheterization in these patients is usually performed to assess hemodynamic profile and to detect structural abnormalities amenable for transcatheter or surgical intervention (such as venovenous or systemic-to-pulmonary collateral coiling/occlusion, angioplasty or stenting for baffle narrowing or branch PA stenosis, intracardiac leak closure, fenestration closure, Fontan conversion). Hemodynamic profile may give relevant insight into the principal modality of TCPC failure and guide important clinical decisions (**Figure 10.5**). Avoidance of pitfalls in TCPC hemodynamic assessment includes: (1) hemodynamic pressure "zeroing" should be obtained with meticulous care because even a few millimeters of mercury pressure error may carry relevant implications in the diagnostic process; (2) pressure within the TCPC baffle should be taken before and after any relevant narrowing to assess for hemodynamic degree of stenosis, although angiographic appearance is often more relevant than pressure drop in this low nonpulsatile flow state; (3) real working pressure of TCPC (ideally hemodynamic evaluation should be reassessed after closure of such decompressing channels); (4) pulmonary capillary wedge pressure measurement is usually not accurate in cases of TCPC. The

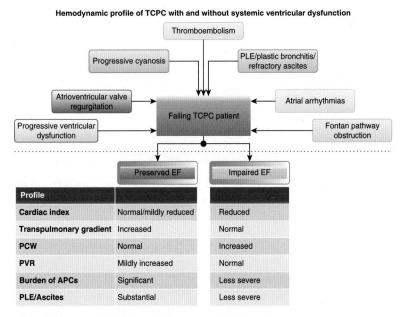

Figure 10.5 Hemodynamic profile of TCPC with and without systemic ventricular dysfunction. Complex features of "failing" Fontan physiology do encompass multiple mechanisms (summarized in the top portion of the figure). However, the presence of severe systolic dysfunction of the single ventricle in these patients is usually characterized by a specific hemodynamic profile that is summarized on the right bottom panel of the picture. Conversely, normal systolic performance of the single ventricle is usually characterized by a moderate increase in the transpulmonary gradient and evidence for splanchnic congestion and lymphatic disease (such as protein-losing enteropathy, plastic bronchitis, refractory ascites). APCs, aortopulmonary collaterals; EF, ejection fraction; PCW, pulmonary capillary wedge; PLE, protein-losing enteropathy; PVR, pulmonary vascular resistance; TCPC, total cavopulmonary connection.

end-diastolic systemic ventricular pressure should be acquired if "true" transpulmonary gradient is of clinical interest; (5) the Ohm law for resistance calculation carries great potential for inaccuracy due to absence of pulsatile flow, the presence of marginal pulmonary blood flow, decompressing channels, and systemic-to-pulmonary collaterals. Thus, PVR calculation may create a spurious sense of safety or concern in these patients. This is particularly important in patients with TCPC considered for heart transplant who can experience (at the time of graft anastomosis and reestablishment of pulsatile pulmonary blood flow) a significant increase in measured PVR beyond expectation based on pretransplant transpulmonary gradient.

CONCLUSION

Accurate planned and coordinated multidisciplinary care is required for the hemodynamic evaluation of young and older patients with congenital heart disease. Increasing survival into adulthood of children with complex congenital heart disease requires specifically trained physicians and interventionalists with thorough understanding of anatomy and physiology of this heterogeneous group of cardiac malformation to provide ready and expert provision of hemodynamic assessment and potential medical, catheter-based, and surgical interventions, as appropriate.

SUGGESTED READINGS

1. Assenza GE, Graham DA, Landzberg MJ, et al. MELD-XI score and cardiac mortality or transplantation in patients after Fontan surgery. *Heart.* 2013;99:491-496.
2. Badesch DB, Abman SH, Simonneau G, Rubin LJ, McLaughlin VV. Medical therapy for pulmonary arterial hypertension: updated ACCP evidence-based clinical practice guidelines. *Chest.* 2007;131(6):1917-1928.
3. Baraona F, Valente AM, Porayette P, Pluchinotta FR, Sanders SP. Coronary arteries in childhood heart disease: implications for management of young adults. *J Clin Exp Cardiolog.* 2012;S8(suppl 8):006-022.
4. Bridges ND, Lock JE, Mayer JE, Burnett J, Castaneda AR. Cardiac catheterization and test occlusion of the interatrial communication after the fenestrated Fontan operation. *J Am Coll Cardiol.* 1995;25(7):1712-1717.
5. Chung T, Burrows PE. Angiography of congenital heart disease. In: Lock JE, Keane JF, Perry SB, eds. *Diagnostic and Interventional Catheterization in Congenital Heart Disease.* 2nd ed. Kluwer; 2000:73.
6. Damilakis J, Theocharopoulos N, Perisinakis K, et al. Conceptus radiation dose and risk from cardiac catheter ablation procedures. *Circulation.* 2001;104(8):893-897.
7. Dasi LP, Pekkan K, de Zelicourt D, et al. Hemodynamic energy dissipation in the cardiovascular system: generalized theoretical analysis on disease states. *Ann Biomed Eng.* 2009;37(4):661-673.
8. Fernandes SM, Newburger JW, Lang P, et al. Usefulness of epoprostenol therapy in the severely ill adolescent/adult with Eisenmenger physiology. *Am J Cardiol.* 2003;91(5):632-635.
9. Flanagan MF, Hourihan M, Keane JF. Incidence of renal dysfunction in adults with cyanotic congenital heart disease. *Am J Cardiol.* 1991;68(4):403-406.
10. Freed MD, Miettinen O, Nadas AS. Oximetric detection of intracardiac left-to-right shunts. *Br Heart J.* 1979;42(6):690-694.
11. Freeman SB, Taft LF, Dooley KI, et al. Population-based study of congenital heart defects in Down syndrome. *Am J Med Genet.* 1998;80:213-217.
12. Galie' N, Humbert M, Vachieri JL, et al. 2015 ESC/ERS guidelines for the diagnosis and treatment of pulmonary hypertension. The Joint Task force for the diagnosis and treatment of pulmonary hypertension of the European Society of Cardiology (ESC) and the European Respiratory Society (ERS): Endorsed by Association for European Paediatric and Congenital Cardiology (AEPC), International Society for Heart and Lung Transplantation (ISHLT). *Eur Heart J.* 2016;37:67-119.
13. Jacobs IN, Tegue WG, Bland JW. Pulmonary vascular complications of chronic airway obstructions in children. *Arch Otolaryngol Head Neck Surg.* 1997;123:700-704.
14. Landzberg MJ. Closure of atrial septal defects in adult patients: justification of the "tipping point". *J Interv Cardiol.* 2001;14(2):267-269.
15. Landzberg MJ. Heart failure in the adult with congenital heart disease. In: Wernovsky G, Shaddy R, eds. *Pediatric Heart Failure.* Taylor and Francis Group; 2005:869-888.
16. Lock JE, Einzig SA, Moller JH. Hemodynamic responses to exercise in normal children. *Am J Cardiol.* 1978;41(7):1278-1284.
17. Marelli AJ, Mackie AS, Ionescu-Ittu R, Rahme E, Pilote L. Congenital heart disease in the general population: changing prevalence and age distribution. *Circulation.* 2007;115(2):163-172.
18. McElhinney DB, Hellenbrand WE, Zahn EM, et al. Short- and medium-term outcomes after transcatheter pulmonary valve placement in the expanded multicenter US Melody valve trial. *Circulation.* 2010;122(5):507-516.
19. McLaughlin VV, Archer SL, Badesch DB, et al. ACCF/AHA 2009 expert consensus document on pulmonary hypertension a report of the American College of Cardiology Foundation Task force on expert Consensus Documents and the American Heart Association developed in collaboration with the American College of Chest Physicians; American Thoracic Society, Inc.; and the Pulmonary Hypertension Association. *J Am Coll Cardiol.* 2009;53:1573-1619.
20. Rosenzweig EB, Kerstein D, Barst RJ. Long term prostacyclin for pulmonary hypertension with associated congenital heart defects. *Circulation.* 1999;99(14):1858-1865.
21. Shim D, Lloyd TR, Cho KJ, Moorehead CP, Beekman RH III. Transhepatic cardiac catheterization in children. Evaluation of efficacy and safety. *Circulation.* 1995;92(6):1526-1530.
22. Van der Stelt F, Siegerink SN, Krings GJ, Molenschot MMC, Breur JMPJ. Three-dimensional rotational angiography in pediatric patients with congenital heart disease: a literature review. *Pediatr Cardiol.* 2019;40(2):257-264.
23. Verma R, Keane JF. Use of cut-off pigtail catheters with intraluminal guide wires in interventional procedures in congenital heart disease. *Cathet Cardiovasc Diag.* 1994;33(1):85-88.
24. Warnes CA, Liberthson R, Danielson GK, et al. Task force 1: the changing profile of congenital heart disease in adult life. *J Am Coll Cardiol.* 2001;37(5):1170-1175.

11 Pressure and Blood Flow Measurement[1]

Force is transmitted through a fluid medium as a pressure wave. A ventricular pressure wave may be considered a complex periodic fluctuation in force per unit area, with 1 cycle consisting of the time interval from the onset of 1 systole to the onset of the subsequent systole. The number of times the cycle occurs in 1 second is termed the fundamental frequency of cardiac pressure generation. Thus, a fundamental frequency of 2 corresponds to a heart rate of 120 beats per minute (bpm). Definitions of terms relevant to the theory and practice of pressure measurement are listed in **Table 11.1**.

Any complex waveform may be considered the mathematical summation of a series of simple sine waves of differing amplitude and frequency (**Figure 11.1**). The sine wave frequencies are usually expressed as harmonics, or multiples of the fundamental frequency. For example, at a heart rate of 120 bpm, the fundamental frequency is 2 cycles per second (Hz) and the first 5 harmonics are sine waves whose frequencies are 2, 4, 6, 8, and 10 Hz. The practical consequence of this analysis is that, to record pressure accurately, a system must respond with equal amplitude for a given input throughout the range of frequencies contained within the pressure wave. If components in a particular frequency range are either suppressed or exaggerated by the transducer system, the recorded signal will be a grossly distorted version of the original physiologic waveform.

PRESSURE MEASURING DEVICES

Key concepts applicable to modern pressure measurement devices include sensitivity, frequency response, natural frequency, damping, and linearity.

Sensitivity

The sensitivity of such a measurement system is the ability to detect small changes in the input signal. It may be defined as the ratio of the amplitude of the recorded signal to the amplitude of the input signal. With the Hurthle manometer illustrated in **Figure 11.2**, the more rigid the sensing membrane, the lower the sensitivity; conversely, the more flaccid the membrane, the higher the sensitivity. This general principle applies to manometers currently in use, where the instrument must be sensitive enough to respond to a small input signal with an adequate output.

Frequency Response

A second crucial property of any pressure measurement system is its frequency response, defined as the ratio of output amplitude to input amplitude over a range of frequencies of the input pressure wave. To measure pressure accurately, the frequency response (amplitude ratio) must be constant over a broad range of frequency variation. Otherwise, the amplitude of major frequency components of the pressure waveform may be attenuated while minor components are amplified, so that the recorded waveform becomes a distorted caricature of the physiologic event.

---

[1]We gratefully acknowledge the *Grossman & Baim's Cardiac Catheterization, Angiography, and Intervention,* 9th edition contributions of Drs. Mauro Moscucci and William Grossman as portions of their chapters, Pressure Measurements and Blood Flow Measurement: Cardiac Output and Vascular Resistance, were retained in this text.

Table 11.1	Definitions of Terms Relevant to the Theory and Practice of Pressure Measurement
Term	**Definition**
Pressure wave	Complex periodic fluctuation in force per unit area Units: dyn/cm²: 1 dyn/cm² = 1 microbar = 10^{-1} N/M² = 7.5 × 10^{-4} mmHg mmHg: 1 mmHg = 1 Torr = 1/760 atmospheric pressure
Fundamental frequency	Number of times the pressure wave cycles in 1 s
Harmonic	Multiple of the fundamental frequency
Fourier analysis	Resolution of any complex periodic wave into a series of single sine waves of differing frequency and amplitude
Sensitivity of pressure measurement system	Ratio of the amplitude of the recorded signal to the amplitude of the input signal
Linearity	Relationship between input and output of the first order
Frequency response of pressure measurement system	Ratio of output amplitude to input amplitude over a range of frequencies of the input pressure wave
Natural frequency	Frequency at which the pressure measurement system oscillates or responds when shock-excited; also, the frequency of an input pressure wave at which the ratio of output/input amplitude of an undamaged system is maximal. Units: cycles/s, Hz
Damping	Dissipation of the energy of oscillation of a pressure measurement system owing to friction Units: damping coefficient, D (see text)
Optimal damping	Damping that progressively blunts the increase in output/input ratio that occurs with increasing frequency of pressure wave input. Optimal damping can maintain frequency response flat (output/input ratio = 1) to 88% of the natural frequency of the system
Strain gauge	Variable-resistance transducer in which the strain ($\Delta L/L$) on a series of wires is determined by the pressure on the transducer's diaphragm. Over a wide range, electrical resistance (R) of the wire is directly proportional to $\Delta L/L$
Wheatstone bridge	Arrangement of electrical connections in a strain gauge such that pressure-induced changes in resistance result in proportional changes in voltage across the bridge
Balancing a transducer	Interpolating a variable resistance across the output of a Wheatstone bridge/strain gauge transducer so that atmospheric pressure at the zero level (eg, midchest) induces an arbitrary voltage output on the monitor/recording device (ie, a voltage that positions the transducer output on the oscilloscopic pressure baseline)

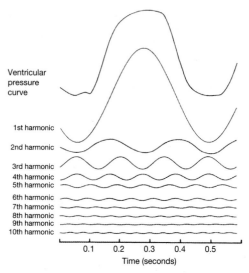

Ventricular
pressure
curve

1st harmonic
2nd harmonic
3rd harmonic
4th harmonic
5th harmonic
6th harmonic
7th harmonic
8th harmonic
9th harmonic
10th harmonic

0.1   0.2   0.3   0.4   0.5
Time (seconds)

Figure 11.1 Resolution of a normal ventricular pressure curve (top) into its first 10 harmonics by Fourier analysis. If components in a particular frequency range (eg, the third harmonic, which in this case is 7 Hz) were either suppressed or exaggerated by the transducer system, the recorded signal would be a grossly distorted version of the original physiologic signal. (Adapted from Wiggers CJ. *The Pressure Pulses in the Cardiovascular System*. Longmans, Green; 1928:1.)

Natural Frequency and Damping

A third important concept is the natural frequency of a sensing membrane and how it determines the degree of damping required for optimal recording. If the sensing membrane were to be shock-excited (like a gong) in the absence of friction, it would oscillate for an indefinite period in simple harmonic motion. The frequency of this motion would be the natural frequency of the system. Any means of dissipating the energy of this oscillation, such as friction, is called damping.

The significance of the natural frequency and the importance of proper damping are illustrated in **Figure 11.3**. The amplitude of an output signal tends to be

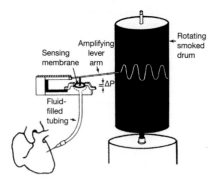

Rotating
smoked
drum

Amplifying
lever
arm

Sensing
membrane

ΔP

Fluid-
filled
tubing

Figure 11.2 Schematic illustration of the original Hurthle manometer. A rubber tambour serves as the sensing membrane and is coupled with an amplifying lever arm that records changes in pressure (ΔP) on a rotating smoked drum. Pressure is transmitted from the heart (*lower left corner*) to the sensing membrane by fluid-filled tubing.

augmented as the frequency of the input signal approaches the natural frequency of the sensing membrane. The physical counterpart of this augmentation is that the sensing membrane of the pressure transducer vibrates with increasing energy and violence. The same mechanism underlies the fracture of a crystal glass when an opera singer vocalizes the appropriate input frequency. Damping dissipates the energy of the oscillating sensing membrane, and optimal damping dissipates the energy gradually, thereby maintaining the frequency response curve nearly flat (constant output/input ratio) as it approaches the region of the pressure measurement system's natural frequency.

Linearity
Linearity is an additional critical component of recording systems, and it exists when the relationship between the input signal and the output signal is of the first order. Linearity allows the use of a single calibration factor for different amplitudes of the input signal.

TRANSFORMING PRESSURE WAVES INTO ELECTRICAL SIGNALS: THE ELECTRICAL STRAIN GAUGE

Pressure measurement systems today generally use electrical strain gauges based on the principle of the Wheatstone bridge. In its simplest form, the strain gauge is a variable resistance transducer whose operation depends on the fact that, when an electrical wire is stretched, its resistance to the flow of current increases. As long as the strain remains well below the elastic limit of the wire, there is a wide range within which the increase in resistance is accurately proportional to the increase in length.

Figure 11.4 illustrates how the Wheatstone bridge uses this principle in converting a pressure signal to an electrical signal.

Because movement of the diaphragm (D) in **Figure 11.4** is necessary to produce current flow in the Wheatstone bridge, a certain volume of fluid must actually move through the catheter and connecting tubing to produce a recorded pressure.

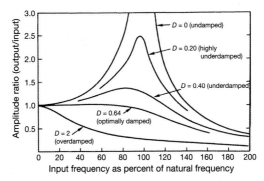

Figure 11.3 Frequency response curves of a pressure measurement system. The amplitude of an input signal tends to be augmented as the frequency of that signal approaches the natural frequency of the sensing membrane. Optimal damping dissipates the energy of the oscillating sensing membrane gradually and thereby maintains a nearly flat natural frequency curve (constant output/input ratio) as it approaches the region of the pressure measurement system's natural frequency (see text). D, damping coefficient.

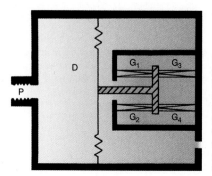

Figure 11.4 Schematic representation of a strain gauge pressure transducer. Pressure is transmitted through port P and acts on diaphragm D, which is vented to atmospheric pressure on its opposite side. Pressure causes the diaphragm to stretch, in turn stretching and therefore increasing the resistance of wires G_1 and G_2, while having the opposite effect on wires G_3 and G_4. The wires are electrically connected as shown in **Figure 11.5**.

Therefore, the use of a low-volume-displacement transducer with a small chamber volume improves the frequency response characteristics of the system.

Balancing a transducer is simply a process whereby a variable resistance is interpolated into the circuit so that at an arbitrary baseline pressure, the voltage across the output terminal, can be reduced to zero. Some amplifiers use an alternating current signal in place of the DC current source shown in **Figure 11.5**. When these carrier current amplifiers are used, a variable capacitor (the C balance) must be used in addition to the variable resistor to balance the bridge.

PRACTICAL PRESSURE TRANSDUCER SYSTEM FOR THE CATHETERIZATION LABORATORY

Incorporating all the principles discussed so far in this chapter, many laboratories have settled on a practical system in which a fluid-filled catheter is attached by means of a manifold to a small-volume-displacement strain gauge-type pressure transducer (**Figures 11.6** and **11.7**).

The system illustrated in **Figure 11.6** is used for pressure measurement from the right side of the heart and for arterial monitor lines. The system used for left-sided heart pressure measurement is more complex because it also incorporates ports for radiographic contrast administration and blood discard, as well as a syringe for

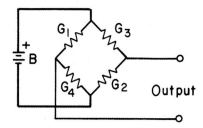

Figure 11.5 Strain gauge connection of the Wheatstone bridge. In this arrangement, if all resistances are equal, then exactly half the voltage of battery B exists at the junction of G_1 and G_4 and half at the junction of G_2 and G_3; therefore, no current will flow between the output terminals. However, when pressure is applied to the diaphragm (see **Figure 11.4**), the resistances are unbalanced, so that the junction of G_1 and G_4 becomes negative and a current flows across the output terminals.

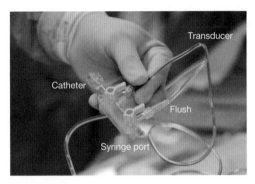

Figure 11.6 A practical system for pressure measurement with excellent frequency response. The catheter is connected to a manifold. The manifold's 2 side arms are connected to a small-volume fluid-filled pressure transducer by fluid-filled tubing and to a pressurized flush solution.

coronary angiography. Virtually all catheterization laboratories use relatively inexpensive, sterile, disposable pressure transducers in which a tiny integrated circuit on a thin silicon diaphragm serves as the sensing element. Fluid pressure is transmitted to this element through a gel medium, bending the circuit and altering the resistance of resistors in the silicon diaphragm.

With this system, a frequency response that is flat (±5%) up to 20 Hz can be achieved routinely. **Figure 11.8** illustrates an alternative set up of the manifold, which includes a separate zero line and which allows keeping the transducer on the table and connected directly to the manifold. With this set up, the exit port of the zero line must be positioned at the appropriate height.

The establishment of a zero reference is an important practical undertaking that must be accomplished as a part of each catheterization procedure. Midchest level is used widely as zero reference. However, the validity of choosing the midchest level for zero reference has been challenged in an excellent study by Courtois et al. They

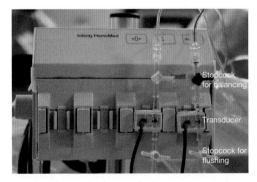

Figure 11.7 Pressure transducers mounted on a metal pole attached to the cardiac catheterization table. The top stopcock is used for zero-pressure reference, and the lower stopcock is used for flushing the transducer.

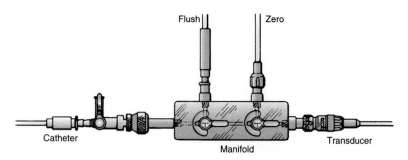

Figure 11.8 Alternative setup for a pressure manifold for pressure measurement. The catheter is connected by a stopcock to a manifold, which is connected at its other end to a small-volume fluid-filled pressure transducer. The manifold's 2 side arms are connected by fluid-filled tubing to a zero-pressure reference level and to a pressurized flush solution. Thus, this setup includes a separate zero line, which should be positioned at the appropriate height as shown in **Figure 11.9**.

examined the influence of hydrostatic forces (caused by the effects of gravity) and concluded that intracardiac pressures should be referenced to an external fluid-filled transducer aligned with the uppermost blood level in the chamber where pressure is being measured. In practical terms, the zero level should be positioned approximately 5 cm below the left sternal border at the fourth left intercostal space (LICS) (**Figure 11.9**). This eliminates the gravitational/hydrostatic effect of a column of blood above the catheter tip and within the ventricular chamber. Although the right ventricle and left atrium (LA) are at different levels in the chest than the left ventricle (LV), Courtois et al. calculated that the error introduced by use of a point 5 cm below the fourth LICS, at the left sternal border, is approximately ±0.8 mmHg for chambers other than the LV.

As illustrated in **Figure 11.7**, the transducers are mounted on the metal pole and their height can be adjusted as needed once the appropriate midchest level (half of the patient's AP diameter below the angle of Louis), or the 5 cm level below the left sternal border at the fourth LICS, has been identified.

It is critical to remove any air bubble, as air bubbles result in an underdamped pressure waveform. Modern pressure transducers are precalibrated, and many manufactures provide electronic devices to validate calibration. Otherwise, the free port of the Morse manifold is left open to air, in communication with the individual zero

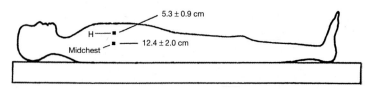

Figure 11.9 Schematic representation of measured heights for an external fluid-filled transducer reference position relative to the anterior chest wall at a midchest level and at the uppermost blood level (H) in the left ventricle in 7 patients. (Reproduced with permission from Courtois M, Fattal PG, Kovacs SJ Jr., Tiefenbrunn AJ, Ludbrook PA. Anatomically and physiologically based reference level for measurement of intracardiac pressures. *Circulation*. 1995; 92:1994-2000.)

lines of the various left- and right-sided heart manifold systems by way of the series of stopcocks that constitute the Morse manifold, thus referencing all the transducer systems to a common zero level.

PHYSIOLOGIC CHARACTERISTICS OF PRESSURE WAVEFORMS
Reflected Waves

As shown in **Figure 11.10**, forward pressure and flow waves, as seen in the central aorta, are intrinsically identical in shape and timing. The pressure wave is modified by summation with a reflected pressure wave ($P_{backward}$), and the resultant measured central aortic pressure wave shows a steady increase throughout ejection (**Figure 11.11**). The flow wave is also modified by summation with a reflected flow wave (F), but because flow is directional, backward F reduces the magnitude of flow in late ejection, giving backward the characteristic F as is seen with aortic flowmeters or measured Doppler signals.

The reflections for pressure occur from many sites within the arterial tree, but the major effective reflection site in humans appears to be the region of the terminal abdominal aorta. Ascending aortic pressure is increased substantially within 1 beat after bilateral occlusion of the femoral arteries by external manual compression.

Various factors influence the magnitude of reflected waves (**Table 11.2**). Pressure reflections are diminished during the strain phase of the Valsalva maneuver, with the result that pressure and flow waveforms become similar in appearance (**Figure 11.12**). After release of the Valsalva strain, reflected waves return and are exaggerated. Therefore, the commonly noted late-peaking appearance of central aortic and left ventricular pressure tracings in humans (**Figure 11.13**), referred to as the type A waveform pattern, is a result of strong pressure reflections in late systole.

Reflected waves can be of substantial magnitude (**Figure 11.11**) and are increased in the patient with heart failure. Laskey and Kussmaul showed that reflected pressure

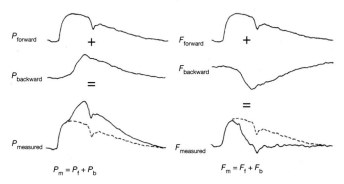

Figure 11.10 Central aortic pressure (*P*) and flow (*F*) measured in a patient during cardiac catheterization. Computer-derived forward and backward pressure and flow components are shown individually: their sum results in the measured waves. (See text for discussion.) (Reprinted with permission from Murgo JP, Westerhof N, Giolma JP, et al. Manipulation of ascending aortic pressure and flow wave reflections with Valsalva maneuver: relationship to input impedance. *Circulation.* 1981;63:122.)

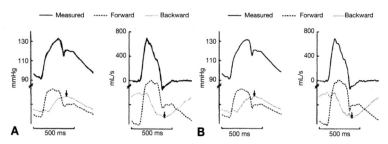

Figure 11.11 Representative ascending aortic pressure and velocity signals from normal subject at rest. The upper panels are the measured pressure (left) and flow (right) pulses, and the lower panels depict the composite forward and reflected components. The superimposed *dashed line* in the upper panels represents the inverse Fourier transformed composite wave (derived from frequency domain analysis). *Arrow* indicates peak of backward wave. **B,** The time domain method of measured wave *(upper panels)* decomposition yields forward and reflected components *(lower panels)* in close agreement with the frequency domain method illustrated in **panel A**. (Reproduced with permission from Laskey WK, Kussmaul WG. Arterial wave reflection in heart failure. *Circulation.* 1987;75:711-722.).

Table 11.2 **Factors that Influence the Magnitude of Reflected Waves**
Factors that augment pressure wave reflections
Vasoconstriction
Heart failure
Hypertension
Aortic or iliofemoral obstruction
Valsalva maneuver—after release
Factors that diminish pressure wave reflections
Vasodilation
Physiologic (eg, fever)
Pharmacologic (eg, nitroglycerin, nitroprusside)
Hypovolemia
Hypotension
Valsalva maneuver—strain phase

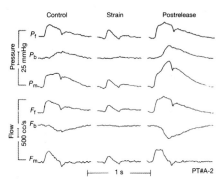

Figure 11.12 Measurements of central aortic pressure (P_m) and flow (F_m) in a patient performing Valsalva maneuver during cardiac catheterization. Control, Valsalva strain, and post-Valsalva release tracings are shown. P_m is the sum of forward (P_f) and backward or reflected (P_b) pressure waves; F_m is the sum of F_f and F_b. (See text for discussion.) (Reprinted with permission from Murgo JP, Westerhof N, Giolma JP, et al. Manipulation of ascending aortic pressure and flow wave reflections with Valsalva maneuver: relationship to input impedance. *Circulation*. 1981;63:122.)

waves were increased in amplitude in 17 patients with heart failure secondary to idiopathic dilated cardiomyopathy, often producing an exaggerated dicrotic wave. Infusion of sodium nitroprusside intravenously markedly reduced the magnitude of the reflected pressure waves and delayed their timing; both these changes were deemed beneficial with regard to left ventricular systolic load.

Wedge Pressures
Broadly stated, a wedge pressure is obtained when an end-hole catheter is positioned in a designated blood vessel with its open end hole facing a capillary bed, with no connecting vessels conducting flow into or away from the designated blood vessel

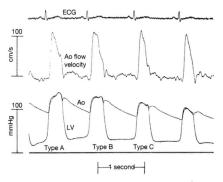

Figure 11.13 Left ventricular (LV) and central aortic (Ao) pressure and aortic flow velocity tracings in a patient at the initiation of the strain phase of a Valsalva maneuver. (See text for details.) (Reprinted with permission from Murgo JP, Westerhof N, Giolma JP, et al. Manipulation of ascending aortic pressure and flow wave reflections with Valsalva maneuver: relationship to input impedance. *Circulation*. 1981;63:122.)

between the catheter tip and the capillary bed. A true wedge pressure can be measured only in the absence of flow. In the absence of flow, pressure equilibrates across the capillary bed so that the catheter-tip pressure is equal to that on the other side of the capillary bed.

NORMAL CONTOURS OF PRESSURE WAVEFORMS

Atrial Pressure

The atrial pressure waveform includes 3 positive waves, the a, c, and v waves, and 3 negative waves or descents, the x, x_1, and y descent (**Figure 11.14**). The a wave corresponds to atrial contraction and occurs within the PR interval. It is followed by the x descent, which corresponds to atrial relaxation, and which is absent in patients with atrial fibrillation. The x descent is followed by the positive c wave, due to a slight increase in atrial pressure following closure of the atrioventricular valve at the beginning of ventricular systole and its bulging into the atrium. During ventricular systole, continuous atrial relaxation and the descent of the atrioventricular valve annulus result in further reduction of atrial pressure and the corresponding x_1 descent. Venous return to the atrium while the atrioventricular valve is closed leads to a progressive increase in atrial pressure (v wave), which is then followed by the y descent after opening of the atrioventricular valve and rapid emptying of the atrium. The left and right atrial pressure contours are similar, with the left atrial pressure being generally higher than the right atrial pressure and with a more prominent V wave in the left atrial pressure contour. Hemodynamic changes secondary to the development of constrictive or tamponade physiology result in characteristic changes in the atrial pressure contour (see Chapter 20).

Pulmonary Wedge Pressure

As shown in **Figure 11.15**, when an end-hole catheter is advanced to a distal branch of the pulmonary artery and occludes forward flow, the corresponding pulmonary veins (PVs), the LA, the open mitral valve, and the LV become an unrestricted vascular bed during diastole. Pressure changes in the LA will be transmitted to the transducer distal to the balloon with a time delay of 0.02 to 0.08 seconds (**Figure 11.16**). Both balloon-tipped and non-balloon-tipped catheters such as the Cournand catheter or a multipurpose catheter can be used, although there is an increased risk of perforation with non-balloon-tipped catheters. Potential artifacts can occur through either "underwedging," thus leading to a hybrid PA/PCWP waveform, or "overwedging." Adequate wedge position can be ensured by observing the pressure

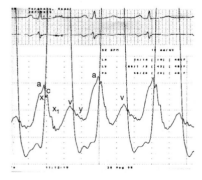

Figure 11.14 Simultaneous left atrial and ventricular pressure recording in a patient with mitral stenosis. See text for the description of the components of the atrial pressure waveform.

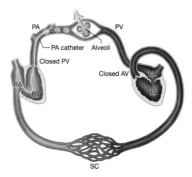

Figure 11.15 Schematic representation of the pulmonary and systemic circulation during pulmonary artery (PA) catheterization and balloon inflation in diastole. There is an unrestricted vascular bed spanning from the distal PA (distal to the transducer) to the pulmonary circulation, the pulmonary veins (PVs), the left atrium (LA), and the left ventricle (LV). AV, aortic valve; RA, right atrium; RV, right ventricle; SC, systemic circulation. (Reproduced with permission from Moscucci M, Maniu C. Pressure measurements. In: Moscucci M, Cohen MG, Chetcuti SJ, eds. *Atlas of Cardiac Catheterization and Interventional Cardiology*. Wolters Kluwer; 2019:130.)

waveform and by obtaining an oxygen saturation in wedge position, which should be above 95%. Examples of pressure waveforms with adequate or inadequate wedge positions are shown in **Figure 11.17**.

Ventricular Pressure

The ventricular pressure waveform is characterized by a systolic and a diastolic phase. As ventricular systole begins, pressure rises and the atrioventricular valve closes. The end diastolic point corresponds to the beginning of ventricular systole, and it is timed to the peak or nadir of the QRS complex. Closing of the atrioventricular valves

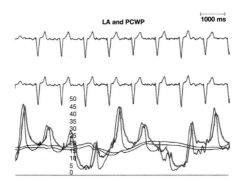

Figure 11.16 Simultaneous left atrial (LA) and pulmonary capillary wedge pressure (PCWP) measurements in a patient with a bioprosthetic mitral valve. Note the time delay of the PCWP tracing (in red) as well as prominent V waves and overall elevated pressures. (Reproduced with permission from Moscucci M, Maniu C. Pressure measurements. In: Moscucci M, Cohen MG, Chetcuti SJ, eds. *Atlas of Cardiac Catheterization and Interventional Cardiology*. Wolters Kluwer; 2019:130.)

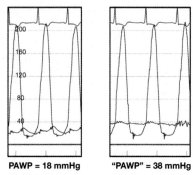

PAWP = 18 mmHg   **"PAWP" = 38 mmHg**

Figure 11.17 The pulmonary artery wedge pressure (PAWP) must be obtained meticulously during cardiac catheterization, optimally performed with a large-bore end-hole catheter. Confirmation of the PAWP examining the pressure contour for respiratory variation and a >95% saturation is recommended to ensure an accurate pressure measurement. Left, PAWP was taken with a large-bore 7F balloon wedge catheter with a 98% saturation confirmation. There is appropriate respiratory variation and a proper contour of the PAWP. Right, the attempt at PAWP was done with a small-lumen thermodilution catheter. This most likely represents a damped pulmonary artery pressure. Confirmation by saturation was not performed. (Reproduced with permission from Nishimura RA, Carabello BA. Hemodynamics in the cardiac catheterization laboratory of the 21st century. *Circulation*. 2012;125:2138-2150.)

is followed by the isovolumic contraction phase, characterized by a raise in intra-ventricular pressure without a change in volume until the opening of the semilunar valve (**Figures 11.18** and **11.19**). The ejection phase then ensues following opening of the semilunar valve and ends with the closing of the valve. This phase is followed by isovolumic relaxation, which ends with opening of the atrioventricular valve and the beginning of diastolic ventricular filling. The ventricular pressure continues to fall at the beginning of rapid filling, reaching a minimum after which the pressure starts raising and ends with a positive wave corresponding to the contribution of atrial systole to ventricular filling. The diastasis corresponds to the phase of diastole characterized by a gradual increase in left ventricular diastolic pressure without a significant increase in volume.

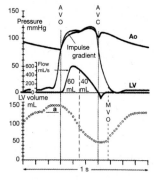

Figure 11.18 Impulse gradient in a normal ventricle and corresponding changes in volumes. Left ventricular (LV) and aortic (Ao) pressure, aortic flow, and volumetric relationship are displayed. Vertical lines indicate aortic valve opening (AVO) and aortic valve closure (AVC) and encompass the systolic ejection period. Dashed lines indicate the midpoint of systole and mitral valve opening (MVO). a, atrial contribution to ventricular filling. (Reproduced with permission from Criley JM, Siegel RJ. Has "obstruction" hindered our understanding of hypertrophic cardiomyopathy? *Circulation*. 1985; 72:1148-1154.)

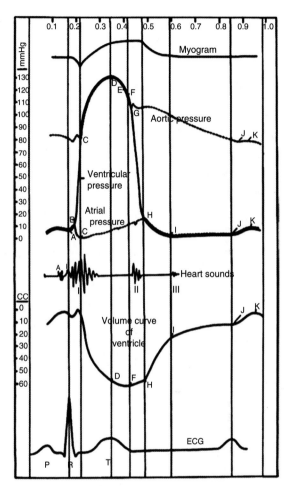

Figure 11.19 Wiggers diagram illustrating the dynamic, mechanical, acoustic, and electrical events during a cardiac cycle. Mechanical systole begins with the rise of pressure at A and ends with the release of tension in all muscle units at F. It is divided into phases of isometric contraction (A-C), maximum ejection (C-D), and reduced ejection (D-F). The subsequent period of diastole is divided into phases of protodiastole, representing the time required for closure of the semilunar valves (F-G), isometric relaxation (G-H), rapid ventricular filling (H-I), diastasis (I-J), and filling by atrial contraction (J-K). (Reproduced with permission from Wiggers CJ. The Henry Jackson memorial lecture dynamics of ventricular contraction under abnormal conditions. *Circulation*. 1952;5:321-348.)

Aortic Pressure

The contour of the aortic pressure is the result of the forward wave and reflected waves. It should be noted that the arterial pressure might rise slightly during isovolumic contraction of the LV, due to bulging of the semilunar valve in the aorta. At the end of the isovolumic ventricular contraction phase, with opening of the aortic valve, the ejections phase begins and the aortic pressure starts rising. The initial steep increase is followed by a peak and then by a decline to the dicrotic notch, which corresponds to closure of the aortic valve and end of ejection.

SOURCES OF ERROR AND ARTIFACT

Common sources of error and artifact include deterioration in frequency response, catheter whip artifact, end pressure artifact, catheter impact artifact, systolic pressure amplification in the periphery, and errors in zero level, balancing, and calibration.

Deterioration in Frequency Response

Although frequency response may be high and damping optimal during setup of the transducers, substantial deterioration in the characteristics can develop during the course of a catheterization study.

Air bubbles may be introduced into the catheters, stopcocks, or tubing or dissolved air may come out of the saline solution used to fill the transducer. Even the smallest air bubbles have a drastic effect on pressure measurement because they cause excessive damping and lower the natural frequency (by serving as an added compliance). When the natural frequency of the pressure measurement system falls, high-frequency components of the pressure waveform (such as those that occur with intraventricular pressure rise and fall) may set the system in oscillation, producing the ventricular pressure overshoot commonly seen in early systole and diastole (**Figure 11.20**). Flushing out the catheter, manifold, and transducer dispels these small air bubbles and restores the frequency response of the pressure measurement system (**Figure 11.21**).

Catheter Whip Artifact

Motion of the tip of the catheter within the heart and great vessels accelerates the fluid contained within the catheter. Such catheter whip artifacts may produce superimposed waves of ±10 mmHg. Catheter whip artifacts are particularly common in tracings from the pulmonary arteries and are difficult to avoid (**Figure 11.22**).

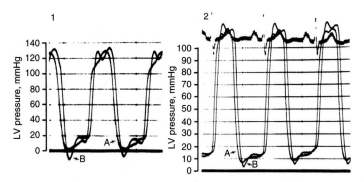

Figure 11.20 Left ventricular (LV) pressure signals as recorded with a micromanometer and with a system using long, fluid-filled tubing and several interposed stopcocks between the pressure transducer and the 7F NIH catheter. The micromanometer tracing is labeled A, and the fluid-filled catheter tracing is labeled B. Note both the early diastolic and the early ejection phase overshoots recorded with the fluid-filled catheter, indicating a poor frequency response, especially in the graph on the left.

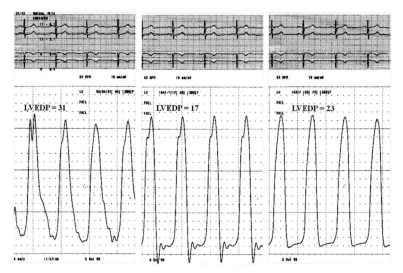

Figure 11.21 Pitfalls in measurements of the left ventricular diastolic pressure (all measurements obtained in the same patient). Left: The left ventricular end-diastolic pressure (LVEDP) is markedly elevated, and there is an abnormal contour of the pressure waveform. The abnormal contour and elevation of LVEDP is due to inappropriate position of the left ventricular pigtail catheter, with a side hole in the ascending aorta. Middle: There is an early diastolic overshoot due to an air bubble in the system. Right: Normal tracing after repositioning and flushing the catheter.

End Pressure Artifact

Flowing blood has a kinetic energy by virtue of its motion, and when this flow suddenly comes to a halt, the kinetic energy is converted in part into pressure. Therefore, an end-hole catheter pointing upstream (eg, radial or femoral arterial pressure monitoring line) records a pressure that is artifactually elevated by the converted kinetic energy. This added pressure may range from 2 to 10 mmHg.

Catheter Impact Artifact

Catheter impact artifact is similar to catheter whip artifact. When a fluid-filled catheter is hit (eg, by valves in the act of opening or closing or by the walls of the ventricular chambers), a pressure transient is created. Catheter impact artifacts are common with pigtail catheters in the left ventricular chamber, where the terminal pigtail may be hit by the mitral valve leaflets as they open in early diastole.

Systolic Pressure Amplification in the Periphery

When radial, brachial, or femoral arterial pressures are measured and used to represent aortic pressure, it must be remembered that peak systolic pressure in these arteries may be considerably higher (eg, by 20-50 mmHg) than peak systolic pressure in the central aorta, although mean arterial pressure will be the same or slightly lower. There is convincing evidence that the change in waveform of arterial pressure as it travels away from the heart is largely a consequence of reflected waves from the

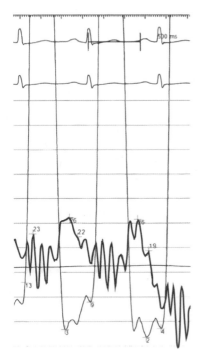

Figure 11.22 Pulmonary artery wedge pressure during nitroprusside (Nipride) infusion in a patient with severe mitral regurgitation. Note the multiple superimposed waves secondary to catheter whip artifact. (Reproduced with permission from Moscucci M, Maniu C. Pressure measurements. In: Moscucci M, Cohen MG, Chetcuti SJ, eds. *Atlas of Cardiac Catheterization and Interventional Cardiology.* Wolters Kluwer; 2019:131.)

aortic bifurcation, arterial branch points, and small peripheral vessels, causing amplification of the peak systolic and pulse pressures (**Figure 11.23**). The pressure amplification in the periphery is particularly marked in the radial artery and may mask and distort pressure gradients across the aortic valve or left ventricular outflow tract. Use of a double-lumen catheter (eg, double-lumen pigtail) allows measurement of left ventricular and central aortic pressures simultaneously, thus avoiding this problem. Other methods include the transseptal technique with a second catheter in the central aorta, the use of a pigtail catheter inserted from the contralateral femoral artery, or the use of a diagnostic catheter inside a guiding catheter.

Errors in Zero Level, Balancing, or Calibration

Error because of improper zero reference is common. All manometers must be zeroed at the same point (and the zero-reference point should be changed if the patient's position is changed during the course of the study, eg, if pillows are placed to prop up the patient). Transducers requiring calibration should be calibrated before each period of use.

MICROMANOMETERS

To reduce the mass and inertia of the pressure measurement system, improve the frequency response characteristics, and decrease artifacts associated with underdamping, overdamping, and catheter whip, miniaturized transducers have been developed

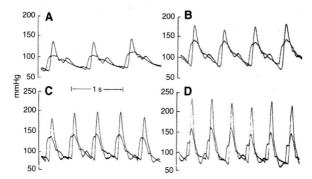

Figure 11.23 A, The pulse wave generated by the heart travels down the arterial tree with a certain velocity (pulse wave velocity), which in turn depends on the distensibility of the arterial wall. Eventually, the pulse wave is reflected at branch points, and travels backward. Peripheral pulse pressure is the summation of the forward and the reflected waves. Thus, pulse pressure depends on the stroke volume, the elasticity and diameter of the aorta, the pulse wave velocity, and effective reflective distance (distance from reflection points to the heart). **B,** The amplitude of pulse pressure increases toward the periphery, especially so in younger people, because these points are closer to the reflection sites and the reflected wave has to travel back a lesser distance. **C,** In individuals with a stiff aorta, the reflected wave returns earlier in systole and superimposes on the forward wave at the inflection point to result in an augmentation of the systolic pressure and pulse pressure. The debate centers on whether the forward wave determined by proximal aortic impedance (and aortic diameter) contributes more to pulse pressure relative to the reflected wave. (Reproduced with permission from Vasan RS. Pathogenesis of elevated peripheral pulse pressure. *Hypertension.* 2008;51:33-36.)

that fit on the distal tip of standard catheters or guidewires and therefore may be used as intracardiac manometers. Measuring pressure directly within the vessel or cardiac chamber with the transducer on the tip of the catheter prevents the distortions associated with fluid-filled systems. In addition, these micromanometers have a flat frequency response up to 1000 Hz, thus allowing accurate recording at high heart rates. Particularly reliable catheter tip manometers are made by Millar Instruments. Variations of these catheters include a pigtail tip, as well as 1 or 2 pressure sensors and as many as 12 electrodes for simultaneous high-fidelity pressure and volume measurements. Disposable versions of Millar catheters and pressure wires are available for clinical use.

For accurate measurement of the rate of ventricular pressure rise (dP/dt) and other parameters of myocardial performance occurring during the first 40 to 50 ms of ventricular systole, high-frequency response characteristics are necessary.

PRESSURE TRACINGS IN VALVULAR AND NONVALVULAR HEART DISEASE

Familiarity with normal and abnormal pressure waveforms is critical for optimal evaluation and management of patients referred to the catheterization laboratory. **Figures 11.24-11.28** provide examples of abnormal pressure tracings in patients with valvular and nonvalvular heart disease.

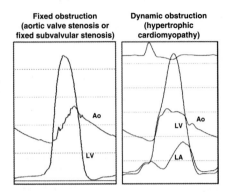

Figure 11.24 A visual assessment of the contour of the aortic (Ao) and left ventricular (LV) pressures is important during cardiac catheterization. Left, Patients with fixed obstruction (either valvular stenosis or fixed subvalvular stenosis) will demonstrate a parvus and a tardus in the upstroke of the aortic pressure, beginning at the time of aortic valve opening. Right, In patients with a dynamic obstruction (such as that found in hypertrophic cardiomyopathy), the aortic pressure will rise rapidly at the onset of aortic valve opening and then develop a spike-and-dome contour as the obstruction occurs in late systole. The LV pressure also has a late peak because of the mechanism of this dynamic obstruction. (Reproduced with permission from Nishimura RA, Carabello BA. Hemodynamics in the cardiac catheterization laboratory of the 21st century. *Circulation*. 2012;125:2138-2150.)

BLOOD FLOW MEASUREMENT

In the absence of major disease of the vascular tree (eg, arterial obstruction), the maintenance of appropriate blood flow to the body depends largely on the heart's ability to pump blood in the forward direction.

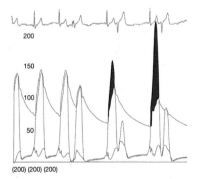

Figure 11.25 Hypertrophic cardiomyopathy. Simultaneous left ventricular and aortic pressure measured in a patient with hypertrophic cardiomyopathy. Note the typical "Brockenbrough-Braunwald-Morrow sign," represented by a marked increase in left ventricular outflow tract gradient accompanied by a reduction in aortic pressure following a premature beat. The postextrasystolic potentiation following the premature beat leads to an increase in dynamic obstruction and resultant reduction in stroke volume and pulse pressure. (Reproduced with permission from Moscucci M, Maniu C. Pressure measurements. In: Moscucci M, Cohen MG, Chetcuti SJ, eds. *Atlas of Cardiac Catheterization and Interventional Cardiology.* Wolters Kluwer; 2019:132.)

Snapshot: PCW : 26/26/17

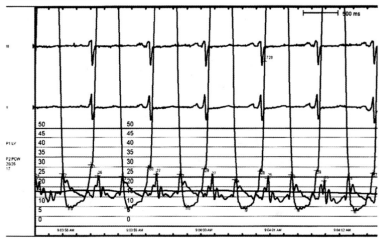

Snapshot: Gradient Measurement: Valve Area Measures

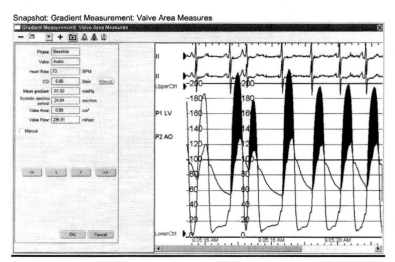

Figure 11.26 Hemodynamic tracing from a patient with severe aortic stenosis. Note the pressure waveform immediately after the premature beat. Contrary to what is shown in Figure 11.25, the postpremature beat is characterized by an increase in both left ventricular and aortic (Ao) pressure, rather than by an increase in gradient associated with a decrease in Ao pressure. (Reproduced with permission from Moscucci M, Maniu C. Pressure measurements. In: Moscucci M, Cohen MG, Chetcuti SJ, eds. *Atlas of Cardiac Catheterization and Interventional Cardiology.* Wolters Kluwer; 2019:137.)

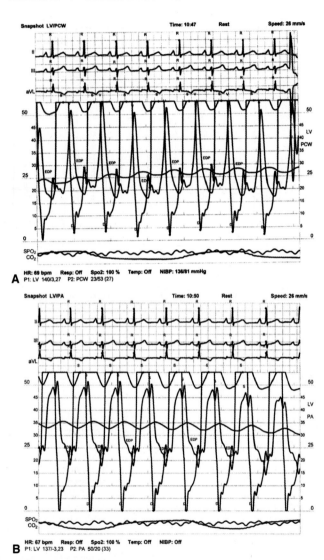

Figure 11.27 Severe mitral regurgitation. Hemodynamic tracings from a patient with severe mitral regurgitation. **Panel A** shows the pulmonary capillary wedge pressure with "giant" V waves. **Panel B** shows the pulmonary artery catheterization (PA) pressure. Note the double peak of the PA pressure tracing. The second positive wave is a manifestation of the V wave transmitted retrograde through the pulmonary vasculature, and it can be seen in the setting of severe mitral regurgitation. (Reproduced with permission from Moscucci M, Maniu C. Pressure measurements. In: Moscucci M, Cohen MG, Chetcuti SJ, eds. *Atlas of Cardiac Catheterization and Interventional Cardiology.* Wolters Kluwer; 2019:139.)

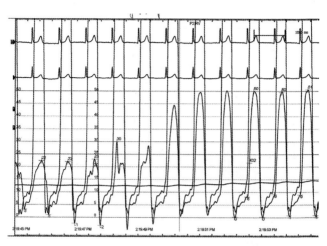

Figure 11.28 Right ventricular (RV) outflow tract obstruction. Pullback of a right-sided heart catheter from the pulmonary artery to the RV inflow tract. Note the significant increase in pressure when the catheter is withdrawn in the RV inflow tract.

EXTRACTION RESERVE AND CARDIAC OUTPUT

The extraction of nutrients by metabolizing tissues is a function not only of the rate of delivery of those nutrients (the cardiac output) but also of the ability of each tissue to extract those nutrients from the circulation. Therefore, tissue viability can be maintained despite a fall in cardiac output as long as there is increased extraction of required nutrients. The extraction of a given nutrient (or of any substance) from the circulation by a particular tissue is expressed as the arteriovenous difference across that tissue, and the factor by which the arteriovenous difference can increase at constant flow (owing to changes in metabolic demand) may be termed the extraction reserve. For example, arterial blood in humans is normally 95% saturated with oxygen; that is, if 1 L of blood has the capacity to carry approximately 200 mL of oxygen when fully saturated, arterial blood will usually be found to contain 190 mL of oxygen per liter (190/200 = 95%). Venous blood returning from the body normally has an average oxygen saturation of 75%; that is, mixed venous blood generally contains 150 mL of oxygen per liter of blood (150/200 = 75%). Thus, the normal arteriovenous difference for oxygen is 40 mL/L (190-150 mL/L).

The normal extraction reserve for oxygen is 3, which means that under extreme metabolic demand, the body's tissues can extract up to 120 mL of oxygen (3 × 40 mL) from each liter of blood delivered. Thus, if arterial saturation remains constant at 95%, full use of the extraction reserve will result in a mixed venous oxygen content of 70 mL/L (190-120 mL/L) or a mixed venous oxygen saturation of 35% (70/200 = 35%). This is essentially the value found for mixed venous (ie, pulmonary artery) oxygen saturation in normal men studied at maximal exercise. The relation between cardiac output and arteriovenous O_2 difference is illustrated in **Figure 11.29**.

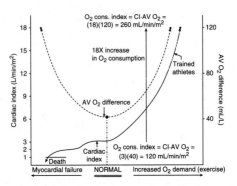

Figure 11.29 Relationship between arteriovenous oxygen (AV O_2) difference (broken line) and cardiac index (solid curve) in normal subjects at rest (center) and during exercise (right), and in the patient with progressively worsening myocardial failure (left). (See text for discussion.)

Lower Limit of Cardiac Output

The value of 3 for the oxygen extraction reserve predicts that, in progressive cardiac decompensation, meeting the basal oxygen requirements of the body demands that oxygen extraction increase as cardiac output falls until the arteriovenous oxygen difference has tripled and cardiac output has fallen to one-third of its normal value (**Figure 11.29**). Because the extraction reserve has now been used fully, any further reduction of cardiac output will result in tissue hypoxia, anaerobic metabolism, acidosis, and, eventually, circulatory collapse. Indeed, for many years it has been observed that a fall in resting cardiac output to below one-third of normal (ie, a cardiac index of <1.0 L/min/m²) is incompatible with life.

Upper Limit of Cardiac Output

Several studies have indicated that the largest increase in cardiac output that can be achieved by a trained athlete at maximal exercise is 600% of the resting output. If a normal 70-kg man has a cardiac output of 5 L/min or 3.0 L/min/m², his maximal cardiac output might be as high as 30 L/min (18 L/min/m²). Because cardiac output increases by approximately 600 mL for each 100 mL increase in oxygen requirements of the body, an increase in cardiac output of 25 L/min with maximal exercise would suggest an increase in total-body oxygen requirements of 4167 mL/min, which is approximately an 18-fold increase over the normal resting value of 250 mL/min. The 18-fold increase in total-body oxygen requirements is met by the combined 6-fold increase in oxygen delivery (ie, cardiac output) and 3-fold increase in oxygen extraction (extraction reserve). These relations are illustrated in **Figure 11.29**.

Factors Influencing Cardiac Output in Normal Subjects

The range of the "normal" cardiac output is difficult to define with precision because it is influenced by several variables. Obviously, body size is important, and for this reason, normalization of the cardiac output for differing body size is considered fundamental. Because cardiac output seems to be predominantly a function of the body's oxygen consumption or metabolic rate and because metabolic rate is thought to correlate best with body surface area (BSA), it has become customary to express cardiac output in terms of the cardiac index ([liters/min]/[BSA, m^2]). BSA is not measured directly but is instead calculated from one of the experimentally developed formulas, such as that of Dubois.

$$\text{Body surface area}\left(m^2\right) = 0.007184 \times \text{weight}^{0.425}\left(kg\right) \times \text{height}^{0.725}\left(cm\right) \qquad (11.1)$$

The normal cardiac output appears to vary also with age, steadily decreasing from approximately 4.5 L/min/m^2 at age 7 years to 2.5 L/min/m^2 at age 70 years. This is not surprising, given that the body's metabolic rate is the highest in childhood and progressively diminishes with age.

Cardiac output is also affected by posture, decreasing by approximately 20% when a person rises (or is tilted) from a lying to a standing position. In addition, body temperature, anxiety, environmental heat and humidity, and a host of other factors influence the normal resting cardiac output, and these must be considered in interpreting any value of cardiac output measured in the clinical setting.

TECHNIQUES FOR DETERMINATION OF CARDIAC OUTPUT

Of the numerous techniques devised over the years to measure cardiac output, 2 have won general acceptance in cardiac catheterization laboratories: the Fick oxygen technique and the indicator dilution technique. Both techniques are similar in that they are based on the theoretical principle enunciated by Adolph Fick in 1870. The principle states that the total uptake or release of any substance by an organ is the product of blood flow to the organ and the arteriovenous concentration difference of the substance. For the lungs, the substance released to the blood is oxygen, and the pulmonary blood flow can be determined by knowing the arteriovenous difference of oxygen across the lungs and the oxygen consumption per minute.

Fick Oxygen Method

In the Fick oxygen method, pulmonary blood flow should be determined by measuring the arteriovenous difference of oxygen across the lungs and the rate of oxygen uptake by blood from the lungs. If there is no intracardiac shunt and pulmonary blood flow is equal to systemic blood flow, the Fick oxygen method also measures systemic blood flow. Thus, cardiac output equals oxygen consumption divided by arteriovenous oxygen difference.

In actual practice, the rate at which oxygen is taken up from the lungs by blood is not measured, but rather the uptake of oxygen from room air by the lungs is measured, because at steady state these 2 measurements are equal. Furthermore, arteriovenous oxygen difference across the lungs is not measured directly. Generally, pulmonary arterial blood (true mixed venous blood) is sampled, but pulmonary venous blood is not sampled. Instead, left ventricular or systemic arterial blood is sampled and assumed to have an oxygen content representative of mixed pulmonary venous blood. Actually, because of bronchial venous and Thebesian venous drainage, the oxygen content of systemic arterial blood is commonly 2 to 5 mL/L of blood lower than that of pulmonary venous blood as it leaves the alveoli.

Oxygen Consumption

Methods for measurement of oxygen consumption have included the Douglas bag method, the polarographic method, and the paramagnetic method. As of today, direct measurements of oxygen consumption are rarely obtained in the cardiac catheterization laboratory. A description of each system and brand is beyond the scope of this chapter.

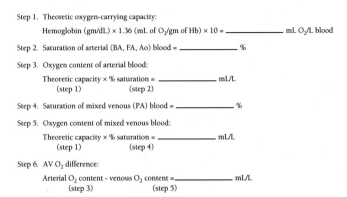

Step 1. Theoretic oxygen-carrying capacity:

Hemoglobin (gm/dL) × 1.36 (mL of O_2/gm of Hb) × 10 = _____ mL O_2/L blood

Step 2. Saturation of arterial (BA, FA, Ao) blood = _____ %

Step 3. Oxygen content of arterial blood:

Theoretic capacity × % saturation = _____ mL/L
   (step 1)   (step 2)

Step 4. Saturation of mixed venous (PA) blood = _____ %

Step 5. Oxygen content of mixed venous blood:

Theoretic capacity × % saturation = _____ mL/L
   (step 1)   (step 4)

Step 6. AV O_2 difference:

Arterial O_2 content - venous O_2 content = _____ mL/L
   (step 3)   (step 5)

Figure 11.30 Calculation of oxygen content and arteriovenous (AV) oxygen difference when using the reflectance oximetry method. Ao, aorta; BA, brachial artery; FA, femoral artery; PA, pulmonary artery.

Arteriovenous Oxygen Difference

The arteriovenous oxygen difference across the lungs must be measured to calculate cardiac output by Fick principle (**Figures 11.30** and **11.31**). Systemic arterial and mixed venous (pulmonary arterial) blood samples are obtained when O_2 consumption is being measured.

A formula for approximating the theoretical oxygen-carrying capacity in humans is as follows:

$$\text{Hemoglobin}(g/dL) \times 1.36(\text{mL } O_2/g \text{ of hemoglobin}) \times 10$$
$$= \text{theoretical } O_2 - \text{carrying capacity}(\text{mL } O_2/\text{liter of blood})$$
(11.2)

In several textbooks, the constant is given as 1.34, but studies on crystalline human hemoglobin suggest that the correct number may be 1.36. Whatever is its correct value, the formula is only an approximation. Current oximeters, such as the AVOXimeter 1000E or 4000 (Instrumentation Laboratory, Bedford, Massachusetts), illuminate a very small sample of heparinized blood (volume, 50 μL) with light of multiple wavelengths and record the optical density of each transmitted wavelength. This approach allows estimation of total hemoglobin concentration as well as the concentrations of its various components: oxyhemoglobin, methemoglobin, and carboxyhemoglobin.

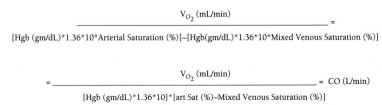

$$\frac{V_{O_2} \text{ (mL/min)}}{[\text{Hgb (gm/dL)}*1.36*10*\text{Arterial Saturation (\%)}]-[\text{Hgb(gm/dL)}*1.36*10*\text{Mixed Venous Saturation (\%)}]} =$$

$$= \frac{V_{O_2} \text{ (mL/min)}}{[\text{Hgb (gm/dL)}*1.36*10]*[\text{art Sat (\%)}-\text{Mixed Venous Saturation (\%)}]} = \text{CO (L/min)}$$

Figure 11.31 Calculation of cardiac output using the Fick oxygen method

Arterial blood may be taken from a systemic artery, the LV, the LA, or the PVs. Theoretically, pulmonary venous blood is preferable to peripheral arterial blood for the arteriovenous oxygen difference calculations. However, except in the presence of a right-to-left intracardiac shunt, pulmonary venous oxygen content may be approximated by systemic arterial oxygen content, ignoring the small amount of venous admixture resulting from bronchial and Thebesian venous drainage. If arterial desaturation (eg, arterial blood oxygen saturation <95%) is present, a central right-to-left shunt should be excluded before accepting systemic arterial oxygen content as representative of pulmonary venous blood.

The most reliable site for obtaining mixed venous blood is the pulmonary artery. Because of streaming and incomplete mixing, using the blood from more proximal sites such as the right atrium or vena cavae as representative of mixed venous blood is less accurate.

Sources of Error

Potential errors in the determination of cardiac output by the Fick oxygen technique may come from a number of sources. Improper collection of the mixed venous blood sample (eg, air bubbles) is a common source of error. Partial contamination of pulmonary arterial blood with pulmonary capillary wedge blood may result in a falsely high mixed venous blood oxygen content. If the mixed venous blood sample is taken from the right atrium, inferior vena cava, coronary sinus, or similar sites, a falsely low or high value for arteriovenous difference may result. Also, care must be taken not to dilute the blood sample with an excessive quantity of heparinized saline solution.

The average error in determining oxygen consumption has been estimated to be approximately 6%. The error for arteriovenous oxygen difference has been estimated at 5%. Narrow arteriovenous oxygen differences are more prone to introduce error than are wide arteriovenous oxygen differences. Thus, the Fick oxygen method is most accurate in patients with low cardiac output, in whom the arteriovenous oxygen difference is wide. The total error in determination of the cardiac output by the Fick oxygen method has been established to be about 10%.

To avoid the technical difficulties and expense associated with measurement of oxygen consumption, most laboratories today assume that O_2 consumption can be predicted from the BSA, with or without a correction for age and sex. Thus, some laboratories assume that resting O_2 consumption is 125 mL/m^2, or 110 mL/m^2 for elderly patients (Dehmer formula).

Additional methods to estimate oxygen consumption that have been proposed include the formula of LaFarge (Eq. 11.3) and the formula of Bergstra (Eq. 11.4):

$$O_2\left(\text{mL/min}\right) = 138.1 - \left(X \times \log_e \text{age}\right) + \left(0.378 \times \text{Heart Rate}\right) \\ \times \text{BSA}\left(\text{Men}: X = 11.49; \text{Women}: X = 17.04\right) \tag{11.3}$$

$$O_2\left(\text{mL/min}\right) = 157.3 \times \text{BSA} + X - \left(10.5 \times \log_e \text{age}\right) + 4.8\left(\text{Men}: X = 10; \text{Women} = 0\right) \tag{11.4}$$

The validity of each formula was evaluated in a study by Narang et al. Oxygen consumption was measured using the Douglas bag technique and compared with estimates derived from each formula. Measured O_2 consumption differed significantly from each estimate, with a mean interquartile of 28.4 mL/min, 37.7 mL/min, and 31.7 mL/min, for the formulae of Dehmer, LaFarge, and Bergstra, respectively ($P < .0001$ for each). Thus, assumed values for O_2 consumption are likely to introduce considerable error, no matter which method is used.

Indicator Dilution Methods

The indicator dilution method is merely a specific application of Fick general principle.

There are 2 general types of the indicator dilution method: the continuous-infusion method and the single injection method. The single-injection method is the most widely used and is discussed here in detail. The fundamental requirements for this method include the following:

1. A bolus of nontoxic indicator substance is injected; the substance mixes completely with blood, and its concentration can be measured accurately.
2. The indicator substance is neither added to nor subtracted from blood during its passage between the injection and the sampling site.
3. Most of the indicator substance must pass the site of sampling before recirculation begins.
4. The indicator substance must go through a portion of the central circulation where all the blood of the body becomes mixed.

The theoretical considerations for the single-injection method may be summarized as follows: An injection of a specified amount of an indicator, I, into a proximal vessel or chamber (eg, the right atrium for the thermodilution method) is followed by continuous measurement of the indicator concentration C in blood as a function of time, t, at a point downstream from the injection (eg, pulmonary artery for thermodilution technique). Because all of the injected indicator, I, must pass the downstream measurement site,

$$I = \dot{Q}\int_0^\infty C(t)\,dt \qquad (11.5)$$

where Q is the volume flow (in milliliters per minute) between the site of injection and the site of measurement. Thus, Q (which is the cardiac output in the methods to be described) may be calculated as

$$\dot{Q} = \frac{I}{\int_0^\infty C(t)\,dt} \qquad (11.6)$$

Numerous indicators have been used successfully. Indocyanine green previously had enjoyed long-standing acceptance in clinical practice but is no longer used today for routine measurement of cardiac output.

Thermodilution Method

A thermal indicator method for measuring cardiac output was first introduced by Fegler in 1954 but was not applied to the clinical situation until the works of Branthwaite and Bradley and Ganz et al. were published. In the initial study by Ganz et al., 2 thermistors were used: one in the superior vena cava at the site at which the cold dextrose solution was injected into the bloodstream and a second downstream thermistor in the pulmonary artery. These 2 thermistors allowed accurate measurement of the temperature of the injectate, T_I, as well as the temperature of blood, T_B, downstream from the injection site. Using the basic indicator dilution equation, the cardiac output by thermodilution CO_{TD} in milliliters is given as

$$CO_{TD} = \frac{V_I \left(T_B - T_I \right) \left(S_I \cdot C_I / S_B \cdot C_B \right) 60 \left(s/min \right)}{\int_0^\infty \Delta T_B \left(t \right) dt}$$ (11.7)

where V_I is the volume of injectate (mL) and S_B, S_I, C_B, and C_I are the specific gravity and specific heat of blood and injectate, respectively. When 5% dextrose is used as the indicator, $S_I \bullet C_I / S_B \bullet C_B = 1.08$. Most of the commercially available thermodilution systems use a single thermistor only, placed at the downstream site, and assume that the temperature of the injectate (measured in a bowl before injection or with a thermometer attached to the bag in a closed system) increases by a predictable amount (catheter warming) during injection. The cardiac output calculated by the thermodilution equation is multiplied by an empirical correction factor (0.825) to correct for the catheter warming.

It has been shown that improved accuracy and precision can be obtained with the thermodilution technique when cardiac output is measured using a dual-thermistor catheter system. The use of a second thermistor positioned to measure temperature at the point where the injectate exits the catheter in the right atrium can take into account any warming of the injectate that occurs as it travels from the injectate syringe to the point of exit from the catheter in the right atrium.

Sources of Error

1. The method is unreliable in the presence of significant tricuspid regurgitation.
2. The baseline temperature of blood in the pulmonary artery usually shows distinct fluctuations associated with respiratory and cardiac cycles. If these fluctuations are large, they may approach the magnitude of the temperature change produced by the cold-indicator injection.
3. Loss of injected indicator (cold) between the injection and the measuring site (pulmonary artery) is not usually a problem, but in low-flow, low-output states, loss of indicator may occur because of warming of blood by the walls of the cardiac chambers and surrounding tissues. This concern is supported by the study of van Grondelle et al., who found that thermodilution cardiac output measurements overestimated cardiac output consistently in patients with low output (<3.5 L/min), and this overestimation was the highest, averaging 35%, in patients whose cardiac output was <2.5 L/min. This is what might be expected from the equation for calculation of cardiac output by thermodilution, since the change in pulmonary artery blood temperature (ATB) will be reduced if cold is lost owing to warming of the injectate during its slow passage through the vena cava, right atrium, and right ventricle. Because ATB is the denominator in the equation for cardiac output calculation, reduction in ATB will result in a rise in calculated cardiac output.
4. The empirical correction factor of 0.825 may be inadequate to correct for deviations of true injectate temperature from the temperature of the injectate in the bowl or reservoir, owing to warming in the syringe by the hand of the individual injecting the dextrose solution from the syringe or by catheter warming.
5. Most laboratories today use room temperature, rather than ice-cold, D5W or saline. The use of room temperature solutions rather than ice-cold solutions reduces the signal-to-noise ratio, and it can introduce additional variability from sample to sample.

In general, indicator dilution cardiac output determinations involve an error of 5% to 10% when performed carefully. The values obtained correlate well with those calculated by the Fick oxygen method. **Table 11.3** summarizes pitfalls of cardiac output determination with the Fick method and with the thermodilution indicator method.

Continuous Cardiac Output Monitoring

The evolution of ICU (intensive care unit) care and invasive hemodynamic monitoring has spearheaded the development of right-sided heart catheters and technology for continuous cardiac output monitoring (Edwards Lifesciences, Irvine, California). These catheters are based on the thermodilution method, with the difference that they use a warm indicator rather than a cold indicator. The catheter includes a proximal thermal filament, located in the right atrium, and a distal thermistor or sensor, located in the pulmonary artery at 4 cm from the tip of the catheter. The thermal filament generates an input signal, which results in warming of the blood. Thus, a "warm" bolus rather than a "cold" bolus is generated. The input signal is detected by the distal sensor in the pulmonary artery and processed by a computer, which creates a washout curve and determines the cardiac output. These catheters are often used for continuous monitoring of critically ill patients in the ICU setting, trauma patients,

Table 11.3	Pitfalls in the Determination of Cardiac Output With the Fick Method and the Thermodilution Method
Fick method	
Inadequate mixing of blood in the right atrium	
Inappropriate sampling (high right atrium, low right atrium, distal PA in partial wedge position)	
Contamination of blood sample with air or heparinized saline	
V_{O_2} usually not measured. There might be significant variation in V_{O_2}, particularly in critically ill patients	
Improper measurement of V_{O_2}	
High-output states with narrow AV O_2 difference	
Thermodilution method	
Low-output states (incomplete mixing of the indicator)	
Atrial fibrillation (incomplete mixing of the indicator)	
Tricuspid regurgitation (indicator abnormally recirculated)	
Intracardiac shunts (indicator abnormally recirculated)	
Simultaneous administration of intravenous fluids	

PA, mean pulmonary arterial pressure.

and cardiac surgery patients in the perioperative period. Several studies have shown that, when compared with the standard intermittent bolus thermodilution technique, continuous cardiac output monitoring with the warm bolus provides more accurate and reproducible measurements.

CLINICAL MEASUREMENT OF VASCULAR RESISTANCE
Poiseuille Law
The French physician Jean Leonard Marie Poiseuille (1799–1869) made many important contributions to the study of hemodynamics. His discoveries, later modified by others, are expressed in what is regarded as Poiseuille law, which may be stated as follows:

$$Q = \frac{\pi \left(P_i - P_o \right) r^4}{8 \eta l} \tag{11.8}$$

where Q is the volume flow, $P_i - P_o$ is inflow pressure − outflow pressure, r is the radius of the tube, l is the length of the tube, and n is the viscosity of the fluid.

This relationship applies in the specific circumstance of steady-state laminar flow of a homogeneous fluid through a rigid tube. Under these conditions, flow, Q, varies directly as the pressure difference, $P_i - P_o$, and the fourth power of the tube's radius, r. It varies inversely as the length, l, of the tube and the viscosity, n, of the fluid.

Hydraulic resistance, R, is defined by analogy to Ohm law as the ratio of mean pressure drop, AP, to flow, Q, across the vascular circuit. The various factors contributing to vascular resistance can be illustrated by rearranging Poiseuille law as follows:

$$R = \frac{P_i - P_o}{Q} = \frac{8 \eta l}{\pi r^4} \tag{11.9}$$

It is apparent from this equation that, in the condition of steady laminar flow of a homogeneous fluid through a rigid cylindrical tube, resistance to flow depends only on the dimensions of the tube and the viscosity of the fluid. In particular, the resistance is remarkably sensitive to changes in the radius of the tube, as it varies inversely with the fourth power of the radius.

Vascular Resistance and Pressure-flow Relationships
The applicability of laws derived from steady-state fluid mechanics in assessing vascular resistance is somewhat ambiguous because blood flow is pulsatile, blood is a nonhomogeneous fluid, and the vascular bed is a nonlinear, elastic, frequency-dependent system. In such a system, resistance varies continuously with pressure and flow and is influenced by inertia, reflected waves, and the phase angle between pulse and flow wave velocities.

To assess both vessel caliber and vessel elasticity, the concept of *vascular impedance* has been used. Vascular impedance has been defined as the instantaneous ratio of pulsatile pressure to pulsatile flow. Because impedance may not be the same for all frequencies, its calculation requires resolution of the harmonic components of both pressure and flow pulsations. The *impedance modulus* so calculated is then expressed as a spectrum of impedance versus frequency. Although measurement of impedance is important in research studies, it is rarely included in routine diagnostic cardiac catheterization, and the reader is referred elsewhere for a full discussion.

As a consequence of the foregoing considerations and the many active and passive factors that influence pressure and flow in blood vessels, the concept of vascular resistance in its pure physical sense is limited in application. In the context of the clinical and physiologic setting, however, pulmonary and systemic vascular resistances calculated from hemodynamic measurements made during cardiac catheterization have acquired empiric pathophysiologic meaning and often become important factors in clinical decision-making.

Estimation of Vascular Resistance in the Clinical Situation

Calculations of vascular resistance are usually applied to both the pulmonary and the systemic circulations. To estimate pulmonary and systemic vascular resistances quantitatively, knowledge of both the driving pressure across the pulmonary and systemic vascular beds and the respective blood flow through them is required.

The formulas generally used are the following:

$$\text{A. Systemic vascular resistance} = \frac{\overline{Ao} - \overline{RA}}{Q_S}$$

$$\text{B. Total pulmonary resistance} = \frac{\overline{PA}}{Q_P} \qquad (11.10)$$

$$\text{C. Pulmonary vacular resistance} = \frac{\overline{PA} - \overline{LA}}{Q_P}$$

where Ao is mean systemic arterial pressure, RA is mean right atrial pressure, PA is mean pulmonary arterial pressure, LA is mean left atrial pressure, Q_s is systemic blood flow, and Q_p is pulmonary blood flow.

In many laboratories, the mean pulmonary capillary wedge pressure is used as an approximation of mean left atrial pressure. The flows are volume flows (as opposed to velocity flows) and are expressed in liters per minute, and the pressures are expressed in millimeters of mercury (mmHg). These equations yield resistance in arbitrary resistance units (R units) expressed in mmHg per liter per minute, also called *hybrid resistance units* (HRUs). These HRUs are sometimes referred to as Wood units because they were first introduced by Dr. Paul Wood. They may be converted to metric resistance units expressed in dynes-sec-cm^{-5} by use of a conversion factor of 80. In this system, resistance is expressed as

$$\text{Resistance} = \frac{\Delta P\left(\text{mmHg}\right) \times 1,332\ \text{dyn/cm}^2/\text{mmHg}}{Q_S\ or\ Q_P\left(\text{L/min}\right) \times 1,000\ \text{mL/L} \div 60\ \text{s/min}}$$

$$= \frac{\Delta P}{Q_S\ or\ Q_S} \times 80\ \text{dyns/cm}^5 \qquad (11.11)$$

In pediatric practice, it is conventional to normalize vascular resistances for BSA, thus giving a resistance index. Although this is not commonly done in adult cardiac catheterization laboratories, the practice makes sense because normal cardiac output and therefore vascular resistance may be substantially different in a 260-lb man and a 110-lb woman. The normalized resistance, however, is not obtained by dividing resistance (as calculated in Eq. 11.8) by BSA. Rather, normalized resistance is calculated by substituting the blood flow index for blood flow in the resistance formula. Thus systemic vascular resistance index (SVRI) is calculated as

$$\text{SVRI} = \frac{\left(\overline{Ao} - \overline{RA}\right) \times 80}{\text{CI}} \qquad (11.12)$$

where CI is the cardiac (or systemic blood flow) index. Therefore, SVRI equals systemic vascular resistance multiplied by BSA.

It is important to realize that, in conditions of intracardiac shunts or shunts between the pulmonary and systemic circulations, pulmonary blood flow and systemic flow may not be equal, and the respective flow through each circuit must be measured and used in the appropriate resistance calculation. Normal values for vascular resistance in adults are given in **Table 11.4**.

Systemic Vascular Resistance

The minute-to-minute control of vascular resistance, at least in the systemic bed, is an amalgam of autonomic nervous system influences and local metabolic factors. Hypotension or reduced cardiac output generally triggers increased systemic resistance by means of the baroreceptors, α-adrenergic neural pathways, and release of humoral vasoconstrictor hormones, but these influences may be opposed by metabolic factors if the hypotension or low cardiac output results in decreased tissue perfusion with local hypoxia and acidosis. This latter circumstance is commonly seen in congestive heart failure or shock.

Knowledge of changes in systemic vascular resistance is also important in evaluating the hemodynamic response to stress tests, such as dynamic or isometric exercise. In this regard, there is ample evidence suggesting that normally systemic vascular resistance falls in response to dynamic exercise, but pulmonary vascular resistance remains unchanged (at least with supine bicycle exercise).

Low systemic vascular resistance may be seen in conditions in which blood flow is abnormally high, such as may occur in patients with arteriovenous fistula, severe anemia, and other high-output states or conditions associated with peripheral vasodilation and high output, such as septic shock. It is important to realize that, in these circumstances, there may well be regional differences in vascular resistance (eg, very low in the arteriovenous fistula but normal or increased in other vascular beds), and calculations based on mean pressure and flow in the entire systemic circulation must be interpreted with caution.

Total Pulmonary Resistance

Calculated as the ratio of mean pulmonary arterial pressure to pulmonary blood flow, total pulmonary resistance expresses the resistance to flow in transporting a volume of blood from the pulmonary artery to the LV in diastole, neglecting left ventricular diastolic pressure. This relationship is obviously influenced by alterations in left atrial pressure and will not consistently provide useful information about the condition of the pulmonary vasculature. Although widely used 25 years ago, this parameter is less

Table 11.4 Normal Values of Vascular Resistance

Systemic vascular resistance	1170 ± 270 dyn s/cm^5
Systemic vascular resistance index	2130 ± 450 dyn s/cm^5 • M^2
Pulmonary vascular resistance	67 ± 30 dyn s/cm^5
Pulmonary vascular resistance index	123 ± 54 dyn s/cm^5 • M^2

Values are expressed as mean ± standard deviation and were derived from 37 subjects without demonstrable cardiovascular disease (17 males, 20 females, age 47 ± 9 y) who underwent diagnostic cardiac catheterization at the Peter Bent Brigham Hospital between July 1, 1975, and June 30, 1978.

commonly used today and in general should be used primarily in the patient in whom measurement of left atrial or pulmonary capillary wedge pressure is not possible.

Pulmonary Vascular Resistance

Pulmonary vascular resistance expresses the pressure drop across the major pulmonary vessels, the precapillary arterioles, and the pulmonary capillary bed and is more precise in assessing the presence and degree of pulmonary vascular disease than is total pulmonary resistance. Simple calculation of pulmonary vascular resistance provides general information about the pulmonary circulation, but this must be interpreted in the context of the clinical situation and other hemodynamic data obtained during cardiac catheterization.

Measured pulmonary vascular resistance may be elevated by hypoxia, hypercapnia, increased sympathetic tone, polycythemia, local release of serotonin, mechanical obstruction by multiple pulmonary emboli, precapillary pulmonary edema, or lung compression (pleural effusion, increased intrathoracic pressure via respirator). On the other hand, pulmonary vascular resistance may be reduced by oxygen, adenosine, isoproterenol, a-antagonists such as phentolamine or tolazoline, inhaled nitric oxide, prostacyclin infusions, nitroprusside, and high doses of calcium channel blockers. These vasodilators may be used to test for fixed, irreversible pulmonary hypertension. Patients with high pulmonary vascular resistance (eg, >600 dyn s/cm^5) in association with a central shunt (eg, ventricular septal defect) should be given 100% oxygen via face mask before concluding that the changes are fixed. Elderly patients with a combination of left-sided heart failure and chronic obstructive lung disease may have considerable pulmonary vasoconstriction owing to alveolar hypoventilation and its resultant hypoxia. Inhalation of 100% oxygen in such cases may result in a dramatic fall in pulmonary arterial pressure and vascular resistance.

PULMONARY VASCULAR DISEASE IN PATIENTS WITH CONGENITAL CENTRAL SHUNTS

The decision as to whether a patient with congenital heart disease would benefit from corrective surgery often hinges on the calculated pulmonary vascular resistance. Although each case must be evaluated based on its own characteristics, many criteria for operability have been proposed. It has been suggested that the ratio between pulmonary vascular resistance and systemic vascular resistance (resistance ratio, PVR/SVR) be used as a criterion for operability in dealing with congenital heart disease. Normally, this ratio is <0.25. Values of 0.25 to 0.50 indicate moderate pulmonary vascular disease, and values higher than 0.75 indicate severe pulmonary vascular disease. When the PVR/SVR resistance ratio is >1.0, surgical correction of the congenital defect is considered contraindicated because of the severity of the pulmonary vascular disease.

In his classic description of the Eisenmenger syndrome, Wood pointed out that attempted surgical repair of the shunt defect was a major cause of death in these patients. He stated that, in patients with a pulmonary blood flow of <1.75 times the systemic flow or with a total pulmonary vascular resistance of >12 Wood or hybrid units (960 dyn s/cm^5), ordinary surgical repair of the defect should not be attempted. Others have suggested similar criteria for special instances or conditions.

PULMONARY VASCULAR DISEASE IN PATIENTS WITH MITRAL STENOSIS

Marked elevations in pulmonary vascular resistance may also be seen in acquired heart disease, notably in mitral stenosis. The effect of mitral valve replacement in patients with mitral stenosis and/or regurgitation associated with pulmonary hypertension has been evaluated. Most patients experience significant reduction in pulmonary vascular resistance following successful repair of the mitral valve lesion. Although some degree of pulmonary hypertension may persist postoperatively, significant palliative benefit usually occurs, and the decision regarding surgery must be made in light of information regarding left and right ventricular function as well as the degree of pulmonary hypertension.

SUGGESTED READINGS

1. Accessed August 3, 2020. https://millar.com/Research/PressureVolume-Loop-System/.
2. Burns AT, La Gerche A, Prior DL, Macisaac AI. Left ventricular untwisting is an important determinant of early diastolic function. *JACC Cardiovasc Imaging*. 2009;2(6):709-716.
3. Cha SD, Roman CF, Maranhao V. Clinical trial of the disposable transducer catheter. *Cathet Cardiovasc Diagn*. 1988;14(1):63-68.
4. Chiu YC, Arand PW, Carroll JD. Power-afterload relation in the failing human ventricle. *Circ Res*. 1992;70(3):530-535.
5. DiSesa VJ, Cohn LH, Grossman W. Management of adults with congenital bidirectional cardiac shunts, cyanosis, and pulmonary vascular obstruction: successful operative repair in 3 patients. *Am J Cardiol*. 1983;51(9):1495-1497.
6. Falsetti HL, Mates RE, Greene DG, Bunnell IL. V_{max} as an index of contractile state in man. *Circulation*. 1971;43(4):467-479.
7. Feneley MP, Skelton TN, Kisslo KB, Davis JW, Bashore TM, Rankin JS. Comparison of preload recruitable stroke work, end-systolic pressure-volume and dp/dtmax-end-diastolic volume relations as indexes of left ventricular contractile performance in patients undergoing routine cardiac catheterization. *J Am Coll Cardiol*. 1992;19(7):1522-1530.
8. Fry DL. Physiologic recording by modern instruments with particular reference to pressure recording. *Physiol Rev*. 1960;40:753-788.
9. Ganz W, Donoso R, Marcus HS, Forrester JS, Swan HJC. A new technique for measurement of cardiac output by thermodilution in man. *Am J Cardiol*. 1971;27(4):392-396.
10. Gersh BJ, Hahn CE, Prys-Roberts C. Physical criteria for measurement of left ventricular pressure and its first derivative. *Cardiovasc Res*. 1971;5(1):32-40.
11. Givertz MM, Andreou C, Conrad CH, Colucci WS. Direct myocardial effects of levosimendan in humans with left ventricular dysfunction: alteration of force-frequency and relaxation-frequency relationships. *Circulation*. 2007;115(10):1218-1224.
12. Gleason WL, Braunwald E. Studies on the first derivative of the ventricular pressure pulse in man. *J Clin Invest*. 1962;41(1):80-91.
13. Hansen AT. Pressure measurement in the human organism. *Acta Physiol Scand*. 1949;19(suppl 68):87.
14. Hurthle K. Beitrage zur hamodynamik. *Arch Ges Physiol*. 1898;72:566.
15. Lange RA, Moore DM Jr, Cigarroa RG, Hillis LD. Use of pulmonary capillary wedge pressure to assess severity of mitral stenosis: is true left atrial pressure needed in this condition? *J Am Coll Cardiol*. 1989;13(4):825-831.
16. Laskey WK, Kussmaul WG. Arterial wave reflection in heart failure. *Circulation*. 1987;75(4):711-722.
17. Levine MJ, Weinstein JS, Diver DJ, et al. Progressive improvement in pulmonary vascular resistance after percutaneous mitral valvuloplasty. *Circulation*. 1989;79(5):1061-1067.
18. Liu CP, Ting CT, Yang TM, et al. Reduced left ventricular compliance in human mitral stenosis. Role of reversible internal constraint. *Circulation*. 1992;85(4):1447-1456.
19. Mcdonald DA. *Blood Flow in Arteries*. 2nd ed. Williams & Wilkins; 1974.
20. Murgo JP, Westerhof N, Giolma JP, Altobelli SA. Manipulation of ascending aortic pressure and flow wave reflections with the Valsalva maneuver: relationship to input impedance. *Circulation*. 1981;63(1):122-132.
21. Narang N, Thibodeau JT, Levine BD, et al. Inaccuracy of estimated resting oxygen uptake in the clinical setting. *Circulation*. 2014;129(2):203-210.
22. Rowell LB, Brengelmann GL, Blackmon JR, Bruce RA, Murray JA. Disparities between aortic and peripheral pulse pressures induced by upright exercise and vasomotor changes in man. *Circulation*. 1968;37(6):954-964.
23. Wood EH, Leusen IR, Warner HR, Wright JL. Measurement of pressures in man by cardiac catheters. *Circ Res*. 1954;2(4):294-303.
24. Wood P. The Eisenmenger syndrome or pulmonary hypertension with reversed central shunt. I. *Br Med J*. 1958;2(5098):701-709.

12 Shunt Detection and Quantification[1]

Detection, localization, and quantification of intracardiac shunts are an integral part of the hemodynamic evaluation of patients with congenital heart disease. In most cases, an intracardiac shunt is suspected on the basis of the clinical evaluation of the patient before catheterization. However, there are several circumstances in which data obtained at catheterization should alert the cardiologist to look for a shunt that had not been suspected previously:

1. Unexplained arterial desaturation should raise the suspicion of a right-to-left intracardiac shunt.
2. Conversely, when the oxygen content of blood in the pulmonary artery is unexpectedly high (ie, if the pulmonary artery [PA] blood oxygen saturation is >80%), the possibility of a left-to-right intracardiac shunt should be considered. It is for these 2 reasons that arterial and PA saturation should be measured routinely *during* cardiac catheterization.
3. When the data obtained at cardiac catheterization do not confirm the presence of a suspected lesion, one should consider the presence of an intracardiac shunt. For example, if left ventricular cineangiography fails to reveal mitral regurgitation in a patient in whom this was judged to be the cause of a systolic murmur, it is prudent to look for evidence of a ventricular septal defect (VSD) with left-to-right shunting.

DETECTION OF LEFT-TO-RIGHT INTRACARDIAC SHUNTS

Many techniques are available for the detection, localization, and quantification of left-to-right intracardiac shunts. The techniques vary in their sensitivity, the type of indicator they use, and the equipment needed to sense and read out the presence of the indicator.

Measurement of Blood Oxygen Saturation and Content in the Right Side of the Heart (Oximetry Run)

In the oximetry run, a basic technique for detecting and quantifying left-to-right shunts, the oxygen content or percentage saturation is measured in blood samples drawn sequentially from the PA, right ventricle (RV), right atrium (RA), superior vena cava (SVC), and inferior vena cava (IVC). A left-to-right shunt may be detected and localized if a significant step-up in blood oxygen saturation or content is found in one of the right heart chambers. A significant step-up is defined as an increase in blood oxygen content or saturation that exceeds the normal variability that might be observed if multiple samples were drawn from that cardiac chamber.

The technique of the oximetry run is based on the pioneering studies of Dexter and his associates in 1947. They found that multiple samples drawn from the RA could vary in oxygen content by as much as 2 volumes percent (vol%). This variability has been attributed to the fact that the RA receives its blood from 3 sources with varying oxygen content: the SVC, IVC, and coronary sinus.

Dexter's study described normal variability and gave the criteria for a significant oxygen step-up only for measurement of blood oxygen content. As of today, cardiac

[1]We gratefully acknowledge the *Grossman & Baim's Cardiac Catheterization, Angiography, and Intervention*, 9th edition contributions of Drs. Mauro Moscucci and William Grossman as portions of their chapter, Shunt Detection and Quantification, were retained in this text.

catheterization laboratories have moved toward the measurement of percentage oxygen saturation by spectrophotometric oximetry as the routine method for oximetric analysis of blood samples. Oxygen content may then be calculated from percent O_2 saturation, the patient's blood hemoglobin concentration, and an assumed constant value for the oxygen-carrying capacity of hemoglobin (1.36 mL O_2/g hemoglobin), as discussed in Chapter 11.

The relationship between oxygen content and oxygen saturation obviously depends on the hemoglobin concentration in the patient's blood, and the potential presence of carboxyhemoglobin or hemoglobin variants with O_2-carrying capacity other than 1.36. Also, systemic blood flow may be an important determinant of oxygen variability in the right heart chambers, because high systemic flow tends to equalize the differences across various tissue beds.

In the context of these considerations, **Table 12.1** lists the criteria for a significant step-up in right-sided heart oxygen content and percentage oxygen saturation associated with various types of left-to-right shunts, based on a study by Antman and coworkers and other investigators. As can be seen from the bottom row ("Any level") of **Table 12.1**, the simplest way to screen for a left-to-right shunt is to sample SVC and PA blood and measure the difference, if any, in percentage O_2 saturation. If the AO_2 saturation between these samples is >8%, a left-to-right shunt may be present at atrial, ventricular, or great vessel level, and a full oximetry run should be done.

Oximetry Run

The blood samples needed to localize a step-up in the right side of the heart are obtained by performing what is called an oximetry run. The samples needed and the recommended order in which they should be obtained are as follows:

Obtain a 2-mL sample from each of the following locations:

1. Left and/or right pulmonary artery
2. Main pulmonary artery[2]
3. Right ventricle, outflow tract[2]
4. Right ventricle, mid[3]
5. Right ventricle, tricuspid valve or apex[2,3]
6. Right atrium, low or near tricuspid valve
7. Right atrium, mid
8. Right atrium, high
9. Superior vena cava, low (near junction with right atrium)
10. Superior vena cava, high (near junction with innominate vein)
11. Inferior vena cava, high (just at or below diaphragm)
12. Inferior vena cava, low (at L4-L5)
13. Left ventricle
14. Aorta (distal to insertion of ductus)

In performing the oximetry run, an end-hole catheter (eg, Swan-Ganz balloon flotation catheter) is positioned in the right or left PA. Cardiac output is measured by the Fick method. As soon as the determination of oxygen consumption is completed, the operator begins to obtain 2 mL blood samples from each of

[2]Confirm location by pressure measurement.
[3]If frequent extrasystoles occur, do not persist. Obtain samples from 3 different locations in RV and RA.

Level of Shunt	Criteria for Significant Step-Up				Approximate Minimal Q_p/Q_s Required for Detection (Assuming SBFI = 3 L/min/M²)	Possible Causes of Step-Up
	Mean of Distal Chamber Samples	Mean of Proximal Chamber Samples	Highest Value in Proximal Chamber	Highest Value in Distal Chamber		
	O₂ %sat	O₂ vol%	O₂ %sat	O₂ vol%		
Atrial (SVC/IVC to RA)	≥7	≥1.3	≥11	≥2.0	1.5-1.9	Atrial septal defect; partial anomalous pulmonary venous drainage; ruptured sinus of Valsalva; VSD with TR; coronary fistula to RA
Ventricular (RA to RV)	≥5	≥1.0	≥10	≥1.7	1.3-1.5	VSD; PDA with PR; primum ASD; coronary fistula to RV
Great vessel (RV to PA)	≥5	≥1.0	≥5	≥1.0	≥1.3	PDA; aortic-pulmonic window; aberrant coronary artery origin
Any level (SVC to PA)	≥7	≥1.3	≥8	≥1.5	≥1.5	All of the above

Note: Table 12.1 header: Detection of Left-to-Right Shunt by Oximetry. The O₂ %sat / O₂ vol% subheadings appear as: Mean of Distal Chamber Samples = O₂ %sat; Mean of Proximal Chamber Samples = O₂ vol%; Highest Value in Proximal Chamber = O₂ %sat; Highest Value in Distal Chamber = O₂ vol%.

ASD, atrial septal defect; PA, pulmonary artery; PDA, patent ductus arteriosus; PR, pulmonic regurgitation; Q_p/Q_s, pulmonary to systemic flow ratio; RA, right atrium; RV, right ventricle; SBFI, systemic blood flow index; SVC and IVC, superior and inferior vena cavae; TR, tricuspid regurgitation; VSD, ventricular septal defect.

the locations indicated, under fluoroscopic control and confirmation by pressure measurement. If a sample cannot be obtained from a specific site because of ventricular premature beats, that site should be skipped until the rest of the run has been completed.

Oxygen saturation and/or content in each of the samples is determined as discussed previously, and the presence and localization of a significant step-up are determined by applying the criteria listed in **Table 12.1**.

An alternative method for performing the oximetry run is to withdraw a fiberoptic catheter from the PA through the right heart chambers and the inferior and superior venae cavae, allowing continuous readout of oxygen saturation.

If the oximetry run reveals that a significant step-up is present, the pulmonary blood flow, systemic blood flow, and magnitude of left-to-right and right-to-left shunts may be calculated according to the following formulas.

Calculation of Pulmonary Blood Flow (Q_p)

Pulmonary blood flow is calculated by the same formula used in the standard Fick equation:

$$Q_p_{(L/min)} = \frac{O_2 \text{ consumption } (mL/min)}{\left[\begin{array}{c} PV\ O_2 \\ \text{content} \\ (mL/L) \end{array}\right] - \left[\begin{array}{c} PA\ O_2 \\ \text{content} \\ (mL/L) \end{array}\right]} \tag{12.1}$$

If a pulmonary vein (PV) has not been entered, systemic arterial oxygen content may be used in the preceding formula if systemic arterial oxygen saturation is >95%. If systemic oxygen saturation is <95%, one must determine whether a right-to-left intracardiac shunt is present. If there is an intracardiac right-to-left shunt, an assumed value of 98% oxygen capacity for the pulmonary venous oxygen content should be used in calculating pulmonary blood flow. If arterial desaturation is present and is not owing to a right-to-left intracardiac shunt, the observed systemic arterial oxygen saturation should be used to calculate pulmonary blood flow.

Example

Let us suppose that a patient is found to have an atrial septal defect (ASD) with a left-to-right shunt clearly detected by oximetry run. Furthermore, the catheter crosses the defect and a PV is entered, from which a blood sample shows O_2 saturation of 98%. Let us further suppose that systemic arterial blood saturation, however, is 90% and that this is owing to chronic pulmonary disease. After ruling out a right-to-left shunt by any of the various methods (eg, inhalation of 100% oxygen, indocyanine green dye injection in IVC, echocardiogram-bubble study), should we use 98% or 90% for pulmonary venous blood O_2 saturation in the calculation of Q? As indicated earlier, because arterial desaturation is not caused by a right-to-left intracardiac shunt, the observed systemic arterial O_2 saturation (90%) should be used because this summates all the PVs draining both lungs, not just the one with 98% O_2 saturation.

Calculation of Systemic Blood Flow (Q_s)

Use the following equation for systemic blood flow:

$$Q_s_{(L/min)} = \frac{O_2 \text{ consumption } (mL/min)}{\left[\begin{array}{c} SA\ O_2 \\ \text{content} \\ (mL/L) \end{array}\right] - \left[\begin{array}{c} MV\ O_2 \\ \text{content} \\ (mL/L) \end{array}\right]} \tag{12.2}$$

The key to proper measurement of systemic blood flow in the presence of an intracardiac shunt is that the mixed venous oxygen content must be measured in the chamber immediately proximal to the shunt, as shown in **Table 12.2**.

Calculation of Left-To-Right Shunt

If there is no evidence of an associated right-to-left shunt, the left-to-right shunt is calculated by

$$L \rightarrow R \text{ shunt} = Q_p - Q_s \text{ (measured in L/min)} \qquad (12.3)$$

Examples of Left-to-Right Shunt Detection and Quantification

Some examples of oximetry runs are presented to illustrate interpretation.

Atrial Septal Defect

In the example seen in **Figure 12.1**, there is a step-up in oxygen saturation in the mid-RA. The average or mean value for the vena caval samples in this patient is calculated as (3[SVC] + 1[IVC]) ÷ 4. SVC is the average of SVC samples (ie, 67.5% in this example), and IVC is the value for the IVC sample taken at the level of the diaphragm only (ie, 73%). Thus the vena caval mean O_2 saturation for the example illustrated in **Figure 12.1** is (3[67.5] + 1[73]) ÷ 4 = 69%. The right atrial mean O_2 saturation for this patient is (74 + 84 + 79) ÷ 3 = 79%. The 10% step-up in mean O_2 saturation from vena cava to RA is higher than the 7% value listed in **Table 12.1** as a criterion for a significant step-up at the atrial level. Note that, for this example, the highest-to-highest approach (highest right atrial O_2 saturation to highest vena caval O_2 saturation) would barely meet the criteria for a significant step-up, because of the high value of IVC saturation (73%) as compared with SVC saturation. Thus, for the detection of a significant step-up at the atrial level using the highest-to-highest approach, it is better to use the highest RA and SVC samples. In this case, the result would be (84%-68%) = 16%, which is clearly above the 11% value listed in **Table 12.1** for detection of a significant step-up. Also, the screening samples that we recommend for all right-sided heart catheterizations (a single sample each from SVC and PA) would have strongly indicated a shunt at some level in the right side of the heart, since AO_2 saturation from SVC to PA is 12% to 13%, well above the 8% value for a significant step-up.

Table 12.2	Calculation of Systemic Blood Flow in the Presence of Left-to-Right Shunt	
Location of Shunt as Determined by Site of O_2 Step-Up	**Mixed Venous Sample to be Used in Calculating Systemic Blood Flow**
1. Pulmonary artery (eg, patent ductus arteriosus)	Right ventricle, average of samples obtained during oximetry run
2. Right ventricle (eg, ventricular septal defect)	Right atrium, average of all samples during oximetry run
3. Right atrium (eg, atrial septal defect)	$$\frac{3(\text{SVC } O_2 \text{ content}) + 1(\text{IVC } O_2 \text{ content})}{4}$$

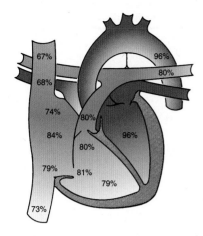

Figure 12.1 Schematic representation of the results of an oximetry run in a patient with a small to moderate atrial septal defect. Values represent percentage O_2 saturation of blood at multiple locations. (See text for details.)

To calculate pulmonary and systemic blood flows for the example given in **Figure 12.1**, we need to know O_2 consumption and blood O_2 capacity. If the patient's O_2 consumption is 240 mL O_2/min and the blood hemoglobin concentration is 14 g%, pulmonary and systemic blood flows may be calculated as follows:

$$Q_p = \frac{O_2 \text{ consumption (mL/min)}}{\left[\begin{array}{c} PV\ O_2 \\ \text{content} \\ (mL/L) \end{array}\right] - \left[\begin{array}{c} PA\ O_2 \\ \text{content} \\ (mL/L) \end{array}\right]} \quad (12.4)$$

PV O_2 content was not measured, but left ventricular and arterial blood O_2 saturation was 96% (effectively ruling out a right-to-left shunt), and therefore, it may be assumed that PV blood O_2 saturation was 96%. Oxygen content of PV blood is calculated as follows:

$$0.96\left(\frac{14\text{ g Hgb}}{100\text{ mL blood}}\right) \times \left(\frac{1.36\text{ mL } O_2}{\text{g Hgb}}\right)$$
$$= 18.3\text{ mL } O_2/100\text{ mL blood} \quad (12.5)$$
$$= 183\text{ mL } O_2/L$$

Similarly, PA O_2 content is calculated as

$$0.80(14)1.36 \times 10 = 152\text{ mL } O_2/L \quad (12.6)$$

Therefore,

$$Q_p = \frac{240\text{ mL } O_2/\text{min}}{[183 - 152]\text{ mL } O_2/L} \quad (12.7)$$
$$= 7.74\text{ L/min}$$

Systemic blood flow for the example illustrated in **Figure 12.1** is calculated as

$$Q_s = \frac{240 \text{ mL O}_2/\text{min}}{\left[\begin{array}{c}\text{systemic}\\\text{arterial}\\\text{O}_2\text{ content}\end{array}\right] - \left[\begin{array}{c}\text{mixed}\\\text{venous}\\\text{O}_2\text{ content}\end{array}\right]}$$

$$= \frac{240}{(0.96 - 0.69)14(1.36)10}$$

$$= 4.7 \text{ L/min}$$

(12.8)

For this calculation, mixed venous O_2 saturation was derived from the formula given in **Table 12.2** as 69%. Thus the ratio of Q_p/Q_s in this example is 7.74/4.7 = 1.65, and the magnitude of the left-to-right shunt is 7.7 − 4.7 = 3 L/min. This patient has a small to moderate ASD.

Ventricular Septal Defect

Figure 12.2 shows another example of findings in an oximetry run. In this case, the patient has a large O_2 step-up in the RV, indicating the presence of a VSD.

In this case, the O_2 saturation of mixed venous blood is calculated by averaging the right atrial O_2 saturations because the RA is the chamber immediately proximal to the O_2 step-up. If O_2 consumption is 260 mL/min and hemoglobin is 15 g%, then:

$$Q_p = \frac{260}{(0.97 - 0.885)15(1.36)10} = 15 \text{ L/min}$$

$$Q_s = \frac{260}{(0.97 - 0.66)15(1.36)10} = 4.1 \text{ L/min}$$

(12.9)

$$Q_p/Q_s = 15/4.1 = 3.7$$

$$\text{L} \rightarrow \text{shunt} = 15 - 4.1 = 10.9 \text{ L/min}$$

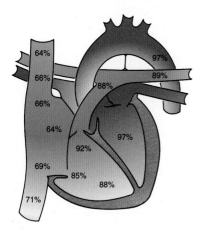

Figure 12.2 Findings from an oximetry run performed in a patient with a large ventricular septal defect. (See text for details.)

Flow Ratio

The ratio Q_p/Q_s gives important physiologic information about the magnitude of a left-to-right shunt. A Q_p/Q_s ratio of <1.5 signifies a small left-to-right shunt and is often a motivation to argue against operative correction, particularly if the patient has an otherwise uncomplicated ASD or VSD. A ratio of >2.0 indicates a large left-to-right shunt and is generally considered sufficient evidence to recommend surgical repair of the defect.

A *simplified formula* for the calculation of flow ratio can be derived by combining the equations for systemic and pulmonary blood flow to obtain

$$\frac{Q_p}{Q_s} = \frac{\left(SA\ O_2 - MV\ O_2\right)}{\left(PV\ O_2 - PA\ O_2\right)} \tag{12. 10}$$

where SA O_2, MV O_2, PV O_2, and PA O_2 are systemic arterial, mixed venous, pulmonary venous, and pulmonary arterial blood oxygen saturations, respectively. For the case illustrated in **Figure 12.1**

$$Q_p/Q_s = \left(96\% - 69\%\ \right)/\left(96\% - 80\%\right) = 1.69.$$

Calculation of Bidirectional Shunts

A simplified approach to the calculation of simultaneous right-to-left and left-to-right (also known as bidirectional) shunts makes use of a hypothetic quantity known as the *effective blood flow*, the flow that would exist in the absence of any left-to-right or right-to-left shunting:

$$Q_{eff} = \frac{O_2\ \text{consumption}\ \left(mL/min\right)}{\left[\begin{array}{c} PV\ O_2 \\ \text{content} \\ \left(mL/L\right) \end{array}\right] - \left[\begin{array}{c} MV\ O_2 \\ \text{content} \\ \left(mL/L\right) \end{array}\right]} \tag{12.11}$$

The approximate left-to-right shunt then equals $Q_p - Q_{eff}$, and the approximate right-to-left shunt equals $Q_s - Q_{eff}$. Actually, this effective blood flow approach is an approximation of the significantly more complex formula shown in Equation (12.12).

$$L \rightarrow R = \frac{Q_p\left(MV\ O_2\ \text{content} - PA\ O_2\ \text{content}\right)}{\left(MV\ O_2\ \text{content} - PV^d\ O_2\ \text{content}\right)}$$

$$R \rightarrow L = \frac{Q_p\left(PV^d\ O_2\ \text{content} - SA\ O_2\ \text{content}\right) \times \left(PA\ O_2\ \text{content} - PV^d\ O_2\ \text{content}\right)}{\left(SA\ O_2\ \text{content} - MV\ O_2\ \text{content}\right) \times \left(MV\ O_2\ \text{content} - PV^d\ O_2\ \text{content}\right)}$$

$$\tag{12.12}$$

Limitations of the Oximetry Method

An important limitation of the oxygen step-up method for detecting intracardiac shunts is that it lacks sensitivity. Most shunts of a magnitude that would lead to a recommendation for surgical closure of a VSD or patent ductus arteriosus are detected by this method. Small shunts, however, are not consistently detected by this technique.

High levels of systemic flow tend to equalize the arterial and venous oxygen values across a given vascular bed. Therefore, elevated systemic blood flow will cause the mixed venous oxygen saturation to be higher than normal, and interchamber variability owing to streaming will be blunted. Even a small increase in right-sided heart oxygen saturation under such conditions might indicate the presence of a significant left-to-right shunt; larger increases would indicate voluminous left-to-right shunting of blood.

Fundamental to the oximetric method of shunt detection is the fact that left-to-right shunting across an intracardiac defect will cause an increase in blood O_2 saturation in the chamber receiving the shunt proportional to the magnitude of the shunt. The increase in blood O_2 content in the chamber receiving the shunt, however, depends not only on the magnitude of the shunt but also on the O_2-carrying capacity of the blood (ie, the hemoglobin concentration).

To minimize errors and maximize the physiologic strengths of the oximetry method for shunt detection and quantification, the guidelines listed in **Table 12.3** should be followed.

Other Indicators

Many other sensitive techniques are available for detecting smaller left-to-right shunts. These include indocyanine green dye curves, radionuclide techniques, contrast angiography, and echocardiographic methods. For discussion of predominantly non-catheter-based methods (eg, echo, radionuclide) and older methods, the reader is referred to textbooks devoted to those techniques.

Angiography

Selective angiography is effective in visualizing and localizing the site of left-to-right shunts. Angiographic demonstration of anatomy has become a routine part of the preoperative evaluation of patients with congenital or acquired shunts and is useful in localizing the anatomic site of the shunt. Actually, the use of angiography in this fashion should be considered an indicator-dilution method, with the radiographic contrast agent being the indicator and the cinefluoroscopy unit serving as the densitometer.

Angiography, however, cannot replace the important physiologic measurements that allow quantitation of flow and vascular resistance. Without quantitative evaluation of pulmonary and systemic flows (Q_p and Q_s) and their associated resistances (PVR and SVR), appropriate decisions regarding patient management cannot be made, nor can prognosis be assessed.

Table 12.3 Guidelines for Optimum of the Oximetric Method for Shunt Detection and Quantification

1. Blood samples at multiple sites should be obtained rapidly.
2. Blood O_2 content data are preferable to identify the presence and location of a shunt.
3. Comparison of the mean of all values obtained in the respective chambers is preferable to comparison of the highest values in each chamber.
4. Because of the significant influence of systemic blood flow on shunt detection, exercise should be used in equivocal cases where a low systemic blood flow is present at rest.

Based on the data of Antman EM, Marsh JD, Green LH, Grossman W. Blood oxygen measurements in the assessment of intracardiac left to right shunts: a critical appraisal of methodology. *Am J Cardiol.* 1980;46:265-271.

DETECTION OF RIGHT-TO-LEFT INTRACARDIAC SHUNTS

The primary indication for the use of techniques to detect and localize right-to-left intracardiac shunts is the presence of cyanosis or, more commonly, arterial hypoxemia. The presence of arterial hypoxemia raises 2 specific questions: first, is the observed hypoxemia owing to an intracardiac shunt, or is it owing to a ventilation/perfusion imbalance secondary to a variety of forms of intrinsic pulmonary disease? This problem is particularly important in patients with coexistent congenital heart disease and pulmonary disease. Second, if hypoxemia is caused by an intracardiac shunt, what is its site and what is its magnitude?

Measurements of right-to-left shunts in patients with cyanotic heart disease date back at least to 1941 and continue to be a challenging task.

Angiography

With appropriate techniques, angiography may be used to detect right-to-left intracardiac shunts. This method is particularly important in detecting right-to-left shunting caused by a pulmonary arteriovenous fistula. In this circumstance, the shunt cannot be detected by indicator-dilution curves on the basis of a shortened appearance time. That is, the difference in transit time when the pulmonary capillaries are bypassed is not perceptible by standard indicator-dilution techniques. Although angiography may localize right-to-left shunts, it does not permit quantification.

Oximetry

The site of right-to-left shunts may be localized if blood samples can be obtained from a PV, the left atrium, left ventricle, and aorta. The pulmonary venous blood of patients with arterial hypoxemia caused by an intracardiac right-to-left shunt is fully saturated with oxygen. Therefore, the site of a right-to-left shunt may be localized by noting which left heart chamber is the first to show desaturation (ie, a step-down in oxygen concentration). Thus, if left atrial blood oxygen saturation is normal but desaturation is present in the left ventricle and in the systemic circulation, the right-to-left shunt is across a VSD.

Echocardiography

Echocardiographic methods have been proved sensitive enough for the detection and localization of left-to-right and right-to-left shunts. The echocardiographic contrast study using agitated saline solution with microbubbles or some of the newer specifically designed echo contrast agents can detect small shunts, and the use of 2-dimensional echocardiographic techniques can localize the site of the shunt to the atrial or ventricular septum. Echo-Doppler techniques can also be used to detect and localize intracardiac shunts. In this regard, color Doppler echocardiography is particularly useful in detecting and localizing small intracardiac shunts without the need for injection of an echo contrast agent.

SUGGESTED READINGS

1. Antman EM, Marsh JD, Green LH, Grossman W. Blood oxygen measurements in the assessment of intracardiac left to right shunts: a critical appraisal of methodology. *Am J Cardiol.* 1980;46(2):265-271.
2. Barratt-Boyes BF, Wood EH. The oxygen saturation of blood in the venae cavae, right heart chambers, and pulmonary vessels of healthy subjects. *J Lab Clin Med.* 1957;50:93-106.
3. Dexter L, Haynes FW, Burwell CS, Eppinger EC, Sagerson RP, Evans JM. Studies of congenital heart disease: technique of venous catheterization as a diagnostic procedure. *J Clin Invest.* 1947;26(3):547-553.
4. Dexter L, Haynes FW, Burwell CS, Eppinger EC, Sagerson RP, Evans JM. Studies of congenital heart disease. II: the pressure and oxygen content of blood in the right auricle, right ventricle, and pulmonary artery in control patients, with observations on the oxygen saturation and source of pulmonary "capillary" blood. *J Clin Invest.* 1947;26(3):554-560.

5. Flamm MD, Cohn KE, Hancock EW. Measurement of systemic cardiac output at rest and exercise in patients with atrial septal defect. *Am J Cardiol*. 1969;23(2):258-265.
6. Freed MD, Miettinen OS, Nadas AS. Oximetric detection of intracardiac left-to-right shunts. *Br Heart J*. 1979;42(6):690-694.
7. Levy AM, Monroe RG, Hugenholtz PG, Nadas AS. Clinical use of ascorbic acid as an indicator of right-to-left shunt. With a note on other applications. *Br Heart J*. 1967;29(1):22-29.
8. Parker JA, Treves S. Radionuclide detection, localization, and quantitation of intracardiac shunts and shunts between the great arteries. *Prog Cardiovasc Dis*. 1977;20(2):121-150.
9. Prinzmetal M. Calculation of the venous arterial shunt in congenital heart disease. *J Clin Invest*. 1941;20(6):705-708.
10. Singleton RT, Dembo DH, Scherlis L. Krypton-85 in the detection of intracardiac left-to-right shunts. *Circulation*. 1965;32:134-137.
11. Swan HJC, Wood EH. Localization of cardiac defects by dye-dilution curves recorded after injection of T-1824 at multiple sites in the heart and great vessels during cardiac catheterization. *Proc Staff Meet Mayo Clin*. 1952;28(4):95-100.

13 Calculation of Stenotic Valve Orifice Area[1]

$\mathbf{F}$or any stenotic orifice size, a stronger flow across the orifice yields a higher pressure gradient. Using 2 fundamental hydraulic formulas, Dr. Richard Gorlin and his father developed a formula for the calculation of cardiac valvular orifices from flow and pressure-gradient data. Today, this formula is usually worked out using computerized pressure monitoring systems, but it is still valuable to understand its derivation and characteristics.

THE GORLIN FORMULA

The first hydraulic formula that the Gorlins used was based on Bernoulli law, which describes flow across a round orifice:

$$F = AVC_c \tag{13.1}$$

where F is the flow rate, A is the orifice area, V is the velocity of flow, and C_c is the coefficient of orifice contraction. The constant C_c compensates for the physical phenomenon that, except for a perfect orifice, the area of a stream flowing through an orifice will be less than the true area of the orifice. Simply stated: Flow = area × velocity and area = flow/velocity.

Rearranging the terms,

$$A = \frac{F}{VC_c} \tag{13.2}$$

The second hydraulic principle used in the derivation of the Gorlin formula relates pressure gradient and velocity of flow according to Torricelli law:

$$V^2 = (C_v)^2 \times 2gh \ or \ V = (C_v)\sqrt{2gh} \tag{13.3}$$

where V is the velocity of flow; C_v is the coefficient of velocity, correcting for the energy loss as pressure energy is converted to kinetic or velocity energy; h is the pressure gradient in cm H_2O; and g is the gravitational constant (980 cm/s^2 for converting mass to units of pressure). In effect it converts pressure differences into flow velocity so that it can be applied to the first formula above.

Combining the 2 equations,

$$A = \frac{F}{C_v\sqrt{2gh} \times C_c} = \frac{F}{C_v C_c \sqrt{2 \times 980 \times h}}$$
$$= \frac{F}{(C)(44.3)\sqrt{h}} \tag{13.4}$$

where C is an empirical constant accounting for C_v and C_c, and the expression of h is in millimeters of mercury (rather than centimeters of water), and correcting the calculated valve area to the actual valve area measured at surgery or autopsy.

---

[1]We gratefully acknowledge the *Grossman & Baim's Cardiac Catheterization, Angiography, and Intervention*, 9th edition contributions of Drs. Blase A. Carabello and William Grossman, as portions of their chapter, Calculation of Stenotic Valve Orifice Area, were retained in this text.

It is obvious that antegrade flow across the mitral and tricuspid valves occurs only in diastole, whereas that across the aortic and pulmonic valves occurs only in systole. Accordingly, the flow, F, in Eq. (13.4) is the total cardiac output expressed in terms of the number of seconds per minute during which there is actually forward flow across the valve. For the mitral and tricuspid valves, this is calculated by multiplying the diastolic filling period (seconds per beat) by the heart rate (beats per minute [bpm]), yielding the number of seconds per minute during which there is diastolic flow. Diastolic flow in milliliters per second is calculated by dividing cardiac output in milliliters per minute (or cubic centimeters per minute) by the number of seconds per minute during which there is flow (diastolic filling period). The diastolic filling period begins at mitral valve opening and continues until end diastole. The systolic ejection period begins with aortic valve opening and proceeds till the dicrotic notch or some other evidence of aortic valve closure **Figure 13.1**.

Thus, the final equation for the calculation of valve orifice area A (in cm²) is

$$A = \frac{CO/(DFP \text{ or } SEP)(HR)}{44.3C\sqrt{\Delta P}} \tag{13.5}$$

where CO is the cardiac output (cm³/min), DFP is the diastolic filling period (seconds/beat), SEP is the systolic ejection period (seconds/beat), HR is the heart rate (beats/min), C is an empirical constant, and P is the pressure gradient. DFP is measured directly from left ventricular (LV) vs pulmonary capillary wedge (PCW) or left atrial pressure tracings as shown in **Figure 13.1**.

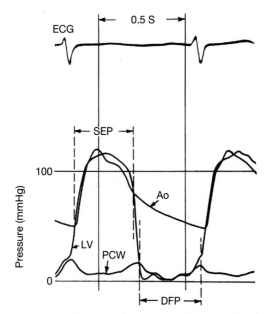

Figure 13.1 Left ventricular (LV), aortic (Ao), and pulmonary capillary wedge (PCW) pressure tracings from a patient without valvular heart disease, illustrating the definition and measurement of diastolic filling period (DFP) and systolic ejection period (SEP). (See text for discussion.)

An empirical constant of 0.7 (later adjusted to 0.85) was derived by comparing the calculated and actual mitral valve areas. With the use of this constant, the maximum deviation of the calculated valve area from the measured valve area was 0.2 cm². The empirical constant for the aortic, tricuspid, and pulmonic valves has never been derived because of lack of data comparing actual with calculated valve areas for these valves; the constant for these valves has been assumed to be 1.0 (ie, 1.0 × 44.3 = 44.3). Nonetheless, the Gorlin formula remains the gold standard for assessing the severity of stenosis in cardiac valves.

MITRAL VALVE AREA

By rearranging the terms of Eq. (13.5), one sees that for the mitral valve,

$$\Delta P = \left[\frac{CO/(HR)(DFP)}{(MVA)(44.3)(0.85)}\right]^2 \tag{13.6}$$

where ΔP is the mean transmitral pressure gradient and MVA is the mitral valve area. Thus, by doubling cardiac output one will quadruple the gradient across the valve, if heart rate and diastolic filling period remain constant. The normal mitral orifice in an adult has a cross-sectional area of 4.0 to 5.0 cm² when the mitral valve is completely open in diastole. Considerable reduction in this orifice area can occur without symptomatic limitation, but when the area is 1.5 cm² or less, a substantial resting gradient will be present across the mitral valve and any demand for increased cardiac output will be met by increases in left atrial and pulmonary capillary pressure that lead to pulmonary congestion and edema.

Figure 13.2 demonstrates that a cardiac output of 5 L/min can be maintained with only a minimal mitral diastolic gradient as the mitral orifice area contracts from its normal 4.0 to 5.0 cm² to a moderately stenotic area of 2.0 cm². After that, the gradient rises so that, at an orifice area of 1.0 cm², a resting gradient of 8 to 10 mmHg is required to maintain the cardiac output at 5 L/min with a normal resting heart rate of 72 bpm (**Figure 13.2**).

Example of Valve Area Calculation in Mitral Stenosis

Figure 13.3 shows PCW and LV pressure tracings in a 40-year-old woman with rheumatic heart disease and severe mitral stenosis. The valve orifice area is calculated with the aid of a form reproduced as in **Table 13.1**. In this patient, 5 beats were chosen from the recordings taken closest in time to the Fick cardiac output determination. Planimetry of the area between PCW and LV pressure tracings (**Figure 13.3**) was done for these 5 beats, and these areas were divided by the length of the diastolic filling periods for each beat, giving an average gradient deflection in millimeters. The mean gradient in millimeters of mercury (**Table 13.1**, part B) was calculated as the average gradient deflection in millimeters multiplied by the scale factor (mmHg/mm deflection). In this case, the mean gradient was 30 mmHg. Next, the average diastolic filling period was calculated (**Table 13.1**, part C) using the average measured length between initial PCW-LV crossover in early diastole and end diastole (peak of the R wave by electrocardiogram [ECG]). This average length in millimeters was divided by the paper speed (millimeters per second) to give the average diastolic filling period, which in this case was 0.40 second. Heart rate and cardiac output (**Table 13.1**, parts D and E) are recorded, ideally from data collected simultaneously with the recording of the PCW-LV pressure gradient. Heart rate was 80 bpm and cardiac output was 4680 cm³/min in the case illustrated in **Figure 13.3**. It should be noted that cardiac output must be expressed in cubic centimeters per minute if valve area is expressed in

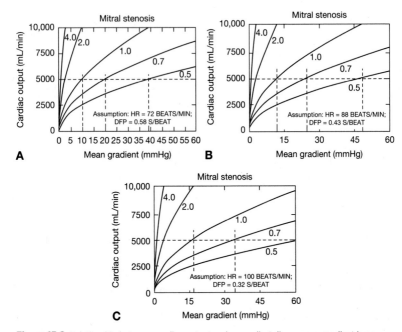

Figure 13.2 Relationship between cardiac output and mean diastolic pressure gradient in patients with mitral stenosis, calculated using Eq. 13.6, derived from the Gorlin formula. Curves represent orifice areas of 4.0, 2.0, 1.0, 0.7, and 0.5 cm². **A-C,** Flow-gradient relations at differing heart rates and diastolic filling periods. (See text for discussion.) (Courtesy of Dr. James J. Ferguson III.)

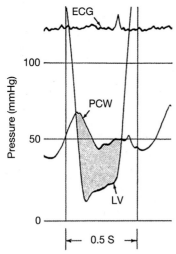

Figure 13.3 Pulmonary capillary wedge (PCW) and left ventricular (LV) pressure tracings in a 40-year-old woman with severe mitral stenosis. This woman also had systemic arterial hypertension and significant elevation of her LV diastolic pressure. (See text for discussion.)

Table 13.1 **Valve Orifice Area Determination**					

Patient _____ Age _____
Unit Number _____ Date _____

A. Complex no.	Area of gradient (mm²)	/	Length of diastolic or systolic period (mm)	=	Average gradient (deflection, mm)
1.	_____	/	_____	=	_____
2.	_____	/	_____	=	_____
3.	_____	/	_____	=	_____
4.	_____	/	_____	=	_____
5.	_____	/	_____	=	_____

B. Mean gradient = average gradient (mm deflection) × scale factor (mmHg/mm deflection)

  = _____ × _____ = _____ mmHg

C. Average diastolic or systolic period = average length (mm)/paper speed (mm/s)

  = _____/_____ = _____ s/beat

D. Heart rate = _____ beat/min

E. Cardiac output (Fick or indicator dilution) = _____ mL/min

F. $$\frac{\text{cardiac output} \left(\text{heart rate} \times \text{avg. diastolic or systolic period} \right)}{\text{valve constant}^a \times \sqrt{\text{mean gradient}}}$$

  _____/(_____ × _____)

  = _____ = _____ cm²

  _____ × $\sqrt{}$

G. Valve area index = valve area/body surface area = _____ cm²/m²

^{a}Valve constants: for mitral valve use 37.7; for aortic, tricuspid, and pulmonic valves use 44.3.

square centimeters of cross-sectional area. Entering these values in the formula given in Table 13.1, part F, and using a constant of 0.85(44.3) = 37.7 for the mitral valve, we get

$$\text{mitral valve area} = \frac{\left(4{,}680 \text{ cm}^3/\text{min}\right)\left(80 \text{ beats}/\text{min}\right)\left(0.40 \text{ s}/\text{beat}\right)}{37.7\sqrt{30 \text{ mmHg}}} \qquad (13.7)$$

$$= 0.71 \text{ cm}^2$$

Pitfalls

Pulmonary Capillary Wedge Tracing

In most cases, PCW pressure is substituted for left atrial pressure under the assumption that a properly confirmed wedge pressure accurately reflects left atrial pressure. Nishimura et al. found that transmitral gradient was overestimated by 3.3 to 3.5 mmHg when a Swan-Ganz catheter was used to measure the wedge pressure in comparison with actual left atrial pressure. Lange et al. measured left atrial pressure directly (transseptal) and compared it with oximetrically confirmed wedge pressure obtained using a stiff woven Dacron catheter. In this study, overestimation of true left atrial pressure was only 1.7 ± 0.6 mmHg. Failure to wedge the catheter properly may cause one to compare a damped pulmonary artery pressure with the LV pressure, yielding a falsely high gradient. To ensure that the right-sided heart catheter is properly wedged, one should verify that

1. The mean wedge pressure is lower than the mean pulmonary artery pressure.
2. Blood withdrawn from the wedged catheter is >95% saturated with oxygen, or at least equal in oxygen saturation to arterial blood.

Alignment Mismatch

Alignment of the PCW and LV pressure tracings does not match alignment of simultaneous left atrial and LV tracings because there is a time delay in the transmission of the left atrial pressure signal back through the pulmonary venous and capillary beds. The resulting pressure mismatch is small when PCW pressure is measured in the distal pulmonary arteries using a 7F or 8F Cournand or Goodale-Lubin catheter but may be larger when wedge pressure is measured more proximally in the pulmonary arterial tree using a balloon-tipped flow-directed catheter. The A and V waves in an optimally damped PCW tracing are delayed typically by 50 to 70 ms as compared with a simultaneous left atrial pressure tracing. Thus, ideally, the wedge pressure should be realigned with the LV pressure by shifting it leftward by 50 to 70 ms.

The V wave, which is normally present in the left atrium (where it represents pulmonary venous return), peaks immediately before the downstroke of the LV pressure tracing. With a wedge pressure measured distally using a 7F Goodale-Lubin catheter (**Figure 13.3**), the peak of the V wave is bisected by the rapid downstroke of LV pressure decline. Realignment of the wedge tracing in such a way that the V wave peak is bisected by (or slightly to the left of) the downstroke of LV pressure is a practical method for achieving better physiologic realignment.

Calibration Errors

Failure to calibrate the pressure transducers properly and adjust them to the same zero reference point may yield an erroneous gradient.

Cardiac Output Determination Cardiac output must be determined accurately and simultaneously with the gradient determination using the techniques described in Chapter 11. The measurement used in the valve area formula is usually the forward cardiac output determined by the Fick method or the thermodilution method. If mitral valvular regurgitation exists, the gradient across the valve will reflect not only the net forward flow but forward plus regurgitant or total transmitral diastolic flow. Therefore, using only the net forward flow to calculate the valve orifice area will *underestimate* the actual anatomic valve area in cases where regurgitation coexists with stenosis. Tricuspid regurgitation may cause the thermodilution technique for measuring cardiac output to be inaccurate.

Early Diastasis

Even when left atrial and LV pressures equalize (diastasis) before the end of diastole, there will generally still be a flow through the mitral valve after the point of diastasis. The diastolic filling period to be used in valve area calculation should include all of nonisovolumic diastole, not just the period during which a gradient is present.

AORTIC VALVE AREA

An aortic valve area (AVA) of 1.0 cm² or less is generally considered severe enough to account for the symptoms of angina, syncope, or heart failure in a patient with aortic stenosis. The American Heart Association/American College of Cardiology Guidelines for the Management of Patients with Valvular Heart Disease define "severe" aortic stenosis as an AVA of <1.0 cm². **Figure 13.4** illustrates the relationship between cardiac output and aortic pressure gradient over a range of values of AVA and at 3 different values of heart rate and systolic ejection period. For the aortic valve, Eq. 13.4 can be rearranged as

$$\Delta P = \left[\frac{CO/(HR)(SEP)}{44.3 AVA} \right]^2 \tag{13.8}$$

As can be seen in **Figure 13.4A**, at a normal resting cardiac output of 5.0 L/min, an aortic orifice area of 0.7 cm² will result in a pressure gradient of approximately

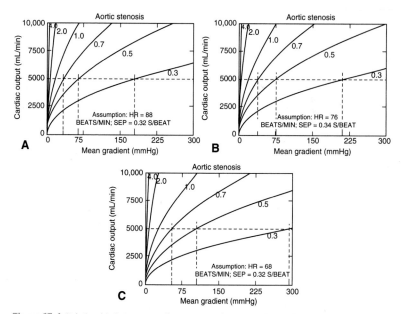

Figure 13.4 Relationship between cardiac output and mean aortic systolic pressure gradient in patients with aortic stenosis, calculated using Eq. (13.7), derived from the Gorlin formula. Curves represent orifice areas of 4.0, 2.0, 1.0, 0.7, 0.5, and 0.3 cm². A–C. Flow-gradient relations at differing heart rates and systolic ejection periods. (Courtesy of Dr. James J. Ferguson III.)

33 mmHg across the aortic valve. Doubling of the cardiac output, as might occur with exercise, would increase the gradient by a factor of 4 to 132 mmHg if the systolic time per minute did not change. This increase in gradient would require a peak LV pressure in excess of 250 mmHg to maintain a central aortic pressure of 120 mmHg. Such a major increase in LV pressure obviously increases myocardial oxygen demand and limits ejection performance. These factors contribute to the symptoms of angina and congestive heart failure, respectively. The limitations in cardiac output imposed by high afterload may contribute to hypotension when peripheral vasodilation occurs during muscular exercise.

Figure 13.4B and C shows that, with decreasing heart rate, the gradient *increases* in aortic stenosis for any value of cardiac output. This is opposite to the effect of heart rate in mitral stenosis and reflects the opposite effects of heart rate on systolic and diastolic time per minute. Viewed another way, as the heart rate slows in aortic stenosis, the stroke volume increases if cardiac output remains constant. Thus, the flow per beat across the aortic valve increases and so does the pressure gradient.

Example

Figure 13.5 demonstrates simultaneous pressure tracings from the left ventricle (LV) and right femoral artery (RFA) in a patient with exertional syncope. Because the pulse wave takes a finite period of time to travel from the LV to the femoral artery (FA), the FA tracing is somewhat delayed (Figure 13.5A). Figure 13.5B shows the LV and RFA tracings realigned to correct for the delay in transmission time. For this example, the average aortic pressure gradient is 40 mmHg, the systolic ejection period is 0.33 second, the heart rate is 74 bpm, and the cardiac output is 5000 mL/min. Using these values together with an aortic valve constant of (1) (44.3) = 44.3 in the equation in Table 13.1 gives

$$\text{aortic valve area} = \frac{\left(5{,}000\ \text{cm}^3/\text{min}\right)\big/\left(74\ \text{beats}/\text{min}\right)\left(0.33\ \text{s}/\text{beat}\right)}{44.3\sqrt{40\ \text{mmHg}}} = 0.7\ \text{cm}^2 \quad (13.9)$$

As discussed in Chapters 11 and 14, peripheral arterial pressure waveforms are distorted in ways other than time delay. These distortions include systolic amplification and spreading out (widening) of the pressure waveform. Figure 13.6 shows LV-central

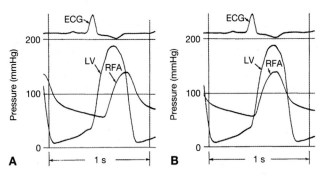

Figure 13.5 Left ventricular (LV) and right femoral artery (RFA) pressure tracings in a patient who presented with exertional syncope owing to aortic stenosis. **A,** The tracings actually recorded, demonstrating the significant time delay for the pressure waveform to reach the RFA. **B,** Realignment using tracing paper. (See text for discussion.)

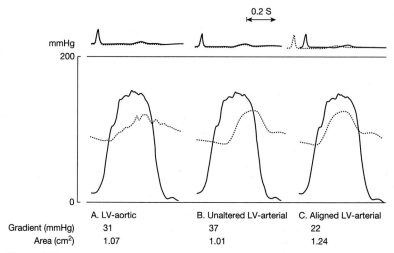

	A. LV-aortic	B. Unaltered LV-arterial	C. Aligned LV-arterial
Gradient (mmHg)	31	37	22
Area (cm²)	1.07	1.01	1.24

Figure 13.6 Pressure gradients in aortic stenosis. **A,** The left ventricular (LV)-central aortic gradient. **B,** LV-femoral artery gradient without alignment. **C,** LV-femoral artery gradient with alignment obtained by moving the femoral artery tracing leftward so that its upstroke coincides with the LV pressure upstroke. (Reproduced with permission from Folland ED, Parisi AF, Carbone C. Is peripheral arterial pressure a satisfactory substitute for ascending aortic pressure when measuring aortic valve gradients? *J Am Coll Cardiol.* 1984;4:1207.)

aortic gradient (A), LV-FA gradient without alignment (B), and LV-FA gradient with alignment (C). Without realignment of the LV-FA gradient, the LV-Ao gradient was overestimated by about 9 mmHg. In contrast, aligned LV-FA gradient underestimated the LV-Ao gradient by about 10 mmHg, because peak systolic arterial pressure is higher in peripheral arterial pressure tracings than in central aortic tracings. A second error in gradient measurement can occur if the LV catheter is placed in the LV outflow tract. As shown in **Figure 13.7**, a gradient usually exists between the body of the LV and the outflow tract, produced as blood accelerates when it enters this relatively narrow portion of the LV. A catheter tip placed in the LV outflow tract will measure a typical LV pressure tracing but can underestimate the true LV-aorta gradient by 30 mmHg.

Assey et al. measured the transaortic valve gradients in 15 patients from 8 different combinations of catheter locations using the schema shown in **Figure 13.8**. The average mean gradient recorded between positions 1 and 3 was the highest, whereas the gradient between positions 1 and 5 recorded using the alignment technique produced the smallest value. In some patients, the differences in gradient among the different measurement sites were as much as 45 mmHg.

The most accurate approach for gradient measurement involves the use of a second catheter positioned in the ascending aorta or the use of dual lumen catheters. In particular, dual-lumen catheters, such as the Langston catheter (Vascular Solutions Inc, Minneapolis, Minnesota), provide today an excellent option for simultaneous and accurate measurements of LV and ascending aortic pressure.

If a second catheter or a dual-lumen catheter is not used to obtain simultaneous LV and peripheral pressures, the gradient may be obtained by recording the LV pressure and superimposing it on the aortic pressure obtained immediately after the LV catheter is pulled back into the aorta.

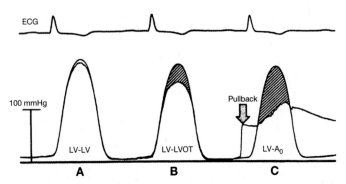

Figure 13.7 A, Pressure tracings recorded from 2 catheters placed within the body of the left ventricular (LV) chamber. Tracings are nearly identical. **B,** Pressures recorded by 2 catheters, one placed in the body of the LV chamber and the other placed in the left ventricular outflow tract (LVOT), proximal to the aortic valve (Ao). Both catheters recorded characteristic LV pressure tracings; however, there is a substantial pressure gradient between the body of the left ventricle and the outflow tract. This is not owing to anatomic subvalvular stenosis but rather to acceleration of blood as it enters the relatively narrow outflow tract. **C,** Pressures recorded from one catheter in the body of the left ventricle and a second catheter in the proximal aorta. These tracings demonstrate the gradient across the aortic valve and outflow tract. (Reproduced from Pasipoularides A. Clinical assessment of ventricular ejection dynamics with and without outflow obstruction. *J Am Coll Cardiol.* 1990;15:859-882, with permission.)

In most practices, aortic stenosis severity is determined by echo-Doppler examination. Thus, direct pressure measurement is used only when noninvasive data including physical examination are discrepant. In such cases extra care must be taken to use the most reliable invasive methods to obtain the most accurate transaortic gradient.

Pitfalls

Transducer Calibration

Attention to cardiac output determination and transducer calibration is critical. Assurance that proper transducer calibration has been accomplished can be obtained by comparing the left-sided heart catheter pressure with the peripheral arterial catheter pressure before insertion of the left-sided heart catheter into the LV.

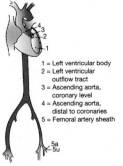

1 = Left ventricular body
2 = Left ventricular outflow tract
3 = Ascending aorta, coronary level
4 = Ascending aorta, distal to coronaries
5 = Femoral artery sheath

Figure 13.8 Two sites for recording left ventricular pressure (1 and 2) and 3 sites for recording distal pressure (3, 4, and 5) are shown. Site 5u represents the actual femoral artery pressure tracing, which is unaligned with the left ventricular pressure tracing. Site 5a represents the recording obtained from the femoral artery, which is then manually aligned to match the left ventricular pressure tracing in time. The following are the potential recording sites for obtaining the transaortic valve pressure gradient in aortic stenosis: 1-3, 1-4, 1-5a, 1-5u, 2-3, 2-4, 2-5a, and 2-5u. Gradients recorded at these different sites may vary widely in any given patient. (Reproduced with permission from Assey ME, Zile MR, Usher BW, Karavan MP, Carabello BA. Effect of catheter positioning on the variability of measured gradient in aortic stenosis. *Cathet Cardiovasc Diagn.* 1993;30:287.)

Pullback Hemodynamics

When the AVA is diminished to 0.6 cm² or less, a 7F or 8F catheter placed retrograde across the valve takes up a significant amount of the residual orifice area, and the catheter may actually increase the severity of stenosis. Conversely, removal of the catheter reduces the severity of stenosis. A rise in peripheral pressure can occur in severe aortic stenosis when the LV catheter is removed from the aortic valve orifice (Carabello sign).

AREA OF TRICUSPID AND PULMONIC VALVES

No general agreement exists as to what constitutes a critical orifice area for tricuspid and pulmonic valves. In general, a mean gradient of 5 mmHg across the tricuspid valve is sufficient to cause symptoms of systemic venous hypertension. Gradients across the pulmonic valve of <50 mmHg are usually well tolerated, but gradients of >100 mmHg indicate a need for surgical correction. Between 50 and 100 mmHg, decision regarding surgical correction depends on the clinical features of each case.

ALTERNATIVES TO THE GORLIN FORMULA

A simplified valve formula for the calculation of stenotic cardiac valve areas was proposed by Hakki et al. The simplified formula is based on their observation that the product of heart rate, SEP or DFP, and the Gorlin formula constant was nearly the same for all patients whose hemodynamics were measured in the resting state and that the value of this product was close to 1.0.

$$\text{Valve area} = \frac{\text{cardiac output}\left(\text{liters/minute}\right)}{\sqrt{\text{pressure gradient}}} \qquad (13.10)$$

For the examples given earlier in this chapter, the simplified formula works reasonably well. Thus for the patient with mitral stenosis (**Figure 13.3**) with a cardiac output of 4680 mL/min and a mitral diastolic gradient of 30 mmHg, mitral valve area is 4.68 divided by the square root of 30, or 0.85 cm², using the simplified formula as opposed to the value of 0.71 cm² calculated using the Gorlin formula. Because the percentage of time per minute spent in diastole or systole changes substantially at higher heart rates, the simplified formula may be less useful in the presence of substantial tachycardia. This point, however, has not been tested adequately.

ASSESSMENT OF AORTIC STENOSIS IN PATIENTS WITH LOW CARDIAC OUTPUT

Valve calculations made using the Gorlin formula are flow dependent: that is, as cardiac output increases, calculated area increases, and as cardiac output decreases, calculated area decreases. Two potential mechanisms exist by which calculated valve orifice area increases with cardiac output: (1) Increased flow through the stenotic aortic valve in conjunction with increased LV pressure physically opens the valve to a larger orifice area, and thus the valve orifice really is wider during increased flow. (2) Inaccuracies in the Gorlin formula cause the calculated area (but not necessarily the actual orifice area) to be flow dependent.

On the one hand, Tardif and coworkers have shown that 2-dimensional transesophageal echocardiographic imaging of the stenotic aortic valve has failed to demonstrate true changes in valve orifice area when increased flow caused calculated area to increase. Their data suggest that the relationship between calculated area and flow resides within the calculation rather than in representing a true change in area.

However, it remains unclear whether the echocardiographic method used is sensitive enough to detect tiny (0.2-0.4 cm^2) changes in actual valve area. On the other hand, Voelker and colleagues working in vitro concluded that changes in calculated orifice area with changes in flow were probably owing to actual changes in valve area. Flow dependence of calculated valve orifice area appears to be less in bicuspid than in tricuspid valves but is more at lower flows than at higher flows.

These problems in assessing stenosis severity have substantial clinical importance. As an example, a patient with a reduced cardiac output and low LV ejection fraction who has both cardiomyopathy and mild aortic stenosis, despite a calculated valve area of 0.7 cm^2, may not benefit from aortic valve replacement because aortic stenosis is not the cause of the LV dysfunction. On the other hand, many patients with low gradients may improve substantially following surgery.

As described in detail in Chapter 17, hemodynamic manipulation in the catheterization laboratory can distinguish between these 2 different clinical entities. In patients with mild aortic stenosis, an infusion of nitroprusside or dobutamine increases forward output substantially but may actually decrease the transvalvular gradient. In such cases, the calculated AVA can increase significantly (**Table 13.2**). On the other hand, in patients with truly severe aortic stenosis, infusion of nitroprusside widens the transvalvular gradient and increases the calculated AVA only slightly, if at all.

Dobutamine, which produces similar changes in cardiac output, can be infused instead of nitroprusside. Importantly, patients with true aortic stenosis in whom stroke volume is augmented by at least 20% during dobutamine infusion have a much lower surgical mortality than observed in patients who fail to show inotropic reserve (see also Chapter 17). It should be noted that inotropic reserve is helpful in risk stratifying low-flow, low-gradient patients for surgical valve replacement but not for transcatheter valve replacement (TAVR). This seems logical since inotropic support is often a key mechanism for separating patients from cardiopulmonary bypass, a need not present in TAVR.

In addition to low flow, low gradient with reduced ejection fraction, low flow and low gradient with normal ejection fraction has also been observed in many patients. Such patients have small concentrically hypertrophied LVs so that a normal ejection from a small LV yields a low stroke volume and thus a low gradient. In these cases, the practitioner may be misled by the low gradient into believing that the aortic stenosis is mild or moderate in severity when in fact it is severe. Severity is confirmed by a low valve area and severe valve calcification.

Table 13.2	Nitroprusside Infusion in a Patient With Mild Aortic Stenosis	
	Baseline	**Nitroprusside (0.5 mg/kg/min)**
Cardiac output (L/min)	3.0	4.5
Left ventricular pressure (mmHg)	130/30	120/20
Aortic pressure (mmHg)	90/60	90/50
Aortic valve area (cm^2)	0.6	1.0
Valve resistance (dyn s/cm^5)	200	160

From Carabello BA, Ballard WL, Gazes PC. *Patient 65. Cardiology Pearls.* Hanley & Belfus; 1994:142.

VALVE RESISTANCE

Valve resistance is simply the mean aortic valve gradient divided by the cardiac output per second of systolic flow. It has the advantage of being calculated from 2 directly obtained pieces of data (output and gradient) and requires no discharge coefficient. A simplified formula for calculating aortic valve resistance has been shown by Cannon et al. to help differentiate patients with severe aortic stenosis from those patients who had similarly small calculated AVA but were subsequently demonstrated to have mild disease. Resistance appears to be less flow dependent than is valve area. Resistance is unlikely to supplant the Gorlin formula in assessing stenosis severity but may be an important adjunct to it in patients with low cardiac output

$$\frac{\left(\begin{array}{c}\text{Mean}\\\text{gradient}\end{array}\right)\left(\begin{array}{c}\text{Systolic ejection}\\\text{period}\end{array}\right)\left(\begin{array}{c}\text{Heart}\\\text{rate}\end{array}\right)}{\text{Cardiac output}\left(\text{liters/minute}\right)} = \times 1.33 \tag{13.11}$$

Acknowledgment

We would like to express our appreciation to Dr. James J. Ferguson III, who supplied **Figures 13.2** and **13.4**, constructed by him through computer simulation.

SUGGESTED READINGS

1. Burwash IG, Thomas DD, Sadahiro M, et al. Dependence of Gorlin formula and continuity equation valve areas on transvalvular volume flow rate in valvular aortic stenosis. *Circulation.* 1994;89(2):827-835.
2. Carabello BA, Barry WH, Grossman W. Changes in arterial pressure during left heart pullback in patients with aortic stenosis: a sign of severe aortic stenosis. *Am J Cardiol.* 1979;44(3):424-427.
3. Clavel MA, Pibarot P, Messika-Zeitoun D, et al. Impact of aortic valve calcification, as measured by MDCT, on survival in patients with aortic stenosis: results of an international registry study. *J Am Coll Cardiol.* 2014;64(12):1202-1213.
4. Cohen MV, Gorlin R. Modified orifice equation for the calculation of mitral valve area. *Am Heart J.* 1972;84(6):839-840.
5. Dumesnil JG, Pibarot P, Carabello BA. Paradoxical low flow and/or low gradient severe aortic stenosis despite preserved left ventricular ejection fraction: implications for diagnosis and treatment. *Eur Heart J.* 2010;31(3):281-289.
6. Gorlin R, Gorlin G. Hydraulic formula for calculation of the area of the stenotic mitral valve, other cardiac valves, and central circulatory shunts. I. *Am Heart J.* 1951;41:1-29.
7. Hachicha Z, Dumesnil JG, Bogaty P, Pibarot P. Paradoxical low-flow, low-gradient severe aortic stenosis despite preserved ejection fraction is associated with higher afterload and reduced survival. *Circulation.* 2007;115(22):2856-2864.
8. Hakki AH, Iskandrian AS, Bemis CE, et al. A simplified valve formula for the calculation of stenotic cardiac valve areas. *Circulation.* 1981;63(5):1050-1055.
9. Maes F, Lerakis S, Barbosa Ribeiro H, et al. Outcomes from transcatheter aortic valve replacement in patients with low-flow, low-gradient aortic stenosis and left ventricular ejection fraction less than 30%: a substudy from the TOPAS-TAVI registry. *JAMA Cardiol.* 2019;4(1):64-70.
10. Marcus R, Bednarz J, Abruzzo J, et al. Mechanism underlying flowdependency of valve orifice area determined by the Gorlin formula in patients with aortic valve obstruction. *Circulation.* 1993;88(suppl I):I-103.
11. Nishimura RA, Rihal CS, Tajik AJ, Holmes DR Jr. Accurate measurement of the transmitral gradient in patients with mitral stenosis: a simultaneous catheterization and Doppler echocardiographic study. *J Am Coll Cardiol.* 1994;24(1):152-158.
12. Shively BK, Charlton GA, Crawford MH, Chaney RK. Flow dependence of valve area in aortic stenosis: relation to valve morphology. *J Am Coll Cardiol.* 1998;31(3):654-660.
13. Tardif JC, Rodrigues AG, Hardy JF, et al. Simultaneous determination of aortic valve area by the Gorlin formula and by transesophageal echocardiography under different transvalvular flow conditions: evidence that anatomic aortic valve area does not change with variations in flow in aortic stenosis. *J Am Coll Cardiol.* 1997;29:1296.
14. Voelker W, Reul H, Nienhaus G, et al. Comparison of valvular resistance, stroke work loss and Gorlin valve area for quantification of aortic stenosis: an in vitro study in a pulsatile aortic flow model. *Circulation.* 1995;91(4):1196-1204.

14 | Pitfalls in the Evaluation of Hemodynamic Data[1]

Modern recording systems have eliminated a slew of mechanical errors introduced by the use of analog pen on paper or even needle on drums (see Chapter 11). Unfortunately, in the wake of automation, accuracy still requires attention to basic concepts in order to avoid the generation of erroneous data.

BASIC CONCEPTS

There are several categories of potential errors in cardiac hemodynamic measurements. First, artifacts can be induced by mechanical or operator errors, including unrecognized transducer failure, incorrect transducer positioning, inadequate balancing, and under- or overdamping. Second, and probably more significant, is misinterpretation of recordings, including failure to recognize catheter location (eg, pulmonary wedge vs pulmonary artery), failure to understand the influence of loading conditions, and failure to understand the implications of incorrectly recorded tracings. Finally, standardized software provided with hemodynamic recording equipment assumes that each laboratory follows the common practices of data acquisition, which may not always be a valid assumption, thus resulting in erroneous reporting.

As an example of the first category, the three hemodynamic tracings in **Figure 14.1** show right atrial (RA) pressure recordings performed within 1 minute of each other in the same patient. The mean RA pressures are 6, 17, and 24 mmHg, and the differences merely reflect zeroing of the transducer at heights above, at, and below the patient's right atrium.

Failure to adequately balance transducers can result in the recording of negative diastolic pressures, largely a physiologic impossibility. Grossly negative diastolic pressures are not possible under ordinary physiological circumstances, and a negative left ventricular (LV) end-diastolic pressure would reflect net reversal of blood flow. **Figure 14.2A-E** shows hemodynamics of a patient with a dilated cardiomyopathy presenting with heart failure and different type of artifacts that can occur during recording of hemodynamic data.

Examples of generic assumptions made by software vendors are the recordings of LV versus systemic pressure in patients with aortic stenosis (**Figures 14.3A and 14.4A**).

TRANSVALVULAR GRADIENT

The common reliance on valve gradients to assess the severity of valve disease ignores the role of loading conditions, systolic and diastolic filling periods, and transvalvular flow on the gradient measurement. Examples in **Figure 14.5** show underestimation of the severity of valvular stenosis in the setting of volume depletion and sedation, corrected by volume infusion and exercise, respectively. The disproportionate rise in gradient associated with increasing heart rates in mitral stenosis reflects the disproportionate fall in the diastolic filling period that occurs simultaneously; this is seen even with mild mitral stenosis and includes rise in

[1]We gratefully acknowledge the Grossman & Baim's *Cardiac Catheterization, Angiography, and Intervention*, 9th edition contributions of Dr. Zoltan G. Turi, as portions of his chapter, Pitfalls in the Evaluation of Hemodynamic Data, were retained in this text.

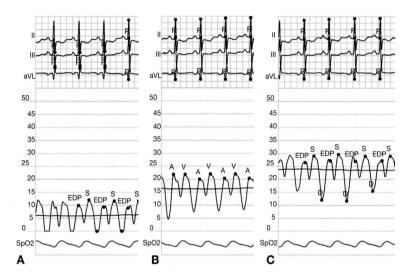

Figure 14.1 **A-C,** Three sets of right atrial pressures in a patient with severe aortic stenosis and radiation-induced pericardial disease s/p pericardiectomy. The panels reveal normal, moderately elevated, and severely elevated right atrial pressures, all recorded on a 50-mmHg scale. The tracings were taken a few seconds apart, with the transducers positioned above, at, and below the level of the patient's heart. Failure to compulsively align the transducer with the level of the patient's heart produces substantial error in hemodynamic recordings. Note the steep Y descent, which falsely appears to have an excursion below zero in the tracing at left **(A).**

left atrial pressure, gradient, and pulmonary artery pressure. With increasing flow across the valve, exponential rises are noted with fixed severe stenosis, whereas in the setting of mild to moderate disease, further opening of the stenotic valve results in blunting of the gradient rise. These findings in turn allow the use of maneuvers that increase transvalvular flow or modify diastolic and systolic filling periods, such as dobutamine infusion, pacing, and vasodilators, to further assess equivocal valve disease severity (see **Figure 14.6**).

EFFECTS OF CATHETER LOCATION

The primary pitfall in aortic stenosis pressure measurement relates to the comparison of pressures at levels other than either side of the aortic valve. Measurement of LV versus femoral artery pressure is particularly common: because of reflected harmonics, the phasic waveform difference between femoral and central aortic pressure is substantial, even though under ordinary circumstances, the mean pressure will be the same (see Chapter 11). **Figure 14.7A and B** shows the effect of measuring LV pressure against central aortic pressure and femoral artery pressure, respectively (see also Chapter 13). The latter remains a common technique along with simple pullback measurement across the aortic valve; both techniques are fraught with errors. **Figure 14.7C-E** was recorded in a patient with no aortic stenosis and merely reflects transducer balancing artifact.

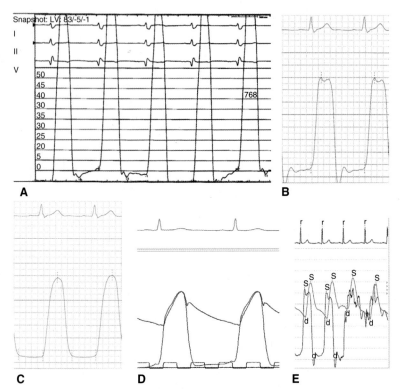

Figure 14.2 A, Left ventricular (LV) pressure tracing of a 63-year-old patient presenting with congestive heart failure with a newly diagnosed cardiomyopathy. The left ventricular end-diastolic pressure of −1 mmHg is an obvious artifact, although it was included in the patient's assessment. This occurred almost certainly owing to the transducer having been mounted well above the patient's heart. In addition to the negative pressures, the hemodynamics are inconsistent with the patient having a newly diagnosed cardiomyopathy. This is an example of a fundamental flaw in modern hemodynamic assessment and reporting: blind repetition of numbers reported by machine. **B and C,** Two other examples of distorted LV pressure recordings (200-mmHg scale). The tracing in panel **(B)** was obtained with overly compliant tubing attached to the diagnostic catheter, whereas for the tracing in panel **(C)**, air was present in the tubing between the catheter and the manifold. (Figures B and C courtesy of Dr. John Hirshfeld, University of Pennsylvania.) **D and E,** LV versus central aortic pressure with high-fidelity pressure recordings using micromanometer catheters **(D)**. In contrast, tracing **(E)** shows the loss of fidelity inherent in using fluid-filled catheters; the last 2 beats reflect a left ventricle to central aortic pullback. The femoral arterial pressure upstroke is delayed, and because of harmonics and possibly the height of the LV transducer, the femoral arterial pressure appears to be substantially higher than LV systolic pressure. Similar to **(B)** above, the LV pressure tracing is underdamped. (B and C, courtesy of Dr. John Hirshfeld, University of Pennsylvania; Tracings courtesy of Dr. Morton Kern, University of California, Irvine.)

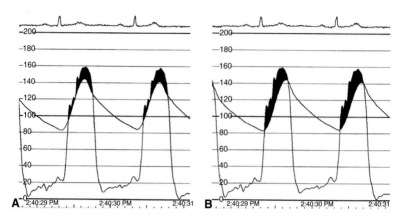

Figure 14.3 A, Inappropriate phase shift seen in pressure tracings. The software used by the cath lab had assumed incorrectly that systemic pressure was being recorded at the level of the femoral/external iliac artery. The aortic pressure tracing was thus moved forward in time, creating the artifact seen, which depicts systemic pressure rise occurring prior to LV contraction, a physiologic impossibility (in the absence of certain types of cardiac assist devices that would have a quite different signature). The gradient was reported as 11 mmHg and the calculated aortic valve area as 1.7 cm². **B,** With the elimination of the phase shift, the gradient is now reported as 20 mmHg and the valve area as 1.3 cm². (Figure courtesy of Dr. John Hirshfeld, University of Pennsylvania.)

The primary pitfalls in mitral stenosis assessment again reflect the importance of pressures measured on either side of the mitral valve. A substantial artifactual gradient results from indirect measurement of left atrial pressure across the pulmonary vascular bed using a wedged pulmonary artery catheter. **Figure 14.8** shows the inherent gradient when left atrial and pulmonary wedge pressures are recorded simultaneously. In the example in **Figure 14.9A**, the gradient between wedge and LV pressures was incorrectly interpreted as showing severe mitral stenosis. Simultaneous recording of left atrial and LV pressures showed early decompression of the left atrium consistent with mild mitral stenosis.

OTHER CONSIDERATIONS

Both heart rate, as already discussed, and heart rhythm can have significant influence on hemodynamics. An example of the effect of paced rhythm is seen in **Figure 14.10**. Other pitfalls of hemodynamic measurement include practices as simple as adequate flushing of the catheter (**Figure 14.11**). Air bubbles, clots, compliance of the tubing, and introduction of contrast (which affects viscosity and therefore resistance) all influence the recordings made through fluid-filled systems. Keeping tubing length short, having the transducer as close to the end of the catheter as possible, and flushing the system adequately and repeatedly are all important elements.

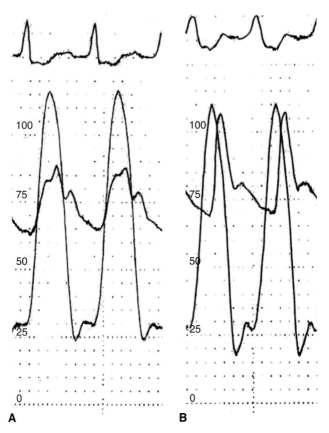

A   **B**

Figure 14.4 Tracings from the first report of transcatheter aortic valve replacement (TAVR) in a human. The results of this first TAVR are actually even better than the tracings would suggest at first glance. The tracing in panel **(A)** depicts systemic pressure rise commencing prior to the rise of left ventricular (LV) pressure, an example of the phenomenon shown in **Figure 14.3**. The tracing thus underestimates the pre-TAVR gradient and overestimates the valve area. The tracing in panel **(B)** demonstrates LV versus femoral pressure, in this case artificially increasing the apparent gradient and underestimating the resultant valve area. Note the late rise in systemic pressure upstroke. At the same time, the severity of aortic stenosis may be underestimated when femoral rather than central aortic pressure is used because of higher systemic peak pressure, reflecting the recruitment of harmonics as the pressure waveform passes through a long area of stiff blood vessels. The systemic pressure will also show a higher dP/dt than if it were recorded in the ascending aorta. Finally, complicating the issue in this particular patient: there was severe peripheral vascular disease, which would also result in overestimating the aortic valve gradient if femoral rather than central aortic pressure is used. (Reproduced from Eltchaninoff H, Tron C, Cribier A. Percutaneous implantation of aortic valve prosthesis in patients with calcific aortic stenosis: technical aspects. *J Interv Cardiol.* 2003;16(6):515-521.)

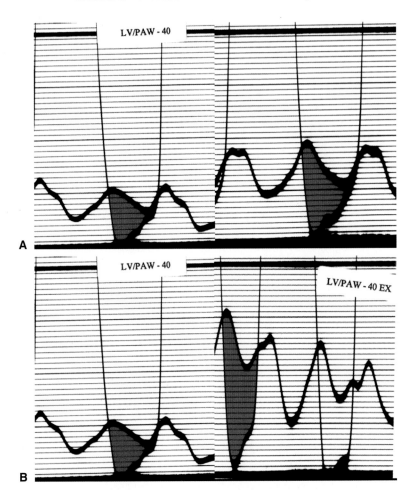

Figure 14.5 Response to 100 cc saline **(A)** and to arm exercise **(B)** in a patient undergoing cardiac catheterization in the late afternoon after having been NPO overnight. In the setting of a compliant left atrium, dehydration can result in substantial underestimation of the severity of mitral stenosis: the gradient on the right side of panel **(A)** has approximately doubled. Because of the disproportionate fall in diastolic filling period with increasing heart rate, and the effect of increasing flow across the valve with exercise, even relatively modest exertion can have a substantial effect on the gradient, which roughly tripled in the right side of panel **(B)**. (See text for discussion.) EX, exercise; LV, left ventricle; PAW, pulmonary artery wedge pressure.

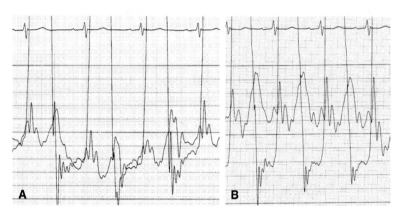

Figure 14.6 Left ventricular versus pulmonary wedge pressure in a patient with mitral stenosis, sedated and somewhat dehydrated (40-mmHg scale). Baseline tracing is shown in panel **(A)** and tracing during dobutamine infusion in **(B)**. This intervention is typically applied for patients with aortic stenosis but can readily be applied to assess all stenotic orifices with variable blood flow.

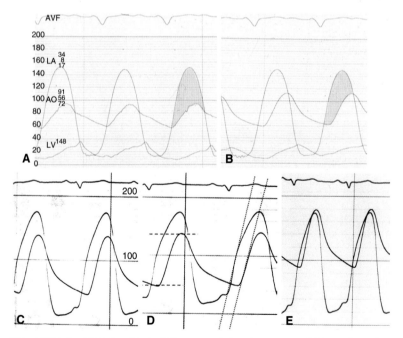

Figure 14.7 **A and B,** Left ventricular (LV) versus central aortic pressure and LV versus femoral artery pressure. The tracings were recorded a few seconds apart. Note the dramatically higher gradient in **(A)** with classic features of severe aortic stenosis. In contrast, tracing **(B)** shows lower peak-to-peak gradient and much higher aortic *dP/dt* and pulse pressure. Using femoral artery

Figure 14.7 *(Continued)*
pressure as a proxy for central aortic pressure can result in substantial underestimation of the severity of aortic stenosis. **C,** LV versus femoral artery pressure in a patient with a systolic ejection murmur billed as having aortic stenosis. A substantial gradient is seen. **D,** However, the *dP/dt* (dotted diagonal lines) of the LV and femoral pressure upstrokes are identical and the pulse pressure (horizontal dashed lines) is high. This tracing is not consistent with aortic stenosis. **E,** Rebalancing of the femoral sheath transducer reveals normal hemodynamics.

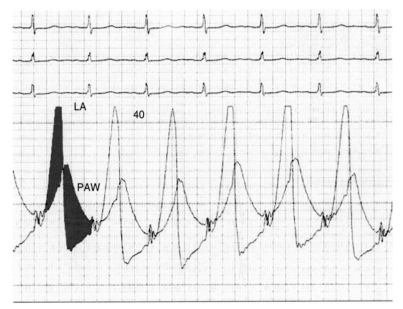

Figure 14.8 Simultaneous left atrial and wedge pressures in a patient with severe mitral insufficiency. The mean pressures are the same, but the A and V waves are blunted when pressures are recorded via a pulmonary catheter wedged in the pulmonary arterial circulation. The gradients shown in blue and red are thus artifactual—the fall in diastolic pressure as the left atrium is decompressed is transmitted with a significant delay. The gradient between wedge and left atrial pressure in diastole results in underestimation of the mitral valve area in mitral stenosis and of the height of the V wave in mitral insufficiency. Note the diastasis by the end of the diastolic cycle.

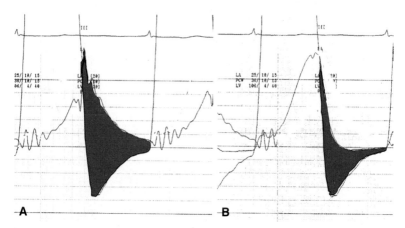

Figure 14.9 This patient was referred for percutaneous balloon mitral valvuloplasty based on echocardiographic findings of severe mitral stenosis and mild mitral insufficiency. The tall V wave and diastasis at late cycle in the left ventricle versus wedge pressure tracing **(A)** are suspicious for severe mitral insufficiency and mild mitral stenosis, respectively. Left ventricle versus left atrial pressure **(B)** shows early decompression of the left atrium consistent with mild mitral stenosis. The patient in fact had severe mitral insufficiency as her primary mitral valve pathology. Note the exaggerated gradient across the mitral valve in A consistent with recording left atrial decompression across the high-resistance pulmonary arteriolar bed.

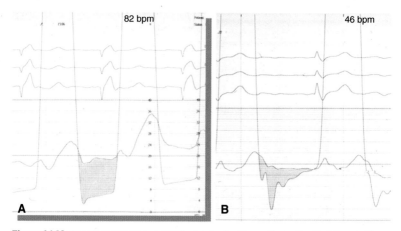

Figure 14.10 The effect of pacing on mitral valve gradient in a patient with mitral stenosis. The tracing in panel **(A)** shows a gradient of approximately 12 mmHg: the effect of the heart rate of 82 bpm. The tracing in panel **(B)** shows the absence of significant gradient with the pacemaker shut off and a much slower heart rate. Note also the establishment of diastasis late in the cardiac cycle.

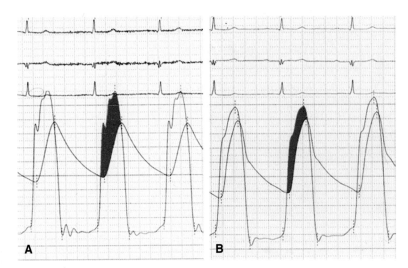

Figure 14.11 A and B, Left ventricular pressure versus aortic pressure taken a few minutes apart. Note the dramatic difference in *dP/dt* and gradient. This patient had aortic sclerosis, not stenosis, with a small gradient. The pressures were recorded through a 6F dual lumen catheter—the aortic pressure lumen is extremely small and damps easily from flow stasis and platelet sludging **(A)**. Flushing the catheter resulted in resolution of most of the gradient **(B)**.

SUGGESTED READINGS

1. Eltchaninoff H, Tron C, Cribier A. Percutaneous implantation of aortic valve prosthesis in patients with calcific aortic stenosis: technical aspects. *J Interv Cardiol.* 2003;16(6):515-521.
2. Folland ED, Parisi AF, Comei C. Simplified method for estimating true aortic valve mean gradient from simultaneous left ventricular and peripheral arterial pressure recordings. *Cathet Cardiovasc Diagn.* 1990;20(4):271-275.
3. Gardner RM. Accuracy and reliability of disposable pressure transducers coupled with modern pressure monitors. *Crit Care Med.* 1996;24(5):879-882.
4. Gordon JB, Folland ED. Analysis of aortic valve gradients by transseptal technique: implications for noninvasive evaluation. *Cathet Cardiovasc Diagn.* 1989;17(3):144-151.
5. Holmes DR Jr, Nishimura R, Fountain R, Turi ZG. Iatrogenic pericardial effusion and tamponade in the percutaneous intracardiac intervention era. *JACC Cardiovasc Interv.* 2009;2(8):705-717.
6. Kern MJ. Hemodynamic rounds series II: pitfalls of right-heart hemodynamics. *Cathet Cardiovasc Diagn.* 1998;43(1):90-94.
7. Nishimura RA, Rihal CS, Tajik AJ, Holmes DR Jr. Accurate measurement of the transmitral gradient in patients with mitral stenosis: a simultaneous catheterization and Doppler echocardiographic study. *J Am Coll Cardiol.* 1994;24(1):152-158.

15 Coronary Angiography, Coronary Artery Anomalies, and Cardiac Ventriculography[1]

Coronary angiography remains the principal component of cardiac catheterization. The goal is to examine the entire coronary tree (both native vessels and any surgically constructed bypass grafts) while recording details of the coronary anatomy, which include the following: the pattern of arterial distribution, anatomic or functional pathology (atherosclerosis, thrombosis, congenital anomalies, or focal coronary spasm), and the presence of collateral connections.

CURRENT INDICATIONS

Current indications for coronary angiography are summarized in the ACCF/SCAI/AATS/AHA/ASE/ASNC/HFSA/HRS/SCCM/SCCT/SCMR/STS Appropriate Use Criteria for Diagnostic Cardiac Catheterization. Although the details of these indications continue to evolve as new applications of catheter-based therapy are developed, they are still best summarized by the principle stated by F. Mason Sones—coronary arteriography is indicated when a problem is encountered whose resolution may be aided by the objective demonstration of the coronary anatomy, provided competent personnel and adequate facilities are available and the potential risks are acceptable to the patient and physician.

GENERAL ISSUES

In the early years, coronary angiography used to be performed using the brachial artery cutdown approach. The development of preshaped catheters and advancements in vascular access techniques have led to the progressive adoption of the percutaneous approach from the femoral, brachial, or radial artery.

THE FEMORAL APPROACH

As described in Chapter 8, the femoral approach to left-sided heart catheterization involves insertion of the catheter either directly over a guidewire or through an introducing sheath. A series of preformed catheters are used, starting with a pigtail catheter for left ventriculography followed by separate catheters (either Judkins or Amplatz shapes) for cannulation of the left and right coronary arteries and any surgical bypass grafts. Coronary catheters are available in 4F, 5F, 6F, 7F, or 8F end-hole designs that may taper further near the tip. They include a soft distal tip to minimize the risk of arterial dissection and steel braid, nylon, or other reinforcing materials (Kevlar, carbon fiber) within the catheter wall to provide the excellent torque control needed for coronary cannulation. Some of the catheters used for native coronary injection via the femoral or brachial approach are shown in **Figure 15.1**.

---

[1]We gratefully acknowledge the *Grossman & Baim's Cardiac Catheterization, Angiography, and Intervention*, 9th edition, contributions of Drs. Mauro Moscucci, Paolo Angelini, Jorge Monge, and Robert Hendel as portions of their chapters, Coronary Angiography; Coronary Artery Anomalies; and Cardiac Ventriculography, were retained in this text.

Insertion and Flushing of the Coronary Catheter

The selected catheter is inserted into the femoral sheath and advanced around the arch and into the ascending aorta before the guidewire is removed. After removal of the guidewire, the catheter is attached to a manifold system that permits the maintenance of a closed system during pressure monitoring, catheter flushing, and contrast agent administration (**Figure 15.2**). The catheter is

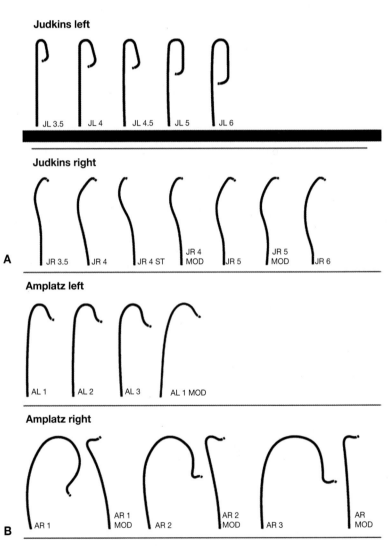

Figure 15.1 Types of catheters currently in wide use for selective native coronary angiography. **A,** Judkins catheters. **B,** Amplatz catheters. (Courtesy of Cordis Corporation, a Cardinal Health Company.)

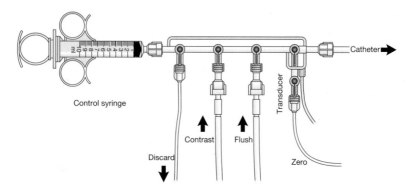

Control syringe

Contrast Flush

Transducer

Discard

Zero

Catheter

Figure 15.2 Four-port coronary manifold. This manifold provides a closed system with which blood can be withdrawn from the catheter and discarded. The catheter can be filled with either flush solution or contrast medium, and the catheter pressure can be observed, all under the control of a series of stopcocks. The fourth port is connected to an empty plastic bag and is used as a discard port (for blood from the double flush, air bubbles) so that the syringe need not be disconnected from the manifold at any time during the procedure.

immediately double-flushed—blood is withdrawn and discarded, after which heparinized saline flush is injected through the catheter lumen. Difficulty in blood withdrawal suggests apposition of the catheter tip to the aortic wall, which can be rectified by slight withdrawal or rotation of the catheter until free blood aspiration is possible. If blood cannot be aspirated despite repositioning the catheter, the catheter should be removed from the body and flushed on a towel, as we have occasionally seen thrombus collected in the catheter during exchanges over a guidewire. The lumen of the introducing sheath should also be flushed immediately before and after each catheter insertion and every 5 minutes thereafter to prevent the formation of thrombus, which is then "collected" by the catheter tip during insertion of the catheter in the sheath. Alternatively, the side arm of the sheath may be connected to a 30-mL/h continuous flow regulator.

Once the catheter has been flushed with saline solution, tip pressure should be displayed on the physiologic monitor at all times (except during actual contrast injections). Next, the catheter lumen should be gently filled with the contrast agent under fluoroscopic visualization. As an alternative to the conventional manifold, several cath labs today use the ACIST | CVi Contrast Delivery System (ACIST Medical Systems, Eden Prairie, Minnesota). The system includes a software-controlled motor-driven pump that delivers contrast media at a user-determined flow rate and volume and a hand controller that allows real-time, variable-flow control of the contrast injection rate. A built-in air column detection sensor alerts the clinician and stops the injection if air is detected in the tubing connected to the catheter, while in-line, hemodynamic monitoring is provided through a pressure transducer included in the syringe kit. The system allows accurate real-time contrast tracking, and it has been shown to reduce significantly the total volume of contrast media used when compared with manual contrast injection using a traditional manifold.

Damping and Ventricularization of the Pressure Waveform

A fall in overall catheter tip pressure (damping) or a fall in diastolic pressure only (ventricularization, **Figure 15.3**) during catheter engagement in a coronary ostium

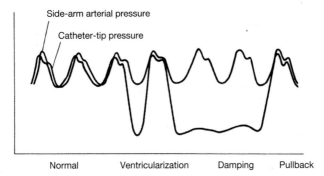

Figure 15.3 Pressure tracings as recorded during coronary angiography. Except for its earlier phase and slightly lower systolic pressure, catheter-tip pressure should resemble the pressure waveform simultaneously monitored by way of the femoral side-arm sheath or other arterial monitor (eg, radial artery). In the presence of an ostial stenosis or an unfavorable catheter position against the vessel wall, the waveform shows either ventricularization (in which systolic pressure is preserved but diastolic pressure is reduced) or frank damping (in which both systolic and diastolic pressures are reduced). In either case, the best approach is to withdraw the catheter immediately until the waveform returns to normal and to attempt to define the cause of the problem by non-selective injections in the sinus of Valsalva. Alternatively, a catheter equipped with side holes near the tip may be used to provide ongoing coronary perfusion.

indicates obstruction of the catheter tip or interference with coronary inflow. The catheter may be reengaged and a cautious small-volume contrast injection made to further clarify the situation. This may disclose a proximal occlusion of the vessel, against which the tip of the coronary catheter is resting. The test injection may also indicate ostial stenosis with absent reflux into the aortic root or retention of the injected contrast in the proximal and mid portion of the vessel. Lack of reflux indicates that the catheter tip is severely restricting or occluding ostial inflow and mandates that only a gentle injection be performed followed by immediate removal of the catheter at the end of a cine run to restore antegrade flow.

Another approach to evaluating such ostial lesions is to perform a nonselective injection into the sinus of Valsalva in an appropriate view (that displays the ostium of the vessel in question with no overlap by the sinus of Valsalva). Vigorous injection despite a damped or ventricularized pressure waveform should be avoided, since it predisposes to ventricular fibrillation or dissection of the proximal coronary artery with major ischemic sequelae. Such a dissection is detected by tracking of contrast down the vessel over the course of the injection and failure of contrast to clear on fluoroscopy after the injection is terminated (**Figure 15.4**).

Cannulation of the Left Coronary Ostium

Engagement of the left coronary ostium is usually quite easy with the Judkins technique. If a left Judkins catheter with a 4-cm curve (commonly referred to as a JL4) is simply allowed to remain en face as it is advanced down into the aortic root, it will engage the left coronary ostium without further manipulation in 80% to 90% of patients (**Figure 15.5**). Engagement should take place with the arm of the catheter traversing the ascending aorta at an angle of approximately 45°, the tip of the catheter in a more or less horizontal orientation, and with no change in the pressure waveform recorded from the catheter tip.

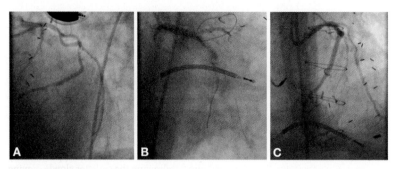

Figure 15.4 Guide catheter–induced coronary dissection and treatment with stent placement. **Panel A** displays a cranial left anterior oblique image showing the aggressive selective cannulation of the left circumflex coronary artery with an extra backup catheter. **Panel B** shows an occlusive dissection and contrast staining in the left circumflex in right anterior oblique. Note that the wire position was preserved throughout the case. **Panel C** shows the final result with complete restoration of flow after stent placement. (Reproduced with permission from: Cohen MG, Rossi JS. Coronary dissection, side branch occlusion and abrupt closure. In: Moscucci M, ed. *Complications of Cardiovascular Procedures: Risk Factors, Management and Bailout Techniques.* Lippincott Williams & Wilkins; 2011.)

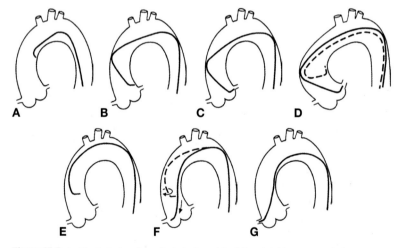

Figure 15.5 Judkins technique for catheterization of the left and right coronary arteries as viewed in the left anterior oblique (LAO) projection. In a patient with a normal-sized aortic arch, simple advancement of the JL4 catheter leads to intubation of the left coronary ostium **(A-C)**. In a patient with an enlarged aortic root **(D)**, the arm of the JL4 may be too short, causing the catheter tip to point upward or even flip back into its packaged shape (dotted catheter). A catheter with an appropriately longer arm (a JL5 or JL6) is required. To catheterize the right coronary ostium, the right Judkins catheter is advanced around the aortic arch with its tip directed leftward, as viewed in the LAO projection, until it reaches a position 2 to 3 cm above the level of the left coronary ostium **(E)**. Clockwise rotation causes the catheter tip to drop into the aortic root and point anteriorly **(F)**. Slight further rotation causes the catheter tip to enter the right coronary ostium **(G)**.

In patients with a widened aortic root owing to aortic valve disease or long-standing hypertension, the 4-cm left Judkins curve may be too short to allow successful engagement: the catheter arm may lie nearly horizontally across the aortic root with the tip pointing vertically against the roof of the left main artery or the catheter may even refold into its packaged shape during advancement into the aortic root (**Figure 15.5D**). In this case, a left Judkins catheter with a larger (JL4.5, JL5, or even JL6) curve should be selected.

In the occasional patient with a short or narrow aortic root, the 4-cm Judkins curve may be too long. When brought down into the aortic root, the catheter arm may lie nearly vertically with the tip pointing downward below the left coronary ostium. The left ostium may still be engaged despite this somewhat unfavorable situation by pushing the catheter down into the left sinus of Valsalva for approximately 10 seconds to tighten the tip angle and then withdrawing the catheter slowly. Having the patient take a deep breath during this maneuver also helps by pulling the heart into a more vertical position to assist in engagement of the left ostium. The most satisfactory approach, however, is to exchange for a JL3.5 catheter with a shorter curve.

On rare occasions, the left coronary ostium lies out of plane (typically high and posterior), as seen in the right anterior oblique (RAO) projection where the ostium is seen to be posterior to the catheter tip. In this case, limited counterclockwise rotation of the left Judkins catheter may help orient the catheter's tip posteriorly and facilitate engagement. Too much rotation of this catheter, however, may result in a refolded catheter that requires guidewire reinsertion to straighten. In that case, it may be helpful to step up to the next larger Judkins curve. Alternately, some operators prefer to switch to a left Amplatz shape (**Figure 15.1**). Amplatz catheters are more tolerant of rotational maneuvering and allow easy engagement of left coronary ostia that lie out of the conventional Judkins plane, as well as subselective engagement of the left anterior descending (LAD) and circumflex coronary arteries in patients with short left main coronary segments or separate left coronary ostia. The technique of cannulation of the left coronary artery using an Amplatz catheter is illustrated in **Figure 15.6**.

Cannulation of the Right Coronary Ostium

After being flushed and filled with contrast in the descending aorta (with the catheter tip directed anteriorly to avoid injection into the intercostal arteries), the right Judkins

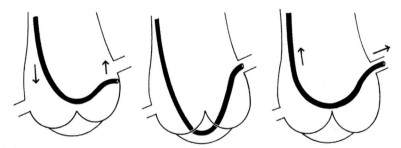

Figure 15.6 Catheterization of the left coronary ostium with an Amplatz catheter. The catheter should be advanced into the ascending aorta with its tip pointing downward so that the terminal catheter configuration resembles a diving duck. As the Amplatz catheter is advanced into the left sinus of Valsalva, its tip initially lies below the left coronary ostium (left). Further advancement causes the tip to ride up the aortic wall and enter the ostium (center). Slight withdrawal of the catheter causes the tip to seat more deeply in the ostium (right).

catheter with a 4-cm curve (JR4) is brought around the aortic arch with the tip facing inward until it comes to lie against the right side of the aortic root with its tip aimed toward the left coronary ostium (**Figure 15.5**). In a left anterior oblique (LAO) projection, the operator slowly and carefully rotates the catheter clockwise by nearly 180° to engage the right coronary artery (RCA). The tip of the right Judkins catheter tends to drop more deeply into the aortic root when the catheter is rotated, as the tertiary curve of the right Judkins shape aligns with the top of the aortic arch. To compensate for this effect, the operator must either begin the rotational maneuver with the tip 2 to 3 cm above the coronary ostium or withdraw the catheter slowly during rotation. Care must be taken to avoid overrotation of the catheter, which tends to cause the catheter tip to engage too deeply into the RCA. To avoid this, the operator should be prepared to apply a small amount of counterclockwise torque immediately as the tip of the catheter enters the ostium. Catheters with smaller (3.5 cm) or larger (5 or 6 cm) Judkins curves or right Amplatz catheters (AR1 or AR2) may be of value if aortic root configuration and proximal right coronary anatomy make engagement difficult.

Sometimes, the right coronary ostium lies high and anterior above the commissure of the left and right aortic valve leaflets rather than in the middle of the right sinus. A nonselective injection performed into the right sinus of Valsalva will show the high anterior origin and trigger a change to a left Amplatz (either AL0.75 or AL1).

The shepherd crook variant of the RCA is characterized by a superior, high course leading to difficult cannulation with Judkins or Amplatz catheters. In those cases, cannulation of the artery might be facilitated by using a left coronary artery bypass catheter or a left internal mammary artery (LIMA) catheter (**Figure 15.7**).

Damping and ventricularization are far more common in the RCA than in the left. The cause may include (1) the generally smaller caliber of the vessel, (2) ostial spasm around the catheter tip, (3) selective engagement of the conus branch, or (4) true ostial stenosis. A nonselective injection into the right sinus of Valsalva or cautious injections in the damped position with immediate postinjection withdrawal of the catheter can usually elucidate the underlying cause.

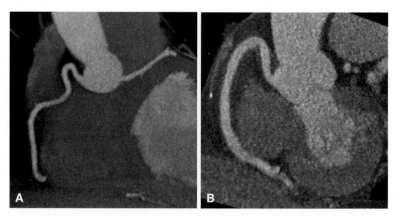

Figure 15.7 Shepherd's crook right coronary artery (RCA) in 2 patients. Oblique coronal CT images show a shepherd's crook RCA with an acute curvature **(A)** and a more obtuse curvature **(B)**. (Reproduced with permission from: Shriki JE, Shinbane JS, Rashid MA, et al. Identifying, characterizing, and classifying congenital anomalies of the coronary arteries. *Radiographics.* 2012;32:453-468.)

Cannulation of Saphenous Vein and Arterial Grafts

The proximal anastomosis of a vein graft or free arterial graft is usually placed on the right or left anterior aortic surface, several centimeters above the sinuses of Valsalva. The operative report always should be obtained before elective angiography on any patient with prior bypass surgery. Searching for proximal anastomosis while not knowing the number of anastomosis or their location increases the risk of stroke, increases the total amount of contrast media needed to perform the procedure, and might result in missing venous or arterial grafts.

Grafts should not be written off as occluded unless a clear stump is demonstrated. If the myocardial territory supplied by a graft assumed to be occluded is still contracting and there is no evident native or collateral blood supply to that territory, there may be a missed graft—the myocardium cannot function without a visible means of support! In that case, it may be valuable to perform an aortogram in an appropriate view to try to demonstrate flow in and locate the origin of such a missed graft.

Left Coronary Artery Grafts

Most commonly, grafts to the left coronary arise from the left anterior surface of the aorta, with grafts to the circumflex system usually placed somewhat higher on the aorta than those to the LAD or diagonal branches. The preferred view for engagement of left coronary artery grafts is the RAO view, with the tip of the catheter pointing anteriorly and to the right of the angiographic view. A right Judkins (JR4) or an Amplatz (AL1) catheter can be used to engage anterior (ie, left) coronary grafts. Special left coronary bypass, internal mammary, or hockey stick catheters may be required for left grafts that originate with an upward trajectory (**Figure 15.8**).

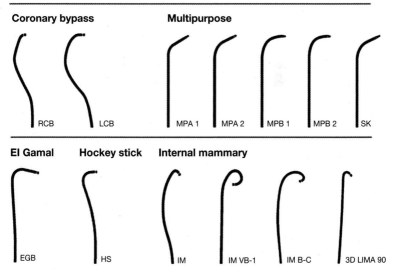

Figure 15.8 Catheters used for bypass graft angiography. Although the right Judkins or Amplatz catheters can be used for many anterior takeoff vein grafts, the catheters shown here may be useful. Top, left to right. Right coronary bypass, left coronary bypass, multipurpose "A" 1 and 2, multipurpose "B" 1 and 2, and multiple SK. Bottom, left to right. El Gamal, hockey stick, and left internal mammary artery.

Right Coronary Artery Grafts

Grafts to the right coronary (or the distal portions of a dominant circumflex) usually originate from the right anterior surface of the aorta, above and somewhat behind the plane of the native right coronary ostium.

For downward-pointing right coronary grafts, a catheter with no primary curve (a multipurpose, Wexler, or JR3.5 short-tip catheter) is preferred, as it provides better alignment with the proximal portion of the graft and better opacification. A preferred view for engagement of RCA grafts is the LAO view, with the tip of the catheter pointing downward and toward the right of the aortic wall (left in the angiographic view).

Internal Mammary Artery Cannulation

Successful cannulation of the LIMA requires knowledge of the left subclavian and brachiocephalic trunk as well as the right subclavian arteries, as shown in **Figure 15.9A**. It is also important to understand some of the common anatomic variants in the internal mammary artery (IMA), including more proximal origin in the vertical portion of the subclavian or origin as a common vessel with the thyrocervical trunk.

In addition, while the Judkins RCA catheter can be used to cannulate the IMA, this approach often does not provide a coaxial and adequate engagement of the artery ostium. Thus, the general preference is to use a dedicated LIMA catheter for cannulation of the IMA.

These grafts can develop significant lesions, although this is uncommon, making it important to evaluate such grafts post bypass catheterization. In patients with early recurrence of angina (within the first 6 months after surgery), most commonly, the lesion is located at the distal mammary-coronary anastomosis. Flow-limiting kinks may also be present in the midgraft, and ostial lesions at the origin of the internal mammary from the subclavian may also occur. It may be important to look for large nonligated side branches that may divert flow from the coronary circulation and occlusion of which (in the occasional patient) may be required for angina relief. It is also important to look for stenoses in the subclavian artery before the takeoff of the internal mammary, which may compromise the inflow to the graft and thereby cause myocardial ischemia.

In the LAO projection, cannulation of the LIMA begins by advancement of this catheter into the aortic arch until it lies just inside the left edge of the wedgelike density formed by the shadow of the upper mediastinum against the lung fields. With 1 to 2 cm of J guidewire protruding from its tip, the mammary catheter is rotated counterclockwise and slowly pulled back until it falls into the subclavian artery origin. From there, the wire can be advanced well out into the axillary artery. The mammary catheter is then advanced over the wire, into the midsubclavian, where the guidewire is then removed, and the catheter is flushed and filled with contrast. A low-osmolar contrast agent should be used to avoid causing central nervous system toxicity by reflux of hyperosmolar ionic contrast up the vertebral arteries. Switching to the straight anteroposterior (AP) projection, the catheter is rotated counterclockwise slightly (to make the tip point slightly anteriorly) as it is withdrawn slowly until the internal mammary is engaged. Intermittent gentle puffs of contrast will help localize the mammary origin during this withdrawal. Great care should be taken to avoid catheter-tip trauma/dissection of the relatively delicate mammary vessel.

If selective cannulation is difficult because of tortuosity or anatomic variations, a variety of super-selective **or** nonselective techniques can be used to permit angiographic evaluation. Inflation of a blood pressure cuff on the ipsilateral arm may help reduce runoff through the axillary artery and improve opacification of the internal mammary in cases where selective cannulation is difficult.

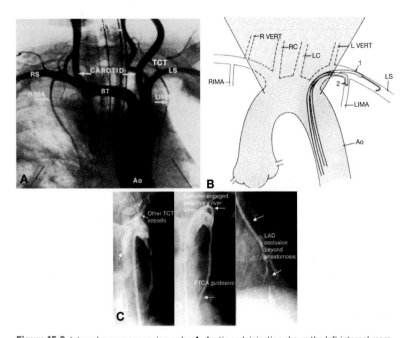

Figure 15.9 Internal mammary angiography. **A,** Aortic arch injection shows the left internal mammary artery (LIMA) originating from the left subclavian (LS), just opposite the thyrocervical trunk (TCT) and distal to the right vertebral artery (VERT). The right internal mammary artery (RIMA) originates from the right subclavian (RS) just distal to the bifurcation of the right carotid from the brachiocephalic trunk (BT). **B,** Schematic diagram shows the corresponding arch vessel origins. Note that the left subclavian originates just inside the patient's leftmost edge of the wedge-shaped shadow cast by the upper mediastinal structures in the left anterior oblique projection. Catheter manipulation in this projection facilitates advancement of a guidewire into the LS (step 1), facilitating selective cannulation of the LIMA during catheter withdrawal and slight counterclockwise rotation (step 2, see text). **C,** Variant in which internal mammary originates in common with the thyrocervical trunk, resulting in poor opacification. An angioplasty guidewire was placed down the internal mammary through a 6F diagnostic catheter and used to advance the tip of the diagnostic catheter selectively down the IMA. From that position, sufficient opacification was obtained to demonstrate occlusion of the distal left anterior descending (LAD) beyond the anastomosis as the cause of the patient's recurrent angina. PTCA, percutaneous transluminal coronary angioplasty.

Cannulation of the right IMA may be slightly more difficult because of the need to avoid the right carotid before entering the right subclavian itself. In the LAO projection, the upper mediastinal wedge is identified. The mammary catheter with protruding J wire is taken to the right edge of this shadow and rotated counterclockwise until it falls into the brachiocephalic trunk. The wire is then advanced toward the right subclavian artery. Predilection for the wire to advance into the right carotid artery may require removing the guidewire and performing a nonselective contrast injection in the brachiocephalic trunk to identify the origin of the subclavian branch. The RAO-caudal projection often gives the best spatial resolution of the right carotid and right subclavian origins, after which a steerable Wholey guidewire (Mallinckrodt) can be used to cannulate the subclavian. Once the wire is firmly out of the subclavian artery, the mammary catheter is advanced as described above. For cannulation of the right IMA, however, the catheter is rotated slightly clockwise during withdrawal to point its tip anteriorly.

Gastroepiploic Graft Cannulation

The effort to perform all-arterial bypass has brought back the right gastroepiploic artery (as an arterial pedicle graft) for anastomosis to the posterior descending or other vessels on the inferior surface of the heart. Angiography of this vessel is possible using standard visceral angiographic catheters (eg, Cobra) designed to enter visceral arteries such as the celiac axis. From there, the catheter can be advanced into the common hepatic (as opposed to the splenic) artery and then turned downward into the gastroduodenal artery (**Figure 15.10**).

THE BRACHIAL OR RADIAL APPROACH

Cannulation of the coronary arteries using the brachial or radial artery approach presents similar challenges. For a detailed description, the reader is directed to Chapters 7 and 9.

ADVERSE EFFECTS OF CORONARY ANGIOGRAPHY

Patients undergoing coronary angiography should always be monitored continuously in terms of clinical status, surface electrocardiogram, and arterial pressure from the catheter tip. In patients with baseline left ventricular dysfunction or marked ischemic instability, when clinically indicated, a right-sided heart catheterization can also be performed to display pulmonary artery pressure continuously on the same scale as that of the arterial pressure, and as an early indicator of procedural problems or progressive decompensation.

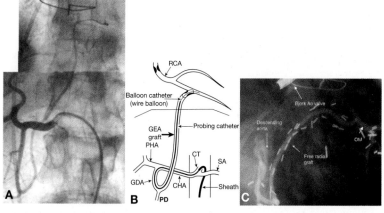

Figure 15.10 A and B, Gastroepiploic graft anatomy. The common hepatic artery (CHA) originates with the splenic artery (SA) from the celiac trunk (CT). The gastroduodenal artery (GDA) originates from the CHA, which then becomes the proper hepatic artery (PHA). The terminal branches of the GDA are the pancreatoduodenal (PD) and the right gastroepiploic artery (GEA), shown here undergoing angioplasty of a lesion at its anastomosis to the right coronary artery (RCA). **C,** Free radial graft from the descending aorta to an obtuse marginal (OM) graft, cannulated using a Cobra visceral angiographic catheter. Localization of the graft ostium was aided by the presence of multiple surgical clips used to ligate small side branches of the radial artery at the time of bypass.

One of the most common adverse effects seen during coronary angiography is the provocation of myocardial ischemia, particularly in patients with unstable angina. When myocardial ischemia does occur, the best course of action is to remove the catheter from the coronary ostium and temporarily suspend injections until angina resolves. Nitroglycerin (200 μg bolus, repeated at 30-second intervals up to a total of 1000 μg) can be administered into either the involved coronary artery or intraarterially. If marked arterial hypertension is present and fails to respond to nitroglycerin, other vasodilators can be administered as needed to bring the blood pressure down. Only rarely (in patients with severe 3-vessel and/or left main coronary disease and those whose ischemia is associated with hypotension) is myocardial ischemia severe enough and refractory to the above management program to prompt placement of an intra-aortic counterpulsation balloon in the contralateral femoral artery before completion of coronary angiography.

Severe allergic reactions are uncommon during coronary angiography and are best prevented by premedication as described in Chapter 4 in patients with a history of prior allergic reaction to radiographic contrast. Acute kidney injury (AKI) may develop after coronary angiography, particularly in patients who are hypovolemic, who receive large volumes of contrast or who have prior renal insufficiency, diabetes, or multiple myeloma. In these patients, every effort should be made to give adequate hydration before and after the procedure (see also Chapters 2 and 4).

Air embolization is a rare complication of coronary angiography, and it occurs always owing to poor technique. Intracoronary administration of nitroglycerin, intracoronary saline flushes, administration of 100% oxygen, and attempts to aspirate the injected air have been proposed as interventions to revert the acute ischemic changes associated with this complication.

INJECTION TECHNIQUE

Timid injections permit intermittent entry of nonopaque blood into the coronary artery and might fail to allow visualization of the coronary ostium and proximal coronary branches. On the other hand, vigorous injections may cause coronary dissection or excessive myocardial blushing, and prolonged injections may contribute to increased myocardial depression or bradycardia.

Injection velocity should be built up gradually during the first second until the injection rate is adequate to completely replace antegrade blood flow into the coronary ostium. The rate and volume of injection required to accomplish this goal have been measured and found to average 7 mL at 2.1 mL/s in the left and 4.8 mL at 1.7 mL/s in the right coronary. In patients with occlusion, much lower rates and volumes are required, and in patients with left ventricular hypertrophy (eg, aortic stenosis, hypertrophic cardiomyopathy), larger volumes and higher rates of injection may be required. In addition, visualization of the RCA can often be achieved with <4 mL of contrast. Thus, the injection should be maintained until the entire vessel is opacified. The injection should then be terminated abruptly by turning the manifold stopcock back to monitor pressure, although cine filming should continue until opacification of distal vessels or late-filling branches is complete. The operator should monitor for excessive bradycardia or hypotension, review the video loop, and set up the gantry angles for the next injection. To avoid problems, each injection should begin with a completely full (and bubble-free) injection syringe, held with the handle slightly elevated so that any microbubbles will drift up toward the plunger. The injection syringe should be managed in such a way as to avoid mixing of blood and contrast because such mixing may promote formation of thrombi (particularly when nonionic contrast agents are used).

Although manual contrast injection is the standard technique in coronary angiography, some operators favor the use of a power injector (as used in left

ventriculography or aortography) to perform coronary injections. This approach allows a single operator to perform injections and move the table and has proved safe in thousands of procedures.

ANATOMY, ANGIOGRAPHIC VIEWS, AND QUANTITATION OF STENOSIS

Coronary Anatomy

The main coronary trunks can be considered to lie in 1 of 2 orthogonal planes (**Figure 15.11**). The anterior descending and posterior descending coronary arteries lie in the plane of the interventricular septum, whereas the right and circumflex coronary trunks lie in the plane of the atrioventricular valves. In the 60° LAO projection, one is looking down the plane of the interventricular septum, with the plane of the AV valves seen en face; in the 30° RAO projection, one is looking down the plane of the AV valves, with the plane of the interventricular septum seen en face. The major segments and branches have each been assigned a numerical identification in the Bypass Angioplasty Revascularization Investigation (BARI) modification of the CASS nomenclature (**Figure 15.12**).

Right-Dominant Circulation

The RCA gives rise to the conus branch (which supplies the right ventricular outflow tract) and 1 or more acute marginal branches (which supply the free wall of the right ventricle), whether or not the circulation is right dominant. In the 85% of patients who have a right-dominant coronary artery, it goes on to form the AV nodal artery, the posterior descending artery, and the posterolateral left ventricular branches that supply the inferior aspect of the interventricular septum (see **Figure 15.11**). After a short (but variable) distance, the left main trunk branches into the LAD and the

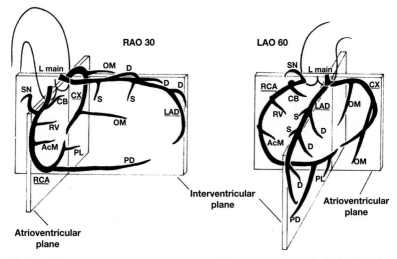

Figure 15.11 Representation of coronary anatomy relative to the interventricular and atrioventricular valve planes. Coronary branches are as indicated—AcM, acute marginal; CB, conus branch; CX, circumflex; D, diagonal; L main, left main; LAD, left anterior descending; LAO, left anterior oblique; OM, obtuse marginal; PD, posterior descending; PL, posterolateral left ventricular; RAO, left anterior oblique; RCA, right coronary artery; S, septal; SN, sinus node.

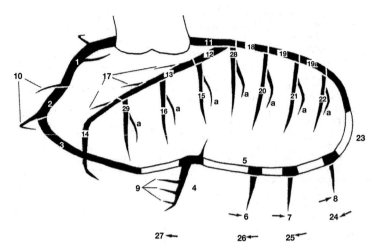

Figure 15.12 The numerical coding system and official names of the coronary segments, as used in the Bypass Angioplasty Revascularization Investigation (BARI) study. Right coronary: 1, proximal; 2, middle; 3, distal; 4, posterior descending; 5, posteroatrioventricular; 6, first posterolateral; 7, second posterolateral; 8, third posterolateral; 9, inferior septals; 10, acute marginals. Left coronary: 11, left main; 12, proximal left anterior descending; 13, middle left anterior descending; 14, distal left anterior descending; 15, first diagonal (a, a branch of first diagonal); 16, second diagonal; 17, septals (anterior septals); 18, proximal circumflex; 19, middle circumflex; 19a, distal circumflex; 20, 21, and 22, first, second, and third obtuse marginals; 23, left atrioventricular; 24, 25, and 26, first, second, and third posterolaterals (in left- or balanced-dominant system); 27, left posterior descending (in left-dominant system); 28, ramus (ramus intermedius); 29, third diagonal. (Reprinted with permission from The BARI Protocol. Protocol for the bypass angioplasty revascularization investigation. *Circulation.* 1991; 84:V1-V27.)

circumflex coronary arteries. The LAD artery gives rise to septal branches that curve down into the interventricular septum, as well as to diagonal branches that wrap over the anterolateral free wall of the left ventricle (LV).

Some patients have a twin LAD system, in which 1 trunk (frequently intramyocardial) supplies the entire septum and the other trunk runs on the surface of the heart supplying all the diagonal branches. The circumflex artery courses clockwise in the AV groove (viewed from the apex) as it gives rise to 1 or more obtuse marginal branches that supply the lateral free wall of the LV but does not reach the crux in patients with a right-dominant circulation. In some patients, a large intermedius or ramus medianus branch (neither a diagonal nor a marginal) may originate directly from the left main trunk, bisecting the angle between the left anterior descending and circumflex arteries, to create a trifurcation pattern of the left main coronary artery. Regardless of whether the patient is right or left dominant, the sinus node originates as a proximal branch of the right coronary in 60% of patients and as a left atrial branch of the circumflex in the remaining 40% of patients.

Left-Dominant Circulation

In 8% of patients, the coronary circulation is left dominant; that is, the posterolateral left ventricular, posterior descending, and AV nodal arteries are all supplied by the terminal portion of the left circumflex coronary artery. In such patients, the RCA is small and supplies only the right atrium and right ventricle. It may be important to visualize this, as a potential source of right-to-left collaterals, but the small diameter of a nondominant RCA predisposes it to damping and catheter-induced spasm, which makes limited injections advisable.

Balanced Dominant Circulation

In about 7% of hearts, there is a codominant or balanced system, in which the RCA gives rise to the posterior descending artery and then terminates and the circumflex artery gives rise to all the posterior left ventricular branches and perhaps also a parallel posterior descending branch that supplies part of the interventricular septum. In some patients, the supply to the inferior wall may be further fractionated among a short posterior descending branch of the right coronary (which supplies the inferobase), branches of the distal circumflex (which supply the midinferior wall), and branches of the acute marginal (which extend to supply the inferoapex).

Angiographic Views

Accurate coronary diagnosis requires coronary injections in multiple views to make sure that all coronary segments are seen clearly without foreshortening or overlapping. The angulation of each view is defined using 2 terms. The first term denotes rotation; for example, the term RAO designates a view where the image intensifier is positioned over the patient's right anterior chest wall (RAO) and LAO designates a view where the image intensifier is positioned over the patient's left anterior chest wall (LAO). The second term denotes skew, that is, the amount of angulation toward the patient's head (cranial) or foot (caudal). Although the full nomenclature of skew specifies first the source of the beam and then the location of the imaging device (eg, caudocranial, to denote that the x-ray tube is toward the patient's feet while the image intensifier is located toward the patient's head), in practice this is simplified to give just the location of the imaging device. The term RAO caudocranial is thus stated as RAO cranial (**Figure 15.13**).

A series of screening views should be used as the foundation of a study, adjusted or supplemented by 1 or more additional X-ray tube views selected to more completely define suspicious areas. This requires the operator to interpret the coronary anatomy as each injection is made or by digital review, and it is not acceptable to simply shoot a series of routine views and hope that the study will prove adequate when reviewed later.

Right Anterior Oblique Projections

The straight 30° RAO projection of the left coronary suffers from overlap and foreshortening of both the left anterior descending and the circumflex vessels. Thus, a suggested initial view of choice is the RAO-caudal projection (0°-10° RAO and 15°-20° caudal), since it provides an excellent view of the left main bifurcation, the proximal left anterior descending artery, and the proximal to mid circumflex artery. The second view is a shallow RAO-cranial projection (0°-10° RAO and 25°-40° cranial), which provides a superior view of the mid and distal LAD artery, with clear visualization of the origins of the septal and diagonal branches. This shallow RAO cranial view is also quite good for examination of the distal RCA or distal circumflex, since it effectively unstacks the posterior descending and posterolateral branches and projects them without foreshortening.

Left Anterior Oblique Projections

The conventional 60° LAO projection is limited by overlap and foreshortening of the left coronary artery, although it is very useful in the evaluation of the proximal and mid RCA. The LAO-cranial view, created by the addition of 15° to 30° of cranial angulation, elongates the left main and proximal LAD arteries while projecting the intermedius

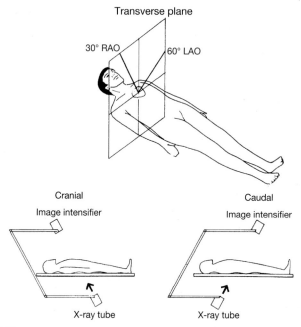

Figure 15.13 Geometry of angulated views. Conventional coronary angiography was performed previously using angulation only in the transverse plane (top), as demonstrated by the 60° left anterior oblique (LAO) and 30° right anterior oblique (RAO) views. Currently, improved x-ray equipment permits simultaneous cranial or caudal angulation in the sagittal plane. Each view is named based on the location of the image intensifier, rather than the older nomenclature specifying the location of both the x-ray tube and intensifier (eg, cranial is equivalent to caudocranial).

or first diagonal branch downward off the proximal circumflex. Performing the angiographic run during a sustained maximal inspiration will usually pull the diaphragm down and improve x-ray penetration. The LAO-caudal view (40°-60° LAO and 10°-20° caudal) projects the left coronary artery upward from the left main in the appearance of a spider (hence the older term, *spider view*) and usually offers improved visualization of the left main, left main bifurcation, proximal LAD, and proximal circumflex arteries. This view can often be enhanced by filming during maximal expiration, which accentuates a horizontal cardiac position and allows a better look from below. A shallow LAO-cranial view will also allow optimal visualization of the distal RCA, its bifurcation into the posterior descending artery and the posterolateral artery, and the complete posterior descending artery and posterolateral artery systems.

Posteroanterior and Left Lateral Projections

The straight posteroanterior (PA, or "0-0") and left lateral projections tend to be underused in the era of complex angulation. Because the left main coronary artery curves from a more leftward to an almost anterior direction along its length, the PA projection (sometimes referred to incorrectly as the AP projection) frequently provides the best view of the left main ostium. On the other hand, the shallow RAO-caudal view frequently provides a better look at the more distal left main artery. The left lateral projection is particularly useful in examining the proximal circumflex and the proximal and distal LAD arteries, particularly when combined with slight (10°-15°) cranial angulation. This projection also provides the best look at the anastomosis of a left internal mammary graft to the mid-distal LAD and offers an excellent look at the midportion of the RCA, free of the excessive motion seen when this portion of the vessel is viewed in the straight RAO projection. The left lateral projection also has the advantage of allowing easy radiographic penetration in most patients when it is performed with both of the patient's hands positioned behind the head, although it generates the highest degree of backscatter given the proximity of the beam entry point on the patient's right side to the operator.

A uniform sequence of these views, adjusting the exact angles slightly in each patient as dictated by test puffs of contrast, can thus be adopted, and it can result in optimum visualization of coronary anatomy while minimizing use of contrast media and radiation exposure. Beginning with the left coronary artery, these views include the following:

1. RAO-caudal to visualize the left main, proximal LAD, and proximal circumflex
2. RAO-cranial to visualize the mid and distal LAD without overlap of septal or diagonal branches
3. LAO-cranial to visualize the mid and distal LAD in an orthogonal projection
4. LAO-caudal to visualize the left main and proximal circumflex

One or more supplemental views (PA, lateral-cranial, lateral-caudal) may then be taken to clarify any areas of uncertainty. The right coronary catheter is then placed, after which 2 screening views are obtained:

1. LAO to visualize the proximal and mid RCA
2. LAO-cranial to visualize the distal RCA and its bifurcation into the posterior descending and posterolateral branches
3. RAO-cranial to visualize the posterior descending and posterolateral branches
4. Lateral to visualize the mid-RCA

Lesion Quantification

To quantify a coronary stenosis accurately, it must be seen in profile, free from artifact related to foreshortening or obfuscation by a crossing vessel. Multiple views are important because many lesions have a markedly eccentric (elliptical rather than round) lumen. Suspicious lesions must be examined in a variety of other projections to reveal their true severity and to distinguish the lucency caused by eccentric stenosis from a similar lucency that may be seen adjacent to an area of denser contrast (caused by tortuosity or overlapping vessels in the absence of any true abnormality at the site) owing to a perceptual artifact known as the Mach effect.

In clinical practice, the degree of lesion stenosis is usually estimated visually from the coronary angiogram rather than by quantitative angiographic analysis (quantitative coronary angiography [QCA]). The operator must thus develop a sense of what constitutes a 50%, 70%, and 90% diameter stenosis. Although the process of visually estimating the degree of coronary stenosis may seem straightforward, it is subject to significant operator variability (the standard deviation for repeat estimates is <18%) as well as a systematic form of "stenosis inflation" that causes operators to estimate a diameter stenosis roughly 20% higher than that measured by QCA.

Features such as eccentricity, ulceration, and thrombus may be associated with unstable clinical patterns, whereas features such as calcification, eccentricity, or thrombus may influence the choice of catheter intervention. Thus, accurate evaluation of lesion morphology from the coronary angiogram has become important.

Coronary Collaterals

In reviewing the coronary angiogram, one basic principle is that there should be evident blood supply to all portions of the LV. Previously occluded vessel branches usually manifest as truncated stumps, but a stump may not be evident if there has been a flush occlusion at the origin of the involved vessel. These occluded or severely stenotic vessels will frequently be seen to fill late in the injection by antegrade (so-called bridging) collaterals or collaterals that originate from the same (intracoronary) or an adjacent (intercoronary) vessel (**Figure 15.14**). Finally, coronary occlusion may present in some patients simply as an angiographically arid area to which there is no evidence of either antegrade or collateral flow and no evident vascular stump. However, if such an area fails to show regional hypokinesis on the left ventriculogram, the operator should search carefully for blood supply by way of anomalous vessels or unopacified collaterals (ie, a separate origin conus branch that was not opacified during the main right coronary injections) because the myocardium cannot continue to function normally with no visible means of support.

Although it is uncommon, what appears as a network of collaterals may be the vascular supply to an organized thrombus (in the LV or left atrium) or a cardiac

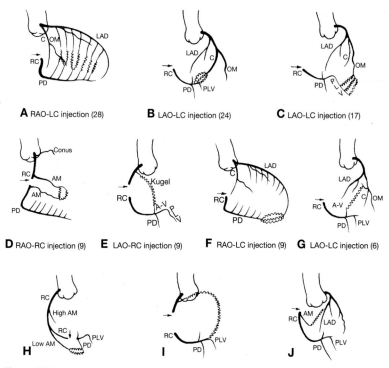

Figure 15.14 A-J, Ten collateral pathways observed in patients with right coronary (RC) obstruction (total occlusion or >90% stenosis). AM, acute marginal branch of right coronary artery; AV, atrioventricular nodal; C, circumflex; LAD, left anterior descending; LC, left coronary; OM, obtuse marginal; PD, posterior descending; PLV, posterior left ventricular branch. Numbers in parentheses represent the number of cases in this series. (Reprinted with permission of American Heart Association, Inc. from Levin DC. Pathways and functional significance of the coronary collateral circulation. *Circulation.* 1974;50:831-837.)

tumor. Those entities should be suspected when filling of an apparent collateral network is seen in the absence of occlusion or severe stenosis of the normal supply to a myocardial territory.

BIPLANE AND ROTATIONAL CORONARY ANGIOGRAPHY

Although advances in technology have resulted in a marked improvement in the safety of coronary angiography, the procedure is still associated with a small risk related to radiation exposure (see Chapter 2). In addition, particularly in high-risk patients with underlying renal insufficiency and other comorbidities, administration of contrast media can result in the development of AKI (see Chapter 4). There have been several studies aimed toward identifying ways to reduce radiation exposure and the total amount of contrast media required for image acquisition. Biplane coronary angiography requires by definition the use of a biplane cardiac cath lab, and it involves obtaining 2 views during a single injection using the frontal and lateral planes positioned in orthogonal views. Usually, the lateral plane is positioned in a left cranial or caudal view and the frontal plane is positioned in the contralateral cranial or caudal view (LAO cranial–RAO caudal and LAO caudal–RAO cranial). This simplifies panning during acquisition of the angiographic images. Biplane angiography can result in a reduction in the amount of contrast media required for angiography, although radiation exposure is the same or can be slightly higher because of the additional fluoroscopy time needed for appropriate positioning of the frontal and lateral planes.

High-speed rotational angiography is an alternative technique that has been evaluated in several small randomized clinical trials. In this technique, the C-arm and the detector rotate around the patient at a high speed during a single contrast injection and the corresponding image acquisition. Two rotations in caudal and cranial angulation (LAO to RAO) are usually performed for the left coronary artery system, while a single rotation (LAO to RAO) is usually performed for the RCA system. The newest technology has the ability to perform dual-axis rotation (dual-axis rotational coronary angiography), in which the C-arm is preprogrammed to make a single-run rotation along a curved trajectory around the patient, acquiring all the views in a single rotation. It has been shown that rotational angiography can result in a significant reduction in contrast dose, radiation exposure, and image acquisition time when compared with conventional angiography, without compromising the quality of imaging. In addition, through the application of 3D reconstruction algorithms, rotational angiography allows the acquisition of 3D images that can be used in planning interventional procedures.

NONATHEROSCLEROTIC CORONARY ARTERY DISEASE

Although atherosclerotic stenosis is far and away the most common pathologic process responsible for myocardial ischemia, the angiographer must be aware of various other potential causes, including congenital anomalies of coronary origin, coronary fistulae, coronary aneurysms, and muscle bridges.

The coronary arteries may also be affected by vasculitis, including polyarteritis nodosa and the mucocutaneous lymph node syndrome (Kawasaki disease).

Although not an arteritis, cardiac allograft vasculopathy is one of the most troublesome long-term complications of heart transplantation.

Patients who have received prior mantle radiation therapy for Hodgkin disease may be at risk for radiation-induced coronary stenosis, particularly of the left and right coronary ostia and the proximal left coronary artery, up to 20 years after completing their course of therapy.

Finally, some patients who come for catheterization have no demonstrable coronary abnormality to account for their clinically suspected ischemic heart disease. The possibility of epicardial or microvascular coronary vasospastic disease might be considered.

Coronary Vasospasm

Vasospasm of an epicardial coronary artery typically presents as variant (or Prinzmetal) angina in which episodes of rest pain occur despite well-preserved effort tolerance at other times. An electrocardiogram recorded during an episode of spontaneous pain usually shows ST elevation in the territory supplied by the vasospastic artery. Absence of a significant coronary lesion in such a patient confirms the diagnosis of variant angina owing to focal coronary spasm (**Figure 15.15**). In these patients, coronary angiography is performed mainly to look at the extent of underlying atherosclerosis. Provocative maneuvers to initiate spasm were once common to confirm the diagnosis and evaluate drug therapy. It is now used mostly when the diagnosis of variant angina is

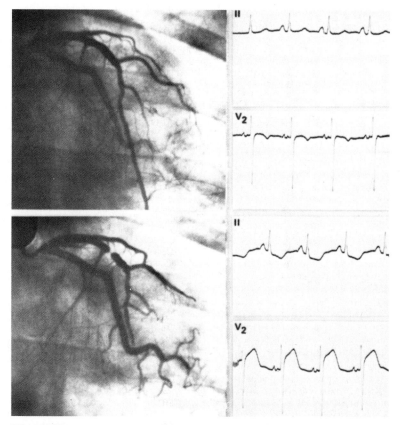

Figure 15.15 True coronary spasm. Intense focal vasospasm of the left anterior descending coronary artery is shown in right anterior oblique projection in a patient with variant angina. Note the absence of a significant underlying atherosclerotic stenosis in the top view, the absence of vasoconstriction of other vessel segments, and the marked ST elevation in the anterior leads during the spontaneous vasospastic episode. (Republished by permission of McGraw-Hill, from Baim DS, Harrison DC. Nonatherosclerotic coronary heart disease. In: Hurst JW, ed. *The Heart*. 5th ed. McGraw-Hill; 1985.)

uncertain and a patient with troublesome chest pain fails to manifest sufficient disease to explain its cause.

If provocative testing for coronary spasm is contemplated, the patient should be withdrawn from calcium channel blockers for at least 24 hours and long-acting nitrates for at least 12 hours before the study and should not be premedicated with either atropine or sublingual nitroglycerin. Ongoing therapy with any of these agents may render provocative tests falsely negative.

Testing for coronary spasm should be performed only after baseline angiographic evaluation of both left and right coronary arteries. It should not be performed in patients with severe hypertension or severe anatomic cardiac pathology (left ventricular dysfunction, left main or multivessel disease, or aortic stenosis). As an example, a protocol for using methylergonovine calls for a total of 0.4 mg (400 mg equals 2 ampules) to be diluted to a total volume of 8 mL in an appropriately labeled 10-mL syringe. The provocative test consists of graded intravenous administration of 1 mL (0.05 mg), 2 mL (0.10 mg), and 5 mL (0.25 mg) of this mixture at 3- to 5-minute intervals. Parenteral nitroglycerin (100-200 µg/mL) must be premixed and loaded in a labeled syringe before the testing begins. It is also advisable to have an intracoronary calcium channel blocker (verapamil 100 µg/mL, diltiazem 250 µg/mL) or nitroprusside (100 µg/mL) close at hand in case nitroglycerin-refractory spasm develops. Temporary pacing and defibrillator equipment should also be available to treat the bradyarrhythmias or tachyarrhythmias that sometimes accompany coronary spasm. At 1 minute before each ergonovine dose, the patient is interrogated about symptoms similar to those of their clinical complaint and a 12-lead electrocardiogram is recorded. After each electrocardiogram, coronary angiography is performed, looking either at both arteries or only at the artery of highest clinical suspicion for vasospasm. In the absence of clinical symptoms, electrocardiographic changes, or focal coronary vasospasm, the next ergonovine dose is administered, and the cycle is repeated until the total dose of 0.4 mg has been given. The provocative test should be considered positive only if focal spasm (>70% diameter stenosis) occurs and is associated with clinical symptoms and/or electrocardiographic changes. Even if there are no symptoms or electrocardiographic changes, both coronary arteries should be opacified at the end of the provocative test, and any generalized vasoconstrictor effect should be terminated by administration of nitroglycerin before documenting the resolution of spasm and the extent of underlying atherosclerotic stenosis. It should be noted that coronary artery spasm may occur in 2 vessels simultaneously, and visualization of only 1 vessel may fail to adequately assess the magnitude of the vasospastic response.

Some operators have used an intracoronary methylergonovine administration protocol, in which a 4-minute intracoronary infusion (10 µg/min in the right and 16 µg/min in the left coronary) is performed. Alternatively, discrete doses of 5 to 10 µg may be administered into a coronary artery, waiting for 3 minutes and imaging between doses (maximal total dose 50 µg per vessel). These intracoronary protocols may be advantageous in that they produce less systemic effect (hypertension, esophageal spasm). The other intracoronary provocative test for coronary spasm uses acetylcholine (ACH) at serial doses of 20 to 50 to 100 µg injected into the left coronary and 20 to 50 to 80 µg injected into the right coronary. Another ACH protocol uses incremental doses of 2, 20, 100, and 200 µg administered over periods of 3 minutes each into the left coronary artery and 80 µg ACH over 3 minutes into the RCA in patients who do not develop symptoms or ischemic electrocardiogram (ECG) changes. Heart rate, blood pressure, and the 12-lead ECG must be continuously monitored during ACH testing. Some investigators have also used hyperventilation as a provocative test for spasm.

When provocative testing produces clinical symptoms but no angiographic evidence of vasospasm in either coronary artery, there may still be scintigraphic evidence of myocardial ischemia owing to microvascular spasm. Both multivessel epicardial and microvascular spasm have been implicated in takotsubo syndrome where extreme emotional stress is followed by chest pain, ST elevation, and a particular pattern of apical hypokinesis extending beyond the usual single coronary territory. If there are no signs of myocardial ischemia, an alternative diagnosis such as esophageal dysmotility, which can also be provoked by methylergonovine, should be considered.

It is also important to distinguish the intense focal spasm seen in patients with variant angina from the normal mild (15%-20%) diffuse coronary narrowing seen as a pharmacologic response to ergonovine in normal patients. True coronary spasm must also be distinguished from spasm induced by mechanical interventions such as rotational atherectomy or catheter-tip spasm (**Figure 15.16**). Catheter-tip spasm is most common in the RCA, is not associated with clinical symptoms or electrocardiographic changes, and

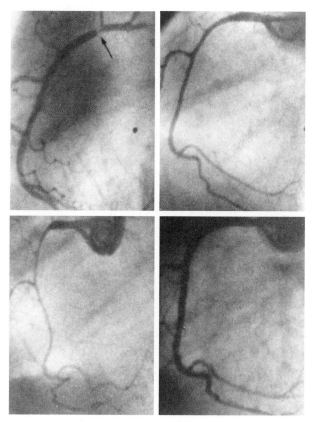

Figure 15.16 Vasomotor changes not representing true coronary spasm. During right coronary catheterization with a Judkins catheter (top left), this patient developed severe catheter-tip spasm (arrow). Recatheterization 24 hours later with an Amplatz catheter (top right) showed neither catheter-tip spasm nor an atherosclerotic stenosis. Following ergonovine 0.4 mg, marked diffuse coronary narrowing was observed (bottom left) without angina or electrocardiographic changes. After the intracoronary administration of nitroglycerin 200 μg (bottom right), there was marked diffuse vasodilation.

does not indicate variant angina. It should be recognized as such, however, and treated by withdrawal of the catheter, administration of nitroglycerin, and nonselective or cautious repeat selective opacification of the involved vessel to avoid mistaking catheter-tip spasm for an atherosclerotic lesion. Spasm should also be distinguished from a "pleating" artifact that may occur when a curved artery is straightened out by a stiff guidewire (**Figure 15.17**), causing folds of the vessel wall to impinge on the lumen. Pleating is refractory to nitroglycerin but resolves immediately when the stiff guidewire is withdrawn.

MISTAKES IN INTERPRETATION

Mistakes in interpretation might be due to inadequate number of projections, inadequate injection of contrast media, or superselective catheterization of the LAD artery or left circumflex artery, which can occur when the left main coronary artery is short and its bifurcation occurs early. To the inexperienced operator, this may give the impression of total occlusion of the nonvisualized vessel.

Selective cannulation of a coronary artery may also fail to detect significant ostial stenosis, particularly if the catheter tip lies beyond the lesion and adequate contrast reflux is not produced. If ostial stenosis is suspected (eg, if there is partial ventricularization or damping), performing a final injection during withdrawal of the catheter from the ostium might be helpful (**Figure 15.18**).

Total Occlusion

If a coronary artery or a branch is totally occluded at its origin, it may not be visualized, and the occlusion may be missed. If the occlusion is flush with the parent vessel, no stump will be seen. Such occlusions are primarily recognized by visualization of the distal segment of the occluded vessel by means of collateral channels or by noting the absence of the usual vascularity seen in a particular portion of the heart.

Complex Stenosis Classification and Risk Stratification

Revascularization planning following diagnostic coronary angiography should include a thorough assessment of potential benefits and risks based on patient's comorbidities, stenosis location, stenosis characteristics, and number of diseased vessels. For example, bifurcation lesions can present different challenges for percutaneous coronary intervention (PCI) depending on location within the main and

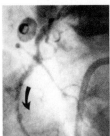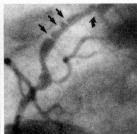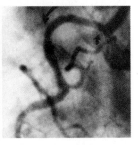

Figure 15.17 Right coronary artery "pleating" artifact. Left. Baseline injection shows diffuse disease in this tortuous right coronary artery selected for rotational atherectomy (arrow). Center. Straightening of the proximal vessel by the stiff type C wire, creating 3 areas of infolding of the vessel wall (arrows) as well as the appearance of ostial stenosis (curved arrow). Right. Immediately on withdrawal of the guidewire, the artery returned to its baseline curvature and these defects were resolved (arrows).

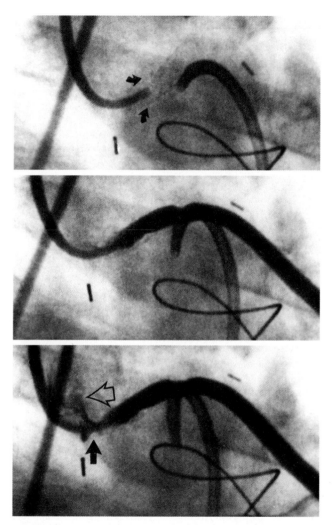

Figure 15.18 Masking of ostial stenosis during superselective cannulation. Ostial stenosis of a previously stented vein graft is not apparent with the tip of the catheter well beyond the stenosis (top and center) (arrows). Continued injection during catheter withdrawal (bottom) causes reflux into the aorta (solid arrow) and clearly shows significant ostial stenosis (arrow).

branch vessels. The Medina classification provides a visual approach that can be used in selecting a suitable technique for the specific bifurcation lesion (**Figure 15.19**).

The SYNTAX score was developed to quantify the extent of coronary artery disease. The score is based on number of lesions, functional importance of the lesion depending on vessel location, and lesion complexity. In the Synergy between PCI with Taxus and Cardiac Surgery (SYNTAX) trial comparing multivessel PCI with

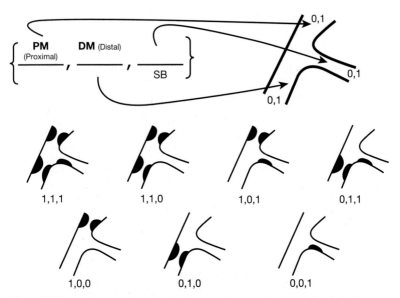

Figure 15.19 Medina Classification of bifurcation stenosis. (Reproduced with permission from: Louvard Y, Medina A. Definitions and classifications of bifurcation lesions and treatment. *EuroIntervention*. 2015;11(suppl V):V23-V26.)

coronary artery bypass grafting (CABG), patients with low (0-22) or intermediate (23-32) SYNTAX scores in the PCI group had outcomes similar to those of patients with low or intermediate scores in the CABG group. However, in patients with high scores (>33), outcomes were significantly worse in the PCI group when compared with CABG. At 5-year follow-up, Major Adverse Cardiovascular and Cerebrovascular Events (MACCE) rates were similar between the 2 treatment groups in low-score patients, while they were significantly higher in the PCI group when compared with CABG in intermediate- (36% vs 25.8%, P = .008) and high-score (44% vs 26.8%, P < .0001) patients. More recently, the Syntax score II has been developed by adding to the anatomical SYNTAX score additional variables including age, female sex, creatinine clearance, left ventricular ejection fraction, presence of unprotected left main coronary artery disease, peripheral vascular disease, and chronic obstructive pulmonary disease. Both calculators can be accessed online and can be used for an assessment of risks and benefits of PCI versus CABG in patients with left main and multivessel disease (http://syntaxscore.org/calculator/syntaxscore/frameset.htm; access date: 06/22/2023).

CORONARY ARTERY ANOMALIES

Given the great variability of coronary anatomy, a general definition of "normal" coronary arteries should be founded on the knowledge of the variations of each of the features used to describe coronary anatomy (eg, the number and location of ostia, the diameter or cross-sectional area of coronary arteries). Generally, each descriptive feature should be considered anatomically normal when it is found in more than 1% of a general population or within 2 standard deviations of the mean value for Gaussian distribution continuous parameters.

Normally, the coronary ostia lead to an orthogonally oriented coronary proximal stem, off the aortic wall (**Figures 15.20** and **15.21**). A popular classification of the coronary anomalies (**Table 15.1**) uses the basic features that describe each anatomic entity, especially the anomalies of origin, according to its course and destination. **Figure 15.22** describes diagrammatically the normal distribution of the 3 primary coronary arteries in a coronal plane, and their multiple possible anomalies of origin and proximal course.

Of the 66 different types of coronary artery anomalies (CAAs) (**Table 15.1**), only 1 subgroup is considered to intrinsically pose any risk of causing coronary dysfunction (ie, ischemia): the anomalous origin of a coronary artery from an "opposite" sinus of Valsalva, with an intramural course (ACAOS). Such anomalies are found in approximately 1% of adult cardiac catheterization laboratory patients. Most of the other CAA variants are not known to cause ischemia by themselves (and these non-ACAOS CAA should not be included in a discussion of clinically important CAA in the adult), but they could have clinical consequences because of clinical uncertainty about their recognition and management and because of occasional complicating factors (the most frequent of which is associated coronary artery atherothrombotic disease).

Table 15.1 Classification of Coronary Anomalies

A. Anomalies of origination and course
1. Absent left main trunk (split origination of LCA)
2. Anomalous location of coronary ostium within aortic root or near proper aortic sinus of Valsalva (for each artery)
   a. High
   b. Low
   c. Commissural
3. Anomalous location of coronary ostium outside normal "coronary" aortic sinuses
   a. Right posterior aortic sinus
   b. Ascending aorta, with anomalous course
      • Intramural (ACAOS)
      • Extramural
   c. Left ventricle
   d. Right ventricle
   e. Pulmonary artery. Variants:
      • LCA arising from posterior-facing sinus (ALCAPA)
      • Cx arising from posterior-facing sinus
      • LAD arising from posterior-facing sinus
      • RCA arising from anterior-right-facing sinus
      • Ectopic location (outside facing sinuses) of any coronary artery from pulmonary artery
      • From anterior left sinus
      • From pulmonary trunk
      • From pulmonary branch
   f. Aortic arch
   g. Innominate artery
   h. Right carotid artery
   i. Internal mammary artery
   j. Bronchial artery
   k. Subclavian artery
   l. Descending thoracic aorta
4. Anomalous origination of coronary ostium from opposite, facing "coronary" sinus (which may involve joint origination or adjacent double ostia). Variants:
   a. RCA arising from left anterior sinus, with anomalous course

Table 15.1 Classification of Coronary Anomalies (Continued)

- Posterior atrioventricular groove or retrocardiac
- Retroaortic[a]
- Between aorta and pulmonary artery,[a] preaortic, intramural (aortic), or ACAOS
- Intraseptal[a]
- Anterior to pulmonary outflow[a] or precardiac
- Posteroanterior interventricular groove[a]
  - b. LAD arising from right anterior sinus, with anomalous course
    - Between aorta and pulmonary artery, preaortic, intramural (aortic), or ACAOS
    - Intraseptal
    - Anterior to pulmonary outflow or precardiac
    - Posteroanterior interventricular groove
  - c. Cx arising from right anterior sinus, with anomalous course
    - Posterior atrioventricular groove
    - Retroaortic
  - d. LCA arising from right anterior sinus, with anomalous course
    - Posterior atrioventricular groove[a] or retrocardiac
    - Retroaortic
    - Between aorta and pulmonary artery,[a] preaortic, intramural (aortic), or ACAOS
    - Intraseptal
    - Anterior to pulmonary outflow[a] or precardiac
    - Posteroanterior interventricular groove[a]
  - e. LCA arising from the "noncoronary" sinus, with anomalous course
    - Intramural (ACAOS)
    - Extramural
  5. Single coronary artery
  B. Anomalies of intrinsic coronary arterial anatomy
  1. Congenital ostial stenosis or atresia (LCA, LAD, RCA, Cx)
  2. Coronary ostial dimple
  3. Coronary ectasia or aneurysm
  4. Absent coronary artery
  5. Coronary hypoplasia
  6. Intramural coronary artery (myocardial bridge)
  7. Subendocardial coronary course
  8. Coronary crossing
  9. Anomalous origination of posterior descending branch or septal penetrating branch
  10. Absent PD or split RCA
    a. Proximal + distal PDs, arising from separate RCA sources
    b. Proximal PD arising from RCA, distal PD arising from LAD
    c. Proximal PD arising from RCA, distal PD arising from Cx
  11. Absent or split LAD
    a. Large first septal branch and small distal LAD
    b. Double LAD
  12. Ectopic origination of first septal branch
  C. Anomalies of coronary termination
  1. Decreased number of arteriolar/capillary ramifications (hypothetical)
  2. Fistulas from RCA, LCA, or infundibular artery to
    a. Right ventricle
    b. Right atrium
    c. Coronary sinus
    d. Superior vena cava
    e. Pulmonary artery
    f. Pulmonary vein
    g. Left atrium
    h. Left ventricle
    i. Multiple microfistulas draining into one or both ventricles
  D. Anomalous collateral vessels

ACAOS, anomalous origin of a coronary artery from an opposite sinus of Valsalva, with intramural course; ALCAPA, anomalous origin of the left coronary artery from the pulmonary artery; Cx, circumflex; LAD, left anterior descending coronary artery; LCA, left coronary artery; PD, posterior descending branch; RCA, right coronary artery.
[a]If a single, common ostium is present, the pattern is considered to represent "single" coronary artery.

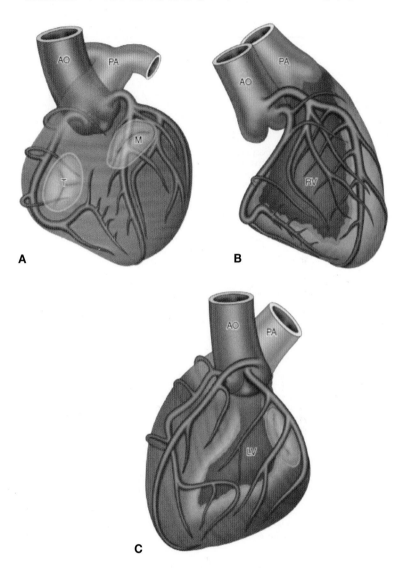

Figure 15.20 Relationship between coronary arteries and cardiac structures as seen in the frontal **(A)**, right anterior oblique **(B)**, and left anterior oblique projections **(C)**. AO, aorta; LV, left ventricle; M, mitral valve; PA, pulmonary artery; RV, right ventricle; T, tricuspid valve. (Reproduced with permission from Angelini P. *Coronary Artery Anomalies: A Comprehensive Approach*. Lippincott Williams & Wilkins; 1999.)

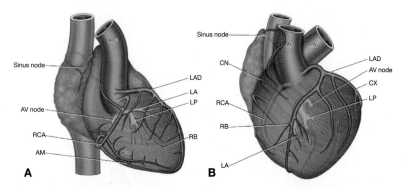

Figure 15.21 Right **(A)** and left **(B)** anterior oblique views of the main coronary branches and related cardiac structures. AM, acute marginal artery; Ao, aorta; AV, atrioventricular; CN, conal branch; Cx, circumflex artery; LA, left anterior fascicle of the left bundle branch; LAD, left anterior descending artery; LP, left posterior fascicle of the left bundle branch; PA, pulmonary artery; PD, posterior descending branch; RB, right bundle; RCA, right coronary artery; SN, sinus node. (Reproduced with permission from Angelini P. *Coronary Artery Anomalies: A Comprehensive Approach.* Lippincott Williams & Wilkins; 1999.)

Anomalous Origin of a Coronary Artery From an Opposite Sinus of Valsalva, With an Intramural Course

As confirmed by most autopsy-based studies on the subject, ACAOS is the only kind of CAA with a clear ischemic potential. This anomaly is especially critical to recognize because of its mortality implications in the young, specifically in athletes and military recruits, as well as because of its potential to cause disabling angina, dyspnea, and syncope. Anatomists have long debated the mechanisms and specific anatomic features of ACAOS that may lead to critical ischemia. Initially, a slitlike orifice, tangential orientation of the origin, a passage between the aorta and the pulmonary artery, or ostial fibrous ridges were implicated in the causation of ischemia in ACAOS cases. More recently, accurate in vivo imaging of such anomalies by intravascular ultrasound (IVUS), as well as some anatomic evidence, has led to the clear conclusion that the intramural proximal course of the ectopic ACAOS coronary artery, inside the aortic wall, is the recurrent and quantifiable mechanism of ACAOS-related ischemia (**Figures 15.23-15.27**).

In the catheterization laboratory, selective coronary angiography in patients with ACAOS can be challenging because of the ectopic location of the coronary artery and its tangential origin from the aortic wall.

The R-ACAOS (ACAOS of the RCA) cases frequently pose particular difficulties in locating and selectively cannulating the ectopic ostium at the left sinus of Valsalva if one is using routine diagnostic catheters. In R-ACAOS cases, the ostium is usually located somewhere between the left coronary ostium (which is usually normal) and the anterior commissure of the aortic valve. Also, the initial coronary course is tangential and located inside the aortic wall ("intramural").

Selective coronary angiography cannot reveal the severity of proximal R-ACAOS (or L-ACAOS) stenosis, but it can clearly indicate to the trained eye the presence of ACAOS. Specifically, angiography can definitely distinguish between the intramural (ie, "between aorta and pulmonary artery" or preaortic) and the intraseptal (or infundibular) course, which is not a type of ACAOS (**Figure 15.28**). The criteria for differentiating the 2 forms by angiography are listed in **Table 15.2**. Coronary angiography is also essential for establishing the important dominance patterns of the coronary arteries (or the origin of the posterior descending branch) and the coexistence of atherosclerotic, acquired coronary artery disease.

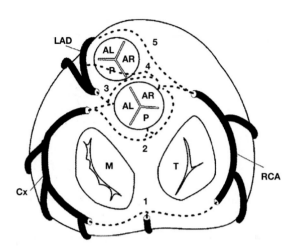

Figure 15.22 Diagrammatic illustration of the locations of the 3 elementary coronary arteries (LAD, Cx, and RCA) in a coronal view from above. The dotted lines represent the connections and courses of each artery, both normal (ie, from the proper aortic sinus) and abnormal. The Arabic numbers indicate the different courses: 1. posterior (to the atrioventricular valves); 2. retroaortic; 3. preaortic (intramural, aortic wall); 4. intraseptal (infundibular); and 5. prepulmonic. AL, antero-left; AR, antero-right; Cx, circumflex artery; LAD, left anterior descending artery; M, mitral valve; P, posterior; RCA, right coronary artery; T, tricuspid valve. (Adapted from Angelini P, Villason S, Chan AV Jr., Diez JG. Normal and anomalous coronary arteries in humans. In: Angelini P, ed. *Coronary Artery Anomalies: A Comprehensive Approach.* Lippincott Williams & Wilkins; 1999:27-150, with permission.)

Computed tomography angiography (CTA) and magnetic resonance imaging (MRI) are excellent methods of establishing confidently the specific type of abnormal courses that an ectopic artery takes (**Figure 15.24A-D**). Evidence suggestive of lateral compression can also be obtained by CTA, especially by using the equivalent view to the RAO projection, which reveals clearly the location of the abnormal proximal trunk "between aorta and pulmonary artery." Unfortunately, this technique is not yet precise enough to detect and measure stenosis in patients with ACAOS.

The main reasons for performing IVUS (or, possibly, optical coherence tomography [OCT]) imaging in a patient with ACAOS are based on the need to establish the severity of the individual case and the type of proximal coronary artery stenosis. **Figures 15.25, 15.26,** and **15.27C-E** illustrate the typical and important findings that IVUS or OCT can reveal in cases of R-ACAOS and L-ACAOS:

1. the length of the intramural segment;
2. the severity of circumferential hypoplasia with respect to the distal epicardial reference vessel;
3. the vessel asymmetry score (or the ratio of transverse to longitudinal diameter in cross-sectional images), which may be a simple marker of the severity of stenosis; and
4. the systolic versus diastolic cross-sectional area of stenosis during a cardiac cycle, measured at baseline and during a simulated exercise explores the changes of the same parameters during infusion of saline [500 mL bolus], atropine [0.5 mg], and dobutamine [40 pg/kg/min]) (Systolic Area versus Diastolic area test [SAD test]).

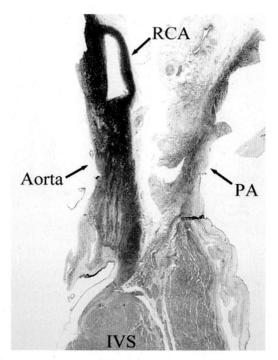

Figure 15.23 Histologic cross section of the anterior wall of the aorta and the posterior wall of the pulmonary artery (PA) at the level of the aortopulmonary "septum" (ie, the closest site between the 2), showing the critical autopsy findings in an athlete with R-ACAOS that resulted in his sudden death. Note that the space between the aorta and the PA is not where the ectopic artery lies; rather, the artery passes within the media of the aorta, where it becomes laterally compressed (intramural). Compare this image with the IVUS (intravascular ultrasound) and OCT (optical coherence tomography) images in Figures 15.25-15.26. IVS, interventricular septum; RCA, right coronary artery. (Photo courtesy of Dwayne A. Wolf, MD, PhD; Office of the Medical Examiner of Harris County, Texas. From Angelini P. Coronary Artery Anomalies-Current Clinical Issues: definitions, classification, incidence, clinical relevance, and treatment guidelines. *Tex Heart Inst J*. 2002;29:271-278. © 2002 by the Texas Heart Institute, Houston.)

At this time, surgical intervention in specialized centers for ACAOS tends to favor unroofing when feasible (especially in view of the possible involvement of the anterior commissure of the aortic valve). Reimplantation of the ectopic artery is also possible and is often successful in expert hands if the proximal intramural segment is removed (**Figure 15.29**). Bypass surgery with the use of IMA grafts is less likely to be successful because of competitive flow and the expected hypoplastic regression of the graft lumen if there is less than critical stenosis at baseline.

Other Coronary Anomalies Frequently Encountered in the Adult Cath Lab: Coronary Fistulae and Myocardial Bridges

Generally, the 2 conditions discussed below are encountered relatively frequently in the catheterization laboratory, but they are not intrinsic causes of coronary dysfunction.

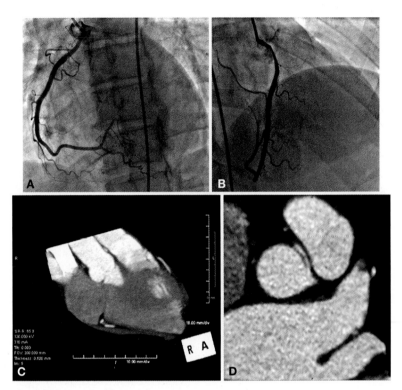

Figure 15.24 Unselective **(A)** and selective **(B)** coronary angiographic frames in a typical case of R-ACAOS. Note that the proximal right coronary artery (RCA) appears mildly ectatic in the left anterior oblique projection but is not obstructed by this diagnostic technique. The RCA is dominant, with an ostium located next to that of the left coronary artery. Computed tomographic angiograms of R-ACAOS (**C**, sagittal plane; **D**, coronal plane). Figures 15.25 and 15.26 show the same case, imaged with different imaging techniques.

Coronary Fistulae

Coronary fistulae are defined as consisting of abnormal connections between a coronary artery and a low-pressure vascular space, such as a systemic vein (eg, the coronary sinus or the superior vena cava) or a cardiac cavity (both in the atrial and in the ventricular sections). The clinical importance of a coronary fistula is related to

1. the amount of fistulous blood flow, which leads to progressive coronary fistulous tract enlargement and vascular wall degeneration, with secondary atherothrombotic changes that include aneurysmatic dilatation;
2. the amount of right- and left-sided cardiac cavity overload, secondary to blood shunting; coronary nutrient flow steal secondary to a parallel, competing, fistulous, low-pressure resistance path and the nutrient high-resistance path, with resulting possible ischemia of the dependent myocardial coronary territory;
3. aortic root distortion secondary to aneurysmatic dilation of the involved coronary artery and sinus of Valsalva, and any resulting regurgitation.

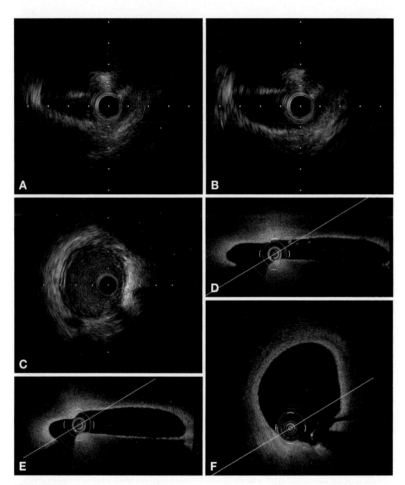

Figure 15.25 Intravascular ultrasound images of the area close to the R-ACAOS ostium. **A,** Systolic frame. **B,** Diastolic frame. **C,** A distal right coronary artery reference site (area of relative stenosis is about 60%). D-F. Optical coherence tomographic images taken at the same sites. Note that the images are much more precise, allowing more accurate assessment of stenosis severity. **D,** Ostium during systole. **E,** Ostium during diastole. **F,** Distal reference; relative stenosis: 65% in systole, 60% in diastole.

At present, most cases of large coronary fistulae are diagnosed initially by echocardiography or CTA. Later, they may become targets of diagnostic and therapeutic catheterization, in laboratory procedures.

In patients considered to require surgical repair, it is essential to ascertain preoperatively whether there is any associated fixed coronary artery disease, the exact course of the fistulous tract, and, especially, the site of origin of important nutrient

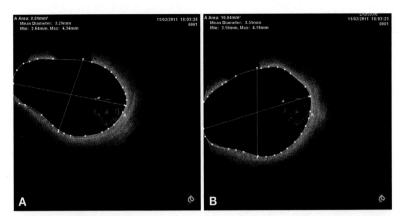

Figure 15.26 Optical coherence tomographic imaging in systole **(A)** and diastole **(B)** of a mild stenosis of the intramural segment in a case of R-ACAOS (of the lowest severity ever seen in our practice). The mean degree of stenosis was 30% (mild).

branches that need to be protected during surgical or catheter-based interventions (**Figure 15.30**).

Ideally, visualization of large fistulae should be performed with a guide catheter (generally size 6F-8F), which can allow both stable selective positioning during angiography and adequate contrast medium injection, depending on blood flow regimens. As a guideline, one should consider that the normal, adult left coronary artery flow is in the range of 150 to 200 mL/min, whereas the "surgical" (large) coronary fistulae have usually much more flow (depending on the diameter, degree of stenosis, length of the fistulous tract, and final destination pressure regimen), typically in the range of 300 to 1500 mL/min. Oxygen saturation–based calculations of shunt are generally not reliable.

Although the indications for closing a coronary fistula are not well established, preventing aneurysmal dilatation is the main consideration. Indeed, even after successful repair, aneurysmal dilatation of the fistulous tract will remain, now in the presence of much reduced blood flow, thus increasing the patient's risk of coronary mural thrombosis. Intervening before adult age is generally recommended, because negative postoperative remodeling of the fistulous artery as indicated by the presence of mural calcification, is not likely in the adult but is common in the young.

Myocardial Bridges

Myocardial bridges are defined as coronary segments that undergo phasic systolic narrowing at sites of intramural course, generally within the left ventricular wall. Administering a vasodilator, such as intracoronary nitroglycerin, during coronary angiography enhances the angiographic appearance of the systolic narrowing. Usually, myocardial bridges are first identified in the catheterization laboratory either because of a chance of association with other disease (especially left ventricular hypertrophy or coronary artery disease) or because a secondary study is performed in view of a positive stress test.

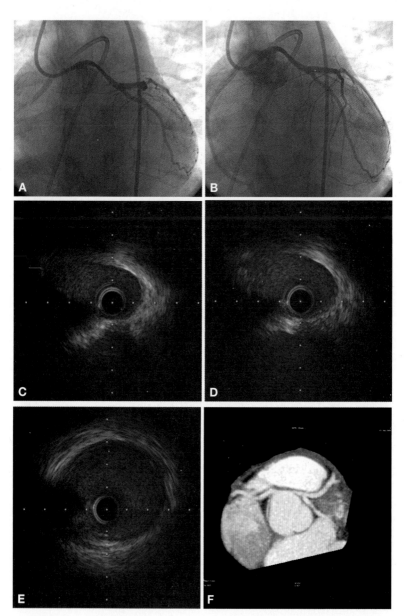

Figure 15.27 Angiographic images of L-ACAOS in systole **(A)** and diastole **(B)**. The left main trunk seen in **(A)** shows the appearance of phasic narrowing relative to **(B)**. Intravascular ultrasound images showing the systolic **(C)** and diastolic **(D)** intramural segment and the distal reference **(E)** cross section of the left main trunk. Area of relative stenosis = 55%. **F,** Computed tomographic angiograms in the same case showing ectopic origin of the left coronary artery adjacent to the normally situated right coronary artery.

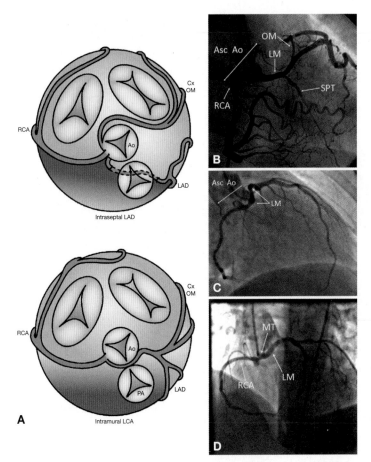

Figure 15.28 Diagrammatic representation of the abnormal proximal courses of ectopic left coronary arteries (LCAs) in 2 similar cases: the intraseptal, infundibular variant (diagram in **A**, with typical angiogram in **B**), and the intramural, preaortic variant (diagram in **A**, typical angiograms in **C** and **D**). Only the intramural case (ACAOS) has intrinsic ischemic potential. In **B** (intraseptal) and **C** (intramural), the 2 variants are shown in the same right anterior oblique projection; note that the intramural variant features a course stuck to the anterior border of the aorta (the one on the right side of the aorta, Ao, in this view), and it is tilted upward. In the opposite case, the intraseptal variant is directed inferiorly and anteriorly in this projection, as it provides a characteristic first branch that is clearly a septal branch (SPT) **(B)**. In the intraseptal case, the distal left main reaches the epicardial surface of the heart at the proximal left anterior descending. **D,** The left anterior oblique projection, of the intramural variety, shows the same uphill course as in **C**, with a "halo" that suggests an intramural course, just below the sinotubular junction. Asc Ao, ascending aorta; Cx, circumflex artery; LAD, left anterior descending artery; LM, left main artery; MT, mixed, short common trunk, joining the origins of the RCA and the LCA; OM, obtuse marginal branch; PA, pulmonary artery; RCA, right coronary artery. See text.

Table 15.2 Differential Angiographic Features in Cases of Preaortic (Intramural, L-ACAOS) and Infundibular (Intraseptal) Varieties of Ectopic Origin of the Left Coronary Artery From the Right Sinus of Valsalva

Feature	Intramural	Intraseptal
Retroaortic course in RAO projection	No	No
Initial course in RAO projection	Preaortic/superior (around aortic root)	Anterior-inferior
First branch off left main	Distal LAD/Cx splitting	First septal branch off mid left main
Left main systolic narrowing	Not usually recognized by angiography; if present, it is at proximal 1 cm (lateral compression)	Frequent, at distal left main (mild concentric myocardial bridge effect)
Distal left main location	Normal (next to left sinus)	LM connects with mid-LAD

Cx, circumflex; LAD, left anterior descending coronary artery; LM, left main; RAO, right anterior oblique.

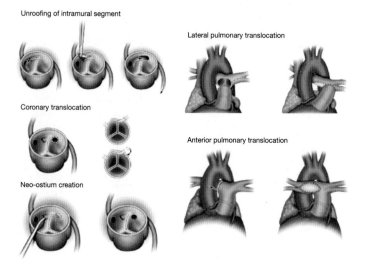

Figure 15.29 Surgical techniques currently used for treatment of patients with AAOCA (anomalous aortic origin of the coronary artery). (Adapted from Mery CM, Lawrence SM, Krishnamurthy R, et al. Anomalous aortic origin of a coronary artery: toward a standardized approach. *Semin Thoracic Surg.* 2014;26:110-122.)

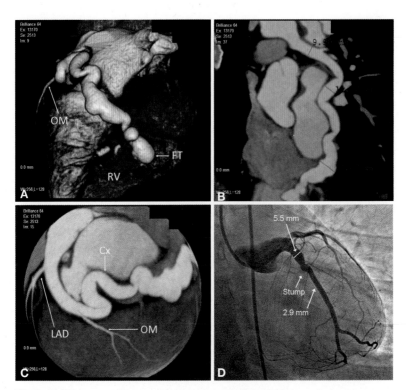

Figure 15.30 Computed tomographic angiograms (CTA) (A-C) of a case of a large coronary fistula from the left main to the posterior part of the right ventricle in a 27-year-old asymptomatic woman. This technique can show in great detail the luminal size, course, site of origin, and final termination of the fistula, as well as any mural aneurysms or clots. **A,** A 3D volume-rendering reconstruction shows clearly the luminal irregularities causing both stenosis and ectasia of different segments. **B,** Measurements of diameters at different levels by a volume-rendering image. The most relevant feature is the location of the branching of nutrient vessels, especially of the obtuse marginal, which is well shown by curved multiplane reformation **(C)**. CTA is probably a better technique than catheter angiography for evaluating coronary fistulae, especially for gathering operational parameters for catheter-based closure. **D,** Coronary angiogram obtained at the time of a scheduled, elective coil embolization, 4 y after the CTA. The fistulous tract, distal to the origin of the OM, was found to be totally occluded by apparent but silent spontaneous thrombosis. Note that the LM and proximal Cx are significantly smaller in this image than on the CTA, suggesting that negative remodeling has occurred. Cx, circumflex; FT, fistulous termination; LAD, left anterior descending; LM, left main; OM, obtuse marginal branch; RV, right ventricle.

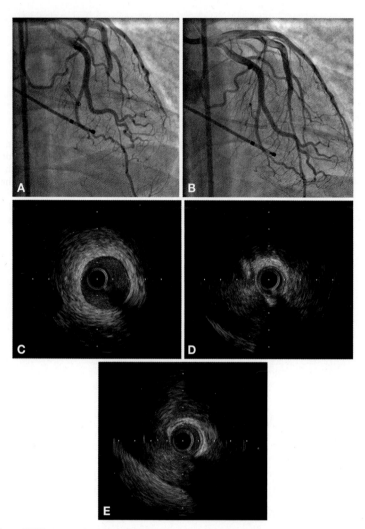

Figure 15.31 A case of atypical chest pain in a patient with hypertrophic cardiomyopathy. The initial angiograms taken during systole **(A)** and diastole **(B)** revealed diffuse diastolic narrowing and systolic obliteration of the mid segment (4 cm long) of the left anterior descending; an intravascular ultrasound (IVUS) study was used to establish the nature of the diastolic narrowing (intimal growth vs hypoplasia). IVUS images obtained after intracoronary nitroglycerine administration show that hypoplasia without intimal thickening was the mechanism of stenosis at the level of the myocardial bridge (**C**, proximal reference cross section; **D**, intramyocardial systolic and **E**, diastolic images). Unroofing of the myocardial bridge was suggested, in case medical treatment (with beta-blockers) was inadequate to relieve the symptoms. This procedure never became necessary.

In patients with a history of acute myocardial infarction or anginalike chest pain, especially if it occurs at rest, evaluation of myocardial bridges should probably include a functional study of endothelial dysfunction, such as acetylcholine challenge. **Figure 15.31** shows the angiographic and IVUS findings at a myocardial bridge in a patient with resting chest pain and hypertrophic cardiomyopathy.

Endothelial dysfunction is particularly frequent in patients with myocardial bridges, and the recent literature supports the notion that endothelial dysfunction may underlie the events of both myocardial infarction and resting angina. Intracoronary infusion of acetylcholine should be carried out according to existing protocols. In particular, progressive intracoronary doses of acetylcholine should be tested (25, 50, 75, and 100 µg administered over 30- to 120-second time intervals) with standby intracoronary infusion of nitroglycerin in case significant spasm or angina occurs. Significant stenosis is generally considered to be a reversible narrowing of more than 70% of the luminal diameter. Temporary right ventricular pacing is mandatory when acetylcholine is administered, because bradycardia is frequently induced.

Empirical indications for intervention on muscular bridges are not supported by any definitive studies at this time, so such interventions should be used prudently, if ever. Coronary stenting, in particular, should be used with caution, because it is associated with a clearly increased restenosis risk secondary to intimal growth, stent crushing, or both.

CARDIAC VENTRICULOGRAPHY

Cardiac ventriculography is used to define the anatomy and function of the ventricles and related structures in patients with congenital, valvular, coronary, or myopathic heart disease. Specifically, left ventriculography may provide valuable information about global and segmental left ventricular function; mitral valvular regurgitation; and the presence, location, and severity of a number of other abnormalities such as ventricular septal defect and hypertrophic cardiomyopathy. As a result, left ventriculography is often included as part of the routine diagnostic cardiac catheterization protocol in a patient being evaluated for coronary artery disease, aortic or mitral valvular disease, unexplained left ventricular failure, or congenital heart disease. Similarly, right ventriculography may provide information about global and segmental right ventricular function and can be especially helpful in patients with congenital heart disease.

INJECTION CATHETERS

To achieve adequate opacification of the left or right ventricle, it is necessary to deliver a relatively large amount of contrast material in a relatively short period of time. This is best done using catheters with multiple side holes to allow rapid delivery of contrast material with the catheter remaining in a stable position in the midventricle. Catheters that have only an end hole (such as multipurpose catheters) are not well suited for left ventriculography, since the contrast jet out of the single end hole can cause the catheter to recoil during contrast delivery, potentially resulting in ventricular ectopic beats, inadequate ventricular opacification, and myocardial staining or even perforation.

Pigtail Catheter

The pigtail catheter (developed by Judkins) and its modification leading to the angled pigtail catheters, which have a 145° to 155° shaft angle at its distal end (just proximal to the side holes), has several advantages over an end-hole-only design for left and right ventriculography (**Figure 15.32**). Its end hole permits its insertion over a J-tipped guidewire so that the pigtail catheter can be advanced safely to the LV from

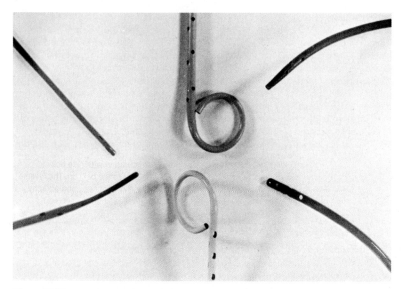

Figure 15.32 Examples of ventriculographic catheters (clockwise from the top): pigtail, 8F (Cook); Gensini, 7F; NIH, 8F; pigtail, 8F (Cordis); Lehman ventriculographic, 8F; Sones, 7.5F tapering to a 5.5F tip (see text for details).

any arterial access site (see Chapter 6). The loop shape keeps the end hole away from direct contact with the endocardium, while the multiple side holes on the catheter shaft located up to several centimeters proximal to the pigtail loop provide numerous simultaneous exit paths for the contrast material. These offset jet directions help stabilize the catheter within the LV during contrast injection and reduce the magnitude of catheter recoil. This virtually eliminates the possibility of endocardial staining, since the end hole usually is not positioned adjacent to ventricular trabeculae and substantially reduces the occurrence of ventricular ectopic beats.

The pigtail usually passes easily across a normal aortic valve, either directly or by prolapsing across the valve leaflets. Passage across a stenotic aortic valve usually requires use of a straight leading guidewire. In patients with porcine aortic valve prosthesis, the pigtail generally passes across the bioprosthesis even more easily than do straight catheters such as the multipurpose, since the pigtail configuration seems to prevent the catheter from sliding down into the lateral sinuses outside the support struts. Pigtail catheters can also be passed retrograde across a ball valve prosthesis (Starr-Edwards), but the resulting interference of the catheter shaft with seating of the ball during diastole may cause significant aortic regurgitation. Of course, no catheter should ever be passed across a tilting-disc aortic valve prosthesis (Bjork-Shiley, Medtronic-Hall, or St. Jude) because of the risk of catheter entrapment.

Straight-Tip Left Ventriculographic Catheters

Several straight-tip ventriculographic catheters were developed and used in the early stage of coronary angiography, when catheterization was performed from the brachial approach, but currently they are rarely if ever used (**Figure 15.32**).

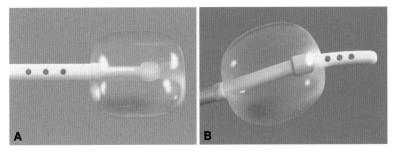

Figure 15.33 The Berman angiographic catheter. **A,** Normal configuration with side holes proximal to the balloon. **B,** Reverse configuration with side holes distal to the balloon. The reverse configuration is used for balloon occlusion pulmonary angiography and peripheral angiography. (Image courtesy of Teleflex Incorporated. ©2020 Teleflex Incorporated. All rights reserved.)

Balloon-Tip Ventriculographic Catheters

The Berman angiographic catheter is a balloon-tip catheter that is available in 4F, 5F, 6F, 7F, and 8F sizes (Teleflex, Morrisville, NC). It is used for right ventriculography, pulmonary angiography, peripheral angiography, and in the reverse configuration for balloon occlusion angiography (**Figure 15.33**). The balloon tip provides the advantage of easier advancement in the right ventricle or in the pulmonary artery, and by keeping the catheter and side holes away from the endocardium, it can reduce the risk of myocardial staining and ventricular arrhythmias.

INJECTION SITE

Adequate opacification of either ventricle is accomplished only if a large amount of contrast material is delivered in a short period of time. Although satisfactory opacification of the LV can sometimes be achieved by injection of contrast material into the left atrium, this requires transseptal catheterization, does not allow evaluation of mitral valvular incompetence, and may obscure the basal portion of the LV and the aortic valve. Similarly, the LV may be opacified by aortography in patients with significant aortic regurgitation and the right ventricle may be opacified by injecting contrast material into the venae cavae or right atrium. The best approach to ventriculography in the adult patient, however, is via injection of contrast material directly into the ventricular chamber in question.

In the LV, the optimal catheter position is the midcavity, provided that ventricular ectopy is not a problem (**Figure 15.34**). The midcavitary position ensures (1) adequate delivery of contrast material to the chamber's body and apex; (2) lack of interference with mitral valvular function, which would have otherwise produced factitious mitral regurgitation; and (3) positioning of the holes through which the contrast material is injected away from ventricular trabeculae (thereby avoiding a possible cause of endocardial staining). In some patients, however, the midcavitary position induces repetitive ventricular ectopy. In that case, the tip of the catheter is best repositioned in such a way that it lies in the left ventricular inflow tract immediately in front of the posterior leaflet of the mitral valve. This position is usually free of ventricular ectopy but may produce mitral regurgitation if the catheter is too close to the mitral valve. In occasional patients with vigorous ventricular contraction, no stable midventricular position can be found for the catheter. The pigtail catheter can

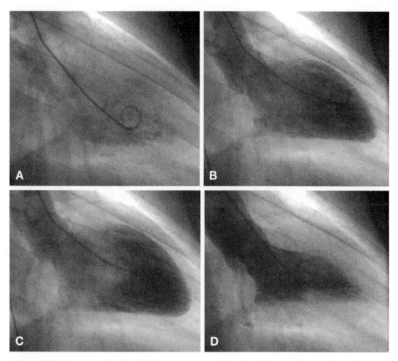

Figure 15.34 An example of midcavitary catheter position for 30° right anterior oblique left ventriculography using an angled pigtail catheter. **A,** Just before the injection of contrast material. **B,** At the end of rapid filling. **C,** At end diastole (post A-wave). **D,** At end systole.

then be advanced to be in continuous contact with the left ventricular apex (assuming that there is no evidence of apical aneurysm of mural thrombus) to allow measurement of left ventricular pressure during stable rhythm and left ventriculography with the rate of contrast injection reduced to 10 mL/s (see below).

When the pigtail catheter is rotated in the LV, it may pass under the chordae. This can be suspected if the catheter shaft passes close to the inferior wall or exhibits an abrupt kink and can be confirmed if the loop of the pigtail opens up as the catheter is withdrawn back to the left ventricular outflow tract. Because the side holes on the catheter shaft are held in close proximity to the myocardial wall by the chordae, this position increases the risk of myocardial staining and should be corrected before ventriculography is performed. If repositioning the catheter would be difficult (as in a patient whose stenotic aortic valve has just been crossed) and ventriculography is required, a reduced injection rate should be used as described above for the Sones catheter.

INJECTION RATE AND VOLUME

Rapid delivery of an adequate amount of contrast material requires the use of a power injector. Flow injectors allow one to select both the volume and the rate of delivery of contrast material. Sufficient pressure to deliver the selected volume of injectate in the selected time period is automatically developed, although a maximal pressure limit of roughly 1000 psi is set to minimize the risk of catheter burst. Of course, this high pressure is not actually delivered to the catheter tip but is dissipated as frictional losses in the shaft of the catheter. Some injectors permit synchronization of the injection of contrast material with the R-wave of the electrocardiogram, so that a set flow rate is delivered in each of several successive diastolic intervals. Although this has been said to be a technique that lessens the incidence of ventricular ectopic beats and minimizes the volume of contrast material required for adequate ventricular opacification, our impression is that it offers no clear advantage over the nonsynchronized methods.

Cine left ventriculography is accomplished using an injection rate and volume that depend on (1) the type and size of the catheter, (2) the size of the ventricular chamber to be opacified, (3) the approximate ventricular stroke volume, and (4) the preventriculography hemodynamics. Different operators use different catheters and different injection parameters for left ventricular injection. In most cases performed with pigtail catheters, the injection parameters are chosen as 30 to 36 mL injected at the rate of 10 to 12 mL/s (ie, a 3-second-long injection). Somewhat higher volume and rate may be used in patients with a high cardiac output or large ventricular chamber, and somewhat smaller volumes and rates may be used in smaller or irritable ventricles. When an end hole (eg, Sones or multipurpose) catheter is used for left ventriculography, the rate of injection of contrast material should not exceed 7 to 10 mL/s to minimize the chance of recoil and staining. Hand injection through the manifold cannot provide adequate volume and flow rate to fill the ventricle and should be avoided.

Low-osmolar contrast media have substantially improved the safety of left ventriculography in patients with depressed myocardial function, severe coronary artery disease, and/or aortic stenosis, as discussed in Chapter 2. Even so, in patients with hemodynamic evidence of severe left ventricular dysfunction and/or if filling pressures are markedly elevated (>25 mmHg), left ventriculography should be performed only after the elevated filling pressure has been reduced by the administration of intravenous nitroglycerin or sodium nitroprusside. With the current radiographic equipment, low-osmolar contrast agents, and techniques using smaller amounts of contrast material, it is a rare case that a patient cannot undergo left ventriculography safely. But failure to take a severely elevated preventriculography pulmonary capillary wedge pressure or left ventricular end-diastolic pressure seriously can lead to disastrous consequences, including intractable pulmonary edema and even death. In any patient with increased risk (LV dysfunction, mural thrombus, renal insufficiency), one should always ask whether noninvasive means of assessing left ventricular function (see below) might not be preferable to contrast ventriculography.

Before performing a power injection of contrast material, one should take appropriate precautions in filling and firing the power injector to prevent air embolism. The injection syringe is made of siliconized plastic so that the contrast medium and any air may be easily visible. This syringe is usually loaded from a contrast bottle through a short U-shaped straw, while the syringe barrel is pointed upward. With the injector still in the vertical position, 30-in-long sterile roentgenography tubing is connected to the syringe and all air is expelled from the syringe and tubing by holding the load switch in the forward position as the operator taps the syringe and its Luer-Lok connector to discharge all air bubbles. Alternatively, some laboratories fill the injector by connecting the sterile roentgenography tubing to the coronary manifold, drawing contrast from that supply (generally a slower process, more prone to bubble formation).

Only after all of the bubbles have been expelled in the nose-up position should the injector head be inverted. A fluid-to-fluid connection is accomplished by touching the meniscus of blood spurting from the hub of the catheter to the meniscus of contrast exiting the roentgenography tubing as the technician slowly advances the syringe plunger of the injector manually. When the connection is made, the injector operator stops advancing and begins retracting the plunger until the interface between contrast material and blood can be seen in the roentgenography tubing and verified to be free of air bubbles. Prior to the left ventriculographic run, a test injection of a small amount of contrast material is often performed under fluoroscopic visualization to enable the physician to assess catheter and patient position and confirm that ventricular ectopy does not occur. If the catheter is repositioned, another test injection is recommended before the definitive injection.

Prior to performing the angiogram, the physician should look closely at the injector syringe to confirm that it is filled with contrast medium, free of air, and oriented in the desired nose-down direction. They should grasp the catheter at its hub so that the catheter can be pulled back instantaneously if ventricular extrasystoles, myocardial staining, or other untoward events develop during injection. The technician or other individual firing the injector should be prepared to abort the injection on command from the physician operator in the event of an untoward occurrence. If extrasystoles develop, we withdraw the ventriculographic catheter a distance of approximately 2 to 3 cm after the first extrasystole, which usually results in a quiet position for the remainder of the 3- to 4-second contrast injection.

Instructions to the patient regarding respiration during contrast ventriculography vary from laboratory to laboratory. Earlier imaging systems were often inadequate to give good definition of the left ventricular silhouette unless ventriculography was performed during deep inspiration to move the diaphragm out of the radiographic field. With modern imaging systems, excellent definition of the ventricular silhouette can be achieved without the restriction that ventriculography be performed during held deep inspiration. Left ventriculography done during normal quiet breathing allows physiologic interpretation of left ventricular volumes, angiographic stroke volume, and calculated left ventricular regurgitant fraction in cases of valvular regurgitation.

FILMING PROJECTION AND TECHNIQUE

Projections should be used that provide maximal delineation of the structure of interest and minimal overlapping of other structures. The 30° RAO projection eliminates overlap of the LV and the vertebral column; allows one to assess anterior, apical, and inferior segmental wall motion; and places the mitral valve in profile to provide a reliable assessment of the presence and severity of mitral regurgitation. The 60° LAO view allows one to assess ventricular septal integrity and motion, lateral and posterior segmental function, and aortic valvular anatomy. To prevent foreshortening of the LV and visualize the entire length of the interventricular septum in profile, 15° to 30° cranial angulation should be added to the 60° LAO view, and the angiogram should be performed during a sustained deep inspiration to minimize obstruction by the diaphragm. This view allows visualization of ventricular septal defects and the associated left-to-right shunting, the septal bulge and systolic anterior motion in hypertrophic obstructive cardiomyopathy, or isolated lateral wall motion abnormalities. For routine left or right ventriculography, 30 frames per second using the 9-in field of view allows the best temporal and spatial imaging, but many laboratories now use 15 frames per second for both ventriculography and coronary angiography to reduce radiation exposure (see Chapter 2).

If both RAO and LAO ventriculograms are indicated, it requires 2 separate injections in a single-plane room. If available, biplane ventriculography is thus preferable to single-plane ventriculography because it allows one to obtain more information at essentially no additional risk to the patient. In the patient with coronary artery disease, biplane left ventriculography provides more information on the location and severity of segmental wall motion abnormalities than does single-plane ventriculography; in the patient with congenital heart disease, biplane right ventriculography allows one to assess accurately the anatomy of the right ventricular outflow tract, the pulmonic valve, and the proximal portions of the pulmonary artery. But biplane ventriculography has several disadvantages, including (1) higher cost of the biplane cineangiographic equipment; (2) reduced quality of cineangiographic imaging in each plane owing to radiation scatter caused by the opposite plane; (3) additional time required to position the biplane equipment appropriately, especially when the brachial approach is used; and (4) additional radiation exposure to personnel in the room. In reality, most laboratories have only 1 biplane laboratory in their imaging suite, so that almost all left ventriculograms are done single plane. Table 15.3 provides a list of preferred left and right ventriculographic views for various conditions. Additional information on preferred angiographic projections for congenital lesions is provided in Chapter 10.

Table 15.3 **Preferred Left and Right Ventriculographic Views for Specific Conditions[13]**

Condition	Left Ventriculography	Right Ventriculography
Assessment of LV and RV function	30° RAO 60° LAO	AP cranial
Membranous VSD	70° LAO 30° cranial RAO	
Muscular VSD	4-chamber projection (45° LAO 45° cranial) 70° LAO 30° cranial RAO	
Atrioventricular septal defects	4-chamber projection (45° LAO 45° cranial) 45° RAO 45° cranial	RAO cranial Lateral
Pulmonic stenosis	AP cranial Lateral	
Left ventricular outflow tract obstruction (including fibromuscular subaortic stenosis)	70° LAO 30° cranial RAO	
Double outlet right ventricle	70° LAO 30° cranial RAO	AP Lateral
L-transposition of the great arteries	RAO cranial/LAO cranial (catheter in the morphologic left ventricle, antegrade)	
Transposition of the great arteries	70° LAO 30° cranial RAO (catheter antegrade, across the foramen ovalis)	

AP, anteroposterior; LAO, left anterior oblique; RAO, right anterior oblique, VSD, ventricular septal defect.

RIGHT VENTRICULOGRAPHY

Although right ventriculography is rarely performed in the adult cardiac catheterization laboratory, it is important to be familiar with optimal views, injection catheters, and indications.

The AP view with cranial angulation and the lateral view are generally preferred for right ventriculography, as they elongate the right ventricular outflow tract and the central pulmonary arteries. The optimal catheter position is the midcavity, provided that repetitive ventricular ectopy does not occur. If ectopy is uncontrollable, the catheter may be positioned in the outflow tract, just below.

ANALYSIS OF THE VENTRICULOGRAM

The left ventriculogram is analyzed both qualitatively and quantitatively on a normal sinus beat that follows a previous normal sinus beat in which the ventricle is well opacified; evaluation of ectopic or postectopic beats will give a false assessment of ventricular function. Overall, ventricular dysfunction is described as hyperdynamic (>70%), normal (50%-69%), mildly hypokinetic (35%-49%), moderately hypokinetic (20%-24%), or severely hypokinetic (<20%). Regional wall motion can be graded qualitatively as normal, hypokinetic, akinetic, or dyskinetic for each of the segments seen in the RAO projection (anterolateral, apical, inferior, posterobasal segments) and in the LAO projection (basal septal, apical septal, apical lateral, basal lateral segments). Quantitative evaluation involves measurement of ejection fraction (the percent of end-diastolic volume that is ejected during systole), the absolute end-diastolic and end-systolic volumes (using the area-length method), and chord-by-chord local shortening.

The degree of mitral regurgitation can be estimated (on a scale of 1+ to 4+) by examining any systolic leakage of contrast from the LV back into the left atrium and the opacification of the left atrium relative to the LV, in the RAO projection. In patients with a markedly enlarged left atrium from chronic mitral regurgitation, however, the dilution of the regurgitant contrast jet within this larger left atrial volume may lead to underestimation of regurgitation severity by the atrial density scale. A more quantitative method involves a comparison of the angiographic stroke volume (end-diastolic volume minus end-systolic volume) with the forward stroke volume (cardiac output divided by heart rate). These should be equal in absent significant left-sided valvular regurgitation, but in patients with mitral (or aortic) regurgitation, the angiographic stroke volume will be larger than the forward stroke volume (by an amount equal to the regurgitant volume). The severity of the regurgitant lesion can then be estimated by calculating the regurgitant fraction (the regurgitant volume divided by angiographic stroke volume), which indicates the percent of the volume ejected during each systole that goes backward into the left atrium rather than forward into the aorta. Mild (1+) mitral regurgitation is usually associated with a regurgitant fraction of <30%, moderate (2+) with a regurgitant fraction of 30% to 39%, moderately severe (3+) with a regurgitant fraction of 40% to 49%, and severe mitral regurgitation with a regurgitant fraction >50%.

Qualitative review of the right and left ventriculogram can also identify specific patterns suggestive of takotsubo heart (**Figure 15.35**), or congenital diseases such as RV dysplasia and left ventricular noncompaction (**Figures 15.36 and 15.37**), which should not be missed on a routine ventriculogram and which can be confirmed by MRI. In addition, in patients with acute myocardial infarction, the qualitative analysis of the left ventriculogram should focus on the identification of potential rare complications such as contained free wall ventricular rupture, ventricular septal defect, and papillary muscle rupture.

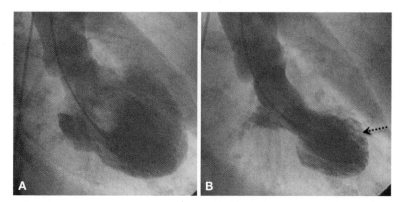

Figure 15.35 Takotsubo heart. **A,** A 71-year-old woman under extreme emotional stress presented with anterior ST-segment elevation, elevated creatine phosphokinase isoenzymes, and diffuse akinesis of the left ventricular apex (including both anterior and inferior aspects), resembling the shape of a Japanese octopus trap (takotsubo; narrow neck and round bottom), despite angiographically normal coronary arteries. **B,** Within 3 wk, left ventricular function had returned to near normal (dotted arrow). The mechanism is believed to be intense sympathetic arteriolar vasoconstriction involving the apical myocardium. (Case provided by Alan Yeung, MD, Stanford University.)

COMPLICATIONS AND HAZARDS

Although complications of cardiac catheterization and angiography are discussed in detail in Chapter 4, certain specific points relevant to ventriculography are presented here.

Arrhythmias

Ventricular extrasystoles occur frequently during ventriculography and are usually caused by mechanical stimulation of the ventricular endocardium by the catheter or a jet of the contrast agent. Such extrasystoles can usually be eliminated or at least min-

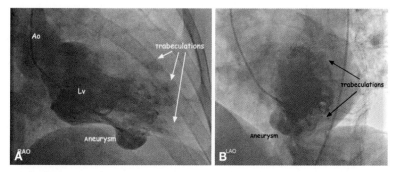

Figure 15.36 Left ventricular noncompaction and aneurysm in a patient with no significant coronary artery disease. **A,** Left ventriculography mid-systolic frame in the right anterior oblique (RAO) view. **B,** End-systolic frame in the left anterior oblique (LAO) view. A large inferior aneurysm and extensive trabeculations of the anterior and lateral wall are seen. (Reproduced with permission from: Ionescu CN, Turcot D. Left ventricular non-compaction and aneurysm revealed by left ventriculography. *Catheter Cardiovasc Interv.* 2012;80:109-111.).

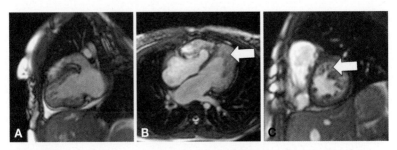

Figure 15.37 Left ventricular noncompaction. Cardiac magnetic resonance images of a 26-year-old patient with heart failure. The images were obtained using steady-state free precession and are displayed in the vertical long axis **(A)**, axial **(B)**, and short axis **(C)** planes and demonstrate marked trabeculations (arrows) of the left ventricle, consistent with left ventricular noncompaction.

imized by repositioning the catheter. Although short runs of ventricular tachycardia occur during an occasional ventriculogram, they almost always cease promptly when the catheter is removed from the ventricle. Rarely, ventricular tachycardia caused by ventriculography is sustained even after catheter removal. It should be treated quickly with a bolus of intravenous lidocaine and, if necessary, direct current countershock. Ventricular fibrillation has been reported to be induced by an improperly grounded power injector.

Intramyocardial Injection (Endocardial Staining)

Deposition of contrast material within the endocardium and myocardium is usually caused by improper positioning of the ventriculographic catheter so that it passes under one of the papillary muscles or a side hole lies firmly against the endocardium. Although a small endocardial stain usually causes no problem, a large stain may lead to medically refractory ventricular tachyarrhythmias, including ventricular tachycardia or fibrillation. Rarely, the power injection of contrast material causes myocardial perforation, with resultant leakage of blood and contrast material into the pericardial space and development of cardiac tamponade. This must be treated by emergency pericardiocentesis and immediate consultation obtained from a cardiothoracic surgeon.

Fascicular Block

Because of the proximity of the anterior fascicle of the left bundle to the left ventricular outflow tract, transient left anterior fascicular block may occur during retrograde left-sided heart catheterization. In the patient with underlying right bundle branch block and left posterior fascicular block, complete heart block may occur as the catheter is advanced into the LV. Although temporary pacing is usually required, catheter-induced fascicular block usually resolves within 12 to 24 hours. Transient complete left bundle branch block is an extremely rare complication of retrograde left-sided heart catheterization.

Embolism

Inadvertent injection of air or thrombus probably poses the greatest risk associated with ventriculography. Nevertheless, the risk of air embolization should be avoidable by following good practices in filling the injector and confirming a bubble-free hookup as described above. The presence of thrombi on or within the ventriculographic catheter is minimized by frequent flushing of the catheter with a solution containing heparin when the ventriculographic catheter is first introduced and just prior to hooking up for the ventriculogram. If there is any suspicion (from noninvasive testing) of a thrombus in the left ventricular apex, great care should be taken to position the ventriculographic catheter in the left ventricular inflow tract, avoiding the apical portion completely, or ventriculography itself should be avoided, relying on noninvasive evaluation. Partially organized thrombi may also be dislodged from the left ventricular wall by the catheter tip or the force of a power injection. Accordingly, the ventricular angiographic catheter should not be advanced to the left ventricular apex except under exceptional circumstances (eg, suspicion of idiopathic hypertrophic subaortic stenosis).

Complications of Contrast Media

With earlier ionic contrast agents, ventriculography produced a modest fall in systemic arterial pressure, a reflex increase in heart rate, and a transient depression of left ventricular contractility that resolved within 1 to 2 minutes. Patients used to experience a hot flash owing to the powerful vasodilation caused by the contrast material as it distributed throughout the arterial tree, and nausea or vomiting could occur in 20% to 30% of cases. With the current low-osmolar contrast agents, these complications are uncommon.

SUGGESTED READINGS

1. Aldridge HE. A decade or more of cranial and caudal angled projections in coronary arteriography – another look. *Cathet Cardiovasc Diagn.* 1984;10(6):539-542.
2. Amplatz K, Formanek G, Stanger P, Wilson W. Mechanics of selective coronary artery catheterization via femoral approach. *Radiology.* 1967;89(6):1040-1047.
3. Angelini P, Cheong B. Left coronary artery from the right coronary sinus: what can CT angiography tell us?. *J Cardiovasc Comput Tomogr.* 2010;4:255-257.
4. Angelini P, Uribe C. Anatomic spectrum of left coronary artery anomalies and associated mechanisms of coronary insufficiency. *Catheter Cardiovasc Interv.* 2018;92(2):313-321.
5. Angelini P, Villason S, Chan AV, Diez JG. Normal and anomalous coronary arteries in humans. In: Angelini P, ed. *Coronary Artery Anomalies—A Comprehensive Approach.* Lippincott Williams & Wilkins; 1999.
6. Angelini P, Walmsley RP, Libreros A, Ott DA. Symptomatic anomalous origination of the left coronary artery from the opposite sinus of Valsalva: clinical presentations, diagnosis, and surgical repair. *Tex Heart Inst J.* 2006;33(2):171-179.
7. Ayres RW, Lu CT, Benzuly KH, Hill GA, Rossen JD. Transcatheter embolization of an internal mammary artery bypass graft sidebranch causing coronary steal syndrome. *Cathet Cardiovasc Diagn.* 1994;31(4):301-303.
8. Bilazarian SD, Shemin RJ, Mills RM. Catheterization of coronary artery bypass graft from the descending aorta. *Cathet Cardiovasc Diagn.* 1990;21(2):103-105.
9. Budoff MJ, Achenbach S, Duerinckx A. Clinical utility of computed tomography and magnetic resonance techniques for noninvasive coronary angiography. *J Am Coll Cardiol.* 2003;42(11):1867-1878.
10. Cannon RO III, Watson RM, Rosing DR, Epstein SE. Angina caused by reduced vasodilator reserve of the small coronary arteries. *J Am Coll Cardiol.* 1983;1(6):1359-1373.
11. Di Serafino L, Turturo M, Lanzone S, et al. Comparison of the effect of dual-axis rotational coronary angiography versus conventional coronary angiography on frequency of acute kidney injury, X-ray exposure time, and quantity of contrast medium injected. *Am J Cardiol.* 2018;121(9):1046-1050.
12. Dorros G, Thota V, Ramireddy K, Joseph G. Catheter-based techniques for closure of coronary fistulae. *Cathet Cardiovasc Diagn.* 1999;46(2):143-150.
13. Elliott LP, Green CE, Rogers WJ, et al. Advantage of the cranial-right anterior oblique view in diagnosing mid left anterior descending and distal right coronary artery disease. *Am J Cardiol.* 1981;48(4):754-764.
14. Empen K, Kuon E, Hummel A, et al. Comparison of rotational with conventional coronary angiography. *Am Heart J.* 2010;160(3):552-563.
15. Farooq V, van Klaveren D, Steyerberg EW, et al. Anatomical and clinical characteristics to guide decision making between coronary artery bypass surgery and percutaneous coronary intervention for individual patients: development and validation of SYNTAX score II. *Lancet.* 2013;381(9867):639-650.

16. Freeman R, O'Donnell M, Share D, et al. Nephropathy requiring dialysis after percutaneous coronary interventions: incidence, risk factors and the critical role of an adjusted contrast dose. *Am J Cardiol.* 2002;90(10):1068-1073.

17. Friedman AC, Spindola-Franco H, Nivatpumin T. Coronary spasm: Prinzmetal's variant angina vs. catheter-induced spasm; refractory spasm vs. fixed stenosis. *Am J Radiol.* 1979;132(6):897-904.

18. Gibson CM, Cannon CP, Daley WL, et al. TIMI frame count: a quantitative method of assessing coronary artery flow. *Circulation.* 1996;93(5):879-888.

19. Grech M, Debono J, Xuereb RG, Fenech A, Grech V. A comparison between dual axis rotational coronary angiography and conventional coronary angiography. *Catheter Cardiovasc Interv.* 2012;80(4):576-580.

20. Harding MB, Leithe ME, Mark DB, et al. Ergonovine maleate testing during cardiac catheterization: a 10-year perspective in 3,447 patients without significant coronary artery disease or Prinzmetal's variant angina. *J Am Coll Cardiol.* 1992;20(1):107-111.

21. Hays JT, Stein B, Raizner AE. The crumpled coronary: an enigma of arteriographic pseudopathology and its potential for misinterpretation. *Cathet Cardiovasc Diagn.* 1994;31(4):293-300.

22. Jennette JC, Falk RJ. Small-vessel vasculitis. *N Engl J Med.* 1997;337(21):1512-1523.

23. Judkins MP. Selective coronary arteriography. I. A percutaneous transfemoral technic. *Radiology.* 1967;89(5):815-824.

24. Khan M, Schmidt DH, Bajwa T, Shalev Y. Coronary air embolism: incidence, severity, and suggested approaches to treatment. *Cathet Cardiovasc Diagn.* 1995;36(4):313-318.

25. Kuntz RE, Baim DS. Internal mammary angiography: a review of technical issues and newer methods. *Cathet Cardiovasc Diagn.* 1990;20(1):10-16.

26. Kurisu S, Sato H, Kawagoe T, et al. Tako-tsubo-like left ventricular dysfunction with ST-segment elevation: a novel cardiac syndrome mimicking acute myocardial infarction. *Am Heart J.* 2002;143(3):448-455.

27. Levin DC. Pathways and functional significance of the coronary collateral circulation. *Circulation.* 1974;50(4):831-837.

28. Liberthson RR. Sudden death from cardiac causes in children and young adults. *N Engl J Med.* 1996;334(16):1039-1044.

29. Louvard Y, Medina A. Definitions and classifications of bifurcation lesions and treatment. *EuroIntervention.* 2015;11(suppl V):V23-V26.

30. Mintz GS, Popma JJ, Pichard AD, et al. Limitations of angiography in the assessment of plaque distribution in coronary artery disease: a systematic study of target lesion eccentricity in 1446 lesions. *Circulation.* 1996;93(5):924-931.

31. Mohr FW, Morice M-C, Kappetein AP, et al. Coronary artery bypass graft surgery versus percutaneous coronary intervention in patients with three-vessel disease and left main coronary disease: 5-year follow-up of the randomised, clinical SYNTAX trial. *Lancet.* 2013;381(9867):629-638.

32. Newburger JW, Takahashi M, Gerber MA, et al. Diagnosis, treatment, and long-term management of Kawasaki disease: a statement for health professionals from the Committee on Rheumatic Fever, Endocarditis and Kawasaki Disease, Council on Cardiovascular Disease in the Young, American Heart Association. *Circulation.* 2004;110(17):2747-2771.

33. Om A, Ellahham S, Vetrovec GW. Radiation-induced coronary artery disease. *Am Heart J.* 1992;124(6):1598-1602.

34. Patel MR, Bailey SR, Bonow RO, et al. ACCF/SCAI/AATS/AHA/ASE/ASNC/HFSA/HRS/SCCM/SCCT/SCMR/STS. 2012 appropriate use criteria for diagnostic catheterization: a report of the American College of Cardiology Foundation Appropriate Use Criteria Task Force, Society for Cardiovascular Angiography and Interventions, American Association for Thoracic Surgery, American Heart Association, American Society of Echocardiography, American Society of Nuclear Cardiology, Heart Failure Society of America, Heart Rhythm Society, Society of Critical Care Medicine, Society of Cardiovascular Computed Tomography, Society for Cardiovascular Magnetic Resonance, and Society of Thoracic Surgeons. *J Am Coll Cardiol.* 2012;59(22):1995-2027.

35. Petersen SE, Selvanayagam JB, Wiesmann F, et al. Left ventricular non-compaction: insights from cardiovascular magnetic resonance imaging. *J Am Coll Cardiol.* 2005;46(1):101-105.

36. Ropers D, Moshage W, Daniel WG, Jessl J, Gottwik M, Achenbach S. Visualization of coronary artery anomalies and their anatomic course by contrast-enhanced electron beam tomography and three dimensional reconstruction. *Am J Cardiol.* 2001;87(2):193-197.

37. Ryan TJ. The coronary angiogram and its seminal contributions to cardiovascular medicine over five decades. *Circulation.* 2002;106(6):752-756.

38. Serota H, Barth CW III, Seuc CA, Vandormael M, Aguirre F, Kern MJ. Rapid identification of the course of anomalous coronary arteries in adults—the "dot and eye" method. *Am J Cardiol.* 1990;65(13):891-898.

39. Shirani J, Roberts WC. Solitary coronary ostium in the aorta in the absence of other major congenital cardiovascular anomalies. *J Am Coll Cardiol.* 1993;21(1):137-143.

40. Sianos G, Morel MA, Kappetein AP, et al. The SYNTAX score: an angiographic tool grading the complexity of coronary artery disease. *EuroIntervention*. 2005;1(2):219-227.
41. Sones FM Jr. *Coronary Arteriography*: Read before the Eighth Annual Convention of the American College of Cardiology; 1959.
42. Sotomi Y, Collet C, Cavalcante R, et al. Tools and techniques - clinical: SYNTAX score II calculator. *EuroIntervention*. 2016;12(1):120-123.
43. Sueda S, Kohno H, Fukuda H, et al. Induction of coronary artery spasm by two pharmacological agents: comparison between intracoronary injection of acetylcholine and ergonovine. *Coron Artery Dis*. 2003;14(6):451-457.
44. Sueda S, Kohno H, Fukuda H, et al. Frequency of provoked coronary spasms in patients undergoing coronary arteriography using a spasm provocation test via intracoronary administration of ergonovine. *Angiology*. 2004;55(4):403-411.
45. Suma H, Wanibuchi Y, Terada Y, Fukuda S, Takayama T, Furuta S. The right gastroepiploic artery graft—clinical and angiographic mid-term results in 200 patients. *J Thorac Cardiovasc Surg*. 1993;105(4):615-622; discussion 623.
46. Tanimoto Y, Matsuda Y, Fujii B, et al. Angiography of right gastroepiploic artery for coronary artery bypass graft. *Cathet Cardiovasc Diagn*. 1989;16(1):35-38.
47. The BARI Protocol. Protocol for the bypass angioplasty revascularization investigation. *Circulation*. 1991;84:V1-V27.
48. Uren NG, Melin JA, De Bruyne B, Wijns W, Baudhuin T, Camici PG. Relation between myocardial blood flow and the severity of coronary artery stenosis. *N Engl J Med*. 1994;330(25):1782-1788.
49. Weis M, von Scheidt W. Cardiac allograft vasculopathy: a review. *Circulation*. 1997;96(6):2069-2077.
50. Yamanaka O, Hobbs RE. Coronary artery anomalies in 126,595 patients undergoing coronary arteriography. *Cathet Cardiovasc Diagn*. 1990;21(1):28-40.
51. Yetman AT, McCrindle BW, MacDonald C, Freedom RM, Gow R. Myocardial bridging in children with hypertrophic cardiomyopathy–a risk factor for sudden death. *N Engl J Med*. 1998;339(17):1201-1209.

16 Angiography of the Aorta, Peripheral, and Pulmonary Arteries[1]

RADIOGRAPHIC IMAGING

Catheter-based angiography has undergone a new level of complexity and sophistication, and remains the gold standard for diagnosis of arterial disease. The techniques of vascular angiography are predicated on maximizing benefit for the patient while minimizing the associated risk.

VASCULAR ACCESS

The most favorable site of access is determined by integrating the clinical history, physical examination, anatomic assessment from noninvasive studies (eg, duplex ultrasound [DUS], magnetic resonance angiogram [MRA], or computed tomography angiogram [CTA]), and the anticipated strategy for endovascular assessment and therapy. The common femoral artery (CFA) remains the most frequently used site for vascular access. However, advances in technology and technique permit consideration of radial, brachial, axillary, and transpedal approaches. In addition, there is now increased utilization of other alternative access sites, such as direct puncture of the superficial femoral artery (SFA), popliteal, or tibial vessels, as well as the carotid artery. These techniques can be particularly useful when angiography is performed in anticipation of intervention. Pre-procedural planning enables careful consideration of optimal access site, both for diagnostic angiography and interventions.

The advent of crossover catheters or "guide-sheaths" has led many operators to adopt crossover techniques from the contralateral femoral artery as the preferred approach for angiography and intervention. Retrograde access enables assessment of aortoiliac inflow as well as bilateral runoff angiography, with subsequent placement of a guide-sheath for contralateral intervention. This approach also has the advantage of more conventional and perhaps easier (eg, retrograde) arterial access and sheath removal. Contralateral access for intervention may be difficult or impossible in certain circumstances, such as that of a very angulated aortic bifurcation or in the case of prior intervention where the aortic bifurcation has been reconstructed and "elevated" by stents or stent grafting. Finally, when considering access for diagnostic angiography that may convert to intervention, one should anticipate whether the contralateral approach will allow for sufficient length of devices; adequate control for manipulation and torque of guidewires; and longitudinal support for advancement of therapeutic devices, such as balloons, stents, and atherectomy catheters.

Antegrade puncture of the ipsilateral CFA provides more support for catheter advancement and better tactile feedback and one-to-one guidewire movement and torque and thus remains a widely used approach to treat superficial femoral, popliteal, or infrapopliteal arterial disease. While it offers a more stable platform for intervention, antegrade access poses greater technical challenge and limits the scope of angiography to the ipsilateral leg. As with retrograde CFA access, the desired site of entry is in the middle of the CFA below the inguinal ligament, but given the relatively shallow angle of approach with the needle to the vessel, the skin puncture is made

---

[1]We gratefully acknowledge the *Grossman & Baim's Cardiac Catheterization, Angiography, and Intervention*, 9th edition contributions of Drs Michael N. Young, Beau M. Hawkins, Kenneth Rosenfield, Douglas E. Drachman, Kyung J. Cho, and Nils Kucher, as portions of their chapters, "Angiography of the Aorta and Peripheral Arteries" and "Pulmonary Angiography," were retained in this text.

at or, more frequently, significantly above the top of the femoral head. A less acute needle angle, generally <45°, facilitates catheter and sheath insertion by avoiding the kinking associated with a steeper-angled entry; it also directs the guidewire and sheath more along the anteromedial course of the SFA, as opposed to the postero-lateral course of the profunda femoris. Arterial puncture is commonly performed with fluoroscopic and ultrasound guidance aiming for the mid-portion of the femoral head. Aids to antegrade access include arterial calcification or prior studies (angio, CTA, or MRA) that define the bifurcation of the CFA in relation to the femoral head. In cases with a known high CFA bifurcation, the antegrade stick should be modified accordingly.

Great care should be exercised while advancing and manipulating catheters and guidewires in the severely diseased peripheral circulation to reduce the chance of dis-section or embolization related to the traumatic disruption of cholesterol-rich athero-sclerotic plaque. The rare but devastating complication of atheroembolism may lead to livedo reticularis, renal failure, stroke, or potential death.

RADIOLOGIC EQUIPMENT

To capture the larger regions of interest (eg, the entire aortic arch, the pelvic vascula-ture, or both legs), a large-field (48 cm) flat-panel detector is recommended. Digital subtraction angiography (DSA) and road mapping are two techniques commonly used in peripheral angiography and intervention. In DSA, subtraction of a precon-trast mask suppresses interfering structures from subsequent projections, thereby enhancing arterial filling and masking fixed structures (bone, calcifications, soft tis-sue, and air densities) (**Figure 16.1**). This allows the use of lower doses or reduced concentrations of iodinated contrast or use of noniodinated contrast including car-bon dioxide or gadolinium. Another useful technique used in DSA is road mapping. This technique is used for selective catheterization and is a useful aid for visualiza-tion of a moving catheter. Prior to moving the catheter, a small amount of contrast

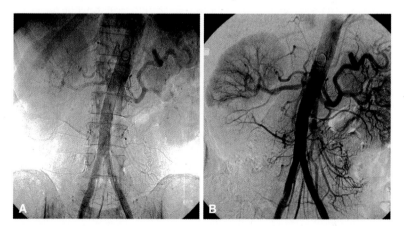

Figure 16.1 A, Normal abdominal aortogram using iodinated contrast material obtained by digital imaging technique. **B,** Same imaging data, but with enhancement of contrast-filled vessels obtained by the subtraction of all background densities (bones, soft tissue, gas) as recorded on a mask immediately prior to contrast injection.

medium is injected. The image with filled vessels is stored in memory as a mask (a road map along which the catheter is to be moved). This mask is then subtracted from the fluoroscopic images that follow, which will display both the vessels and the catheter with its tip.

CATHETERS AND GUIDEWIRES

Traditional peripheral angiography guidewires are made of a stainless-steel coil surrounding a tapered inner core that runs the length of the wire for additional strength. A central safety wire filament is incorporated to prevent separation if the wire coil ever fractures. More contemporary guidewires with a nitinol core are less susceptible to distortion of the shaft or permanent "fouling" of the steerable tip. Standard wires vary in diameter from 0.012 to 0.052 in, with 0.035 and 0.038 in being the most commonly used sizes for diagnostic angiography. The length of most standard wires is between 120 and 200 cm; longer exchange length guidewires (measuring 260-300 cm, and recently up to 400 cm) allow the operator to maintain the tip of the wire at a selected position in the body during catheter exchange. Tip configurations include straight tip, angled tip, and J-shaped tip. Special features may include the ability to move the wire's inner core to vary the length of the floppy tip, deflect the wire tip, or transmit torque from the shaft to the tip so that it can be steered within the vascular tree. Varying degrees of shaft stiffness (eg, extra-support wires) allow advancement of stiff devices through tortuous vessels. Low-friction wires with a hydrophilic coating (GLIDEWIRE) have revolutionized peripheral work and made it possible to perform superselective catheterization and to traverse complex stenoses and long occlusions. An ever-increasing number of specialty wires in various diameters are available for use in peripheral artery disease (PAD); in addition, the full array of coronary guidewires are currently employed in the periphery, especially in complex anatomy and for challenging revascularization procedures (eg, carotid, renal, tibial, and pedal arch vessels).

Peripheral angiographic catheters are constructed of polyurethane, polyethylene, Teflon, or nylon with a wire braid in the wall of the catheter to impart torqueability. An ideal catheter has good shape memory; is nonthrombogenic; has sufficient torque control to facilitate rotational detectability; can accommodate high-pressure injection; and tracks well with longitudinal advancement, frequently aided by hydrophilic polymer coating.

For catheters designed to be positioned in the abdominal aorta from the CFA, a length of 60 to 80 cm is sufficient; in the thoracic or carotid areas, a length of 100 to 120 cm (similar to those of left heart catheters) may be required. The most common diagnostic catheter sizes are 4F to 7F. Alternative access sites may alter the requirements for length and French size.

Several catheter shapes have been designed, and each ultimately determines a specific function (**Figure 16.2**). While there are a very large number of specific catheter configurations and curves, they may be categorized according to the following general types.

- Straight catheters with multiple side ports that are used for power injection of contrast into large vessels and for exchange.
- Pigtail, Omni Flush, or tennis racquet catheters that are used for nonselective angiography in large vessels (ie, aorta, pulmonary artery, or cardiac chambers). Multiple side holes along the distal shaft allow rapid delivery of contrast instead of a single forceful jet that could cause catheter whipping or subintimal dissection as might be seen with contrast exiting the end-hole alone.

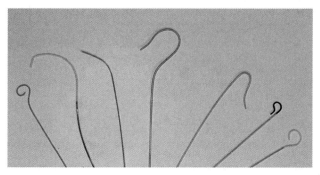

Figure 16.2 Peripheral angiographic catheters. Left to right. Pigtail, cobra, multipurpose, head-hunter, Simmons, SOS Omni, and tennis racquet.

- Simple curved catheters (eg, Berenstein, cobra, headhunter, Judkins right) that are used for vessel selection.
- Complex reverse-curve catheters (eg, Simmons, sidewinder, Vitek, SOS Omni) that are used for selective catheterization of certain aortic branches.

End-hole catheters, ideally with a 0.035″ lumen (eg, 4F or 5F straight glide catheter or equivalent) that may be advanced to selective or supraelective locations to approach the desired vascular territory; judicious hand injection of contrast (or contrast diluted with saline) may provide highest resolution imaging of the target segments. Smaller lumen catheters (eg, 0.018″ or even 0.014″) can also be used for superselective injection, albeit with a reduced volume of contrast. Adequate visualization of the target vessel can often be obtained by diluting of contrast (to reduce viscosity) and using subtraction imaging techniques.

THORACIC AORTA
Disorders of the Thoracic Aorta
Aortic Coarctation

Coarctation of the aorta occurs in 0.02% to 0.06% of the population and may be associated with bicuspid aortic valve (33% of cases), patent ductus arteriosus, ventricular septal defect, or Turner syndrome. To bypass the resulting bandlike narrowing of the aorta, collateral flow occurs retrograde into the posterior intercostal branches of the descending aorta. The resultant enlargement and tortuosity of these intercostal arteries are responsible for the "rib notching" seen in chest radiographs.

The classical findings by aortography or MRA are of a high-grade, discrete narrowing of the aorta at the level of the isthmus, with associated dilatation of the ascending aorta and enlargement of the internal thoracic and intercostal arteries. Aortography assumes a significant role in differentiating the wide variety of abnormal patterns, including complete aortic interruption, hypoplastic aorta, and the most common type—a stenosis at the site of the isthmus, distal to the origin of the left subclavian artery. Both anteroposterior (AP) and lateral (right anterior oblique [RAO]/left anterior oblique [LAO]) aortography should be initially undertaken, with contrast injection performed proximal to the presumed site of coarctation using either large-film or cineangiographic technique. When attempting to traverse the site of narrowing in retrograde fashion, care must be taken to avoid inadvertent perforation of the thin-walled poststenotic segment. Entry to the prestenotic aorta from the brachial or axillary arteries may hence be preferred.

Thoracic Aortic Aneurysms

Thoracic aortic aneurysms (TAAs) and pseudoaneurysms may have various causes, including those that are degenerative, atherosclerosis-related, or congenital (aneurysms of the Valsalva sinus); other causes include trauma, infection (syphilitic, bacterial), cystic medial degeneration, connective tissue disorders, vasculitis, and chronic dissection. Degenerative aneurysms involving the descending aorta account for approximately 75% of TAAs. Cystic medial degeneration (as seen in the Marfan syndrome) may also result in aneurysms of the ascending aorta. Aneurysms caused by blunt or penetrating trauma often involve the proximal descending thoracic aorta where the mobile arch segment joins the descending segment fixed to the spine. These may present as pseudoaneurysms-contained ruptures that lack intimal and medial components and are contained only by adventitia and periaortic tissue.

The natural history of untreated TAA is less understood as compared with the extensive data available on untreated infrarenal abdominal aortic aneurysm (AAA). Many patients with TAA are asymptomatic at the time of diagnosis, with the aneurysm incidentally detected during testing for an unrelated disorder. Thoracic aneurysms appear to enlarge at a more rapid rate than that observed in abdominal aneurysms (0.42 vs 0.28 cm/y), and aneurysms larger than 5 to 6 cm in diameter progress even more rapidly and have a higher likelihood of rupture. The cumulative 5-year risk of rupture is increased fivefold in aneurysms >6 cm in diameter. Symptoms tend to develop late in the course of the enlargement of the aorta and are usually related to impingement on adjacent structures. In addition to presenting with catastrophic rupture, patients with TAA may report dyspnea, hoarseness, dysphagia, stridor, and plethora with edema from superior vena cava compression. Neck or jaw pain may also be present in patients with aneurysms of the aortic arch. Dilatation of the aortic valve annulus and aortic valve may produce aortic regurgitation and congestive heart failure. Aneurysms of the descending thoracic aorta may produce pleuritic left-sided or interscapular pain, whereas thoracoabdominal aortic aneurysms may induce complaints of abdominal pain and left shoulder discomfort from irritation of the left hemidiaphragm.

The primary treatment for TAA is surgical repair when the diameter reaches more than 5 to 6 cm or symptoms develop. The standard procedure is to use a Dacron graft to replace the diseased segment. In most patients undergoing elective thoracic aorta surgical repair, aortography is required to provide information about the location of the aneurysm and its relationship to major aortic branches in the chest and abdomen. Stent graft devices have been successfully used as an alternative to surgical grafting for both thoracic and aortic degenerative TAA and posttraumatic descending TAA. Although early experience was plagued by incomplete aneurysm thrombosis, graft leak, and failure, advances in the technology are rapidly expanding the role of endovascular stent grafts in TAA treatment.

Aortic Dissection

Aortic dissection is a longitudinal cleavage of the aortic media by a dissecting column of blood. An intimal tear allows the passage of blood into the aortic wall, separating the inner and outer layers of the aortic wall and creating a "double barrel lumen." Men are affected about twice as frequently as women. Most patients are between 50 and 70 years of age and have arterial hypertension. Other risk factors include cystic medial degeneration, Marfan syndrome, bicuspid aortic valve, aortic coarctation, blunt trauma, pregnancy, connective tissue disorders, and thoracic aorta operative procedures. The dissection may extend proximally from its origin to the aortic annulus or distally to involve the entire length of the aorta and any or all of its major branches, until terminated by an aortic branch or atherosclerotic plaque.

Associated peripheral and visceral patterns of arterial obstructions may be owing to direct extension of the dissection plane into the affected arterial orifice (static dissection) or compromise of the visceral artery origin by the expanded false lumen (dynamic dissection).

Dissection is usually heralded by the sudden onset of excruciating pain described as tearing, throbbing, lacerating, ripping, or burning in the anterior chest, neck, or intrascapular region. Similar pain may occur with rupture or sudden expansion of a chronic dissection. If the acute dissection results in compression of aortic branches, symptoms and signs of acute myocardial infarction, stroke or transient ischemic attack (TIA), paraparesis, mesenteric ischemia, renal failure, paraplegia, and extremity ischemia may result. Most patients with ascending aortic extension who are treated medically die within 3 months, usually from dissection into the pericardium, mediastinum, or pleural cavity.

Once considered the gold standard for diagnosis of aortic dissection, aortography (which has a sensitivity of 80% and specificity of 95%) has largely been replaced by computed tomography (CT), MRA, and transesophageal echocardiography (TEE). Visualization of an intimal flap is the only direct aortographic sign that is pathognomonic of dissection. This occurs frequently in association with delayed or sluggish filling of a second lumen, although about 20% of patients with aortic dissection have only one visible aortic channel. The presence of a false lumen may still be suspected, however, if that single channel shows evidence of diminished caliber and absent branching owing either to extrinsic compression by a hematoma in the false lumen or to intrinsic luminal collapse consequent to loss of wall elastin. The false lumen of an aortic dissection is distinguished angiographically by its anterolateral ascending and posterolateral descending position, differential reduced flow, and a generally larger caliber than that of the true lumen. Beyond documenting the dissection, aortography provides information about aortic insufficiency and branch vessel or coronary artery involvement, particularly in cases where CT or magnetic resonance imaging findings are equivocal, and there is a strong clinical suspicion of aortic dissection.

Two classification systems of aortic dissection are widely used: the DeBakey classification and the Stanford classification. The DeBakey classification is based on the anatomical extent of the dissection. In type I, the tear originates in the ascending aorta and extends distally. Type II dissections are confined to the ascending aorta. In type III, the dissection may be confined to the descending aorta (type IIIa) or extend into the abdominal aorta and iliac arteries (type IIIb). The Stanford classification is based solely on the location of the origin of the dissection. Type A includes all cases where the ascending aorta is involved, and type B includes those where the ascending aorta is not involved.

When performing aortography in a patient with suspected aortic dissection, the preferred entry point is the femoral artery that demonstrates the best pulse. An atraumatic diagnostic catheter (eg, pigtail, Omni Flush, or tennis racquet) with a soft J-tipped or 5 to 15 cm floppy-tipped guidewire should be advanced under fluoroscopic guidance with frequent test injections. Since the entry to the false lumen is commonly on the greater (outer) curve of the aorta, the catheter may be used to direct the wire toward the inner curve to maximize the chance of remaining in the true lumen. If this is performed successfully, structures such as the aortic leaflets and coronary arteries will be visible, and it will be possible to enter the left ventricle. It is not uncommon, though, to enter the false lumen during initial catheter advancement. When this becomes apparent on test injections, care should be taken to avoid extending the false lumen, pulling the catheter back and using the techniques discussed above to reenter the true lumen. It should also be noted that dissection of the ascending aorta can track retrograde to involve the ostium of one of the coronary arteries, so visualization of a coronary artery does not guarantee that the catheter location is within the true lumen.

Surgical repair of Stanford type A aortic dissections entails Dacron graft placement of the ascending aorta. If the aortic valve is abnormal, it is replaced. Similarly, if there is involvement of the coronary artery ostia, bypass is performed. In contrast, patients with type B acute aortic dissections can be initially treated with medical therapy, reserving surgical intervention for those with signs of impending rupture (persistent pain and hypotension), ischemia of legs, malperfusion of mesenteric or renal arteries, or paraparesis/paraplegia. In cases of chronic dissection, interventional or operative treatment should be considered if the diameter of the descending aorta exceeds 5 to 6 cm or symptoms develop. Endovascular stents and balloon fenestration have been successfully used in the past for treatment of ischemic complications associated with aortic dissection. Increasingly, stent grafting has become recognized as a preferred primary treatment for acute dissection of the descending aorta and/or abdominal aorta.

Vasculitides

Vasculitis, highlighted by inflammation of the vessel wall, has two forms that commonly affect the aorta and its branches. These produce dilation of the proximal aorta, narrowing or occlusion of large aortic branches, or both. Takayasu arteritis is characterized by irregularity of the ascending aorta, narrowing of the descending aorta, obstructions of arch vessels, and aortic insufficiency or dissection. There may also be associated stenoses in the pulmonary arterial bed as a distinguishing feature. Therapeutic options include surgical bypass or balloon angioplasty demonstrating adjunctive stenting in patients with end-organ ischemia. Importantly, intervention should generally be reserved until acute inflammation has subsided.

Giant cell or temporal arteritis is a vasculitis of large and medium arteries. Angiographic evidence of aortic branch involvement shows long, smooth stenoses alternating with relatively normal segments. The intracranial carotid artery and its branches, or the distal subclavian arteries, are usually involved, with aortic disease being relatively uncommon.

ABDOMINAL AORTA
Abdominal Aortography

Abdominal aortography is typically performed via the femoral approach but is also readily performed from transradial access. A 4F to 6F multiside-hole pigtail catheter may be used, or an Omni Flush diagnostic catheter may be preferred from transfemoral access in order to limit proximal propagation of contrast injection, limiting which visceral vessels are opacified and optimizing contrast opacification. If transfemoral or radial access is not feasible, alternative vascular access options include via translumbar, axillary, or brachial arteries. The tip of the catheter should be positioned at the T12 or L1 level, thus placing the side holes adjacent to the first and second lumbar vertebrae. Contrast medium may be diluted with saline if digital subtraction protocols are utilized; a 70% strength represents a reasonable compromise for vessel opacification, injectate viscosity, vessel opacification, and contrast volume minimization. Volume and rate of contrast injection may vary based on location of injection, desired vascular distribution imaged, patient habitus, catheter style and caliber, and patient clinical parameters; many operators select rates between 10 and 20 mL/s and total volumes between 10 and 50 mL per injection. Image acquisition should be performed at 3 frames per second or greater when evaluating the mesenteric or renal arteries. When performing arteriography in an aorta with suspected or known aneurysmal disease or severe atherosclerotic involvement, meticulous care should be taken to avoid dislodging mural thrombus or protruding atherosclerotic plaque which could precipitate distal embolization. In the patient with a known "friable" aorta, overly high-pressure injection should be avoided to minimize the chance of penetrating the plaque with contrast (eg, "staining" the aortic wall).

Selective Mesenteric Angiography

After nonselective abdominal aortography has been performed in AP, lateral, and/or RAO with caudal angulation, selective imaging of the celiac axis, superior mesenteric artery (SMA), and inferior mesenteric artery may be considered. Many diagnostic catheters may be effective for selective cannulation of these vessels. However, the reverse curve inherent to SOS Omni (Omni Flush) selective-type catheters may offer strategic advantage for engaging the 3 vessels from transfemoral access, given the downward angulation of the origins. Depending on the location of the potential lesions and specific mesenteric vessel engagement, a combination of AP, lateral, and RAO caudal angulation may enable optimal visualization of the origins and proximal segments. Distal portions of the celiac and SMA are better evaluated in AP angulation, with adjustment of the cranial-caudal angle as necessary.

SUBCLAVIAN AND VERTEBRAL ARTERIES
Manifestations of Subclavian Disease

Atherosclerosis of the proximal subclavian artery may manifest clinically as arm claudication, subclavian steal syndrome, or (in patients with previous internal mammary grafting) coronary ischemia. In classic subclavian steal, stenosis or occlusion of the proximal subclavian artery causes blood from the contralateral vertebral artery to flow antegrade up to the basilar system and then retrograde down the ipsilateral vertebral artery, filling the subclavian artery distal to the lesion. In rare cases, this may cause cerebral ischemia during upper extremity exercise or with certain changes of the position of neck (eg, tilting the head and looking skyward). In patients who have undergone internal mammary artery bypass grafting to a coronary artery (mostly the left anterior descending [LAD]), a proximal subclavian obstruction may result in retrograde flow in the graft, leading to coronary ischemia (coronary-subclavian steal) (**Figure 16.3A and B**). Ischemia may be exacerbated by activity, such as arm exertion, that increases the retrograde graft flow and the associated steal or diversion of blood from the coronary bed. Stenosis of the vertebral origin is relatively common, particularly at its origin from the subclavian artery.

Subclavian and Vertebral Arteriography

A nonselective aortic arch arteriogram with a 5F/6F pigtail catheter, with injection of 20 to 40 mL at a rate of 15 to 20 mL/s in the LAO projection 20° to 50°, can visualize the origin of the great vessels to evaluate for atherosclerotic occlusive disease. The optimum catheter for selective catheterization of the innominate or subclavian artery depends on the configuration of the great vessels of the neck. For the simple origin takeoff, angiography can generally be performed with a 5F/6F Davis, headhunter, Berenstein, JR4, hockey stick, or VTK catheter. If the arch aortogram demonstrates an elongated arch, a reverse-curve catheter such as a VTK or Simmons may be required. A 30° to 45° LAO projection is useful for selecting each of the branches, with the catheters formed and oriented in the ascending aorta and withdrawn sequentially

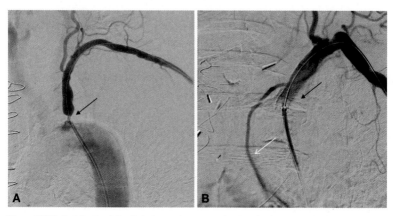

Figure 16.3 A, Selective left subclavian angiogram under digital subtraction depicting severe ostial stenosis (arrow). **B,** Postintervention angiogram following successful covered stenting (black arrow) of an ostial left subclavian stenosis with improved antegrade flow into a left internal mammary artery (LIMA) graft (white arrow).

from the innominate through the left common carotid to the left subclavian artery. So as to avoid raising a plaque during withdrawal from the ascending aorta, configuring the curve in the descending aorta and then advancing to the point of engagement may be preferred for the "reverse-curve" VTK and Simmons catheters. Angiography of the innominate with 30° to 40° RAO and mild caudal angulation will enable visualization of the bifurcation of the right common carotid and subclavian arteries. Subclavian and vertebral angiography can generally be performed in the AP view, with the addition of an oblique view (RAO or LAO) if there is suspicion of an eccentric lesion. If a proximal vertebral artery stenosis is expected, selective injection of the ipsilateral subclavian artery in the AP projection is usually diagnostic. Often, cranial or caudal angulation is required to open up and clearly define the origin of the vertebral arteries. The origins of the internal mammary arteries are frequently defined best in the RAO cranial angulation, a point of particular importance in subclavian intervention.

Carotid Arteries

Extracranial Carotid Atherosclerosis

Approximately 795,000 new or recurrent strokes occur annually in the United States, accounting for 1 of every 19 deaths. Nearly 90% are ischemic and while the majority of these are likely cardioembolic, an estimated 25% to 30% are believed to be attributable to extracranial carotid artery disease. Patients with carotid artery disease frequently have concomitant severe coronary artery disease. Even patients with asymptomatic carotid artery stenosis have an increased risk of coronary events. Just the finding of increased carotid intima media thickness on duplex ultrasonographic images predicts a higher risk of myocardial infarction or stroke, as much as 3.87 times that observed in patients with minimal thickness. Importantly, according to NHLBI tabulations, the age-adjusted stroke rates declined by 13.6% between 2007 and 2017, presumably due to increased statin use, better blood pressure control, and appropriate treatment with antiplatelet and antithrombotic agents for those at high risk. Despite the reduction in age-adjusted risk, the actual number of stroke deaths increased by 7.7%. While the majority of extracranial carotid disease is asymptomatic, carotid artery stenosis remains a significant cause of stroke. There is great controversy regarding optimal management. The result is significant variation in treatment.

Most patients with extracranial carotid artery disease are identified by the presence of a carotid bruit on physical examination, with no referable symptoms. Estimates of the prevalence of asymptomatic carotid bruits in adults range from 1% to 2.3% in patients in the age group of 45 to 54 years and 8.2% in patients older than 75 years. Absence of a bruit, however, does not imply absence of significant carotid disease. In a substudy of the North American Symptomatic Carotid Endarterectomy Trial (NASCET), 1268 patients with recent transient cerebral ischemia or nondisabling stroke were examined for the presence of a carotid bruit. Fifty-eight percent of patients had a bruit localized to the ipsilateral carotid artery; 31% had a carotid bruit involving the contralateral vessel; and 24% had bilateral carotid bruits. The sensitivity and specificity of a focal bruit for predicting high-grade ipsilateral carotid stenosis were 63% and 61%, respectively.

Many carotid lesions are discovered only after the patient begins to experience symptoms, which may vary from transient monocular blindness (amaurosis fugax) to expressive or receptive aphasia, hemiparesis/hemiplegia, and mental status changes. Although these episodic symptoms last a few minutes to a few hours and then completely resolve, they are harbingers of recurrent and potentially nonreversible events and thus warrant urgent evaluation and therapy in an attempt to prevent a catastrophic stroke.

The first study in this evaluation is typically carotid DUS, which provides 2-dimensional images of the extracranial carotid arteries and may provide information about plaque morphology. Color-coded images can detect increased velocities of blood flow, which correlate to higher degrees of stenosis, while Doppler waveforms and velocities can also be measured to evaluate stenosis severity when performed by skilled vascular ultrasonographers. Once a significant stenosis is identified, contrast or MRA is commonly performed to corroborate the ultrasound study findings. A strategy of DUS followed by CTA yielded a sensitivity of 100% and specificity of 84%. In cases in which there is discordance between DUS and cross-sectional imaging techniques, catheter angiography is warranted.

Carotid Arteriography

To completely evaluate cerebral circulation, arch aortography and selective carotid and vertebral (eg, "4-vessel") angiography should be performed. Arch aortography defines the disease state of the aorta and the configuration and the orientation of the great vessel origins, thus enabling optimal catheter choice for selective cannulation. Anatomical variations of the typical aortic arch include origin of the left common carotid from the innominate (bovine arch), seen in 10% of patients; origin of the left vertebral from the aorta in 3%, and origin of the right subclavian as the distal-most vessel in 1% (arteria lusoria).

Prior to selective cannulation, careful assessment of the cervical vessels and their origins and course as they arise from the aorta is prudent in order to choose catheter shapes that will minimize the need for manipulation. For normal arch anatomy, a Davis, Berenstein, Judkins right, or headhunter catheter can be used. For elongated arch anatomy or in the case where the great vessels arise from the ascending aorta, a retroflexed catheter such as a VTK or Simmons may be required to selectively engage. Having engaged the carotid ostium, the catheter can be advanced over a 0.035-in or 0.038-in GLIDEWIRE.

Once the diagnostic catheter is advanced to or beyond the aortic arch, careful double flushing is mandatory to minimize risk of embolization. Injections of diluted

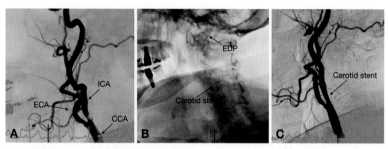

Figure 16.4 A, Carotid angiogram confirming severe stenosis involving the ostium of the left ICA. **B,** Fluoroscopic image demonstrating carotid stenting via a transfemoral approach. **C,** Angiogram of the carotid bifurcation following successful stenting of the stenotic left ICA with a 9 to 7 × 40 mm bare-metal self-expanding stenting using a distal embolic protection device. CCA, common carotid artery; ECA, external carotid artery; EDP, embolic distal protection; ICA, internal carotid artery.

contrast can be performed by hand or by automated injection at 4 to 6 mL/s for a total of 8 mL in the common carotid artery with digital subtraction at 4 or 6 frames per second, and at 3 to 4 mL/s for a total of 5 to 6 mL in the vertebral artery. In general, lower rates and volumes of contrast are initially used in the cerebral circulation, and adjustments are made as needed for subsequent injections.

Multiple oblique projections are necessary, including AP, lateral, and oblique views, to optimally visualize narrowing at the carotid bifurcation and proximal internal carotid artery (ICA). The lateral projection is often the best to visualize the proximal ICA and carotid siphon. Ipsilateral oblique views also are useful for delineating disease at the carotid bifurcation and proximal ICA (**Figures 16.4** and **16.5**).

The angiographic views commonly used to delineate the intracerebral course of the ICAs include the Towne view (AP cranial to bring the petrous ridge over the roof of the orbit) and the straight lateral view (with the pinnae of the ears superimposed). To calculate the percent diameter stenosis, the projection that demonstrates the highest degree of stenosis should be used. Many methods of calculating carotid artery stenosis have been used in previous trials; however, the NASCET methodology is the most widely accepted. It compares the minimum lumen diameter at the stenotic site in the ICA with that of the normal appearing segment of vessel distal to the stenosis, where the vessel walls become parallel.

RENAL ARTERIES
Atherosclerotic Renal Artery Stenosis

Atherosclerotic renal artery stenosis (ARAS) is clearly more common than was previously believed, with increasing prevalence in certain patient populations. In one series of 395 arteriograms performed in patients with AAA, aortoiliac atherosclerosis, or infrainguinal atherosclerosis, 33% to 50% had a renal artery stenosis of >50%. The presence of coronary artery atherosclerosis is also a marker for ARAS. In a prospective study of 1302 patients undergoing coronary arteriography, concurrent abdominal aortography demonstrated significant RAS in 15% of patients.

Several clinical clues may suggest the presence of ARAS. Patients who develop diastolic hypertension after 55 years of age, who have exacerbation of previously well-controlled hypertension, who demonstrate refractory hypertension (uncontrolled hypertension despite treatment with 3 antihypertensive medications of

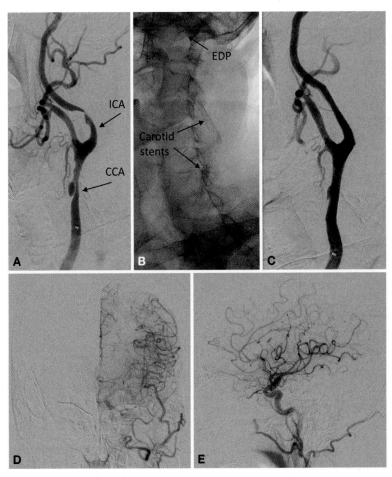

Figure 16.5 A, Extensive calcified and ulcerated atherosclerotic disease of the left CCA and ICA secondary to late effects of radiation injury. **B,** Deployment of 10 to 8 × 40 mm (CCA) and 8 to 6 × 40 mm bare-metal stents (ICA) using an EDP. **C,** Successful revascularization of the left cervical carotid artery. **D and E,** Postintervention cerebral angiograms show improved filling of A1 segment and anterior communicating artery and absence of distal embolization. CCA, common carotid artery; EDP, embolic distal protection; ICA, internal carotid artery.

synergistic classes at maximal doses), who develop azotemia after treatment with an angiotensin-converting enzyme inhibitor, or who present with malignant hypertension (severe hypertension and papilledema, acute myocardial infarction, acute stroke or TIA, aortic dissection, acute renal failure) should all be suspected of having renal artery stenosis.

A number of noninvasive diagnostic tests have been used to determine if renal artery stenosis is present. Renal artery DUS can be an excellent test to diagnose renal artery stenosis if performed by a skilled operator. Using peak systolic velocity (PSV) within the renal artery of >180 cm/s as the criterion, duplex scanning was able to discern between normal and diseased renal arteries with a sensitivity of 95% and specificity of 90%. The ratio of PSV in the area of renal artery stenosis to the PSV within the aorta (renal-to-aortic ratio, RAR) of >3.5 predicts the presence of >60% renal artery stenosis with a sensitivity of 92%.

Renal Arteriography

Access for renal angiography is most commonly achieved via the femoral approach. However, a brachial approach may be advantageous if there is significant infrarenal aortic atheroma or aneurysmal disease or an extreme downward angulation of the renal arteries detected by preprocedural noninvasive testing.

The first stage of renal angiography is an abdominal aortogram, allowing for identification of ostia of the bilateral renal arteries and location of any accessory renal arteries, which is seen in as many as 25% of the population. Frequently, an aortogram will suffice in ruling out significant renal artery stenosis. As with abdominal aortography described above, a 4F to 5F multiholed catheter placed at the L1-L2 interspace for power injection using DSA is generally sufficient to provide adequate opacification. In the setting of renal insufficiency, carbon dioxide can be used as a surrogate contrast agent. In this setting, a bolus dose of 40 to 50 mL of carbon dioxide delivered by hand injection during breathholding using DSA (at least 4 frames per second) should be sufficient for adequate localization of the renal artery origins to allow for selective angiography.

Commonly used catheters for selective engagement include 5F Judkins right, internal mammary, hockey stick, or renal double-curve catheters. From the femoral approach, catheter lengths should be shorter than those selected for standard coronary angiography. For downward angulated renal arteries, a reverse-curve catheter such as an Omni selective catheter may be more appropriate from the femoral approach or a 5F multipurpose catheter from an upper extremity approach. Renal artery engagement is generally favored from the left upper extremity due to its shorter distance to the target vessels compared to the right side.

Occasionally, renal angiography will yield an equivocal or indeterminate angiographic result, particularly in complex conditions such as fibromuscular dysplasia, Takayasu arteritis, radiation, aneurysms, or vasculitis. In this setting, measurement of a trans-stenotic gradient may provide useful information regarding the hemodynamic significance of a stenosis. Pressure measurement is most accurately performed using a specialized 0.014-in pressure wire but alternatively can be performed by measuring the differential pressure between a 4F catheter placed beyond the lesion and a 5F or 6F catheter placed in the aorta. Gradients higher than 10 mmHg mean or 20 mmHg systolic are considered significant.

PELVIC AND LOWER EXTREMITIES

Tibial anatomy is distinctly important for vascular interventionalists who perform endovascular revascularization for patients with chronic limb-threatening ischemia (CLTI). The blood supply to the foot can be divided into 3 major angiosomes, that is, areas of the foot that receive direct blood supply from one of the 3 tibial arteries. The dorsum of the foot is perfused by the anterior tibial artery, the heel predominantly by the peroneal artery, and the plantar surface is supplied by the posterior tibial artery. Since patients with CLTI often have tissue loss, performing direct revascularization of the affected angiosome by treating the corresponding tibial theoretically increases perfusion to the area of tissue loss to facilitate wound healing. Angiosome-guided revascularization has been shown in observational studies to augment wound healing and increase limb salvage rates.

Lower Extremity Peripheral Artery Disease

Patients with asymptomatic PAD are at minimal risk of developing critical limb ischemia that threatens limb survival. In general, patients first manifest intermittent claudication before progressing to develop rest pain, a nonhealing ischemic ulcer, or gangrene. The currently accepted methods of determining the presence of PAD include an historical review of patient symptoms and atherosclerotic risk factors, physical examination, and the use of noninvasive vascular tests. Clinical history is often quite unreliable for confirming the diagnosis of PAD, as <50% of patients actually have classic symptoms of intermittent claudication.

A simple noninvasive test is the ankle-brachial index (ABI) test. This test compares the blood pressure obtained with a handheld Doppler in the DP or PT artery (whichever is higher) to the blood pressure in the higher of the two brachial pressures. Generally, an ABI of >0.9 is considered normal, >0.4 to <0.9 reflects mild to moderate PAD, and <0.4 suggests severe PAD. The addition of treadmill walking to obtain a postexercise ABI adds significantly to the sensitivity of the resting ABI in detecting PAD.

The most common symptom described by patients with PAD is intermittent claudication. The discomfort is usually brought on by walking and alleviated by rest. The discomfort generally pertains to the muscle groups immediately distal to the arterial segments involved (eg, SFA stenosis causes calf discomfort). In classic intermittent claudication, the onset of discomfort is quite predictable and occurs at similar distances, provided the speed, incline, and terrain have remained unchanged. Patients generally stop, stand, and wait for 1 to 5 minutes for relief prior to resumption of walking. Depending upon the level(s) of obstruction, the discomfort can involve the buttocks, hips, calves, or ankles. Occasionally, very proximal disease (eg, of the aorta, iliac, or common femoral arteries) can result in thigh claudication. Not infrequently, symptoms of vascular insufficiency are mistaken for arthritis, especially in the case of hip and ankle claudication.

Progression to critical limb ischemia manifests as ischemic pain at rest, generally in the arch of the foot or toes. Discomfort occurs when the patient is lying supine and is relieved by hanging the foot over the bedside or getting up and walking. Patients may resort to sleeping in a reclining chair to provide a dependent position to the foot. Ischemic ulcerations may occur spontaneously or as a result of trauma to toes or areas where bony prominences are exposed. The presence of ischemic rest pain or ulceration warrants a prompt and aggressive strategy for imaging and revascularization.

Once the ABI test—preferably at rest and post treadmill exercise—has been performed to provide objective evidence of the overall severity of PAD, more specific information can be obtained noninvasively in the vascular laboratory. The addition of segmental limb pressures can aid in localizing stenoses or occlusions.

Pulse volume recordings (PVRs) are plethysmographic tracings that detect the changes in the volume of blood flowing through a limb. Cuffs are inflated to 65 mmHg, and a plethysmographic tracing is recorded at various levels. The normal PVR is similar to the normal arterial pulse-wave tracing and consists of a rapid systolic upstroke and a rapid downstroke with a prominent dicrotic notch. With increasing severity of disease, the waveform becomes more attenuated, with a wide downslope, and in extreme cases, the waveform is virtually absent.

Of the patients who have undergone surgical bypass graft revascularization, particularly with saphenous vein, 21% to 33% will develop graft stenosis. Once the graft becomes thrombosed, secondary patency rates are dismal, so early detection of a graft stenosis is important and should lead to its repair prior to graft thrombosis. If this is done, an estimated 80% of grafts can be salvaged. A well-organized graft surveillance program is thus crucial to preserving patency of bypass grafts. In one series of 170 saphenous vein bypass grafts, 110 stenoses were detected over a 39-month period. In those grafts that underwent surgical revision once a stenosis was detected, the 4-year patency was 88%, whereas in those grafts that did not undergo revision despite the detection of a stenosis, the 4-year patency was 57%.

PULMONARY ANGIOGRAPHY

Hemodynamic Monitoring

Patients who need pulmonary angiography are often acutely ill and may require continuous blood pressure measurement monitoring. An important part of the procedure is formal hemodynamic measurements (both pressures and oxygen saturation) during catheter pullback. The coronary sinus is occasionally entered while trying to access the right ventricular (RV) outflow tract (particularly from jugular or brachial access route). To minimize the risk of perforation, catheter advancement should be halted if a right atrial pressure waveform continues to be present as the catheter is advanced across the spine into what should fluoroscopically be the right ventricle. Catheter position in the coronary sinus can be confirmed or excluded by a hand injection of a contrast medium under fluoroscopy. Damping of the pressure in the main pulmonary artery may indicate the presence of massive pulmonary embolism (PE), with the catheter holes embedded in the embolus. In that situation, a hand injection of contrast can confirm the diagnosis.

Percutaneous Venous Catheterization

The veins used for catheterization of the pulmonary artery are the femoral, jugular, and upper extremity vein. Of these, the right femoral vein is preferable because it provides a relatively straight course to the inferior vena cava (IVC) and right heart. In patients with suspected proximal deep vein thrombosis (DVT), ultrasound examination may be considered prior to vascular entry. The procedure is performed with mild conscious sedation. It is important that the patient be alert during the procedure so that he or she can cooperate with breath holding during imaging. In case heparin has been administered for suspected PE, it should be continued during the examination.

To minimize the risk of dislodging thrombi during catheter advancement, manual injection of 10 mL of contrast into the femoral vein may help to exclude massive iliac vein or cava thrombosis prior to advancing the guidewire and the catheter to the right heart.

Occasionally, because of femoral or iliac vein thrombosis, IVC occlusion, or groin infection, the femoral vein cannot be used. The vein of choice then becomes the jugular or an upper extremity vein. The right heart may be approached easily with a balloon-directed catheter when gaining vascular access via the internal jugular vein.

Pulmonary Artery Catheterization

Most catheters used for diagnostic pulmonary angiography are between 5F and 7F pigtail catheters to provide a lumen that will accommodate contrast injection rates of 15 to 20 mL/s. A 4F nylon pulmonary pigtail catheter allows flow rates of 20 mL/s at 1050 psi and may reduce access-site complications. The 3 common approaches for pulmonary artery catheterization are shown in **Figure 16.6**. The presence of a properly placed IVC filter does not necessarily preclude a transfemoral approach. Safe transfilter angiography has been reported by passing straight or J-tipped guidewires followed by catheters through stainless-steel Greenfield, VenaTech, and Bird's Nest filters. After the guidewire is passed through the IVC filter, a long sheath is placed across the filter, with its leading tip beyond the filter to prevent filter dislodgment.

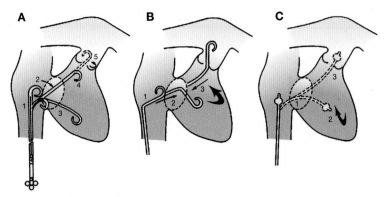

Figure 16.6 Techniques for pulmonary artery catheterization. **A,** Straight-body pigtail catheter and tip-deflecting wire. The pigtail catheter is placed in the right atrium (1). The wire is deflected to point toward the right ventricle (2). The wire is fixed, and the catheter is advanced over it into the right ventricle (3). The tip deflection is released (4). Counterclockwise rotation of the catheter swings the pigtail anteriorly (5). Simultaneous advancement of the catheter places it into the main pulmonary artery. Advancing the catheter farther usually takes it into the left main pulmonary artery. The tip-deflecting wire is used to direct the catheter downward and to the right for right main pulmonary artery catheterization. **B,** Grollman pulmonary artery catheter. The pigtail catheter is placed in the right atrium (1). The anteromedial portion of the right atrium is probed to facilitate catheter entry into the right ventricle (2). The catheter is then slightly withdrawn and rotated counterclockwise to allow entry into the right ventricular outflow tract and main pulmonary artery (3). **C,** Balloon-tipped catheter. The balloon is inflated under fluoroscopic guidance in the common iliac vein, and the catheter is advanced under observation into the right atrium (1). The catheter is then rotated anteromedially to facilitate direct entry into the right ventricle (2). As soon as the tricuspid valve is passed, documented by a right ventricular pressure waveform, the catheter is rotated to point the balloon tip cranially toward the right ventricular outflow tract before advancing it further (3). Deep inspiration of the patient may facilitate flow-directed entry of the balloon tip from the outflow tract into the main pulmonary artery, with a preference to enter the left pulmonary artery.

Catheters used for pulmonary angiography are of 2 basic designs: the pigtail type and balloon-tipped type. The pigtail type catheters have multiple side holes, whereas the curled catheter tip allows safe passage through the right heart. While being removed from the pulmonary arteries, all pigtail catheters must be straightened with a floppy-tip guidewire or a J-tipped guidewire in the main pulmonary artery under fluoroscopic observation, since the catheter tip may otherwise engage a papillary muscle, chordae tendineae, or tricuspid valve leaflet during withdrawal. The balloon-tipped catheters are assisted by blood flow through the right heart chambers and into the pulmonary arteries. Side holes in the catheter shaft allow power injection into the main branches, whereas the catheter end-hole makes balloon occlusion angiography possible with the same catheter (**Figure 16.7**). Balloon catheters are first deflated and can then be removed without fluoroscopy.

Catheter Exchange

The curved pigtail catheter can be easily advanced into the right or left descending pulmonary artery for selective and superselective angiograms of the right middle lobe, left lingular segment, and lower lobes. When superselective catheterization of the segmental or subsegmental pulmonary arteries is required for evaluation of the peripheral pulmonary vasculature or to perform therapeutic embolization or stent

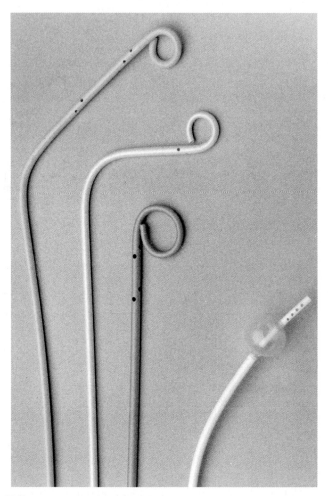

Figure 16.7 Catheters for pulmonary angiography. Left to right. The Nyman, Grollman, and straight pigtail catheters (Eppendorf type) and the balloon occlusion catheter with side holes distal to the balloon (Berman type).

placement, the catheter exchange method is used to exchange the pigtail catheter for a sheath, a guiding catheter, or an end-hole selective catheter. An exchange guidewire such as Rosen wire guide (0.035 in × 260 cm, 2 cm flexible tip and tightened "J" tip configuration, Cook Medical) is introduced into the catheter and gently advanced through the pigtail as far into the pulmonary artery branch as possible. Then, while the guidewire is held stationary, the catheter is slowly withdrawn over the guidewire until it exits from the puncture site. A new catheter or introducer is then advanced over the guidewire. When the catheter has been advanced the desired distance, the guidewire can be removed and the catheter tip is further manipulated into the desired branch using a steerable guidewire such as the angle-tipped GLIDEWIRE (Terumo Interventional Systems, Somerset, NJ).

Contrast Agent Injection Rates

The contrast injection rate is determined by the rate of blood flow in the selected vessel and pulmonary artery pressure. Contrast medium should be injected at a rate that approximates as closely as possible the rate of blood flow in the artery being opacified. The left and right pulmonary arteries have a blood flow of 20 to 25 mL/s in most patients without lung disease and pulmonary hypertension. The injection rate is adjusted according to the flow rate estimated at the test injection. The usual injection rates in patients with normal pulmonary artery pressure are 20 to 25 mL/s for a total volume of 40 to 50 mL. In general, the rate of injection for superselective pulmonary angiograms should be slightly more than the expected blood flow of the artery being injected to, to ensure complete filling of the vascular bed. Depending on the size of the pulmonary artery being injected to, the injection rate for superselective angiogram is 5 to 10 mL/s for a total volume of 15 to 20 mL (**Table 16.1**). In the presence of pulmonary hypertension, the amount of contrast medium should be reduced to minimize the adverse hemodynamic impact of a full contrast injection under such circumstances. The rate of injection in this condition should be reduced to 15 to 20 mL/s for a total volume of 30 to 40 mL. Even though the rate of injection is reduced, the total volume of contrast should be at least 30 mL to ensure complete filling of the central pulmonary arteries for the evaluation of pulmonary thromboembolic disease. With the use of nonionic low-osmolar or iso-osmolar contrast agents, tailored pulmonary angiography with lower flow rates and more distal injections has proved to be safe even in the presence of severe pulmonary hypertension. Contrast injection should be performed using an automated injector system at a pressure of at least 600 psi (42 kg/cm^2). For balloon occlusion angiography of segmental vessels, a hand injection of 5 to 10 mL is used.

Imaging Modes

Pulmonary angiography is performed using the digital subtraction technique. The digital technique allows rapid image acquisition and flexible display format. Images can be viewed individually or in cine format on the monitor, in either the subtracted or the unsubtracted mode. In addition, DSA may even allow satisfactory opacification of pulmonary arteries when contrast is injected into the superior vena cava or right atrium. The major disadvantage of DSA is that it requires motionless image acquisition. This may be especially difficult in evaluation of patients with severe cardiopulmonary symptoms, who may not be able to hold their breath during image acquisition.

Complications and Contraindications

The complications observed during the Prospective Investigation of Pulmonary Embolism Diagnosis (PIOPED) study were tabulated according to these definitions

Table 16.1 Injection Factors for Pulmonary Angiography

Artery	Injection Rate (mL/s)	Quantity of Contrast Medium (mL)
Right/left pulmonary artery	20-25	40-50
Right/left pulmonary artery (pulmonary hypertension)	15-20	30-40
Lobar pulmonary arteries	15-20	30-40
Segmental pulmonary arteries	5-10	15-20

(**Table 16.2**). Three of the 5 deaths reported occurred owing to severe baseline cardiopulmonary compromise rather than catheterization or angiography. In another study, 3 deaths occurred in the presence of a RV end-diastolic pressure of >20 mmHg. Unlike in previous large series studies, no myocardial perforations occurred in PIOPED, which can be attributed to the exclusive use of pigtail type rather than straight catheters.

There are no absolute contraindications to pulmonary angiography, although risk clearly increases with severe pulmonary hypertension, allergy to iodine contrast, renal insufficiency, left bundle branch block, or severe congestive heart failure. With the use of nonionic, low-osmolar contrast, and prophylactic oxygen administration, the risks in these conditions may be reduced.

Table 16.2 Complications of Pulmonary Angiography in the Prospective Investigation of Pulmonary Embolism Diagnosis (PIOPED) Study ($N = 1111$)	
Major	
Death	5 (0.5%)
Cardiopulmonary resuscitation, ventilation	4 (0.4%)
Renal failure (dialysis)	3 (0.3%)
Hematoma (2-unit transfusion)	2 (0.2%)
Total	14 (1.3%)
Minor	
Respiratory distress	4 (0.4%)
Renal dysfunction	10 (0.9%)
Angina	2 (0.2%)
Hypotension	2 (0.2%)
Pulmonary congestion	4 (0.4%)
Urticaria, itching, or periorbital edema	16 (1.4%)
Hematoma	9 (0.81%)
Arrhythmia	6 (0.54%)
Subintimal contrast (dissection)	4 (0.4%)
Narcotic overdose	1 (0.1%)
Nausea and vomiting	1 (0.1%)
Right bundle branch block	1 (0.1%)
Total	60 (5.4%)

Data from Baum S, ed. *Abrams Angiography*. Little, Brown and Co; 1997.

PULMONARY EMBOLISM

The annual incidence of venous thromboembolism—DVT and PE—exceeds 1 per 1000. The main cause of early death is acute RV failure, although most deaths beyond 30 days are owing to underlying disease (eg, cancer, congestive heart failure, or chronic lung disease). The overall 3-month mortality is approximately 15%.

Noninvasive Imaging Tests

Ventilation Perfusion Scanning

Lung scanning has been the principal imaging test for suspected PE. However, an increasing number of hospitals obtain lung scans only in patients with clinical situations such as allergy to radiographic contrast agents, severe renal insufficiency, or pregnancy. Normal and high-probability lung scans are themselves diagnostic. However, most patients with suspected PE have ventilation perfusion scan results that are nondiagnostic (low- or intermediate- or indeterminate-probability scans). The diagnostic accuracy may be improved when scans are interpreted in conjunction with clinical pretest probability, but additional imaging studies are usually required.

Contrast-Enhanced Chest Computed Tomography

Chest CT has virtually replaced lung scanning as the initial imaging test for PE. The latest generation of multidetector CT scanners permits image acquisition of the entire chest with 1 mm resolution and a single breath hold of <10 seconds, enabling accurate imaging of the complete pulmonary vasculature. At the same time, the deep veins can be examined for proximal DVT by obtaining additional images from the pelvic and femoropopliteal regions. Chest CT also helps detect alternative diagnoses, such as aortic dissection, pneumonia, or pericardial tamponade. As compared with first-generation single-slice scanners, the sensitivity of multirow detector CT increases from about 70% to >90%.

In patients with confirmed PE, chest CT may also provide prognostic information in the presence of RV enlargement if identified in a reconstructed CT 4-chamber view. In a study of 63 patients with PE, a ratio of right to left ventricular dimension of >0.9 identified patients at risk for adverse clinical events. In a study of 260 patients with acute PE with CT signs of RV dysfunction, 3D ventricular volume measurement was a predictor of early death in patients with acute PE.

Venous Ultrasonography

Compression ultrasound study of the deep veins is noninvasive and accurate in diagnosing symptomatic proximal DVT. If it confirms DVT in patients with symptoms suggestive of PE, the diagnosis can be made without further workup. However, approximately half of the PE patients have no ultrasound evidence of DVT because the entire clot has already embolized to the lungs. Therefore, patients suspected of PE who have no evidence of DVT still require further investigation for PE.

Contrast Venography

Venography is required for catheter-directed thrombolysis, catheter embolectomy, percutaneous angioplasty with or without stent placement, and insertion of an IVC filter. Inferior vena cavography with iodinated contrast medium or medical grade carbon dioxide (30-40 mL CO_2) is performed to evaluate patency of the IVC and exclude cava duplication or renal vein anomaly prior to filter placement. CO_2 has no nephrotoxicity or allergic reaction and is safe in both the arterial (below the diaphragm) and the venous circulations if air contamination can be prevented.

Retrievable vena cava filters have largely replaced permanent filters to protect against PE in patients who have time-limited contraindication to anticoagulation.

Therefore, the filters should be removed once protection from PE is no longer needed to avoid the long-term risk of IVC filter placement.

Echocardiography

Transthoracic echocardiography has emerged as an important tool for risk stratification of patients with acute PE. The presence of RV dysfunction on the echocardiogram is an independent predictor of early death, but echocardiography cannot be recommended to diagnose or exclude PE routinely because about half of the patients with confirmed PE have normal echocardiogram. However, bedside echocardiography facilitates discrimination of patients suspected of having either PE or left-sided cardiogenic shock. Potentially lifesaving therapy, including thrombolysis, catheter intervention, or surgical embolectomy, can be initiated based on echocardiographic evidence of RV dysfunction without necessarily performing time-consuming PE imaging tests. **Figure 16.8** illustrates suggested diagnostic strategy for patients with suspected PE without cardiogenic shock.

Interpretation and Validity of Pulmonary Angiograms

Angiographic studies have validated the angiographic criteria for acute PE. Primary angiographic criteria for PE are persistent central or marginal intraluminal radiolucency

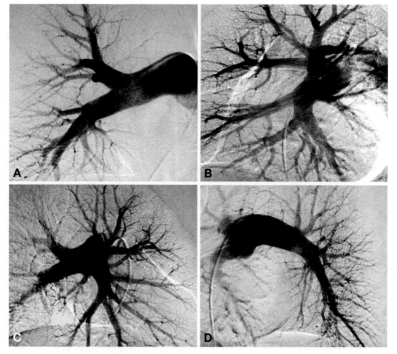

Figure 16.8 Normal pulmonary DSA. Prospective Investigation of Pulmonary Embolism Diagnosis (PIOPED) II study has adopted the following oblique projections for the right and left pulmonary angiography. **A,** Right pulmonary DSA (30° RAO). **B,** Right pulmonary DSA (40° LAO). **C,** Left pulmonary DSA (50° RAO). **D,** Left pulmonary DSA (40° LAO). DSA, digital subtraction angiography; LAO, left anterior oblique; RAO, right anterior oblique.

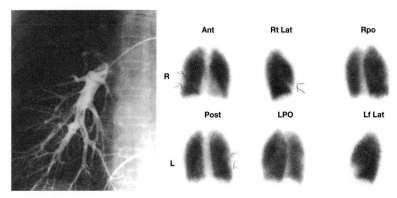

Figure 16.9 Primary evidence of acute pulmonary embolism. Selective cut-film angiogram of the right lower lobe pulmonary artery with multiple intraluminal radiolucencies, almost completely outlined by contrast (left), and the corresponding segmental perfusion defects (arrows) of the right lower lobe (right). Ant, anterior; Lf lat, left lateral; LPO, left posterior oblique; Post, posterior; Rpo, right posterior; Rt lat, right lateral.

and the trailing edge of an intraluminal radiolucency obstructive to contrast flow (**Figure 16.9**). Complete obstruction showing abrupt vessel cutoff with a concave border of the contrast column is also considered primary evidence of acute PE (**Figure 16.10**).

Hemodynamic Characteristics

Many PE patients without cardiopulmonary disease have normal hemodynamics. Systolic RV pressure rarely exceeds 50 mmHg in patients without preexisting cardiopulmonary disease. Instead, an acute increase in RV afterload with a systolic pressure above 50 to 60 mmHg will result in acute RV dilatation and systolic failure. Patients with recurrent PE may tolerate higher systolic pressure values prior to the

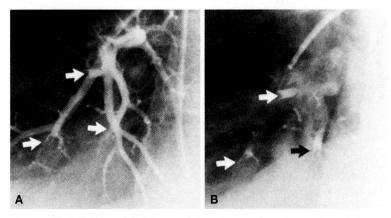

Figure 16.10 A, Right lower lobe balloon occlusion pulmonary cineangiogram demonstrates multiple vessels "cut off" (arrows). **B,** Balloon deflation facilitated distal contrast distribution, with a visible trailing edge of a thrombus (arrows).

development RV failure. As a result of RV diastolic dysfunction, the RV diastolic pressure approximates pulmonary artery diastolic pressure and typically shows a prominent dip and rapid rise (square root sign). Right atrial pressure is elevated, with a prominent A wave and a steep x-descent. As RV dilatation and dysfunction evolve, reduced RV output impairs left ventricular filling. Left ventricular distensibility may be further compromised owing to a shift of the interventricular septum toward the left ventricle. In PE patients, increased myocardial load can be quantified with brain natriuretic peptide levels; elevated troponin levels indicate increased RV strain.

Endovascular Therapy for Acute Pulmonary Embolism

In patients with massive PE, catheter intervention with or without embolectomy is an alternative to systemic thrombolysis or surgical embolectomy (**Figures 16.11** and **16.12**).

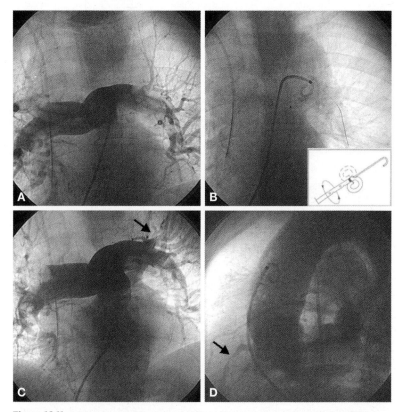

Figure 16.11 Catheter fragmentation in combination with a continuous systemic infusion of 100 mg alteplase over 2 hours in a 64-year-old woman with massive pulmonary embolism and cardiogenic shock. **A,** Frontal view demonstrating subtotal filling defects in both main pulmonary arteries. **B,** Catheter thrombus fragmentation in the left pulmonary artery (pars superior) using a pigtail rotational catheter. **C,** Following catheter fragmentation, improved flow in the left upper lobe pulmonary arteries (arrow) was accompanied by a prompt increase in systemic arterial pressure from 70 to 95 mmHg. **D,** Lateral view demonstrating a significant proximal stenosis of the right coronary artery approximately 7 seconds after nonselective injection of 40 mL contrast into the main pulmonary artery (arrow).

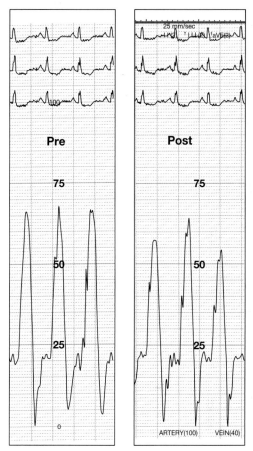

Figure 16.12 Right ventricular pressure curves pre and post catheter fragmentation in the patient from Figure 16.11. Despite rapid clinical improvement, there was only a mild decrease in right ventricular systolic pressure following catheter fragmentation.

Catheter intervention may be combined with local or systemic thrombolysis. Most of the devices appear to be effective, safe, and potentially lifesaving in the presence of large fresh clots, but none has been investigated in a controlled clinical trial.

The endovascular technique proceeds as follows: the right femoral vein or right internal jugular vein (if the femoral vein approach is not available due to DVT) is accessed using the micropuncture technique under ultrasound guidance. A 7F sheath is inserted in the femoral vein, and a 7F APC or MONT-1 catheter is advanced into the right atrium and manipulated through the tricuspid valve and right ventricle into the pulmonary artery. Contrast medium is injected under fluoroscopy to assess pulmonary artery blood flow and the severity of pulmonary emboli. Right and left pulmonary arteriograms are then obtained at reduced contrast injection rates and quantities. The pulmonary artery with the largest central embolus is cannulated, and a 7F-long sheath is placed over a heavy-duty guidewire such as Rosen wire guide (Cook Medical) or an Amplatz Super Stiff guidewire (Boston Scientific Corp). Catheter-directed mechanical thrombo-fragmentation and aspiration with intrathrombic injection of 10 mg of tissue plasminogen activator (tPA; alteplase, Genentech Inc) is performed to debulk central clot and achieve restoration of pulmonary artery blood flow. Any mechanical thrombectomy device can be used to remove clots. This initial intervention may be followed by catheter-directed thrombolysis with central infusion of tPA at 1 to 2 mg/h. The treatment of submassive PE may begin with catheter-directed thrombolysis with 1 to 2 mg/h of tPA infusion into the right and left pulmonary arteries using 2 infusion catheters for 18 to 24 hours. An IVC filter is usually put in place before or at the end of the intervention.

SUGGESTED READINGS

1. Adler J, Fan V, Edelman J, et al. Pulmonary vein stenosis after atrial fibrillation ablation. *Adv Pulm Hypertens*. 2018;16:149-151.
2. Albrecht MH, Bickford MW, Nance JW Jr., et al. State-of-the art pulmonary CT angiography for acute pulmonary embolism. *AJR Am J Roentgenol*. 2017;208(3):495-504.
3. Anaya-Ayala JE, Loebe M, Davies MG. Endovascular management of early lung transplant-related anastomotic pulmonary artery stenosis. *J Vasc Interv Radiol*. 2015;26(6):878-882.
4. Aronberg DJ, Glazer HS, Madsen K, Sagel SS. Normal thoracic aortic diameters by computed tomography. *J Comput Assist Tomogr*. 1984;8(2):247-250.
5. Baikoussis NG, Apostolakis E, Papakonstantinou NA, Sarantitis I, Dougenis D. Safety of magnetic resonance imaging in patients with implanted cardiac prostheses and metallic cardiovascular electronic devices. *Ann Thorac Surg*. 2011;91(6):2006-2011.
6. Batra K, Chamarthy MR, Reddick M, Roda MS, Wait M, Kalva SP. Diagnosis and interventions of vascular complications in lung transplant. *Cardiovasc Diagn Ther*. 2018;8(3):378-386.
7. Bhatt A, Al-Hakim R, Benenati JF. Techniques and devices for catheter-directed therapy in pulmonary embolism. *Tech Vasc Interv Radiol*. 2017;20(3):185-192.
8. Brown AH. Coronary steal by internal mammary graft with subclavian stenosis. *J Thorac Cardiovasc Surg*. 1977;73(5):690-693.
9. Cambria RP, Brewster DC, Gertler J, et al. Vascular complications associated with spontaneous aortic dissection. *J Vasc Surg*. 1988;7(2):199-209.
10. Cambria RA, Gloviczki P, Stanson AW, et al. Outcome and expansion rate of 57 thoracoabdominal aortic aneurysms managed non-operatively. *Am J Surg*. 1995;170(2):213-217.
11. Crawford ES, Svensson LG, Coselli JS, Safi HJ, Hess KR. Aortic dissection and dissecting aortic aneurysms. *Ann Surg*. 1988;208(3):254-273.
12. Creager MA, Gornik HL, Gray BH, et al. COCATS 4 Task Force 9: training in vascular medicine. *J Am Coll Cardiol*. 2015;65(17):1832-1843. doi:doi:10.1016/j.jacc.2015.03.025.
13. Cronin P, Dwamena BA. A clinically Meaningful Interpretation of the prospective investigation of pulmonary embolism diagnosis (PIOPED) scintigraphic data. *Acad Radiol*. 2017;24(5):550-562.
14. Dake MD, Miller DC, Semba CP, Mitchell RS, Walker PJ, Liddell RP. Transluminal placement of endovascular stent-grafts for the treatment of descending thoracic aortic aneurysms. *N Engl J Med*. 1994;331(26):1729-1734.
15. De Gregorio MA, Guirola JA, Lahuerta C, Serrano C, Figueredo AL, Kuo WT. Interventional radiology treatment for pulmonary embolism. *World J Radiol*. 2017;9(7):295-303.
16. Dunn KL, Wolf JP, Dorfman DM, Fitzpatrick P, Baker JL, Goldhaber SZ. Normal D-dimer levels in emergency department patients suspected of acute pulmonary embolism. *J Am Coll Cardiol*. 2002;40(8):1475-1478.
17. Fields JM, Davis J, Girson L, et al. Transthoracic echocardiography for diagnosing pulmonary embolism: a systematic review and meta-analysis. *J Am Soc Echocardiogr*. 2017;30(7):714-723.e4.
18. Gabella G. Cardiovascular system. In: Williams PL, Bannister LH, Berry MM, eds. *Gray's Anatomy*. Churchill Livingstone; 1995:1505-1546.
19. Glower DD, Speier RH, White WD, Smith LR, Rankin JS, Wolfe WG. Management and long-term outcome of aortic dissection. *Ann Surg*. 1991;214(1):31-41.
20. Hawkins IF. Carbon dioxide digital subtraction arteriography. *AJR Am J Roentgenol*. 1982;139(1):19-24.
21. Hirose Y, Hamada S, Takamiya M, Imakita S, Naito H, Nishimura T. Aortic aneurysms: growth rates measured with CT. *Radiology*. 1992;185(1):249-252.

22. Huang IKH, Nadarajah M, Teo LT, Ahmed DBAA, Pua U. Percutaneous coil embolization of traumatic juxtacardiac right inferior pulmonary vein pseudoaneurysm. *J Vasc Interv Radiol.* 2015;26(5):755.e1-757.e1.

23. Jahromi AS, Cina CS, Liu Y, Clase CM. Sensitivity and specificity of color duplex ultrasound measurement in the estimation of internal carotid artery stenosis: a systematic review and meta-analysis. *J Vasc Surg.* 2005;41(6):962-972.

24. Kaatee R, Beek FJ, de Lange EE, et al. Renal artery stenosis: detection and quantification with spiral CT angiography versus optimized digital subtraction angiography. *Radiology.* 1997;205(1):121-127.

25. Kuo WT. Endovascular therapy for acute pulmonary embolism. *J Vasc Interv Radiol.* 2012;23(2):167. e4-179.e4; quiz 179.

26. Lee JS, Moon T, Kim TH, et al. Deep vein thrombosis in patients with pulmonary embolism: prevalence, clinical significance and outcome. *Vasc Specialist Int.* 2016;32(4):166-174.

27. Lewis VD III, Meranze SG, McLean GK, O'Neill JA Jr., Berkowitz HD, Burke DR. The midaortic syndrome: diagnosis and treatment. *Radiology.* 1988;167(1):111-113.

28. Marsalese DL, Moodie DS, Vacante M, et al. Marfan's syndrome: natural history and long-term follow-up of cardiovascular involvement. *J Am Coll Cardiol.* 1989;14(2):422-428; discussion 429-431.

29. Mihai G, Simonetti OP, Thavendiranathan P. Noncontrast MRA for the diagnosis of vascular diseases. *Cardiol Clin.* 2011;29(3):341-350.

30. Moriarty JM, Edwards M, Plotnik AN, et al. Intervention in massive pulmonary embolus: catheter thrombectomy/thromboaspiration versus systemic lysis versus surgical thrombectomy. *Semin Intervent Radiol.* 2018;35(2):108-115.

31. Napel S, Marks MP, Rubin GD, et al. CT angiography with spiral CT and maximum intensity projection. *Radiology.* 1992;185(2):607-610.

32. Olin JW, Piedmonte MR, Young JR, DeAnna S, Grubb M, Childs MB. The utility of duplex ultrasound scanning of the renal arteries for diagnosing significant renal artery stenosis. *Ann Intern Med.* 1995;122(11):833-838.

33. Onteddu NK, Palumbo A, Kalva SP. Pulmonary vein varix with pulmonary vein stenosis. *J Vasc Interv Radiol.* 2017;28(1):147.

34. Ouwendijk R, de Vries M, Stijnen T, et al. Multicenter randomized controlled trial of the costs and effects of noninvasive diagnostic imaging in patients with peripheral arterial disease: the DIPAD trial. *AJR Am J Roentgenol.* 2008;190(5):1349-1357.

35. Park HS, Chamarthy MR, Lamus D, Saboo SS, Sutphin PD, Kalva SP. Pulmonary artery aneurysms: diagnosis and endovascular therapy. *Cardiovasc Diagn Ther.* 2018;8(3):350-361.

36. Saboo SS, Chamarthy M, Bhalla S, et al. Pulmonary arteriovenous malformations: diagnosis. *Cardiovasc Diagn Ther.* 2018;8(3):325-337.

37. Sharma A, Gulati GS, Parakh N, Aggarwal A. Pulmonary arteriovenous malformation in chronic thromboembolic pulmonary hypertension. *Indian J Radiol Imaging.* 2016;26(2):195-197.

38. Soto B, Harman MA, Ceballos R, Barcia A. Angiographic diagnosis of dissecting aneurysm of the aorta. *Am J Roentgenol Radium Ther Nucl Med.* 1972;116(1):146-154.

39. Srivastava A, Troop B, Peick A, Kanne A. Inferior vena cava filter placement at bedside using computed tomography scan information: a new technique for accurate deployment. *Am J Surg.* 2016;211(1):172-178.

40. Stein PD, Goldhaber SZ, Henry JW, Miller AC. Arterial blood gas analysis in the assessment of suspected acute pulmonary embolism. *Chest.* 1996;109(1):78-81.

41. Torikai H, Hasegawa I, Jinzaki M, Narimatsu Y. Preliminary Experience of endovascular embolization using N-butyl cyanoacrylate for hemoptysis due to infectious pulmonary artery pseudoaneurysms via systemic arterial approach. *J Vasc Interv Radiol.* 2017;28(10):1438.e1-1442.e1.

42. Tsuchiya N, van Beek EJR, Ohno Y, et al. Magnetic resonance angiography for the primary diagnosis of pulmonary embolism: a review from the international workshop for pulmonary functional imaging. *World J Radiol.* 2018;10(6):52-64.

43. Tsukada J, Hasegawa I, Torikai H, Sayama K, Jinzaki M, Narimatsu Y. Interventional therapeutic strategy for hemoptysis originating from infectious pulmonary artery pseudoaneurysms. *J Vasc Interv Radiol.* 2015;26(7):1046.e1-1051.e1.

44. Wahlers T, Laas J, Alken A, Borst HG. Repair of acute type A aortic dissection after cesarean section in the thirty-ninth week of pregnancy. *J Thorac Cardiovasc Surg.* 1994;107(1):314-315.

45. Wang TJ, Nam BH, D'Agostino RB, et al. Carotid intima-media thickness is associated with premature parental coronary heart disease: the Framingham Heart Study. *Circulation.* 2003;108(5):572-576.

46. Weaver FA, Pentecost MJ, Yellin AE, Davis S, Finck E, Teitelbaum G. Clinical applications of carbon dioxide/digital subtraction arteriography. *J Vasc Surg.* 1991;13(2):266-272; discussion 272-273.

47. Wible BC, Buckley JR, Cho KH, Bunte MC, Saucier NA, Borsa JJ. Safety and efficacy of acute pulmonary embolism treated via large-bore aspiration mechanical thrombectomy using the Inari FlowTriever device. *J Vasc Interv Radiol.* 2019;30(9):1370-1375.

17 Stress Testing During Cardiac Catheterization: Exercise and Dobutamine Challenge[1]

Patients with significant heart disease may have entirely normal hemodynamics when assessed in the resting state during cardiac catheterization. Because most cardiac symptoms are precipitated by exertion or some other stress, however, it may also be important to assess hemodynamic performance during some form of stress such as muscular exercise, pharmacologic intervention (eg, dobutamine infusion), or pacing-induced tachycardia. Such an evaluation enables the physician to assess the *cardiovascular reserve* and the relationship (if any) between specific symptoms and hemodynamic impairment. Physiologic information so obtained is often valuable in prescribing specific medical therapy, selecting patients for corrective cardiac surgery, and estimating prognosis.

Muscular exercise, particularly dynamic exercise, has been studied extensively in the cardiac catheterization laboratory, and the normal hemodynamic responses are reasonably well understood. There are major differences between the hemodynamic responses to dynamic exercise using either the arms or the legs, and these 2 types of exercises are discussed separately.

DYNAMIC EXERCISE

During dynamic exertion, skeletal muscles actively contract and develop force that is translated into motion and work. This is accompanied by an increase in both oxygen (O_2) consumption and carbon dioxide production by skeletal muscle and a corresponding increase in alveolar gas exchange needed to support the higher metabolic rate. In normal sedentary individuals, the level of O_2 consumption during maximal exercise (max) can increase about 12-fold in comparison with that during the resting state. In Olympic-class athletes, max may represent an 18-fold increase in O_2 consumption. The increased oxygen requirements of muscular exercise are met by both an increase in the cardiac output and an increased extraction of oxygen from arterial blood by skeletal muscle, which causes widening of the arteriovenous oxygen difference (AV O_2 difference).

The need for the heart to increase cardiac output appropriately for the increase in O_2 consumption resulting from exercise is met by an increase in *heart rate* and an increase in *stroke volume*. The relative contributions of these increases to the rise in cardiac output depend on the type of exercise (supine vs upright), the intensity of exercise, the limitation of diastolic filling at high heart rates, and the response to sympathetic stimulation. Metabolic adaptations of exercising muscle include a switch from use of free fatty acids at rest to an enhanced uptake of glucose. Because carbohydrate metabolism produces more carbon dioxide than fat metabolism does, the *respiratory quotient* (ratio of carbon dioxide production to O_2 consumption) rises from a resting value of 0.7 toward 1.0. The delivery of bloodborne oxygen and glucose to working skeletal muscle is enhanced by a reduction in skeletal muscle vascular resistance mediated by metabolic by-products and by sympathetically mediated vasoconstriction elsewhere, which causes a redistribution of blood away from the renal and splanchnic beds to the exercising muscle.

[1]We gratefully acknowledge the *Grossman & Baim's Cardiac Catheterization, Angiography, And Intervention*, 9th edition contributions of Drs. Marc D. Feldman, William Grossman, and Mauro Moscucci, as portions of their chapters, Stress Testing During Cardiac Catheterization: Exercise, Pacing and Dobutamine Challenge, were retained in this text.

Exercise depends on the adequacy of pulmonary function to increase oxygen supply. During progressive exercise, there is a linear increase in minute ventilation relative to the increase in O_2 consumption. When the intensity and duration of exercise are such that oxygen delivered to the exercising muscle is insufficient, anaerobic metabolism of glucose develops, causing metabolic acidosis and an increase in respiratory quotient to values >1.0; minute ventilation increases out of proportion to O_2 consumption. Beyond this *anaerobic threshold*, the accumulation of hydrogen ions and lactate usually causes skeletal muscle weakness, pain, and severe breathlessness. Thus, it is best to conduct exercise studies in the catheterization laboratory in such a way that the patient reaches a *steady-state level of submaximal exercise* below the anaerobic threshold and exercise can be sustained for greater than 6 minutes. This approach permits estimation of cardiovascular reserve and allows the physician to determine whether the increase in cardiac output is appropriate for the increase in O_2 consumption occurring at that particular level of exercise.

Oxygen Uptake and Cardiac Output

There is a linear relationship between O_2 consumption and increasing workload. Oxygen uptake increases steadily over a few minutes to reach a new steady state that is directly related to the intensity or level of exercise. Simultaneously, the mixed venous blood oxygen saturation decreases to a lower steady level related to the intensity of exercise, producing an increase in the AV O_2 difference.

The cardiac output increases linearly with increasing workload during both supine and upright exercise in normal subjects. As can be seen from the regression equation

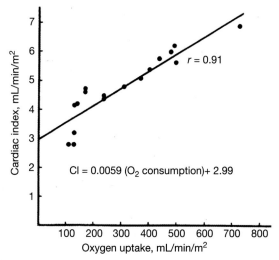

Figure 17.1 The relationship between cardiac output and oxygen consumption (both indexed for body surface area) during supine dynamic exercise of varying intensity in normal subjects, based on the data supplied by Dexter. As can be seen from the regression equation for this relationship, for each increment of 100 mL/min/m² of oxygen consumption, there is an increase in cardiac output of 590 mL/min/m². CI, cardiac index. (Data from Dexter L, Whittenberger JL, Haynes FW, Goodale WT, Gorlin R, Sawyer CG. Effect of exercise on circulatory dynamics of normal individuals. *J Appl Physiol*. 1951;3:439-453.)

for this relationship (**Figure 17.1**), for each increment of 100 mL/min/m² of O_2 consumption during exercise, there is an increase in cardiac output of 590 mL/min/m².

Exercise Index

The linear relationship between oxygen uptake and cardiac output during exercise, illustrated in **Figure 17.1**, may be used to assess whether the cardiac output response measured in an individual patient is appropriate to the level of exercise and increased oxygen uptake. The regression formula is CI = 0.0059X + 2.99, where CI is the cardiac index in liters per minute per square meter of body surface area (BSA) and X is the O_2 consumption in milliliters per minute per square meter BSA. This formula may be used to calculate the *predicted cardiac index* for a given level of O_2 consumption (X), and the predicted cardiac index may then be compared with the *measured cardiac index*.

This equation can be used to calculate a predicted cardiac index by measuring O_2 consumption during dynamic exercise. The patient's actual measured cardiac index during exercise is then divided by the predicted cardiac index to determine the deviation from normal:

$$\text{Exercise index} = \frac{\text{Measured cardiac index}\left(L/min/m^2\right)}{\text{Predicted cardiac index}\left(L/min/m^2\right)} \qquad (17.1)$$

We have termed this ratio the *exercise index*, since it allows expression of exercise capacity as a percentage of the normal response. An exercise index of 0.8 or higher indicates a normal cardiac output response to exercise.

Systemic and Pulmonary Arterial Pressure and Heart Rate

Systolic arterial pressure and mean arterial pressure also increase linearly in relation to O_2 consumption during dynamic exercise in normal subjects. Despite this increase in arterial pressure, systemic vascular resistance decreases substantially during dynamic exercise, indicating that the elevated arterial blood pressure is secondary to increased cardiac output. Patients who are unable to generate an adequate increase in cardiac output during dynamic exercise may also increase their arterial pressure; that is, in this circumstance, systemic vascular resistance does not decline and may actually increase.

The behavior of the pulmonary circulation in response to dynamic exercise is different from that of the systemic circulation in normal individuals. Mean pulmonary artery (PA) pressure increases almost proportionally with cardiac output (pulmonary blood flow), so that there is only a slight decrease in pulmonary vascular resistance, in contrast to the normal substantial decrease in the resistance of the systemic vasculature.

Heart rate increases consistently during both supine and upright dynamic exercise and tends to increase linearly in relation to O_2 consumption. During dynamic supine exercise in the catheterization laboratory, tachycardia is the predominant factor in increasing cardiac output. Tachycardia exerts a positive inotropic effect (treppe phenomenon), but increased sympathetic nervous system activity appears to be the most significant factor leading to enhanced myocardial contractility. In most normal subjects, supine bicycle exercise is accompanied by an increase in ejection fraction and other ejection indices off left ventricular (LV) systolic function with a decrease in LV end-systolic volume.

Upright vs Supine Exercise

The contributions of heart rate and stroke volume to cardiac output differ in supine and upright bicycle exercise. End-diastolic volumes at rest are near maximum when normal subjects are supine, smaller when they are sitting, and smallest when they are standing. When subjects are in the upright position, LV end-diastolic volume, cardiac output, and stroke volume are lower than when they are in the supine position. During erect bicycle exercise, most normal subjects demonstrate an increase in ejection fraction and reduction in end-systolic volume, some enhancement of LV end-diastolic volume, and an increase in stroke volume as well as heart rate. LV end-diastolic volume and stroke volume tend to increase up to about 50% of peak O_2 consumption and then to plateau or actually decrease at high levels of exercise. At high levels of exercise and fast heart rates, recruitment of the Frank-Starling mechanism may be blunted by the effects of tachycardia and limitation of diastolic filling owing to shortening of diastole. At high levels of upright exercise, the stroke volume is preserved by a progressive decrease in end-systolic volume and increase in ejection fraction in the presence of a constant or decreased LV end-diastolic volume. Studies of the effect of dynamic supine bicycle exercise in young adults have shown no changes or a fall in LV end-diastolic pressure (LVEDP) and volume during exercise. In contrast, studies of older normal subjects or patients with atypical chest pain and normal coronary arteries have generally shown that both dynamic supine and upright bicycle exercise are associated with an increase in LVEDP, which is consistent with an age-dependent reliance on an increase in preload during exercise. For example, in a group of 10 sedentary men whose average age was 46 years, there was a rise in LVEDP from 8 ± 1 to 16 ± 2 mmHg during supine bicycle exercise and a rise from 4 ± 1 to 11 ± 1 mmHg during upright bicycle exercise. The diminished heart rate and contractility responses during exercise and the resultant increased dependence on the Frank-Starling mechanism with aging may reflect an age-related decrease in responsiveness to adrenergic stimulation.

Left Ventricular Diastolic Function

In normal subjects, multiple adjustments occur to accommodate an increased transmitral flow into the left ventricle in the face of an abbreviated diastolic filling period and to maintain low pressures throughout diastole. Exercise is associated with a progressive acceleration of isovolumetric relaxation so that enhanced diastolic filling occurs with minimal change in mitral valve opening pressure. The exercise-induced enhancement of diastolic relaxation and filling is probably modulated by both adrenergic stimulation and increased heart rate.

In normal subjects, there is either no change or a downward shift in the LV diastolic pressure-volume relation during exercise (**Figure 17.2**). However, presence of ischemia or cardiac hypertrophy and heart failure with preserved ejection fraction may provoke an upward shift in the LV diastolic pressure-volume relationship, so that any level of LV end-diastolic volume is associated with a much higher LVEDP during exercise. In such patients, the left ventricle may be regarded as exhibiting increased chamber stiffness (decreased distensibility) during exercise. In patients with coronary artery disease, a transient but striking upward shift in the LV diastolic pressure-volume relation is common during episodes of ischemia. Patients with coronary artery disease who develop angina during dynamic exercise in the catheterization laboratory commonly show a marked rise in LVEDP. A careful study of the dynamics of LV diastolic filling during exercise in patients with coronary artery disease has been reported. LV diastolic pressure-volume relations in 34 patients with

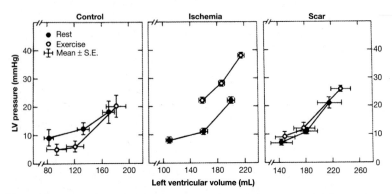

Figure 17.2 Left ventricular (LV) diastolic pressure-volume relations at rest and during exercise in patients without heart disease (control), as compared with patients with coronary disease who developed ischemia during exercise (ischemia) and patients with akinetic areas owing to previous infarction but no active ischemia during exercise (scar). Pressure and volume are averaged at 3 diastolic points: early diastolic pressure nadir, mid diastole, and end diastole. The control group had a downward shift of the early diastolic pressure-volume relation, but the ischemia group showed an upward and rightward shift. (From Carroll JD, Hess OM, Hirzel HO, Krayenbuehl HP Dynamics of left ventricular filling at rest and during exercise. *Circulation*. 1983; 68:59-67, with permission.)

coronary disease who developed ischemia during exercise were compared with those from 5 patients with minimal cardiovascular disease (control) and 5 patients with an akinetic area at rest from a prior infarction but no active ischemia during exercise (the scar group). There was an upward shift in the LV diastolic pressure-volume relationship during exercise-induced ischemia, which was not seen in either the scar or the control group (**Figure 17.2**). Therefore, interpretation of an exercise-induced rise in LVEDP in patients with coronary artery disease is complex and may be related to both a decrease in LV chamber distensibility and an increase in LV end-diastolic volume secondary to a reduction in ejection fraction.

The presence of cardiac hypertrophy is frequently characterized by depression of the rates of LV relaxation and diastolic filling at rest, and this depression profoundly impedes LV filling during exercise-induced tachycardia. In patients with conditions such as hypertrophic cardiomyopathy, in whom baseline LV end-systolic volumes are small, there is no reserve to further enhance systolic shortening, and abnormal diastolic properties limit the capacity to recruit the Frank-Starling mechanism during exercise. Furthermore, tachycardia may provoke ischemia (owing to impaired coronary vasodilator reserve), accompanied by an upward shift in the diastolic pressure-volume relationship.

Marked abnormalities in LV diastolic function occur with exercise in patients with clinical evidence of heart failure but normal resting systolic function (heart failure with preserved ejection fraction, or HFpEF). Patients with New York Heart Association class III or IV heart failure with 1 or more documented episodes of pulmonary edema and no significant coronary artery disease have been studied. These patients typically have LV ejection fractions of >50%, without echocardiographic evidence of regional wall motion abnormalities, or valvular or pericardial disease, and increased LV wall thickness and mass. Patients were studied by symptom limited upright exercise with simultaneous hemodynamic and radionuclide measurements, and the data were compared with those seen in age- and sex-matched healthy volunteers who served as controls. As can be seen in **Figure 17.3**, maximum exercise capacity was reduced, and the cardiac output increased primarily as a result of tachycardia, with no change in stroke volume. **Figure 17.4** shows that LV ejection fraction was normal at rest and with exercise for both patients and control subjects, but there was a striking rise in pulmonary capillary wedge pressure in patients with diastolic heart failure, as compared with the control subjects. Accordingly, these patients clearly have "pure" diastolic heart failure. As seen in **Figure 17.5**, diastolic distensibility markedly decreased with exercise in these patients. More recently, it has been demonstrated that exercise hemodynamics of patients who presented with exertional dyspnea of unknown etiology are helpful in making a diagnosis of diastolic dysfunction. These patients typically have EF of >50%, no significant coronary disease, normal brain natriuretic peptide, and normal resting hemodynamics (mean PA pressure <25 mmHg and PA

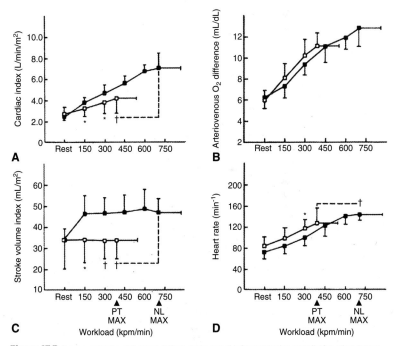

Figure 17.3 Seven patients with heart failure and normal left ventricular systolic function (open symbols) were compared with 10 age- and gender-matched healthy volunteers (solid symbols) who served as controls. All subjects underwent upright bicycle exercise with hemodynamic evaluation. Cardiac index increased for the patients with heart failure (A) as a result of an increase in initial stroke volume index (C), and heart rate (D), with fixed arteriovenous O_2 difference (B). NL MAX, normal subject maximum exercise; PT MAX, patient maximum exercise. (Reprinted from Kitzman D, Higginbotham MB, Cobb FR, et al. Exercise intolerance in patients with heart failure and preserved left ventricular systolic function: failure of the Frank-Starling mechanism. *J Am Coll Cardiol.* 1991;17:1065-1072. Copyright © 1991 Elsevier, with permission.)

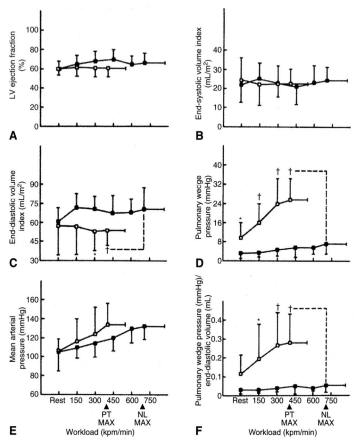

Figure 17.4 Response of left ventricular function to upright bicycle exercise in the patients with diastolic heart failure (□) and healthy controls (■) illustrated in **Figure 17.3**. Pulmonary wedge pressure increases dramatically (D), but left ventricular end-diastolic volume fails to increase in the patients with heart failure (C), as compared with healthy age- and gender-matched controls, as well as their ratio (F). LV ejection fraction remains normal (A) and end-systolic volume index and mean arterial pressure do not change (B and E). The intolerance to exercise is probably the result of increased pulmonary capillary wedge pressure and the resultant increased lung stiffness rather than decreased cardiac output or oxygen delivery to metabolizing tissues. NL MAX, normal subject maximum exercise; PT MAX, patient maximum exercise. (Reprinted from Kitzman D, Higginbotham MB, Cobb FR, et al. Exercise intolerance in patients with heart failure and preserved left ventricular systolic function: failure of the Frank-Starling mechanism. *J Am Coll Cardiol*. 1991;17:1065-1072. Copyright © 1991 Elsevier, with permission.)

wedge pressure [PCWP] < 15 mmHg; n = 55). On the basis of exercise hemodynamics, 32 of 55 patients were classified as having HFpEF (PCWP > 25 mmHg; n = 32) and 23 patients were classified as having noncardiac dyspnea (PCWP < 25 mmHg; **Figure 17.6**). These data support the value of exercise hemodynamics in reaching the correct diagnosis in selected patients with unexplained dyspnea.

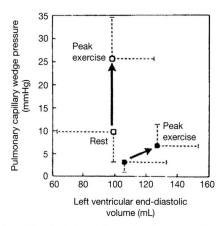

Figure 17.5 Plot of the relationship between changes in pulmonary capillary wedge pressure and left ventricular end-diastolic volume in the patients illustrated in **Figures 17.3** and **17.4**. In patients with diastolic heart failure, the stiff left ventricle cannot dilate normally (□) in response to the increased venous return during exercise, leading to a marked rise in left ventricular filling pressure, as compared with normal controls (■). (Reprinted from Kitzman D, Higginbotham MB, Cobb FR, et al. Exercise intolerance in patients with heart failure and preserved left ventricular systolic function: failure of the Frank-Starling mechanism. *J Am Coll Cardiol*. 1991;17:1065-1072. Copyright © 1991 Elsevier, with permission.)

Examples of the Use of Exercise to Evaluate Left Ventricular Failure in the Cardiac Catheterization Laboratory

A suggested supine bicycle exercise protocol for the cardiac catheterization laboratory is illustrated in **Table 17.1**. Examples of the hemodynamic changes that can occur during supine bicycle exercise are shown in **Tables 17.2** and **17.3**. Table 17.2 illustrates the response to 6 minutes of supine bicycle exercise of a 36-year-old woman with idiopathic dilated cardiomyopathy (ejection fraction 40%) whose major symptom was exertional dyspnea. Because her ejection fraction was only moderately depressed and her hemodynamic values were almost normal at rest, resting hemodynamic data alone did not clarify whether her cardiovascular reserve was impaired and whether her exertional dyspnea was likely to be cardiac in origin. During exercise, the cardiac index increased appropriately in relation to the increase in O_2 consumption, yielding an exercise index of 1.1.

$$\frac{\Delta \text{ cardiac index}}{\Delta O_2 \text{ consumption index}} = \frac{3,300}{387} = 8.5 \tag{17.2}$$

The increase in cardiac output, however, was accomplished at the cost of a substantial increase in mean pulmonary capillary wedge pressure, which rose from 11 to 27 mmHg. These data suggest that the patient had some limitation of inotropic reserve and that her ability to increase cardiac output depended heavily on use of the Frank-Starling mechanism. Therefore, her dyspnea can be considered to be of cardiac origin.

The case of a patient with more severe impairment of cardiovascular reserve is illustrated in **Table 17.3**, which shows the response to 6 minutes of supine bicycle

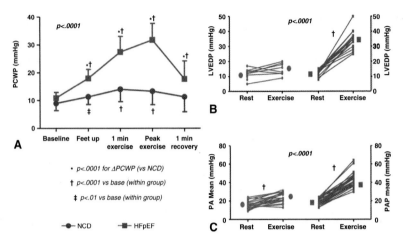

Figure 17.6 Exercise hemodynamics in patients with exertional dyspnea and preserved ejection fraction. Pulmonary capillary wedge pressure (PCWP) increased to a larger extent in patients with heart failure with preserved ejection fraction (HFpEF) as compared with patients with noncardiac dyspnea (NCD) with leg elevation and during exercise (A). PCWP returned to baseline almost immediately in recovery. Left ventricular end-diastolic pressure (LVEDP) (B) and mean pulmonary artery pressure (PAP) (C) also rose with exercise more dramatically in the HFpEF group (P for exercise change between groups). (Reproduced with permission from: Borlaug BA, Nishimura RA, Sorajja P, Lam CSP, Redfield MM. Exercise hemodynamics enhance diagnosis of early heart failure with preserved ejection fraction. *Circ Heart Fail*. 2010;3:588-595.)

exercise of a 60-year-old man with idiopathic dilated cardiomyopathy and symptoms of marked fatigue and dyspnea with minimal exertion. His chest radiograph showed cardiomegaly with no evidence of pulmonary edema, and his rest hemodynamics were almost normal. Supine bicycle exercise was associated with a marked rise in both left- and right-sided heart filling pressures and a marginal ability to increase cardiac output appropriately in relation to his increase in O_2 consumption. His exercise index was 0.85.

$$\frac{\Delta \text{ cardiac index}}{\Delta \text{ } O_2 \text{ consumption index}} = \frac{1700}{341} = 4.9 \tag{17.3}$$

Table 17.1 **Supine Bicycle Exercise Protocol**

Exercise	60 rpm
Initial workload	20 W
Increments	10 W/3 min
Hemodynamics	a. Baseline with leg elevation b. At 1.5 min into exercise (20 W) c. At peak exercise d. At 1 min into recovery

Table 17.2	Response to Supine Bicycle Exercise in a 36-Year-Old Woman With Dilated Cardiomyopathy	
Hemodynamic Parameter	**Resting**	**Exercise (6 min)**
Oxygen consumption index (mL/min/m²)	117	504
Atrioventricular oxygen difference (mL/L)	34	75
Cardiac index (L/min/m²)	3.4	6.7
Heart rate (beats/min)	80	140
Systemic arterial pressure (mmHg), systolic/diastolic (mean)	130/70 (95)	142/83 (110)
Right atrial mean pressure (mmHg)	6	7
Pulmonary capillary wedge mean pressure (mmHg)	11	27
Left ventricular pressure (mmHg)	130/17	142/28
Exercise index	—	1.1
Exercise factor	—	8.5

The cause of exercise intolerance in some patients with LV failure is diminished cardiovascular reserve, so that oxygen delivered to the working skeletal muscle is inadequate to meet the demands of aerobic metabolism. Some other patients are limited not by the inability to deliver oxygen to working skeletal muscle but by the rise in pulmonary capillary wedge pressure associated with exercise (**Table 17.2**).

Table 17.3	Response to Supine Bicycle Exercise in a 60-Year-Old Man With Dilated Cardiomyopathy	
Hemodynamic Parameter	**Resting**	**Exercise (6 min)**
Oxygen consumption index (mL/min/m²)	128	469
AV O_2 difference (mL/L)	40	96
Cardiac index (L/min/m²)	3.2	4.9
Heart rate (beats/min)	90	141
Systemic arterial pressure (mmHg), systolic/diastolic (mean)	91/62 (73)	107/67 (88)
Right atrial mean pressure (mmHg)	5	20
Pulmonary capillary wedge mean pressure (mmHg)	12	34
Left ventricular pressure (mmHg)	91/16	107/34
Exercise index	—	0.85
Exercise factor	—	4.9

As illustrated in these examples, the relative contributions of the inability of the heart to augment cardiac output versus an exercise-induced rise in pulmonary capillary wedge pressure that could impair gas exchange are controversial. Exercise tolerance in patients with congestive heart failure is highly variable and correlates poorly with ejection fraction. Studies of the hemodynamic and ventilatory response to exercise have shown that, as the clinical severity of congestive heart failure worsens, there is a progressive decrease in maximal O_2 consumption, premature onset of the anaerobic threshold, and decline in both maximal cardiac output and the cardiac output achieved at levels of submaximal O_2 consumption. Studies of brief exercise performed by patients with chronic congestive heart failure have shown that arterial oxygen saturation usually increases (presumably as a result of increased ventilation) despite elevation of the pulmonary capillary wedge pressure; maximal oxygen extraction is normal; and ventilatory mechanisms do not limit maximum O_2 consumption, so that both symptomatic limitation and the inability to normally increase oxygen delivery are caused by the failure to increase cardiac output adequately. Conversely, in patients with depressed LV ejection fraction who can achieve normal levels of exercise, factors that contribute to normal exercise capacity include normal augmentation of heart rate, the ability to increase cardiac output through further increases in LV end-diastolic volume and stroke volume, and tolerance of a high pulmonary venous pressure, possibly because of enhanced lymphatic drainage.

Therefore, in patients with severe depression of LV ejection fraction, the failure to increase cardiac output normally appears to be related both to the inability to increase stroke volume and to the inability to increase heart rate, as compared with age-matched subjects. This *impaired chronotropic response* appears to be caused by an impaired response to adrenergic stimulation that may be related to several defects, including a reduced cardiac receptor density, "uncoupling" of the receptor and adenylate cyclase activity, and deficient production of cyclic adenosine monophosphate.

Evaluation of Valvular Heart Disease

Valvular Stenosis

Exercise may also be used in the cardiac catheterization laboratory to evaluate valvular heart disease. Gradients across the atrioventricular and semilunar valves may become apparent during exercise and may reach levels that account for the clinical symptoms of the patient. Exercise hemodynamics are especially useful when the resting transvalvular gradient or estimated valve area has borderline significance.

An example of the hemodynamic changes during supine dynamic exercise in a patient with moderate mitral stenosis is shown in **Figure 17.7** and **Table 17.4**. As the result of increased mitral valve flow and a decreased diastolic filling period, the pressure gradient increased significantly, producing left atrial pressures of sufficient magnitude to cause symptoms. Cardiac output increased normally, yielding an exercise index of 1.2.

$$\frac{\Delta \text{ cardiac output}}{\Delta O_2 \text{ consumption}} = \frac{2,800}{481} = 5.8 \qquad (17.4)$$

These data are compatible with mild mitral stenosis and illustrate the changes in the diastolic pressure gradient across the mitral valve required to produce an increase in cardiac output appropriate to the increased oxygen requirements of strenuous exercise.

In evaluating hemodynamic changes across stenotic valves during exercise, it is often found that the calculated valve area during exercise varies somewhat from that

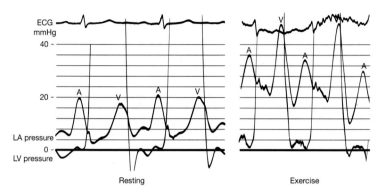

Figure 17.7 Simultaneous pressure recordings from left atrium and left ventricle at rest and at 5 minutes of bicycle ergometer exercise in a patient with mitral stenosis. The hemodynamic data for this patient are presented in **Table 17.4**.

calculated on the basis of resting data (it is usually slightly larger). This variance is usually small and may be related to actual changes in the degree of valvular obstruction (ie, a higher gradient and greater flow may force the stenotic leaflets to open wider), deficient data, or computational errors inherent in the assumptions applied to the equation for calculating valve orifice size.

Table 17.4 Hemodynamic Changes During Supine Dynamic Exercise in a Patient With Mitral Stenosis[a]

Parameter	Resting	Exercise (5 min)
Left atrial pressure (mmHg)		
A wave	20	34
V wave	18	46
Mean	10	26
Left ventricular mean diastolic pressure (mmHg)	1	4
Oxygen consumption (mL/min)	207	688
Atrioventricular oxygen difference (mL/L)	31	74
Cardiac output (L/min)	6.5	9.3
Heart rate (beats/min)	72	108
Mitral value area (cm^2)	1.6	1.8
Exercise index	—	1.2
Exercise factor	—	5.8

[a]Same patient as in **Figure 17.7**.

Valvular Insufficiency

The hemodynamic consequences of valvular insufficiency with ventricular volume overload may be subtle at rest. Dynamic exercise, by calling on the heart to substantially augment its forward cardiac output, may elicit changes in LVEDP and volume (preload) and in systemic vascular resistance (afterload) that are useful in assessing the cardiovascular limitations imposed by the valve lesion. Of particular importance, here is the inability of many patients with valvular insufficiency to increase forward cardiac output in an appropriate manner, resulting in a low exercise index. Dynamic exercise testing is especially valuable in such patients because the qualitative assessment of valvular insufficiency from angiograms may be unreliable and does not correlate well with the extent of functional impairment.

Figure 17.8 shows the hemodynamic response to dynamic bicycle exercise of a 55-year-old man with rheumatic heart disease and mitral regurgitation. The patient was able to increase cardiac output normally, but mean pulmonary capillary wedge pressure increased from 18 to 30 mmHg, with V-waves rising to 60 mmHg, during 6 minutes of supine bicycle exercise. This patient had successful mitral valve replacement with relief of symptoms.

Performing a Dynamic Exercise Test

Dynamic exercise during cardiac catheterization is easily performed with a bicycle ergometer while the patient is supine. A protocol detailing the exercise test should be prepared beforehand to ensure that all essential data are obtained (**Table 17.1**). Pressures should be obtained so that the appropriate valve gradients can be evaluated, and LV pressure should be monitored if LV performance is in question.

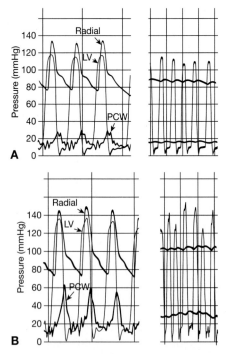

Figure 17.8 Hemodynamic findings during exercise in a 55-year-old man with mitral regurgitation. Left ventricular (LV), pulmonary capillary wedge (PCW), and radial artery pressure tracings are shown before (A) and during (B) the 6th minute of supine bicycle exercise. PCW mean pressure and V-wave increased substantially with exercise.

Supine bicycle exercise tests are performed most easily when catheterization is done via the arm (eg, brachial, radial) and/or neck (eg, jugular, brachial vein) approach.

We usually carry out a supine bicycle exercise test immediately after baseline hemodynamic values and cardiac output have been measured, before contrast angiography. The patient's feet are secured in the bicycle stirrups, and the right-sided heart, left-sided heart, and systemic arterial catheters and attached manifolds are positioned in such a way that they are not kinked or under tension and will not be disturbed during the exercise. Next, the system for measuring O_2 consumption is put in place (see Chapter 11). Alternatively, cardiac output can be assessed with the use of an indicator dilution technique (eg, thermodilution), and O_2 consumption can be estimated as the quotient of cardiac output and AV O_2 difference.

Before beginning exercise, the patient is instructed that they will be coached to achieve a certain level of submaximal exercise over the first 1 minute that can be sustained for an additional 4 to 6 minutes. A sufficient number of syringes for measuring systemic arterial and mixed venous (PA) blood oxygen saturation content should be at hand.

With the patient resting quietly and feet positioned on the bicycle, all manometers are zeroed, phasic and mean pressures are recorded, and cardiac output measurements are repeated to obtain an accurate pre-exercise baseline with legs elevated in the stirrups. Exercise is then begun with all pressures displayed continuously on the monitor. We generally record LV phasic pressure, systemic arterial (eg, radial or femoral artery) mean pressure, and pulmonary capillary mean pressure simultaneously. At each 1-minute interval, a brief recording of all 3 phasic pressures is done. Continuous observation and recording of pressures is important because it permits accurate monitoring of any rise in filling pressure or fall in arterial pressure during exercise and ensures that catheters remain in correct position for measurements at peak exercise.

After the patient has achieved a steady-state level of exercise for 4 minutes, simultaneous LV-systemic arterial, LV-PCW, and PCW-to-PA pullback pressures are recorded during minutes 4 to 6, without attempting to re-zero the transducers. The right-sided heart catheter is pulled back to the PA, and exercise cardiac output is measured by the Fick or thermodilution technique, at which time systemic arterial and PA blood samples are drawn for measurement of oxygen saturation.

Dynamic Arm Exercise

An excellent alternative to dynamic leg exercise is arm exercise during cardiac catheterization. In an era when maximum efficiency and rapid patient turnover are priorities, arm exercise offers many advantages. It does not require preloading of the bike apparatus before placement of the patient on the catheterization laboratory table. Furthermore, the risk to the femoral vessels and maintenance of the sterile field during leg exercise are also not issues. Most important is that, when performing arm exercise to exhaustion, it is just as relevant to making clinical decisions as dynamic leg exercise.

Dynamic arm exercise is associated with higher afterload due to the generation of higher arterial pressures than leg exercise. However, due to the smaller muscle mass, there is lower augmentation of SV. Why then does arm exercise at maximum intensity generate higher MVO_2 than leg exercise? The explanation is the presence of more efferent motor neurons in the arms than in the legs, resulting in greater sympathetic nerve activation. Consistent with these findings is greater release of plasma noradrenaline during arm exercise. Furthermore, arm and legs working at the same relative intensities result in greater utilization of glycogen and secondary release of lactate during arm exercise. Finally, there are no differences in end-tidal oxygen, end-tidal CO_2, or Hgb saturation with oxygen all as a function of a percentage of O_2 consumption, between arm and leg exercise.

Dynamic arm exercise has been used successfully to evaluate many clinical conditions. The severity of stenotic valves with minimal gradients at rest can be evaluated due to the increase in venous return and rise in filling pressures provided by arm exercise. Publications differentiating dyspnea on exertion due to HFpEF from other causes have always equally used dynamic arm or leg exercise and observe similar exercise hemodynamics with both forms of exercise. The differentiation of pulmonary hypertension due to a pulmonary disorder from a secondary disorder such as LV diastolic dysfunction has been successful with arm exercise as well. Finally, arm exercise had similar findings with leg exercise in post-heart transplant patients. The conclusion is that dynamic arm exercise is a very robust form of exercise and offers an alternative to leg exercise.

DOBUTAMINE STRESS TESTING

Dobutamine is a racemic mixture of 2 enantiomers that activates α1, β1, and β2 adrenergic receptors. The (−) enantiomer has strong α-agonist properties, the effect of which is counteracted by the partial agonism of the (+) enantiomer and by vasodilation secondary to activation of β2 receptors. At doses commonly used, dobutamine has a predominant positive inotropic effect resulting in increased myocardial contractility and stroke volume. Higher doses lead to an increase in heart rate and to a modest peripheral vasodilation. The vasodilation is mediated by stimulation of β2 receptors that antagonizes the α-effects of the (−) enantiomer. It should be noted that, in patients who are on β-blockers, administration of dobutamine can increase peripheral vascular resistance, possibly owing to the unopposed α-effect.

Dobutamine stress testing is commonly used in conjunction with other imaging modalities for the evaluation of ischemia and myocardial viability, and it has been used in the cardiac catheterization laboratory to assess contractile reserve in patients with reduced LV systolic function. In addition, dobutamine stress testing has emerged as a useful tool for assessing patients with low-flow, low-gradient aortic stenosis (AS). The definition of severe AS includes an aortic valve area (AVA) of <1 cm², a peak transalvular aortic valve velocity of >4 m/s, and a mean gradient of >40 mmHg. However, there is a subset of patients who exhibit a discrepancy in these hemodynamic parameters. In these patients, the AVA is <1 cm², but the mean gradient can be <30 mmHg (low-flow, low-gradient AS). This discrepancy has been described in patients with LV systolic dysfunction. The proposed mechanism for this discrepancy is that, in patients with reduced ejection fraction, contractility and stroke volume are inadequate to lead to full opening of the aortic valve, thus resulting in underestimation of the actual AVA. Inaccuracies related to the flow dependency of valve area calculations using the Gorlin formula have also been proposed. Studies have evaluated with dobutamine challenge 32 patients who had a calculated AVA of <1 cm², ejection fraction of <40%, and a mean gradient of <40 mmHg. Dobutamine infusion was started at 5 µg/kg/min, with increments of 3 to 10 µg/kg/min every 5 minutes. Contractile reserve was defined as an increase in stoke volume of >20% following dobutamine infusion. Endpoints used during dobutamine infusion were (1) maximum dose of 40 µg/kg/min, (2) mean gradient of >40 mmHg, (3) 50% increase in cardiac output, (4) a peak heart rate of >140 beats/min, or (5) development of symptoms. The average mean gradient was 27 ± 7 mmHg, and it increased to 41 ± 13 mmHg with dobutamine. Three patients who had a final AVA of >1.2 cm² and 4 patients who had a final mean gradient of <30 mmHg were not referred for surgery. On the basis of the results of the dobutamine test, 21 patients underwent aortic valve replacement. Severe calcific AS was found at the time of surgery in all the patients referred for surgery who had a final AVA of <1.2 cm² at peak dobutamine infusion and a mean gradient of >30 mmHg. Among the patients who underwent surgery, the survival rate at follow-up was 80% (12/15) in the group with contractile reserve and 33% (2/6) in a small group without contractile reserve (**Figure 17.9**). These data suggest that, in the setting of low-flow AS, dobutamine challenge can aid in the identification of patients with true AS and it can further provide risk stratification on the basis of contractile reserve. The likelihood of true anatomic valvular stenosis is low when dobutamine challenge results in an increase in valve area without an increase in gradient (**Figure 17.10**). In addition, the poor prognosis in patients without contractile reserve has been confirmed by other studies that have assessed the value of dobutamine echocardiography in this patient population. While patients with contractile reserve tend to do significantly better with surgery when compared with medical therapy, patients without contractile reserve have a very poor prognosis with either surgery or medical therapy (**Figure 17.11**). Thus, the assessment of contractile reserve can be used for further risk stratification and, in conjunction with other factors, for triaging patients toward the appropriate therapy. On the basis of these and other studies, current guidelines for the management of patients with valvular heart disease list dobutamine echocardiography or cardiac catheterization with dobutamine challenge as a class IIA indication for the evaluation of patients with low-flow, low-gradient AS.

More recently, the classification of AS has been expanded to paradoxical low-flow low-gradient AS, where the SV is less than 35 mL/m², the LVEF is greater than 50%, the AVA is less than 1.0, but the gradient is also less than 40 mmHg. These patients characteristically are predominantly women, have small LV cavities, severe concentric remodeling, and restrictive physiology. The application of dobutamine to these patients who have diastolic dysfunction similar to HFpEF is not currently recommended. However, operators need to rule out other causes for low-flow states when making a diagnosis of paradoxical low-flow low-gradient AS. These include restrictive LV physiology, mitral regurgitation, mitral stenosis, atrial fibrillation, right ventricle dysfunction, tricuspid

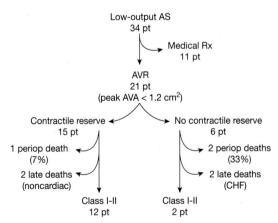

Figure 17.9 Clinical outcome of patients (pt) with low-output aortic stenosis (AS) who underwent aortic valve replacement (AVR). Contractile reserve was defined as an increase in stroke volume of >20% during dobutamine infusion. AVA, aortic valve area; CHF, congestive heart failure; periop, perioperative; Rx, treatment. (Reproduced with permission from: Nishimura RA, Grantham JA, Connolly HM, et al. Low-output, low-gradient aortic stenosis in patients with depressed left ventricular systolic function: the clinical utility of the dobutamine challenge in the catheterization laboratory. *Circulation*. 2002;106:809-813.)

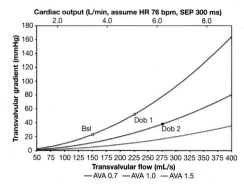

Figure 17.10 Plot of the relationship between mean gradient (*y*-axis) and transvalvular flow x-axis, bottom) according to the Gorlin formula for 3 different values of aortic valve area (AVA; 0.7, 1.0, and 1.5 cm²). Cardiac output (*x*-axis, top) is also shown, assuming a heart rate of 75 bpm and an SEP of 300 ms. At low transvalvular flows, mean gradient is low at all 3 valve areas. Two different responses to dobutamine challenge are illustrated for a hypothetical patient (O; Bsl) with a baseline flow of 150 mL/s, mean gradient of 23 mmHg, and calculated AVA of 0.7 cm². In one scenario (O; Dob 1), flow increases to 225 mL/s, mean gradient increases to 52 mmHg, and AVA remains at 0.7 cm², consistent with fixed aortic stenosis (AS). In the second scenario (•; Dob 2), flow increases to 275 mL/s, mean gradient increases to 38 mmHg, and AVA increases to 1.0 cm². This patient has changed to a different curve, consistent with relative or pseudo-AS. HR, heart rate; SEP, systolic ejection period. (Reproduced with permission from: Grayburn PA. Assessment of low-gradient aortic stenosis with dobutamine. *Circulation.* 2006;113:604-606.)

regurgitation, and decreased arterial compliance as in hypertension. Thus, other means are needed to confirm the diagnosis of paradoxical low-flow low-gradient AS. These include the severity of aortic valve deformity including thickening and calcification seen on echo. More recently, computed tomography scan has been used for a modified Agatston method to quantitate the degree of aortic valve calcification. A score greater than 1200 Agatston units (AU) for women and greater than 2000 AU for men is consistent with significant AS.

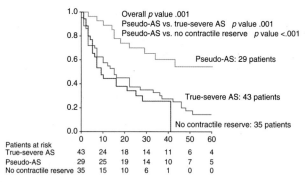

Figure 17.11 Kaplan-Meier survival estimates in low-flow/low-gradient aortic stenosis under conservative treatment according to the results of dobutamine testing. (Reproduced with permission from: Fougeres E, Tribouilloy C, Monchi M, et al. Outcomes of pseudo-severe aortic stenosis under conservative treatment. *Eur Heart J.* 2012:33:2426-2433.)

SUGGESTED READINGS

1. Adda J, Mielot C, Giorgi R, et al. Low-flow, low-gradient severe aortic stenosis despite normal ejection fraction is associated with severe left ventricular dysfunction as assessed by speckle-tracking echocardiography: a multicenter study. *Circ Cardiovasc Imaging.* 2012;5(1):27-35.

2. Ahlborg G, Jensen-Urstad M. Metabolism in exercising arm vs. leg muscle. *Clin Physiol.* 1991;11(5):459-468.

3. Balady GJ, Jacobs AK, Faxon DP, Ryan TJ. Dynamic arm exercise during cardiac catheterization in the assessment of stenotic valvular disease. *Clin Cardiol.* 1990;13(9):632-637.

4. Barry WH, Brooker JZ, Alderman EL, Harrison DC. Changes in diastolic stiffness and tone of the left ventricle during angina pectoris. *Circulation.* 1974;49(2):255-263.

5. Borlaug BA, Nishimura RA, Sorajja P, Lam CSP, Redfield MM. Exercise hemodynamics enhance diagnosis of early heart failure with preserved ejection fraction. *Circ Heart Fail.* 2010;3(5):588-595.

6. Borlaug BA, Jaber WA, Ommen SR, Lam CS, Redfield MM, Nishimura RA. Diastolic relaxation and compliance reserve during dynamic exercise in heart failure with preserved ejection fraction. *Heart.* 2011;97(12):964-969.

7. Braunwald E, Sonnenblick EH, Ross J Jr, et al. An analysis of the cardiac response to exercise. *Circ Res.* 1967;20(suppl I):44.

8. Bristow MR, Ginsburg R, Minobe W, et al. Decreased catecholamine sensitivity and beta-adrenergic-receptor density in failing human hearts. *N Engl J Med.* 1982;307(4):205-211.

9. Calbet JAL, Gonzalez-Alonso J, Helge JW, et al. Central and peripheral hemodynamics in exercising humans: leg vs arm exercise. *Scand J Med Sci Sports.* 2015;25(suppl 4):144-157.

10. Carroll JD, Hess OM, Krayenbuehl HP. Diastolic function during exercise-induced ischemia in man. In: Grossman W, Lorell BH, eds. *Diastolic Relaxation of the Heart.* Martinus Nijhoff; 1986:217.

11. Clavel M-A, Burwash IG, Pibarot P. Cardiac imaging for assessing low-gradient severe aortic stenosis. *JACC Cardiovasc Imaging.* 2017;10(2):185-202.

12. Colucci WS, Ribeiro JP, Rocco MB, et al. Impaired chronotropic response to exercise in patients with congestive heart failure. Role of postsynaptic beta-adrenergic desensitization. *Circulation.* 1989;80(2):314-323.

13. Dexter L, Whittenberger JL, Haynes FW, Goodale WT, Gorlin R, Sawyer CG. Effect of exercise on circulatory dynamics of normal individuals. *J Appl Physiol.* 1951;3(8):439-453.

14. Donald KW, Bishop JM, Cumming G, Wade OL. The effect of exercise on the cardiac output and circulatory dynamics of normal subjects. *Clin Sci.* 1955;14(1):37-73.

15. Feldman MD, Alderman JD, Aroesty JM, et al. Depression of systolic and diastolic myocardial reserve during atrial pacing tachycardia in patients with dilated cardiomyopathy. *J Clin Invest.* 1988;82(5):1661-1669.

16. Feldman MD, Ayers CR, Lehman MR, et al. Improved detection of ischemia-induced increases in coronary sinus adenosine in patients with coronary artery disease. *Clin Chem.* 1992;38(2):256-262.

17. Fifer MA, Borow KM, Colan S, Lorell BH. Early diastolic left ventricular function in children and adults with aortic stenosis. *J Am Coll Cardiol.* 1985;5:1147-1154.

18. Fougeres E, Tribouilloy C, Monchi M, et al. Outcomes of pseudo-severe aortic stenosis under conservative treatment. *Eur Heart J.* 2012;33(19):2426-2433.

19. Grayburn PA. Assessment of low-gradient aortic stenosis with dobutamine. *Circulation.* 2006;113(5):604-606.

20. Grossman W, McLaurin LP, Saltz SB, Paraskos JA, Dalen JE, Dexter L. Changes in the inotropic state of the left ventricle during isometric exercise. *Br Heart J.* 1973;35(7):697-704.

21. Grossman W. Diastolic dysfunction in congestive heart failure. *N Engl J Med.* 1991;325(22):1557-1564.

22. Higginbotham MB, Morris KG, Williams RS, McHale PA, Coleman RE, Cobb FR. Regulation of stroke volume during submaximal and maximal upright exercise in normal man. *Circ Res.* 1986;58(2):281-291.

23. Hoffman BB. Catecholamines, sympathomimetic drugs, and adrenergic receptor antagonists. In: Hardmon JG, Limbert LE, eds. *Goodman and Gilman: The Pharmacological Basis of Therapeutics.* McGraw Hill; 2001.

24. Karliner JS, LeWinter MM, Mahler F, Engler R, O'Rourke RA. Pharmacologic and hemodynamic influences on the rate of isovolumic left ventricular relaxation in the normal conscious dog. *J Clin Invest.* 1977;60(3):511-521.

25. Keteyian S, Marks CRC, Levine AB, et al. Cardiovascular responses of cardiac transplant patients to arm and leg exercise. *Eur J Appl Physiol.* 1994;68(5):441-444.

26. Kitzman D, Sullivan MJ. Exercise intolerance in patients with heart failure: role of diastolic dysfunction. In: Lorell BH, Grossman W, eds. *Diastolic Relaxation of the Heart.* 2nd ed. Kluwer; 1994:295.

27. Mann T, Brodie BR, Grossman W, McLaurin L. Effect of angina on the left ventricular diastolic pressure-volume relationship. *Circulation.* 1977;55(5):761-766.

28. Mann T, Goldberg S, Mudge GH Jr, Grossman W. Factors contributing to altered left ventricular diastolic properties during angina pectoris. *Circulation*. 1979;59(1):14-20.
29. McLaughlin DP, Beller GA, Linden J, et al. Hemodynamic and metabolic correlates of dipyridamole-induced myocardial thallium 201 perfusion abnormalities in multivessel coronary artery disease. *Am J Cardiol*. 1994;73(16):1159-1164.
30. Monin JL, Monchi M, Gest V, Duval-Moulin AM, Dubois-Rande JL, Gueret P. Aortic stenosis with severe left ventricular dysfunction and low transvalvular pressure gradients: risk stratification by low-dose dobutamine echocardiography. *J Am Coll Cardiol*. 2001;37(8):2101-2107.
31. Monin JL, Quere JP, Monchi M, et al. Low-gradient aortic stenosis: operative risk stratification and predictors for long-term outcome. A multicenter study using dobutamine stress hemodynamics. *Circulation*. 2003;108(3):319-324.
32. Murgo JP, Craig WE, Pasipoularides A. Evaluation of time course of left ventricular isovolumic relaxation in man. In: Grossman W, Lorell BH, eds. *Diastolic Relaxation of the Heart*. Martinus Nijhoff; 1986:217.
33. Nishimura RA, Grantham JA, Connolly HM, Schaff HV, Higano ST, Holmes DR Jr. Low-output, low-gradient aortic stenosis in patients with depressed left ventricular systolic function: the clinical utility of the dobutamine challenge in the catheterization laboratory. *Circulation*. 2002;106(7):809-813.
34. Otto CM, Nishimura RA, Bonow RO, et al. 2020 ACC/AHA guideline for the management of patients with valvular heart disease: a report of the American College of Cardiology/American Heart Association Joint Committee on Clinical Practice Guidelines. *J Am Coll Cardiol*. 2021;77(4):e25-e197. doi:10.1016/j.jacc.2020.11.018.
35. Paulus WJ. Upward shift and outward bulge: divergent myocardial effects of pacing angina and brief coronary occlusion. *Circulation*. 1990;81(4):1436-1439.
36. Plotnick GD, Becker LC, Fisher ML, et al. Use of the Frank-Starling mechanism during submaximal versus maximal upright exercise. *Am J Physiol*. 1986;251(6 Pt 2):H1101-H1105.
37. Powers SK, Dodd S, Woodyard J, Beadle RE, Church G. Haemoglobin saturation during incremental arm and leg exercise. *Br J Sports Med*. 1984;18(3):212-216.
38. Ricci D, Orlick A, Alderman E, et al. Role of tachycardia as an inotropic stimulus in man. *J Clin Invest*. 1979;63(4):695-703.
39. Schwammenthal E, Vered Z, Moshkowitz Y, et al. Dobutamine echocardiography in patients with aortic stenosis and left ventricular dysfunction: predicting outcome as a function of management strategy. *Chest*. 2001;119(6):1766-1777.
40. Tarantini G, Covolo E, Razzolini R, et al. Valve replacement for severe aortic stenosis with low transvalvular gradient and left ventricular ejection fraction exceeding 0.50. *Ann Thorac Surg*. 2011;91(6):1808-1815.
41. Weiner DA. Normal hemodynamic, ventilatory, and metabolic response to exercise. *Arch Intern Med*. 1983;143(11):2173-2175.
42. Weiss JL, Frederiksen JW, Weisfeldt ML. Hemodynamic determinants of the time-course of fall in canine left ventricular pressure. *J Clin Invest*. 1976;58(3):751-760.

18 Measurement of Ventricular Volumes, Ejection Fraction, Mass, Wall Stress, and Regional Wall Motion[1]

Direct measurement of ventricular dimension, area, and wall thickness allows calculation of volume, ejection fraction, mass, and wall stress. Assessment of pressure-volume relationships provides additional information regarding systolic and diastolic function of the ventricular chambers. Finally, the techniques developed to assess *regional* left ventricular wall motion have proved useful in the evaluation of patients with coronary artery disease.

VOLUMES
Technical Considerations

Ventriculograms are generally recorded in digital format at 15 to 30 frames per second (fps), and radiographic contrast material is usually injected into the left ventricle at rates of 7 to 15 mL/s for a total volume of 25 to 45 mL. Alternatively, the left ventricle may be visualized from contrast injections into the pulmonary artery, the left atrium (by the transseptal technique), or, in cases of severe aortic insufficiency, the aortic root.

With the widespread availability of computer systems, the technique of determining ventricular volumes has evolved from a handheld planimeter with pencil and paper (or a calculator) to semiautomated or fully automated software packages.

In the first step in assessing left ventricular chamber volume, the left ventricular outline or silhouette is traced. The ventricular silhouette should be traced at the *outermost margin of visible radiographic contrast* so as to include trabeculations and papillary muscles within the perimeter (**Figure 18.1**). The aortic valve border is defined as a line connecting the inferior aspects of the sinuses of Valsalva. More recent systems incorporate a semiautomated edge-detection algorithm, wherein some points on the ventricular silhouette are entered manually and others are supplied by the computer software, or a fully automated edge-detection algorithm.

To facilitate the calculation of left ventricular volume, the ventricle is often approximated by an ellipsoid. Alternatively, techniques based on Simpson rule, which is independent of assumptions regarding ventricular shape, may be used. According to this rule, the volume of any object is equal to the sum of the volumes of individual slices of known thickness composing the object. Thinner slices will result in more accurate measurements. Contemporary software programs may allow the user to choose between these 2 techniques. Because the x-rays emanate from a point source, they are nonparallel; correction must therefore be made for magnification of the ventricular image onto the detector. Finally, ventricular volumes calculated by most mathematical techniques overestimate true ventricular chamber volume, so that regression equations must be used to correct for the overestimation.

Biplane Formula

Biplane left ventriculography may be performed in the anteroposterior (AP) and lateral projections, the 30° right anterior oblique (RAO) and 60° left anterior oblique

---

[1]We gratefully acknowledge the *Grossman & Baim's Cardiac Catheterization, Angiography, and Intervention*, 9th edition contributions of Drs. Michael A. Feifer and William Grossman as portions of their chapter, Measurement of Ventricular Volumes, Ejection Fraction, Mass, Wall Stress, and Regional Wall Motion, were retained in this text.

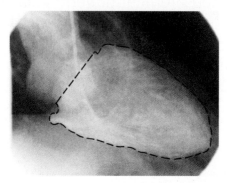

Figure 18.1 Left ventriculogram in the 30° right anterior oblique projection. The ventricular outline has been traced, as indicated by the broken line.

(LAO) projections, or angulated projections (eg, 45° RAO and 60° LAO/25° cranial). Although it has a complex geometric shape, the left ventricle can be approximated with considerable accuracy by an ellipsoid (**Figure 18.2**). The volume of an ellipsoid is given by the equation:

$$V = \frac{4}{3}\pi\frac{L}{2}\frac{M}{2}\frac{N}{2} = \frac{\pi}{6}LMN \qquad (18.1)$$

where V is the volume, L is the long axis, and M and N are the short axes of the ellipsoid. The long axis, L, is taken practically to be L_{max}, the longest chord that can be drawn within the ventricular silhouette in either projection. To determine M and N, each of the biplane projections of the left ventricle is approximated by an ellipse. M and N are taken to be the minor axes of these ellipses. They are calculated by the *area-length method*, as introduced by Dodge et al. from the silhouette areas and long-axis lengths in each projection, using the standard geometric formula for the area of an ellipse as a function of its major and minor axes. For biplane oblique

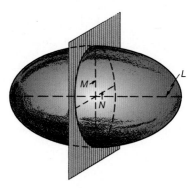

Figure 18.2 Ellipsoid used as a reference figure for the left ventricle. The long axis, L, and the short axes, M and N, are shown.

(RAO/LAO) left ventriculography, for example, the areas of the 2 ventricular silhouettes are given as:

$$A_{RAO} = \pi \frac{L_{RAO}}{2} \frac{M}{2} \text{ and } A_{LAO} = \pi \frac{L_{LAO}}{2} \frac{N}{2} \qquad (18.2)$$

L_{RAO} and L_{LAO} are the longest chords that can be drawn in the RAO and LAO silhouettes, respectively. The area of each traced silhouette (**Figure 18.1**) is obtained by planimetry, and M and N are calculated by rearrangement as follows:

$$M = \frac{4A_{RAO}}{\pi L_{RAO}} \text{ and } N = \frac{4A_{LAO}}{\pi L_{LAO}} \qquad (18.3)$$

Combining Eqs. (18.1) to (18.3):

$$V = \frac{\pi}{6} L_{max} \left(\frac{4A_{RAO}}{\pi L_{RAO}} \right) \left(\frac{4A_{LAO}}{\pi L_{LAO}} \right) = \frac{8}{3\pi} \frac{A_{RAO} A_{LAO}}{L_{min}} \qquad (18.4)$$

where L_{min} is the shorter of L_{RAO} and L_{LAO}. Because L_{RAO} is almost always longer than L_{LAO}, L_{LAO} is usually substituted for L_{min}.

Equation (18.4) is derived for projections at right angles, or *orthogonal* projections, and is applicable to biplane oblique ventriculography in the 30° RAO and 60° LAO views, as just described, or for the older AP and lateral format. Although it is not valid theoretically for nonorthogonal projections (eg, RAO and angulated LAO), it has been demonstrated empirically to be useful in those situations as well.

Right ventricular volumes have been calculated from biplane AP and lateral images using a modification of the Dodge area-length technique or Simpson rule. Because right ventricular volumes are rarely calculated from cineangiographic studies today, the reader is referred elsewhere for methodologic details.

Single-Plane Formula

The area-length ellipsoid method for estimating left ventricular chamber volume has been modified for use in the usual situation in which only single-plane measurements obtained in the AP or RAO projection are available. Inherent in single-plane methods is the assumption that the left ventricular shape may be approximated by a prolate spheroid—that is, an ellipsoid in which the 2 minor axes are equal. It is assumed that the minor axis of the ventricle in the projection used is equal to the minor axis in the orthogonal plane, which was not imaged. Recalling Eq. (18.1) for the general case of an ellipsoid:

$$V = \frac{\pi}{6} LMN \qquad (18.5)$$

If only single-plane (eg, RAO) ventriculography is done, we assume that $M = N$ and that L in the plane presented is the true long axis of the ellipsoid. M is calculated from the single-plane silhouette area (A) and L by the area-length method as $M = 4A/L$. Therefore, the single-plane volume calculation becomes:

$$V = \frac{\pi}{6} LM^2 = \frac{\pi}{6} L \left(\frac{4A}{\pi L} \right)^2 = \frac{8A^2}{3\pi L} \qquad (18.6)$$

Magnification Correction: Single Plane

Correction may be accomplished by imaging a calibrated grid at the estimated level of the ventricle and submitting the grid to the same magnification process as that to which the ventricle is subjected. Use of x-ray systems in which the center of the ventricle can be positioned at a fixed point (isocenter), around which the x-ray tubes and image intensifiers rotate, allows for magnification correction without the use of grids. The use of catheters with radiopaque markers separated by 1 cm can also yield accurate correction factors. In addition, an approximation of the magnification correction may be obtained by considering the diameter of the catheter used for left ventriculography. However, there is a large potential percentage error in measurement of this small dimension, and the percentage error in volumes derived from it is roughly triple that in the linear correction factor. In the single-plane formula, the cube of the linear correction factor adjusts the volume for magnification:

$$V = \frac{8}{3\pi}(CF)^3 \frac{A^2}{L} \qquad (18.7)$$

Magnification Correction: Biplane

In biplane studies, a correction factor (CF) must be calculated separately for each projection, yielding, in the case of biplane oblique cineangiography, CF_{RAO} and CF_{LAO}. The linear correction factor is multiplied by the measured lengths, and the square of this correction factor is multiplied by planimetered areas to convert to true lengths and areas. Accordingly, the corrected volume of the ventricle is:

$$V = \frac{8}{3\pi} \frac{(CF_{RAO})^2 (CF_{LAO})^2}{CF_{LAO}} \frac{A_{RAO} A_{LAO}}{L_{LAO}} = \frac{8 CF_{RAO}{}^2 CF_{LAO}}{3\pi} \frac{A_{RAO} A_{LAO}}{L_{LAO}} \qquad (18.8)$$

Regression Equations

Postmortem studies of hearts injected with contrast material have demonstrated that angiographic volumes calculated by Eq. (18.8) overestimate true left ventricular cavity volumes. This overestimation results in large part from the papillary muscles and trabeculae carneae, which do not contribute to blood volume but are nevertheless included within the traced left ventricular silhouette. Regression equations derived from these studies are used to adjust the calculated volumes. For cine studies in the 60° RAO/30° LAO projections, Wynne et al. used postmortem casts, as shown in **Figure 18.3**, to derive a regression equation. Single-plane techniques tend to overestimate volume significantly, as compared with biplane methods, and this is reflected in the single-plane regression equations. Regression equations are incorporated into commercial catheterization laboratory packages.

EJECTION FRACTION AND REGURGITANT FRACTION

Visual inspection of the cine images allows selection of frames depicting the maximum (end-diastolic) and minimum (end-systolic) ventricular volumes. The ejection fraction (EF) is then calculated as follows:

$$EF = \frac{EDV - ESV}{EDV} = \frac{SV}{EDV} \qquad (18.9)$$

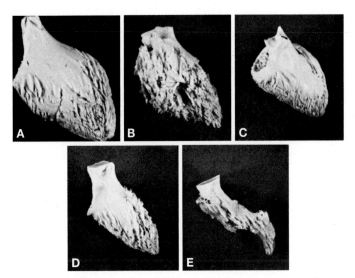

Figure 18.3 Left ventricular (A-E) casts made from fresh postmortem specimens of human hearts, using an encapsulant mixed with barium sulfate powder. The shape of the left ventricle only roughly approximates an ellipsoid of revolution; nevertheless, amazingly good correlation was obtained between true volume of these casts (measured by water displacement of the actual cast) and calculated volume. (From Wynne J, Green LH, Grossman W, et al. Estimation of left ventricular volumes in man from biplane cineangiograms filmed in oblique projections. *Am J Cardiol* 1978;41:726-732, with permission.)

where EDV is the end-diastolic ventricular volume, ESV is the end-systolic ventricular volume, and SV is the angiographic stroke volume.

In patients with aortic and/or mitral regurgitation, comparison of the angiographically determined stroke volume with the forward stroke volume determined by the Fick technique or (in the absence of concomitant tricuspid regurgitation) the thermodilution technique yields the regurgitant stroke volume, that portion of the ejected volume that is regurgitated, and therefore does not contribute to the net cardiac output. The regurgitant fraction (RF) is defined as follows:

$$RF = \frac{SV_{angiographic} - SV_{forward}}{SV_{angiographic}} \quad (18.10)$$

In cases of combined aortic and mitral regurgitation, estimation of the relative contribution of the 2 lesions must be made from the cineangiograms.

OTHER TECHNIQUES FOR MEASURING VENTRICULAR VOLUME AND EJECTION FRACTION

Image enhancement by computerized digital subtraction techniques can be used to obtain left ventriculograms after peripheral intravenous administration of contrast material. Peripheral injection of the contrast agent eliminates the problem of ventricular extrasystoles sometimes associated with direct injection of contrast material into the ventricular chamber. The image enhancement provided by the digital subtraction process permits also direct left ventricular injections with small volumes of contrast agents.

Alternatively, ventricular volume may be assessed noninvasively through the use of computed tomography, radionuclide ventriculography, or magnetic resonance imaging. Among these modalities, MRI has emerged as the accepted gold standard for measurement of left ventricular volumes.

The development of multielectrode catheters capable of measuring intracavitary electrical impedance has provided an additional tool for the measurement of ventricular volumes and ejection fraction without the use of contrast agents, and for the assessment of left ventricular performance through the evaluation of the end-systolic pressure-volume relationship. An illustration of the potential usefulness of this catheter in assessing left ventricular pressure-volume relationships is shown in **Figure 18.4**. Newer catheters, 5F to 7F in diameter, combine volume and micromanometer pressure measurements (**Figure 18.5**).

LEFT VENTRICULAR MASS

Measurement of left ventricular wall thickness, in addition to the parameters measured for volume determination, allows calculation of left ventricular wall volume and estimation of left ventricular mass (LVM). For these calculations, it is assumed that wall thickness is uniform throughout the ventricle. Wall thickness (h) is measured at end-diastole at the left ventricular free wall roughly two-thirds of the distance from the aortic valve to the apex in the AP or RAO projection. Appropriate magnification correction is applied. For biplane methods, the total volume of the left ventricular chamber and wall, V_{c+w}, is approximated by that of the corresponding ellipsoid:

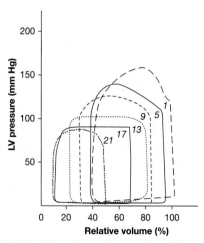

Figure 18.4 Use of multielectrode impedance catheter to obtain left ventricular pressure-volume loops every fourth beat during inhalation of amyl nitrate. (From McKay RG, Spears JR, Aroesty JM, et al. Instantaneous measurement of left and right ventricular stroke volume and pressure-volume relationships with an impedance catheter. *Circulation* 1984;69:703-710, with permission.)

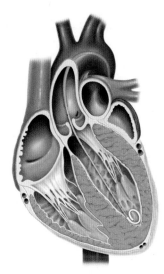

Figure 18.5 Pressure-volume catheter. This catheter includes 2 pressure sensors and 12 electrodes for simultaneous high-fidelity pressure and volume measurements. The pressure sensors are between the 4th and 5th electrodes, and 5 cm proximal to the 12th electrode. (Copyright © Miguel de la Flor, PhD, CMI.)

$$V_{c+w} = \frac{4}{3}\pi\left(\frac{L+2h}{2}\right)\left(\frac{M+2h}{2}\right)\left(\frac{N+2h}{2}\right)$$

$$= \frac{\pi}{6}(L+2h)\left(\frac{4A_{RAO}}{\pi L_{RAO}}+2h\right)$$

$$\cdot\left(\frac{4A_{LAO}}{\pi L_{LAO}}+2h\right) \tag{18.11}$$

As with h, appropriate correction for magnification must be applied to A and L so that V_{c+w} represents the total volume of the left ventricular chamber and wall corrected for magnification. For single-plane methods, it is assumed that $M = N$, yielding the single-plane formula:

$$V_{c+w} = \frac{\pi}{6}(L+2h)\left(\frac{4A}{\pi L}+2h\right)^2 \tag{18.12}$$

The volume of the chamber is calculated by the biplane or single-plane technique. To exclude the volume of the papillary muscles and trabeculae from the chamber volume (and thus include their mass in LVM), the appropriate regression equation is applied, so that V_c is the regressed value for chamber volume. LVM, then, is calculated as follows:

$$LVM = 1.050V_w$$
$$= 1.050(V_{c+w} - V_c) \tag{18.13}$$

where V_w is wall volume, and 1.050 is the specific gravity of heart muscle. This method has been validated by postmortem examination of hearts; however, it may not be accurate in the presence of marked right ventricular hypertrophy or pericardial effusion or thickening, where accurate measurement of wall thickness from the RAO silhouette may be impossible.

WALL STRESS

Consideration of ventricular pressure and volume is useful for the assessment of *ventricular* performance, whereas direct evaluation of *myocardial* function requires attention to forces acting at the level of the individual myocardial fiber. In particular, correction must be made for differences in ventricular wall thickness (h) and chamber radius (R), which modify the extent to which intraventricular pressure (P) is borne by the individual fiber; this is especially important in disease states characterized by ventricular hypertrophy or dilation or both. Such a correction may be achieved by consideration of wall stress (σ). Several formulas are commonly used to calculate stress, all related to the basic Laplace relation:

$$\sigma = \frac{PR}{2h} \tag{18.14}$$

Assumptions regarding the shape of the ventricular chamber and the properties of the ventricular wall have led to a number of such formulas for wall stress components in the circumferential, meridional, and radial directions (**Figure 18.6**). Consideration of circumferential and meridional stress has been particularly useful for clinical applications. A representative formula for calculation of circumferential stress, σ, is:

$$\sigma_c = \frac{Pb}{h}\left(1 - \frac{h}{2b}\right)\left(1 - \frac{hb}{2a^2}\right) \tag{18.15}$$

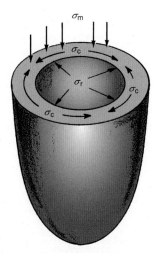

Figure 18.6 Circumferential (a_c), meridional (a_m), and radial (a_r) components of left ventricular wall stress for an ellipsoid model. The 3 components of wall stress are mutually perpendicular.

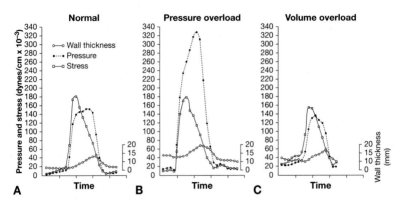

Figure 18.7 A comparison of changes in left ventricular pressure, wall thickness, and meridional stress throughout the cardiac cycle for representative normal (A), pressure-overloaded (B), and volume-overloaded (C) ventricles. These parameters are plotted at 40-ms intervals. In all 3 types of ventricles, peak stress occurs earlier than peak pressure. In the pressure-overloaded ventricle, peak pressure is markedly elevated but peak systolic stress and end-diastolic stress are normal. In the volume-overloaded ventricle, peak systolic stress is normal but end-diastolic stress is elevated. (From Grossman W, Jones D, McLaurin LP. Wall stress and patterns of hypertrophy in the human left ventricle. *J Clin Invest* 1975;56:56-64, with permission.)

where a and b are the major and minor semiaxes, respectively, at the midwall. Meridional stress, σ_m, may be calculated as follows:

$$\sigma_m = \frac{PR}{2h\left(1 + h/2R\right)} \qquad 18.16$$

where R is the internal chamber radius as bounded by the endocardial surface.

Calculation of wall stress in disease states has provided information not apparent from consideration of pressure and volume data alone. For example, it has been demonstrated that peak stress does not necessarily occur at the same time in the cardiac cycle as does peak pressure and that, in compensated pressure overload, the increase in ventricular pressure is offset by a proportional increase in wall thickness, so that wall stress remains normal (**Figure 18.7**).

PRESSURE-VOLUME CURVES

Simultaneous measurement of ventricular pressure and volume allows construction of the pressure-volume diagram (**Figure 18.4**). The position and slope of the diastolic portion of the pressure-volume curve provide information regarding diastolic properties of the ventricle. Construction of the systolic portion of the curve is useful for analysis of the end-systolic pressure-volume relation, a measure of ventricular contractile function.

REGIONAL LEFT VENTRICULAR WALL MOTION

The recognition that left ventricular regional dyssynergy is a more sensitive marker of coronary artery disease than is depression of global function has led to attempts to quantify abnormalities of regional wall motion. Left ventriculography is performed in the RAO or RAO and LAO projections. The ventricle is divided into regions by 1 of

2 methods: (1) construction of lines perpendicular to the major axis that divide the major axis into equal segments or (2) construction of lines drawn from the midpoint of the major axis to the ventricular outline at intervals of a fixed number of degrees. The extent of inward (or outward) movement of individual segments can then be measured, usually with the aid of computer techniques, providing quantitative measures of hypokinesis, akinesis, and dyskinesis.

SUGGESTED READINGS

1. Arcilla RA, Tsai P, Thilenius O, Ranniger K. Angiographic method for volume estimation of right and left ventricles. *Chest.* 1971;60(5):446-454.
2. Bunnell IL, Grant C, Greene DG. Left ventricular function derived from the pressure-volume diagram. *Am J Med.* 1965;39(6):881-894.
3. Dodge HT, Sandler H, Ballew DW, LORD JD Jr. The use of biplane angiocardigraphy for the measurement of left ventricular volume in man. *Am Heart J.* 1960;60:762-776.
4. Dodge HT, Hay RE, Sandler H. Pressure-volume of the diastolic left ventricle of man with heart disease. *Am Heart J.* 1962;64:503-511.
5. Fujita M, Sasayama S, Kawai C, Eiho S, Kuwahara M. Automatic processing of cine ventriculograms for analysis of regional myocardial function. *Circulation.* 1981;63(5):1065-1074.
6. Greene DG, Carlisle R, Grant C, Bunnell IL. Estimation of left ventricular volume by one-plane cineangiography. *Circulation.* 1967;35(1):61-69.
7. Grossman W, Jones D, McLaurin LP. Wall stress and patterns of hypertrophy in the human left ventricle. *J Clin Invest.* 1975;56(1):56-64.
8. Hood WP Jr, Rackley CE, Rolett EL. Wall stress in the normal and hypertrophied human left ventricle. *Am J Cardiol.* 1968;22(4):550-558.
9. Jones JW, Rackley CE, Bruce RA, Dodge HT, Cobb LA, Sandler H. Left ventricular volumes in valvular heart disease. *Circulation.* 1964;29:887-891.
10. Kass DA, Midei M, Graves W, Brinker JA, Maughan WL. Use of a conductance (volume) catheter and transient inferior vena caval occlusion for rapid determination of pressure-volume relationships in man. *Cathet Cardiovasc Diagn.* 1988;15(3):192-202.
11. Kasser IS, Kennedy JW. Measurement of left ventricular volumes in man by single-plane cineangiocardiography. *Invest Radiol.* 1969;4(2):83-90.
12. Kennedy JW, Reichenbach DD, Baxley WA, Dodge HT. Left ventricular mass: a comparison of angiocardiographic measurements with autopsy weight. *Am J Cardiol.* 1967;19(2):221-223.
13. Kennedy JW, Trenholme SE, Kasser IS. Left ventricular volume and mass from single-plane cineangiocardiogram: a comparison of anteroposterior and right anterior oblique methods. *Am Heart J.* 1970;80(3):343-352.
14. McKay RG, Aroesty JM, Heller GV, et al. Left ventricular pressurevolume diagrams and end-systolic pressure-volume relations in human beings. *J Am Coll Cardiol.* 1984;3(2 Pt 1):301-312.
15. McKay RG, Spears JR, Aroesty JM, et al. Instantaneous measurement of left and right ventricular stroke volume and pressure-volume relationships with an impedance catheter. *Circulation.* 1984;69(4):703-710.
16. Miller GAH, Brown R, Swan HJC. Isolated congenital mitral insufficiency with particular reference to left heart volumes. *Circulation.* 1964;29:356-365.
17. Nissen SE, Elion JL, Grayburn P, Booth DC, Wisenbaugh TW, DeMaria AN. Determination of left ventricular ejection fraction by computer densitometric analysis of digital subtraction angiography: experimental validation and correlation with area-length methods. *Am J Cardiol.* 1987;59(6):675-680.
18. Rackley CE, Dodge HT, Coble YD Jr, Hay RE. A method for determining left ventricular mass in man. *Circulation.* 1964;29:666-671.
19. Sandler H, Dodge HT. The use of single plane angiocardiograms for the calculation of left ventricular volume in man. *Am Heart J.* 1968;75(3):325-334.
20. Sasayama S, Nonogi H, Kawai C, Fujita M, Eiho S, Kuwahara M. Automated method for left ventricular volume measurement by cineventriculography with minimal doses of contrast medium. *Am J Cardiol.* 1981;48(4):746-753.
21. Sasayama S, Nonogi H, Kawai C. Assessment of left ventricular function using an angiographic method. *Jpn Circ J.* 1982;46(10):1127-1137.
22. Sheehan FH, Bolson EL, Dodge HT, Mathey DG, Schofer J, Woo HW. Advantages and applications of the centerline method for characterizing regional ventricular function. *Circulation.* 1986;74(2):293-305.

23. Sheehan FH, Schofer J, Mathey DG, et al. Measurement of regional wall motion from biplane contrast ventriculograms: a comparison of the 30 degree right anterior oblique and 60 degree left anterior oblique projections in patients with acute myocardial infarction. *Circulation*. 1986;74(4):796-804.

24. Sievers B, Schrader S, Rehwald W, Hunold P, Barkhausen J, Erbel R. Left ventricular function assessment using a fast 3D gradient echo pulse sequence: comparison to standard multi-breath hold 2D steady state free precession imaging and accounting for papillary muscles and trabeculations. *Acta Cardiol*. 2011;66(3):349-357.

25. Takx RAP, Moscariello A, Schoepf UJ, et al. Quantification of left and right ventricular function and myocardial mass: comparison of low-radiation dose 2nd generation dual-source CT and cardiac MRI. *Eur J Radiol*. 2012;81(4):e598-e604.

26. Wynne J, Green LH, Mann T, Levin D, Grossman W. Estimation of left ventricular volumes in man from biplane cineangiograms filmed in oblique projections. *Am J Cardiol*. 1978;41(4):726-732.

27. Yin FCP. Ventricular wall stress. *Circ Res*. 1981;49:829-842.

28. Zhong L, Ghista DN, Tan RS. Left ventricular wall stress compendium. *Comput Methods Biomech Biomed Engin*. 2012;15(10):1015-1041.

19 Evaluation of Systolic and Diastolic Function of the Ventricles and Myocardium[1]

A critical aspect of most cardiac catheterization procedures is the evaluation of myocardial function. At its simplest, this consists of a visual assessment of the left ventricular (LV) contractile pattern from the left ventriculogram, together with measurement of LV end-diastolic pressure (LVEDP). In laboratories where patients have right-sided heart catheterization and cardiac output measurement as part of the standard cardiac catheterization procedure, additional information about LV function may be gleaned from cardiac output, stroke volume, and pulmonary capillary wedge pressure, whereas right ventricular (RV) function is reflected by the values of right ventricular end-diastolic pressure (RVEDP) and right atrial pressure.

SYSTOLIC FUNCTION
Preload, Afterload, and Contractility

Systolic function of the myocardium is a reflection of the interaction of myocardial preload, afterload, and contractility. *Preload* is the load that stretches myofibrils during diastole and determines the end-diastolic sarcomere length. For the left ventricle, this load is often quantified as the LVEDP. This pressure (P), together with LV wall thickness (h) and radius (R), determines LV end-diastolic *wall stress ($\sigma \approx PR/h$)*, which is an estimate of the force stretching the myocardial fibers at end diastole. The end-diastolic stress or stretching force is resisted by the intrinsic stiffness or elasticity of the myocardium, and the interaction of end-diastolic stretching force and myocardial stiffness determines the extent of end-diastolic sarcomere stretch. If the myocardium is diffusely fibrotic or infiltrated with amyloid, a very high end-diastolic stretching force may be required to produce even a normal end-diastolic sarcomere length. In such a case, LVEDP may be very high (eg, >25 mmHg), and attempts to lower it by diuretic or venodilator therapy may lead to reduction in end-diastolic sarcomere stretch to subnormal values and a concomitant fall in cardiac output.

Increased preload augments the extent and velocity of myocardial shortening at any given afterload. In the intact heart, the relationship is more complex because increases in preload generally produce increases in LV chamber size and LV systolic pressure. Therefore, *afterload* (the force resisting systolic shortening of the myofibrils) also increases, and this increase tends to blunt the increases in the extent and velocity of myocardial shortening caused by increased diastolic fiber stretch.

Afterload varies throughout systole as the ventricular systolic pressure rises and blood is ejected from the ventricular chamber. LV systolic stress approximates the force resisting myocardial fiber shortening within the wall of the ventricle. End-systolic wall stress is considered by many to be the final afterload that determines the extent of myocardial fiber shortening when preload and contractility are constant. An increase in end-systolic wall stress results in a decrease in myocardial fiber shortening. For the intact ventricle, an increase in afterload (end-systolic wall stress) therefore results in a fall in stroke volume and ejection fraction (EF).

[1]We gratefully acknowledge the *Grossman & Baim's Cardiac Catheterization, Angiography, and Intervention*, 9th edition contributions of Drs. William Grossman and Mauro Moscucci, as portions of their chapter, Evaluation of Systolic and Diastolic Function of the Ventricles and Myocardium, were retained in this text.

Contractility refers to the property of heart muscle that accounts for alterations in performance induced by biochemical and hormonal changes; it has classically been regarded to be independent of preload and afterload. Contractility is generally used as a synonym for *inotropy*: both terms refer to the level of activation of cross-bridge cycling during systole. Contractility changes are assessed in the experimental laboratory by measuring myocardial function (extent or speed of shortening, maximum force generation) while preload and afterload are held constant. In contrast to skeletal muscle, the strength of contraction of heart muscle can be increased readily by a variety of biochemical and hormonal stimuli, some of which are listed in **Table 19.1**.

Assessment of systolic function requires consideration of the simultaneous influence of afterload, preload, and contractility. Systolic function should *not* be regarded as synonymous with contractility. Major depression of systolic function can occur with normal contractility, as in conditions with the so-called afterload excess (see later discussion).

Table 19.1 Hormones and Drugs That Influence Myocardial Contractility

Agent	Presumed Mechanism	Influence on Contractility
Catecholamines with β-agonist activity	β-Receptor stimulation →↑ adenylate cyclase activity →↑ cyclic AMP →↑ Ca^{++} influx through sarcolemma →↑ cytosolic Ca^{++}	+
Digitalis glycosides	Inhibition of Na^+/K^+ ATPase →↑ intracellular Na^+ →↑ Na^+/Ca^{++} exchange →↑ cytosolic Ca^{++}	+
Calcium salts	↑ Extracellular Ca^{++} →↑ Ca^{++} influx via slow channels and Na^+/Ca^{++} exchange →↑ cytosolic Ca^{++}	+
Caffeine	Multiple actions: Local release of catecholamines Inhibition of sarcoplasmic reticular Ca^{++} uptake Inhibition of phosphodiesterase →↑ cyclic AMP ↑ Sensitivity of contractile proteins of Ca^{++}	+
Milrinone, amrinone, other bipyridines	Phosphodiesterase inhibition →↑ cyclic AMP →↑ cytosolic Ca^{++}	+
Thyroid hormone	Increases myosin ATPase activity by altering production of certain myosin isozymes	+
Calcium sensitizers (Levosimendan, Pimobendan, EMD-57033, MCI-154)	Augmentation of Ca^{++}-Troponin C binding Activation of myosin Effect on cross-bridge association and dissociation rates	
Calcium-blocking agents (verapamil, nifedipine, D600, diltiazem)	Block Ca^{++} entry via slow channels	−
Barbiturates, ethanol	Depress contractility by unknown mechanism	−

Isovolumic Indices

One of the oldest and most widely used measures of myocardial contractility is the maximum rate of rise of LV systolic pressure, dP/dt. In 1962, Gleason and Braunwald first reported measurement of dP/dt in humans. They studied 40 patients with micromanometer catheters. Maximum dP/dt in those patients without hemodynamic abnormalities ranged from 841 to 1696 mmHg/s in the left ventricle and 223 to 296 mmHg/s in the right ventricle. Interventions known to increase myocardial contractility, such as exercise and infusion of norepinephrine or isoproterenol, caused major increases in dP/dt. Increased heart rate produced by intravenous atropine also caused a rise in maximum dP/dt, and the authors attributed this to the *Treppe phenomenon* described by Bowditch and characterized by a gradual increase in contractility following rapid sequential stimulation. This phenomenon, also known as the staircase effect, is felt to be secondary to accumulation of intracellular Na^+, leading to a reduction in Na^+/Ca^{++} exchange (3 inward Na^+ exchanged for one outward Ca^{++}) during the repolarization phase of the action potential and a corresponding increase in cytosolic Ca^{++}. In the study by Gleason and Braunwald, acute increases in arterial pressure and afterload produced by infusion of the a-adrenergic vasoconstricting agent methoxamine produced little change in dP/dt. These points are illustrated in **Figures 19.1** and **19.2**.

In normal subjects and in patients with no significant cardiac abnormality, maximum dP/dt increases significantly in response to isometric exercise, dynamic exercise, tachycardia by atrial pacing or atropine, β-agonists, and digitalis glycosides. Relatively, few studies have been done in humans to assess the changes in dP/dt induced by alterations in afterload and preload, but some studies do indicate that maximum positive dP/dt tends to increase slightly (6%-8%) with moderate increases in LV preload and shows little change with methoxamine-induced increases or nitroprusside-induced decreases in mean arterial pressure of 25 to 30 mmHg. Extensive studies in animals have examined the influence of changes in afterload, preload, and contractility on maximum dP/dt. These studies generally show that maximum dP/dt rises with increases in afterload and preload, but the changes were quite small (<10%) in the physiologic range.

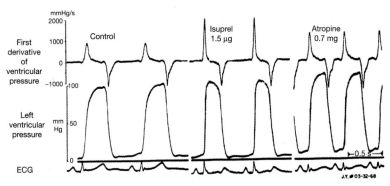

Figure 19.1 Micromanometer recordings of left ventricular pressure and its first derivative, dP/dt, in a patient with normal left ventricular function. Isoproterenol markedly increases contractility with large increments in positive dP/dt. Atropine produces tachycardia, which results in a Treppe effect and a rise in +dP/dt above control. ECG, electrocardiography. (From Gleason WL, Braunwald E. Studies on the first derivative of the ventricular pressure pulse in man. *J Clin Invest.* 1962;41:80-91, with permission.)

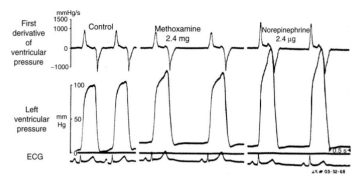

Figure 19.2 Micromanometer recordings of left ventricular (LV) pressure and dP/dt, as in **Figure 19.1**. Methoxamine raises arterial and LV systolic pressure but does not increase +dP/dt. In contrast, the combined α- and β-adrenergic effects of norepinephrine increase LV systolic pressure and +dP/dt. ECG, electrocardiography. (From Gleason WL, Braunwald E. Studies on the first derivative of the ventricular pressure pulse in man. *J Clin Invest.* 1962;41:80, with permission.)

Accurate measurement of dP/dt requires a pressure measurement system with excellent frequency-response characteristics. Micromanometer catheters are usually required to achieve this frequency-response range.

In addition to dP/dt, several other isovolumic indices have been introduced in an attempt to obtain a "pure" contractility index, completely independent of alterations in preload and afterload. These indices include the maximum value of (dP/dt)/P, where P is LV pressure (the maximum value of (dP/dt)/P is sometimes called V_{PM}); (peak dP/dt)/IIT, where IIT is the integrated isovolumic tension; (dP/dt)/CPIP, where CPIP is the common peak isovolumic pressure; V_{max}, the extrapolated value of (dP/dt)/P versus P when $P = 0$; (dP/dt)/P_D when the developed LV pressure, P_D, equals 5, 10, or 40 mmHg; and the fractional rate of change of power, which involves the second derivative of LV pressure.

Although changes in dP/dt reflect acute changes in inotropy in a given individual, the usefulness of dP/dt is reduced in comparisons between individuals, especially when there has been chronic LV pressure or volume overload. Peak dP/dt generally increases in patients with chronic aortic stenosis, even though contractility is normal or decreased in most of these patients. To account for chronic changes in LV geometry and mass that occur with chronic LV overload, some investigators have examined the rate of rise of systolic wall stress. The peak value of dσ/dt may be used as a contractility index, as may be the spectrum plot that relates dσ/dt to instantaneous σ (**Figure 19.3**).

Pressure-Volume Analysis

Since the time of Frank and Starling, pressure-volume (PV) diagrams have been used to analyze ventricular function. The normally contracting left ventricle ejects blood under pressure and, as shown in **Figure 19.4**, the relationship between its pressure generation and ejection can be expressed in a plot of LV pressure against volume.

Stroke Work

The area ABCD enclosed within the PV diagram in **Figure 19.4** is the external left ventricular stroke work (LVSW), represented mathematically as $\int P dV$. The calculation of LVSW is most accurate when it is derived by integrating the area within a complete PV diagrams.

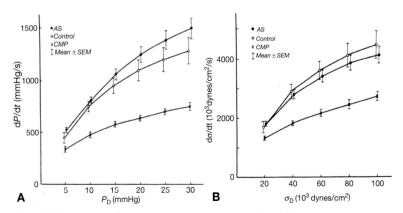

Figure 19.3 Left ventricular (LV) isovolumic indices of contractility. **A,** Rate of pressure development (dP/dt) as a function of LV-developed pressure (P_D). Mean values in control subjects (open circles), patients with aortic stenosis (AS, filled circles), and patients with dilated cardiomyopathy (CMP, crosses) are shown. Brackets represent standard errors of the mean (SEM). **B,** Rate of wall stress development (ds/dt) as a function of LV-developed stress (σ_D) for the same groups. There are no significant differences for patients with AS as compared with controls, although patients with CMP clearly show depressed values for dP/dt and dσ/dt at all levels of P_D and σ_D. (From Fifer MA, Gunther S, Grossman W, Mirsky I, Carabello B, Barry WH. Myocardial contractile function in aortic stenosis as determined from the rate of stress development during isovolumic systole. *Am J Cardiol.* 1979;44:1318-1325, with permission.)

LVSW is a reasonably good measure of LV systolic function in the absence of volume or pressure overload conditions, both of which may substantially increase calculated LVSW. The normal LVSW in adults is approximately 90 ± 30 cJ (mean ± SD); in adult patients with dilated cardiomyopathy or heart failure from extensive prior myocardial infarction, LVSW is often <40 cJ. Values <25 cJ indicate severe LV systolic failure, and when LVSW is <20 cJ, the prognosis is grave.

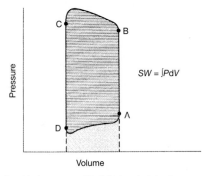

Figure 19.4 Diagram of ventricular pressure *(P)* plotted against simultaneous ventricular volume *(V)* for a single cardiac contraction. For the left ventricle (LV), point A represents end-diastole; segment AB, isovolumic contraction; point B, aortic valve opening; segment BC, LV ejection; point C, aortic valve closure and end ejection; segment CD, isovolumic relaxation; point D, mitral valve opening; and segment DA, LV filling. LV stroke work (SW) is represented by the cross-hatched area, and the stippled area represents diastolic work done on the left ventricle by the right ventricle and left atrium (see text for details)

LVSW is a measure of total LV chamber function and can be considered to reflect myocardial contractility only when the ventricle is reasonably homogeneous in its composition, as in most patients with dilated cardiomyopathy. For patients with coronary artery disease and extensive myocardial infarction, LVSW may be depressed even though well-perfused areas of the myocardium with normal contractility remain.

Because power is the rate at which work is done, LV power in the normal heart is the integral of the product of LV pressure during ejection and aortic flow. LV power may be regarded as a measure of overall LV contractile function; with refinement (such as the measurement of preload-adjusted maximal power), it can be used as a measure of the inotropic state.

Ejection Phase Indices

LV systolic function can be assessed using only the volume data from the *P-V* diagram. One of the most widely used indices of LV systolic performance is the EF, which is defined as follows:

$$EF = (LVEDV - LVESV)/LVEDV \qquad (19.1)$$

where LVEDV and LVESV are the LV end-diastolic and end-systolic volumes, respectively. In the cardiac catheterization laboratory, left ventricular EF (LVEF) is most often derived from the LV angiogram. If the EF is divided by the ejection time (ET), measured from the aortic pressure tracing, the quotient is called *mean normalized systolic ejection rate (MNSER)*.

$$MNSER = \frac{(LVEDV - LVESV)}{(LVEDV)(ET)} \qquad (19.2)$$

Finally, another ejection phase index of LV systolic function is the velocity of circumferential fiber shortening, V_{CF}. This is calculated as the rate of shortening of a theoretic LV myocardial fiber in a circumferential plane at the midpoint of the long axis of the ventricle. For convenience, mean V_{CF} is used most often, rather than instantaneous or peak V_{CF}. Mean V_{CF} is obtained by subtracting the end-systolic endocardial circumferential fiber length (nD_{ES}) from the end-diastolic endocardial circumferential fiber length (nD_{ED}) and then dividing by ET and normalizing for end-diastolic circumferential fiber length:

$$V_{CF} = (\pi D_{ED} - \pi D_{ES})/\pi D_{ED}(ET)$$
$$= (D_{ED} - D_{ES})/D_{ED}(ET) \qquad (19.3)$$

D_{ED} and D_{ES} are end-diastolic and end-systolic minor axis dimensions. Although V_{CF} can be calculated from angiographic data using the area-length method ($D = 4 A/\pi L$), it is most commonly calculated from the values of D measured by M-mode echocardiography. Normal values for isovolumic and ejection phase indices are given in **Table 19.2**.

Ejection indices depend heavily on preload and afterload and cannot be regarded as reliable indices of contractility in conditions associated with altered loading conditions. For example, increases in preload cause the EF (and other ejection indices) to rise; consequently, LVEF may be increased in patients with mitral or aortic regurgitation, severe anemia, or other causes of increased diastolic LV inflow and may mask underlying deterioration of myocardial contractility. Conversely, increases in afterload cause the EF to fall; consequently, LVEF

Table 19.2 Evaluation of Left Ventricular Systolic Performance: Normal Values of Some Isovolumic and Ejection Phase Indices

Contractility Indices	Normal Values (Mean ± SD)
Isovolumic indices	
Maximum dP/dt	1610 ± 290 mmHg/s
	1670 ± 320 mmHg/s
	1661 ± 323 mmHg/s
Maximum $(dP/dt)/P$	44 ± 8.4 s^{-1}
	1.47 ± 0.19 ML/s
$(dP/dt)/P_D$ at P_D = 40 mmHg	37.6 ± 12.2 s^{-1}
Ejection phase indices	
LVSW	81 ± 23 cJ
LVSWI	53 ± 22 cJ/m^2
	41 ± 12 cJ/m^2
EF (angiographic)	0.72 ± 0.08
MNSER	
Angiographic	3.32 ± 0.84 EDV/s
Echographic	2.29 ± 0.30 EDV/s
Mean V_{CF}	
Angiographic	1.83 ± 0.56 ED circ/s
	1.50 ± 0.27 ED circ/s
Echographic	1.09 ± 0.12 ED circ/s

circ, circumference; dP/dt, rate of rise of left ventricular pressure; ED, end-diastolic; EDV, end-diastolic volumes; EF, ejection fraction; LVSW, left ventricular stroke work; LVSWI, left ventricular stroke work index; ML, muscle length; MNSER, mean normalized systolic ejection rate; P_D, developed left ventricular pressure; SD, standard deviation; V, volume; V_{CF}, velocity of circumferential fiber shortening.

may be low in patients with severe aortic stenosis or other causes of increased resistance to systolic ejection and may falsely suggest underlying depression of myocardial contractility.

An LVEF of <0.40 indicates depressed LV systolic pump function, and if there is no abnormal loading to account for it, an LVEF of <0.40 can be taken to signify depressed myocardial contractility. An LVEF < 0.20 corresponds to severe depression of LV systolic performance and is usually associated with a poor prognosis. Interpretation of EF and other ejection indices improves by consideration of the ventricular preload and afterload, and the latter values are defined most precisely by end-diastolic and end-systolic wall stresses, respectively.

End-Systolic Pressure-Volume and σ-Length Relations

Over the past 40 years, several groups have shown that the LV end-systolic P-V, pressure-diameter, and σ-length relationships accurately reflect myocardial contractility, independent of changes in ventricular loading. This has been established in a series of studies in animals and humans. The fundamental principle of end-systolic P-V analysis is that at end-systole, there is a single line relating LV chamber pressure to volume, unique for the level of contractility and independent of loading conditions. The LV end-systolic P-V line can be generated by producing a series of P-V loops (such as the one in **Figure 19.4**) over a range of loading conditions (**Figure 19.5**). The line connecting the upper left corners of the individual P-V diagrams is the end-systolic P-V line (**Figure 19.5A**), characterized by a slope and by an x-axis intercept called V_0 (the extrapolated end-systolic volume when end-systolic pressure is zero). Current evidence indicates that an increase in contractility shifts the end-systolic P-V line to the left with a steeper slope, and a depression in contractility is associated with a displacement of the line downward and to the right, with a reduced slope. Although there is some uncertainty as to the meaning of V_0, it is generally agreed that an increase in slope of the end-systolic P-V line is a sensitive indicator of an increase in contractility. However, the technique of end-systolic analysis may not be as useful in comparisons among subjects as it is in comparisons of values in a single subject measured before and after an intervention. The end-systolic P-V lines for groups of patients with normal, intermediate, and depressed LV contractility are shown in **Figure 19.6**.

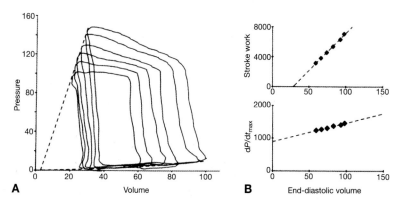

Figure 19.5 A, Left ventricular (LV) pressure-volume loops obtained during rapid LV unloading achieved by inferior vena cava (IVC) balloon occlusion in a patient undergoing cardiac catheterization. Volume was obtained by a conductance catheter technique. **B,** Relationships between stroke work, maximum rate of rise of LV systolic pressure, dP/dt$_{max}$, and LV end-diastolic volume. (From Kass DA, Maughan WL. From E_{max} to pressure-volume relations: a broader view. *Circulation.* 1988;77:1203, with permission.)

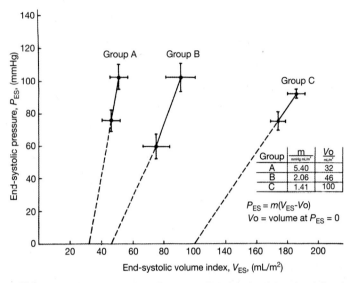

Figure 19.6 Left ventricular (LV) end-systolic pressure (P_{ES}) plotted against end-systolic volume index (V_{ES}) at 2 levels of loading for each of 3 patient groups: Group A, patients with normal LV contractile function; Group B, patients with moderate depression of LV contractile performance; Group C, patients with marked depression of LV contractility. Depressed contractility shifts the P_{ES}-V_{ES} relation to the right, with a reduced slope (m) and increased intercept (V_0). (From Grossman W, Braunwald E, Mann JT, McLaurin LP, Green LH. Contractile state of the left ventricle in man as evaluated from end-systolic pressure relations. *Circulation*. 1977;45:845-852, with permission.)

Relationship Between Peak dP/dt and End-Diastolic Volume

Little and coworkers examined the relationship between LV dP/dt *max* and end-diastolic volume and have proposed the slope of this relationship as an index of contractile state. They showed that, on theoretical grounds, this relationship can be derived from the LV end-systolic P-V relationship; both provide estimates of maximal myocardial elastance. This relationship is simpler to derive because both LV end-diastolic volume and dP/dt max are more readily defined than either end-systolic pressure or volume. One need not be concerned about a lack of coincidence between end-systole and maximal elastance, as with the end-systolic P-V relationship. The dP/dt–end-diastolic max volume relationship, however, is yet to be evaluated extensively in the clinical setting. Also, the end-systolic P-V relationship can be estimated clinically by entirely noninvasive methods. Nevertheless, the relationship between dP/dt max and end-diastolic volume represents an intriguing concept and may prove to be a valuable index of contractile state.

Stress-Shortening Relationships

Another approach to the assessment of LV systolic performance and myocardial contractility involves measuring the extent of cardiac muscle shortening and relating this shortening to the systolic wall stress (σ) resisting shortening.

If a ventricle is presented with progressively increasing resistance to ejection, σ rises while the extent of myocardial shortening declines. Therefore, a plot of systolic σ on the horizontal axis against myocardial shortening expressed as EF, VC_p or percent fractional shortening (%Δ*D*) on the vertical axis yields a tight inverse relationship (**Figure 19.7**). Data from studies of individual patients may then be compared with these normal values. In **Figure 19.7**, if the point relating end-systolic σ (σ) and %Δ*D* for a given patient lies within the confidence lines of the normal population, myocardial contractility is likely to be normal; however, if the σ_{es}-%Δ*D* point lies below the normal range, contractility is depressed even if %Δ*D* is normal.

Plots of systolic wall stress against LVEF have been analyzed for patients with a variety of conditions, including LV pressure overload. In these plots, comprising multiple individual data points (each point relating LV wall σ and EF for an individual patient), an inverse systolic σ-EF relationship is apparent for patients with chronic LV pressure overload. This suggests that the depressed LVEF in some of these individuals is caused by excessive systolic σ; that is, the load-resisting systolic shortening is abnormally high and is responsible for a reduced extent of shortening. This combination of high σ and low EF is sometimes referred to as *afterload* mismatch, and it implies that hypertrophy has been inadequate to return systolic wall stress to its relatively low normal level. Patients in whom LVEF is diminished out of proportion to any increase in systolic wall stress can be assumed to have depressed myocardial contractility (**Figure 19.8**).

A refinement of this approach involves measuring the relation between end-systolic LV wall stress and the heart rate–corrected velocity of fiber shortening. This approach was found to be sensitive and preload independent in an assessment of LV response to nitroprusside and dopamine infusions in patients with dilated cardiomyopathy. In that study, this approach was more sensitive to detecting increased contractility than was LV d*P*/d*t*.

The advantage of σ-shortening analysis over *P-V* diagram analysis is that wall σ takes into consideration changes in LV geometry and muscle mass that occur in response to chronic alterations in loading.

Myocardial Deformation Analysis—Left Ventricular Strain

Recently, left ventricular strain analysis has emerged as a valid and sensitive method to assess left ventricular systolic performance. A simple definition of strain is the

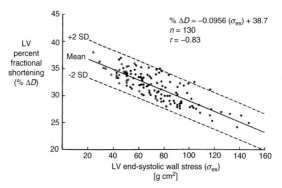

Figure 19.7 Relationship between left ventricular (LV) end-systolic wall stress (σ_{es}) and % fractional shortening (%Δ*O*) measured by echocardiography for 130 control points, at rest (open circles) or during methoxamine infusion (solid circles). The inverse relationship defines normal LV myocardial contractility. (From Borow KM, Green LH, Grossman W, et al. Left ventricular end-systolic stress-shortening and stress-length relations in humans. *Am J Cardiol.* 1982;50:1301-1308, with permission.)

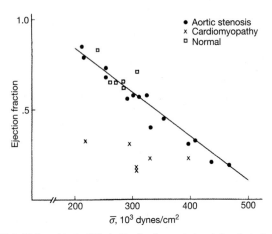

Figure 19.8 Plot of left ventricular (LV) ejection fraction against systolic σ, including patients with aortic stenosis (solid circles), dilated cardiomyopathy (*crosses*), and normal ventricular function (open squares). The regression line was constructed from the patients with normal LV function and those with aortic stenosis (see text for discussion). (From Gunther S, Grossman W. Determination of ventricular function in pressure overload hypertrophy in man. *Circulation*. 1979;5:679-688, with permission.)

measure of the amount of change in dimension (deformation) of an object when a force is applied. When applied to myocardial fiber, the following parameters are defined:

$$L_0 = \text{Baseline length}$$
$$L = \text{Final length}$$

The corresponding strain measurement will be the solution of the equation:

$$\varepsilon = (L - L_0)/L_0 \qquad (19.4)$$

Thus, the measurement of strain is dimensionless, and it is expressed as percentage. Positive values correspond to myocardial segments lengthening, and negative values correspond to myocardial segments shortening. The application of strain analysis involves a thorough understanding of the 3-dimensional deformation of the left ventricle during systole, which includes longitudinal shortening (negative strain), circumferential shortening (negative strain), radial thickening (positive strain), and the additional "torsion/twist" clockwise/counterclockwise rotation of the base and of the apex (**Figure 19.9**). Strain rate is the local rate of deformation per unit time and it is determined according to the equation:

$$(\Delta L/L_0)\Delta t = (\Delta L/\Delta t)L_0 = \Delta V L_0. \qquad (19.5)$$

Tissue Doppler imaging (TDI) and speckle tracking echocardiography (STE) are the echocardiographic techniques that have been developed to measure left ventricular strain. The reliability of TDI depends on a parallel position of the ultrasound beam with respect to the myocardial movement (with an angle that should be no greater than 15°-20°). TDI is limited to the velocity component toward or away from

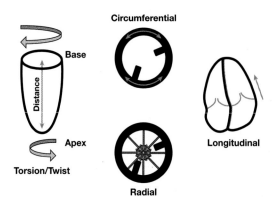

Figure 19.9 Mechanics of the left ventricle. According to the myocardial fiber orientation, the left ventricle contracts longitudinally, circumferentially, or radially. In addition, the base rotates clockwise, while the apex rotates counterclockwise. (Reproduced with permission from Narang A, Addetia K. An introduction to left ventricular strain. *Curr Opin Cardiol.* 2018;33:455-463.)

the probe, and therefore, it is used from an apical view for the measurement of longitudinal strain and occasionally from a short-axis view for circumferential strain assessment. Speckle tracking echocardiography is based on the principle of tracking (during the cardiac cycle) the motion of "speckles" created by the ultrasound beam scatter. In contrast to TDI, STE is generally independent from the angle of the ultrasound beam, and it can measure motion in any direction within the image plane. Therefore, STE can be used for the assessment of two-dimensional left ventricular strain and with further modification of 3-dimensional left ventricular strain. Longitudinal strain can be obtained as global longitudinal strain (GLS) from the apical view or as segmental strain according to the 17 segments. Several studies have evaluated the clinical value of GLS in assessing left ventricular systolic function in patients with aortic and mitral valve disease, in patients with cardiomyopathies, and its ability to detect even subclinical myocardial dysfunction. Overall, GLS has been shown to be a reliable and sensitive method for assessing left ventricular systolic function. Further discussion of left ventricular strain assessment is beyond the scope of this textbook, and our readers are directed to excellent published reviews and subspecialty textbooks.

DIASTOLIC FUNCTION
Left Ventricular Diastolic Distensibility: Pressure-Volume Relationship

Analysis of diastolic function today requires appreciation that diastolic compliance is variable and may change substantially in a given patient from 1 minute to the next. Diastolic function is summated physiologically in the relation between LV pressure and volume during diastole (**Figure 19.4**, segment DA). Traditionally, an upward shift in this diastolic *P-V* relation is regarded as indicating increased LV diastolic chamber stiffness, and a downward shift indicates decreased stiffness or increased LV diastolic chamber compliance. In the terminology of physics and engineering, stiffness, and its opposite, compliance, relate a change in pressure (*AP*) to a change in volume (*AV*); therefore, some investigators have restricted these terms to refer to the slope of the diastolic *P-V* relation. In this regard, as seen in segment DA of

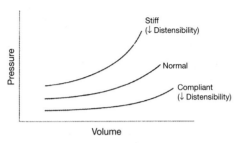

Figure 19.10 Diagrammatic representation of ventricular diastolic pressure-volume relations for normal, stiff, and compliant ventricles (see text for discussion).

Figure 19.4, LV diastolic stiffness (AP/AV) is low early in diastole and rises steadily throughout diastolic filling.

Figure 19.10 shows theoretical LV diastolic *P-V* plots for patients with normal, stiff, and compliant ventricular chambers.

Various formulas have been developed for analyzing the curvature of the LV diastolic *P-V* plot. These generally assume that the curvature is exponential, an assumption that is often but not always reasonable. Diastolic *P-V* and P-segment length (SL) plots constructed from a series of end-diastolic points have been used in animal experiments to assess LV diastolic compliance, and this technique has been applied to clinical studies. When a series of end-diastolic *P-V* or P-SL points are plotted, the relation is more strictly exponential, and application of mathematical models and analysis is more easily justified by the good agreement of measured data and mathematical predictions.

Clinical Conditions Influencing Diastolic Distensibility

Factors that influence the position of the LV diastolic *P-V* plot (ie, factors that influence LV diastolic *distensibility*) are listed in **Table 19.3**. *Constrictive pericarditis* and *pericardial tamponade* are associated with a striking upward shift in the diastolic *P-V* relation. This upward shift is a parallel shift without substantial change in curvature. Pericardial restraint is also important in the mechanism whereby altered RV loading can alter the LV diastolic *P-V* relation. When distended, the right ventricle can decrease LV diastolic distensibility by exerting an extrinsic pressure on the LV chamber in diastole through the shared interventricular septum, which may actually bulge into the LV chamber. *Acute RV infarction* causes dilatation of the RV chamber that, in the presence of an intact, previously unstressed pericardium, may lead to extrinsic compression of the LV in diastole with a hemodynamic pattern resembling that of cardiac tamponade. The effect of increased RV loading on LV diastolic distensibility is an example of ventricular interaction, which is more prominent in the presence of an intact and relatively snug pericardium. In animal experiments, it is difficult to demonstrate diastolic ventricular interaction once the pericardium has been opened wide.

Coronary vascular turgor can influence LV diastolic chamber stiffness. The LV wall has a rich blood supply, and engorgement of the capillaries and venules with blood makes the wall relatively stiff: for obvious reasons, this has been referred to as the erectile effect. Although the erectile effect is probably not of much importance when coronary blood flow and pressure (the two components determining the degree of turgor) are in the physiologic range, a marked fall in coronary flow and pressure

Table 19.3	**Factors That Influence Left Ventricular (LV) Diastolic Chamber Distensibility**

I. Factors extrinsic to the LV chamber
   A. Pericardial restraint
   B. Right ventricular loading
   C. Coronary vascular turgor (erectile effect)
   D. Extrinsic compression (eg, tumor, pleural pressure)
II. Factors intrinsic to LV chamber
   A. Passive elasticity of LV wall (stiffness or compliance when myocytes are completely relaxed)
      1. Thickness of LV wall
      2. Composition of LV wall (muscle, fibrosis, edema, amyloid, hemosiderin) including both endocardium and myocardium
      3. Temperature, osmolality
   B. Active elasticity of LV wall owing to residual cross-bridge activation (cycling and/or latch state) through part or all of diastole
      1. Slow relaxation affecting early diastole only
      2. Incomplete relaxation affecting early-, middle-, and end-diastolic distensibility
      3. Diastolic tone, contracture, or rigor
   C. Elastic recoil (diastolic suction)
   D. Viscoelasticity (stress relaxation, creep)

(as occurs distal to a coronary occlusion when collateral flow is poor or absent) is associated with a decrease in stiffness of the affected myocardium and an increase in LV diastolic distensibility.

Extrinsic *compression of the heart by tumor* may cause decreased LV diastolic distensibility and may mimic cardiac tamponade.

When an upward shift in the diastolic *P-V* relation is present and the extrinsic factors listed in **Table 19.3** cannot clearly explain the altered distensibility, a change in one of the intrinsic determinants of LV distensibility is likely to be present. Altered passive elasticity caused by *amyloidosis*, edema, or diffuse fibrosis may cause a restrictive cardiomyopathic pattern, with high LV diastolic pressure relative to volume in the presence of reasonably well-preserved systolic function. Clinically, heart failure may be present in such a scenario. Endomyocardial biopsy of the right or left ventricle may be needed to establish the diagnosis. Finally, in heart failure with reduced ejection fraction (HFrEF), the reduction in contractility is associated with an impairment in relaxation secondary to a combination of factors including abnormal calcium handling, abnormal loading conditions, and alteration in passive elasticity.

Myocardial Ischemia

During *angina pectoris*, a 10 to 15 mmHg rise in average LV diastolic pressure may occur with little or no change in diastolic volume; if this persists for a sufficient duration (>10-20 minutes), pulmonary edema may occur. Such episodes of *flash pulmonary edema* in patients with essentially normal LV systolic function and normal LV chamber size generally indicate a large mass of ischemic myocardium and suggest 3-vessel or left main coronary artery obstruction. The mechanism of impaired myocardial relaxation during the ischemia of angina pectoris is not understood completely but may be associated with diastolic Ca^{++} overload of the ischemic myocytes, in part related to ischemic dysfunction of the sarcoplasmic reticulum. During the ischemia of acute coronary occlusion, an upward shift of the diastolic *P-V* relation may occur if sufficient collateral blood flow is present to permit continued systolic contraction of the ischemic segment. If ischemia is sufficiently severe to cause complete akinesis of the affected myocardium, however, altered distensibility does not occur: *incomplete relaxation* can occur only in myocytes when there has been systolic cross-bridge activation. Also, the marked decrease in coronary vascular turgor distal to a coronary occlusion with poor or absent collaterals, together with local accumulation of hydrogen ions (H^+), contributes to an increase in regional distensibility, so that the net effect on the ventricular diastolic P-V relation may be one of no change.

Cardiac Hypertrophy

Impaired relaxation with decreased LV diastolic distensibility is also seen in patients with *hypertrophic cardiomyopathy*, during angina pectoris in patients with *aortic stenosis* and normal coronary arteries, and in patients with cardiac hypertrophy secondary to hypertension.

Indices of Left Ventricular Diastolic Relaxation Rate

Much attention has been given to measures of LV diastolic relaxation during the isovolumic relaxation period and during early, middle, and late diastolic filling. These indices may be considered as either pressure-derived or volume flow-derived and may assess either global or regional diastolic relaxation. A listing of some of these indices and their normal values is given in **Table 19.4**.

Isovolumic Pressure Decay

The time course of LV pressure decline after aortic valve closure is altered in conditions known to be associated with abnormalities of myocardial relaxation. One of the simplest ways of quantifying the time course of LV pressure decline is to measure the maximum rate of pressure fall, peak negative dP/dt. Although peak negative dP/dt is altered by conditions that change myocardial relaxation, it is also altered by changes in loading conditions. For example, LV peak negative dP/dt increases (ie, rises in absolute value) when aortic pressure rises. An increase in peak negative dP/dt when aortic pressure is unchanged or declining, however, signifies an improvement of LV relaxation. LV peak negative dP/dt decreases during the myocardial ischemia of either angina pectoris or infarction and increases in response to β-adrenergic stimulation and the phosphodiesterase inhibitor milrinone. It is not increased by digitalis glycosides.

Time Constant of Relaxation

Because of the load dependency of peak negative dP/dt and the fact that it uses information from only 1 point on the LV pressure-time plot, other indices have been introduced that analyze the time course of LV isovolumic pressure fall more completely. In 1976, Weiss and coworkers introduced the time constant T (or tau) of LV isovolumic pressure decline. First, LV isovolumic pressure decline is fit to the equation:

$$P = e^{At+B} \qquad (19.6)$$

where P is LV isovolumic pressure, e is a mathematical constant (natural logarithm base), t is time after peak negative dP/dt, and A and B are constants. This can also be expressed as:

$$\ln P = At + B \qquad (19.7)$$

Then, the natural logarithm of LV pressure versus time is plotted to allow calculation of the slope A, a negative number the units of which are seconds^{-1}. The time constant T of isovolumic pressure fall is then defined as $-1/A$ (expressed in ms) representing the time that it takes for P to decline to 1/e times its value.

Not only slow myocardial relaxation but also asynchrony of the relaxation process within the ventricular chamber results in prolongation of T. In addition, T is probably

Table 19.4 Evaluation of Left Ventricular Diastolic Performance: Normal Values for Some Indices of Relaxation and Filling

Parameter	Normal Values
Peak $-dP/dt$	2660 ± 700 mmHg/s
	2922 ± 750 mmHg/s
	1864 ± 390 mmHg/s
	1825 ± 261 mmHg/s
T (logarithmic method, Equation 19.7)	38 ± 7 ms
	33 ± 8 ms
	31 ± 3 ms
T (derivative method)	55 ± 12 ms
	47 ± 10
P_B (derivative method)	−25 ± 9 mmHg
PFR	3.3 ± 0.6 EDV/s
Time-to-PFR	136 ± 23 ms
Peak $-dh/dt$ (posterior wall)	8.4 ± 3.0 cm/s
	8.2 ± 3.7 cm/s

EDV, end-diastolic volumes; LV, left ventricular; peak $-dh/dt$, maximum rate of posterior wall thinning, measured by echocardiography; peak $-dP/dt$, maximum rate of left ventricular isovolumic pressure decline; PFR, left ventricular peak filling rate, from radionuclide ventriculography, normalized to end-diastolic volumes per second; T, time constant of left ventricular isovolumic relaxation, calculated assuming both zero pressure intercept (Eq. 19.7) and variable pressure (P_B) intercept.

not completely independent of loading conditions, although the influence of altered loading is relatively small. Measurement of T should be attempted only from LV pressure tracings obtained with high-fidelity, micromanometer-tipped catheters, or from fluid-filled systems with demonstrated optimal damping and high (>25 Hz) natural frequencies.

Volume-Derived Indices of Relaxation

Peak Filling Rate After mitral valve opening, ventricular filling usually proceeds briskly with an initial rapid filling phase, a middle slow filling phase, and a terminal increase in filling rate associated with atrial systole. The rapid filling phase may be characterized by a maximum or peak filling rate (PFR) and time-to-PFR. PFR is usually determined by plotting LV volume against time, fitting the initial portion of this plot after mitral valve opening to a third- (or higher) order polynomial and solving for the first derivative of this polynomial. LV volume for this calculation may be obtained from the LV cineangiogram or by radionuclide techniques.

As one might expect, PFR is preload dependent: interventions that raise left atrial pressure increase PFR, and interventions that reduce pulmonary venous return and left atrial pressure cause PFR to decrease. However, an increase in PFR that occurs when LV filling pressure (pulmonary capillary wedge pressure, left atrial pressure, or LV diastolic pressure) is unchanged or falling can reasonably be taken as an indication that LV relaxation has improved. For example, PFR has been shown to decrease during angina pectoris when LV filling pressure is increasing. Because the rise in LV filling pressure by itself would cause an increase in PFR, the fall in PFR that is actually observed most likely indicates slowed relaxation of the myocardium, consistent with the other findings in this condition (fall in peak negative dP/dt, prolongation of T) that suggest impaired relaxation of the ischemic myocardium. PFR is reduced in patients with coronary stenoses, even in the absence of overt ischemia, and improves after coronary angioplasty. PFR is also reduced in patients with hypertrophic cardiomyopathy and improves after administration of a calcium-blocking agent. PFR is usually normalized for end-diastolic volumes (EDV) and expressed as EDV/s. Cardiac dilatation by itself tends to depress PFR, exaggerating its preload dependence.

Regional Diastolic Dysfunction Diastolic dysfunction of specific regions of the left ventricle may be difficult to assess solely by examination of a global parameter of LV diastolic function such as the time constant of relaxation or the PFR. As pointed out by Pouleur and Rousseau, the time course of LV isovolumic pressure decline underestimates the severity of regional impairment in the rate of relaxation. Marked slowing of regional relaxation in an area of myocardial ischemia is partially masked by normal or enhanced rates of relaxation in adjacent normal regions of the myocardium. Regional wall stress measurements have been proposed as an ideal way to assess regional rates of relaxation, but these can be made only by having knowledge of simultaneous LV pressure wall thickness and geometry.

Rate of Wall Thinning Another index of diastolic function, similar in some ways to PFR, is the peak rate of diastolic LV wall thinning. This can be measured echocardiographically by plotting posterior or septal wall thickness against time, fitting the data to a polynomial, and taking the first derivative. The posterior wall thickness, h, and its first derivative, dh/dt, reflect regional diastolic function of the posterior wall myocardium. An advantage of peak negative dh/dt over PFR is that the former assesses regional myocardial function, whereas PFR describes behavior of the whole ventricle and is insensitive when equal and opposite changes in diastolic function are occurring in different parts of the LV chamber. Peak negative dh/dt decreases during angina, even though LV filling pressure rises.

Rate of Myocardial Motion Tissue Doppler has emerged as a useful, noninvasive method to assess diastolic function. It is based on the Doppler principle according to which a target moving away from or toward an ultrasound source will backscatter the ultrasound waves with a wavelength higher (moving toward) or lower (moving away) than the wavelength of the source. The relationship between the velocity of the target and the Doppler shift in frequency is expressed by the Doppler equation.

TDI allows measurement of myocardial tissue velocities by focusing on the high-amplitude, low-frequency signals reflected by the myocardium. The region of interest (ROI) of tissue Doppler is placed on myocardial tissue at the level of the mitral annulus on the basal septum or the basal lateral wall. Acquisition is performed from either the four-chamber or the two-chamber acoustic window (apical approach), as the ventricular apex remains virtually fixed during the cardiac cycle. Three waveforms are recorded per cardiac cycle during apnea to minimize motion artifacts. The tissue Doppler waveform is characterized by a positive *Sm* wave corresponding to the movement of the mitral annulus toward the apex during ventricular systole, a negative *Em* wave corresponding to early diastolic relaxation, and a negative *Am* wave corresponding to atrial contraction (**Figure 19.11**). Tissue Doppler measurements are generally load independent when compared to mitral flow velocities, although experimental studies have suggested that they might be affected by early diastolic lengthening load, in addition to translation movements and tethering. Several studies have assessed *Em* velocities and *Em/Am* ratios in different age groups, disease states, and loading conditions.

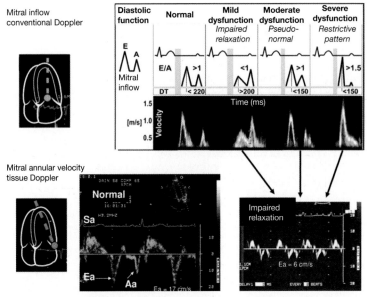

Figure 19.11 The upper panel illustrates the conventional Doppler interrogation of mitral inflow. The normal mitral valve inflow pattern is characterized by $E > A$ and an E wave deceleration time of 150 to 220 ms. Impaired left ventricular (LV) relaxation or decreased LV compliance is associated with a reversal of E and A waves and prolongation of E-wave deceleration to >220 ms. Pseudonormalization of the E/A ratio can occur when increased left atrial pressure results in an increased driving pressure and a consequent increased E-wave velocity across the mitral valve into a noncompliant LV. With severe diastolic dysfunction, the mitral valve inflow pattern can become restrictive, reflecting rapid equilibration of elevated left atrial and LV diastolic pressures in the noncompliant LV. The lower panel illustrates the 3 basic waveforms of tissue Doppler interrogation: Sa (systolic myocardial motion, or *Sm*), Ea (early diastolic motion, or *Em*), and Aa (atrial contraction, or *Em*). (Reproduced with permission from Ho CY, Solomon SD. A clinician's guide to tissue Doppler imaging. *Circulation.* 2006;113:e396-e398.)

Em velocities of >12 cm/s and *Em/Am* ratios of >1 are associated with normal diastolic function, while *Em* velocities of <8 cm/s and *Em/Am* ratios of <1 have been used as cutoffs for diastolic dysfunction and impaired relaxation. It has also been shown that the ratio of early transmitral peak LV inflow velocity E to early myocardial velocity *Em* (*E/Em ratio*) correlates well with invasive measurements of LV stiffness and diastolic function (**Figure 19.12**), and that a ratio of >8 can be used as a parameter to identify patients with heart failure with preserved ejection fraction (HFpEF) and diastolic dysfunction (**Figure 19.13**).

Various other indices of diastolic myocardial relaxation have been proposed. Most are imperfect, as are the ones discussed here. However, important information about diastolic relaxation and distensibility can usually be gleaned from examination of the parameters discussed in this chapter, taken in the context of the clinical setting and other hemodynamic findings in an individual patient.

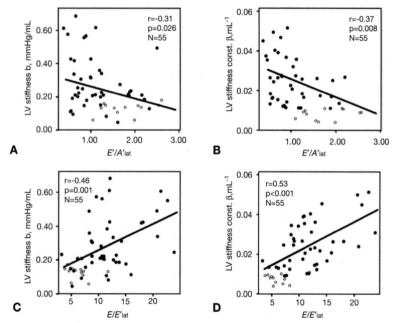

Figure 19.12 Linear regression between the LV stiffness (b and β) and tissue Doppler indices. *Blank spots* represent controls. **A and B,** Linear regression lines $E'/A'^{∧}$. $b = -0.08$ (95% confidence interval: -0.15 to -0.02) $× E'/A'_{lat} + 0.37$, $r = -0.31$, $P = .026$; and $b = -0.008$ (95% confidence interval: -0.014 to -0.002) $× E'/A'_{lat} + 0.032$, $r = -0.37$, $P = .008$; **C and D,** Linear regression lines E/E'_{lat}: $b = 0.016$ (95% confidence interval: 0.008-0.023) $× E/E_{lat} + 0.10$, $r = 0.46$, $P < .001$; and $b = 0.0014$ (95% confidence interval: 0.001-0.002) $× E/E_{lat} + 0.008$, $r = 0.53$, $P < .001$. E/A_{lat}, ratio of early to late diastolic velocity of mitral annulus at lateral site; E/E'_{lat}, LV filling index at lateral site; *P*, descriptive significance level. const., constant. (Reproduced with permission from Kasner M, Westerman D, Steendijk P, et al. Utility of Doppler echocardiography and tissue Doppler imaging in the estimation of diastolic function in heart failure with normal ejection fraction: a comparative Doppler-conductance catheter study. *Circulation.* 2007;116:637-647.)

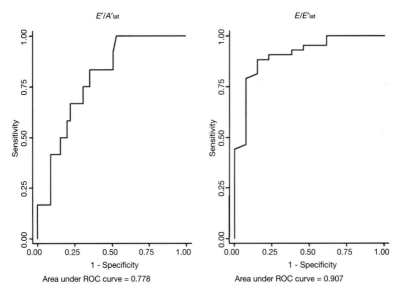

Figure 19.13 Receiver operating characteristic (ROC) analysis for TDI (tissue Doppler imaging) indices E'/A'_{lat} and E/E'_{lat}. The sensitivity/specificity ratio for E'/A'_{lat} (<1) is 67%/84% and for E/E'_{lat} (>8) is 83%/92%. E'/A'_{lat}, early to late diastolic velocity ratio of mitral annulus at lateral site; E/E'_{lat}, LV filling index at lateral site. LV, left ventricular. (Reproduced with permission from Kasner M, Westerman D, Steendijk P, et al. Utility of Doppler echocardiography and tissue Doppler imaging in the estimation of diastolic function in heart failure with normal ejection fraction: a comparative Doppler-conductance catheter study. *Circulation.* 2007;116:637-647.)

SUGGESTED READINGS

1. Borow KM, Neumann A, Wynne J. Sensitivity of end-systolic pressure-dimension and pressure-volume relations to the inotropic state in humans. *Circulation.* 1982;65(5):988-997.

2. Borow KM, Neumann A, Marcus RH, Sareli P, Lang RM. Effects of simultaneous alterations in pre-load and afterload on measurements of left ventricular contractility in patients with dilated cardio-myopathy: comparisons of ejection phase, isovolumetric and end-systolic force-velocity indexes. *J Am Coll Cardiol.* 1992;20(4):787-795.

3. Broughton A, Korner PI. Steady-state effects of preload and afterload on isovolumic indices of contractility in autonomically blocked dogs. *Cardiovasc Res.* 1980;14(5):245-253.

4. Burkhoff D, Sugiura S, Yue DT, Sagawa K. Contractility-dependent curvilinearity of end-systolic pressure-volume relations. *Am J Physiol.* 1987;252(6 Pt 2):H1218-H1227.

5. Carroll JD, Hess OM, Hirzel HO, Krayenbuehl HP. Exercise-induced ischemia: the influence of altered relaxation on early diastolic pressures. *Circulation.* 1983;67(3):521-528.

6. Feldman MD, Alderman J, Aroesty JM, et al. Depression of systolic and diastolic myocardial reserve during atrial pacing tachycardia in patients with dilated cardiomyopathy. *J Clin Invest.* 1988;82(5):1661-1669.

7. Fifer MA, Gunther S, Grossman W, Mirsky I, Carabello B, Barry WH. Myocardial contractile function in aortic stenosis as determined from the rate of stress development during isovolumic systole. *Am J Cardiol.* 1979;44(7):1318-1325.

8. Gaasch WH, Battle WE, Oboler AA, Banas JS Jr, Levine HJ. Left ventricular stress and compliance in man: with special reference to normalized ventricular function curves. *Circulation.* 1972;45(4):746-762.

9. Gersh BJ, Hahn CEW, Prys-Roberts C. Physical criteria for measurement of left ventricular pressure and its first derivative. *Cardiovasc Res.* 1971;5(1):32-40.

10. Geyer H, Caracciolo G, Abe H, et al. Assessment of myocardial mechanics using speckle tracking echocardiography: fundamentals and clinical applications. *J Am Soc Echocardiogr*. 2010;23(4):351-369; quiz 453-355.

11. Glantz SA, Misbach GA, Moores WY, et al. The pericardium substantially affects the left ventricular diastolic pressure-volume relationship in the dog. *Circ Res*. 1978;42(3):433-441.

12. Grossman W, Haynes F, Paraskos J, Saltz S, Dalen JE, Dexter L. Alterations in preload and myocardial mechanics in the dog and in man. *Circ Res*. 1972;31(1):83-94.

13. Grossman W, McLaurin LP, Paraskos JA, Saltz S, Dalen JE, Dexter L. Changes in the inotropic state of the left ventricle during isometric exercise. *Br Heart J*. 1973;35(7):697-704.

14. Grossman W, Braunwald E, Mann T, McLaurin LP, Green LH. Contractile state of the left ventricle in man as evaluated from end-systolic pressure-volume relations. *Circulation*. 1977;56(5):845-852.

15. Hayashida W, Kumada T, Kohno F, et al. Left ventricular regional relaxation and its nonuniformity in hypertrophic nonobstructive cardiomyopathy. *Circulation*. 1991;84(4):1496-1504.

16. Hirota Y. A clinical study of left ventricular relaxation. *Circulation*. 1980;62(4):756-763.

17. Kass DA, Solaro RJ. Mechanisms and use of calcium-sensitizing agents in the failing heart. *Circulation*. 2006;113(2):305-315.

18. Kass DA, Yamazaki T, Burkhoff D, Maughan WL, Sagawa K. Determination of left ventricular end-systolic pressure-volume relationships by the conductance (volume) catheter technique. *Circulation*. 1986;73(3):586-595.

19. Kass DA, Midei M, Graves W, Brinker JA, Maughan WL. Use of a conductance (volume) catheter and transient inferior vena caval occlusion for rapid determination of pressure-volume relationships in man. *Cathet Cardiovasc Diagn*. 1988;15(3):192-202.

20. Konstam MA, Cohen SR, Salem DN, et al. Comparison of left and right ventricular end-systolic pressure-volume relations in congestive heart failure. *J Am Coll Cardiol*. 1985;5(6):1326-1334.

21. Krayenbuehl HP, Rutishauser W, Wirz P, Amende I, Mehmel H. High-fidelity left ventricular pressure measurements for the assessment of cardiac contractility in man. *Am J Cardiol*. 1973;31(4):415-427.

22. McKay RG, Spears JR, Aroesty JM, et al. Instantaneous measurement of left and right ventricular stroke volume and pressure volume relationships with an impedance catheter. *Circulation*. 1984;69(4):703-710.

23. McKay RG, Aroesty JM, Heller GV, Royal HD, Warren SE, Grossman W. Assessment of the end-systolic pressure-volume relationship in human beings with the use of a time-varying elastance model. *Circulation*. 1986;74(1):97-104.

24. McLaurin LP, Rolett EL, Grossman W. Impaired left ventricular relaxation during pacing induced ischemia. *Am J Cardiol*. 1973;32(6):751-757.

25. Monrad ES, McKay RG, Baim DS, et al. Improvement in indexes of diastolic performance in patients with congestive heart failure treated with milrinone. *Circulation*. 1984;70(6):1030-1037.

26. Mor-Avi V, Lang RM, Badano LP, et al. Current and evolving echocardiographic techniques for the quantitative evaluation of cardiac mechanics: ase/eae consensus statement on methodology and indications endorsed by the Japanese society of echocardiography. *Eur J Echocardiogr*. 2011;12(3):167-205.

27. Narang A, Addetia K. An introduction to left ventricular strain. *Curr Opin Cardiol*. 2018;33(5):455-463.

28. Ng ACT, Delgado V, Bax JJ. Application of left ventricular strain in patients with aortic and mitral valve disease. *Curr Opin Cardiol*. 2018;33(5):470-478.

29. Nikitin NP, Witte KKA, Thackray SDR, de Silva R, Clark AL, Cleland JGF. Longitudinal ventricular function: normal values of atrioventricular annular and myocardial velocities measured with quantitative two-dimensional color Doppler tissue imaging. *J Am Soc Echocardiogr*. 2003;16(9):906-921.

30. Nishimura RA, Schwartz RS, Tajik AJ, Holmes DR Jr. Noninvasive measurement of rate of left ventricular relaxation by Doppler echocardiography: validation with simultaneous cardiac catheterization. *Circulation*. 1993;88(1):146-155.

31. Ommen SR, Nishimura RA, Appleton CP, et al. Clinical utility of Doppler echocardiography and tissue Doppler imaging in the estimation of left ventricular filling pressures: a comparative simultaneous Doppler-catheterization study. *Circulation*. 2000;102(15):1788-1794.

32. Peterson KL, Skloven D, Ludbrook P, Uther JB, Ross J Jr. Comparison of isovolumic and ejection phase indices of myocardial performance in man. *Circulation*. 1974;49(6):1088-1101.

33. Pouleur H, Rousseau M. Regional diastolic dysfunction in coronary artery disease: clinical and therapeutic implications. In: Grossman W, Lorell BH, eds. *Diastolic Relaxation of the Heart: Basic Research and Current Applications for Clinical Cardiology*. Martinus Nijhoff; 1988:245.

34. Poulsen SH, Andersen NH, Ivarsen PI, Mogensen CE, Egeblad H. Doppler tissue imaging reveals systolic dysfunction in patients with hypertension and apparent "isolated" diastolic dysfunction. *J Am Soc Echocardiogr*. 2003;16(7):724-731.

35. Rankin LS, Moos S, Grossman W. Alterations in preload and ejection phase indices of left ventricular performance. *Circulation*. 1975;51(5):910-915.
36. Ross J Jr, Braunwald E. The study of left ventricular function in man by increasing resistance to ventricular ejection with angiotensin. *Circulation*. 1964;29:739-749.
37. Sagawa K, Suga H, Shoukas AA, et al. The end-systolic pressure-volume relation of the ventricle: definition, modifications and clinical use. *Circulation*. 1981;63(6):1223-1227.
38. Sharir T, Feldman MD, Haber H, et al. Ventricular systolic assessment in patients with dilated cardiomyopathy by preload-adjusted maximal power. Validation and noninvasive application. *Circulation*. 1994;89(5):2045-2053.
39. Sohn DW, Chai IH, Lee DJ, et al. Assessment of mitral annulus velocity by Doppler tissue imaging in the evaluation of left ventricular diastolic function. *J Am Coll Cardiol*. 1997;30(2):474-480.
40. Starling MR, Walsh RA, Dell'Italia LJ, Mancini GB, Lasher JC, Lancaster JL. The relationship of various measures of end-systole to left ventricular maximum time-varying elastance in man. *Circulation*. 1987;76(1):32-43.
41. Suga H, Sagawa K, Shoukas AA. Load independence of the instantaneous pressure-volume ratio of the canine left ventricle and effects of epinephrine and heart rate on the ratio. *Circ Res*. 1973;32(3):314-322.
42. Thompson DS, Waldron CB, Juul SM, et al. Analysis of left ventricular pressure during isovolumic relaxation in coronary artery disease. *Circulation*. 1982;65(4):690-697.
43. Vogel WM, Apstein CS, Briggs LL, Gaasch WH, Ahn J. Acute alterations in left ventricular diastolic chamber stiffness: role of the "erectile" effect of coronary arterial pressure and flow in normal and damaged hearts. *Circ Res*. 1982;51(4):465-478.
44. Watanabe J, Levine MJ, Bellotto F, Johnson RG, Grossman W. Effects of coronary venous pressure on left ventricular diastolic distensibility. *Circ Res*. 1990;67(4):923-932.
45. Yamada H, Oki T, Mishiro Y, et al. Effect of aging on diastolic left ventricular myocardial velocities measured by pulsed tissue Doppler imaging in healthy subjects. *J Am Soc Echocardiogr*. 1999;12(7):574-581.
46. Zimpfer M, Vatner SF. Effects of acute increases in left ventricular preload on indices of myocardial function in conscious, unrestrained and intact, tranquilized baboons. *J Clin Invest*. 1981;67(2):430-438.

20 Evaluation of Tamponade, Constrictive, and Restrictive Physiology[1]

The pericardium separates the heart from the surrounding structures, and it has important mechanical, membranous, biofeedback, and barrier functions. As a relatively inelastic sac, it contributes to maintenance of normal atrial and ventricular compliance and optimal ventricular shape, provides protection against excessive ventricular-atrial valve regurgitation, and limits excessive acute dilation or mismatch between right- and left-side chamber volume. A small amount of pericardial fluid is usually present and has the important role of reducing friction during cardiac contraction, while mechanoreceptors in the pericardium may provide biofeedback regulating heart rate and blood pressure. In addition, the negative pericardial pressure and its changes during respiratory cycles contribute to enhancing venous return to the right atrium to aid filling during inspiration.

While the diagnosis of pericardial tamponade is relatively straightforward, the differentiation between constrictive pericardial disease and restrictive physiology often presents challenges requiring the integration of hemodynamic measurements, imaging, and occasionally an endomyocardial or pericardial biopsy.

NORMAL HEMODYNAMICS DURING THE RESPIRATORY CYCLE AND THE ROLE OF THE PERICARDIUM

The normal pericardial pressure is subatmospheric, and it tracks intrapleural pressure during the respiratory cycle. The negative pericardial pressure has the important role of maintaining a positive transmyocardial pressure gradient (intracavitary pressure - pericardial pressure), resulting in a net chamber-distending pressure that is slightly higher than the intracavitary pressure. This transmyocardial pressure gradient facilitates diastolic filling, particularly in the low-pressure right heart. During inspiration, there is a reduction in intrapleural pressure that affects all structures within the thorax, associated with a fall in chamber pressures and pulmonary wedge pressure. The reduction in intrapericardial pressure tends to be larger than the fall in systemic venous pressure, and with descent of the diaphragm, intra-abdominal pressure increases, resulting in an increase in the pressure gradient from extrathoracic veins to the right atrium. These forces collectively serve to enhance right atrial and right ventricular (RV) filling during inspiration. Because the decrease in intrapleural pressure with inspiration is more effectively transmitted to the pulmonary venous bed than to the left ventricle, the pressure *gradient* from pulmonary vein to left atrium decreases slightly, resulting in a slight drop in the transmitral pressure gradient and a mild reduction of left ventricular (LV) diastolic volume and stroke volume. Hence, the mild decrease in systemic arterial pressure observed during normal inspiration is attributable to the slight reduction in left ventricular preload and transmission of the negative intrathoracic pressure to the aorta and peripheral arteries. As ventricular systole begins, the rapid reduction in ventricular volume causes a drop in pericardial pressure, which increases atrial transmyocardial gradients to further enhance atrial filling.

The right and left ventricles share the intraventricular septum and are contained in the relatively indistensible pericardial sac, creating the substrate for the hemodynamic phenomenon known as diastolic ventricular interaction when the pericar-

[1]We gratefully acknowledge the Grossman & Baim's *Cardiac Catheterization, Angiography, and Intervention*, 9th edition contributions of Drs. Mauro Moscucci and Barry A. Borlaug as portions of their chapter, "Evaluation of Tamponade, Constrictive, and Restrictive Physiology," were retained in this text.

dium becomes diseased or when the heart becomes enlarged to the pericardial limits. Within the setting of this enhanced ventricular interaction, an increase in volume of one ventricle (in the setting of a compliant septum and an intact pericardium) will affect filling and volume of the other ventricle. As described below, the compliance of the septum can explain at least in part the differences in ventricular interdependence observed with pericardial tamponade, pericardial constriction, and restrictive physiology.

TAMPONADE PHYSIOLOGY

Under normal conditions, the pericardial sac contains 15 to 35 mL of fluid. Given the relatively inelastic characteristics of the pericardium, rapid accumulation of pericardial fluid leads to a marked increase in intrapericardial pressure. In contrast, over a prolonged period of time (as with eccentric cardiac remodeling or slowly growing malignant effusion), the pericardium can stretch and accommodate larger volumes, shifting the pressure-volume curve to the right (**Figure 20.1**). Tamponade physiology develops when the size of the effusion becomes sufficient to increase total pericardial volume from the shallow, compliant portion of the pericardial pressure-volume relationship to the steep, noncompliant portion (*arrows*, **Figure 20.1**). If venous return remains unchanged, an increase in intrapericardial pressure will decrease transmural diastolic filling pressures in all heart chambers, resulting in typical changes in the atrial pressure waveform. As described in Chapter 11, the normal atrial waveform is characterized by 3 positive deflections (*a*, *c*, and v waves) and 3 negative deflections (*x*, *X*, and *y* descents). The *x* descent corresponds to atrial relaxation. During ventricular systole, continuous atrial relaxation and the descent of the atrioventricular valve annulus result in further reduction of atrial pressure and in the corresponding *X* descent. After the nadir of the *X* descent, the atrium fills during ventricular systole while the atrioventricular valve is closed (*v* wave). This phase is followed by the *y* descent, which corresponds to opening of the atrioventricular valve and rapid emptying of the atrium. In pericardial tamponade, as intrapericardial pres-

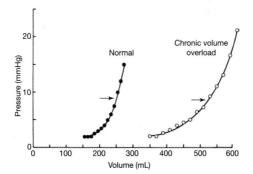

Figure 20.1 Pericardial pressure-volume relations determined in the pericardium obtained from a normal experimental animal and from an animal with chronic cardiac dilation produced by volume loading. The pericardial pressure-volume relation is shifted to the right in the volume-loaded animal, demonstrating that the pericardium can dilate to accommodate slowly increasing volume. The arrows indicate the steep, noncompliant portion of the pericardial volume-pressure relationship. (Reproduced with permission from Freeman GL, LeWinter MM. Pericardial adaptations during chronic cardiac dilation in dogs. *Circ Res.* 1984;54:294-300.)

sure increases, an increase in venous return will initially serve to maintain cardiac filling and prevent diastolic collapse of cardiac chambers. Further increase in pericardial pressure will lead to a progressive impairment in atrial emptying and ventricular filling, with blunting or disappearance of the y descent while the x descent is typically preserved or enhanced (**Figure 20.2**). There is also loss of the early dip in minimal LV diastolic pressure and equalization between right atrial and LV pressure at the onset of diastole (**Figure 20.3**).

As pericardial pressure continues to increase, diastolic filling pressures will equalize across the 4 cardiac chambers, eventually culminating in diastolic compression of the right-side and then the left-side cardiac chambers. Diastolic filling dynamics throughout the cardiac cycle essentially become a zero-sum game—for any increase in ventricular volume, there is an obligate decrease in atrial volume; and conversely when right-side filling volume increases (as during inspiration), there is a matched drop in left-side volume. This enhancement of ventricular interdependence explains the pathophysiology and most physical findings in tamponade. As described above, under normal conditions inspiration causes a decrease in intrapericardial and intrathoracic pressure, which is coupled with an increase in systemic venous return to the right heart. There is also an increase in the capacitance of the pulmonary vasculature and reduction in the pressure gradient from pulmonary vein to left atrium, which results in a decrease in left ventricular filling, stroke volume, and systolic pressure. In pericardial tamponade, these effects are magnified dramatically, and

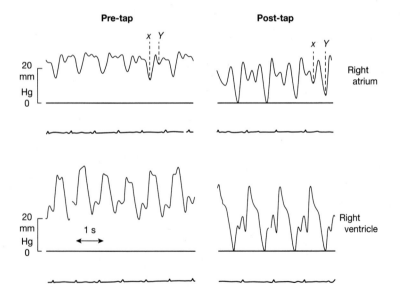

Figure 20.2 Right atrial and right ventricular pressure pulses, before and after removal of pericardial fluid, in a patient with subacute effusive-constrictive pericarditis that followed radiotherapy. The right atrial pulse shows a predominant systolic descent (X > Y) initially and a predominant diastolic descent (X < Y) after removal of fluid. The diastolic dip-plateau pattern in the right ventricular pulse is prominent only after removal of fluid, in association with the X < Y right atrial pulse. (Reproduced with permission from Hancock EW. Subacute effusive-constrictive pericarditis. *Circulation.* 1971;43:183-192.)

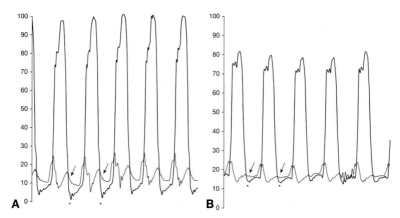

Figure 20.3 A, Left atrial (red) and left ventricular (black) tracings in a patient with mitral stenosis prior to percutaneous balloon valvotomy. Note the *y* descent (arrows) and low minimal LV diastolic pressure (*). **B,** After balloon inflation, LV systolic pressure is reduced, the *y* descent is absent (arrows), and the LV minimal diastolic pressure has increased substantially (*), findings related to cardiac perforation and cardiac tamponade. LV, left ventricular.

increased systemic venous return to the right side of the heart is coupled with acute reduction in left-side filling owing to reduction in the pulmonary capillary to LV diastolic gradient (**Figure 20.4**). The converse then occurs during expiration, when left-side filling is augmented at the cost of right heart filling—such that the diastolic volumes, stroke volumes, and accordingly developed pressures within one ventricle

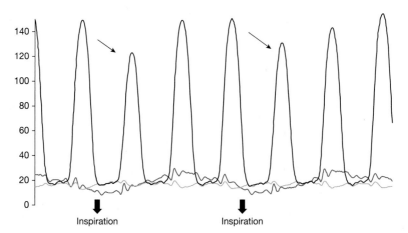

Figure 20.4 Mechanism of the pulsus paradoxus in cardiac tamponade. During inspiration (thick arrows), the pulmonary wedge pressure (red) drops below the right atrial pressure (which approximates pericardial pressure, blue) and the LV diastolic pressure (black), resulting in a reduction in transmural filling pressure, acute "underfilling" of the LV, reduced LV stroke volume, and reduced LV systolic pressure (thin arrows). LV, left ventricular.

are 180° out of phase with those in the other ventricle (**Figure 20.5**). The reduction in left ventricular filling and thus stroke volume reduces aortic systolic blood pressure by >10 mmHg during inspiration.

Cardiac tamponade is a clinical diagnosis based upon typical symptoms including fatigue, dyspnea, and air hunger together with physical findings including elevated venous pressure, sinus tachycardia, and pulsus paradoxus. The diagnosis can be confirmed by echocardiography, which typically shows pericardial effusion, right atrial and right ventricular diastolic collapse, abnormal increase in blood flow velocity across the tricuspid valve and corresponding decrease in flow velocity across the mitral valve during inspiration, and dilated inferior vena cava without collapse during inspiration. Confirmation of tamponade physiology is obtained through hemodynamic measurements during cardiac catheterization and through documentation of elevation of pericardial pressure above atmospheric pressure, its equalization with right atrial pressure, and its decrease to subatmospheric levels following pericardiocentesis. Detailed understanding of the hemodynamic changes in tamponade and a high index of suspicion are especially important in the evolving era of advanced percutaneous treatments for structural heart disease and cardiac arrhythmias, where cardiac perforations may be more commonly observed.

Constrictive-Effusive Physiology

In rare cases, following pericardiocentesis the pericardial pressure returns to subatmospheric (<0 mmHg) levels, while the right atrial pressure and the right ventricular diastolic pressures remain elevated, with a typical dip and plateau pattern in the right ventricular pressure tracing. This pattern is consistent with effusive-constrictive physiology, and it has been suggested that this represents evolution of acute pericarditis with pericardial effusion toward pericardial constriction.

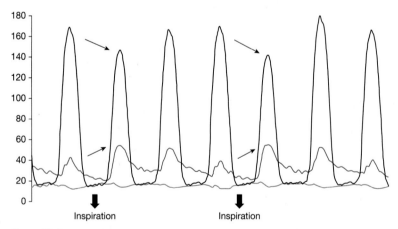

Figure 20.5 In tamponade, enhanced LV and RV diastolic filling are 180° out of phase with each other (thin arrows) as the septum bows from right to left during inspiration (thick arrows) (increase in pulmonary artery pressure [red], coupled with decrease in LV systolic pressure [black]) and then back from left to right during expiration (decrease in PA pressure and increase in LV systolic pressure). LV, left ventricular; PA, pulmonary artery; RV, right ventricular.

Low-Pressure Tamponade

A clinical syndrome characterized by low pericardial pressure leading to cardiac compression because of low filling pressures, without the typical clinical findings associated with tamponade, has also been described. In an analysis of 279 patients undergoing pericardiocentesis at a single institution, 29 patients met the criteria for low-pressure tamponade (defined as intrapericardial pressure of <7 mmHg before pericardiocentesis and right atrial pressure of <4 mmHg after pericardiocentesis, group 1), whereas 114 patients met the criteria for classic tamponade (intrapericardial pressure of >7 mmHg before pericardiocentesis and right atrial pressure of >4 mmHg after pericardiocentesis, group 2). Typical findings of tamponade were present in only 24% of patients in group 1, as compared to 71% in group 2.

Both patient groups had a significant increase in cardiac index following pericardiocentesis. Overall, these data support the importance of transmural or transmyocardial pressure as the primary determinant of atrial filling and highlight the importance of a high degree of suspicion in patients who might have symptoms or findings consistent with hemodynamic compromise and in whom classic findings of tamponade might be absent.

Regional Cardiac Tamponade

In the setting of large, circumferential pericardial effusions, cardiac tamponade presents with typical clinical and echocardiographic findings. In contrast, following cardiac surgery, cardiac tamponade is frequently secondary to a loculated effusion characteristically localized in the posterior wall, and in such patients the typical findings of tamponade are absent. Echocardiography may reveal evidence of regional left ventricular diastolic collapse in the setting of these loculated pericardial effusions (**Figure 20.6**). It has been suggested that loculated effusion develops because of posterior adherence of the anterior right ventricular and atrial walls and anterior pericardium to the chest wall, and adhesions in the surrounding area. Common hemodynamic findings in these patients include elevated right atrial and right ventricular diastolic pressure, elevated pulmonary capillary wedge pressure, and equalization of right atrial and pulmonary capillary wedge pressure within 5 mmHg.

CONSTRICTIVE PHYSIOLOGY

Pericardial constriction is the result of inflammatory processes of the pericardium leading to progressive fibrosis, thickening, and in some cases calcification of pericardial layers (**Figure 20.7**). While prior cardiac surgery and radiation therapy are common etiologies, the most frequent cause remains idiopathic. The hemodynamic changes associated with constrictive pericarditis are similar to those observed with pericardial tamponade and are often difficult to distinguish from restrictive cardiomyopathy. In constrictive pericarditis, ventricular filling occurs predominantly during early diastole, as the ventricles cannot expand further during mid to late diastole owing to the pericardial constraint. Accordingly, the ventricular diastolic pressure tracing is characterized by an early dip followed by a positive "rapid filling wave" and plateau phase (dip and plateau pattern or square root sign; **Figure 20.8**). It has been suggested that this early dip is secondary to a "rubber bulb" effect or "spring back" of the pericardial layer during early diastole. This rapid filling corresponds to the pericardial knock often appreciated on physical examination. The right atrial waveform will show steep x and y descents related to atrial relaxation and rapid early filling, creating the so-called M or W sign (**Figure 20.9**),

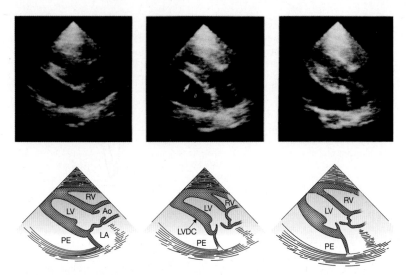

Figure 20.6 Serial echocardiographic images in the parasternal long-axis view from a postoperative patient with cardiac tamponade show a large posterior pericardial effusion (PE). Right ventricle (RV) is adherent to the anterior chest wall. Contour of the left ventricular (LV)-free wall is normal at end systole. During early diastole, however, LV posterior wall invaginates inward, which is identified by the arrow as LV diastolic collapse (LVDC). This LVDC is only transient; by late diastole, LV has assumed its normal contour. Ao, aorta; LA, left atrium. (Reproduced (top) and redrawn from (bottom) Chuttani K, Pandian NG, Mohanty PK, et al. Left ventricular diastolic collapse: an echocardiographic sign of regional cardiac tamponade. *Circulation*. 1991;83:1999-2006, with permission.)

and the mean right atrial pressure will often increase during deep inspiration (Kussmaul sign, **Figures 20.10** and **20.11**). As described above, inspiration normally decreases left-side filling slightly because the pressure gradient from pulmonary vein to left atrium and left ventricle is reduced. In constriction, the rigid, fibrotic pericardium further "insulates" the left ventricle from the inspiratory drop in intrathoracic

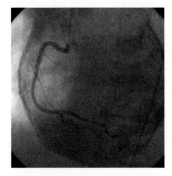

Figure 20.7 Still-frame fluoroscopic image showing marked pericardial calcification during contrast injection in the right coronary artery.

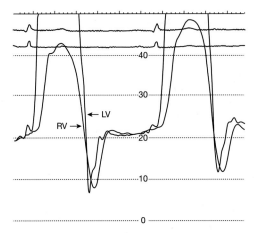

Figure 20.8 Simultaneous right ventricular (RV) and left ventricular (LV) pressure recordings demonstrating equalization of diastolic pressures and characteristic "dip and plateau" contour. (Reproduced with permission from Vaitkus PT, Cooper KA, Shuman WP, Hardin NJ. Images in cardiovascular medicine. Constrictive pericarditis. *Circulation.* 1996;93:834-835.)

pressure—exaggerating this normal drop in the pulmonary vein to left ventricle gradient. This phenomenon, termed intrathoracic-intracardiac dissociation, can be identified by a variation in pulmonary wedge to left ventricular diastolic pressure gradient of >5 mmHg from inspiration to expiration (**Figure 20.12**). Thus, the left ventricle becomes acutely underfilled during inspiration, accounting for the drop in LV and aortic systolic pressure (pulsus paradoxus, **Figure 20.13**). Because of the markedly enhanced ventricular interaction mediated by pericardial restraint, the right ventricle then takes advantage of this left-side underfill-

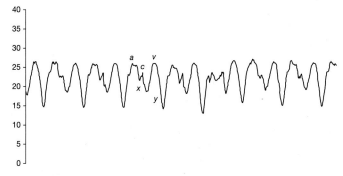

Figure 20.9 Right atrial pressure tracing in a patient with constrictive pericarditis. Mean central venous pressure is markedly elevated (23 mmHg) with prominent *x* and particularly *y* descents giving the sawtooth appearance known as the "M" or "W" sign.

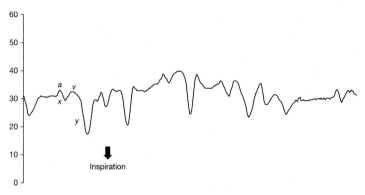

Figure 20.10 Elevation in right atrial pressure during inspiration (Kussmaul sign) in a patient with constrictive pericarditis.

ing. The septum bows from right to left, and right ventricular diastolic volume increases with acute increases in RV stroke volume, and RV systolic pressure will increase during inspiration. This discordant change in LV and RV systolic pressures (or pressure-time area) is the key hemodynamic finding of enhanced ventricular interdependence (**Figure 20.14**).

Additional "classical" hemodynamic findings associated with constrictive physiology include equalization of diastolic pressures across the 4 cardiac chambers

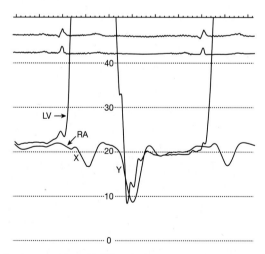

Figure 20.11 Simultaneous right atrial (RA) and LV pressure recordings demonstrating equalization during diastole and prominent X and Y descents in the RA tracing. (Reproduced with permission from Vaitkus PT, Cooper KA, Shuman WP, Hardin NJ. Images in cardiovascular medicine. Constrictive pericarditis. *Circulation*. 1996;93:834-835.)

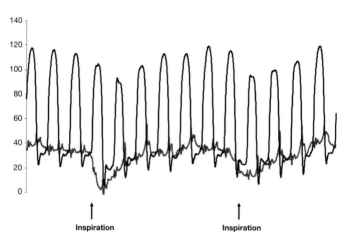

Figure 20.12 Dynamic criteria for pericardial constriction: Simultaneous recording of left ventricular (black tracing) and pulmonary capillary wedge pressure (red tracing) showing intrathoracic-intracavitary dissociation during inspiration.

(left ventricular end-diastolic pressure [LVEDP]—right ventricular end-diastolic pressure [RVEDP] < 5 mmHg), the absence of significant pulmonary hypertension (pulmonary artery systolic pressure < 55 mmHg), and a RVEDP to right ventricular systolic pressure (RVEDP/RVSP) ratio of >1/3 (**Figure 20.15**). While these findings are generally of high sensitivity, they are poorly specific for constriction and are often seen in restrictive disease or "garden variety" heart failure (**Table 20.1**).

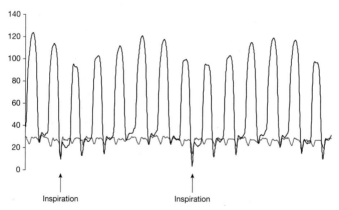

Figure 20.13 During inspiration, there is marked drop in LV systolic pressure (pulsus paradoxus, black tracing) with no reduction in right atrial pressure (Kussmaul sign, blue tracing) in a patient with constrictive pericarditis. Note the prominent *y* descent in the right atrial tracing superimposed on the prominent "dip and plateau" in the LV tracing, which is in contrast to the absent *y* descent and minimal diastolic pressure in tamponade. LV, left ventricular.

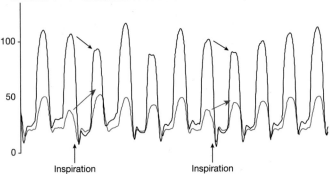

Figure 20.14 Ventricular discordance. During inspiration, the increase in right ventricular pressure (red tracing, red arrows) is associated with a reduction in left ventricular pressure (black tracing, black arrows).

The hemodynamic findings of pericardial constriction are preload dependent, and the equalization of diastolic pressures might be absent in the setting of intravascular volume depletion. Thus, volume loading should be part of the cardiac catheterization protocol in those cases where initial filling pressures are low and the initial hemodynamic data are nondiagnostic (**Figure 20.16**). However, the latter group of occult constriction should also display a low cardiac output, and as a general rule of thumb, hemodynamically important constrictive pericarditis is virtually excluded in patients with normal right atrial pressure and normal cardiac output, even if pericardial disease is present.

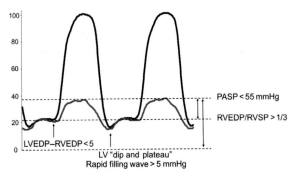

Figure 20.15 Left (black) and right ventricular (red) pressure tracings showing classical hemodynamic findings observed in constriction including near equalization in LV and RV end-diastolic pressures (LVEDP, RVEDP), a prominent "dip and plateau" with elevated rapid filling wave, ratio of RVEDP to RV systolic pressure of >0.33, and absent pulmonary hypertension (PA systolic pressure, PASP, <55 mmHg). LV, left ventricular; LVEDP, left ventricular end-diastolic pressure; PA, pulmonary artery; PASP, pulmonary artery systolic pressure; RV, right ventricular; RVSP, right ventricular systolic pressure.

Table 20.1 Sensitivities, Specificities, Positive Predictive Values, and Negative Predictive Values as a Function of Criteria for the Diagnosis of Constrictive Pericarditis

Criteria	Sensitivity (%)	Specificity (%)	PPV (%)	NPV (%)
Conventional				
LVEDP – RVEDP ≤ 5 mmHg	60	38	4	57
RVEDP/RVSP > 1/3	93	38	52	89
PASP < 55 mmHg	93	24	47	25
LV RFW ≥ 7 mmHg	93	57	61	92
Respiratory change in RAP < 3 mmHg	93	48	58	92
Dynamic respiratory				
PCWP – LV respiratory gradient ≥ 5 mmHg	93	81	78	94
LV-RV interdependence	100	95	94	100

LV, left ventricular; LVEDP, left ventricular end-diastolic pressure; NPV, negative predictive value; PASP, pulmonary artery systolic pressure; PCWP, pulmonary capillary wedge pressure, PPV, positive predictive value; RAP, right atrial pressure; RFW, rapid filling wave; RV, right ventricular; RVEDP, right ventricular end-diastolic pressure; RVSP, right ventricular systolic pressure.
Reproduced with permission from Hurrell DG, Nishimura RA, Higano ST, et al. Value of dynamic respiratory changes in left and right ventricular pressures for the diagnosis of constrictive pericarditis. *Circulation*. 1996;93:2007-2013.

RESTRICTIVE PHYSIOLOGY

As with constrictive pericarditis, restrictive cardiomyopathy is characterized by severe diastolic dysfunction and preserved ejection fraction. The fundamental difference is that diastolic filling is restricted by the myocardium in restriction rather than by the pericardium. Both constrictive pericarditis and restrictive cardiomyopathy are commonly associated with rapid x and y descents, the Kussmaul sign, and with typical right and left ventricular "dip and plateau" patterns during diastole. Restrictive cardiomyopathy typically involves the entire myocardium, including the interventricular septum, which impedes the septal shift toward the left during inspiration. Thus, left ventricular pressure tracks right ventricular pressure during systole with respiration in a concordant fashion.

In addition to restrictive cardiomyopathy and constrictive pericarditis, other cardiovascular diseases can also cause similar hemodynamics. In particular, patients with right-side heart failure and severe tricuspid regurgitation also may display numerous classical findings and even some elements of enhanced interdependence. This is because right-side chamber enlargement increases pericardial restraint, even in the absence of pericardial pathology. However, in contrast to constriction, patients with severe tricuspid insufficiency will frequently display an increase in RV diastolic pressure above that of the LV during inspiration.

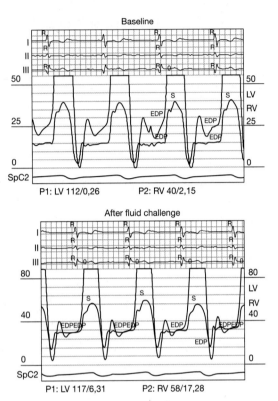

Figure 20.16 Pressure curves showing increased left and right ventricular diastolic pressures (top) with dip and plateau (square root sign), consistent with constriction physiology, and equalization of diastolic pressures after volume loading (bottom). EDP, end diastolic pressure; LV, left ventricular; RV, right ventricular. (Reproduced with permission from Sharif D, Radzievsky N, Rosenschein U. Images in cardiovascular medicine. Recurrent pericardial constriction: vibrations of the knock, the calcific shield, and the evoked constrictive physiology. *Circulation.* 2008;118:1685-1688.)

SUGGESTED READINGS

1. Atherton JJ, Moore TD, Thomson HL, Frenneaux MP. Restrictive left ventricular filling patterns are predictive of diastolic ventricular interaction in chronic heart failure. *J Am Coll Cardiol.* 1998;31(2):413-418.
2. Bogaert J, Francone M. Cardiovascular magnetic resonance in pericardial diseases. *J Cardiovasc Magn Reson.* 2009;11(1):14.
3. Boltwood CM, Lee PY, Tei C, Shah PM. Low-pressure cardiac tamponade. *N Engl J Med.* 1983;309(11):667-668.
4. Bush CA, Stang JM, Wooley CF, Kilman JW. Occult constrictive pericardial disease. Diagnosis by rapid volume expansion and correction by pericardiectomy. *Circulation.* 1977;56(6):924-930.
5. Chuttani K, Pandian NG, Mohanty PK, et al. Left ventricular diastolic collapse. An echocardiographic sign of regional cardiac tamponade. *Circulation.* 1991;83(6):1999-2006.
6. Dwivedi SK, Saran R, Narain VS. Left ventricular diastolic collapse in low-pressure cardiac tamponade. *Clin Cardiol.* 1998;21(3):224-226.

7. Farrar DJ, Chow E, Brown CD. Isolated systolic and diastolic ventricular interactions in pacing-induced dilated cardiomyopathy and effects of volume loading and pericardium. *Circulation.* 1995;92(5):1284-1290.

8. Freeman GL, LeWinter MM. Pericardial adaptations during chronic cardiac dilation in dogs. *Circ Res.* 1984;54(3):294-300.

9. Frenneaux M, Williams L. Ventricular-arterial and ventricular-ventricular interactions and their relevance to diastolic filling. *Prog Cardiovasc Dis.* 2007;49(4):252-262.

10. Garcia MJ, Rodriguez L, Ares M, Griffin BP, Thomas JD, Klein AL. Differentiation of constrictive pericarditis from restrictive cardiomyopathy: assessment of left ventricular diastolic velocities in longitudinal axis by Doppler tissue imaging. *J Am Coll Cardiol.* 1996;27(1):108-114.

11. Ha JW, Oh JK, Ling LH, Nishimura RA, Seward JB, Tajik AJ. Annulus paradoxus: transmitral flow velocity to mitral annular velocity ratio is inversely proportional to pulmonary capillary wedge pressure in patients with constrictive pericarditis. *Circulation.* 2001;104(9):976-978.

12. Hancock EW. Subacute effusive-constrictive pericarditis. *Circulation.* 1971;43(2):183-192.

13. Hancock EW. A clearer view of effusive-constrictive pericarditis. *N Engl J Med.* 2004;350(5):435-437.

14. Hayes SN, Freeman WK, Gersh BJ. Low pressure cardiac tamponade: diagnosis facilitated by Doppler echocardiography. *Br Heart J.* 1990;63(2):136-140.

15. Hurrell DG, Nishimura RA, Higano ST, et al. Value of dynamic respiratory changes in left and right ventricular pressures for the diagnosis of constrictive pericarditis. *Circulation.* 1996;93(11):2007-2013.

16. Jaber WA, Sorajja P, Borlaug BA, Nishimura RA. Differentiation of tricuspid regurgitation from constrictive pericarditis: novel criteria for diagnosis in the cardiac catheterisation laboratory. *Heart.* 2009;95(17):1449-1454.

17. Labib SB, Udelson JE, Pandian NG. Echocardiography in low pressure cardiac tamponade. *Am J Cardiol.* 1989;63(15):1156-1157.

18. Little WC, Warner JG Jr., Rankin KM, Kitzman DW, Cheng CP. Evaluation of left ventricular diastolic function from the pattern of left ventricular filling. *Clin Cardiol.* 1998;21(1):5-9.

19. Myers RB, Spodick DH. Constrictive pericarditis: clinical and pathophysiologic characteristics. *Am Heart J.* 1999;138(2 pt 1):219-232.

20. Sagrista-Sauleda J, Angel J, Sanchez A, Permanyer-Miralda G, Soler-Soler J. Effusive-constrictive pericarditis. *N Engl J Med.* 2004;350(5):469-475.

21. Sagrista-Sauleda J, Angel J, Sambola A, Alguersuari J, Permanyer-Miralda G, Soler-Soler J. Low-pressure cardiac tamponade: clinical and hemodynamic profile. *Circulation.* 2006;114(9):945-952.

22. Spodick DH. Physiology of the normal pericardium: functions of the pericardium. In: Spodick DH, ed. *The Pericardium: A Comprehensive Textbook.* Marcel Dekker, Inc; 1997:15-26.

23. Spodick DH. Constrictive pericarditis. In: Spodick DH, ed. *The Pericardium: A Comprehensive Textbook.* Marcel Dekker, Inc; 1997:214-259.

24. Talreja DR, Edwards WD, Danielson GK, et al. Constrictive pericarditis in 26 patients with histologically normal pericardial thickness. *Circulation.* 2003;108(15):1852-1857.

25. Vaitkus PT, Cooper KA, Shuman WP, Hardin NJ. Images in cardiovascular medicine. Constrictive pericarditis. *Circulation.* 1996;93(4):834-835.

21 Evaluation of Myocardial and Coronary Blood Flow and Metabolism[1]

CONTROL OF MYOCARDIAL BLOOD FLOW: THE MYOCARDIAL OXYGEN SUPPLY AND DEMAND RELATIONSHIP

The heart requires a sufficient quantity (supply) of oxygen for any given oxygen need (demand), to prevent ischemia or infarction. The heart is an aerobic organ that relies almost exclusively on the real-time oxidation of substrates for energy generation, with little ability to accumulate an oxygen debt as is seen with skeletal muscle. In the steady state, cardiac metabolic activity is thus accurately measured by myocardial oxygen demand (MVO_2). The total metabolism of an arrested, quiescent heart is approximately 1.5 mL O_2/100 g myocardium/min, to support the physiologic processes not associated with contraction. In contrast, a beating canine heart has MVO_2 ranging from 8 to 15 mL O_2/100 g myocardium/min.

Under normal aerobic conditions, several substrates contribute simultaneously to meeting myocardial energy needs: free fatty acid (65%), glucose (15%), lactate and pyruvate (12%), and amino acids (5%), whereas glycolysis plays only a minor role. In fact, lactate is extracted by the myocardium, converted into pyruvate, and oxidized by way of the Krebs cycle. In the fasting state, when serum fatty acids are high, myocardial glucose uptake tends to be suppressed in favor of fatty acid utilization. But after an oral glucose load, or when a fall in myocardial blood flow or oxygen supply leads to a reduction or loss in mechanical function, glucose uptake is enhanced and fatty acid oxidation declines. Although glucose metabolism is preferentially aerobic, decreasing oxygen availability decreases high-energy phosphate and leads to the accumulation of ATP breakdown products (ADP, AMP, and other nucleosides). The myocardium then turns toward enhancing glycogenolysis and glycolysis to augment ATP production. In doing so, the pyruvate-lactate equilibrium is shifted toward lactate formation, causing net transmyocardial lactate production rather than extraction.

At rest, the rate of force development and the frequency of force generation per unit time accounts for approximately 60% of myocardial energy use; myocardial relaxation accounts for approximately 15% of energy use; electrical activity accounts for 4%; and basal cellular metabolism accounts for the remaining 20% of energy use. As workload increases, myocardial contractile function consumes an even larger fraction of high-energy phosphate availability. Any compromise in substrate availability causes the myocardium to minimize energy expenditure on mechanical work and divert the remaining high-energy substrates for the continued maintenance of cellular integrity, thus setting the stage for myocardial "hibernation" or worse leads to complete cessation of energy production with irreversible cellular injury.

---

[1]We gratefully acknowledge the Grossman & Baim's *Cardiac Catheterization, Angiography, and Intervention*, 9th edition contributions of Drs. Morton J. Kern, Arnold H. Seto, and Michael J. Lim as portions of their chapter, Evaluation of Myocardial and Coronary Blood Flow and Metabolism, were retained in this text.

Determinants of Myocardial Oxygen Supply

The 3 major physiologic determinants of MVO_2 are heart rate, myocardial contractility, and myocardial wall tension or stress.

1. Heart rate is the most important determinant of MVO_2. When heart rate doubles, myocardial oxygen uptake approximately doubles. Heart rate is a dominant factor in the O_2 supply-demand ratio for 2 reasons: Increases in heart rate increases oxygen consumption, and increases in heart rate reduce subendocardial coronary flow owing to shortening of the diastolic filling period. Subendocardial ischemia may thus occur during tachycardia because of simultaneously increasing demand (tachycardia) and compromised flow for the subepicardium.

2. Myocardial contractility is related to myocardial oxygen consumption by the degree of pressure work per heartbeat. The net effect of positive inotropic stimuli (eg, Ca^{++} and catecholamines) on MVO_2 is the result of myocardial contractility, which is increased by inotropic stimuli.

3. Myocardial wall tension is proportional to increased aortic pressure, myocardial fibril length, and ventricular volume. Myocardial oxygen consumption doubles as mean aortic pressure increases from 75 to 175 mmHg, at constant heart rate and stroke volume. Comparing the relative effects of ventricular pressure, stroke volume, and heart rate on MVO_2, ventricular pressure development is a key determinant of MVO_2.

MEASUREMENT OF MYOCARDIAL METABOLISM

Measurement of myocardial metabolism (MVO_2) may be performed noninvasively (eg, positron emission tomography scanning) or invasively by coronary blood flow x (arterial O_2 content – coronary sinus O_2 content). In studies involving ischemic myocardial metabolism, the most accurately measured products are lactate, adenosine, and oxygen.

Regulation of Coronary Blood Flow and Resistance

Coronary arterial resistance is the sum of the resistances of the epicardial coronary conduit ($R1$) and the precapillary arteriolar ($R2$) and intramyocardial capillary ($R3$) resistance circuits (**Figure 21.1**). Normal epicardial coronary arteries in humans typically taper from the base of the heart with diameters of 5 to 6 mm to the apex where the vessel diameter is approximately 0.3 mm. The epicardial vessels do not offer appreciable resistance to blood flow ($R1$) in their normal state until atherosclerotic obstructions develop. Most of the epicardial vessel wall consists of a muscular media that responds to changes in aortic pressure and flow, modulating coronary tone by responding to flow-mediated endothelium-derived relaxing factors. Large-conduit arteries can produce episodic increases in resistance during severe focal or diffuse contraction (vasospasm) in the absence of significant atherosclerosis. One exception is myocardial bridging, in which intramyocardial vessel segments may offer increased resistance during systole and more seriously diastole owing to mechanical compression of the bridged segment during ventricular contraction and relaxation.

Precapillary arterioles are resistive vessels ($R2$) that are the principal controllers of coronary blood flow. Precapillary arterioles (100-500 μm in size) contribute approximately 25% to 35% of total coronary resistance. The precapillary arteriolar resistance function autoregulates the driving pressure at the origin of the precapillary arterioles within a finite pressure range. This regulatory function is also influenced by myogenic and flow-dependent vasodilatation related to shear stress.

The microcirculatory resistance ($R3$) circuit consists of a dense network of about 4000 capillaries per square millimeter, which ensures that each myocyte is adjacent

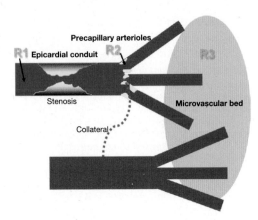

Figure 21.1 Diagram of coronary resistances. The epicardial arteries (*R*1) normally have negligible resistance until an atherosclerotic narrowing occurs (top artery). The precapillary arterioles (*R*2) regulate most of the coronary flow to the microvascular bed (*R*3).

to a capillary. Capillaries are not uniformly patent because precapillary sphincters regulate flow according to oxygen demand. Several conditions, such as left ventricular (LV) hypertrophy, myocardial ischemia, or diabetes, can increase the microcirculatory resistance (R3) and blunt the normal maximal increases in coronary flow.

As in any vascular bed, blood flow to the myocardium depends on the coronary artery driving (aortic) pressure and the resistance produced by the serial vascular components. Coronary vascular resistance, in turn, is regulated by several interrelated control mechanisms that include myocardial metabolism (metabolic control), endothelial (and other humoral) control, autoregulation, myogenic control, extravascular compressive forces, and neural control. These control mechanisms may be impaired in diseased states, thereby contributing to the development of myocardial ischemia.

Coronary vasodilatory reserve (CVR) is the ability of the coronary vascular bed to increase flow from a basal level to a maximal hyperemic level in response to a mechanical or pharmacologic stimulus. Such stimuli include the reactive hyperemia that follows transient ischemia (eg, coronary occlusion/release), exercise, and the administration of various pharmacologic agents. CFR is expressed as the ratio of maximal hyperemic flow to resting coronary flow—a ratio that averages from 2 to 5 in patients. In experimental animal studies, increasing conduit stenosis (R1) produces a predictable decline in CFR, beginning at about a 60% epicardial coronary artery stenosis.

At diameter stenoses of ≥90%, all available coronary reserve has been exhausted and resting flow begins to decline (**Figure 21.2**). This relationship between increasing stenosis severity and reduced available CFR has been used in assessing the effective physiologic severity of any given coronary stenosis and forms the basis of many noninvasive test modalities for ischemia.

In clinical practice, the influence of a stenosis on coronary blood flow is principally related to the morphologic features of the stenosis, with resistance to flow changing exponentially with lumen cross-sectional area and linearly with lesion length (**Figure 21.3**). Additional factors contributing to stenosis resistance include the shape of the entrance and exit orifices, vessel stiffness, distensibility of the diseased segment (permitting active or passive vasomotion), and the variable lumen obstruction that may be superimposed by platelet aggregation and thrombosis compromising lumen area, a process active in acute coronary syndromes.

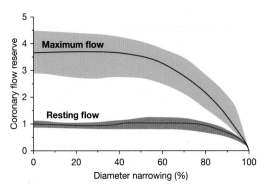

Figure 21.2 Coronary flow reserve expressed as ratio of maximum to resting flow plotted as a function of percent diameter narrowing. With progressive narrowing, resting flow does not change (red line), whereas maximum potential increase in flow and coronary flow reserve begin to be impaired at approximately 60% diameter narrowing. (Reproduced with permission from Gould KL, Lipscomb K, Hamilton GW. Physiologic basis for assessing critical coronary stenosis: instantaneous flow response and regional distribution during coronary hyperemia as measures of coronary flow reserve. *Am J Cardiol.* 1974;33:87-94.)

As blood traverses a diseased arterial segment, turbulence, friction, and separation of laminar flow cause energy loss, resulting in a pressure gradient (ΔP) across the stenosis.

Using a simplified Bernoulli formula for fluid dynamics, pressure loss across a stenosis can be estimated from blood flow,

$$\Delta P = fQ + sQ^2 \tag{21.1}$$

$$\Delta P = \frac{1.8Q}{d_{\text{sten}}^4} + \frac{6.1Q^2}{d_{\text{sten}}^4} \tag{21.2}$$

where ΔP is the pressure drop across a stenosis in millimeters of mercury, Q is the flow across the stenosis in milliliters per second, and d is the minimal diameter

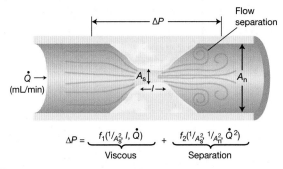

$$\Delta P = \underbrace{f_1(^1/_{A_s^2}, I, \dot{Q})}_{\text{Viscous}} + \underbrace{f_2(^1/_{A_s^2}, ^1/_{A_n^2}, \dot{Q}^2)}_{\text{Separation}}$$

Figure 21.3 Diagrammatic illustration of the Bernoulli equation. ΔP, pressure gradient; A_s, area of the stenosis; A_n, area of the normal segment; L, stenosis length; Q, flow; f_1, viscous friction factor (f); f_2, separation coefficient (s).

of the stenosis lumen in millimeters. In Eq. (21.1), the first term (f) accounts for energy losses owing to viscous friction between the laminar layers of fluid and the second term (s) reflects energy loss when normal arterial flow is transformed first to high-velocity flow in the stenosis and then to the turbulent nonlaminar distal flow eddies at the exit from the stenosis (inertia and expansion).

It is important to note that the separation energy loss term (s) increases with the square of the flow while viscous energy loss (f) becomes negligible. Thus, increases in coronary blood flow increase the associated pressure gradient in an exponential manner. Despite augmentation of coronary blood flow, the increasing pressure loss across the stenotic segment reduces myocardial perfusion pressure and lowers the threshold for myocardial ischemia relative to demand.

From Eq. (21.2), the transstenotic pressure drop is inversely proportional to the fourth power of the lumen radius. As a consequence, in a severe stenosis, relatively small change in luminal diameter (such as that caused by active or passive vasomotion or transient obstruction by thrombus) can produce marked hemodynamic effects. For example, when the diameter stenosis increases from 80% to 90%, the resistance of a stenosis rises nearly 3-fold. For most stenoses, the length of the narrowing has only a modest effect on its physiologic significance. However, in very long narrowed segments, significant turbulence occurs along the walls of the stenotic segment and energy is dissipated as heat when eddies form and impact on the vessel wall. In addition, a preserved arc of vascular smooth muscle in some diseased arteries may be compliant and subject to dynamic changes that can alter luminal caliber and stenosis resistance. Dynamic changes in stenosis severity and resistance can also occur passively in response to changes in intraluminal distending pressure or selective dilation of distal resistance vessels. Thus, for a given stenosis, there is a family of pressure-flow relationships reflecting altered stenosis diameter and variable distending pressure.

MEASUREMENTS OF INTRACORONARY PRESSURE AND FLOW VELOCITY USING SENSOR-TIPPED GUIDEWIRES

Measurements of intracoronary (IC) blood flow velocity or pressure can be used to describe the coronary physiologic responses to mechanical or pharmacologic interventions, determine the functional significance of a coronary stenosis, and assess the microcirculation and collateral flow. Directly measured physiologic data provide critical information, complementary to the anatomic findings and highly useful for clinical decision making.

Technique of Angioplasty Sensor Guidewire Use

After diagnostic angiography or during angioplasty, the sensor angioplasty (0.014″) guidewire is passed through a standard Y-connector attached to the guiding catheter (6F catheters are suitable). Standard anticoagulation is given (eg, 70-100 units of unfractionated heparin per kg) before introducing the guidewire. IC nitroglycerin (100-200 pg) is given before guidewire introduction to reduce guidewire-induced vasospasm.

To measure Doppler coronary flow velocity (**Figure 21.4**), the Doppler sensor, located at the very distal guidewire tip, is advanced at least >2 cm beyond the stenosis to measure laminar flow (otherwise the turbulent flow close to the stenosis may underestimate true velocity). Resting flow velocity is recorded, and then coronary hyperemia is induced by IC or intravenous (IV) adenosine with continuous recording of the flow velocity signals. CFR is computed as the ratio of maximal hyperemic to basal average peak velocity (**Figure 21.5**). Because of the highly position-dependent signal, poor signal acquisition may occur in 15% of patients, requiring the operator to adjust the guidewire position in order to optimize the velocity signal.

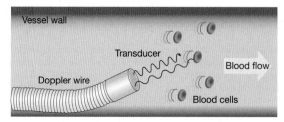

Figure 21.4 Schematic depiction of a Doppler flow wire emitting ultrasound signals along the direction of the vessel with return of the signals after interacting with flowing red blood cells to produce a Doppler-derived blood flow velocity in a coronary artery.

The **pressure wire sensor** is located approximately 3 cm from the distal wire tip designed to permit movement of the sensor across stenotic areas without losing position in the distal vessel. To measure translesional pressure for the calculation of the resting (eg, P_d/P_a, diastolic pressure ratios) or hyperemic pressure-derived lesion assessment indices (eg, FFR), the following steps are recommended:

1. Set both the fluid filled guide catheter and micromanometer sensor wire pressures to zero (ie, atmospheric pressure) on the table.
2. Introduce the pressure wire through the guide catheter to the coronary ostium. Match the guide catheter and wire pressures by electronically equalizing or normalizing the 2 pressures. (Note: matching central aortic and guidewire pressures can occur in the guide catheter, outside the guide, or even when the guide is seated in the coronary ostium provided there is no ostial obstruction to flow.)
3. Advance the guidewire into the artery with the sensor beyond the stenosis by a distance of >2 cm (enough distance to permit reestablishment of laminar flow).

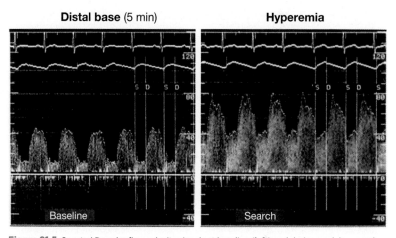

Figure 21.5 Spectral Doppler flow velocity signals at baseline **(left)** and during peak hyperemia **(right)**. "S" and "D" labels associated with the systolic and diastolic portions of the cardiac cycle. The average peak velocity (APV) at baseline was 27 cm/s, and the APV at hyperemia was 53. Coronary flow reserve = 53/27 = 2.1.

4. Record baseline pressures. For FFR, continue pressure recordings during induction of coronary hyperemia. Baseline resting distal/aortic pressure ratios, also known as nonhyperemic pressure ratios, are discussed below. FFR can be obtained after observing response to IV or IC adenosine injection or FFR measured at maximal hyperemia as the lowest ratio of distal coronary to aortic pressure (**Figure 21.6**).

5. After measurements are completed, signal drift can be detected by the matched pressure waveforms on wire pullback to the guide catheter.

The safety of IC sensor-wire measurements is excellent, with benign problems related mostly to adenosine. Severe transient bradycardia after IC adenosine occurs in <2.0% of patients, coronary spasm during passage of the Doppler guidewire in 1%, and ventricular fibrillation during the procedure in 0.2% of patients.

Coronary Hyperemia for Stenosis Assessment

At maximal hyperemia, autoregulation is abolished and microvascular resistance is constant and minimal. Under these conditions, coronary blood flow is linearly related to the driving pressure. Therefore, maximal hyperemic coronary blood flow is closely dependent on the coronary arterial pressure at the time of the measurement.

The most widely used pharmacologic agent to induce coronary hyperemia is adenosine. Adenosine is a potent short-acting hyperemic stimulus with the total duration of hyperemia only 25% that of papaverine or dipyridamole. Adenosine is benign at appropriate dosages (50-100 µg in the right coronary artery [RCA] and 100 to 200 µg in the left coronary artery [LCA], or infused intravenously at 140 µg/kg/min). IV and IC adenosine produce equal levels of hyperemia. In 30 patients without stenoses, Doppler wire measurements demonstrated that maximal hyperemia occurred with 60 µg

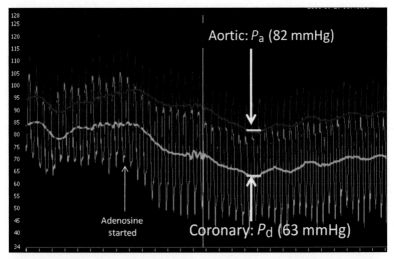

Figure 21.6 Pressure tracings depicting the fluid-filled aortic phasic and mean pressure **(red)** as well as the distal coronary micromanometer phasic and mean pressure **(green)**. There is a resting gradient between the mean pressures prior to adenosine administration. After adenosine, the pressure gradient widens. The largest pressure difference at steady hyperemia is then used to determine fractional flow reserve. In this case, it is calculated as 63/82, or 0.77.

of IC adenosine in the RCA and 160 µg in the LCA. The duration of the plateau reached 12 ± 13 s after injection of 100 µg in the RCA and 21 ± 6 s after the injection of 200 µg in the LCA. Adenosine IV is preferable for pressure wire pullback assessment. IC adenosine provides more rapid results with fewer adverse systemic symptoms.

Iodinated contrast media produce partial submaximal hyperemia. Nitrates increase volumetric flow, but since these agents also dilate epicardial conductance vessels, the increase in coronary flow velocity is less than those with adenosine or papaverine. IC papaverine (8-12 mg) increases coronary blood flow velocity 4 to 6 times over resting values in patients with normal coronary arteries and produces a response equal to that of an IV infusion of dipyridamole in a dose of 0.56 to 0.84 mg/kg of body weight, and can cause QT prolongation and, rarely, ventricular tachycardia or fibrillation.

Translesional Pressure-Derived Fractional Flow Reserve

Using the ratio translesional coronary pressures at maximal hyperemia, Pijls et al. derived an estimate of the percentage of normal coronary blood flow expected to go through a stenotic artery, called the fractional flow reserve (FFR). Using hyperemia to abolish autoregulation, the FFR is linearly correlated with coronary flow.

Pijls and colleagues described 3 components of the flow contributions: (1) the coronary artery, (2) the myocardium, and (3) the collateral supply. FFR of the coronary artery (FFR_{cor}) is defined as the maximum coronary artery flow in the presence of a stenosis divided by the maximum flow in that artery if no stenosis were present. Similarly, FFR of the myocardium (FFR_{myo}) is defined as maximum myocardial (artery and myocardial bed) flow distal to an epicardial stenosis divided by its value if no epicardial stenosis were present. The difference between FFR myo and FFR cor is FFR of the collateral flow.

The following equation is used to calculate the FFR of a coronary artery and its subtended myocardium:

$$FFR_{cor} = \left(P_d - P_w\right)/\left(P_a - P_w\right)$$
$$FFR_{myo} = \left(P_d - P_v\right)/\left(P_a - P_v\right)$$
$$FFR_{collateral} = FFR_{myo} - FFR_{cor} \tag{21.3}$$

where Pa, Pd, Pv, and P_w are the aortic, distal arterial, venous (or right atrial), and coronary wedge (during balloon occlusion) pressures, respectively; because FFR_{cor} uses P_w, it can be calculated only during coronary angioplasty.

FFR myo can be readily calculated during either diagnostic or interventional procedures. In most clinical circumstances P_v is negligible relative to aortic pressure and hence omitted from the calculations. FFR reflects both antegrade and collateral (or bypass graft) myocardial perfusion rather than merely the transstenotic pressure loss (ie, a stenosis pressure gradient). Because it is calculated only at peak hyperemia and excludes the microcirculatory resistance from the computation, FFR is differentiated from CVR as being largely independent of basal flow, driving pressure, heart rate, systemic blood pressure, and status of the microcirculation.

In contrast to the resting or hyperemic absolute pressure gradient (AP), FFR is strongly related to inducible myocardial ischemia as demonstrated by comparisons with different clinical stress testing modalities in patients with stable angina. The clinical nonischemic threshold value of FFR is >0.80, while <0.75 is the best cutoff value for ischemic stress testing. In patients with an abnormal microcirculation, a normal FFR indicates that the epicardial conduit resistance (eg, a stenosis) is not a major contributing factor to perfusion impairment and that focal conduit enlargement (eg, stenting) would not restore normal perfusion. FFR is thus specific for stenosis resistance and by design excludes the assessment and influence of the microcirculation. **Table 21.1** lists several potential pitfalls that can produce erroneous coronary pressure measurements. In particular, recognition of guide catheter damping or ventricularization due to deep catheter seating should prompt correction.

Coronary Pulse Wave Analysis

Davies et al. reported on the use of coronary pulse wave analysis to better understand the relationship between myocardial contraction, myocardial resistance, aortic and coronary pressures, and their reflected pressure waves. The pulse analysis begins with the acquisition of simultaneous high-fidelity IC pressure and flow velocity signals obtained from sensor-tipped angioplasty guidewires. Normal coronary perfusion is the net result of pressure waves and flow generated initially in the proximal aorta and those counterbalancing pressure waves moving back toward the aorta originating in the distal end of the coronary flow path. The cycle of cardiac contraction and relaxation produces 6 pressure waves having different magnitude (intensity), direction, and velocity owing to competing accelerations and decelerations. Coronary blood flow into the myocardium is largely determined by the prominent coronary suction wave of LV relaxation at the beginning of diastole (wave 5), increasing coronary flow from the aorta into the epicardial coronary artery and into the myocardium. During systolic ejection, LV and aortic pressures are coupled, with LV pressure being the major determinant of intramyocardial stress. As pressures at each end of the coronary artery (aortic and LV-myocardial) are similar during systole, the net change in coronary flow during systole is normally minimal. In diastole, the aortic valve closure uncouples aortic from LV pressure producing an aortic-LV myocardial pressure gradient accelerating coronary blood flow (via the diastolic suction wave) into the epicardial artery and myocardium.

NONHYPEREMIC PRESSURE RATIOS

The use of FFR in interventional cardiology is <20% of cases worldwide. Some operators cite cost, time, complexity of technique, and side effects from use of adenosine (eg, dyspnea, heart block). Nonhyperemic indices have promoted the incorporation of physiology into the catheterization laboratory through simplicity and avoiding the need for adenosine hyperemia.

Table 21.1 Pitfalls of Fractional Flow Reserve

1. **Equipment factors**:
   - Erroneous zero (tubing/connector leaks)
   - Faulty electric wire connection
   - Pressure signal drift, miscalibration, ECG
2. **Procedural factors**
   - Guide catheter damping
   - Incorrect sensor position
   - Inadequate hyperemia
   - Changing basal flow
3. **Physiological factors**
   - Serial lesion
   - LM/collateral myocardial bed size
   - STEMI
   - Left ventricular hypertrophy
   - Elevated left ventricular or right atrial pressure

Instantaneous Wave-Free Ratio

Using the wave-intensity analysis described previously, Sen and Davies identified a period of diastole in which equilibrium is reached between pressure waves from the aorta and distal microcirculatory reflection. This wave-free period (WFP) occurs 75% of the way through diastole to 5 ms before systole and is a period during which the resistance is relatively low and stable, also suggesting a period wherein there is a direct relationship between pressure and flow. The P_d/P_a during the WFP was called the instantaneous wave-free pressure ratio (iFR) (**Figure 21.7**). In contrast to FFR, which abolishes autoregulation, iFR may represent the extent to which autoregulatory vasodilatory responses maintain resting coronary flow in the presence of a coronary stenosis, but at the cost of pressure loss across the epicardial stenosis.

CLINICAL APPLICATIONS OF CORONARY BLOOD FLOW AND PRESSURE MEASUREMENTS

The physiologic criteria for a hemodynamically significant coronary lesion include a poststenotic absolute coronary flow reserve (CVR) of <2.0 and an FFR of <0.80 or iFR of <0.89 when using pressure-sensor guidewires.

Validation and Threshold of Ischemia

FFR values of <0.75 are associated with ischemic stress testing in numerous comparative studies, with high sensitivity (88%), specificity (100%), positive predictive value (100%), and overall accuracy (93%). FFR values of >0.80 are associated with negative ischemic results with a predictive accuracy of 95%. Single stress testing comparisons with variations in testing methods and patient cohorts have produced a zone of FFR with overlapping positive and negative results (0.75-0.80). The use of FFR in this

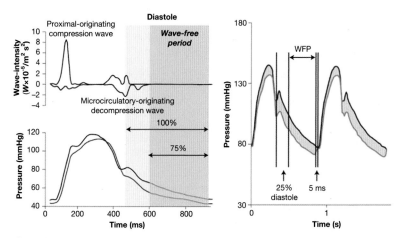

Figure 21.7 Instantaneous wave-free pressure ratio (iFR). **(Left)** Wave-free period (WFP) is demonstrated by the absence of reflected backward and forward traveling waves during diastole. **(Right)** Use of aortic (red line) and distal coronary pressure (green line) across a lesion to compute iFR. (Modified from Sen S, Escaned J, Malik IS, et al. Development and validation of a new adenosine-independent index of stenosis severity from coronary wave-intensity analysis: results of the ADVISE (ADenosine Vasodilator Independent Stenosis Evaluation) study. *J Am Coll Cardiol.* 2012;59:1392-1402.)

zone requires clinical judgment. A meta-analysis of 31 studies comparing the results of FFR with that of quantitative coronary angiography (QCA) and/or noninvasive imaging of the same lesions reported (18 studies, 1522 lesions) found that QCA had a sensitivity of 78% and specificity of 51% against FFR (<0.75 cutoff). As compared with noninvasive imaging (21 studies, 1249 lesions), receiver/operator characteristic estimates were similar for comparisons of FFR with perfusion scintigraphy (976 lesions, sensitivity 75%, specificity 77%) and dobutamine stress echocardiography (273 lesions, sensitivity 82%, specificity 74%). Given the variances in sensitivity, specificity, positive and negative predictive accuracy among patients, and methods of stress testing, it is not surprising that, unlike the initial validation study comparing FFR with 3 different stress tests in the same patient before and after percutaneous coronary intervention (PCI), this meta-analysis showed only modest concordance of FFR with noninvasive imaging tests. Furthermore, because perfusion scintigraphy compares relative and not absolute myocardial flow in different coronary beds, scintigraphy, although considered the clinical "gold standard" of ischemia, has limitations in identifying the hemodynamic significance of individual lesions in patients with multivessel coronary artery disease (CAD). Similarly, in stress echocardiography, severe ischemia in one region may mask the consequences of a less severe albeit hemodynamically significant lesion in another region. In contrast to noninvasive tests, FFR is a vessel-specific index of ischemia.

Coronary Flow Reserve and Fractional Flow Reserve

Although no longer routinely used for stenosis assessment, a Doppler-tipped sensor guidewire can measure CFR. An abnormal CFR (<2.0) corresponded to reversible myocardial perfusion imaging defects with high sensitivity (86%-92%), specificity (89%-100%), predictive accuracy (89%-96%), and positive and negative predictive values (84%-100% and 77%-95%, respectively). The microcirculatory contribution to an abnormal CFR makes CFR alone less useful for epicardial lesion assessment unless normal. Combined pressure and flow data have produced a novel set of invasive physiologic tools for microvascular assessment, such as index of microcirculatory resistance and hyperemic myocardial resistance.

Instantaneous Wave-Free Ratio Compared With Fractional Flow Reserve

Providing clinical data to support the "wave-free period" iFR measurement was carried out by comparing iFR and FFR values in the same stenosis across many groups of patients and by multiple investigators. There were no correlations performed of iFR to noninvasive references for myocardial ischemia. However, the ADVISE study was representative of the body of work, demonstrating that, across 157 stenoses, there was a good comparison between iFR and FFR assessment and a very good ability to reproduce iFR measurement.

Clinical Studies of Fractional Flow Reserve for Lesion Assessment

The DEFER study randomized 325 patients scheduled for PCI into 3 groups and has reported the 15-year long-term outcomes. If FFR was >0.75, patients were randomly assigned to the deferral group (n = 91, medical therapy [MT] for CAD) or the PCI performance group (n = 90, PCI with stents). If FFR was <0.75, PCI was performed as planned and patients were entered into the reference group (n = 144). After 15 years, the event-free survival was not different between the deferred and the performed group and both were significantly better than in the reference PCI group (63%, P = .03). After 15 years, the overall death rates were not different among the 3 groups: 33.0% in the Defer group, 31.1% in the Perform group, and 36.1% in the Reference group (Defer vs Perform, RR 1.06, 95%

confidence interval [CI]: 0.69 to 1.62, P = .79). The rate of myocardial infarction (MI) was significantly lower in the Defer group (2.2%) compared with the Perform group (10.0%; RR 0.22, 95% CI: 0.05-0.99, P = .03). Treating patients guided by FFR is associated with a low event rate, comparable with those in patients with normal noninvasive testing.

In a large prospective randomized, multicenter trial, Tonino et al., on behalf of the FAME (FFR vs Angiography for Multivessel Evaluation study) investigators, tested the outcomes for 2 PCI strategies in patients with multivessel CAD: a physiologically guided PCI approach (FFR-PCI) as compared with the conventional angiographic-guided PCI (Angio-PCI). After identifying which of the multiple lesions required treatment, 1005 patients undergoing PCI with drug-eluting stents were randomly assigned to 1 of the 2 strategies; 496 patients were assigned to the Angio-PCI group, and 509 to the FFR-PCI group. For the FFR-PCI group, all lesions had FFR measurements and were only stented if the FFR was <0.80. The primary endpoints of death, MI, and repeat revascularization (coronary artery bypass grafting [CABG] or PCI) were obtained at 1 year.

As compared with the Angio-PCI group, the FFR-PCI group used fewer stents per patient (1.9 ± 1.3 vs 2.7 ± 1.2, P < .001) and less contrast (272 vs 302 mL, P < .001) and had lower procedure cost ($5332 vs $6,007, P < .001) and shorter hospital stay (3.4 vs 3.7 days, P = .05). More importantly, at 2-year follow-up, the FFR-PCI group presented with fewer major adverse cardiovascular events (MACE; 13.2% vs 18.4%, P = .02), fewer combined death or MI (7.3% vs 11%, P = .04), and a lower total number of MACE (76 vs 113, P = .02) as compared with the Angio-PCI group.

To better address the benefits of angioplasty in lesions with an abnormal FFR, the FAME2 study randomized 888 patients with stable angina and FFR <0.80 to optimal MT alone or with stenting. The primary endpoint was a composite of death, MI, or urgent revascularization. At 5 years, the rate of the primary endpoint was lower in the PCI group than in the MT group (13.9% vs 27.0%; hazard ratio, 0.46; 95% CI, 0.34-0.63; P < .001). The difference was driven by urgent revascularizations (**Figure 21.8**), which occurred in 6.3% of the patients in the PCI group as compared with 21.1% of those in the MT group (hazard ratio, 0.27; 95% CI, 0.18-0.41). There was no significant difference in the rate of the primary endpoint between the PCI group and a registry cohort. Angina was significantly less severe in the PCI group at all follow-up points to 3 years. These data suggest that, in contrast to other studies of stable angina (COURAGE), PCI can be a reasonable and cost-effective therapy that may reduce clinically significant events.

PHYSIOLOGIC LESION ASSESSMENT FOR CORONARY INTERVENTIONS
Left Main Stenosis

The correct clinical assessment of left main (LM) CAD lesions is of pivotal importance. Decisions based on angiography alone, especially in the absence of ischemia, are questionable and can be supported by adjunctive lesion assessment modalities. Nonischemic FFR values (>0.80) in LM lesions are associated with excellent long-term outcomes. For example, multiple single-center studies and 1 multicenter trial have consistently found a low incidence of MACE including cardiac death or MI in groups with FFR >0.80 (treated medically) as compared with those undergoing CABG when FFR was <0.80. Hamilos et al. reported on 5-year outcome of the use of FFR to triage patients with LM narrowing to medical or surgical therapy based on the criterion of FFR <0.80. FFR can identify the physiologic significance of intermediate LM disease and the suitability of surgical revascularization or continued MT with excellent survival and low event rates. See **Table 21.2** for additional trials.

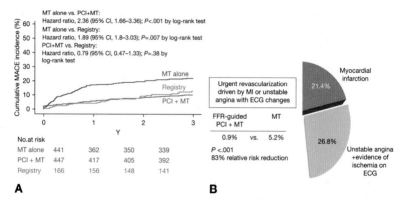

Figure 21.8 **A,** Kaplan-Meier curves are shown for the cumulative incidence of the major adverse cardiovascular *events* (MACE) of death, myocardial infarction, or urgent revascularization in the group randomly assigned to percutaneous coronary intervention (PCI) plus medical therapy (MT), the group randomly assigned to MT alone, and the group who did not undergo randomization and were enrolled in a registry. CI indicates confidence interval. **B,** Breakdown of events classified as Urgent Revascularization from the FAME 2 trial. About 21.4% of patients in this group were diagnosed with myocardial infarction (MI) and 26.8% of them had unstable angina with electrocardiogram (ECG) evidence of ischemia. In these patients, there was an 83% relative risk reduction with PCI compared with MT during the follow-up period.

However, because the pressure sensor is either in the LAD or Left Circumflex (LCX), the FFR will be artificially increased because the myocardium supplied by the LM will be reduced. Understanding the LM FFR in the setting of LAD and/or LCX disease requires further explanation. An accurate LM FFR reflects maximal flow through both the LAD and the LCX, and a second significant stenosis in the LAD or LCX will prevent obtaining maximal flow through the LM and underestimate the severity of the LM.

Fractional Flow Reserve and Ostial Branch Assessment

Ostial narrowings, especially in side branches within stents (called "jailed" branches), are particularly difficult to assess by angiography because of the overlap orientation relative to the parent branch, stent struts across the branch, and image foreshortening. Koo et al. compared FFR with QCA in 97 jailed side branch lesions (vessel size >2.0 mm, percent stenosis >50% by visual estimation) after stent implantation (no lesion with <75% stenosis had FFR <0.75). Among 73 lesions with >75% stenosis, only 20 lesions (27%) were functionally significant. Koo et al. also reported the 9-month outcome of FFR-guided side branch PCI strategy for bifurcation lesions. Among 91 patients, side branch intervention was performed in 26 of 28 patients with FFR <0.75. In this subgroup FFR increased to >0.75 despite residual stenosis of 69 ± 10%. At 9 months, functional restenosis was 8% (5 of 65) with no difference in events as compared with 110 side branches treated by angiography alone (4.6% vs 3.7%, P = .7). Measurement of FFR for ostial and side branch assessment identifies even the minority of lesions that are functionally significant.

Fractional Flow Reserve and Saphenous Vein Graft Assessment

Considerations regarding use of FFR in assessing lesions in the saphenous vein graft (SVG) involve 3 sources of coronary blood flow to the distal myocardial region: the competing flows (and pressure) from (1) the native and (2) conduit vessels and (3)

Table 21.2 Left Main Coronary Artery Revascularization Outcomes and Fractional Flow Reserve

First Author	N		FFR Cutoff Value	FU Mean Duration (Mo)	Overall Survival	
	Total	DEFER Group	Surgical Group			DEFER Group (%)	Surgical Group (%)
Bech	54	24	30	0.75	29 ± 15	100	97
Jasti	51	37	14	0.75	25 ± 11	100	100
Jimenez-Navarro	27	20	7	0.75	26 ± 12	100	86
Legutko	38	20	18	0.75	24 ± 12	100	89
Suemaru	15	8	7	0.75	33 ± 10	100	100
Lindstaedt	51	24	27	0.75	29 ± 16	100	81
Hamilos	213	138	75	0.80	35 ± 12	90	86
Total (or mean)	449	271	178	–	28 ± 13	95[a]	89

FFR, fractional flow reserve; FU, duration of follow-up.
Reproduced with permission from Puri R, Kapadia SR, Nicholls SJ, et al. Optimizing outcomes during left main percutaneous coronary intervention with intravascular ultrasound and fractional flow reserve the current state of evidence. *J Am Coll Cardiol Interv.* 2012;5:697-707.
[a]*P* = nonsignificant compared with surgical group.

the collateral flow induced from long-standing native coronary occlusion. In the most uncomplicated situation of an occluded native vessel with minimal distal collateral supply, the theory of FFR should apply just as much to a lesion in an SVG to the RCA feeding a normal myocardial bed as to a lesion in the native right coronary. For more complex situations, the FFR will reflect the summed responses of the 3 supply sources and yield a net FFR, with a value <0.80 indicating potential ischemia in that region and vice versa.

FFR may provide insight into the fate of SVG conduits implanted distal to hemodynamically insignificant lesions. Surgeons and cardiologists recognize that in such vessels late patency is reduced and native CAD can be accelerated. Even though most surgical consultations recommend "bypass all lesions with >50% diameter narrowing in patients with multivessel disease," the patency rate of SVGs on vessels with hemodynamically nonsignificant lesions has rarely been questioned. Theoretically, coronary blood flow could favor the lower resistance path through the native (relatively) nonobstructed arteries rather than through vein grafts, with slower or competitive graft flow promoting premature graft closure.

Assessment of Diffuse Atherosclerosis

A diffusely diseased atherosclerotic coronary artery can be viewed as reducing perfusion pressure along the length of the conduit. Diffuse atherosclerosis, in contrast to a focal narrowing, is characterized by a continuous and gradual pressure recovery as the sensor moves from the distal to proximal arterial region without a localized abrupt increase in pressure related to an isolated stenosis. Diffusely diseased anatomy is ideally identified by an iFR pullback. DeBruyne et al. examined FFR in normal and diffusely atherosclerotic nonstenotic arteries. FFR in the normal group was 0.97 ± 0.02 and was significantly lower, 0.89 ± 0.08, in the diffuse disease group. In 8% of arteries in the diffuse disease group without a focal narrowing, FFR was <0.75, a value below the ischemic threshold. For diffuse atherosclerosis, mechanical therapy to treat impaired flow would be futile.

Serial Epicardial Lesions

An essential prerequisite for the calculation of FFR is the achievement of maximum transstenotic flow. In the case of 2 consecutive stenoses, the blood flow interaction between the stenoses limits the applicability of the simple FFR ratio (P_d/P_a) derived for a single stenosis. When a second stenosis is present in the same epicardial vessel, flow through 1 stenosis will be submaximal because of the second stenosis. The extent to which both stenoses influence each other is somewhat unpredictable. In this case, the simple FFR does not predict to what extent a proximal lesion will influence myocardial flow until complete relief of the second stenosis and restoration of maximal hyperemia. However, the simple FFR can assess the *summed* effect across any series of stenoses, but individual lesions in the series will be more difficult to appreciate without special calculations—see case example in **Figure 21.9**.

The most practical technique to assess serial lesions involves 2 steps with 2 different measurements:

1. Pass the pressure wire distal to the last lesion and measure the summed FFR across all lesions. For example, if the FFR = 0.84, then none of the lesions would need treatment and nothing further needs to be done.
2. If the summed FFR in step 1 is <0.80, the next step is to determine which of the lesions contributes the maximum resistance to flow (ie, the largest pressure gradient). This is accomplished by performing a pressure pullback during IV adenosine hyperemia or iFR pullback without the need for hyperemia. The pressure

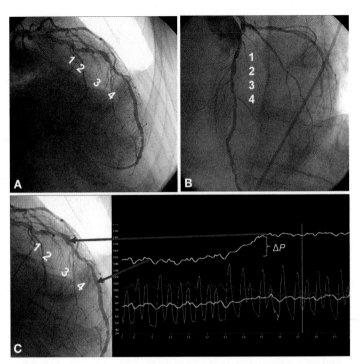

Figure 21.9 A, Right anterior oblique angiogram of the left anterior descending artery (LAD) with multiple serial lesions (1-4). **B,** Left anterior oblique angiogram of the same LAD with serial lesions (1-4). **C,** A pressure wire was advanced distal to lesion #4; maximal hyperemia was induced by intravenous adenosine; and the wire was slowly pulled from the distal LAD to a position proximal to lesion #1 as visualized by fluoroscopy. As identified on the pressure curve, a focal change in pressure gradient was observed (ΔP). The location of this change in pressure was at lesion #3. Given this information, 1 stent was placed at that location.

gradient (ΔP) between lesions indicates the degree of lesion severity. Treatment with stenting should then start with the lesion exhibiting the most significant gradient (largest ΔP). After treating this lesion, the remaining lesion(s) should be reassessed by repeating the standard FFR technique. If the FFR still remains ischemic, then treatment should progress to the next largest ΔP.

Individual FFR of each stenosis can be separately predicted by different equations using P_a, pressure between the 2 stenoses (P_m), P_d, and P_w, recorded during maximum hyperemia, thus reducing the error of FFR calculation in the presence of a second stenosis. The serial FFR formula requires P_w obtained during coronary balloon occlusion and thus is not applicable for purely diagnostic studies.

CLINICAL STUDIES OF INSTANTANEOUS WAVE-FREE RATIO

The DEFINE-FLAIR trial was a randomized, multicenter trial that aimed to determine if iFR was noninferior to FFR in terms of MACE at 1-year follow-up. Patients included in the study had CAD and either stable angina or ACS with at least 1 native coronary vessel with "questionable physiologic severity," defined as 40% to 70% stenosis by visual, angiographic assessment. A total of 2492 patients were randomized to have revascularization guided by either iFR or FFR, but not both. The patient and follow-up caregivers were blinded to the group assignment. The prespecified PCI treatment threshold for FFR was <0.80 and iFR <0.89. The measured primary outcome was MACE, a composite of death, nonfatal MI, or unplanned revascularization. The noninferiority margin was prespecified as a 3.4% difference in risk, based on an assumed annual rate of 8.5%, in line with other major cardiovascular outcome trials. The primary endpoint of MACE was not significantly different between the iFR group versus the FFR group, with difference in risk of −0.2% points (95% CI, −2.3-1.8 vs 95% CI, −2.9-2.5) respectively, $P = .83$). The hazard ratio for MACE with iFR was 0.95 (95% CI 0.68-1.33, $P = .78$).

The iFR-SWEDEHEART trial was also an open-label randomized study of design similar to that of the DEFINE-FLAIR trial. A total of 2037 patients across 15 hospitals in Sweden, Denmark, and Iceland were enrolled into the trial. The iFR group had significantly more lesions evaluated per patient compared with the FFR group (1.55 ± 0.86 vs 1.43 ± 0.70, $P = .002$). However, as in DEFINE-FLAIR, there were significantly fewer hemodynamically significant lesions as assessed by iFR compared with FFR (29.1% vs 36.8%, $P < .001$), leading to fewer stents placed per patient (1.58 ± 1.08 vs 1.73 ± 1.19, $P = .05$). The primary endpoint occurred in 6.7% in the iFR group compared with 6.1% in the FFR group. The difference in event rates between treatments was 0.7% (95% CI of −1.5-2.8, $P = .007$ for noninferiority), which corresponds to a hazard ratio of 1.12 (95% CI 0.79-1.58, $P = .53$).

The iFR-SWEDEHEART and DEFINE-FLAIR studies were designed to have similar designs and endpoints to facilitate a pooled analysis. Across both studies, PCI was deferred more frequently in the iFR group compared with the FFR group (50% vs 45%, $P < .01$). At 1 year, the MACE rate in the deferred population was similar between the iFR and FFR groups (4.12% vs 4.05%; fully adjusted hazard ratio, 1.13; 95% CI, 0.72-1.79; $P = .60$).

Given the results of these studies, iFR can be concluded to be clinically noninferior to FFR in lesion assessment, even as iFR is not concordant with FFR in a significant proportion of cases. The potential advantages to iFR include reductions in procedure time and costs and avoidance of the minor adverse effects of adenosine hyperemia.

Instantaneous Wave-Free Ratio and Fractional Flow Reserve in Stable Ischemic Heart Disease

The ORBITA trial intensively applied optimal MT to 230 patients with stable, single vessel coronary disease to evaluate the effect of PCI in this cohort. During angiography, lesions underwent physiologic assessment with FFR or iFR with the clinical operator blinded to the results. If the patient was randomized to PCI, FFR or iFR was again measured following the procedure with continued blinding of the results. Dobutamine stress echocardiography was also performed in all patients. In evaluating the physiologic data, the investigators found a strong relationship between treatment differences in stress echo score and prerandomized FFR/iFR (**Figure 21.10**). These data strongly suggest that, even in a contemporary study with aggressive antianginal therapy, coronary physiologic data are reflective of noninvasive stress testing of myocardial ischemia.

Instantaneous Wave-Free Ratio in Clinical Multivessel Disease

The DEFINE-REAL study investigated the effects of iFR in treatment decision making of 484 patients with angiographic multivessel disease. A total of 828 of 1097 vessels were investigated with FFR ($n = 324$) or iFR ($n = 160$). There was a high level of cor-

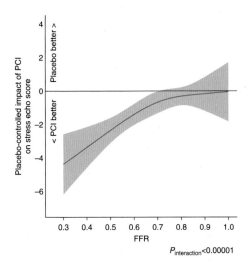

Figure 21.10 Relationship of treatment difference in stress echo score and prerandomization fractional flow reserve (FFR) and instantaneous wave-free ratio (iFR) by the randomization arm. At the right, with FFR « 1.0, the curve is »0, indicating that there is no difference between percutaneous coronary intervention (PCI) and placebo. The shaded area represents the 95% confidence interval (CI) for the estimate of this mean effect. At progressively lower FFR values, there is a progressively larger difference between PCI and placebo on the endpoint. This progressive tendency for larger effects on stress echo score with lower prerandomization FFR has P interaction <0.00001. (Reproduced with permission from Al-Lamee R, Howard JP, Shun-Shin MJ, et al. Fractional flow reserve and instantaneous wave-free ratio as predictors of the placebo-controlled response to percutaneous coronary intervention in stable single-vessel coronary artery disease. *Circulation.* 2018;138(17):1780-1792.)

relation between iFR and FFR assessment of these lesions within the study (92%), and the use of prospective, routine invasive physiology was shown to result in a high rate of lesion reclassification (26%). This translated into a change in clinical management strategy for 45% of the lesions assessed compared with the angiographically derived strategy originally identified. The use of iFR was associated with the interrogation of more vessels and a higher overall management reclassification (57.5% vs 39.9%) as compared with FFR. Thus, this clinical observational study suggests that the "ease" of iFR measurement facilitated a more complete physiologic assessment in a cohort of patients with multivessel disease.

Instantaneous Wave-Free Ratio in Serial Lesions

iFR may have particular accuracy in predicting pre- and post-PCI hemodynamic values compared with FFR, as hyperemia increases the risk of "cross talk" between serial stenoses, while resting coronary flow values tend to be more constant. iFR-GRADIENT was a multicenter trial that examined the performance of iFR-pullback in serial and diffuse lesions to predict physiologic outcomes post-PCI. A total of 159 patients with 168 coronary vessels indicated for PCI were enrolled and had pullback recordings. Post-PCI iFR was predicted from the iFR gradient across the lesion to be treated. The predicted post-PCI iFR correlated moderately well with the observed post-PCI iFR (0.93 ± 0.05 vs 0.92 ± 0.06, $r = 0.73$, $P < .001$), with an average difference of 1.4%. Compared with conventional angiography alone, the addition of real-time iFR-pullback data changed revascularization planning in 43 of 159 (30%) patients and 52 of 168 (31%) vessels. There was a significant decrease in the number ($P = .0001$) and length ($P < .0001$) of hemodynamically significant lesions planned for revascularization.

Other Nonhyperemic Pressure Ratios

Although iFR requires a proprietary algorithm, multiple other resting pressure indices (resting full-cycle ratio, diastolic flow ratio, dPR) have been developed and do not. Aside from the whole-cycle averaged P_d/P_a ratio, these have in common a measurement of the lowest P_d/P_a ratio over a portion (or all) of the cardiac cycle and a best cutoff value of <0.89. An analysis of 257 pressure waveforms by Van't Veer and colleagues found that multiple diastolic resting indices (entire dPR, 25%-75% of diastole [dPR_{25-75}], midpoint of diastole [dPR_{mid}]) were numerically identical to iFR, with correlations >0.99. These results imply that the WFP may not have practical importance above that of any other diastolic period and that other nonhyperemic indices with similar characteristics can be substituted for iFR in clinical practice.

Post–Percutaneous Coronary Intervention Coronary Hemodynamic Measurements

Evolving data support FFR and iFR use following PCI to screen for stent underexpansion, diffuse disease, or angiographically occult lesions that were not revascularized. Normalization or near-normalization of hemodynamic parameters would be expected to result in the optimal clinical outcome.

FFR has been studied the most in the post-PCI setting. In a study by Agarwal, 574 patients received FFR assessment following PCI and 21% were found to have a post-PCI FFR <0.81 despite an adequate angiographic result. Following subsequent interventions including further postdilatation or stenting, FFR in this subgroup increased from 0.78 ± 0.08 to 0.87 ± 0.06 ($P < .0001$). Patients who achieved final FFR >0.86 had significantly lower MACE compared with the final FFR <0.86 group (17% vs 23%; log-rank $P = .02$). Final FFR <0.86 had incremental prognostic value over clinical and angiographic variables for MACE prediction (**Figure 21.11**).

Acute Coronary Syndromes

The pathophysiology of the infarct-related artery and microvascular bed after MI is complex. Because of the dynamic nature of patients with ACS, particularly MI, the predictive ability of FFR has some theoretic limitations. In ACS, the microvascular bed in the infarct zone may not have uniform, constant, or minimal resistance. The stenosis may also evolve as thrombus and vasoconstriction abate. FFR measurements are not meaningful when angiographic reperfusion (ie, TIMI 3 flow) has not been achieved in the artery. FFR has limited utility in the infarct-related artery in the acute setting. However, FFR has value in lesion assessment in the recovery phase of MI and in the assessment of lesions in the remote non-infarct-related vessels.

The utility of FFR in the nonculprit artery was established in the DANAMI-3-PRIMULTI study, which randomized 627 patients with ST segment elevation myocardial infarction (STEMI) to either no further invasive treatment after primary PCI of the culprit artery or complete FFR-guided revascularization. The primary endpoint was a composite of all-cause mortality, nonfatal reinfarction, and ischemia-driven revascularization (**Figure 21.12**). This endpoint occurred in 68 (22%) patients who had PCI of the infarct-related artery only and in 40 (13%) patients who had complete revascularization (hazard ratio 0-56, 95% CI 0-38-0-83; $P = .004$).

To address the utility of measurements days after MI, DeBruyne et al. compared single-photon emission computerized tomography (SPECT) myocardial perfusion

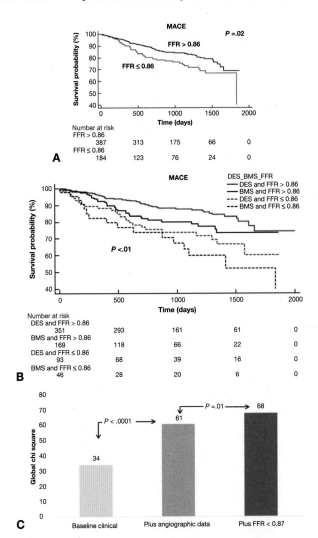

Figure 21.11 Prognostic value of post–percutaneous coronary intervention fractional flow reserve (FFR). **A,** Kaplan-Meier curve showing significantly higher survival free of major adverse cardiovascular events (MACE) in the patients with final FFR >0.86 in comparison with the final FFR ≤0.86 group. **B,** Kaplan-Meier curve showing significantly higher survival free of MACE in the patients with drug-eluting stents (DES) and final FFR >0.86 followed by patients with bare-metal stents (BMS) and final FFR >0.86, followed by patients with DES and final FFR ≤0.86 and followed by patients with BMS and final FFR ≤0.86, respectively. **C,** Incremental prognostic value of final FFR. The addition of final FFR <0.87 added incremental value for prediction of MACE over baseline clinical and angiographic data (all *P* < .05). (Adapted from Agarwal SK, Kasula S, Hacioglu Y, Ahmed Z, Uretsky BF, Hakeem A. Utilizing post-intervention fractional flow reserve to optimize acute results and the relationship to long-term outcomes. *JACC Cardiovasc Interv.* 2016;9:1022-1031, with permission.)

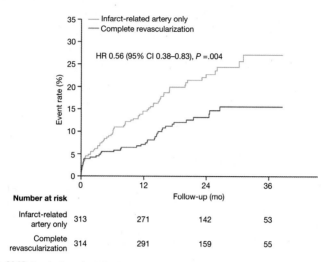

Figure 21.12 Results from the DANAMI-3-PRIMULTI study, demonstrating a lower composite event rate of all-cause mortality, nonfatal reinfarction, and ischemia-driven revascularization with complete fractional flow reserve-guided revascularization rather than culprit-only intervention. (Reproduced with permission from Engstrom T, Kelbsk H, Helqvist S, et al. Complete revascularization versus treatment of the culprit lesion only in patients with ST-segment elevation myocardial infarction and multivessel disease: an open-label, randomized controlled trial. *Lancet.* 2015;386(9994):665-671.)

imaging and FFR obtained before and after PCI in 57 patients with MI >6 days (mean 20 days) prior to evaluation. Patients with positive SPECT before PCI had a significantly lower FFR than patients with negative SPECT (0.52 ± 0.18 vs 0.67 ± 0.16; P = .0079). The sensitivity and specificity of FFR of <0.75 to detect a defect on SPECT were 82% and 87%, respectively. When only truly positive or negative SPECT imaging was considered, the corresponding values were 87% and 100% (P < .001). The best FFR cutoff for determining peri-infarct ischemia was 0.78.

For patients with non-STEMI (NSTEMI), the extent of changes of the microvasculature of the infarct-related artery likely is a function of the size of the infarction, extent of microvascular injury, and time since the infarction. Patients with moderate-sized infarctions (total creatine kinase <1000 U/L) were eligible for inclusion in the FAME study and constituted 32.6% of the total cohort. Using FFR to guide PCI resulted in similar risk reductions of MACE in patients with unstable angina or NSTEMI, compared with patients with stable angina (absolute risk reduction of 5.1% vs 3.7%, respectively, P = .92). The FAMOUS-NSTEMI trial focused exclusively on the NSTEMI population and found in 350 patients that the proportion of patients treated initially by MT was higher in the FFR-guided group than in the angiography-guided group (40 [22.7%] vs 23 [13.2%], difference 95% [95% CI: 1.4%, 17.7%], P = .022). **Table 21.3** lists key trials of FFR in STEMI and other ACSs.

EVOLVING TECHNOLOGIES FOR IMAGING ASSESSMENT OF CORONARY STENOSIS HEMODYNAMICS

Advances in computer processing and computational fluid dynamic models have enabled the estimation of FFR from imaging data (**Figure 21.13**). FFR derived from coronary computed tomography (FFR$_{CT}$, HeartFlow) has had the most extensive val-

Table 21.3 **Key Trials of Fractional Flow Reserve (FFR) in ST Segment Elevation Myocardial Infarction and Other Acute Coronary Syndromes (ACSs)**

	PRAMI	CvLPRIT	DANAMI-3-PRIMULTI	Compare-Acute	PRIME-FFR
Study design	Single-blind randomized	RCT	RCT	Prospective randomized trial	Prospective study
N	465	296	627	885	1983
Follow-up period	23 mo	296 mo	27 mo	36 mo	12 mo
Long-term mortality	Complete revascularization better	Complete revascularization better	Complete revascularization better	Complete revascularization better	Deferral based on FFR is safe in ACS
Assessment of nonculprit lesion	Angiography	Angiography	FFR	FFR	FFR
Timing	Immediate complete revascularization	Immediate complete revascularization or staged PCI	Staged PCI	Immediate complete revascularization or staged PCI	–

PCI, percutaneous coronary intervention; RCT, randomized controlled trial.

idation and is now commercially available. In a prospective randomized trial of 254 patients, FFR_{CT} was superior to computed tomography angiography (CTA) alone and invasive coronary angiography in predicting ischemia as determined by invasive FFR values, with sensitivity and specificity of 86% and 79% for FFR_{CT}, 94% and 34% for coronary CTA, and 64% and 83% for invasive angiography. However, the maximal spatial resolution of CTA data is 0.5 mm, limiting the accuracy of the results.

Estimation of FFR from invasive coronary angiography, which has a spatial resolution of 0.1 to 0.2 mm and high temporal resolution at 15 to 30 frames per second is already captured in the catheterization laboratory. Three commercial and proprietary software algorithms have been tested for angiography-based FFR, all with computation times of <10 minutes. In the FAST-FFR study, 319 vessels from 310 subjects received invasive and angiography-based FFR (FFR, CathWorks). FFRangio values correlated moderately well with FFR measurements ($r = 0.80$, $P < .001$) with Bland-Altman 95% confidence limits between −0.14 and 0.12. Similarly, in the FAVOR II study, an angiographically derived FFR called the quantitative flow ratio (QFR, Medis) showed per-vessel correlation ($r = 0.83$; $P < .001$) and agreement (mean difference, 0.01 ± 0.06) with FFR. Finally, the FAST study found that another version of angiographic FFR (vFFR, Pie Medical) had a correlation with FFR of 0.88. Future studies will determine the extent to which such technologies can replace wire-based hemodynamic measurements.

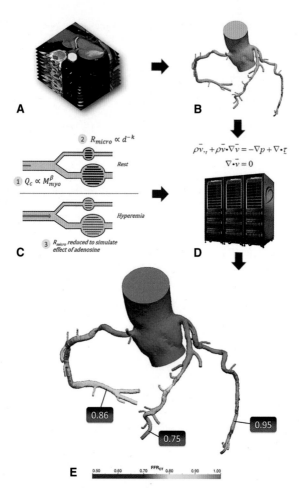

Figure 21.13 Derivation of fractional flow reserve (FFR) from CT angiography. **A,** Routine coronary computed tomography angiography data are received. **B,** A quantitative 3-dimensional anatomic model is generated. **C,** A physiological model of the coronary microcirculation is derived from patient-specific data with 3 main principles: (1) resting coronary flow proportional to myocardial mass, (2) microvascular resistance inversely proportional to vessel size, and (3) microvascular resistance reduced to simulate maximal hyperemia. **D,** Physical laws of fluid dynamics are applied to compute coronary blood flow. **E,** Fractional flow reserve derived from standard acquired coronary computed tomography angiography datasets (FFR$_{CT}$) is calculated for each point in the coronary tree. (Reproduced with permission from Norgaard J, Leipsic J, Gaur S, et al. Diagnostic performance of noninvasive fractional flow reserve derived from coronary computed tomography angiography in suspected coronary artery disease: the NXT trial [Analysis of Coronary Blood Flow Using CT Angiography—Next Steps]. *J Am Coll Cardiol.* 2014;63(12):1145-1155.)

CORONARY PHYSIOLOGIC TOOLS LESS COMMONLY UTILIZED IN ROUTINE CLINICAL PRACTICE

Angiographic Blood Flow Estimation—Thrombolysis in Myocardial Infarction Flow and Thrombolysis in Myocardial Infarction Frame Count

Since its introduction by the Thrombolysis in Myocardial Infarction (TIMI) investigators in 1985, the TIMI frame count (a simple, qualitative grading of angiographic coronary flow rates) has been widely used to gauge the restoration of perfusion in clinical trials. Improved TIMI flow grades are associated with improved outcomes (**Table 21.4**).

A quantitative method of TIMI flow counts the number of cine frames from the introduction of contrast in the coronary artery at the guide to a predetermined distal landmark. Cineangiography was performed with 6F catheters and filming at 30 frames per second. The TIMI frame count (TFC) for each major vessel is thus standardized according to specific distal landmarks. The distal landmarks commonly used in analysis are the following: (1) for the LAD, the distal bifurcation of the left anterior descending artery at the apex; (2) for the CFX system, the distal bifurcation of the branch segments with the longest total distance; (3) for the RCA, the first branch of the posterolateral artery.

The TFC can be further corrected (corrected TIMI frame count, or CTFC) by normalizing for the length of the LAD coronary artery in comparison with the 2 other major arteries; CTFC thus accounts for the greater distance the contrast has to travel in the LAD coronary artery relative to the other arteries. The average LAD coronary artery is 14.7 cm long; the right, 9.8 cm; and the circumflex, 9.3 cm. CTFC divides the absolute frame count in the LAD coronary artery by 1.7 to standardize the distance of contrast travel in all 3 arteries. Normal TFC and CTFC for LAD coronary artery is 36 ± 3; for the LCX, TFC is 22 ± 4; and for the RCA, TFC is 20 ± 3; but LCX and RCA each have a CTFC of 21 ± 2. A high CTFC may be associated with microvascular dysfunction despite an open artery, whereas CTFCs of <20 frames are

Table 21.4 Thrombolysis in Myocardial Infarction Flow Grades

Flow Grade	Description
TIMI 3	Normal distal runoff, contrast material flows briskly into and clears rapidly from the distal segment
TIMI 2	Good distal runoff, contrast material opacifies the distal segment, but flow is perceptibly slower than in more proximal segments and/or contrast material clears from the distal segment slower than from a comparable segment in another vessel
TIMI 1	Poor distal runoff, a portion of contrast material flows through the stenosed arterial segment, but the distal segment is not fully opacified
TIMI 0	Absence of distal runoff, no contrast material flows through the stenosis

TIMI, thrombolysis in myocardial infarction.
Adapted with permission from Gibson CM, Cannon CP, Daley WL, et al. TIMI frame count: a quantitative method of assessing coronary artery flow. *Circulation.* 1996;93:879-888.

associated with normal microvascular function and a low risk for adverse events in patients following MI.

The TFC method has several limitations. Visual estimates of TIMI flow in the usual clinical setting bear little relationship to the quantitative TFC or measured Doppler flow velocity. Even non-infarct-related coronary arteries may show prolonged frame counts during ACS as compared with normal values. TIMI frame counting can be especially challenging in the digital imaging laboratory with routine use of small-diameter catheters (<6F) and image acquisition rates of <15 frames/s.

Thrombolysis in Myocardial Infarction Blush Score

Angiographic successful reperfusion in acute MI has been defined as TIMI 3 flow. However, TIMI 3 flow does not always result in effective myocardial reperfusion. Myocardial blush grade (MBG) is an angiographic measure of myocardial perfusion at the capillary level and thought to be related to microvascular resistance.

MBG is defined as follows: 0 indicates no myocardial blush or contrast density; 1 indicates minimal myocardial blush or contrast density; 2 indicates moderate myocardial blush or contrast density, but less than that obtained during angiography of a contralateral or ipsilateral non-infarct-related coronary artery; and 3 indicates normal myocardial blush or contrast density, comparable with that obtained during angiography of a contralateral or ipsilateral non-infarct-related coronary artery. When myocardial blush is persistent (staining), it suggests leakage of contrast medium into the extravascular space and is also graded 0. To determine blush grading, the length of the angiographic run needs to be extended in order to visualize the venous phase of the contrast passage. When the LCA is involved, use of the left lateral view is preferred, and for the RCA, the right oblique view. MBG after primary angioplasty for acute MI appears to be an important prognostic feature and should be added to the commonly used TIMI flow grading to define successful angiographic reperfusion following primary angioplasty for acute MI.

SUGGESTED READINGS

1. Adjedj J, Toth GG, Johnson NP, et al. Intracoronary adenosine: dose-response relationship with hyperemia. *JACC Cardiovasc Interv.* 2015;8(11):1422-1430.
2. Agarwal SK, Kasula S, Hacioglu Y, Ahmed Z, Uretsky BF, Hakeem A. Utilizing post-intervention fractional flow reserve to optimize acute results and the relationship to long-term outcomes. *JACC Cardiovasc Interv.* 2016;9(10):1022-1031.
3. Al-Lamee R, Howard JP, Shun-Shin MJ, et al. Fractional flow reserve and instantaneous wave-free ratio as predictors of the placebo-controlled response to percutaneous coronary intervention in stable single-vessel coronary artery disease. *Circulation.* 2018;138(17):1780-1792.
4. Botman CJ, Schonberger J, Koolen S, et al. Does stenosis severity of native vessels influence bypass graft patency? A prospective fractional flow reserve-guided study. *Ann Thorac Surg.* 2007;83(6):2093-2097.
5. Christou MA, Siontis GC, Katritsis DG, Ioannidis JPA. Meta-analysis of fractional flow reserve versus quantitative coronary angiography and noninvasive imaging for evaluation of myocardial ischemia. *Am J Cardiol.* 2007;99(4):450-456.
6. Cook CM, Jeremias A, Petraco R, et al. Fractional flow reserve/instantaneous wave-free ratio discordance in angiographically intermediate coronary stenoses: an analysis using Doppler-derived coronary flow measurements. *JACC Cardiovasc Interv.* 2017;10(24):2514-2524.
7. Davies JE, Whinnett ZI, Francis DP, et al. Evidence of a dominant backward-propagating "suction" wave responsible for diastolic coronary filling in humans, attenuated in left ventricular hypertrophy. *Circulation.* 2006;113(14):1768-1778.
8. Davies JE, Sen S, Dehbi HM, et al. Use of the instantaneous wave-free ratio or fractional flow reserve in PCI. *N Engl J Med.* 2017;376(19):1824-1834.
9. De Bruyne B, Bartunek J, Sys SU, Pijls NH, Heyndrickx GR, Wijns W. Simultaneous coronary pressure and flow velocity measurements in humans: feasibility, reproducibility, and hemodynamic dependence of coronary flow velocity reserve, hyperemic flow versus pressure slope index, and fractional flow reserve. *Circulation.* 1996;94(8):1842-1849.

10. De Bruyne B, Hersbach F, Pijls NH, et al. Abnormal epicardial coronary resistance in patients with diffuse atherosclerosis but "normal" coronary angiography. *Circulation*. 2001;104(20): 2401-2406.

11. de Waard GA, Di Mario C, Lerman A, Serruys PW, van Royen N. Instantaneous wave-free ratio to guide coronary revascularisation: physiological framework, validation and differences from fractional flow reserve. *Eurointervention*. 2017;13(4):450-458.

12. DeBruyne B, Pijls NHJ, Bartunek J, et al. Fractional flow reserve in patients with prior myocardial infarction. *Circulation*. 2001;104(2):157-162.

13. Engstr0m T, Kelbæk H, Helqvist S, et al., DANAMI-3 - PRIMULTI Investigators. Complete revascularisation versus treatment of the culprit lesion only in patients with ST-segment elevation myocardial infarction and multivessel disease (DANAMI-3 - PRIMULTI): an open-label, randomized controlled trial. *Lancet*. 2015;386(9994):665-671.

14. Escaned J, Flores A, Garcia-Pavia P, et al. Assessment of microcirculatory remodeling with intracoronary flow velocity and pressure measurements: validation with endomyocardial sampling in cardiac allografts. *Circulation*. 2009;120(16):1561-1568.

15. Everaars H, de Waard GA, Driessen RS, et al. Doppler flow velocity and thermodilution to assess coronary flow reserve: a head-to-head comparison with [15O]H2O PET. *JACC Cardiovasc Interv*. 2018;11(20):2044-2054.

16. Fearon WF, Low AF, Yong AS, et al. Prognostic value of the index of microcirculatory resistance measured after primary percutaneous coronary intervention. *Circulation*. 2013;127(24):2436-2441.

17. Fearon WF, Nishi T, De Bruyne B, et al. Clinical outcomes and cost-effectiveness of fractional flow reserve-guided percutaneous coronary intervention in patients with stable coronary artery disease: three-year follow-up of the FAME 2 trial (fractional flow reserve versus angiography for multivessel evaluation). *Circulation*. 2018;137(5):480-487.

18. Feldman MD, Ayers CR, Lehman MR, et al. Improved detection of ischemia-induced increases in coronary sinus adenosine in patients with coronary artery disease. *Clin Chem*. 1992;38(2):256-262.

19. Fournier S, Colaiori I, Di Gioia G, Mizukami T, De Bruyne B. Hyperemic pressure-flow relationship in a human. *J Am Coll Cardiol*. 2019;73(10):1229-1230.

20. Gibson CM, Cannon CP, Daley WL, et al. TIMI frame count: a quantitative method of assessing coronary artery flow. *Circulation*. 1996;93(5):879-888.

21. Gotberg M, Christiansen EH, Gudmundsdottir IJ, et al; iFR-SWEDEHEART Investigators. Instantaneous wave-free ratio versus fractional flow reserve to guide PCI. *N Engl J Med*. 2017;376(19):1813-1823.

22. Gould KL, Kirkeeide RL, Buchi M. Coronary flow reserve as a physiologic measure of stenosis severity. *J Am Coll Cardiol*. 1990;15(2):459-474.

23. Hakeem A, Uretsky BF. Role of postintervention fractional flow reserve to improve procedural and clinical outcomes. *Circulation*. 2019;139(5):694-706.

24. Hamilos M, Muller O, Cuisset T, et al. Long-term clinical outcome after fractional flow reserve-guided treatment in patients with angio-graphically equivocal left main coronary artery stenosis. *Circulation*. 2009;120(15):1505-1512.

25. Johnson NP, Jeremias A, Zimmermann FM, et al. Continuum of vasodilator stress from rest to contrast medium to adenosine hyperemia for fractional flow reserve assessment. *JACC Cardiovasc Interv*. 2016;9(8):757-767.

26. Kern MJ, Moore JA, Aguirre FV, et al. Determination of angiographic (TIMI grade) blood flow by intracoronary Doppler flow velocity during acute myocardial infarction. *Circulation*. 1996;94(7):1545-1552.

27. Kikuta Y, Cook CM, Sharp ASP, et al. Pre-angioplasty instantaneous wave-free ratio pullback predicts hemodynamic outcome in humans with coronary artery disease: primary results of the international multicenter iFR GRADIENT registry. *JACC Cardiovasc Interv*. 2018;11(8):757-767.

28. Koo BK, Park KW, Kang HJ, et al. Physiological evaluation of the provisional side-branch intervention strategy for bifurcation lesions using fractional flow reserve. *Eur Heart J*. 2008;29(6):726-732.

29. Layland J, Oldroyd KG, Curzen N, et al; FAMOUS–NSTEMI Investigators. Fractional flow reserve vs. angiography in guiding management to optimize outcomes in non-ST-segment elevation myocardial infarction: the British Heart Foundation FAMOUS-NSTEMI randomized trial. *Eur Heart J*. 2015;36(2):100-111.

30. Lee JM, Shin ES, Nam CW, et al. Clinical outcomes according to fractional flow reserve or instantaneous wave-free ratio in deferred lesions. *JACC Cardiovasc Interv*. 2017;10(24):2502-2510.

31. Matsumoto H, Nakatsuma K, Shimada T, et al. Effect of caffeine on intravenous adenosine-induced hyperemia in fractional flow reserve measurement. *J Invasive Cardiol*. 2014;26(11):580-585.

32. Meuwissen M, Siebes M, Chamuleau SAJ, et al. Hyperemic stenosis resistance index for evaluation of functional coronary lesion severity. *Circulation*. 2002;106(4):441-446.

33. Norgaard BL, Leipsic J, Gaur S, et al. Diagnostic performance of noninvasive fractional flow reserve derived from coronary computed tomography angiography in suspected coronary artery disease: the NXT trial (Analysis of Coronary Blood Flow Using CT Angiography—next Steps). *J Am Coll Cardiol*. 2014;63(12):1145-1155.

34. Ofili EO, Kern MJ, Labovitz AJ, et al. Analysis of coronary blood flow velocity dynamics in angiographically normal and stenosed arteries before and after endolumen enlargement by angioplasty. *J Am Coll Cardiol.* 1993;21(2):308-316.
35. Pijls NH, Bech GJ, el Gamal MI, et al. Quantification of recruitable coronary collateral blood flow in conscious humans and its potential to predict future ischemic events. *J Am Coll Cardiol.* 1995;25(7):1522-1528.
36. Pijls NH, Van Gelder B, Van der Voort P, et al. Fractional flow reserve: a useful index to evaluate the influence of an epicardial coronary stenosis on myocardial blood flow. *Circulation.* 1995;92(11):3183-3193.
37. Pijls NHJ, de Bruyne B, Bech GJ, et al. Coronary pressure measurement to assess the hemodynamic significance of serial stenoses within one coronary artery: validation in humans. *Circulation.* 2000;102(19):2371-2377.
38. Pijls NH, De Bruyne B, Smith L, et al. Coronary thermodilution to assess flow reserve: validation in humans. *Circulation.* 2002;105(21):2482-2486.
39. Rentrop KP, Thornton JC, Feit F, Van Buskirk M. Determinants and protective potential of coronary arterial collaterals as assessed by an angioplasty model. *Am J Cardiol.* 1988;61(10):677-684.
40. Salcedo J, Kern MJ. Effects of caffeine and theophylline on coronary hyperemia induced by adenosine or dipyridamole. *Cathet Cardiovasc Interv.* 2009;74(4):598-605.
41. Sels JW, Tonino PA, Siebert U, et al. Fractional flow reserve in unstable angina and non-ST-segment elevation myocardial infarction experience from the FAME (Fractional flow reserve versus Angiography for Multivessel Evaluation) study. *JACC Cardiovasc Interv.* 2011;4(11):1183-1189.
42. Seto AH, Tehrani D, Kern MJ. Limitations and pitfalls of fractional flow reserve measurements and adenosine-induced hyperemia. *Interv Cardiol Clin.* 2015;4(4):419-434.
43. Thuesen AL, Riber LP, Veien KT, et al. Fractional flow reserve versus angiographically-guided coronary artery bypass grafting. *J Am Coll Cardiol.* 2018;72(22):2732-2743.
44. Tonino PAL, DeBruyne B, Pijls NHJ, et al. Fractional flow reserve versus angiography for guiding percutaneous coronary intervention. *N Engl J Med.* 2009;360(3):213-224.
45. Van Belle E, Gil R, Klauss V, et al. Impact of routine invasive physiology at time of angiography in patients with multivessel coronary artery disease on reclassification of revascularization strategy: results from the DEFINE REAL study. *JACC Cardiovasc Interv.* 2018;11(4):354-365.
46. Van't Veer M, Pijls NHJ, Hennigan B, et al. Comparison of different diastolic resting indexes to iFR: are they all equal? *J Am Coll Cardiol.* 2017;70(25):3088-3096.
47. Wilson RF, Marcus ML, White CW. Prediction of the physiologic significance of coronary arterial lesions by quantitative lesion geometry in patients with limited coronary artery disease. *Circulation.* 1987;75(4):723-732.
48. Xaplanteris P, Fournier S, Pijls NHJ, et al; FAME 2 Investigators. Five-year outcomes with PCI guided by fractional flow reserve. *N Engl J Med.* 2018;379(3):250-259.
49. Zimmermann FM, Ferrara A, Johnson NP, et al. Deferral vs. performance of percutaneous coronary intervention of functionally nonsignificant coronary stenosis: 15-year follow-up of the DEFER trial. *Eur Heart J.* 2015;36(45):3182-3188.

22 Intravascular Imaging Techniques[1]

The advanced catheter-based imaging tools described in this chapter—intravascular ultrasound (IVUS), optical coherence tomography (OCT), angioscopy, and spectroscopy—provide unique insights into vascular disease and the mechanism of therapeutic intervention.

INTRAVASCULAR ULTRASOUND

Intravascular ultrasound catheters use reflected sound waves to visualize the arterial wall in a 2-dimensional, tomographic format, analogous to a histologic cross section. They utilize significantly higher frequencies than employed in noninvasive echocardiography (20-60 MHz as compared with 2-5 MHz). This provides high resolution (40-200 μm) at the expense of beam penetration (limited to 4-8 mm from the catheter tip). This technique has gained acceptance both as a research method and as a clinical tool for situations in which the angiogram is unclear.

Imaging Systems

There are 2 approaches to IVUS imaging: solid-state and mechanical scanning. Both approaches generate a 360°, cross-sectional image plane perpendicular to the catheter tip. In the solid-state approach, the individual elements of a circumferential array of multiple transducers mounted near the tip of the catheter are activated with different time delays to create an ultrasound beam that sweeps the circumference of the vessel. Complex miniaturized integrated circuits in the catheter tip control the timing and integration of the transducer activation and route the resulting echo information is displayed in real time. In the mechanical approach, a single transducer element is rotated inside the tip of a catheter via a torque cable spun by an external motor attached to the proximal end of the catheter. Signals from each angular position of the transducer are collected by a computerized image array processor, which synthesizes a cross-sectional ultrasound image of the **vessel**.

The latest solid-state coronary catheter system (Philips, San Diego, CA) has 64 transducer elements arranged around the catheter tip and uses a center frequency of 20 MHz. The current coronary catheters in a rapid-exchange configuration are 3.5F at the transducer assembly and thus compatible with a 5F guide catheter. Larger peripheral imaging catheters are produced in both over-the-wire and rapid-exchange configurations.

Mechanical IVUS systems operate at a center frequency of 40 to 60 MHz with a distal crossing profile of 2.4F to 3.2F, compatible with a 5F guide catheter. Larger catheters with lower center frequencies are also available for peripheral and intracardiac echocardiography (ICE) imaging. The catheters are advanced over a guidewire using a short rail section at the catheter tip, located beyond the imaging-window segment within which the spinning transducer may be advanced or withdrawn. To improve the trackability and pushability, one manufacturer (Terumo) provides an imaging catheter with a second long rail section located proximally in addition to the standard short rail section at the catheter tip. In all mechanical systems, the fact that the guidewire runs outside the catheter parallel to the imaging segment results in a shadow artifact in the image.

[1]We gratefully acknowledge the Grossman & Baim's *Cardiac Catheterization, Angiography, and Intervention*, 9th edition contributions of Drs. Yasuhiro Honda, Peter J. Fitzgerald, and Paul G. Yock, as portions of their chapter, "Intravascular Imaging Techniques," were retained in this text.

In head-to-head comparisons, mechanical systems have traditionally offered advantages in terms of image quality, as compared to the solid-state systems, owing to their higher center frequencies and the larger effective aperture of the transducer element. Particularly, near-field resolution is excellent with mechanical catheters so that digital subtraction of the ring-down artifact is not required. In addition, a stationary outer sheath of mechanical catheters allows the transducer to be moved through a segment of interest in a precise and controlled manner. On the other hand, the longer rapid-exchange design of the solid-state catheter may track better than the short rail design of mechanical systems in complex coronary anatomy. The distance from the transducer to the catheter tip is shorter than that of mechanical systems, which may also be beneficial in IVUS-guided intervention of chronic total occlusion (CTO) lesions. The solid-state catheter includes no moving parts and thus is free of nonuniform rotational distortion (NURD). This artifact can occur with mechanical systems when bending, causing a wedge-shaped, smeared image to appear in 1 or more segments of the image (**Figure 22.1**). With both systems, serial cross-sectional images can be reconstructed into a longitudinal display mode, and both still frames and video images can be digitally archived on local storage memory. Both systems can be installed directly into the cine angiogram system, enabling operators to quickly and easily incorporate IVUS interrogations into their interventional procedures.

Image Acquisition Procedures

IVUS examination should be performed with intravenous administration of heparin or equivalent anticoagulation (an activated clotting time of >250 seconds is recommended). Intracoronary nitroglycerin (100-200 μg) should also be routinely administered prior to the delivery of the IVUS catheter in order to induce maximal vasodilation and to prevent vasospasm. Using a 0.014-in angioplasty guidewire, the imaging probe is advanced at least 10 mm distal to the area of interest under fluoroscopic guidance. The length of the target vessel is then scanned by retracting the transducer within a stationary outer sheath (mechanical IVUS) or by moving the catheter itself (solid-state IVUS). Automated pullback devices withdraw the imaging element at a steady rate (0.5 or 1.0 mm/s with conventional systems), allowing accurate axial registration of each cross

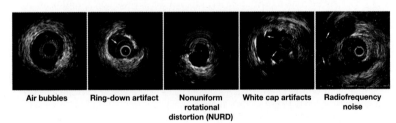

| Air bubbles | Ring-down artifact | Nonuniform rotational distortion (NURD) | White cap artifacts | Radiofrequency noise |

Figure 22.1 Common IVUS image artifacts. **Air bubbles** can cause a high echoic noise around the imaging catheter with image deterioration. **Ring-down** artifacts seen as a series of bright rings around the mechanical IVUS catheter (arrow) can also be caused by air bubbles, which need to be flushed out. **Nonuniform rotational distortion (NURD)** results in a wedge-shaped, smeared appearance in one or more segments of the image (between 9 and 4 o'clock in this example). **White cap** artifacts caused by side-lobe echoes (arrows) originate from a strong reflecting surface, such as metal stent struts or calcification. Smearing of the strut image can lead to the mistaken impression that the struts are protruding into the lumen. **Radiofrequency noise** (arrows) appears as alternating radial spokes or random white dots in the far field. The interference is usually caused by other electrical equipment in the cardiac catheterization laboratory. IVUS, intravascular ultrasound.

section for precise longitudinal distance measurements. The latest generation systems (Terumo and ACIST Medical Systems) offer faster pullback at up to 10 mm/s, which is enabled by the higher image acquisition rates (60 or 90 fps) compared to conventional IVUS systems (16-30 fps). Unless the patient complains of chest discomfort, the image acquisition is recommended to include distal vessel, lesion site, and the entire proximal vessel, back to the aorta. An accurate evaluation of the aorto-ostial segment requires that the guide catheter be disengaged slightly from the ostium.

Image Interpretation

Interpretation of the images begins with the identification of 2 key landmarks: the blood-intima (luminal) border and the media-adventitia interface (**Figure 22.2**). The luminal border is the first bright interface beyond the catheter and is generally easy to locate on IVUS images. However, blood within the lumen exhibits a speckled low-intensity pattern, which is more prominent at higher ultrasound frequencies and may make recognition of the intimal border more difficult. Signal processing software can color code or subtract the blood signal so that it does not obscure the intimal interface. If the blood signal is still confusing, saline can be injected through the guide catheter to reduce blood speckle and help delineate the true lumen border.

The second key IVUS landmark is the media-adventitia border. In muscular arteries such as the coronary tree, the media may stand out as a thin dark band, since it contains much less echo-reflective material (collagen and elastin) than contained by the neighboring intima and adventitia. This provides a characteristic 3-layered (bright-dark-bright) appearance on IVUS images. However, the stronger echo-reflectivity of the intimal layer

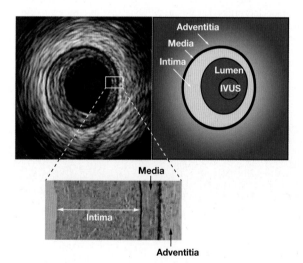

Figure 22.2 Cross-sectional format of a typical IVUS image. The bright-dark-bright, 3-layered appearance is seen in the image with corresponding anatomy as defined. "IVUS" represents the imaging catheter in the blood vessel lumen. Histologic correlations with intima, media, and adventitia are shown. The media has lower ultrasound reflectance owing to less collagen and elastin as compared with the neighboring layers. Because the intimal layer reflects ultrasound more strongly than does the media, there is a spillover in the image, which results in a slight overestimation of the thickness of the intima and a corresponding underestimation of the medial thickness. IVUS, intravascular ultrasound.

often causes a spillover effect, known as *blooming*, resulting in a slight overestimation of the intimal thickness with a corresponding underestimation of the medial thickness. Also, several deviations can be encountered in practice. For instance, the 3-layered appearance may be undetectable in truly normal coronary arteries wherein the intimal thickness is below the effective resolution of IVUS. In atherosclerotic disease where the media has been destroyed, the media may not appear as a distinct layer around the full circumference of the vessel.

In most cases, the IVUS beam penetrates beyond the arterial wall, providing images of perivascular structures such as the cardiac veins, myocardium, and pericardium (**Figure 22.3**). These structures have characteristic appearances when viewed from different positions within the arterial tree and can provide useful landmarks regarding the position of the imaging plane. Recent technical advances that allow coregistration of the IVUS image with contrast angiography can also facilitate localization of the IVUS findings on the angiogram.

Quantitative Assessment

IVUS has an intrinsic distance calibration, provided as a grid on the image. Electronic caliper (diameter) and tracing (area) measurements can be performed at the tightest cross section (maximum stenosis), as well as at reference segments located proximal and distal to the lesion (**Figure 22.4**). In general, the reference segment is selected as the most normal looking (largest lumen with smallest plaque burden) cross section within 10 mm from the lesion with no intervening major side branches.

Vessel and lumen diameter measurements are important in everyday clinical practice where accurate sizing of devices is needed. The maximum and minimum diameters (the major and minor axes of an elliptical cross section) are the most widely used. The ratio of maximum to minimum diameter defines a measure of symmetry. Area measurements are performed with computer planimetry. Lumen area is determined by tracing the leading edge of the blood-intima border, whereas total

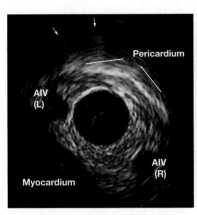 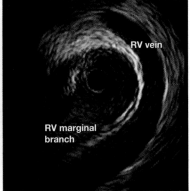

Left anterior descending artery   **Right coronary artery**

Figure 22.3 Perivascular landmarks. On a distal cross section of the left anterior descending artery **(left)**, the right (R) and left (L) branches of the anterior interventricular vein (AIV) are seen framing the coronary artery. The pericardium appears as a bright arc with spokes (arrows) emitting from it. On a cross section of the mid-right coronary artery **(right)**, bridging veins arch over the artery, typically at a position adjacent to the right ventricular (RV) marginal branches.

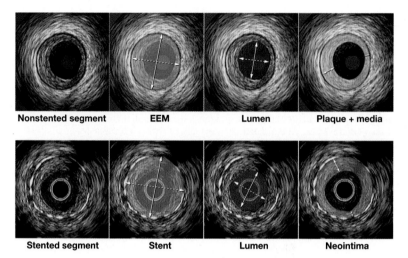

| Nonstented segment | EEM | Lumen | Plaque + media |

| Stented segment | Stent | Lumen | Neointima |

Figure 22.4 Quantitative IVUS measurements for nonstented **(upper)** and stented **(lower)** segments. Area measurements are performed with computer planimetry. EEM area is defined as the area enclosed by the outermost interface between media and adventitia, while lumen area is determined by tracing the leading edge of the blood/intima border. Plaque + media area is calculated as the difference between EEM and lumen areas. Stent area is measured by tracing the leading edge of the stent struts, and neointimal area is calculated as the difference between stent and lumen areas. For EEM, lumen, and stent, the maximum (solid arrows) and minimum (dashed arrows) diameters are determined. For plaque + media and neointima, the maximum (solid arrows) and minimum (dashed arrows) thickness are measured. EEM, external elastic membrane; IVUS, intravascular ultrasound.

vessel (or external elastic membrane, EEM) area is defined as the area enclosed by the outermost interface between media and adventitia. Plaque area (or more accurately, the plaque-plus-media area) is calculated as the difference between vessel and lumen areas; the ratio of plaque area to total vessel area is termed the percent plaque area, plaque burden, or percent cross-sectional narrowing. Metal struts of stents are seen as bright, focal points in a circular-arrayed pattern on the IVUS scan, and the stent measurement is performed at the leading edge of stent struts in the same way as done in nonstented segments. Neointimal hyperplasia within the stent generally has low echo-reflectivity at follow-up IVUS imaging, and the area is calculated as the difference between stent area and lumen area.

Arterial remodeling, originally described by Glagov et al from necropsy specimens, is a bidirectional vessel response represented as the increase or decrease in vessel size that occurs during the development of atherosclerosis. In clinical settings, direct evidence of remodeling can be derived from serial changes in the EEM cross-sectional area (CSA) in 2 or more IVUS measurements obtained at different times. In single time-point studies, measurements of reference sites are used as a surrogate for the original vessel size before the artery became diseased. The reference segment(s) used for such purpose should be measured without any major intervening side branches. Classification of arterial remodeling includes positive (or adaptive), no or intermediate, and negative (or constrictive) remodeling. A remodeling index (the ratio of EEM CSA at the lesion site vs the reference site) as a continuous variable may also be used, in combination with the categorical classifications (positive remodeling = remodeling index >1.0 or 1.05; negative remodeling = remodeling index <1.0 or 0.95).

Serial change of intima or plaque measured by IVUS has been increasingly used as a surrogate endpoint in clinical trials of pharmacologic interventions or transplant vasculopathy. In a meta-regression analysis of 17 prospective studies, a 1% reduction in mean percent plaque volume as induced by dyslipidemia therapies was associated with a 20% reduction in the odds of major adverse cardiovascular events (MACEs). In heart-transplant studies, maximum intimal thickness (MIT) has been widely used as a surrogate marker for long-term outcomes since a rapid increase in MIT (>0.5 mm during the first year post transplant) is associated with an increased risk of a MACE or subsequent development of severe allograft vasculopathy.

Qualitative Assessment

Plaque Characterization

In grayscale IVUS, atheromatous plaques are classified into soft (echogenicity less than the surrounding adventitia), fibrous (intermediate echogenicity between those of soft plaques and highly echogenic calcified plaques), calcified (echogenicity higher than that of the adventitia with acoustic shadowing), and mixed plaques (more than 1 subtype contained within the plaque) (**Figure 22.5**). Calcium deposits are described qualitatively as superficial or deep according to the location of the leading edge of acoustic shadowing within the inner versus outer half of the plaque-plus-media thickness. The shadowing precludes determination of the thickness of a calcific deposit as well as visualization of vessel structures behind the calcium.

Since visual interpretation of conventional grayscale IVUS images has limitations in the precise detection and quantification of specific plaque components, several advanced signal analysis techniques have been developed. To date, 3 different systems have been commercialized based on computer-assisted analysis of raw radiofrequency (RF) signals in the reflected ultrasound beam: Virtual Histology IVUS, the iMap system, and the Integrated Backscatter system. The Virtual Histology (VH) IVUS system (Philips) employs spectral RF analyses with a classification tree algorithm developed from ex vivo coronary data sets and classifies plaques as 4 types: fibrous, necrotic, calcific, and fibrofatty. The iMap system (Boston Scientific) identifies and quantifies 4 different types of atherosclerotic components (fibrotic, necrotic, lipidic, and calcified tissues) based on the degree of spectral similarity between the backscattered signal and a reference library of spectra from

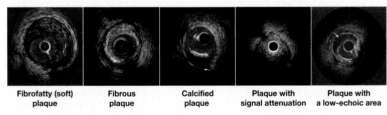

| Fibrofatty (soft) plaque | Fibrous plaque | Calcified plaque | Plaque with signal attenuation | Plaque with a low-echoic area |

Figure 22.5 Plaque characterization by grayscale IVUS. The brightness of the adventitia can be used as a gauge to discriminate between predominantly fatty and fibrous plaque (plaque that appears darker than the adventitia is considered fatty). Regions of calcification are strongly echo-reflective and create a dense shadow peripherally from the catheter, known as acoustic shadowing, with reverberation (arrow in the middle image). Large plaque burden with deep ultrasound signal attenuation despite absence of bright calcium and plaques with a large low-echoic region suggesting a lipid pool (arrow in the right image) are susceptible to distal emboli during balloon dilatation or stenting. IVUS, intravascular ultrasound.

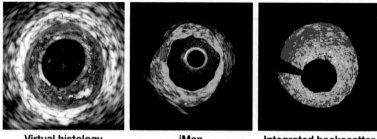

| **Virtual histology** | **iMap** | **Integrated backscatter** |

Figure 22.6 Examples of advanced plaque characterization by radiofrequency IVUS analysis. **Virtual Histology:** Plaque components are determined using spectral radiofrequency signal analyses with a classification algorithm. Dark green = fibrous; light green = fibrofatty; white = calcium; red = necrotic core. **iMap:** Classification of tissue is made based upon the degree of similarity between the sample and a reference frequency spectrum. This method enables confidence-level assessment of each plaque component along with a color-mapped presentation superimposed on the corresponding grayscale image. Green = fibrotic; yellow = lipidic; pink = necrotic; light blue = calcified. **Integrated backscatter IVUS:** A color-mapped presentation of integrated backscatter values (IB-IVUS). Blue = lipid pool; green = fibrous; yellow = dense fibrous; red = calcification. IVUS, intravascular ultrasound.

preserved histological data. Integrated backscatter (IB) IVUS (Terumo) utilizes integrated backscatter values, calculated as the average power of the backscattered ultrasound signal from a sample tissue volume, to differentiate 4 tissue types: calcification, fibrosis, dense fibrosis, and lipid pool. All systems generate color-mapped images of the vessel wall, with a distinct color for each plaque component category (**Figure 22.6**).

Abnormal Lesion Morphology

Thrombus Thrombus is usually recognized as an intraluminal mass, often with a layered, lobulated, or pedunculated appearance (**Figure 22.7**). Acute thrombus may appear as a relatively echodense mass with speckling or scintillation, while old

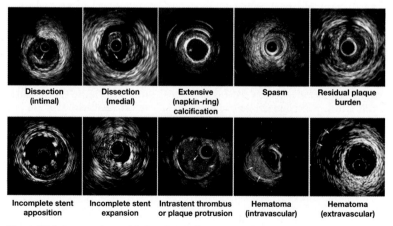

| **Dissection (intimal)** | **Dissection (medial)** | **Extensive (napkin-ring) calcification** | **Spasm** | **Residual plaque burden** |
| **Incomplete stent apposition** | **Incomplete stent expansion** | **Intrastent thrombus or plaque protrusion** | **Hematoma (intravascular)** | **Hematoma (extravascular)** |

Figure 22.7 Common abnormal findings detected by IVUS. IVUS, intravascular ultrasound.

organized thrombus often has a darker ultrasound appearance. Thrombus is also more likely than soft plaque to have the appearance of blood flow in microchannels. However, none of these IVUS features is pathognomonic for thrombus, and slow blood flow, air bubbles, stagnant contrast, or an echolucent plaque should be considered as a differential diagnosis.

Dissection Dissection appears as a fissure or separation within the intima or plaque (**Figure 22.7**). The severity of a dissection can be quantified based on its depth (intimal, medial, or adventitial) and extent (circumferential or longitudinal).

Hematoma Intramural hematoma is recognized as an accumulation of blood within the medial space, displacing the internal elastic membrane (IEM) inward and EEM outward (**Figure 22.7**). On the IVUS image, it is observed typically as a homogeneous, hyperechoic, crescent-shaped (helmet sign) area but may present with a heterogeneous and/or layered appearance when contrast dye or saline is trapped in the false lumen. Entry and/or exit points may or may not be observed.

Vulnerable Plaque

Hypoechoic plaques without a well-formed fibrous cap are presumed to represent potentially vulnerable atherosclerotic lesions. Plaque rupture is diagnosed when a hypoechoic cavity within the plaque is connected with the lumen. Ruptured plaques are often eccentric, less calcified, large in plaque burden, positively remodeled, and associated with thrombus.

Among the IVUS characteristics suggesting plaque instability, extensive positive remodeling represents the most consistent feature reported in grayscale IVUS studies. Pathological studies support this clinical IVUS finding by demonstrating that lesions with positive remodeling frequently exhibit large, soft, lipid-rich plaques with increased inflammatory cell infiltrate. Although current IVUS has limited spatial resolution for the detection of thin fibrous caps, a clinical study with synergy of IVUS and OCT has linked positive remodeling with thinning of the fibrous cap in serial coronary examinations. Other morphologic features associated with clinical instability include noncalcified plaque with ultrasound attenuation, an echolucent zone within plaque, and scattered spotty calcification.

There is increasing interest in the ability of IVUS to predict future coronary events. One of the largest natural history studies is the Providing Regional Observations to Study Predictors of Events in the Coronary Tree (PROSPECT) trial, which employed 3-vessel imaging with VH-IVUS in 697 acute coronary syndrome (ACS) patients. In this trial, a fibroatheroma (defined by VH-IVUS as the presence of >10% confluent necrotic core) was classified as a thin-cap fibroatheroma (TCFA) if >30° of the necrotic core abutted the lumen in 3 or more consecutive frames. Multivariate analysis identified 3 baseline IVUS characteristics that independently predicted events: (1) plaque burden >70% (hazard ratio [HR] = 5.03); (2) VH-determined TCFA (HR = 3.35); and (3) minimum lumen area (MLA) <4.0 mm^2 (HR = 3.21). MACEs occurred in 18% of lesions that had all 3 of these characteristics and in <1% of lesions with none of them.

Interventional Applications

Angiographic Intermediate Lesions

A considerable number of angiographic intermediate lesions referred for elective percutaneous coronary intervention (PCI) are, in fact, hemodynamically insignificant and can be successfully managed with medical treatment alone. In early studies of proximal coronary lesions, MLA measured by IVUS demonstrated reasonable correlation with physiologic assessment results. However, later studies with expanded study populations indicated that the diagnostic accuracies and the optimal cutoff values of the MLA can vary depending on lesion location, vessel size, and the amount of myocardium supplied by the target segment. Overall, a meta-analysis of 11 clinical studies comparing IVUS and fractional flow reserve (FFR) identified the best MLA cutoff value to define the functional significance as 2.61 mm^2 for non–left main coronary artery (LMCA) lesions but with limited sensitivity and specificity (0.79 and 0.65, respectively). In contrast, the IVUS-determined MLA appears to have better accuracy in predicting significant FFR in LMCA lesions (MLA cutoff = 5.35 mm^2; pooled sensitivity 0.90 and specificity 0.90 in the meta-analysis cited above).

Left Main Lesions

In the assessment of LMCA disease, angulations, calcification, or spasm in this location can lead to poor catheter engagement and confound angiographic interpretation. Less than half of patients with angiographically ambiguous LMCA stenosis have a significant stenosis. This is especially true for ostial LMCA disease where only one-third of the lesions have a significant stenosis when evaluated by IVUS.

The ischemic MLA threshold for the LMCA is considered 6 mm^2 based on physiologic assessment with FFR (see above). This cutoff value was validated in a prospective multicenter study (LITRO) where the predefined IVUS criterion of an MLA >6 mm^2 was used for deferred revascularization in patients with intermediate LMCA disease. In a 2-year follow-up period, both cardiac death and event-free survivals were comparable between the deferred and the revascularized groups. Another study has also shown the safety of IVUS-guided deferral of revascularization for intermediate LMCA disease, but using a larger MLA cutoff (7.5 mm^2) predetermined based on the lower range of normal left main MLA from their clinical database. Assessment using IVUS-determined MLA may be particularly useful when significant stenosis coexists in the left anterior descending (LAD) artery and/or circumflex artery, since FFR for the LMCA lesion could be overestimated in the setting of additional lesions in the downstream branches.

Calcified Lesions

It is important to identify calcified plaque since the presence, degree, and location of calcium within the target vessel can substantially affect the delivery and subsequent deployment of coronary stents. One important advantage of IVUS guidance is its ability to assess the extent and distance from the lumen of calcium deposits within a plaque. For example, lesions with extensive superficial calcium may require rotational atherectomy or lithotripsy prior to stenting to avoid underexpansion. Conversely, lesions with deep calcium, which cannot be reached with atherectomy alone, may be successfully treated by lithotripsy.

High-Risk Lesions for Distal Embolization

Evaluation of plaque composition by preinterventional IVUS may predict the occurrence of distal emboli during balloon dilatation or stenting that may result in the "no-reflow" phenomenon leading to periprocedural myocardial infarction (MI). In grayscale IVUS, predictive findings include large plaque burden with (noncalcium-related) signal attenuation, a large low-echoic region suggesting a lipid pool, and thrombus-containing plaque (**Figure 22.5**). Studies with VH-IVUS or IB-IVUS have also demonstrated that the amount of lipid or necrotic core at preintervention was related to findings suggesting distal emboli.

Chronic Total Occlusion Lesions

IVUS is useful in several aspects during intervention on CTO lesions. In lesions with abrupt-type occlusion, the entry point at the CTO ostium is often difficult to identify by angiography. If there is a side branch located near the entrance of the CTO, the IVUS catheter can be inserted into the side branch to examine the target for wire penetration. In addition, the IVUS catheter can possibly be inserted into the subintimal space to determine the direction of the true lumen. Theoretically, true lumen is surrounded by all 3 layers of the vessel. Side branches may offer another clue since they should communicate with the true but not with the false lumen. It is important to note, however, that insertion of the IVUS catheter into the subintimal space has the potential risk of enlarging the subintimal space. IVUS is also useful in retrograde CTO procedures to guide retrograde guidewire crossing and reverse controlled antegrade/retrograde tracking (CART) technique. Intramural or extramural hematoma can occur, and early detection and precise assessment of these conditions are crucial for safe and effective treatment of patients with CTOs.

Restenotic Lesions

The primary mechanism of restenosis can be accurately identified by IVUS, which significantly affects the treatment strategy in patients with restenotic lesions. In an IVUS study of drug-eluting stent (DES) restenosis, 21% of lesions had a minimum stent area (MSA) of <5.0 mm^2, 38% of which were not associated with significant neointimal hyperplasia. A more recent IVUS study of in-stent restenosis (ISR) including second-generation DES demonstrated that stent underexpansion (MSA <5.0 mm^2) was more frequent in DESs than in bare-metal stents (BMSs; 32% vs 22%, respectively). For this type of ISR, mechanical optimization is the first priority, and IVUS can differentiate mechanical issues from exaggerated neointimal proliferation that may truly require DES implantation within the original restenotic stent.

IVUS-Guided Selection of Device Size and Length

When assessed by IVUS, less than 10% of angiographically "normal" reference segments are truly normal. In a DES trial of complex lesions (Angiography vs IVUS Optimization: AVIO study), the size of the postdilatation balloon was selected based on the average of the media-to-media diameters at multiple sites within the stented segment. The precise vessel size measurement is also critically important for size selection of self-expanding or bioresorbable scaffolds (BRSs) because undersizing of these devices is not amendable once deployed in the lesion.

Assessment of true lesion length by IVUS dictates the exact length of stent necessary to appropriately scaffold a lesion. A number of IVUS studies of DESs have identified greater reference plaque burden as an independent predictor of subsequent stent edge restenosis or thrombosis. The STLLR (The Impact of Stent Deployment Techniques on Clinical Outcomes of Patient Treated with the CYPHER Stent) trial also demonstrated that geographic miss, defined as injured or diseased segment uncovered by DESs, had a significant negative impact on both clinical efficacy and safety at 1 year following implantation. Another IVUS study of second-generation DESs reported cutoff values of residual plaque burden to predict subsequent edge restenosis as 54% to 57%. Therefore, complete coverage of the reference disease is currently recommended. Importantly, however, longer stent length has also been reported to be independently associated with DES restenosis and thrombosis. Online IVUS guidance can facilitate the determination of appropriate stent length for anchoring the stent ends in relatively plaque-free vessel segments while minimizing the stent length for complete lesion coverage.

IVUS Guidance for Optimal Stent Expansion

The most consistent risk factor for DES restenosis and thrombosis is underexpansion of the stent, the incidence of which has been reported as 60% to 80% of current DES failures. In the BMS era, the predicted risk of restenosis was reported to decrease 19% for every 1 mm^2 increase in MSA. In the Can Routine Ultrasound Influence Stent Expansion (CRUISE) trial, IVUS guidance by operator preferences increased MSA, leading to a 44% relative reduction in target vessel revascularization at 9 months as compared with angiographic guidance. In another clinical IVUS study of sirolimus-eluting stents, the only independent predictors of angiographic restenosis were post-procedural final MSA of <5.5 mm^2 and IVUS-measured stent length of >40 mm.

IVUS Assessment of Acute Stent Problems

Postinterventional IVUS can identify several stent deployment issues. Incomplete expansion occurs when a portion of the stent is inadequately expanded as compared with the distal and proximal reference dimensions, especially when dense fibrocalcific plaque is present (**Figure 22.7**). Incomplete strut apposition (or malapposition) occurs when part of the stent structure is not fully in contact with the vessel wall. After stent implantation, tears at the edge of the stent can occur, which may be recognized as haziness by angiography. The stent edge tears have been attributed to the shear forces created at the junction between the metal edge of the stent and the adjacent, more compliant, tissue, or to the effect of balloon expansion beyond the edge of the stent. When investigated by IVUS, angiographic hazy lesions can represent a spectrum of anatomic morphologies, such as calcium, dissection, thrombus, hematoma, spasm, and excessive plaque burden with extreme remodeling at the reference segment (**Figure 22.7**).

IVUS Assessment of Chronic Stent Problems

Several IVUS studies have demonstrated that late-acquired incomplete strut apposition (LISA) is frequently observed in lesions of late DES thrombosis (**Figure 22.8**). A literature based meta-analysis also suggested a significantly higher risk of late or very late DES thrombosis in patients with incomplete stent apposition at follow-up (OR 6.51, P = .02). The main mechanism of LISA after DES is often focal, positive vessel remodeling, whereas plaque regression or thrombus resolution is the predominant mechanism of LISA after BMS. In LISA with positive vessel remodeling, incompletely apposed struts are seen primarily in eccentric plaques, and gaps develop mainly on the disease-free side of the vessel wall. Thus, the combination of mechanical vessel injury during stent implantation and biologic vessel injury with pharmacological agents or polymer in the setting of little underlying plaque may predispose the vessel wall to chronic, pathologic dilation.

Other IVUS-detected conditions in DES include stent fractures. By IVUS, strut fracture is defined as longitudinal strut discontinuity and can be categorized based upon its morphological characteristics: (1) strut separation, (2) strut subluxation, or (3) strut intussusceptions. Another proposed classification focuses on potential mechanisms of the strut fracture, categorizing them based upon the presence and absence of aneurysm at the fracture site (type I and II, respectively). Angiographic or IVUS studies have reported the incidence of DES fracture as 0.8% to 7.7%, wherein ISR or stent thrombosis occurred in 22% to 88%, respectively.

Long-Term Clinical Impact of IVUS-Guided Stent Implantation

Numerous clinical studies have provided evidence for the long-term benefits of IVUS in both BMS and DES implantation. In the DES era, the clinical impact of IVUS

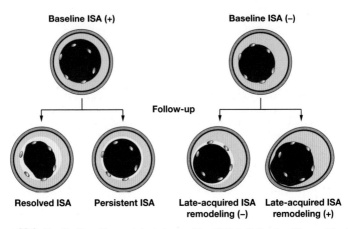

Figure 22.8 Classification of incomplete strut apposition (ISA). **Left.** Baseline ISA can either be resolved (resolved ISA) or remain (persistent ISA) at follow-up. **Right.** Late-acquired ISA without vessel expansion is typically seen in thrombus-containing lesions, whereas late-acquired ISA with focal, positive vessel remodeling is more characteristic of brachytherapy and drug-eluting stents.

guidance was assessed for complex lesions (eg, unprotected LMCA, bifurcation, long lesions, CTO, and ACS). The largest randomized controlled trial for complex lesions was the IVUS-XPL study (Impact of Intravascular Ultrasound Guidance on Outcomes of Xience Prime Stents in Long Lesions), which randomized 1400 patients with long coronary lesions to receive IVUS-guided or angiography-guided everolimus-eluting stent implantation. IVUS guidance resulted in a significantly lower MACE rate at 1 year (2.9% vs 5.8%, HR 0.48, P = .007) driven by a lower risk of ischemia-driven target lesion revascularization. The difference diverged beyond 1 year, with the improvement by IVUS sustained up to 5 years (5.6% vs 10.7%, HR 0.50, P = .001). The largest prospective multicenter registry (8582 patients) including unselected patients treated with second-generation DES was the ADAPT-DES study, in which IVUS guidance was associated with significantly lower incidences of definite or probable stent thrombosis (0.6% vs 1.2%, HR 0.4, P = .003), MI (3.5% vs 5.6%, HR 0.65, P = .0006), and MACE (4.9% vs 7.5%, HR 0.72, P = .003) at 2 years. This study showed continuous divergences of the differences beyond 1 year, and the number needed to treat with IVUS guidance to prevent 1 MACE was reduced from 64 at 1 year to 41 at 2 years.

IVUS Assessment of Bioresorbable Scaffolds

The IVUS appearance of polymeric BRSs is considerably different from that of metallic stents, owing to the penetration of ultrasound beam through the polymer material. Specifically, IVUS often identifies the BRS strut as double-layered bright stripes, suggestive of endoluminal and abluminal strut surfaces. Most BRS devices have unique mechanical properties compared with conventional metallic stents (eg, relatively thick struts and expansion limits) so that accurate evaluation of lesion characteristics and vessel size prior to implantation is considered essential to guide appropriate lesion preparation, to avoid severe vessel-device size mismatch and ultimately to achieve optimal scaffold expansion and apposition. In particular, a higher rate of scaffold thrombosis and its association with inadequate scaffold expansion were reported in Absorb Bioresorbable Vascular Scaffold (Abbott

Vascular, Santa Clara, CA), which has the largest clinical experience in patients with complex lesions. Multiple studies also reported that postprocedural nonuniform scaffold expansion, device-vessel mismatch, and implantation in small vessels were associated with adverse clinical events.

OPTICAL COHERENCE TOMOGRAPHY

OCT generates real-time tomographic images from backscattered reflections of infrared light. This use of optical echoes can thus be regarded as an optical analogue of IVUS. The greatest advantage of this light-based imaging technology is its significantly higher resolution (10 times or more) than that of conventional pulse-echo, ultrasound-based approaches.

Imaging Systems

The intravascular OCT imaging system consists of an optical engine emitting and receiving infrared light signals; a catheter interface unit including a motor drive; a fiberoptic imaging catheter; and a computer processor and display console. The optical engine includes a superluminescent diode as a source of low-coherence, infrared light, with a wavelength of approximately 1300 nm to minimize light absorption by vessel wall and blood cell components. Unlike IVUS, which directly measures the time-of-flight of acoustic reflections, the high propagation speed of light requires OCT to use interferometric techniques to determine the depth of the reflector. In the current second-generation frequency domain (FD)-OCT systems, also known as Fourier domain OCT or optical frequency domain imaging (OFDI), interference is generated using a rapidly swept wavelength source and a stationary reference arm. Each frequency component of the detected interference signal is associated with a discrete depth location within the tissue. To generate an A-line, a technique called the Fourier transform converts the interference information to depth-resolved reflectance. In both approaches, rotation of the imaging lens allows circumferential data to be collected and passed to the processor for reconstruction of a cross-sectional image (B-scan).

Intravascular OCT catheters consist of a fiberoptic core encapsulated in an optically transparent imaging sheath. For the latest FD-OCT systems (Abbott Vascular; Terumo; Gentuity), the imaging probes are integrated in a short-monorail catheter (profile varies currently from 1.8F to 3.2F) compatible with conventional 0.014-in angioplasty guidewires and 6F guide catheters. FD-OCT systems are capable of obtaining A-lines at much higher imaging speeds, achieving significantly higher frame rates (160-250 fps). Current FD-OCT systems offer an axial resolution of 10 to 20 μm and a lateral resolution of 25 to 30 μm at the focus. Pullback of the imaging core enables a longitudinal or 3-dimensional image reconstruction.

Image Acquisition Procedures

The imaging procedure of intravascular OCT is similar to that of IVUS, except that blood must be displaced by an optically transparent liquid (contrast media, saline, or low-molecular-weight dextrose [Dextran 40]) while imaging, since red blood cells scatter near-infrared light, resulting in very large signal loss. Continuous-flushing technique is the standard for FD-OCT, since its high-speed image acquisition enables rapid pullback (up to 100 mm/s) to scan a long coronary segment during short flushing for <2 seconds. Image acquisition is performed with automated pullback during continuous flushing through the guide catheter, either automatically with a power injector (typically at a flow rate of 3-6 mL/s) or manually with a syringe. For the same reason, any blood inside the imaging catheter should be flushed out completely for optimal image quality.

Image Interpretation

Similar to that seen by IVUS, the normal vessel wall is characterized by a 3-layered architecture on OCT images, comprising a highly backscattering (signal-rich) intima, a media with low backscattering (signal-poor), and a heterogeneous and frequently highly backscattering adventitia (**Figure 22.9**). The higher resolution of OCT, however, can often provide superior delineation of each structure with visualization of IEM and EEM as separate thin high-intensity layers. The periadventitial tissues may present an appearance consistent with adipocytes, characterized by large clear structures resembling cells and/or vessels. In calcified lesions, OCT has the advantage of being able to image through calcium without shadowing as seen with IVUS. On the other hand, signal penetration through the diseased arterial wall is more limited (up to 2 mm), making it difficult to investigate deeper portions of the artery or to track the entire circumference of the media-adventitia interface.

Several common image artifacts should be noted (**Figure 22.10**). As seen with mechanical IVUS, NURD can occur with OCT systems caused by a defective catheter or increased friction on the rotating components. The FD-OCT catheter results in the guidewire always being seen as a point artifact with shadowing. Eccentric catheter position within the lumen may result in an artifact termed as "sunflower" or "merry-go-round," where stent struts form a pinwheel pattern, appearing to face the imaging probe. If the catheter has moved significantly with respect to the vessel during the time of a single cross-sectional image acquisition (due to cardiac motion or rapid pullback), an axial discontinuity, termed a "seam line," may appear at the location of the transition between the first and the last A-line. In FD-OCT systems, a portion of the vessel may appear to fold over in the image. This can occur when the vessel is larger than the ranging depth (8-9 mm in current systems) and should not be interpreted as real tissue structure. Residual blood from inadequate vessel flushing can result in significant deterioration of image quality.

Quantitative Assessment

Diameter and area measurements by OCT can be performed in a similar fashion to quantitative IVUS analyses, whereas a few technical considerations specific to OCT

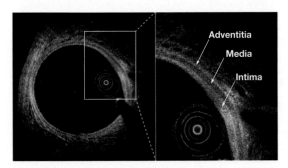

Figure 22.9 Cross-sectional format of a typical OCT image. Similar to that seen by IVUS, the normal vessel wall is characterized by a 3-layered architecture, comprising a highly backscattering intima, a media with low backscattering, and a heterogeneous and frequently highly backscattering adventitia. The periadventitial tissues may present an appearance consistent with adipocytes, characterized by large clear structures. IVUS, intravascular ultrasound; OCT, optical coherence tomography.

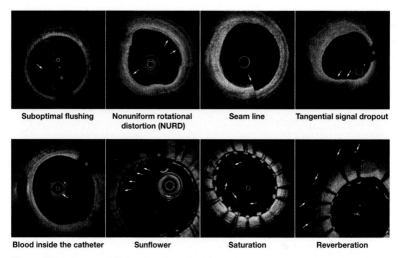

Figure 22.10 Common OCT image artifacts. A guidewire is seen as a point artifact with shadowing (*). **Suboptimal flushing** can result in residual blood inside the vessel lumen (arrow) leading to deterioration of image quality. **Nonuniform rotational distortion (NURD)** results in a wedge-shaped, smeared appearance in one or more segments of the image (arrows). **Seam line** or "sew up" artifact appears as an axial discontinuity (arrow) caused by a catheter motion during the single cross-sectional image acquisition. **Tangential signal dropout** can occur when the optical beam is directed nearly parallel to the tissue surface, which can resemble OCT appearance of thin-cap fibroatheroma (arrows). **Blood inside the catheter** presents as a high-intensity area (arrow) within the imaging sheath, possibly affecting image quality. **Sunflower** or "merry-go-round" artifacts appear as smeared stent struts (arrows) facing the OCT probe, which are usually more pronounced when the imaging catheter is off-centered within the artery. In this example, the image is also blurred owing to blood inside the catheter. **Saturation** artifacts are linear streaks (arrows) of high and/or low intensities along the axial direction. This phenomenon can occur when a strong reflector, such as a guidewire or metal stent struts, backscatters at too high an intensity to be accurately detected by the system. Highly reflective objects can also produce a series of ghost reflections, or **reverberation**, that appear as a replica at a fixed distance from the primary image of an object (arrows). OCT, optical coherence tomography.

should be noted. For accurate measurements, the OCT image should be correctly calibrated for refractive index and Z-offset. Refractive index is a property of a material that governs the speed of light through the material. Because the speed of light is slower in flushing media and tissue than in air, the distances in the images need to be corrected for this delay. OCT manufacturers provide a correction for refractive index by dividing the distances in the axial direction in the OCT image by the estimated refractive index of the flushing media and tissue. Z-offset refers to slight variations in optical path length of the optical fiber within the catheter. Calibration can be achieved by adjusting the optical path length in the sample and/or reference arm, which can be performed automatically or manually before each OCT examination. Since the fiber length can also change during a single pullback, resulting in a varying Z-offset across the OCT data set, OCT images should be evaluated to verify the Z-offset and adjust it, if necessary, before quantitative analysis.

Qualitative Assessment

Plaque Characterization

In OCT, fibrous plaques exhibit homogeneous, signal-rich (highly backscattering) regions; calcified plaques exhibit signal-poor regions with sharply delineated upper and lower borders; and lipid-rich plaques exhibit signal-poor regions (lipid pools) with poorly defined, diffuse borders (**Figure 22.11**). Artifacts such as tangential signal dropout, blood, red thrombus, or macrophage accumulations may also create a lipid pool–like appearance, thus requiring careful interpretation (**Figure 22.10**). A fibrous cap generally appears as a signal-rich band overlying a lipid pool (or necrotic core) or calcium as defined above. Macrophage accumulations may be found within the fibrous cap as signal-rich, distinct, or confluent punctate regions that exceed in intensity the background speckle noise, often accompanied by signal attenuation behind the regions. Cholesterol crystals appear as thin, linear regions of high intensity, usually associated with a fibrous cap or necrotic core (**Figure 22.12**). Microvessels in the coronary plaque present as signal-poor voids that are sharply delineated and are usually followed in multiple contiguous frames. A thrombus is recognized as a mass attached to the luminal surface or floating within the lumen: an erythrocyte-rich thrombus (red thrombus) has high backscattering with high signal attenuation, whereas a platelet-rich thrombus (white thrombus) shows less backscattering and a homogeneous appearance with low attenuation (**Figure 22.12**).

Vulnerable Plaque

The unique capabilities of OCT for the assessment of a lipid pool, a thin fibrous cap, macrophage accumulations, and other detailed surface morphologies suggest OCT

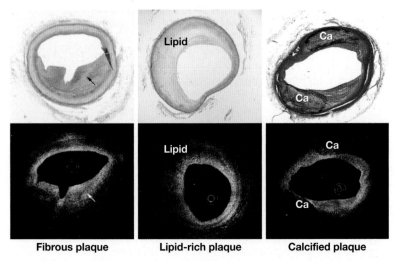

Fibrous plaque   **Lipid-rich plaque**   **Calcified plaque**

Figure 22.11 OCT images and corresponding histology for fibrous, lipid-rich, and calcified plaques. In fibrous plaques, the OCT signal is observed to be strong and homogeneous (arrow). In contrast, both lipid-rich and calcific (Ca) regions appear as a signal-poor region within the vessel wall. Lipid-rich plaques have diffuse or poorly demarcated borders, whereas the borders of calcific plates are sharply delineated (histologic stainings: Elastica Van Gieson for left, hematoxylin and eosin for middle and right, respectively). OCT, optical coherence tomography.

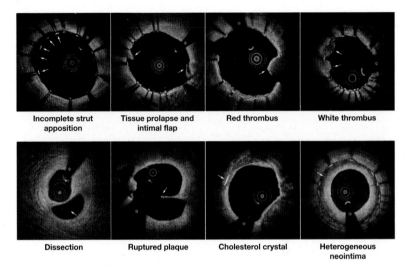

| Incomplete strut apposition | Tissue prolapse and intimal flap | Red thrombus | White thrombus |

| Dissection | Ruptured plaque | Cholesterol crystal | Heterogeneous neointima |

Figure 22.12 Common abnormal findings detected by OCT. All images have guidewire artifact (*).

as a suitable research and clinical tool for vulnerable-plaque investigation. In OCT, TCFA is defined as an OCT-delineated lipid or necrotic core with an overlying fibrous cap where the minimum thickness of the fibrous cap is less than 65 μm.

The fibrous-cap thickness measured by OCT has been shown to correlate well with that obtained from histological examination. The most commonly used threshold is 65 μm based on histopathologic studies, although this cutoff may need to be adjusted when applied to in vivo OCT images, accounting for considerable tissue shrinkage (10%-20%) that occurs during histopathologic processing. A clinical OCT study of ACS patients reported that one-third of plaque ruptures occurred in thick fibrous caps of >70 μm (up to 160 μm). In this study, the broken fibrous-cap thickness correlated positively with activity at the onset of ACS, and the plaques ruptured more frequently at the shoulder in the exertion-triggered ACS (rest 57% vs exertion 93%, $P = .014$). In another clinical study that enrolled ACS and stable angina patients, the thinnest cap thickness was <80 μm in 95% of ruptured plaques. These results suggest that the cap thickness alone may be insufficient to identify lesions at the risk of plaque rupture.

In OCT diagnosis of TCFA, several investigators have used an additional parameter: the lipid core should subtend an arc of >90° or comprise more than one quadrant of the vessel circumference. With these definitions, multiple studies have shown a correlation of OCT-determined TCFA or plaque rupture with clinical presentations. OCT-TCFAs are also observed to cluster in the proximal LAD artery but are more evenly distributed throughout the left circumflex artery and right coronary artery, consistent with previous histopathological reports. As another mechanism for thrombotic events, plaque erosions can also be evaluated in vivo by OCT, typically defined as OCT evidence of thrombus, an irregular luminal surface, and no evidence of cap rupture evaluated in multiple adjacent frames. In a clinical study of acute MI patients examined by multimodality imaging, fibrous-cap erosion was detected in 23% by OCT. Finally, plaques with superficial calcified nodules may also be assumed vulnerable. In an OCT study of 889 de novo culprit lesions (48% ACS), 30% of ACS culprit lesions contained a calcified nodule, and its presence was associated with ACS presentation independent of other vulnerable plaque morphologies.

With respect to the prognostic value of OCT-defined plaque vulnerability features, one large prospective multicenter registry (CLIMA: Relationship Between OCT Coronary Plaque Morphology and Clinical Outcome) has recently demonstrated the potential of OCT to identify patients at higher risk for subsequent coronary events. In 1003 patients enrolled, primary endpoint events occurred in 3.7% (cardiac deaths in 2.5% and target-segment MI in 1.3%) at 1 year. Prespecified 4 high-risk OCT features observed in the untreated proximal LAD were all individually associated with the primary end point: MLA <3.5 mm² (HR 2.1), fibrous cap thickness <75 μm (HR 4.7), maximum lipid arc >180° (HR 2.4), and macrophage infiltration (HR 2.7). The simultaneous presence of the 4 features in the same plaque was observed in 18.9% of the event patients, and the patients with all 4 features had a 7-fold higher risk of subsequent cardiac mortality or MI (HR 7.5, $P < .001$). Importantly, several other clinical studies also suggested that lipid-lowering therapy with statins can significantly increase the fibrous-cap thickness as measured by OCT. Whether these OCT findings can be used as surrogate end points of plaque stabilization therapies remains to be investigated.

Interventional Applications

Preinterventional Plaque Assessment

In addition to the standard morphometrics on the target and reference lumens, preinterventional OCT can offer unique information on lesion characteristics, such as the thickness of superficial calcification, TCFA, plaque rupture, or presence and type of thrombus, that may help guide the procedure. Unlike in IVUS, the OCT signal can penetrate calcium without shadowing. This allows operators to access the thickness of superficial calcification, suggesting the need for plaque modification with rotational atherectomy or lithotripsy prior to stenting. In particular, lesions with calcium deposits with maximum angle >180°, maximum thickness >0.5 mm, and length >5 mm at prestent OCT may be at risk of stent underexpansion. Conversely, even with wide circumferential extension, a calcium crack enabling adequate stent expansion may be successfully created by balloon angioplasty alone if the minimum thickness of the calcium deposit is less than 0.5 mm as measured by OCT.

OCT-Guided Selection of Device Size and Length

As in the case of IVUS, precise quantitative lesion assessment by OCT can guide the optimal sizing of devices to be employed. Unlike EEM-based vessel sizing typically performed with IVUS, reference lumen diameters are often used for OCT-guided PCI because of limited OCT signal penetration for complete EEM visualization. This methodological difference can lead to the selection of smaller stent and balloon sizes with OCT guidance, which may in part account for significantly smaller MSA achieved under OCT guidance, as compared with IVUS guidance, reported in several comparative clinical studies. Based on these results, an EEM-based OCT-guided sizing strategy was recently proposed in the ILUMIEN III: OPTIMIZE PCI (Optical Coherence Tomography Compared to Intravascular Ultrasound and Angiography to Guide Coronary Stent Implantation: A Multicenter Randomized Trial in Percutaneous Coronary Intervention) study. Specifically, the stent diameter in this trial was chosen by the smaller EEM diameter of the proximal or distal reference if the EEM circumference was visualized at >180°; otherwise, the stent size was determined based on reference lumen diameters. Combined with the prespecified poststent optimization strategy, this protocol allowed OCT-guided stenting to achieve comparable MSA results to IVUS-guided stenting.

Appropriate device length can also be defined by OCT. PCI-planning software with automated lumen contour detection facilitates the determination of appropriate landing zones and stent length for optimal lesion coverage. In particular, multiple OCT studies have identified residual stenosis at reference segments (defined as reference lumen area <4.1 or 4.5 mm) as an independent predictor of stent edge restenosis or long-term adverse events. Additionally, a retrospective study of everolimus-eluting stents reported that OCT-defined lipidic plaque (lipidic arc >185°) in the stent edge segment was significantly associated with subsequent edge restenosis.

OCT Assessment of Acute Stent Problems

Appearances of dissections and tissue (plaque or thrombus) protrusions are essentially similar between OCT and IVUS. However, the higher resolution as well as the higher contrast between the lumen and the vessel wall often allows OCT to visualize those entities in greater detail than possible with IVUS (**Figure 22.12**). For instance, in the multicenter CLI-OPCI (Centro per la Lotta Contro l'Infarto Optimization of Percutaneous Coronary Intervention) registry, major dissection at poststenting was defined as a linear rim of tissue with a width >200 μm and a clear separation from the vessel wall or underlying plaque. The presence of major dissection at the distal stent edge was an independent predictor of MACE (HR 2.03, P = .004) at a median follow-up of 833 days.

With respect to in-stent tissue protrusions, at least a certain type of OCT-defined protrusions may also be associated with subsequent adverse events. In the CLI-OPCI registry, while in-stent tissue protrusion was not associated with worse clinical outcomes in the overall population, it was identified as an independent predictor of device-oriented cardiovascular events (HR 2.83, P = .008) when the subjects were limited to ACS patients.

Unlike IVUS, strut apposition is assessed by OCT with direct measurement of the distance between the adluminal reflection of the strut and that of the vessel wall (**Figure 22.13**). Incomplete apposition is then defined as a strut-vessel distance longer than the nominal strut thickness (including polymer if present). Some investigators

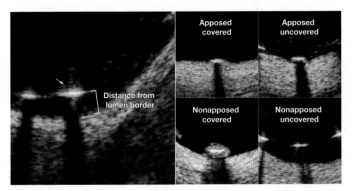

Figure 22.13 OCT assessment of metal stent struts in relation to the arterial wall. Strut apposition to the vessel wall is determined by measuring the distance from the stent strut surface to the vessel wall as compared to the nominal strut thickness. Due to a blooming effect of metal struts (arrow), the highest intensity point within the strut image should be used for the measurement. Stent struts at follow-up are classified into 4 categories, based upon the apposition and tissue coverage of the struts. OCT, optical coherence tomography.

have also proposed further classification of apposed struts as either embedded or protruded. In multimodality imaging studies using both IVUS and OCT, incomplete strut apposition was detected by OCT 2 to 3 times more frequently than by IVUS.

OCT Assessment of Chronic Stent Problems

OCT can offer unique observations of the stented vessel at a chronic phase, particularly in the context of DES. Given the precision with which OCT visualizes the stent struts and their relationships with the vessel wall, the degrees of stent strut apposition and tissue coverage at long-term follow-up are being extensively explored using OCT. Combined with the binary definitions of strut apposition described above, stent struts at follow-up are classified as (1) apposed and covered, (2) apposed and uncovered, (3) nonapposed (protruded) but covered, or (4) nonapposed and uncovered (see **Figure 22.13**).

OCT Assessment of Bioresorbable Scaffolds

Unlike metallic stent struts that appear on OCT as a reflective leading structure with abluminal shadowing, polymeric BRS struts appear as a "black box" area surrounded by bright reflecting frames without significant shadowing. The optical transparency of the polymer struts allows visualization of the vessel wall behind the struts as well as direct assessment of the strut apposition to the vessel wall, rather than based on the distance measurement as required in metallic stents. In a chronic phase, the polymer struts may appear on OCT as preserved box, open box, dissolved bright box, or dissolved black box, presumably reflecting the various stages of strut degradation and resorption in the vessel wall. Since tracing of the back of struts as well as the area occupied by the struts is technically possible, quantitative OCT studies of polymeric BRSs often include more detailed parameters than in metallic stents, such as abluminal and endoluminal device areas, flow area, and total strut and strut core areas.

Similar to metallic stents, suboptimal deployment, such as underexpansion and incomplete lesion coverage, has been shown to be associated with adverse events after BRS implantation. In addition, the unique biomechanical properties of BRS may contribute to a novel failure mode, so-called intraluminal scaffold dismantling, that has been reported by OCT in cases with late or very late scaffold thrombosis. Theoretically, scaffold dismantling, observed as late scaffold discontinuity on OCT, is a programmed phenomenon of no clinical consequence if the discontinuous struts are embedded in neointima. Conversely, degradation of the struts protruding into the lumen may expose the highly thrombogenic remnant scaffold material to the blood flow with subsequent activation of the coagulation cascade. While complete embedment of BRS struts in the vessel wall assured by OCT at the time of implantation may help reduce the risk of this complication, the intraluminal scaffold dismantling can also occur in cases with LISA.

SPECTROSCOPY AND OTHER OPTICAL IMAGING

When tissues are exposed to a light beam containing a broad mixture (spectrum) of wavelengths, wavelengths absorbed by the illuminated molecules will be missing from the spectrum of the original light after it has traversed the tissue. Diffuse reflectance near-infrared spectroscopy (NIRS) analyzes the amount of this absorbance as a function of wavelengths within the near-infrared window (700-2500 nm).

Imaging Systems and Procedures

Diffuse reflectance NIRS shows the ability to identify the lipid component of atherosclerotic plaques in clinical settings. The commercially available coronary spectroscopy system incorporates a dual-modality imaging catheter that provides simultaneous NIRS and IVUS imaging for coregistered acquisition of compositional and structural information (Infraredx). The 3.2F imaging catheter contains, within a protective outer sheath, fiberoptic bundles for delivery and collection of light. The catheter with a rapid exchange design is compatible with a 6F guide catheter and can be advanced to the coronary segment of interest using a standard interventional technique. Unlike other light-based imaging techniques, this system does not require removal of blood from the imaging field. The catheter directs the light to the vessel wall with a mirror located at the tip to acquire spectra within 20 milliseconds, through flowing blood. This configuration allows not only circumferential data collection but also a complete longitudinal scan of the target segment using controlled pullback of the probe. The collected light is analyzed by a spectrometer; using a diagnostic algorithm, the processed data are color-coded and displayed in a 2-dimensional map of the vessel called a "chemogram" with the spatial (circumferential and longitudinal) information (**Figure 22.14**). The current system is specifically designed for the detection of lipid-rich plaque, which is seen in yellow color on the chemogram. A color scale from red to yellow indicates increasing algorithmic probability of a lipid component in the vessel wall. The extended bandwidth (center frequency 50 MHz; range 35-65 MHz) IVUS transducer is mounted adjacent to the NIRS probe, and the chemogram data are laid in a halo surrounding the cross-sectional IVUS image in a real-time manner. A summary of the results for each 2 mm section of artery is displayed as a block chemogram, which also is portrayed in the cross-sectional IVUS image.

Image Interpretation

The chemogram is a 2-dimensional, color-coded map of the location and intensity of lipid viewed from the luminal surface. The x-axis represents millimeters of pullback in the artery, and the y-axis represents degrees of the probe rotation, displayed as if the vessel had been split open along its longitudinal axis. The extent of lipid-rich area in a given segment is quantified as a lipid core burden index (LCBI) with a scale of 0 to 1,000, computed as the fraction of valid pixels within the scanned region that

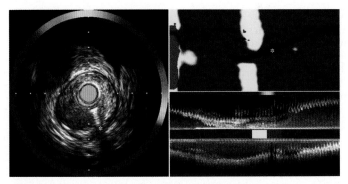

Figure 22.14 Example images obtained with a dual-modality NIRS-IVUS system. A color scale from red to yellow indicates increasing algorithmic probability of lipid content. The spectroscopy data are laid in a halo surrounding the cross-sectional IVUS image in a real-time manner **(left)**. In a 2-dimensional map of the vessel called a chemogram **(upper right)**, the x-axis represents millimeters of pullback in the artery and the y-axis represents degrees of rotation. A summary of the results for each 2 mm section of artery is displayed as a block chemogram, which is portrayed in the cross-sectional **(left)** and longitudinal IVUS images **(lower right)**. (*) indicates a guidewire shadow. NIRS-IVUS, near-infrared spectroscopy intravascular ultrasound.

exceed a lipid probability of 0.6, multiplied by 1000. The maximum value of LCBI for any of the 4-mm segments (maxLCBI$_{4mm}$) within the region is also calculated automatically.

Several ex vivo studies have confirmed the ability of intravascular NIRS to identify the lipid component of human coronary arteries or aortic samples through blood. On the other hand, one technical limitation to note when interpreting NIRS data is that the depth of lipid cannot be estimated due to the lack of axial resolution in the current technique. Therefore, LCBI and maxLCBI$_{4mm}$ primarily represent the geographic extent of lipid accumulation rather than the actual amount (or volume) of the lipid component in the vessel wall. Also, since the y-axis on the chemogram indicates the arc of lipid in degrees as centered on the NIRS probe, the extent of lipid shown in this direction can be affected by the distance from the probe to the vessel wall. For instance, a small superficial lipid pool can display a relatively large lipid arc (and thus an exaggerated LCBI) if the NIRS probe, as the center of the arc, is located close to the lipid pool due to lumen narrowing or off-centered catheter position in the lumen. These facts support the rationale of the NIRS-IVUS hybrid imaging to supplement the chemogram data with coregistered cross-sectional IVUS information.

Diagnostic Applications

The utility of NIRS is being investigated most actively as a diagnostic tool of vulnerable plaque (**Figure 22.15**). A clinical study of acute ST-elevation MI (STEMI) reported that maxLCBI$_{4mm}$ was 4.4-fold higher in culprit segments than in nonculprit segments; a threshold of maxLCBI$_{4mm}$ >400 differentiated STEMI culprit from nonculprit segments with 64% sensitivity and 85% specificity. An ex vivo imaging study also showed that maxLCBI >323 was able to identify TCFA exhibiting 80% sensitivity and 85% specificity, although this data set included only 10 TCFAs out of 271 lesions examined. In another ex vivo study, false negatives for detection of histological fibroatheromas were primarily attributed to the limited sensitivity of NIRS in detecting small necrotic cores, while false positives were seen most often in patho-

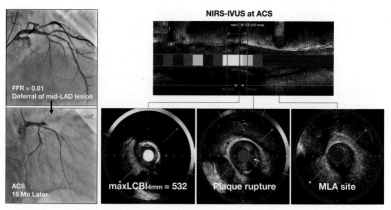

Figure 22.15 A case of acute coronary syndrome that occurred 15 months after FFR-based deferral of mid-LAD artery lesion. NIRS-IVUS at the event shows lipid-rich plaque (maxLC-BI$_{4mm}$ > 400) and plaque rupture (arrow) at the segment adjacent to the minimum lumen area (MLA) site. FFR, fractional flow reserve; LAD, left anterior descending; NIRS-IVUS, near-infrared spectroscopy-intravascular ultrasound.

logical intimal thickening including increased lipid components. Some investigators suggested that combined assessment of maxLCBI with conventional IVUS-derived plaque characteristics, such as plaque burden and ultrasound signal attenuation, could further improve the diagnostic accuracy in detecting histopathologic vulnerable plaque.

The ability of NIRS to predict future adverse events has been evaluated in several longitudinal clinical studies. At present, the largest natural history trial is the LRP (Lipid-Rich Plaque) study, which prospectively enrolled 1563 stable angina or ACS patients for multivessel NIRS-IVUS imaging of nonculprit coronary segments. At 2-year follow-up, the cumulative incidence of nonculprit MACE was 9%, and the unadjusted HR for each 100-unit increase in maxLCBI was 1.21 (P = .0004) on a patient level and 1.45 (P < .0001) on a plaque level. The prespecified threshold of $maxLCBI_{4mm}$ >400 also identified high-risk patients (HR 2.18, P < .0001) and plaque (HR 4.22, P < .0001) for nonculprit MACE. In PROSPECT 2, highly lipidic lesions by combined NIRS-IVUS were independent predictors of patient-level non–culprit lesion-related MACE. Lesions with both large plaque burden by IVUS and large lipid-rich cores by NIRS had a 4-year non–culprit lesion-related MACE of 7%, consistent with nonobstructive lesions with a high lipid content and large lipid burden being at increased risk for future cardiac outcomes.

Interventional Applications

Preinterventional NIRS imaging may offer unique guidance for PCI. In particular, multiple clinical studies have suggested that detection of lipid-rich plaques by NIRS may identify an increased risk of periprocedural MI, presumably caused by embolization of the lipid core content and/or thrombi associated with the mechanical disruption of lipid-rich plaques by PCI. An early substudy of the COLOR (Chemometric Observations of Lipid Core Plaques of Interest in Native Coronary Arteries) registry reported that PCI of lesions with a large lipid core, defined as >500 $maxLCBI_{4mm}$ by preinterventional NIRS, was associated with a 50% risk of periprocedural MI, compared with only a 4.2% risk for lesions without a large lipid core (P = .0002). This preliminary finding was further evaluated in a prospective multicenter CANARY (Coronary Assessment by Near-infrared of Atherosclerotic Rupture-prone Yellow) trial that randomized PCI patients with NIRS-determined high-risk lipid-rich plaques (defined as >600 maxLCBI) to standard PCI versus stent implantation with an embolic protection device in place prior to any angioplasty. This trial confirmed the correlation between greater plaque lipid content and periprocedural MI, although the use of a distal protection filter did not reduce myonecrosis after PCI of lipid-rich plaques.

SUGGESTED READINGS

1. Ali ZA, Maehara A, Genereux P, et al. Optical coherence tomography compared with intravascular ultrasound and with angiography to guide coronary stent implantation (ILUMIEN III: OPTIMIZE PCI). A randomised controlled trial. *Lancet*. 2016;388(10060):2618-2628.
2. Bhindi R, Guan M, Zhao Y, Humphries KH, Mancini GBJ. Coronary atheroma regression and adverse cardiac events: a systematic review and meta-regression analysis. *Atherosclerosis*. 2019;284:194-201.
3. Castagna MT, Mintz GS, Leiboff BO, et al. The contribution of "mechanical" problems to in-stent restenosis: an intravascular ultrasonographic analysis of 1090 consecutive in-stent restenosis lesions. *Am Heart J*. 2001;142(6):970-974.
4. Chieffo A, Latib A, Caussin C, et al. A prospective, randomized trial of intravascular-ultrasound guided compared to angiography guided stent implantation in complex coronary lesions: the AVIO trial. *Am Heart J*. 2013;165(1):65-72.
5. Costa MA, Angiolillo DJ, Tannenbaum M, et al. Impact of stent deployment procedural factors on long-term effectiveness and safety of sirolimus-eluting stents (final results of the multicenter prospective STLLR trial). *Am J Cardiol*. 2008;101(12):1704-1711.

6. Danek BA, Karatasakis A, Karacsonyi J, et al. Long-term follow-up after near-infrared spectroscopy coronary imaging: insights from the lipid cORe plaque association with CLinical events (ORACLE-NIRS) registry. *Cardiovasc Revascularization Med.* 2017;18(3):177-181.

7. Doi H, Maehara A, Mintz GS, et al. Classification and potential mechanisms of intravascular ultrasound patterns of stent fracture. *Am J Cardiol.* 2009;103(6):818-823.

8. Doi H, Maehara A, Mintz GS, et al. Impact of post-intervention minimal stent area on 9-month follow-up patency of paclitaxel-eluting stents: an integrated intravascular ultrasound analysis from the TAXUS IV, V, and VI and TAXUS ATLAS Workhorse, Long Lesion, and Direct Stent Trials. *JACC Cardiovasc Interv.* 2009;2(12):1269-1275.

9. Fitzgerald PJ, Oshima A, Hayase M, et al. Final results of the can routine ultrasound influence stent expansion (CRUISE) study. *Circulation.* 2000;102(5):523-530.

10. Fujii K, Mintz GS, Kobayashi Y, et al. Contribution of stent underexpansion to recurrence after sirolimus-eluting stent implantation for in-stent restenosis. *Circulation.* 2004;109(9):1085-1088.

11. Fujino A, Mintz GS, Lee T, et al. Predictors of calcium fracture derived from balloon angioplasty and its effect on stent expansion assessed by optical coherence tomography. *JACC Cardiovasc Interv.* 2018;11(10):1015-1017.

12. Fujino A, Mintz GS, Matsumura M, et al. A new optical coherence tomography-based calcium scoring system to predict stent underexpansion. *EuroIntervention.* 2018;13(18):e2182-e2189.

13. Goto K, Zhao Z, Matsumura M, et al. Mechanisms and patterns of intravascular ultrasound in-stent restenosis among bare metal stents and first- and second-generation drug-eluting stents. *Am J Cardiol.* 2015;116(9):1351-1357.

14. Hassan AK, Bergheanu SC, Stijnen T, et al. Late stent malapposition risk is higher after drug-eluting stent compared with bare-metal stent implantation and associates with late stent thrombosis. *Eur Heart J.* 2010;31(10):1172-1180.

15. Honda Y. Drug-eluting stents. Insights from invasive imaging technologies. *Circ J.* 2009;73(8):1371-1380.

16. Hong MK, Mintz GS, Lee CW, et al. Intravascular ultrasound predictors of angiographic restenosis after sirolimus-eluting stent implantation. *Eur Heart J.* 2006;27(11):1305-1310.

17. Hong SJ, Kim BK, Shin DH, et al. Effect of intravascular ultrasound-guided vs angiography-guided everolimus-eluting stent implantation: the IVUS-XPL randomized clinical trial. *J Am Med Assoc.* 2015;314(20):2155-2163.

18. Hong SJ, Mintz GS, Ahn CM, et al. Effect of intravascular ultrasound-guided drug-eluting stent implantation: 5-year follow-up of the IVUS-XPL randomized trial. *JACC Cardiovasc Interv.* 2020;13(1):62-71.

19. Inaba S, Mintz GS, Burke AP, et al. Intravascular ultrasound and near-infrared spectroscopic characterization of thin-cap fibroather-oma. *Am J Cardiol.* 2017;119(3):372-378.

20. Ino Y, Kubo T, Matsuo Y, et al. Optical coherence tomography predictors for edge restenosis after everolimus-eluting stent implantation. *Circ Cardiovasc Interv.* 2016;9(10):e004231.

21. Kang SJ, Mintz GS, Park DW, et al. Mechanisms of in-stent restenosis after drug-eluting stent implantation: intravascular ultrasound analysis. *Circ Cardiovasc Interv.* 2011;4(1):9-14.

22. Kang SJ, Cho YR, Park GM, et al. Intravascular ultrasound predictors for edge restenosis after newer generation drug-eluting stent implantation. *Am J Cardiol.* 2013;111(10):1408-1414.

23. Kang SJ, Mintz GS, Pu J, et al. Combined IVUS and NIRS detection of fibroatheromas: histopathological validation in human coronary arteries. *JACC Cardiovasc Imaging.* 2015;8(2):184-194.

24. Kasaoka S, Tobis JM, Akiyama T, et al. Angiographic and intravascular ultrasound predictors of in-stent restenosis. *J Am Coll Cardiol.* 1998;32(6):1630-1635.

25. Kobayashi N, Mintz GS, Witzenbichler B, et al. Prevalence, features, and prognostic importance of edge dissection after drug-eluting stent implantation: an ADAPT-DES intravascular ultrasound substudy. *Circ Cardiovasc Interv.* 2016;9(7):e003553.

26. Kubo T, Imanishi T, Takarada S, et al. Assessment of culprit lesion morphology in acute myocardial infarction: ability of optical coherence tomography compared with intravascular ultrasound and coronary angioscopy. *J Am Coll Cardiol.* 2007;50(10):933-939.

27. Kubo T, Shinke T, Okamura T, et al. Optical frequency domain imaging vs. intravascular ultrasound in percutaneous coronary intervention (OPINION trial): one-year angiographic and clinical results. *Eur Heart J.* 2017;38(42):3139-3147.

28. Lee T, Mintz GS, Matsumura M, et al. Prevalence, predictors, and clinical presentation of a calcified nodule as assessed by optical coherence tomography. *JACC Cardiovasc Imaging.* 2017;10(8):883-891.

29. Madder RD, Husaini M, Davis AT, et al. Large lipid-rich coronary plaques detected by near-infrared spectroscopy at non-stented sites in the target artery identify patients likely to experience future major adverse cardiovascular events. *Eur Heart J Cardiovasc Imaging.* 2016;17(4):393-399.

30. Madder RD, Puri R, Muller JE, et al. Confirmation of the intracoronary near-infrared spectroscopy threshold of lipid-rich plaques that underlie ST-segment-elevation myocardial infarction. *Arterioscler Thromb Vasc Biol.* 2016;36(5):1010-1015.

31. Maehara A, Mintz GS, Witzenbichler B, et al. Relationship between intravascular ultrasound guidance and clinical outcomes after drug-eluting stents. *Circ Cardiovasc Interv.* 2018;11:e006243.

32. Meneveau N, Souteyrand G, Motreff P, et al. Optical coherence tomography to optimize results of percutaneous coronary intervention in patients with non-ST-elevation acute coronary syndrome: results of the multicenter, randomized DOCTORS study (Does Optical Coherence Tomography Optimize Results of Stenting). *Circulation.* 2016;134(13):906-917.

33. Nascimento BR, de Sousa MR, Koo BK, et al. Diagnostic accuracy of intravascular ultrasound-derived minimal lumen area compared with fractional flow reserve-Meta-analysis: pooled accuracy of IVUS luminal area versus FFR. *Catheter Cardiovasc Interv.* 2014;84(3):377-385.

34. Nicholls SJ, Puri R, Anderson T, et al. Effect of evolocumab on coronary plaque composition. *J Am Coll Cardiol.* 2018;72(17):2012-2021.

35. Okada K, Kitahara H, Mitsutake Y, et al. Assessment of bioresorbable scaffold with a novel high-definition 60 MHz IVUS imaging system: comparison with 40-MHz IVUS referenced to optical coherence tomography. *Catheter Cardiovasc Interv.* 2018;91(5):874-883.

36. Prati F, Di Vito L, Biondi-Zoccai G, et al. Angiography alone versus angiography plus optical coherence tomography to guide decisionmaking during percutaneous coronary intervention: the Centro per la Lotta contro l'Infarto-Optimisation of Percutaneous Coronary Intervention (CLI-OPCI) study. *EuroIntervention.* 2012;8(7):823-829.

37. Prati F, Romagnoli E, Burzotta F, et al. Clinical impact of OCT findings during PCI: the CLI-OPCI II study. *JACC Cardiovasc Imaging.* 2015;8(11):1297-1305.

38. Prati F, Romagnoli E, Gatto L, et al. Relationship between coronary plaque morphology of the left anterior descending artery and 12 months clinical outcome: the CLIMA study. *Eur Heart J.* 2020;41(3):383-391.

39. Puri R, Madder RD, Madden SP, et al. Near-infrared spectroscopy enhances intravascular ultrasound assessment of vulnerable coronary plaque: a combined pathological and in vivo study. *Arterioscler Thromb Vasc Biol.* 2015;35(11):2423-2431.

40. Ramasubbu K, Schoenhagen P, Balghith MA, et al. Repeated intravascular ultrasound imaging in cardiac transplant recipients does not accelerate transplant coronary artery disease. *J Am Coll Cardiol.* 2003;41(10):1739-1743.

41. Russo RJ, Silva PD, Teirstein PS, et al. A randomized controlled trial of angiography versus intravascular ultrasound-directed bare-metal coronary stent placement (the AVID Trial). *Circ Cardiovasc Interv.* 2009;2:113-123.

42. Sakurai R, Ako J, Hassan AH, et al. Neointimal progression and luminal narrowing in sirolimus-eluting stent treatment for bare metal in-stent restenosis: a quantitative intravascular ultrasound analysis. *Am Heart J.* 2007;154(2):361-365.

43. Schuurman AS, Vroegindewey MM, Kardys I, et al. Prognostic value of intravascular ultrasound in patients with coronary artery disease. *J Am Coll Cardiol.* 2018;72(17):2003-2011.

44. Sonoda S, Morino Y, Ako J, et al. Impact of final stent dimensions on long-term results following sirolimus-eluting stent implantation: serial intravascular ultrasound analysis from the SIRIUS trial. *J Am Coll Cardiol.* 2004;43(11):1959-1963.

45. Stone GW, Maehara A, Lansky AJ, et al. A prospective naturalhistory study of coronary atherosclerosis. *N Engl J Med.* 2011;364(3):226-235.

46. Tanaka A, Imanishi T, Kitabata H, et al. Morphology of exertion-triggered plaque rupture in patients with acute coronary syndrome: an optical coherence tomography study. *Circulation.* 2008;118(23):2368-2373.

47. Tearney GJ, Regar E, Akasaka T, et al. Consensus standards for acquisition, measurement, and reporting of intravascular optical coherence tomography studies: a report from the International Working Group for Intravascular Optical Coherence Tomography Standardization and Validation. *J Am Coll Cardiol.* 2012;59(12):1058-1072.

48. van der Sijde JN, Karanasos A, van Ditzhuijzen NS, et al. Safety of optical coherence tomography in daily practice: a comparison with intravascular ultrasound. *Eur Heart J Cardiovasc Imaging.* 2017;18(4):467-474.

49. Yonetsu T, Kakuta T, Lee T, et al. In vivo critical fibrous cap thickness for rupture-prone coronary plaques assessed by optical coherence tomography. *Eur Heart J.* 2011;32(10):1251-1259.

23 Endomyocardial Biopsy[1]

Disorders of the myocardium remain one of the most challenging areas in modern cardiology. Although echocardiography and magnetic resonance imaging (MRI), right heart catheterization, left heart catheterization, and angiography can provide substantial amounts of information on various causes of heart failure, more than half of the patients presenting with new-onset heart failure remain classified as idiopathic. In a relatively small subset of this group of patients, myocardial biopsy can allow a more precise characterization of the underlying primary myocardial pathology.

MODERN BIOPTOMES

Currently used biopsy forceps are single-use and disposable devices that eliminate the risk of patient-to-patient disease transmission, pyrogen reaction, need for retooling and resharpening of the cutting edges, and mechanical malfunction sometimes seen in the earlier reusable devices. They follow either a preshaped or a flexible (long-sheath) format (**Figure 23.1**).

The unshaped flexible bioptomes are inserted through a preformed sheath that directs the head of the instrument toward the desired portion of the right ventricular septum or left ventricular wall. The preformed sheath is generally advanced over an angled pigtail or balloon flotation catheter and remains in the ventricular cavity throughout the biopsy procedure. This increases the risk for ventricular arrhythmia or perforation and reduces the operator control of the site and direction of the bioptome's path.

In contrast, the preshaped bioptomes are introduced through a short venous sheath and maneuvered as independent catheters to access the right ventricle. They are stiffer and allow greater control of the course and direction of the instrument by the operator. The degree of curvature of the preshaped bioptome can be modified by the operator to suit the angulation required to traverse the tricuspid valve. For the rare patient in whom the relatively stiff preshaped bioptome fails to enter the right ventricle, biopsy can still be performed by advancing a preformed sheath into the

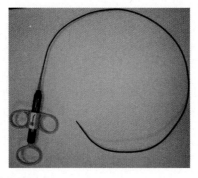

Figure 23.1 Flexible bioptome.

[1]We gratefully acknowledge the Grossman & Baim's *Cardiac Catheterization, Angiography, and Intervention*, 9th edition contributions of Drs Sandra V. Chaparro and Mauro Moscucci as portions of their chapter, "Endomyocardial Biopsy," were retained in this text.

ventricle over either a guidewire or a balloon-tipped catheter. Disposable bioptomes and sheaths are available and vary in length, shape, jaw size, and diameter.

VASCULAR ACCESS FOR ENDOMYOCARDIAL BIOPSY

Right ventricular heart biopsy can be performed percutaneously from the right internal jugular vein, left internal jugular vein, right subclavian, or right or left femoral vein. Left ventricular biopsy is usually performed from the right or left femoral artery; however, it can also be accomplished from the right or left brachial artery and the radial artery.

Internal Jugular Access

Right ventricular endomyocardial biopsy procedures are most commonly performed via the right internal jugular vein. Monitoring during the procedure includes continuous electrocardiogram, pulse oximetry, and blood pressure.

The patient's head is turned 30° to 45° to the left to facilitate evaluation and preparation of the venous cannulation site. The internal jugular is located lateral to the carotid artery, within the anterior triangle formed by the sternal and clavicular head of the sternocleidomastoid muscle and top of the clavicle (**Figure 23.2**). If the location of the internal jugular vein is not readily apparent, the neck vasculature can be evaluated echocardiographically using an ultrasound transducer encased in a sterile sheath. The jugular vein can be distinguished from the more medial carotid artery by location, the pulsatility of the artery, and the compressibility of the vein (**Figure 23.3**).

After the patient's landmarks have been identified, the neck field is prepped and isolated using sterile towels and/or plastic drapes. Successful puncture of the internal jugular is facilitated by distension of the vein—in patients with low venous pressure or a small internal jugular vein, this can be achieved by placing the patient in a head-down Trendelenburg position,

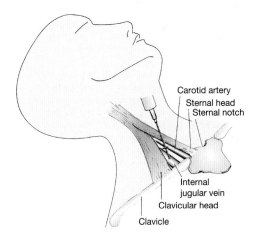

Carotid artery
Sternal head
Sternal notch
Internal jugular vein
Clavicular head
Clavicle

Figure 23.2 Regional anatomy for internal jugular puncture. With the patient's head rotated to the left, the sternal notch and clavicle, as well as the sternal and clavicular heads of the sternocleidomastoid muscle, are identified. A skin nick is made between the 2 heads of this muscle, and 2 fingerbreadths above the top of the clavicle (near the top of the anterior triangle). The needle is inserted at an angle of 30°- 40° from vertical, at 20°-30° right of sagittal, aiming the needle away from the more medially located carotid artery.

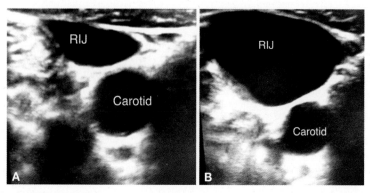

Figure 23.3 Two-dimensional echo of the carotid artery and the right internal jugular (RIJ) vein at rest **(A)** and during Valsalva maneuver **(B)**, showing the marked enlargement in jugular venous caliber with increased distending pressure by elevating the legs on a wedge, or having the patient perform a Valsalva maneuver during needle advancement.

A 25-gauge needle is used to apply a small intradermal bleb of 2% lidocaine at the site of planned sheath entry. A 22-gauge needle is then used to anesthetize the area from the superficial bleb toward the internal jugular vein. After the area is successfully anesthetized, a small (2 mm) incision is made at the superficial site of initial infiltration with a no. 11 surgical blade. The incision is then expanded with the tip of a mosquito clamp to ensure that the skin will accommodate the 7F venous sheath. In the classic approach, the 22-gauge anesthesia needle is directed toward the anticipated venous pathway at an angle of approximately 30° to 40° from vertical and 20° right of the sagittal plane and is advanced in small increments, aspirating before infiltration of small amounts of lidocaine to provide local anesthesia. Excess lidocaine infiltration should be avoided, since it may result in venous compression or infiltration of vocal cords or carotid sheath, resulting in transient hoarseness or Horner syndrome.

Once venous blood is aspirated, indicating entry into the internal jugular vein, the operator notes the position and direction of the needle, and a second 18-gauge single-wall puncture needle with syringe is advanced parallel to the "finder" needle. Continuous aspiration is applied as the needle is advanced in small increments, particularly in individuals with small internal jugular veins or a low central venous pressure. Usually the "give" of the vein wall is palpable, even before blood return is evident. A J-tip guidewire is then introduced, followed by the necessary sheath.

A more recent and common approach today is to use a 21-gauge micropuncture needle and a micropuncture kit (**Figure 23.4**) as the deep anesthesia, probing, and definitive entry device for internal jugular vein cannulation.

Continuous aspiration is applied as the needle is advanced under ultrasound guidance to avoid puncture of the carotid artery.

Should arterial puncture occur, the probing needle and syringe will spontaneously fill with well-oxygenated blood, and the needle must be removed and compression applied for 5 minutes or until hemostasis is achieved. As described above, this problem can be avoided by using ultrasound guidance.

The 21-gauge micropuncture needle is very atraumatic and accepts a 0.018-in stainless-steel or nitinol guidewire over which a special 4 or 5F coaxial hydrophilic-coated double dilator is advanced. Once this has entered the jugular vein and superior

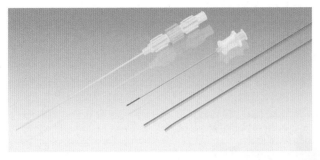

Figure 23.4 Micropuncture apparatus: 21-gauge micropuncture needle, 0.018-in guidewire, 5F guiding sheath, and obturator. (GLIDEACCESS System Image - ©2020 Terumo Medical Corporation. All rights reserved.)

vena cava, the inner cannula and 0.018-in guidewire are removed and a conventional 0.035-in guidewire is inserted through the outer cannula. The cannula is then removed, and a 7F self-sealing sheath is inserted over the guidewire. This is facilitated by passing the wire from the superior vena cava, across the right atrium, and into the inferior vena cava, avoiding runs of ventricular ectopy seen when the wire tip enters the right ventricle. Once the sheath is in the appropriate position, the guidewire and the dilator are removed, the sheath is aspirated and flushed, and the heart biopsy procedure can be carried out. To minimize blood losses and the risk of air aspiration, the needle hub and the hub of the dilator sheaths should be occluded with a gloved finger during guidewire and sheath exchanges.

A further alternative approach is to use a micropuncture vascular access Glidesheath kit, which includes a 21-gauge needle, a 0.021-in hydrophilic-coated or nitinol guidewire, and a 6F sheath (Terumo Interventional Systems, Ann Arbor, MI). The use of sheaths with hemostatic valves is preferred, as they reduce the risk of air aspiration.

Right Subclavian Vein Access

Rarely, the right subclavian vein is used when patient's anatomic factors make the internal jugular and femoral veins inappropriate for access. The entry site into the subclavian vein should be somewhat more lateral than is routinely the case for subclavian venous catheterization, as too acute a superior vena cava/subclavian vein angle will prevent the relatively stiff bioptome from negotiating this angle into the right heart. The standard site of entry for subsequent heart biopsy is the infraclavicular region, lateral to the area of the bend of the clavicle. The needle is directed medially in a plane virtually parallel to the surface of the x-ray table toward the region of the supraclavicular notch. If this is unsuccessful, approaches more inferior or at a steeper angle to the chest wall can be attempted. The standard single-wall or micropuncture technique is used, as noted above. All intravascular catheters should move without obstruction and fluoroscopy should be used to ensure that the guidewire is directed downward toward the inferior vena cava or right atrium rather than upward toward the head.

Femoral Vein and Femoral Artery Access

Femoral vein and femoral artery access have been described in Chapter 8. Left ventricular biopsies are occasionally indicated in patients with specific left ventricular masses or local pathology, isolated ventricular dysfunction, or an infiltrative process specific to the left ventricle. The risks of embolization and perforation are somewhat higher for patients submitted to left ventricular endomyocardial biopsy as opposed to right, ventricular endomyocardial biopsy. After femoral sheath insertion, a constant infusion drip should be maintained through the sheath to avoid clot formation within the lengthy catheters and air embolization.

BIOPSY METHODS

Fluoroscopic guidance has proven most beneficial in the performance of endomyocardial biopsies. Nonetheless, several investigators have described the use of 2-dimensional echocardiography, as opposed to fluoroscopy, which the authors believe reduces the risk of perforation. Visualization of the biopsy forceps is technically difficult and requires considerable operator and technician experience. Echocardiography has been used to biopsy intracardiac masses in the right or left heart.

Right Internal Jugular Venous Approach—Preshaped Bioptome

The preshaped 50-cm bioptome is inserted through the venous sheath with the tip of the bioptome pointing toward the anterior wall of the right atrium. In the mid-right atrium, the bioptome is advanced slowly as it is turned counterclockwise. This is facilitated by the fact that the direction of the bioptome head is concordant with that of the handle; nevertheless, free motion and the desired orientation should always be confirmed fluoroscopically. The anterior rotation of the bioptome head allows the tip to cross the tricuspid valve while it avoids the coronary sinus and tricuspid apparatus. Continued advancement and counterclockwise rotation then allow the bioptome to advance farther into the right ventricle and orient toward the septum (**Figure 23.5**) Extreme care must be exercised during this maneuver to avoid perforation of the vena cava, right atrium, or right ventricular free wall by the relatively stiff bioptome. If resistance is encountered, the bioptome should be pulled back and a different angle of entry attempted—the biopsy forceps should *never* be forced or prolapsed into the ventricle. If entry into the right ventricle remains difficult, a Swan-Ganz catheter or other balloon flotation device may be used to define the pathway across the tricuspid valve into the right ventricle.

Once in the right ventricle, the bioptome should lie against the mid-portion of the interventricular septum. On fluoroscopy, the bioptome should lie across the patient's spine and is usually directed inferiorly below the plane of the tricuspid valve. If there is any question as to the bioptome's position, fluoroscopy in the 30° right anterior oblique and 60° left anterior oblique projections will confirm whether the catheter is on the ventricular side of the atrioventricular groove and pointed toward the septum. The correct position is also marked by ventricular ectopy; absence of such ectopy and fluoroscopy showing the catheter as lying in the atrioventricular groove suggests that the bioptome has entered the coronary sinus or the infradiaphragmatic venous system. It must be withdrawn and repositioned before the jaws are opened and an attempt is made to retrieve tissue.

Even within the right ventricle, it is important to avoid the relatively thin right ventricular free wall by directing the head of the biopsy forceps toward the interventricular septum. The interventricular septum lies in a plane approximately 45° diagonal to the plane of the patient's chest wall and corresponds to orientation of the instrument handle leftward and posteriorly. In patients with cardiomyopathy, especially those with elevated pulmonary pressure or right ventricular enlargement, the orientation of the handle may be straight posterior.

Contact with the interventricular septum is confirmed by the appearance of premature ventricular contractions. The biopsy forceps are then withdrawn 1 to 2 cm,

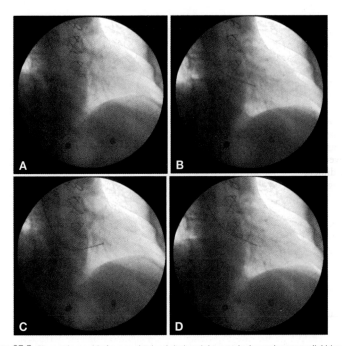

Figure 23.5 Cineangiographic frames obtained during right ventricular endomyocardial biopsy using the Stanford bioptome. From left to right, the top row shows **A,** the bioptome in the right atrium and **B,** then in the right ventricle after crossing the tricuspid valve. In the bottom row, **C,** the jaws are open and **D,** the jaws are closed and the bioptome is withdrawn from the septum with the sample contained.

opened, and advanced slowly to engage the septum. The biopsy head is slowly closed to encapsulate the endomyocardial specimen. Because of the trabeculated nature of the endomyocardial surface, gentle forward pressure should be maintained while the jaws are being closed, to ensure myocardial contact. Patients with restrictive heart disease or following transplant often demonstrate a pulsatile transmission of ventricular contractility through the course of the bioptome, whereas those with idiopathic dilated cardiomyopathy are often "soft" and engagement of the ventricular septum is confirmed only by premature ventricular contractions.

After the biopsy has been secured, the operator must maintain pressure on the forceps closure device to make sure the jaws remain closed while the specimen is withdrawn from the right ventricle, right atrium, and superior vena cava. There may be some slight "give" as the specimen is released from the myocardium. Specimens that require excessive force to remove suggest entrapment of the tricuspid apparatus, transmural biopsy, or biopsy of a scar focus. In these circumstances, the bioptome head is released by opening the jaws, the bioptome is withdrawn, and another biopsy site selected. Once removed, the specimen must be scooped from the forceps and placed in an appropriate preservative.

Patients not infrequently experience a pulling or tugging sensation as the specimen is withdrawn from the heart surface. Sharp chest pain during bioptome insertion or during the performance of an endomyocardial biopsy implies cardiac perforation. Other clues to possible perforation include persistent premature ventricular contractions, excessive retraction of the ventricular wall during biopsy withdrawal, and a biopsy specimen that floats in formalin (suggesting epicardial fat content). Any of these markers should prompt blood pressure checks and fluoroscopy of the heart borders to detect signs of pericardial tamponade. This risk is lowest in patients with prior cardiac surgery or advanced cardiomyopathy and highest in nonsurgical patients with relatively normal chamber size and systolic function.

Patients with heart transplantation who undergo repeated heart biopsies may require variation in the direction of the biopsy forceps to avoid scarred areas of prior biopsy. This may include some anterior or posterior angulation or alteration of the degree of curvature in the bioptome. The number of specimens taken per biopsy procedure is variable and depends on the patient's clinical status. The operator must balance the pathologist's desire to have adequate tissue and the risks involved with performance of the procedure.

At the conclusion of the procedure, the heart border should be examined fluoroscopically to exclude tamponade before the venous sheath is removed and the puncture site is dressed. Patients who have had serial biopsies (eg, transplant patients) can be discharged home within 10 minutes of uncomplicated biopsy.

Right Internal Jugular Vein Approach—Preformed Sheath

The disposable preformed sheath technique can also be used from the internal jugular approach. It differs from the preformed bioptome technique as described above in that the sheath (rather than the bioptome itself) is advanced into the right ventricle. This directs the bioptome, which is very flexible and lacking in inherent shape. A 6F 45-cm preformed sheath can be inserted into the superior vena cava and right atrium. The preformed sheath is guided into the right ventricle by use of a guidewire. Once the sheath is in the right ventricle, the guidewire is removed while the sheath remains in position. If there is any question as to the right ventricular placement, the side arm of the sheath can be attached to a pressure monitor and right ventricular pressure demonstrated, or a gentle contrast injection can be performed. The tip of the preformed sheath should be free floating rather than positioned against the ventricular myocardium or trabeculated portion of the right ventricle muscle. Once in a stable position, the sheath should be aspirated and flushed with heparinized solution.

The bioptome is then inserted through the disposable sheath. The distal portion of the biopsy forceps can be manually curved before entry into the sheath to avoid straightening of the sheath during insertion of the bioptome and thus disturbing the appropriate angle for biopsy performance. The jaws of the bioptome should be opened immediately on exiting the sheath to increase cross-sectional area and thereby reduce the risk of perforating the myocardial wall. The bioptome is directed posteriorly and perpendicular to the plane of the septum. Gentle pressure is applied as the jaws are slowly closed. Once the bioptome has been removed from the sheath, the jaws are opened and the specimen removed. The bioptome jaws are flushed with saline, and repeated biopsies are taken as indicated clinically. Repeated biopsy attempts may require alteration in the direction of the sheath or angulation of the bioptome.

Left Internal Jugular Vein Approach—Flexible Sheath

This technique differs from the right internal jugular approach in the type of sheath used. After the 6F 10-cm sheath is introduced in the left internal vein in the regular fashion, the sheath is exchanged over a 0.035-in wire for a 6F flexible-destination 45-cm sheath. Under careful fluoroscopy guidance, the 45-cm sheath is placed in the right atrium, the wire is removed, and then the bioptome is advanced into the right ventricle.

Femoral Vein Approach—Preformed Sheath

As with the right internal jugular venous approach, we prefer to insert a 5F Ansel Cook 75 cm guiding sheath into the femoral vein. The guiding sheath has an angle of curvature and it is inserted into the right ventricular cavity with the assistance of an internal dilator and guidewire. The femoral approach allows the operator less control over the site and location of the endomyocardial biopsy, which may increase the risk for perforation.

As with the internal jugular approach using a preformed sheath, insertion of the bioptome may straighten the sheath, altering the ideal angle for performance of the biopsy. If this is the case, the distal portion of the otherwise unformed 104-cm bioptome can be manually preshaped before insertion, into a curve similar to that of the sheath to decrease the chance of losing the ideal biopsy angle. Out-of-plane posterior angulation of the tip of the bioptome relative to the broad, more proximal curve can help direct the tip toward the ventricular septum as it exits the sheath.

Once the preformed sheath is inserted, it should be continuously flushed to avoid clot formation, thromboembolic complications, and air embolism. If there is a question as to the biopsy sheath tip location, a hand flush of contrast dye may be helpful. The 104-cm bioptome is inserted through the disposable sheath. The biopsy jaws should be opened just as the bioptome exits the preformed sheath, decreasing the potential for perforation by the bioptome. The biopsy forceps are advanced to the myocardial border with the jaws open. The jaws are slowly closed while gentle pressure is maintained against the septum. If the tip of the preformed sheath lies against the septum, the biopsy forceps can be unsheathed by retracting the sheath while maintaining the biopsy forceps in a stable position. This decreases the potential for perforation. After the specimen is obtained, the biopsy forceps are withdrawn, the sheath is advanced slightly to restore its original position in the ventricle. Once the biopsy specimen has been removed from the preformed sheath, the forceps are opened, and the specimen scooped from the jaws and placed in an appropriate preservative.

Left Ventricular Biopsy—Femoral Artery Preformed Sheath

As with the femoral venous approach, the femoral artery approach requires insertion of a larger preformed short sheath to maintain artery patency and allow biopsy sheath manipulation. Both the short and the long (98-cm) femoral artery disposable sheaths must be maintained under constant pressurized infusion with a heparinized solution to maintain patency and avoid embolic phenomenon. The preformed sheath is inserted into the left ventricular cavity using a guidewire and a pigtail catheter. The wire, pigtail catheter, and preformed sheath are gently manipulated to cross the aortic valve and enter the left ventricular cavity. Once in the left ventricle, an area of acceptable irritability is established. The inferior posterior portions of the left ventricular cavity as well as areas of previous myocardial infarction should be avoided to reduce the risk of perforation because of the relatively thin muscle in these sites.

The sheath is cleared of debris by aspirating and flushing before the 104-cm bioptome is inserted through the sheath and into the left ventricular cavity. The biopsy forceps should be directed away from the mitral valve apparatus. The jaws are opened and directed to the left ventricular wall, the specimen is encapsulated, and the jaws are closed firmly with extraction of the sample. Because of the increased contraction of the left ventricle, less forward pressure is applied while performing the biopsy. The sheath is maintained in the left ventricular cavity and its position adjusted to ensure sampling from several sites.

Left Ventricular Biopsy—Femoral Artery Guiding Catheter Approach

A retrograde left ventricular biopsy can also be performed using a 7F JR4 guiding catheter, which is passed through the aortic valve into the left ventricle using a standard J-tip guide wire. To reach the inferior, posterior, lateral, and apical walls, the JR4 guiding catheter is the best option. For the anterior segments, the recommended guiding catheter is the AL1, and for the left ventricular septum, the JL4. The disposable 105 cm bioptome is advanced through the guiding catheter into the left ventricle under biplane-fluoroscopic or echocardiographic guidance.

Another option, instead of using the guiding catheter, is to use a 7F-long guiding sheath with a straight tip. After each biopsy, aspiration of blood from the guiding catheter and rinsing with heparinized sodium chloride are performed to prevent clotting. Anticoagulation with heparin during the procedure (target activated clotting time 150 seconds) has also been recommended.

Left Ventricular Biopsy—Radial Artery Sheathless Approach

With lower-profile bioptomes, new sheathless techniques have been developed specifically for radial access. After heparinization and nitroglycerin pretreatment are given, a previously inserted 6F Terumo sheath is exchanged over the wire for a 7.5F sheathless multipurpose guiding catheter. A biopsy forceps is then carefully inserted via a Y-connector.

BIOPSY COMPLICATIONS

Virtually all complications associated with endomyocardial biopsy occur during the procedure itself, that is, while the patient is still in the catheterization laboratory. Potential complications include ventricular perforation and pericardial tamponade, malignant ventricular arrhythmias, transient complete heart block, pneumothorax, carotid artery puncture, supraventricular arrhythmias, nerve paresis, and venous hematoma. A large series of right ventricular biopsies via the femoral approach found major complications in only 0.12% and minor complications in 0.2% to 5.5% among 3048 procedures. Another study among heart transplant recipients undergoing femoral-approach biopsy showed an overall complication rate of 0.7% in 2117 procedures. The largest study comparing the right versus the left approach showed that complication rates for left ventricular (0.33%) and right ventricular (0.45%) endomyocardial biopsy were comparable.

Perforation

The greatest risk to patients from the performance of endomyocardial biopsy is ventricular perforation. Perforation is usually a complication of injury to the right ventricular free wall, which is only 1 to 2 mm thick. Patients with pulmonary hypertension, a bleeding diathesis, or right ventricular enlargement may be at increased risk for right ventricular perforation. Any patient complaining of sharp pain during the performance of the endomyocardial biopsy should be considered to have experienced cardiac perforation. Patients in whom perforation occurs immediately complain of visceral pain and within 1 to 2 minutes may develop bradycardia and hypotension. No further biopsy attempts should be made until the significance of the patient's complaints has been fully investigated. This may include fluoroscopy of the heart border, measurement of the right atrial pressure waveform, or performance of a portable echocardiogram. Loss of pulsation of heart borders on fluoroscopy and increased right atrial pressure are strong indicators for pericardial tamponade.

Echocardiography should be obtained immediately to determine the presence and severity of pericardial blood accumulation, and it is a preferred method for assessing and monitoring patients with suspected perforation. Because of the risk of tamponade, a pericardiocentesis tray should always be available in the procedure room where biopsies are performed.

Malignant Ventricular Arrhythmias

Premature ventricular contractions are anticipated when the right or left ventricular cavities are entered, and in fact are an indication of appropriate placement of the bioptome or sheath. Rarely, in patients with cardiomyopathy and preexistent ventricular arrhythmias, sustained malignant ventricular arrhythmia may occur. This can usually be terminated by removing the biopsy sheath or forceps from the ventricular cavity. If this does not stop the ventricular ectopy, medical therapy with antiarrhythmic agents or cardioversion may be necessary.

Supraventricular Arrhythmias

During cannulation of the right atrium, the atrial wall may be stimulated, causing atrial arrhythmias, particularly in those who have had a history of these rhythm disturbances in the past.

Heart Block

Patients with preexistent left bundle branch block may be at risk for complete heart block during manipulation of catheters or bioptomes in the right heart. Pressure against the septum near the tricuspid apparatus may stun the right bundle, delay conduction through the interventricular septum (a new right bundle branch block), or cause progression of prior left bundle branch block to complete heart block. Removal of the offending bioptome or catheter usually resolves the complete heart block. If this is not the case, a temporary pacing catheter can be inserted after removal of the biopsy forceps. For patients with preexisting left bundle branch block, a temporary pacing should be immediately available in the catheterization laboratory for emergency use if needed.

Pneumothorax

Laceration of the lung pleura during performance of the right internal jugular or right subclavian venous entry may result in a pneumothorax. Patients who complain of shortness of breath should be investigated immediately with fluoroscopy of the lung margins and urgent pneumothorax evacuation performed if needed.

Puncture of the Carotid Artery or Subclavian Artery

The internal jugular and subclavian veins lie adjacent to both the carotid and the subclavian arteries. Even with sonographic guidance, occasional arterial puncture may occur. Puncture of an artery caused by the guiding needle, micropuncture needle, or even an 18-gauge needle can be addressed by immediate recognition of the complication, withdrawal of the needle, and compression until hemostasis is obtained. Cannulation of an artery with a large (7-9F) sheath is a more serious error that requires urgent surgical consultation.

Pulmonary Embolization

Patients undergoing biopsy with preformed sheaths may develop clot within the sheath during the performance of the endomyocardial biopsy if not continuously flushed. This may result in recurrent thromboembolic phenomena (pulmonary embolization or potentially paradoxical embolization into the systemic arterial circuit). Air embolism has also been described, with the risk enhanced by a low right atrial pressure, and with the use of a transfemoral vein approach. It can be prevented by meticulous management of the sheath and by asking the patient to hold breath while inserting the bioptome into the sheath or during sheath exchanges.

Nerve Paresis

Excessive or ill-directed infiltration of lidocaine in and around the jugular vein and carotid sheath may result in Horner syndrome, vocal cord paresis, and, though rarely, diaphragmatic weakness. These complications are short lived, lasting 1 to 2 hours, if owing to lidocaine infiltration rather than direct nerve trauma.

Venous Hematoma

A venous hematoma may form as a result of excessive movement of the venous sheath during the procedure, inadequate compression of the venous entry site after the procedure, or late venous bleeding owing to a transient or sustained increase in right atrial pressure or coagulopathy.

Arterial Venous Fistula

Occasionally, arterial fistulas develop between small branches of the coronary artery and the right ventricle in a heart transplant patient. These are caused by biopsy of a septal coronary branch with subsequent arterial communication into the cavity from which the biopsy was performed. A multitude of long-term studies have demonstrated that such coronary AV fistulae are of no hemodynamic or clinical consequence and can be followed up conservatively.

POSTPROCEDURE CARE

Patients undergoing biopsy by jugular venous access can usually be discharged from the biopsy suite or recovery room immediately if no bleeding occurs within 5 to 10 minutes. Patients with femoral venous entry require 2 to 3 hours of supine bed rest before attempting ambulation. Patients with arterial entry require several hours of bed rest with or without arterial closure devices.

Patients should be monitored for bleeding and any change in hemodynamics. Chest radiographs are not routinely obtained post procedure, unless there is a suggestion of pneumothorax during the procedure.

TISSUE PROCESSING

It is generally recommended that at least 5 separate specimens be obtained to minimize sampling error. Most myocardial diseases affect both ventricles, so either chamber may be sampled, depending on operator experience and preference. Selective left ventricular involvement may be present in certain diseases (endomyocardial fibrosis, scleroderma, left heart radiation, and cardiac fibroelastosis of infants and newborns). Left ventricular biopsy may be performed in these conditions or in patients in whom right ventricular biopsy has been unsuccessful or nondiagnostic. In the remaining patients, right (rather than left) ventricular biopsy is generally preferred because of greater ease and speed and less likelihood of morbidity.

The availability of a cardiac pathologist who is fully trained in the evaluation of biopsy-obtained tissue and conversant with the latest classification schemes is mandatory in any biopsy program. Artifacts such as crushing or contraction bands are frequently present in endomyocardial biopsy specimens and may be overinterpreted by an inexperienced pathologist or one used to evaluate only postmortem specimens. The operator may assist the pathologist by appropriate handling of the tissue in the catheterization laboratory. The specimen should be removed gently from the jaws of the bioptome with a fine needle and placed immediately in an appropriate fixative. Frozen specimens may be prepared in the catheterization laboratory by placing the samples in a suitable fluid-embedding medium and immersing them in a liquid nitrogen and dry ice–isopentane mixture to allow immediate interpretation. Additional special sample preparation or staining (iron, amyloid) may be indicated for evaluation for specific disease states (**Table 23.1**).

It is the operator's responsibility to ensure that the heart biopsy specimens obtained are delivered to the appropriate laboratory for analysis. Preferably, the operator should review the slide material obtained and assist the pathologist with an appropriate history to ensure that special studies are conducted as needed.

Patients with idiopathic dilated cardiomyopathy display a specific pathologic pattern including myocyte hypertrophy and interstitial fibrosis. These findings may allow the clinician to rule out other entities and help define the severity and judge the duration of the patient's cardiomyopathic condition. In large-series studies of 4221 patients undergoing myocardial biopsy, the diagnostic yield of left ventricular endomyocardial biopsy was 97.8% compared with 53% for right ventricular biopsy.

Myocardium should always be collected for light microscopy and placed in room temperature in 10% buffered formalin. In certain clinical situations, tissue for electron microscopy should be placed in a glutaraldehyde fixative. Tissue for immunofluorescence should be frozen in optimal cutting temperature compound or placed in Zeus solution, and tissue for viral nucleic acid studies should be frozen or placed in RNAlater RNA stabilizing solution. Taking the biopsy and clinical information together, a diagnosis can be made on virtually all patients presenting with heart failure (**Table 23.2**). Molecular techniques are becoming increasingly available and will dramatically enhance the value of endomyocardial biopsy performance, above and beyond the simple histologic, immunohistochemical, and biochemical analyses that have been available till now. Polymerase chain reaction techniques allow pathologists to determine whether or not the patient's myopathic process is associated with a preexistent or ongoing viral

Table 23.1 **Myocardial Biopsy Processing**

Clinical Indication	Stain
Amyloidosis	Congo red, thioflavin T, methyl violet, modified sulfated Alcian Blue
Endocardial fibroelastosis	Movat pentachrome, Verhoeff Van Gieson
Fibrosis	Masson trichrome, Azan-Mallory, or Sirius red
Glycogen storage disease	Periodic acid-Schiff
Hemochromatosis	Prussian blue
Myocarditis	Lymphocyte marker CD3, CD8
Transplant	C4d and/or C3d staining
Tumor	Immunohistochemical
Viral myocarditis	Viral nucleic acid

Table 23.2 **Myocardial Biopsy Indications and Findings**

Current indications

Cardiac allograft rejection monitoring

Cardiomyopathy of unknown cause

Severe ventricular arrhythmias of unknown cause

Drug-induced cardiomyopathy (anthracycline)

Restrictive or constrictive heart disease

Research interests

Cardiac disorders with specific findings (see also Table 23.4)

Immune/inflammatory disease states

Myocarditis

Cardiac allograft rejection

Sarcoidosis

Cytomegalovirus infection

Toxoplasmosis

Rheumatic carditis

Chagas disease

Kawasaki disease

Degenerative

Idiopathic cardiomyopathy

Anthracycline cardiomyopathy

Radiation cardiomyopathy

Infiltrative

Amyloidosis

Gaucher disease

Hemochromatosis

Fabry disease

Table 23.2	**Myocardial Biopsy Indications and Findings (Continued)**
Glycogen storage disease	
Ischemic	
Acute myocardial infarction	
Chronic ischemic cardiomyopathy	
Schönlein-Henoch purpura	
Cancer	
Primary cardiac cancer	
Metastatic cardiac cancer	

infection. Similarly, other immune markers, such as human leukocyte antigen upregulation and immune deposition, will help identify those patients who suffer from some form of an autoimmune process that may be perpetuating ventricular dysfunction.

The Standards and Definitions Committee of the Society for Cardiovascular Pathology and the Association for European Cardiovascular Pathology have released a consensus statement with recommendations for processing cardiovascular surgical pathology specimens, which is summarized in **Table 23.1**.

BIOPSY IN MYOCARDIAL DISEASE

The utility and findings of endomyocardial biopsy in specific disease states and current indications are summarized below.

Transplant Rejection

Surveillance biopsies are performed frequently during the first 6 months after transplantation because of the high incidence of rejection during this early period. No methodology thus far investigated has demonstrated a sensitivity or predictive accuracy high enough to replace endomyocardial biopsy in the detection of rejection in adults, although this might change with new tests such as donor-derived cell-free DNA. Because immunologic transplant rejection is a diffuse process, sampling errors are rare. The light-microscopic histologic features of rejection include interstitial edema, inflammatory infiltration, and immunoglobulin deposition. More severe rejection is marked by myocytolysis and even interstitial hemorrhage.

The newer (2004) grading scale of the International Society for Heart and Lung Transplantation (ISHLT) distinguishes 4 grades of rejection (**Table 23.3**; **Figures 23.6-23.9**). The ISHLT worked toward a pathological grading system for antibody-mediated rejection (AMR) in heart transplantation based on the results of histologic and immunopathologic studies. Examples of AMR are illustrated in **Figures 23.10** and **23.11**.

Adriamycin Cardiotoxicity

Doxorubicin hydrochloride (Adriamycin) is a potent anthracycline antibiotic that is active against many tumors, but its usefulness is limited by its tendency to cause progressive and irreversible dose-related cardiotoxicity. The incidence is 4% at doses of <500 mg/m², 18% at doses between 500 and 600 mg/m², and 36% at doses of >600 mg/m². One approach to safe clinical use has thus been to limit the

Table 23.3 International Society for Heart and Lung Trans-plantation Standardized Cardiac Biopsy Grading

Grade	Grade	Histopathological Findings
2004 Nomenclature	**1990 Nomenclature**	
0R	0	No rejection
1R	1A	Focal perivascular and/or interstitial infiltrate without myocyte damage
–	1B	Diffuse infiltrate without necrosis
–	2	Single focus of infiltrate with associated myocyte damage
2R	3A	Multifocal infiltrate with myocyte damage
3R	3B	Diffuse infiltrate with myocyte damage
–	4	Diffuse, polymorphous infiltrate with extensive myocyte damage with edema, hemorrhage, or vasculitis

Modified from Stewart S, Winters GL, Fishbein MC, et al. Revision of the 1990 working formulation for the standardization of nomenclature in the diagnosis of heart rejection. *J Heart Lung Transpl.* 2005;24:1710-1720.

total cumulative dose to 500 mg/m², but this constitutes an unnecessary limitation in patients who can tolerate substantially higher doses without cardiotoxicity and who depend on the drug for tumor control. At the same time, this approach fails to protect patients with preexisting heart disease, prior radiotherapy, or cyclophosphamide administration; who are older than 70 years; and who may develop cardiac toxicity at substantially lower doses. Because overt impairment of cardiac function is a relatively late finding in Adriamycin toxicity, noninvasive testing may fail to disclose whether additional doses of Adriamycin can be given safely.

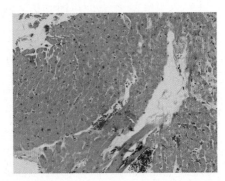

Figure 23.6 Grade 0R rejection in a cardiac biopsy: No inflammation or myocyte injury is noted in this field. Artifactual accumulation of red blood cells in spaces between myocytes, secondary to biopsy and processing procedure. The absence of inflammation and cell injury/necrosis also supports this interpretation.

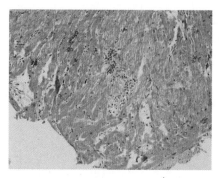

Figure 23.7 Grade 1R rejection in a cardiac biopsy: A single focus of perivascular inflammation with very rare sparse inflammatory cells. No myocyte injury/necrosis is present.

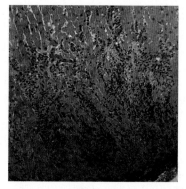

Figure 23.8 Grade 3R rejection in a cardiac biopsy. Diffuse infiltrate with myocyte damage.

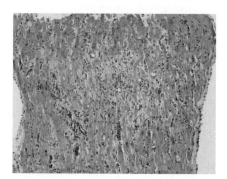

Figure 23.9 Grade 2R rejection in a cardiac biopsy: Focal widening of the interstitium with moderate inflammation of mononuclear cells in close contact with myocyte borders and myocyte loss/injury.

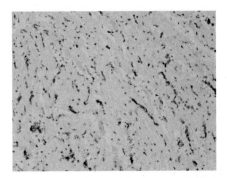

Figure 23.10 C4d humoral rejection in a cardiac biopsy.

Bristow and coworkers, however, have demonstrated that a progressive series of histologic changes (including electron microscopic evidence of myofibrillar loss and cytoplasmic vacuolization) takes place during the development of Adriamycin cardiotoxicity. The extent of these changes can predict whether a patient is likely to develop clinical cardiotoxicity during the subsequent chemotherapy cycle. The 5-step grading system relates grades to the percentage of cells that show these histology changes (1 = <5%, 1.5 = 5%- 15%, 2 = 16%-25%, 2.5 = 26%-35%, and 3 = >35%). A biopsy score of >2.5 indicates that doxorubicin therapy should be terminated, whereas lower scores allow administration of the next cycle of therapy followed by rebiopsy, thus permitting maximal yet safe dosing with Adriamycin while substantially decreasing the incidence of morbidity and mortality from Adriamycin cardiotoxicity.

Dilated Cardiomyopathy

Dilated cardiomyopathy—primary myocardial failure in the absence of underlying coronary, valvular, or pericardial disease—affects about 1 per 2500 people in the United States. The prevalence is 2.5 times higher in blacks and males.

By the time of clinical presentation, most patients with dilated cardiomyopathy already have well-established cardiac damage. Since dilated cardiomyopathy carries a substantial mortality, an approach to any young or middle-aged patient who presents with dilated cardiomyopathy consists of an invasive evaluation that includes both coronary

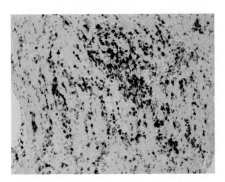

Figure 23.11 Severe CD3 and CD68 humoral rejection in a cardiac biopsy.

angiography and endomyocardial biopsy. The former may be helpful, because clinical signs and symptoms are neither sensitive nor specific for distinguishing idiopathic dilated cardiomyopathy from ischemic cardiomyopathy.

Unfortunately, endomyocardial biopsy in patients with dilated cardiomyopathy generally displays only the monotonous histologic findings of myocyte hypertrophy, interstitial and replacement fibrosis, and endocardial thickening. Occasional small clusters of lymphocytes (<5 per high-power [300× to 400×] field) may be present, without meeting the criteria for diagnosing myocarditis. The amount of collagen—particularly rigid type I collagen—is increased, potentially accounting for an increase in diastolic stiffness. As such, the histologic findings in dilated cardiomyopathy generally do not aid in establishing cause, long-term prognosis, or appropriate specific therapy. However, clearly there are patients with otherwise garden-variety dilated cardiomyopathy, in whom *specific processes* can be diagnosed by endomyocardial biopsy (**Tables 23.2** and **23.4**). The yield of endomyocardial biopsy findings that will significantly alter either therapy or long-term prognosis in dilated cardiomyopathy, however, is admittedly low.

Myocarditis

Myocarditis is an acute or subacute inflammatory illness in which there is variable lymphocytic infiltration in conjunction with myocardial cell damage (**Figure 23.12**). Epidemiologic studies suggest that approximately 5% of a Coxsackie B virus–infected population showed some evidence of cardiac involvement, and replicating enteroviral RNA may be recovered from myocardial samples. Infection and inflammation may resolve spontaneously or may become chronic with perpetuation of an autoimmune process that causes ongoing myocardial damage. Similar processes can result from various viral, protozoal, metazoal, or bacterial infections. Patients with myocarditis typically present with symptoms of chest pain, arrhythmias, or heart failure, with a clinical course that may vary from days to months. Newer noninvasive tests such as cardiac MRI can help identify cases of myocarditis, but they have low sensitivity when compared with endomyocardial biopsy. In patients in whom myocarditis is strongly suspected but not confirmed by cardiac MRI, biopsy should still be performed.

Much of the confusion in this field stemmed from use of various definitions for myocarditis, some of which (eg, more than 5 lymphocytes per high-power field) were fairly liberal. In contrast, the Dallas criteria adopted in 1986 require that infiltrating lymphocytes be adjacent to myocyte necrosis or degeneration to diagnose active myocarditis. If lymphocyte infiltration is present without adjacent myocyte damage, the diagnosis is borderline myocarditis. Roughly 9% of biopsies done for the evaluation of dilated cardiomyopathy will show myocarditis (about two-thirds active and one-third borderline). Biopsy samples that were previously read as showing myocarditis may now be read as borderline or even frankly negative using the Dallas criteria. If the biopsy shows nondiagnostic abnormalities (particularly if borderline changes are present), the patient may still turn out to have active myocarditis on a repeat biopsy. If confirmation of active myocarditis is clinically relevant, repeat right ventricular biopsy is generally sufficient, since the incidence of right versus left ventricular discordance in myocarditis is apparently low.

Using both clinical and histopathologic criteria, the Hopkins group has classified myocarditis as fulminant (intense infiltration, acute onset with progression to death or recovery within 1 month, poor response to immunosuppressives); subacute (less distinct onset, active inflammation, potentially good response to immunosuppressives); chronic active (progressive decline in cardiac function, a biopsy that shows mixed inflammation and fibrosis, and only a brief response to immunosuppressives); or chronic persistent myocarditis (histologic evidence of myocarditis, near-normal ventricular function, unaffected by immunosuppressives). Positive biopsies for myocarditis may thus be found in patients presenting with new- or recent-onset congestive heart failure, including patients with peripartum cardiomyopathy during the last month of pregnancy or within the 5 months

Table 23.4 Final Clinical Plus Biopsy Diagnosis From 1278 Patients With Dilated Cardiomyopathy

Diagnosis	Frequency	%
Idiopathic dilated cardiomyopathy	654	51.2
Myocarditis (two-thirds active, one-third borderline)	117	9.2
Coronary artery disease	98	7.7
Peripartum cardiomyopathy	58	4.5
Hypertension	54	4.2
Human immunodeficiency virus infection	46	3.6
Amyloidosis	41	3.2
Connective tissue disease (mostly scleroderma/lupus)	40	3.1
Drug-induced (mostly Adriamycin)	30	2.3
Chronic alcohol abuse	30	2.3
Familial cardiomyopathy	25	2.0
Valvular heart disease	19	1.5
Sarcoid	16	0.9
Endocrine (mostly thyroid)	11	0.9
Hemochromatosis	9	0.7
Neoplastic	6	0.5

Modified from Felker GM, Hu W, Hare JM, et al. The spectrum of dilated cardiomyopathy. The Johns Hopkins experience with 1278 patients. *Medicine (Baltimore)*. 1999;78:270.

after delivery and in survivors of cardiac arrest who have no other evident organic heart disease. Several studies involving series of patients with human immunodeficiency virus have shown serious clinical cardiac abnormalities associated with myocarditis.

Given this high apparent prevalence of myocarditis among patients with both acute and chronic illness, uncontrolled use of immunosuppressive treatment was common; however, immunosuppressive therapy also caused significant complications, and it was not clear whether the frequency of improvement exceeded that seen spontaneously in many patients with myocarditis.

This general confusion about the prevalence of and optimal treatment for myocarditis led to the conduct of the Myocarditis Treatment Trial. Between October 1986 and October 1990, 2233 patients who underwent nontransplant endomyocardial biopsy within 2 years of symptom onset at any one of 30 participating centers were screened. Histopathologic evidence of myocarditis was found in 214 (10%), of whom 111 with a left ventricular ejection fraction of <45% and no medical contraindication were randomized to either placebo or 24 weeks of cyclosporine/prednisone (after an

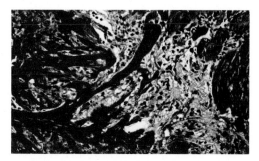

Figure 23.12 Cardiac biopsy in severe myocarditis. A 31-year-old male presented with cardiogenic shock, shock liver, and acute renal failure. Endomyocardial biopsy performed on arrival, revealed diffuse round cell inflammation–associated inflammatory infiltrates, and fibroblastic proliferation consistent with myocarditis.

initial azathioprine/prednisone arm was dropped). There was no significant benefit in the primary end point (improvement in left ventricular ejection fraction from baseline to 28 weeks) in the patients receiving immunosuppression versus those receiving conventional stepped drug therapy for congestive heart failure. Only 66% of baseline biopsies met rigorous Dallas criteria for active myocarditis when overread by the core laboratory, and the trial was seriously underpowered to detect even substantial clinical benefit. Some physicians thus still consider use of immunosuppressives in patients with biopsy-proven myocarditis and a deteriorating clinical picture, particularly in the clinical setting of active myocarditis.

A study by Frustaci has raised questions about the validity of the Dallas criteria as the exclusive marker of myocarditis. In a series of patients with dilated cardiomyopathy and presumed myocarditis who failed to improve with standard medical therapy, those who responded to immunosuppressives with an improvement in ejection fraction had antiheart antibodies and no viral persistence by polymerase chain reaction (see Suggested Reading Frustaci et al 2003). Therefore, the presence of immune upregulation by antiheart antibodies may better define a population with immune-related heart dysfunction responsive to immunosuppressive therapy.

Restrictive Versus Constrictive Disease

Heart failure caused by impaired diastolic functioning of a normal-sized or mildly dilated left ventricle is an uncommon but important clinical entity. In some cases, this may be owing to pericardial constriction, in which instance endomyocardial biopsy would offer no further information. A restrictive pattern may be seen in some patients with hypertrophic myopathy, associated with a pattern of myocyte fiber disarray. More importantly, diastolic dysfunction may also be caused by any one of a series of diseases that can be readily diagnosed with endomyocardial biopsy, thus sparing the patient from inappropriate medical or surgical therapy (e.g., pericardial stripping). These disorders include primary amyloidosis (see **Figure 23.13**), sarcoidosis (see **Figure 23.14**), Loeffler endomyocardial fibrosis, carcinoid-related damage, Fabry disease, glycogen storage diseases, and tumors affecting the heart. Of these, amyloidosis (AL type) is one of the most common (1000-3000 new cases per year in the United States). It also has one of the worst prognoses (typical survival for amyloidosis patients is 12 months, which is reduced to 5 months in patients with cardiac involvement). Although most patients with cardiac amyloidosis have evidence on biopsy of more accessible organs or

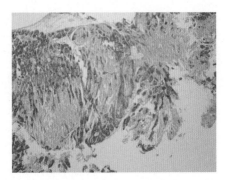

Figure 23.13 Cardiac biopsy in amyloidosis. Congo red staining shows interstitial, pink deposits of amyloid with separation of myocardial fibers.

urinary light chain excretion, about 10% do not. Cardiac biopsy should be performed in patients with thick walls and a small hypokinetic ventricle, particularly if the myocardium has the characteristic speckled appearance on echocardiography.

Sarcoidosis is also relatively common (>10,000 new cases per year in the United States). About half of the patients have electrocardiographic abnormalities of conduction, or repolarization, whereas some have papillary muscle dysfunction, infiltrative cardiomyopathy, or pericarditis.

Hemochromatosis may present with either a dilated or a restrictive pattern. It is found in roughly 1% of endomyocardial biopsies but is important to identify given the benefits of iron chelation therapy.

Other infiltrative diseases that can be diagnosed with endomyocardial biopsy include Fabry disease, which may be responsive to enzyme replacement therapy; fibrosis of the myocardium; and eosinophilic cardiomyopathy, which can be responsive to corticosteroid therapy.

A set of clinical scenarios from which a practical decision to proceed with endomyocardial biopsy can be arrived at has been published jointly by the American Heart Association, the American College of Cardiology, and the European Society of Cardiology, based on case-control series and expert opinion, which is summarized in **Table 23.5.**

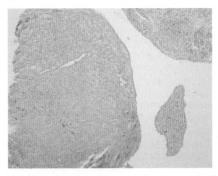

Figure 23.14 Cardiac biopsy in sarcoidosis. There are several noncaseating granulomas with prominent giant cells infiltrating the myocardium.

Table 23.5 **The Role of Endomyocardial Biopsy in 14 Clinical Scenarios**

Class of Recommendation and Level of Evidence	Clinical Scenario
I B	New-onset heart failure of 2 wk duration associated with a normal-sized or dilated left ventricle and hemodynamic compromise
I B	New-onset heart failure of 2 wk to 3 mo duration associated with a dilated left ventricle and new ventricular arrhythmias, second- or third-degree heart block, or failure to respond to usual care within 1-2 wk
IIa C	Heart failure of 3 mo duration associated with a dilated left ventricle and new ventricular arrhythmias, second- or third-degree heart block, or failure to respond to usual care within 1-2 wk
IIa C	Heart failure associated with a DCM of any duration associated with suspected allergic reaction and/or eosinophilia
IIa C	Heart failure associated with suspected anthracycline cardiomyopathy
IIa C	Heart failure associated with unexplained restrictive cardiomyopathy
IIa C	Suspected cardiac tumors
IIa C	Unexplained cardiomyopathy in children
IIb B	New-onset heart failure of 2 wk to 3 mo duration associated with a dilated left ventricle, without new ventricular arrhythmias or second- or third-degree heart block, that responds to usual care within 1-2 wk
IIb C	Heart failure of 3 mo' duration associated with a dilated left ventricle, without new ventricular arrhythmias or second- or third-degree heart block, that responds to usual care within 1-2 wk
IIb C	Heart failure associated with unexplained HCM
IIb C	Suspected ARVD/C
IIb C	Unexplained ventricular arrhythmias
III C	Unexplained atrial fibrillation

• Class I: conditions for which there is evidence for and/or general agreement that the procedure or treatment is beneficial, useful, and effective.
• Class II: conditions for which there is conflicting evidence and/or a divergence of opinion about the usefulness/efficacy of a procedure or treatment.
• Class IIa: weight of evidence/opinion is in favor of usefulness/efficacy.
• Class IIb: usefulness/efficacy is less well established by evidence/opinion.
• Class III: conditions for which there is evidence and/or general agreement that the procedure/treatment is not useful/effective and in some cases may be harmful.
The weight of evidence in support of the recommendation is listed as follows:
• Level of evidence A: data derived from multiple randomized clinical trials.
• Level of evidence B: data derived from a single randomized trial or nonrandomized studies.
• Level of evidence C: only consensus opinion of experts, case studies, or standard of care.
ARVD/C, arrhythmogenic right ventricular dysplasia/cardiomyopathy; DCM, dilated cardiomyopathy; HCM, hypertrophic cardiomyopathy.
Modified from Cooper LT, Baughman KL, Feldman AM, et al. The role of endomyocardial biopsy in the management of cardiovascular disease: a scientific statement from the American Heart Association, the American College of Cardiology, and the European Society of Cardiology. Endorsed by the Heart Failure Society of America and the Heart Failure Association of the European Society of Cardiology. *J Am Coll Cardiol.* 2007;50:1914-1931.

SUGGESTED READINGS

1. Anderson JL, Marshall HW. The femoral venous approach to endomyocardial biopsy: comparison with internal jugular and transarterial approaches. *Am J Cardiol.* 1984;53(6):833-837.
2. Arad M, Maron BJ, Gorham JM, et al. Glycogen storage diseases presenting as hypertrophic cardiomyopathy. *N Engl J Med.* 2005;352(4):362-372.
3. Aretz HT, Billingham ME, Edwards WD, et al. Myocarditis. A histopathologic definition and classification. *Am J Cardiovasc Pathol.* 1987;1:3-14.
4. Berry GJ, Angelini A, Burke MM, et al. The ISHLT working formulation for pathologic diagnosis of antibody-mediated rejection in heart transplantation: evolution and current status (2005-2011). *J Heart Lung Transpl.* 2011;30(6):601-611.
5. Bozkurt B, Colvin M, Cook J, et al. Current diagnostic and treatment strategies for specific dilated cardiomyopathies: a scientific statement from the American Heart Association. *Circulation.* 2016;134(23):e579-e646.
6. Bristow MR, Mason JW, Billingham ME, Daniels JR. Doxorubicin cardiomyopathy: evaluation by phonocardiography, endomyocardial biopsy, and cardiac catheterization. *Ann Intern Med.* 1978;88(2):168-175.
7. Brooksby IA, Jenkins BS, Coltart DJ, Webb-Peploe MM, Davies MJ. Left-ventricular endomyocardial biopsy. *Lancet.* 1974;2(7891):1222-1225.
8. Caves PK, Stinson EB, Graham AF, Billingham ME, Grehl TM, Shumway NE. Percutaneous transvenous endomyocardial biopsy. *J Am Med Assoc.* 1973;225(3):288-291.
9. Caves PK, Schulz WP, Dong E Jr., Stinson EB, Shumway NE. New instrument for transvenous cardiac biopsy. *Am J Cardiol.* 1974;33(2):264-267.
10. Caves P, Coltart J, Billingham M, Rider A, Stinson E. Transvenous endomyocardial biopsy-application of a method for diagnosing heart disease. *Postgrad Med J.* 1975;51(595):286-290.
11. Cooper LT, Baughman KL, Feldman AM, et al. The role of endomyocardial biopsy in the management of cardiovascular disease: a scientific statement from the American Heart Association, the American College of Cardiology, and the European Society of Cardiology. Endorsed by the Heart Failure Society of America and the Heart Failure Association of the European Society of Cardiology. *J Am Coll Cardiol.* 2007;50(19):1914-1931.
12. Cooper LT Jr., Hare JM, Tazelaar HD, et al. Usefulness of immunosuppression for giant cell myocarditis. *Am J Cardiol.* 2008;102(11):1535-1539.
13. Corley DD, Strickman N. Alternative approaches to right ventricular endomyocardial biopsy. *Cathet Cardiovasc Diagn.* 1994;31(3):236-239.
14. Denys BG, Uretsky BF, Reddy PS, Ruffner RJ, Sandhu JS, Breishlatt WM. An ultrasound method for safe and rapid central venous access. *N Engl J Med.* 1991;324(8):566.
15. Denys BG, Uretsky BF, Reddy PS. Ultrasound-assisted cannulation of the internal jugular vein. A prospective comparison to the external landmark-guided technique. *Circulation.* 1993;87(5):1557-1562.
16. Dubrey SW, Hawkins PN, Falk RH. Amyloid diseases of the heart: assessment, diagnosis, and referral. *Heart.* 2011;97(1):75-84.
17. Eng CM, Guffon N, Wilcox WR, et al. Safety and efficacy of recombinant human alpha-galactosidase A—replacement therapy in Fabry's disease. *N Engl J Med.* 2001;345(1):9-16.
18. Fawzy ME, Ziady G, Halim M, Guindy R, Mercer EN, Feteih N. Endomyocardial fibrosis: report of eight cases. *J Am Coll Cardiol.* 1985;5(4):983-988.
19. Fitchett DH, Forbes C, Guerraty AJ. Repeated endomyocardial biopsy causing coronary arterial-right ventricular fistula after cardiac transplantation. *Am J Cardiol.* 1988;62(10 pt 1):829-831.
20. Frustaci A, Chimenti C, Ricci R, et al. Improvement in cardiac function in the cardiac variant of Fabry's disease with galactose-infusion therapy. *N Engl J Med.* 2001;345(1):25-32.
21. Frustaci A, Chimenti C, Calabrese F, Pieroni M, Thiene G, Maseri A. Immunosuppressive therapy for active lymphocytic myocarditis: virological and immunologic profile of responders versus nonresponders. *Circulation.* 2003;107(6):857-863.
22. Hauck AJ, Kearney DL, Edwards WD. Evaluation of postmortem endomyocardial biopsy specimens from 38 patients with lymphocytic myocarditis: implications for role of sampling error. *Mayo Clin Proc.* 1989;64(10):1235-1245.
23. Holzmann M, Nicko A, Kuhl U, et al. Complication rate of right ventricular endomyocardial biopsy via the femoral approach: a retrospective and prospective study analyzing 3048 diagnostic procedures over an 11-year period. *Circulation.* 2008;118(17):1722-1728.
24. Kasper EK, Agema WR, Hutchins GM, Deckers JW, Hare JM, Baughman KL. The causes of dilated cardiomyopathy: a clinicopathologic review of 673 consecutive patients. *J Am Coll Cardiol.* 1994;23(3):586-590.
25. Kreher SK, Ulstad VK, Dick CD, DeGroff R, Olivari MT, Homans DC. Frequent occurrence of occult pulmonary embolism from venous sheaths during endomyocardial biopsy. *J Am Coll Cardiol.* 1992;19(3):581-585.

26. Kuhl U, Lauer B, Souvatzoglu M, Vosberg H, Schultheiss HP. Antimyosin scintigraphy and immu-nohistologic analysis of endomyocardial biopsy in patients with clinically suspected myocardi-tis—evidence of myocardial cell damage and inflammation in the absence of histologic signs of myocarditis. *J Am Coll Cardiol.* 1998;32(5):1371-1376.
27. Kushwaha SS, Fallon JT, Fuster V. Restrictive cardiomyopathy. *N Engl J Med.* 1997;336(4):267-276.
28. Lieberman EB, Hutchins GM, Herskowitz A, Rose NR, Baughman KL. Clinicopathologic descrip-tion of myocarditis. *J Am Coll Cardiol.* 1991;18(7):1617-1626.
29. Lurz P, Luecke C, Eitel I, et al. Comprehensive cardiac magnetic resonance imaging in patients with suspected myocarditis: the MyoRacer-trial. *J Am Coll Cardiol.* 2016;67(15):1800-1811.
30. Mason JW, O'Connell JB, Herskowitz A, et al. A clinical trial of immunosuppressive therapy for myocarditis. The Myocarditis Treatment Trial Investigators. *N Engl J Med.* 1995;333(5):269-275.
31. Mason JW. Endomyocardial biopsy and the causes of dilated cardiomyopathy. *J Am Coll Cardiol.* 1994;23(3):591-592.
32. McCarthy RE III, Boehmer JP, Hruban RH, et al. Long-term outcome of fulminant myocarditis as compared with acute (nonfulminant) myocarditis. *N Engl J Med.* 2000;342(10):690-695.
33. Miller LW, Labovitz AJ, McBride LA, Pennington DG, Kanter K. Echocardiography-guided endo-myocardial biopsy. A 5-year experience. *Circulation.* 1988;78(5 pt 2):III99-III102.
34. Muchtar E, Gertz MA, Kumar SK, et al. Improved outcomes for newly diagnosed AL amyloidosis between 2000 and 2014: cracking the glass ceiling of early death. *Blood.* 2017;129(15):2111-2119.
35. Newman LS, Rose CS, Maier LA. Sarcoidosis. *N Engl J Med.* 1997;336(17):1224-1234.
36. Ntusi N. HIV and myocarditis. *Curr Opin HIV AIDS.* 2017;12(6):561-565.
37. Olson LJ, Edwards WD, Holmes DR Jr., Miller FA Jr., Nordstrom LA, Baldus WP. Endomyo-cardial biopsy in hemochromatosis: clinicopathologic correlates in six cases. *J Am Coll Cardiol.* 1989;13(1):116-120.
38. Pauschinger M, Phan MD, Doerner A, et al. Enteroviral RNA replication in the myocardium of patients with left ventricular dysfunction and clinically suspected myocarditis. *Circulation.* 1999;99(7):889-895.
39. Pauschinger M, Bowles NE, Fuentes-Garcia FJ, et al. Detection of adenoviral genome in the myocar-dium of adult patients with idiopathic left ventricular dysfunction. *Circulation.* 1999;99(10):1348-1354.
40. Pham MX, Teuteberg JJ, Kfoury AG, et al. Gene-expression profiling for rejection surveillance after cardiac transplantation. *N Engl J Med.* 2010;362(20):1890-1900.
41. Richardson P, McKenna W, Bristow M, et al. Report of the 1995 World Health Organization/Inter-national Society and Federation of Cardiology task force on the definition and classification of cardiomyopathies. *Circulation.* 1996;93(5):841-842.
42. Saraiva F, Matos V, Goncalves L, Antunes M, Providência LA. Complications of endomyocardial biopsy in heart transplant patients: a retrospective study of 2117 consecutive procedures. *Transpl Proc.* 2011;43(5):1908-1912.
43. Schoenfeld MH, Supple EW, Dec GW Jr., Fallon JT, Palacios IF. Restrictive cardiomyopathy versus constrictive pericarditis: role of endomyocardial biopsy in avoiding unnecessary thoracotomy. *Cir-culation.* 1987;75(5):1012-1017.
44. Singal PK, Iliskovic N. Doxorubicin-induced cardiomyopathy. *N Engl J Med.* 1998;339(13):900-905.
45. Stewart S, Winters GL, Fishbein MC, et al. Revision of the 1990 working formulation for the standardization of nomenclature in the diagnosis of heart rejection. *J Heart Lung Transpl.* 2005;24(11):1710-1720.
46. Stone JR, Basso C, Baandrup UT, et al. Recommendations for processing cardiovascular surgical pathology specimens: a consensus statement from the standards and definitions Committee of the Society for Cardiovascular Pathology and the Association for European Cardiovascular Pathology. *Cardiovasc Pathol.* 2012;21(1):2-16.
47. Yazaki Y, Isobe M, Hiramitsu S, et al. Comparison of clinical features and prognosis of cardiac sar-coidosis and idiopathic dilated cardiomyopathy. *Am J Cardiol.* 1998;82(4):537-540.

24 Percutaneous Mechanical Circulatory Support[1]

Morbidity and mortality of cardiogenic shock (CS) remain unacceptably high, and conventional pharmacotherapy not infrequently fails to reverse CS. As a result, clinicians often turn to percutaneous mechanical circulatory support (pMCS). This chapter will review 5 major forms of pMCS (**Table 24.1**):

1. Transvalvular left ventricular to aortic pumps
2. Intra-aortic balloon pumps
3. Left atrial to aortic pumps
4. Extracorporeal bypass
5. Right ventricular support devices

pMCS utilization increases in parallel with the rising incidence of CS, and novel forms of pMCS are replacing older devices. For example, intra-aortic balloon pump (IABP) counterpulsation, once the dominant form of mechanical support, accounts for an overall smaller proportion of pMCS devices inserted. This trend coincides with multiple studies,—most notably the landmark IABP-SHOCK II (Intra-aortic Balloon Support for Myocardial Infarction with Cardiogenic Shock) trial, which did not show a benefit in patients with CS. In its stead, percutaneous left ventricular assist devices like the Impella family of devices (Abiomed Inc., Danvers, Massachusetts, USA) and venoarterial extracorporeal membrane oxygenation (VA ECMO) account for a growing share of the pMCS market.

Choosing the right form of pMCS first requires a sound understanding of the patient's hemodynamics. In critically ill patients with CS who are often mechanically ventilated, sedated, and receiving vasoactive medications, right-sided heart catheterization (RHC) with a pulmonary artery catheter (PAC) is considered essential for guiding the decision to initiate pMCS and, equally important, which type of pMCS to use. Although some studies call into question the routine use of PACs in patients with CS, the subgroup of patients with CS refractory to medical therapy requires evaluation with an RHC to identify the ideal pMCS device and optimize the level of device support.

HEMODYNAMIC PRINCIPLES OF CARDIOGENIC SHOCK

The pressure-volume loop (PVL) provides a foundation for understanding cardiac and vascular properties, myocardial energetics, and the impact of different pMCS devices (**Figure 24.1**). This framework allows representation of ventricular preload, afterload, lusitropy, and contractility and their respective roles in determining CO, blood pressure, and pulmonary venous pressures. The normal PVL is a plot of instantaneous ventricular pressure and volume throughout the cardiac cycle. The 4 major phases of the cardiac cycle are readily identified, and they are as follows (starting at end-diastole in the bottom right corner): isovolumic contraction, ejection, isovolumic relaxation, and filling. The PVL is bounded inferiorly by the end-diastolic pressure-volume relationship (EDPVR) and superiorly by the end-systolic pressure-volume relationship (ESPVR). The EDPVR uniquely defines the passive diastolic properties of the left ventricle (LV), and the slope (E_{es}) and volume axis intercept

---

[1]We gratefully acknowledge the Grossman & Baim's *Cardiac Catheterization, Angiography, and Intervention,* 9th edition contributions of Drs Michael I. Brener and Daniel Burkhoff as portions of their chapter, Impella, Intra-aortic Balloon Counterpulsation, TandemHeart, Extracorporeal Bypass, and Right Ventricular Support Devices, were retained in this text.

Table 24.1 Percutaneous Mechanical Circulatory Support Device Characteristics

Device	IABP	Impella 2.5	Impella CP	Impella 5.0 LD/LP	TandemHeart	VA ECMO	Impella RP	Protek Duo
Pump mechanism	Pneumatic	Axial flow	Axial flow	Axial flow	Centrifugal	Centrifugal	Axial	Centrifugal
Cannula size	8F	13F[a]	14F[a]	22F[a]	Inflow: 21F Outflow: 15F-17F	Inflow: 15F-22F Outflow: 18F21F	23F	29F-31F
Insertion technique	Descending aorta via the femoral a.	Retrograde across the AoV via the femoral a.	Retrograde across the AoV via the femoral a.	Retrograde across the AoV from the subclavian a. (LP) or asc. aorta (LD) via surgical cutdown	Inflow cannula into LA via transseptal puncture from femoral v. Outflow cannula into femoral a.	Inflow cannula into the right atrium via the femoral v. Outflow cannula into descending aorta via femoral a.	Femoral v. with inflow in the IVC and outflow across pulmonic valve	Right IJ v. and positioned past pulmonic valve
FDA-approved duration of use	Not specified	6 h for HR-PCI 4 d for CS	6 h for HR-PCI 4 d for CS	6 d (CS only)	6 h	6 h	14 d	6 h
Pump capacity	0.5-1.0 L/min[b]	2.5 L/min	3.5 L/min	5.0 L/min	3.5 (15F) and 5.0 (17F) L/min	3-6 L/min	>4.0 L/min	>4.5 L/min
Hemodynamic support	LV	LV	LV	LV	BiV	BiV	RV	RV
Effect on afterload	↓	↕	↕	↕	↑	↑	↕	↕
Effect on LVEDP	↓	↓	↓	↓	↓	↑	↕	↕

(Continued)

Table 24.1 Percutaneous Mechanical Circulatory Support Device Characteristics (Continued)

Device	IABP	Impella 2.5	Impella CP	Impella 5.0 LD/LP	TandemHeart	VA ECMO	Impella RP	Protek Duo
Effect on coronary perfusion	↑	Unknown; may ↑	Unknown; may ↑	Unknown; may ↑	Unknown; may ↓	Unknown; may ↓	↔	↔
Implantation time	+	++	++	+++	+++	++	++	++
Risk of limb ischemia	+	++	++	++	+++	+++	–	–
Hemolysis	+	++	++	++	++	++	++	++
Anticoagulation	+	+	+	+	+++	+++	+	+++
Requires stable heart rhythm	Yes	No	No	No	No	No	No	No
Management complexity	+	++	++	++	+++	+++	++	+++

↑, increase; ↓, decrease; ↔, neutral; +, limited; ++, intermediate; +++, substantial; a., artery; AoV, aortic valve; asc., ascending; BiV, biventricular; CP, cardiac power; CS, cardiogenic shock; F, French size; FDA, Food and Drug Administration; HR-PCI, high-risk percutaneous coronary intervention; IABP, intra-aortic balloon pump; IJ, internal jugular; LA, left atrium; LD, left direct; LP, left percutaneous; LV, left ventricular; RP, right power; RV, right ventricle; v., vein; VA ECMO, venoarterial extracorporeal membrane oxygenation.
a Size of sheath.
b Indirect support provided by augmentation of intrinsic cardiac output.
Adapted from Combes A, Brodie D, Chen YS, et al. The ICM research agenda on extracorporeal life support. *Intensive Care Med.* 2017;43:1306-1318.

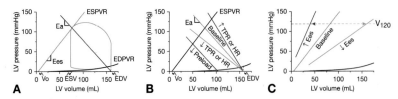

Figure 24.1 A, The normal pressure-volume loop is shaped like a rectangle and bound by 2 important curves: the end-systolic pressure-volume relationship (ESPVR) and end-diastolic pressure-volume relationship (EDPVR). ESPVR is approximately linear and is characterized by its slope (end-systolic elastance, E_{es}) and the volume-axis intercept, V_0. The slope of the line extending from the end-diastolic volume (EDV) point on the volume axis through the end-systolic pressure-volume point of the loop reflects effective arterial elastance (E_a). **B,** The slope of the E_a line, often considered a surrogate of afterload, depends on total peripheral resistance (TPR) and heart rate (HR), and its position along the volume-axis depends on EDV. **C,** The ESPVR shifts with changes in ventricular contractility, which is reflected both by E_{es} and V_0. Changes in contractility can be indexed by V_{120}, the volume at which the ESPVR intersects 120 mmHg. ESV, end-systolic volume; LV, left ventricular. (From Burkhoff D, Sayer G, Doshi D, et al. Hemodynamics of mechanical circulatory support. *J Am Coll Cardiol.* 2015;66:2663-2674.)

of the ESPVR provide a load-independent index of ventricular contractility. In this construct, ventricular preload is indexed by end-diastolic volume (EDV). Ventricular afterload is indexed by effective arterial elastance (E_a), which is the slope of the line connecting the point on the volume axis at the EDV to the point of end-systole on the PVL. E_a is mainly determined by total peripheral arterial resistance and the duration of the cardiac cycle (T) or heart rate.

The PVL also provides a helpful platform for representing the determinants of myocardial oxygen consumption (MVO_2, **Figure 24.2**). MVO_2 is linearly related on a beat-to-beat basis with the ventricular pressure-volume area (PVA), which is the sum of the external stroke work (the area inside the PVL) and the potential energy (PE). PE is the area bounded by the ESPVR, the EDPVR, and the diastolic portion of the PVL; it represents the residual energy stored in the myofilaments at the end of systole that was not converted to external work. Changes in contractility increase myocardial oxygen consumption by increasing the area encapsulated by the PVA, and vice versa. Since PVA correlates with MVO_2 on a beat-to-beat basis for a given contractile state, loading conditions and heart rate profoundly affect overall myocardial oxygen consumption as well, even without changing the contractile properties of the heart.

The PVL in CS differs dramatically from the PVL under normal conditions (**Figure 24.3**). The PVL is shifted down and to the right. An initial insult renders the ESPVR flatter, signifying the abrupt reduction of ventricular contractility. This reduction is accompanied by a profound decline in systolic blood pressure (indexed by the height of the PVL), stroke volume (SV), and CO, along with small elevations of left ventricular EDP (LVEDP) and pulmonary capillary wedge pressure (PCWP). A compensatory response to maintain mean arterial pressure concomitantly shifts the PVL further to the right as catecholamine release precipitates an increase in autonomic tone, causing vasoconstriction and an increase in stressed volume to enhance preload. The dramatic rightward shift of the PVL translates into a marked increase in the PVA and beat-to-beat MVO_2.

High-risk percutaneous coronary intervention (HR-PCI) identifies a subset of coronary revascularization procedures where patients have numerous comorbidities (ie, heart failure with reduced ejection fraction, chronic kidney disease), complex culprit artery anatomy (ie, chronic total occlusion, proximal bifurcation lesions), or a ten-

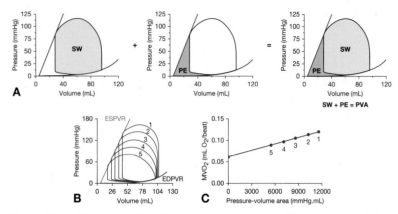

Figure 24.2 A, The pressure-volume loop can also represent myocardial oxygen consumption, which is proportional to the pressure-volume area (PVA). PVA is the sum of external stroke work (SW) and end-systolic potential energy (PE). **B,** PVA varies with loading conditions, including changes in arterial elastance. **C,** A linear relationship between PVA and myocardial oxygen consumption (MVO_2) exists on a per beat basis. EDPVR, end-diastolic pressure-volume relationship; ESPVR, end-systolic pressure-volume relationship. (From Burkhoff D. Hemodynamic support: science and evaluation of the assisted circulation with percutaneous assist devices. *Interv Cardiol Clin*. 2013;2:407-416.)

uous clinical status entering the procedure (ie, CS or acutely decompensated heart failure). In patients with these comorbidities and coronary anatomy, every aspect of a routine PCI, from guide catheter engagement to iodinated contrast exposure to occlusion of the lumen with a coronary balloon, carries the potential of hemodynamic collapse and worsening of the patient's condition prior to realizing any benefits of revascularization. The degree of systemic arterial pressure decline during coronary

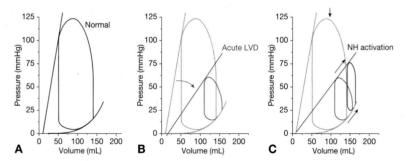

Figure 24.3 A, The pressure-volume loop (PVL) under normal conditions. **B,** The PVL immediately following an acute myocardial infarction causing left ventricular dysfunction (LVD) shifts rightward and downward along the volume axis, reflecting a dramatic increase in left ventricular end-diastolic volume (EDV), and declines in systolic blood pressure and stroke volume. **C,** Changes to the PVL occur as a result of catecholamine surges that lead to changes in stressed volume, which help maintain higher systolic blood pressures at the expense of increased EDV. (From Furer A, Wessler J, Burkhoff D. Hemodynamics of cardiogenic shock. *Interv Cardiol Clin*. 2017;6:359-371.)

interventions depends on multiple factors, including the territory supplied by the artery, the presence and degree of prior infarction in that territory, the degree of collaterals from neighboring vascular beds, global ventricular contractility, the starting blood pressure, and the duration of balloon inflation. Use of pMCS during such procedures is intended to maintain blood pressure and flow during balloon inflations, and in the event of adverse events (ie, dissections, acute thrombosis) that would otherwise result in hemodynamic compromise.

TRANSVALVULAR LEFT-VENTRICLE-TO-AORTIC PUMPS

The Impella class of devices are now widely used on a routine basis and have become the first line of treatment for CS in many centers. Four left ventricular basic models are currently available—Impella 2.5, Impella Cardiac Power (CP) with Smart Assist, Impella 5.0, and Impella 5.5 with Smart Assist; additionally, the Impella Left Direct (LD) is a version of the 5.0 that does not have a pigtail and is intended for placement during surgical procedures (**Figure 24.4**). Each device has its own maximum pumping capacity of approximately 2.5, 4.3, 5.0, and 6.2 L/min, respectively.

The Impella devices are fashioned as an "Archimedes screw" with a catheter-mounted, nonpulsatile microaxial flow pump. Impella 2.5 has a 9F catheter shaft and a 12F pump head and is placed percutaneously via a 13F peel-away femoral arterial sheath. Impella CP also has a 9F catheter shaft but requires a 14F peel-away sheath for a 14F pump head. Both Impella 5.0 and LD models have a 9F catheter shaft with a 21F pump head, which are inserted by direct cutdown to the femoral or axillary artery (5.0) or introduced into the LV (LD) via a 10-mm Dacron graft in the ascending aorta. The Impella 5.5 with Smart Assist is smaller in diameter with a 19F pump head on a 9F catheter shaft and exclusively designed for the axillary artery access. In each of the Impella pumps, the blood inlet lies distal on the cannula and resides within the ventricular chamber. The pump motor is proximal on the cannula and resides in the aorta. In this way, blood is directly aspirated from LV into the aorta in parallel with physiological flow. This configuration has important implications for the effect of these pumps on patient hemodynamics, as discussed below. There are pMCS devices with reduced diameter to decrease vascular complications. The Impella device profile is being reduced, as well as 2 new pMCS devices being developed by CSI (Minneapolis) and Magenta (Israel).

The Impella is powered and controlled by a console (Automated Impella Controller, AIC) that allows the user to monitor performance and adjust pump speed. The user can select a performance level (P0-P8 for Impella 2.5, and P0-P9 for Impella

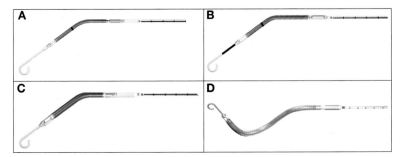

Figure 24.4 Images of the Impella family of device. **A,** Impella 2.5, **B,** Impella 5.0, **C,** Impella CP, and **D,** Impella RP. (Courtesy of Abiomed.)

CP and 5.0 5.5/LD) or use the Auto-Flow feature that allows the catheter to run at the maximum sustained speed while automatically avoiding suction conditions. Under normal operating conditions and typical arterial pressures, the rotor spins at maximum of 33,000 RPMs for the Impella 5.0, 5.5, and LD; at 46,000 RPMs for the Impella CP; and at 51,000 RPMs for the Impella 2.5. The controlling console is also used to manage a purge system designed to keep the corrosive plasma from entering the motor compartment.

Impella Hemodynamics

It is relevant for clinicians to understand the basic concepts that underlie the determinants of flow generated by an Impella device. Every pump has a characteristic relationship between the pressure gradient across its inflow and outflow ports (also referred to as the pressure head, H), the rotational speed (RPMs), and pump flow (Q). In general, at a constant rotational speed, increasing or decreasing the pressure head will result in an increased or decreased flow, respectively. Also, when rotational speed is increased or decreased, flow for a given pressure head will increase or decrease, respectively (**Figure 24.5**). The Impella was designed as a constant-speed pump, such that at any given P-level, the RPM is maintained. Since the inflow for the Impella resides in the LV and the outflow is across the valve in the proximal aorta, the pressure head of the pump is variable throughout the cardiac cycle. Accordingly, pump flow will vary directly with the pressure head. Flow is maximal during systole when the pressure gradient is minimum, and flow is minimum during diastole when the pressure gradient is the largest. Thus, while these devices are *continuous* flow devices, their flow rate is *not constant*. This accounts for the pulsatile flow waveform that is displayed on the Impella console.

The impact of LV-to-aorta pumping on the PVL is illustrated in **Figure 24.6**, with pumping at low (magenta), medium (blue), and high (green) RPMs. Since these devices pump blood continuously out of the LV into the aorta independent of the phase of the cardiac cycle, there is loss of the isovolumic contraction and relaxation

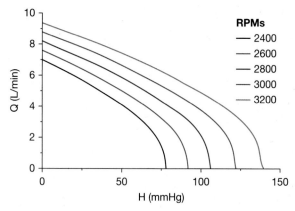

Figure 24.5 Pump flow (Q) is a function of the pump's revolutions per minute (RPMs) and the pressure gradient between the pump's inflow and outflow ports (H). For a given gradient, H, increasing device RPMs will increase flow, Q. (Reprinted with permission from Rich JD, Burkhoff D. HVAD flow waveform morphologies: theoretical foundation and implications for clinical practice. *ASAIO J.* 2017;63:526-535.)

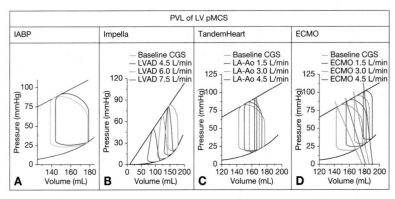

Figure 24.6 A, The impact of counterpulsation on the pressure-volume loop (PVL) shows a reduction in peak ventricular systolic pressure and relatively small effect on stroke volume and left ventricular end-diastolic volume. **B,** Triangularization of the PVL as a result of Impella and continuous left ventricular to aortic pumping. With increasing pump flow, the PVL shifts leftward, reflecting a greater degree of ventricular unloading. **C,** PVL reflecting the effects of a left atrial to aortic pump (LA-Ao, ie, TandemHeart) showing reduced end-diastolic pressures, increased end-systolic volume, and decreasing left ventricular stroke volume. **D,** PVL reflecting the effects of a right atrial to aortic pump like extracorporeal membrane oxygenation (ECMO), which increases end-diastolic pressures, increases effective arterial elastance, and decreases left ventricular stroke volume. IABP, intra-aortic balloon pump; CGS, cardiogenic shock; LVAD, left ventricular assist device; pMCS, percutaneous mechanical circulatory support. (From Burkhoff D, Sayer G, Doshi D, et al. Hemodynamics of mechanical circulatory support. *J Am Coll Cardiol*. 2015;66:2663-2674 and Burkhoff D. Hemodynamic support: science and evaluation of the assisted circulation with percutaneous assist devices. *Interv Cardiol Clin*. 2013;2:407-416.)

phases. The loop transforms from a more or less rectangular shape to a triangular shape, with the degree of triangulation dependent on flow rate. Also, as pumping speed is increased, there is a progressively greater leftward shift of the loop toward lower ventricular EDVs and EDPs, corresponding with progressively lower levels of myocardial oxygen demand. This illustrates the direct unloading effect of the Impella pump on the LV.

On time-domain pressure curves, it can be appreciated that as pump flow increases, peak LV pressure generation decreases due to the reduction in LVEDP. Simultaneously, aortic diastolic, mean, and, to a much lesser extent, systolic pressures increase. The rise in diastolic pressure is due to the continuous pumping of blood from the LV to aorta during diastole, which counteracts the normal diastolic runoff of blood from the capacitance of the larger arteries to the periphery when the heart is not ejecting. Such increases in aortic diastolic and mean pressures have the potential to improve coronary artery flow and myocardial perfusion of ischemic myocardium in which autoregulation has been exhausted. Pulse pressure decreases as pump flow increases, indicating progressively lesser degrees of aortic valve opening and ejection. Under extreme conditions, unloading can lead to a left shift of the LVEDP such that peak LV pressure generation is lower than aortic pressure, and the aortic valve remains closed. This condition is referred to as aortic-ventricular pressure uncoupling.

As noted above, pump flow increases with increasing device RPMs, but output from the native heart itself decreases. On balance, total flow to the body (the sum of pump and heart output) increases, but the increase of total flow does not equal pump flow. For example, if the original CO is 3 L/min and a pump is introduced that is flowing 2 L/min, the total flow is not 5 L/min but rather ~3.3 L/min. Thus, at the lower range of RPMs, part of the total flow is derived from the LV and part from the pump; this condition is referred to as *partial support*.

With progressive increases of RPMs, there are greater degrees of LV unloading. LV peak pressure decreases, aortic pressure increases, the aortic valve remains closed, and there is no output from the LV. This condition is referred to as *full support*; all flow to the body is provided by the pump.

Insertion, Routine Care, and Weaning

Impella 2.5 and CP are inserted using a monorail technique under direct fluoroscopic control. First, the femoral artery is cannulated and then the peel-away sheath is inserted. A 0.018-inch wire is advanced across the aortic valve with the use of a guiding catheter (usually a 4F-5F pigtail catheter), and the Impella catheter is threaded over the wire into the LV. The inlet area of the catheter should be positioned approximately 4 cm below the aortic valve. Once the device is positioned in the ventricle, the wire is removed, and pumping is initiated at the minimum level allowed by the Impella console. At this point, pressure waveforms displayed on the console screen can be utilized to confirm that the device placement is proper and stable. Once proper position is confirmed, pumping speed is typically adjusted to a higher performance level. As the aspirated blood from the Impella can act like a jet on the pump, it is common for Impella to move into the ventricle during the first few minutes of use. It is therefore advisable to wait 5 to 10 minutes before accepting final position. Excessive slack should be removed from the catheter system so that the catheter lies along the "lesser curve" of the aorta, thus minimizing the tendency of the catheter to migrate into the LV.

Care of the patient with an Impella device in situ requires an understanding of routine device monitoring, knowledge of and vigilance for potential complications, as well as an ability to troubleshoot the alarms associated with device malfunction. If the inlet and outlet pressure measurements appear ventricularized, then the Impella is advanced too deep into the LV. Similarly, if the motor current signal flatlines, it reflects a diminished pressure head and the device inlet and outlet are in the same chamber, either both in the aorta or both in the LV. Abnormalities in either the motor current or placement signal will trigger a "position wrong" alarm on the AIC. Whenever a "position wrong" or "position unknown" alarm appears on the AIC, immediate echocardiographic evaluation should proceed to assess the placement of the device, and any device repositioning should occur with echocardiographic guidance.

The strategy for weaning a patient off Impella support depends on the original indication for support. When used to provide prophylactic support for an uncomplicated HR-PCI, for example, the device can simply be turned off and removed. Thus, weaning in this application can be rapid and can take place over minutes. In the patient with hemodynamic compromise, weaning can begin when clinical signs of sufficient native heart recovery are observed. The pump speed can be gradually reduced (ie, to half that used to support the patient), and after a sufficient duration of demonstrated stability, the device can be turned off and removed. Depending on the patient status, device weaning can be an iterative process over several days. However, the Impella performance level should never be set to P0 while the device is in the LV, as there is an open communication between the ascending aorta and the LV that can result in functional regurgitation into the LV. Thus, the minimal allowed support occurs at the P1 or P2 level.

Indications, Contraindications, and Complications

The Impella devices are indicated for 2 primary use settings (**Table 24.2**): HR-PCI and CS. In the context of elective or emergent HR-PCI, the Impella 2.5 and CP are approved by the US Food and Drug Administration (FDA) for temporary (<6 hours) ventricular support in stable patients to prevent hemodynamic deterioration. In the

Table 24.2	**Impella 2.5 and CP Indications and Contraindications**
Indications	
High-risk percutaneous coronary intervention (HR-PCI)	
Acute myocardial infarction complicated by cardiogenic shock (AMICS)	
Acutely decompensated chronic heart failure	
Hemodynamic support during ventricular tachycardia ablation	
Postcardiotomy cardiogenic shock	
Contraindications	
Left ventricular thrombus	
Critical aortic stenosis (valve area < 0.6 cm^2)	
Moderate to severe aortic insufficiency	
Severe peripheral arterial disease	
Significant right-sided heart failure	
Combined cardiorespiratory failure	
Atrial or ventricular septal defects	
Left ventricular rupture	
Cardiac tamponade	
Ongoing cardiopulmonary resuscitation	

context of CS from acute MI, after open-heart surgery, or other cardiomyopathies, all Impella devices are approved for short-term ventricular support (<4 days for Impella 2.5 and CP, and <14 days for Impella 5.0/LD).

Impella devices are contraindicated according to current labeling in any of the following circumstances (**Table 24.2**): LV thrombus, mechanical aortic valve, critical aortic stenosis (aortic valve area < 0.6 cm^2), at least moderate aortic insufficiency, severe peripheral arterial disease, right-sided heart failure, presence of an atrial or ventricular septal defect, LV rupture, cardiac tamponade, or inability to tolerate anticoagulation. However, many of the contraindications stem from the fact that the device has not been specifically studied under these circumstances.

Regarding intolerance to anticoagulation, it is important to note that the Impella motor chamber malfunctions in the presence of clotted blood; accordingly, a partial thromboplastin time (PTT) goal 60 to 80 seconds should be achieved. Unfractionated heparin is routinely added to the purge solution, and the PTT goal should be achieved by additive systemic dosage to target.

Complications related to Impella use fall into 2 major categories: hematologic and vascular. Anemia manifesting after Impella insertion occurs from groin and retroperitoneal hematomas as well as red blood cell hemolysis. The latter complication occurs because of mechanical damage to erythrocytes from the Impella's axial flow pump. It is postulated that a sharp bend in the Impella at the site of the mitral apparatus may contribute to hemolysis. Serum haptoglobin, free hemoglobin, lactate dehydrogenase, or indirect bilirubin (or combinations of these tests) should be monitored at least daily to assess for hemolysis. While laboratory studies are helpful in diagnosing this complication, it can be detected promptly by observing an abrupt darkening of the urine due to the presence of hemoglobin pigment. Prompt reduction of performance level and an immediate check of device positioning should be undertaken, and device removal should proceed if acute kidney injury manifests from pigment nephropathy. Regarding renal function, it is noteworthy that recent clinical data have suggested that Impella support during HR-PCI leads to lower rates of acute kidney injury.

Vascular complications occur with Impella devices because of the large arterial access required for insertion. These complications include acute limb ischemia, pseudoaneurysm formation, distal embolization of plaque and other atherosclerotic material resulting in stroke, and hematomas. There is also concern that the pigtail catheter in the LV from the Impella can also be a nidus for stroke. The PROTECT II trial, which compared intra-aortic balloon counterpulsation with Impella 2.5, found equivalent rates of vascular access complications in a patient population undergoing HR-PCI. In contrast, the IMPRESS analysis randomized 48 patients to receive either pMCS device and found a numerically higher rate of serious vascular complications in the Impella group, but the overall small study population of the trial precluded formal comparison.

Clinical Results

The Impella devices have been evaluated in 2 major clinical scenarios: (1) to prevent or treat hemodynamic compromise in the setting of HR-PCI and (2) in acute MI complicated by CS (AMICS). Data from the cVAD registry showed that the former scenario, HR-PCI, accounts for 47% of Impella use, while 40% of Impella use is for AMICS. Other clinical situations include prophylactic support during ventricular tachycardia ablations and balloon-assisted valvuloplasty procedures, nonischemic cardiomyopathy with acute decompensation, and postcardiotomy shock.

The feasibility of Impella in HR-PCI was first demonstrated in the PROTECT I study. This was a prospective, multicenter study that included 20 patients treated with Impella 2.5. These patients were considered high risk because of poor left ventricular function with ejection fraction <35%, and the intervention was being performed on an unprotected left main coronary artery or the last patent coronary conduit. The mean duration of circulatory support was 1.7 ± 0.6 hours. Mean pump flow during PCI was 2.2 ± 0.3 L/min. None of the patients developed hemodynamic compromise during PCI, which was the primary efficacy objective of the study. The incidence of major adverse cardiovascular events at 30 days (which was the primary safety endpoint) was 20%: 2 patients had a periprocedural MI and 2 patients died (at days 12 and 14, respectively).

Similar findings were obtained in the Europella registry, which was a retrospective multicenter registry of the use of Impella 2.5 that included 144 consecutive patients who underwent HR-PCI. In this study, a PCI was considered high risk if the patient had left main disease (53%), last remaining vessel disease (17%), multivessel coronary artery disease (81%), or low LV ejection fraction (35%). Mortality at 30 days was 5.5%. Rates of MI, stroke, bleeding requiring transfusion or surgery, and vascular complications at 30 days were 0%, 0.7%, 6.2%, and 4.0%, respectively.

These studies set the stage for the prospective, randomized PROTECT II study of HR-PCI in which patients were randomized to prophylactic use of IABP or Impella 2.5. The study was designed to randomize 654 patients at up to 150 sites. The primary endpoint was a composite of major adverse events (MAEs) at 30 days including death, MI, stroke, any repeat revascularization post index procedure, need for cardiac or vascular operation, acute renal dysfunction, increase in aortic insufficiency by more than 1 grade, hypotension, cardiopulmonary resuscitation (CPR) or ventricular arrhythmia requiring cardioversion, and angiographic failure to dilate the target vessel(s). The study's primary endpoint was assessed at 90 days. After review of the data at the interim mark (with follow-up data for 327 patients obtained), the Data Safety Monitoring Board recommended termination of the study owing to futility of the 30-day primary analysis. At the time of the recommendation, the study had reached 69% of the planned enrollment ($n = 447$). Although there was no significant difference in outcomes at 30 days, the prespecified 90-day data showed a significant reduction in MAEs in favor of Impella ($P = .03$). Thus, PROTECT II was (erroneously) terminated early.

Regarding the effect of Impella in CS, the prospective ISAR-SHOCK trial investigated the hemodynamic impact and clinical outcomes in patients randomized to receive IABP support ($n = 12$) versus pMCS with Impella 2.5 ($n = 13$). The primary endpoint was a change in cardiac index (CI), which was met in all patients randomized to receive support with Impella 2.5. Impella increased CI by an average of 0.49 ± 0.46, while CI increased by only 0.11 ± 0.31 L/min/m^2 with IABP support. Overall mortality was 46% in both groups, but conclusions regarding the benefits of Impella over IABP were limited by the small patient population.

IMPRESS in Severe Shock was the first randomized study to assess the effects of Impella CP relative to IABP support. The primary endpoint was 30-day mortality, and no statistically significant difference emerged between either therapy (Impella CP 46% vs IABP 50%). Only those patients who were mechanically ventilated before enrollment were eligible, and while the investigators did not intend to exclusively enroll patients with cardiac arrest, 92% of the study cohort ended up suffering an arrest. Of these patients, only half achieved return of spontaneous circulation after 20 minutes of CPR. Many of the patients died of anoxic brain damage despite successful support by Impella. Accordingly, the high overall mortality and lack of treatment effect with Impella in this underpowered analysis qualify any conclusions drawn from the study. These retrospective and small prospective studies highlight the challenges of performing studies in patients with CS.

In-hospital mortality for patients suffering CS has remained at an estimated 50% for nearly 2 decades. The concept of early initiation of support during PCI has been demonstrated to lead to more complete revascularization and improved survival. The concept of early initiation (prior to PCI) of Impella support was initially investigated in a registry study of 287 consecutive patients enrolled in the cVAD study undergoing PCI for treatment of CS. Survival in patients when support was initiated within 1.25 hours of the onset of shock and prior to PCI was 66%, and initiation of hemodynamic support prior to PCI was independently associated with improved survival. Basir et al. followed up on this analysis by conducting a 5-center pilot study that protocolized the initiation of support prior to PCI in all patients treated for CS in these centers. The Detroit Cardiogenic Shock Initiative (Detroit CSI) demonstrated in-hospital survival of 80%. This study has henceforth been expanded nationally to 35 independent sites and has thus far enrolled 171 patients. In the National CSI study, patients with CS receiving Impella support prior to PCI had a 72% survival-to-discharge rate, an improvement of more than 20% over historic values. These results are encouraging and demonstrate the need for protocolized care in CS and the importance of early hemodynamic support.

Growing interest in this concept of ventricular unloading prior to revascularization has also emerged for the treatment of patients with acute MI. Numerous preclinical studies have examined the potential for unloading to reduce infarct size, and a recently published study investigating the effect of LV unloading with Impella for 30 minutes prior to revascularization in a swine model showed that it triggered a "cardioprotective signaling program." This cascade has the potential to limit reperfusion injury following revascularization and prevent the development of heart failure after acute MI. These findings facilitated the Door-To-Unload ST elevation myocardial infarction (STEMI) safety and feasibility study, which randomized 50 patients with anterior wall acute MI to Impella support with immediate revascularization versus delayed revascularization after 30 minutes of unloading with Impella. The overall size of mean infarct as a percentage of LV mass did not differ between groups (15% ± 12% vs 13% ± 11%), but the study demonstrated feasibility of delayed revascularization, did not compromise the 90-minute door-to-balloon time standard, and showed that infarct size in the delayed revascularization tended to be independent of the area at risk. These findings have set the stage for the initiation of a fully powered pivotal trial. Results from these studies have the potential to significantly change the treatment paradigm for acute MI from a primary "door-to-balloon" time to a novel "door-to-unload time" metric with pMCS.

INTRA-AORTIC BALLOON PUMP

Historically, the IABP has been the most commonly used form of pMCS. The IABP system consists of a catheter with a balloon mounted at the tip that inflates during diastole to generate a positive pressure wave in the ascending aorta that improves coronary flow and then deflates immediately before systole to reduce resistance to systolic ejection (**Figure 24.7**). The device was first implemented in 1968 by Kantrowitz and colleagues and has since then been a key component of the pMCS armamentarium given its ease of insertion, easy operation, and safety profile.

Intra-Aortic Balloon Pump Hemodynamics

IABP deflation immediately before ventricular systole reduces effective afterload, in principle improving forward flow from the LV to the systemic circulation. This translates to an approximate 0.5 to 1.0 L/min (~10%) increase in CO. In patients with chronic heart failure and reduced forward flow, this slight increase in CO may have a more substantial impact as 0.5 to 1.0 L/min represents a considerable fraction of their CO prior to decompensation. The opposite holds true for patients with preserved LV function prior to an acute insult (ie, acute MI or myocarditis), where the augmented CO from the IABP lends marginal support. Returning to the PVL framework, counterpulsation reduces peak LV pressure and slightly increases SV. However, the overall PVL with support is not substantially changed from baseline or presupport, and myocardial oxygen demand is not significantly reduced (**Figure 24.6**). That being said, counterpulsation does exert a significant effect on coronary perfusion by increasing aortic diastolic pressures, and this may be the key factor driving its hemodynamic benefits and perceived clinical benefits.

Deriving maximal benefit depends on proper timing of balloon inflation and deflation. When appropriately timed, the intended effect of the IABP is to reduce ventricular afterload, reduce systolic blood pressure, increase diastolic blood pressure, and increase CO (**Figure 24.8**). Current IABP systems, however, use a fiber optic pressure sensor at the catheter tip to set proper timing automatically and require little, if any, manipulation of the console controls by the operator to maintain correct timing. An alternate means of automatic timing is provided by the surface electrocardiogram. With this approach, balloon inflation during diastole occurs concurrently with ventricular repo-

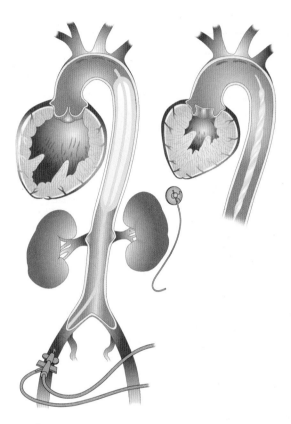

Figure 24.7 Illustration showing correct position of the intra-aortic balloon pump. The balloon inflates during diastole to increase central aortic pressure during ventricular diastole (increasing pressure gradient for coronary blood flow) and deflates during systole, reducing the pressure against which the ventricle ejects.

larization, represented by the peak of the T wave on the ECG. Balloon deflation should occur right before the onset of ventricular systole, which is marked by the peak of the R-wave on the ECG. Other triggering options are also available, such as a fixed internal trigger for patients in ventricular fibrillation or on cardiopulmonary bypass. The console allows for adjustment of the timing of balloon inflation and deflation to optimize the hemodynamic effect, as reflected in the arterial pressure waveform.

Earlier inflation should be avoided because it increases aortic pressure during left ventricular ejection, resulting in increased afterload and decreased SV. Premature inflation can be detected on the arterial pressure tracing by loss of the dicrotic notch, with the augmented pressure waveform overlaying the native systolic pressure waveform.

Late inflation compromises the beneficial hemodynamic effects of the IABP too. Blood transits through the aorta unimpeded during early diastole such that diastolic augmentation is minimized and, thus, coronary perfusion pressures are not maximized. This effect can be spotted on the arterial pressure tracing as an augmented

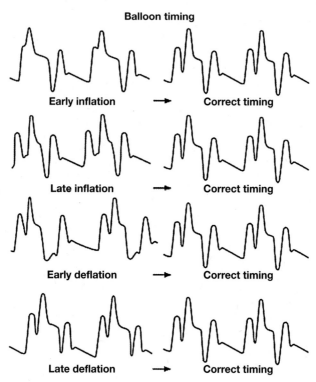

Figure 24.8 Examples of early, late, and correct inflation are shown in the top 2 tracings. Similarly, the deflation knob is moved leftward (earlier) and then slowly advanced toward the right (later in the cardiac cycle) until the end-diastolic pressure dips 10 to 15 mmHg below the patient's unassisted diastolic pressure. This will produce a maximal lowering of the patient's unassisted systolic pressure. Examples of early, late, and correct deflation timing are shown in the bottom 2 traces. When properly timed, balloon inflation occurs at the dicrotic notch and diastolic pressure is augmented as compared with the normal beat. Balloon deflation occurs just prior to ejection, and there is a drop in aortic pressure, signifying reduction of the impedance to ejection.

pressure waveform that arises distinctly apart from the normal systolic pressure waveform. The dicrotic notch is preserved, creating 3 distinct upstrokes on the arterial pressure tracing.

Early balloon deflation, like late balloon inflation, prevents a patient from experiencing the maximal hemodynamic benefit from the diastolic augmentation provided by the IABP. The EDP is unchanged from baseline, and the patient experiences less afterload reduction from the pump. This can be assessed on the arterial pressure tracing as a distinct upstroke toward the end of diastole, creating a parabolic shape in the arterial pressure tracing.

Late balloon deflation implies that the LV contracts during systole against an inflated balloon. Naturally, this increases afterload dramatically and consequently increases myocardial oxygen demand. The decline in pressure typically observed during diastole is blunted, and the EDP is increased above the patient's prior baseline.

Insertion, Routine Care, and Weaning

IABPs consist of a 7.5F to 8F catheter with a cylindrical polyurethane balloon attached at the proximal tip of the catheter. The balloon inflates with 30 to 50 mL of helium gas, which rapidly transits in and out of the balloon because of its low molecular weight and viscosity. The catheter has 2 lumens: an internal lumen through which a guiding wire passes and an external lumen, which connects the balloon with the console's pneumatic pump via extracorporeal tubing. The balloon is typically advanced through an 8F femoral arterial sheath, but a sheathless insertion technique has also been described. The brachial, axillary, and subclavian arteries can be used as alternative access sites but may require surgical cutdown if percutaneous placement cannot be performed. Once arterial access is obtained, the balloon-mounted catheter is advanced to a level 1 to 2 cm distal to the origin of the left subclavian artery. Placement is ideally confirmed fluoroscopically in real time, but it can also be done by chest radiography after emergent bedside insertion; with both modalities, the balloon tip should appear at the level of the carina. Care should be taken to avoid balloon placement too proximally in the aortic arch as well as too distally such that the balloon obstructs the renal arteries.

Clotting parameters (prothrombin time, PTT, and platelet count) should be checked, and a clinical evaluation to identify possible peripheral vascular disease should be performed prior to IABP insertion. Immediately before the IABP is inserted, air is evacuated from the balloon using a large syringe (30-60 mL) attached to a 1-way valve to maintain the lowest possible profile during introduction. If the patient is not already anticoagulated, unfractionated heparin (5000 U) should be given intravenously as soon as the balloon is inserted, followed by continuous intravenous heparin titrated to maintain an activated clotting time (ACT) of 1.5 to 2.0 times the normal. The IABP is then introduced over the wire, and its radiopaque tip is brought to the appropriate position. The guidewire is removed, and blood is aspirated from the guidewire lumen to ensure that no air is trapped. The guidewire lumen is then connected to a pressurized flushing device that delivers 3 mL/h to maintain lumen patency. Special care must be taken to prevent inadvertent injection of air bubbles or thrombi through the guidewire lumen since its tip is only a short distance below the aortic arch. The balloon shaft may be equipped with a protective plastic outer sleeve that can be advanced to mate with the hub of the introducer sheath to maintain sterility if subsequent adjustment is required. If a long sheath has been used to negotiate a tortuous iliac artery, the sheath must be partially withdrawn prior to initiation of counterpulsation so that the distal end of the sheath does not overlie and trap the distal end of the balloon.

Patients on IABP support require intensive care unit (ICU) level care. During counterpulsation, it is particularly important that patients undergo specific evaluations at least daily for evidence of sepsis, thrombocytopenia, hemolysis, and vascular complications like access-site hematoma, pseudoaneurysm formation, and acute limb ischemia. Evaluation of the circulation to the involved limb should be done regularly and documented. Dorsalis pedis and posterior tibial pulses should be palpated at least every 6 to 8 hours. Use of a Doppler probe to confirm presence of distal pulses is mandatory if they are not palpable, as patients might develop acute limb ischemia secondary to arterial thrombosis, distal embolization, or plaque rupture in the setting of severe aortoiliac atherosclerotic disease.

The level of heparin anticoagulation should be monitored closely, with PTT maintained at 50 to 70 seconds to prevent complications from thrombosis or embolization. However, growing clinical experience and some data suggest that a strategy of selective use of heparin (ie, administration of heparin only for a clinical indication) might be associated with a lower bleeding complications rate without an increase in ischemic complications when compared with routine heparin use. Thus, the use of routine full anticoagulation with heparin in low-risk patients has been questioned, as long as the IABP is maintained at 1:1 and when support is needed for a short period of time, particularly in the postoperative state. Mild to moderate thrombocytopenia may occur owing to platelet destruction, but the platelet count rarely falls below 50,000 to 100,000/mL and should rapidly return to normal following balloon removal.

The IABP is usually removed once the patient's condition has stabilized after the acute event. Before removal of an IABP, patients are weaned from support by decreasing the ratio of counterpulsation-supported heart beats to total heart beats from 1:1 to 1:2 and then 1:3. The decision to discontinue counterpulsation depends on the original indication for placement. For patients who received an IABP in the setting of unstable coronary artery disease, they should remain free of angina, arrhythmia, or hemodynamic deterioration with declining levels of support from the IABP. Similarly, for patients with acutely decompensated heart failure, blood pressure, mentation, urine output, and freedom from arrhythmia with lessening IABP support should reassure the clinician that the device can be removed. Once heparin has been stopped, the IABP should be set back to 1:1 counterpulsation and the device removed when the PTT falls below 50 seconds.

Indications, Contraindications, and Complications

The overall indications for IABP use are summarized in **Table 24.3**. In light of the landmark findings from IABP-SHOCK II, the ACC/AHA downgraded the use of an IABP in the context of STEMI complicated by CS from a class I to class IIa recommendation, while the European Society of Cardiology went a step further, actively recommending against its routine use (class III).

The key contraindications for IABP are summarized in **Table 24.3**. The main contraindications to IABP use are moderate to severe aortic regurgitation and peripheral vascular access issues that preclude placement of the catheter and increase the risk of complications with the catheter in place.

Data on 16,909 patients undergoing IABP therapy collected by the Benchmark Counterpulsation Outcomes Registry (sponsored by Datascope Corp.) between 1996 and 2000 showed the incidence of major complications resulting from the use of an IABP to be 2.8%. The incidence of minor complications was 4.2%. Major complications were defined as limb ischemia resulting in a loss of pulse or sensation, or abnormal limb temperature or pallor requiring surgical intervention; severe bleeding requiring transfusion or surgical intervention; balloon leak; and death directly attributable to IABP insertion or failure. Minor complications included limb ischemia (evidenced by a diminished pulse), which resolved after catheter removal, and nonsevere bleeding involving either a minor hematoma or some degree of puncture site oozing. Independent predictors of a major complication were female gender, age (75 years or older), and peripheral vascular disease. IABP-related mortality was 0.5%. IABP treatment in the setting of high-risk STEMI has also been reported to be associated with an absolute 2% increase in stroke rate. Fuchs and colleagues also studied 9662 patients undergoing PCI, the majority of whom presented with unstable angina, to identify risk factors for stroke. The prevalence of stroke was 0.38%, and emergent IABP insertion emerged as the single most powerful predictor. Despite the significant decline in balloon-related complication rates, complications can still be serious and require careful periprocedural assessment and monitoring for prevention.

Clinical Results

The clinical evidence basis justifying the widespread adoption of IABP in the prior decades is slim. A number of cohort studies in the AMICS patient population demonstrated mortality reductions associated with IABP use in specific settings, ie, patients

Table 24.3	Intra-aortic Balloon Pump Indications and Contraindications
Indications	
Acute myocardial infarction complicated by cardiogenic shock	
Mechanical complications following acute myocardial infarction	
Acutely decompensated chronic heart failure	
Ischemia refractory to medical therapy	
Ventricular arrhythmia (ischemia related), refractory to medical therapy	
Postcardiotomy cardiogenic shock	
High-risk percutaneous coronary intervention	
Contraindications	
Significant aortic insufficiency	
Abdominal aortic aneurysm	
Aortic dissection	
Severe peripheral arterial disease (especially with bypass grafts of femoral arteries)	
Bleeding diathesis	

treated with thrombolytics rather than PCI, but did not demonstrate benefit in the majority of patients with STEMI with CS. More recently, a meta-analysis of patients treated with prophylactic IABP prior to coronary artery bypass surgery showed a modest mortality reduction, and another analysis of patients with out-of-hospital cardiac arrest treated with IABP postresuscitation showed improved neurological outcomes. However, when IABP support was studied in randomized clinical trials in patients with ACS, repeated studies failed to demonstrate a clear benefit across a wide range of outcomes. In an early study of 57 patients with acute MI randomized to IABP versus the standard of care, 6-month mortality was unchanged but trended toward a significant reduction in the subgroup of patients presenting with Killip III and IV MIs. The CRISP AMI global multicenter randomized trial investigated the effect of IABP support versus normal therapy in 337 patients with large anterior acute MI. The primary endpoint was infarct size measured by magnetic resonance imaging 3 to 5 days post intervention. The study showed no benefit for IABP therapy; in fact, a nonsignificant trend toward larger infarct size was observed with IABP treatment.

Most importantly, IABP SHOCK II demonstrated that routine usage of IABP in the setting of AMICS treated with PCI did not reduce mortality at 30 days. A total of 600 patients with CS were randomized and 30-day mortality was 39.7% in the IABP group and 41.3% in the control group. There were no significant differences in secondary endpoints or in process-of-care measures, including the time to hemodynamic stabilization, the length of stay in the ICU, serum lactate levels, the dose and duration of catecholamine therapy, and renal function. Timing of IABP insertion also did not affect clinical outcome. Long-term outcomes were recently published from the IABP-SHOCK II study confirming a lack of mortality or quality-of-life benefit with IABP support.

LEFT-ATRIAL-TO-AORTIC PUMPS

The TandemHeart percutaneous ventricular assist device (LivaNova-TandemLife, Pittsburgh, PA, USA) is the only commercially available left-atrial-to-aortic pump available on the market (**Figure 24.9**). The TandemHeart system utilizes a 21F transseptal cannula inserted through the femoral vein to the inferior vena cava (IVC), into the right atrium (RA), and with fluoroscopic and intra cardiac echo guidance, across the atrial septum into the left atrium (LA). Blood is withdrawn via 14 side holes and end holes on the catheter tip from the LA by an extracorporeal, nonpulsatile centrifugal continuous flow pump. The motor operates at speeds between 3500 and 7500 RPMs, is lubricated by a continuous saline infusate, and pumps blood back into the femoral artery via 15F or 17F cannulas, achieving flow rates of 3.5 L/min (15F cannula) to 5.0 L/min (17F cannula) of cardiac support.

Since TandemHeart pumps blood from the LA, there are significant reductions in LA pressure and, therefore, reductions in LVEDP and EDV (**Figure 24.6**). The increased total blood flow is accompanied by increases in systemic arterial pressure,

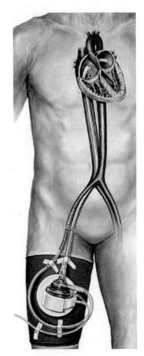

Figure 24.9 Schematic of the TandemHeart system, which uses an extracorporeal centrifugal pump connected to a transseptal catheter to withdraw blood from the left atrium and pump it back to the femoral artery.

during systole and more significantly during diastole because of the continuous, asynchronous pumping throughout the cardiac cycle. With the decrease in preload and the increase in afterload pressure, intrinsic CO decreases, and this is reflected as a decrease in the width of the PVL and possibly a loss of pulsatility on the arterial waveform if the pump overwhelms intrinsic cardiac function.

The only parameter that can be controlled on the system is pump speed (at 50 RPM increments), and change of speed will cause a change of flow as indicated in the controller display screen. Although maximal support is often desirable, this cannot always be achieved under circumstances where blood return to the LA is diminished (ie, right ventricular failure, pulmonary hypertension, hypovolemia, or hemorrhage). If reduced LA filling is traced to one of these conditions, pump speed can be reduced until that condition is corrected, with the understanding that optimal pump performance occurs with LA pressure or PCWP in the range between 10 and 20 mmHg. Specific signs of inadequate blood supply to the pump from the LA include unusual vibrations of the transseptal cannula or the pump, low infusion pressures or infusion pressure alarms, and kinking of the transseptal cannula. The general practice is to adjust the pump speed to a level that still allows a minimum of pulsatile flow across the native aortic valve in order to prevent stasis of blood in the LV and aortic root, which could result in thrombus formation and subsequent embolization.

Patients should be anticoagulated with a PTT goal between 65 to 80 seconds or ACT of 180 to 220 seconds, and pump speed should not be reduced such that flow rates fall under 1 L/min, as pump thrombosis can occur even with appropriate anticoagulation. Importantly, the controller will alarm to alert when flow goes below 1 L/min, with critically high or low infusion rates or pressures below 50 mmHg or above 750 mmHg.

The main complications associated with use of the TandemHeart system include bleeding, complications associated with transseptal puncture (ie, accidental puncture of aorta, myocardial perforation, arrhythmias), dislocation of the transseptal cannula, stroke, vascular access complications, dislocation of the arterial cannulas, leg ischemia, and hemolysis.

The TandemHeart system is generally used to provide temporary circulatory support in conditions such as AMICS or decompensated chronic heart failure, pulmonary edema, and postcardiotomy shock. It has been used successfully as a bridge to recovery in patients with AMICS, acute myocarditis, or end-stage cardiomyopathy. The system is generally contraindicated for patients with any of the following: primary right-sided heart failure, severe aortic regurgitation, or any condition that prevents extracorporeal blood circulation. As with any extracorporeal support system, caution should be exercised in cases of mitral or aortic mechanical heart valves.

TandemHeart has been evaluated in a number of different scenarios. In a single-arm trial of 117 patients with CS refractory to inotropes and IABP, TandemHeart produced impressive improvements in hemodynamic parameters. With the device implanted for a mean of roughly 6 days, the CI improved from 0.5 to 3.0 L/min/m². Two small randomized studies comparing TandemHeart with IABP were conducted over a decade ago, and both demonstrated significant hemodynamic improvements without concomitant improvement of 30-day outcomes. TandemHeart was also associated with numerically higher complications than IABP, and this was driven not just by lower extremity digit ischemia, which occurred in over 20% of patients, but also by infection, bleeding, and arrhythmia.

EXTRACORPOREAL MEMBRANE OXYGENATION/ EXTRACORPOREAL CIRCULATORY LIFE SUPPORT

Extracorporeal membrane oxygenation (ECMO) was developed out of the modern-day heart-lung bypass machine. Since then, ECMO circuits have been refined such that they are quickly assembled, percutaneously inserted, and durable enough for patients to be supported for prolonged periods of time. In 2017, over 10,000 ECMO runs were performed, representing a quadrupling from only a decade prior. Unlike the previously discussed forms of pMCS, the venoarterial configuration of ECMO not only supports flow and pressure within the systemic circulation but also can oxygenate blood and remove carbon dioxide in order to supplement lung function. This is in contradistinction with the venovenous configuration (VV ECMO), which supports lung function and will not be discussed in this chapter. Also, the 2 major forms of VA ECMO are peripheral ECMO (with cannulation via percutaneous routes such as femoral, axillary, subclavian, or jugular vessels) and central ECMO (with cannulation of the RA and ascending aorta performed surgically). This chapter will focus on peripheral ECMO.

A typical VA ECMO circuit comprises 6 critical elements (**Figure 24.10**): (1) inflow and outflow cannulas, (2) 3/8-inch or 1/4-inch tubing, (3) a centrifugal pump, (4) a heat exchanger, (5) a membrane oxygenator, and (6) a console to monitor pump flows and circuit pressures. The inflow cannula resides in a central vein and terminates in the RA. Although multiple veins may support a VA ECMO configuration, the most commonly used vessel is the femoral vein. Inflow catheters in the femoral vein are 50 to 60 cm in length and range in size from 18 to 21F and may have a single end hole or multiple ports to promote more effective venous drainage. While several companies manufacture centrifugal pumps, including LivaNova (TandemHeart), Abbott (Centrimag), and Getinge (CardioHelp), their use in the context of ECMO is considered off-label by the FDA. All pumps operate similarly, rotating at 3000 to 5000 RPMs and supplying 3 to 6 L/min of circulatory support. In most ECMO configurations, once blood exits the pump, it passes through a heat exchanger to be rewarmed. Blood then transits from the heat exchanger to a membrane oxygenator, where gas exchange occurs. Membrane oxygenators are hollow fiber devices made from biopolymers like polymethylpentene. A "sweep" gas passes within the hollow fibers while the patient's blood flows around the fibers, allowing oxygen and carbon dioxide to diffuse in or out across the fibers depending on the diffusion gradient. Increasing the flow rate of the sweep gas will promote carbon dioxide clearance, and vice versa. The F_DO_2 is the fraction of delivered oxygen in the blood returned to the patient, and it is typically 100%. With time, the membrane oxygenator may become inefficient as clot and fibrin adhere to the membrane, effectively reducing the area for gas exchange. The difference in pressure of blood entering and exiting the membrane oxygenator, AP, is one of many variables that can be used to evaluate the membrane oxygenator's performance. Normally this pressure difference is on the order of 5 to 20 mmHg, and the oxygenator should be replaced when it exceeds 60 mmHg or the AP changes rapidly (n.b. these values are specific to the oxygenator structure and membrane surface area). An outflow cannula then returns the oxygenated blood to the patient and is typically positioned in the femoral artery, pumping blood retrograde through the aorta. 15F catheters are the standard size, but 17F catheters are used occasionally to provide additional support.

A trained perfusionist should set up the ECMO circuit, and this can be done in as quickly as 10 to 15 minutes. The earlier ECMO systems required a surgical approach, whereas today, with current devices, percutaneous cannulation of the femoral artery and vein is readily achieved. The venous inflow cannula is advanced to the level of the RA, while the arterial outflow cannula extends to the aortoiliac junction. Once a patient is cannulated onto ECMO support, it is imperative to have a multidisciplinary team of perfusionists, nurses, surgeons, and cardiologists to provide close monitoring of various parameters including arterial blood pressure, pulmonary artery pressures, PCWP, central venous pressure (CVP), and CO. An arterial catheter should be placed in the right hand to monitor blood pressure (noting not only absolute pressures but also the pulsatility of the arterial waveform, which reflects underlying cardiac activ-

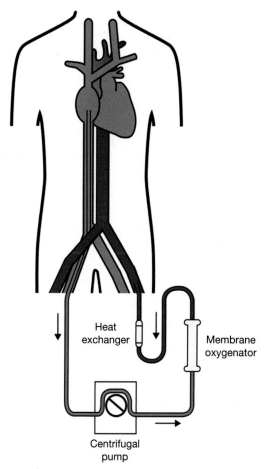

Figure 24.10 A typical configuration of a venoarterial extracorporeal membrane oxygenation circuit. An inflow cannula is positioned in the femoral vein. Blood is drawn through a centrifugal flow pump, then into a membrane oxygenator for gas exchange, and returned via an outflow cannula, positioned in the femoral artery. (From Abrams D, Combes A, Brodie D. Extracorporeal membrane oxygenation in cardiopulmonary disease in adults. *J Am Coll Cardiol.* 2014;63:2769-2778.)

ity) as well as blood oxygenation. As described below in greater detail, VA ECMO increases afterload dramatically to potentially create a "watershed" region in the aortic arch where highly oxygenated blood flowing retrograde from the ECMO circuit intersects with less oxygenated blood that passed through the lungs and is ejected out of the LV. If native cardiac function is sufficient such that the less oxygenated blood from the LV supplies the majority of the blood supply for the brachiocephalic and carotid arteries, creating a "Harlequin syndrome" or "north/south" physiology, then cerebral perfusion will depend on the oxygen content of the blood in the ventricle and not on that of the blood flowing through the ECMO circuit. Accordingly, sampling blood from the right radial artery provides the most conservative estimate of oxygenation to the brain.

Extracorporeal Membrane Oxygenation Hemodynamics

The hemodynamic response to VA ECMO is complex and depends on the nature of the insult and underlying ventricular function. A circuit that pumps blood from the RA or another central vein to the arterial system can technically offload the RV but overload the LV, first by causing significant increases in LV afterload, which subsequently lead to increases in preload and PCWP. LV afterload increases substantially because ECMO can significantly increase blood pressure, which is beneficial to the systemic circulation and end-organ perfusion but taxes an already compromised LV. As a result, the PVL shifts rightward and upward along the EDPVR and SV decreases. Consequently, LVEDP, LA pressure, and PCWP can increase; these increases in LV preload and PCWP can be detrimental to blood oxygen saturation and markedly increase myocardial oxygen demand. These factors can paradoxically worsen LV function, especially in the setting of acute myocardial ischemia or infarction, forcing clinicians to choose a "venting" strategy, which unloads the LV (**Figure 24.7**, discussed further below). Patient characteristics that predispose to the need for LV venting are not fully understood, but theoretical considerations suggest that hearts with worse LV contractility are more likely to require venting. Regardless, many experts strongly advocate the need for continuous hemodynamic monitoring with a PAC to rapidly identify patients in whom PCWP increases with the initiation of ECMO.

Insertion, Monitoring, and Weaning

Patients on ECMO should be monitored in an ICU setting with frequent checks to assess for complications. A perfusionist should evaluate the circuit daily, observing for any malfunction in the membrane oxygenator and for the formation of clot within the circuit's tubing. Shortly after cannulation and the onset of ECMO, many patients vasodilate as cytokine release is triggered by blood components passing through the ECMO circuit. As such, aggressive early resuscitation with intravenous fluid and packed red blood cells (pRBCs) as indicated by the hemoglobin level is critical. Patients should be anticoagulated with a PTT goal between 50 and 75 seconds. Hematologic and clotting parameters need to be monitored frequently as well. Patients on ECMO frequently require many pRBC transfusions and are transfused to a goal hemoglobin between 12 and 14 g/dL in order to maintain adequate circuit volume. Destructive thrombocytopenia is common as well, caused by the shearing effect of the centrifugal pump and the circuit tubing. Mechanical ventilation should only be instituted for patients who cannot protect their airway on account of altered mental status or neurological compromise. When patients are mechanically ventilated, high levels of positive end-expiratory pressure (PEEP) are typically required to prevent atelectasis and injury from being bedbound. This needs to be counterbalanced with the deleterious effects of high PEEP, and some centers favor low tidal volume ventilation for a lung-protective strategy that minimizes ventilator-associated lung injury.

ECMO weaning can commence when patients begin recovering from the initial insult. If patients are supported with multiple modalities (ie, ECMO, Impella, and inotropes), ECMO weaning and decannulation is generally prioritized given the greatest risk of adverse events associated with the device. When ready to wean, the RPMs on the device console are decreased such that flow rates are reduced, typically in increments of 0.25 to 0.5 L/min. Patients should tolerate flow decrements without changes in systemic arterial pressures, pulmonary pressures, or PCWP. The device can be removed when patients tolerate flows as low as 1 L/min. Ideally, the cannulas are removed in the catheterization laboratory or operating room.

Indications, Contraindications, and Complications

The individual components that comprise ECMO circuits are approved for temporary circulatory support for varying durations (**Table 24.4**). Pumps used in ECMO circuits are generally FDA cleared for up to 6 hours of use, although in routine clinical practice, they are used off-label for much longer durations. There is no complete ECMO circuit that is approved by the FDA. Accordingly, there are no formal indications for use as there are for other devices. AMICS, acute left ventricular dysfunction from conditions like stress cardiomyopathy or myocarditis, or acutely decompensated chronic heart failure, right ventricular failure, incessant ventricular arrhythmias, postcardiotomy syndrome, extra-corporeal cardiopulmonary resuscitation, and primary graft failure after orthotopic heart transplantation (OHT) account for the common uses of ECMO. Contemporary guide-lines emphasize that ECMO is not a definitive treatment but rather a bridge, be it to OHT, durable MCS implantation, recovery, or more time for a decision to be made. ECMO is not recommended in patients with irreversible, noncardiac organ failure and in those with irreversible cardiac dysfunction who are not eligible for advanced therapies.

Complications related to ECMO are wide ranging and frequent. The most common complication is bleeding, both from the femoral access sites as well as from the gastrointestinal tract. Bleeding relates partly to concurrent anticoagu-lation being administered, as well as to destruction of critical clotting factors in the blood. Thrombosis is another frequent occurrence from the benign (ie, clot in tubing, which can be replaced) to the catastrophic (ie, cerebrovascular accident).

Despite a venous inflow cannula extracting blood from the RA, the LV continues to fill with blood return from the bronchial circulation and Thebesian coronary veins. Combined with the increased afterload created by retrograde aortic blood flow from

Table 24.4 Extracorporeal Membrane Oxygenation Indications and Contraindications

Indications
Acute myocardial infarction complicated by cardiogenic shock
Acutely decompensated chronic heart failure
Ventricular arrhythmia (ischemia-related), refractory to medical therapy
Postcardiotomy cardiogenic shock
Primary allograft dysfunction after heart transplantation
Severe right ventricular dysfunction
Cardiopulmonary resuscitation
Contraindications
Irreversible end-organ dysfunction
Unrepaired aortic dissection
Severe peripheral vascular disease (peripheral cannulation only)

the ECMO circuit, the LV is prone to distend and overfill, leading to pulmonary edema, hypoxemia, and worsening LV function. When the PCWP is elevated, the aortic valve does not open with each cardiac cycle, oxygenation is poor, and the ventricle appears distended on echocardiography, such that a venting strategy to unload the LV is recommended. A number of different options exist, including IABP support, percutaneous or surgical septostomy to create a left atrial vent, TandemHeart, and Impella.

When an ECMO circuit is combined with an Impella CP device to unload the LV, the configuration is referred to by the moniker, "ECPella." The Impella is set to provide between 1.5 and 2.0 L/min of cardiac support (ie, partial support), which unloads the LV and increases aortic root blood flow to also prevent blood clots from forming and embolizing. When LV function begins to recover, the Impella can be used to not only vent the LV but also expedite ECMO decannulation by increasing the performance level to supply 3.5 to 4 L/min of output.

Clinical Results

ECMO use in the setting of AMICS has been described in multiple cohort studies. A single-center analysis of 18 patients treated with VA ECMO for AMICS demonstrated a short median duration of circulatory support (3.2 days) and a 67% survival to hospital discharge. In a propensity-matched investigation of in-hospital cardiac arrest where 59 patients received ECMO, ECMO outperformed conventional CPR with respect to 30-day survival (hazard ratio [HR] 0.47, 95% confidence interval 0.28-0.77), survival to discharge (HR 0.51, 95% confidence interval 0.35-0.74), and 1-year outcomes (HR 0.53, 95% confidence interval 0.33-0.83). A meta-analysis of 20 studies conducted between 2005 and 2015 with 833 patients reported a 22% survival to discharge and 13% discharge with good neurologic recovery. Extracorporeal life support (ECLS) demonstrated an overall mortality rate of 22% for out-of-hospital cardiac arrest. Despite these positive findings, ECLS remains resource intensive, further limiting more widespread adoption.

RIGHT VENTRICULAR SUPPORT DEVICES

Similar principles govern RV and LV mechanics, and absolute volumes and SVs are very similar in the 2 chambers. However, important distinctions between the 2 exist. First, the RV and LV geometries are different. The RV is crescent shaped, while the LV is ellipsoidal. Second, the relative pressures differ significantly. Under normal conditions RV pressures are one-fifth to one-seventh those of the LV. The peak systolic pressure of the LV normally ranges between 110 and 130 mmHg, while normal peak RV systolic pressure ranges between 15 and 25 mmHg. Qualitative differences in the right- and left-sided heart circulations exist in addition to these quantitative pressure differences. For example, pulmonary arterial pulse pressure is large compared with mean pulmonary arterial pressure, and the diastolic pulmonary artery pressure can decay to nearly equal the end-diastolic right ventricular pressure. This varies from the left-sided heart circulation where aortic EDP is often an order of magnitude higher than that of the LVEDP.

The PVL of a normal RV (**Figure 24.11**) differs from that of the LV in several ways. First, the RV has its own ESPVR and EDPVR that provide the boundaries for its PVL. The slope of the right ventricular ESPVR (E_{es}) is normally one-fifth to one-seventh that of the LV, reflecting the same absolute volumes but differing peak pressures. Despite the marked differences in chamber geometries between the RV and LV, their EDPVRs are similar since the 2 chambers are of similar size. Second, RV PVLs do not exhibit prominent isovolumic periods because diastolic pulmonary pressure can decay nearly to right ventricular EDP. Third, compared with the LV, the RV PVL has a more dome-shaped top and the left upper region of the loop does not form a sharp corner. As a result, the point of first contact between the loop and the ESPVR has a volume (which

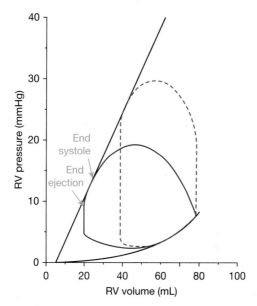

Figure 24.11 The normal right ventricular (RV) pressure-volume loop (PVL; solid blue line). The slope of the RV end-systolic pressure-volume relationship is shallower and systolic pressures are less than those seen in the left ventricular PVL. However, the right and left ventricular end-diastolic pressure-volume relationships are similar. The PVL of RV failure is highlighted as well (dashed red line). (Images generated from the Harvi simulator [http://harvi.online] with permission from PVLoops LLC.)

is technically designated as the end-systolic volume) that is usually significantly higher than the lowest volume (which is technically designated as the end-ejection volume) that determines SV.

The PVL of the failing RV shifts in 2 fundamental ways that depend on the etiology and duration of disease. In the circumstance of acute MI involving the RV free wall or interventricular septum, the loss of contractile tissue is reflected as a decreased slope of the E_{es} (**Figure 24.11**). Over time, with persistent RV dysfunction and elevations of CVP, the RV will also remodel by dilating, shifting the EDPVR rightward. In the face of a primary increase of pulmonary vascular resistance (such as pulmonary arterial hypertension), the RV will similarly remodel. However, the slope of the E_{es} will increase, reflecting the increased pressure present in the pulmonary circuit that the RV must eject against. The overall increase in the area of the PVL reflects the increased workload of the RV in these conditions. Without intervention, these hemodynamic forces will force the RV to continue to remodel, ultimately resulting in decompensation, loss of RV function, and clinical signs of right-sided heart failure. The RV will respond similarly in situations where pulmonary pressures are elevated because of LV failure (World Health Organization group 2 pulmonary hypertension) because pulmonary venous pressure contributed disproportionally to effective RV afterload.

Impella RP

The Impella RP (**Figure 24.12**), like the other devices belonging to the Impella family, is a catheter-mounted microaxial nonpulsatile pump. The Impella RP has an 11F guide catheter and a 21F pump head and is placed percutaneously via the femoral

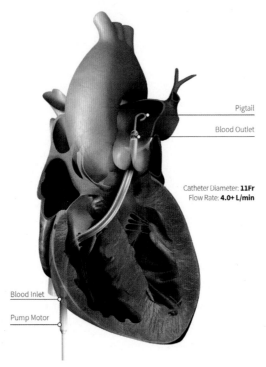

Pigtail

Blood Outlet

Catheter Diameter: **11Fr**
Flow Rate: **4.0+ L/min**

Blood Inlet

Pump Motor

Figure 24.12 Depiction of the Impella RP positioned with its inlet in the inferior vena cava, the pump traversing the tricuspid valve, right ventricle, and pulmonic valve, and its outlet positioned in the pulmonary trunk. (Courtesy of Abiomed.)

vein using a 23F peel-away sheath. The impeller of the Impella RP rotates at up to 33,000 RPMs and can generate >4.0 L/min of flow. Like the other Impella devices, the Impella RP has a range of 0 to 9 performance levels. The device has a special 3-dimensional S-shape such that the inlet sits in the IVC. The pump traverses the tricuspid and pulmonic valves, and it ends with the outlet situated in the pulmonary trunk, at least 3 cm distal to the pulmonic valve. Accordingly, the Impella RP must be placed with fluoroscopic guidance, and catheter maneuvering requires a strong rail provided by a 0.027-inch stiff wire.

Cheung and colleagues conducted the initial hemodynamic study of patients receiving the Impella RP or a larger, surgically inserted counterpart, the Impella RD (Right Direct). They showed that the devices improved CO (2.1 ± 0.1-2.6 ± 0.2 L/min) and reduced CVP (22 ± 5-15 ± 4 mmHg). The RECOVER RIGHT study, published a year later, evaluated 30 patients with RV failure (the majority from post-cardiotomy shock) and reported feasibility of Impella RP implantation (29 of 30 cases successful). Hemodynamics improved (CO 1.8 ± 0.2-3.3 ± 0.2 L/min), and the authors reported an impressive 30-day survival rate of 73.3% with 100% survival among discharged patients at 180 days.

The Impella RP is indicated for right ventricular failure due to acute MI or after open-heart surgery, heart transplantation, or left ventricular assist device insertion in adult and pediatric patients (body surface area >1.5 m^2) for up to 14 days. Contraindications include abnormalities of the femoral vein or IVC (ie, mural thrombus, IVC filter) and right-sided valvular issues (ie, mechanical tricuspid or pulmonic valve, severe tricuspid or pulmonic stenosis or regurgitation). Complications related to Impella RP use are not well described in large registries. The RECOVER RIGHT clinical trial reported a 60% overall bleeding rate, 13.3% hemolysis rate, 0% pulmonary embolism, and 3.3% tricuspid or pulmonary value dysfunction. Early postmarketing studies report 12% major bleeding rate, 10% hemolysis rate, 0% pulmonary embolism, and 7% device malfunction.

BiPella Support

The arrival of the Impella RP created an opportunity to provide biventricular support when paired with an LV Impella device. Commonly referred to as "BiPella" support, this pMCS strategy combines the RV support from an Impella RP with the LV support from an Impella 2.5, CP, or 5.0, with the Impella CP being the most commonly selected device. This form of biventricular support addresses many of the shortcomings of VA ECMO. First, it unloads both ventricles and, in so doing, theoretically increases the chances of LV recovery. This is in contradistinction to ECMO, which abruptly increases ventricular afterload and loads the LV. Second, circuit thrombosis is less common with Impella than with ECMO such that less intensive anticoagulation is required. Last, the BiPella strategy allows more individualized titration of support for the RV and LV, unlike ECMO, which unloads the RV and bypasses (but does not support) the LV. One particular advantage of BiPella support is that, unlike ECMO, the BiPella configuration can be deescalated 1 ventricle at a time. Emerging clinical evidence has suggested that BiPella support in patients with CS promotes better patient outcomes.

Protek Duo

The Protek Duo (CardiacAssist, Pittsburgh, PA, USA) has emerged as another option to provide patients with percutaneous right ventricular support after it obtained 510(k) clearance for use from the FDA in 2014. It is approved for temporary (defined as less than 6 hours) cardiopulmonary bypass, and not actually for right ventricular failure. The device consists of a single cannula with 2 lumens designed for bidirectional flow, which optimizes venous drainage and prevents recirculated blood from returning through the inflow lumen. The cannula removes blood from the RA with the 29F outer lumen of the cannula and then returns it to the pulmonary artery through the 16F inner lumen. A larger 31F outer cannula with an 18.5F inner cannula is also available. Blood withdrawn from the outer cannula is circulated by a TandemHeart centrifugal pump, which can provide 4.5 to 5.0 L/min of RV support. For patients in hypoxic respiratory failure, an oxygenator can be spliced into the circuit after the TandemHeart pump to provide VV ECMO.

The Protek Duo is inserted through the right internal jugular vein over a stiff wire that is advanced into a distal pulmonary arteriole in order to provide an adequate rail for insertion of the large-bore cannula. Proper positioning requires fluoroscopic guidance such that the distal tip of the Protek Duo is positioned at least 3 to 5 cm past the pulmonic valve. Once the correct position has been confirmed, the TandemHeart flows are gradually increased until the desired filling pressure and/or flow is achieved, the circuit begins to chatter as venous return to the RA diminishes, the interventricular septum becomes midline, or flow remains constant despite increased pump speeds. If chatter is encountered at less than desired flow rates, it is recommended to reduce RPMs until the source of chatter is identified and corrected. Anticoagulation with heparin is advised during device insertion with an ACT of 180 to 220 seconds or PTT 65 to 80 seconds during routine use with flow rates above 2.0 L/min.

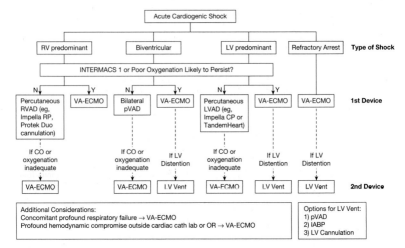

Figure 24.13 An example of an institutional shock algorithm used at NewYork Presbyterian Hospital-Columbia University Irving Medical Center, which highlights the thought process behind primary device choice and device escalation. (From Garan AR, Takeda K, Salna M, et al. Prospective comparison of a percutaneous ventricular assist device and venoarterial extracorporeal membrane oxygenation for patients with cardiogenic shock following acute myocardial infarction. *J Am Heart Assoc.* 2019;8:e012171.)

SUMMARY

Despite significant advances in medical care, more than 4 of every 10 patients with CS die during the index hospitalization. pMCS has not been shown to reduce mortality in randomized trials, but observational data and anecdotal experience support the notion that pMCS can reverse CS when clinicians select the most appropriate device and implant it at the optimal time. Questions remain regarding device selection, timing of support, and escalation of support, and they have collectively focused attention on developing algorithms for managing severe CS requiring pMCS (**Figure 24.13**). Such standardization is essential for optimizing patient care in this field and conducting high-quality research to identify when, where, and in whom to use pMCS.

SUGGESTED READINGS

1. Akanni OJ, Takeda K, Truby LK, et al. EC-VAD: combined use of extracorporeal membrane oxygenation and percutaneous micro-axial pump left ventricular assist device. *ASAIO J.* 2019;65(3):219-226.
2. Anderson MB, Goldstein J, Milano C, et al. Benefits of a novel percutaneous ventricular assist device for right heart failure: the prospective RECOVER RIGHT study of the Impella RP device. *J Heart Lung Transpl.* 2015;34(12):1549-1560.
3. Basir MB, Schreiber TL, Grines CL, et al. Effect of early initiation of mechanical circulatory support on survival in cardiogenic shock. *Am J Cardiol.* 2017;119(6):845-851.
4. Basir MB, Kapur NK, Patel K, et al. Improved outcomes associated with the use of shock protocols: updates from the National Cardiogenic Shock Initiative. *Catheter Cardiovasc Interv.* 2019;93(7):1173-1183.
5. Binanay C, Califf RM, Hasselblad V, et al. Evaluation study of congestive heart failure and pulmonary artery catheterization effectiveness: the ESCAPE trial. *J Am Med Assoc.* 2005;294(13):1625-1633.
6. Burkhoff D, Cohen H, Brunckhorst C, O'Neill WW; TandemHeart Investigators Group. A randomized multicenter clinical study to evaluate the safety and efficacy of the TandemHeart percutaneous ventricular assist device versus conventional therapy with intraaortic balloon pumping for treatment of cardiogenic shock. *Am Heart J.* 2006;152(3):469.e1-469.e8.

7. Burkhoff D, Sayer G, Doshi D, Uriel N. Hemodynamics of mechanical circulatory support. *J Am Coll Cardiol.* 2015;66(23):2663-2674.
8. Cevasco M, Takayama H, Ando M, Garan AR, Naka Y, Takeda K. Left ventricular distension and venting strategies for patients on venoarterial extracorporeal membrane oxygenation. *J Thorac Dis.* 2019;11(4):1676-1683.
9. Cheung AW, White CW, Davis MK, Freed DH. Short-term mechanical circulatory support for recovery from acute right ventricular failure: clinical outcomes. *J Heart Lung Transplant.* 2014;33(8):794-799.
10. Cooper HA, Thompson E, Panza JA. The role of heparin anticoagulation during intra-aortic balloon counterpulsation in the coronary care unit. *Acute Card Care.* 2008;10(4):214-220.
11. Deppe AC, Weber C, Liakopoulos OJ, et al. Preoperative intra-aortic balloon pump use in high-risk patients prior to coronary artery bypass graft surgery decreases the risk for morbidity and mortality-a meta-analysis of 9,212 patients. *J Card Surg.* 2017;32(3):177-185.
12. Dixon SR, Henriques JP, Mauri L, et al. A prospective feasibility trial investigating the use of the Impella 2.5 system in patients undergoing high-risk percutaneous coronary intervention (The PROTECT I Trial): initial U.S. experience. *JACC Cardiovasc Interv.* 2009;2:91-96.
13. Esposito ML, Zhang Y, Qiao X, et al. Left ventricular unloading before reperfusion promotes functional recovery after acute myocardial infarction. *J Am Coll Cardiol.* 2018;72(5):501-514.
14. Flaherty MP, Pant S, Patel SV, et al. Hemodynamic support with a microaxial percutaneous left ventricular assist device (impella) protects against acute kidney injury in patients undergoing high-risk percutaneous coronary intervention. *Circ Res.* 2017;120(4):692-700.
15. Fried JA, Nair A, Takeda K, et al. Clinical and hemodynamic effects of intra-aortic balloon pump therapy in chronic heart failure patients with cardiogenic shock. *J Heart Lung Transpl.* 2018;37(11):1313-1321.
16. Fuchs RM, Brin KP, Brinker JA, Guzman PA, Heuser RR, Yin FC. Augmentation of regional coronary blood flow by intra-aortic balloon counterpulsation in patients with unstable angina. *Circulation.* 1983;68(1):117-123.
17. Garan AR, Takeda K, Salna M, et al. Prospective comparison of a percutaneous ventricular assist device and venoarterial extracorporeal membrane oxygenation for patients with cardiogenic shock following acute myocardial infarction. *J Am Heart Assoc.* 2019;8(9):e012171.
18. Guglin M, Zucker MJ, Bazan VM, et al. Venoarterial ECMO for adults: JACC scientific expert panel. *J Am Coll Cardiol.* 2019;73(6):698-716.
19. Gurbel PA, Anderson RD, MacCord CS, et al. Arterial diastolic pressure augmentation by intra-aortic balloon counterpulsation enhances the onset of coronary artery reperfusion by thrombolytic therapy. *Circulation.* 1994;89(1):361-365.
20. Harjola VP, Lassus J, Sionis A, et al. Clinical picture and risk prediction of short-term mortality in cardiogenic shock. *Eur J Heart Fail.* 2015;17(5):501-509.
21. Hoeper MM, Tudorache I, Kuhn C, et al. Extracorporeal membrane oxygenation watershed. *Circulation.* 2014;130(10):864-865.
22. Ibanez B, James S, Agewall S, et al. 2017 ESC Guidelines for the management of acute myocardial infarction in patients presenting with ST-segment elevation: the task force for the management of acute myocardial infarction in patients presenting with ST-segment elevation of the European Society of Cardiology (ESC). *Eur Heart J.* 2018;39(2):119-177.
23. Iqbal MB, Al-Hussaini A, Rosser G, et al. Intra-aortic balloon pump counterpulsation in the post-resuscitation period is associated with improved functional outcomes in patients surviving an out-of-hospital cardiac arrest: insights from a dedicated heart attack centre. *Heart Lung Circ.* 2016;25(12):1210-1217.
24. Kapur NK, Alkhouli MA, DeMartini TJ, et al. Unloading the left ventricle before reperfusion in patients with anterior ST-segment- elevation myocardial infarction. *Circulation.* 2019;139(3):337-346.
25. Khalid N, Rogers T, Shlofmitz E, et al. Adverse events and modes of failure related to impella RP: insights from the manufacturer and user facility device experience (MAUDE) database. *Cardiovasc Revasc Med.* 2019;20(6):503-506.
26. Londono JC, Martinez CA, Singh V, O'Neill WW. Hemodynamic support with impella 2.5 during balloon aortic valvuloplasty in a high-risk patient. *J Interv Cardiol.* 2011;24(2):193-197.
27. McCabe JC, Abel RM, Subramanian VA, Guy WA Jr. Complications of intra-aortic balloon insertion and counterpulsation. *Circulation.* 1978;57(4):769-773.
28. Millar JE, Fanning JP, McDonald CI, McAuley DF, Fraser JF. The inflammatory response to extracorporeal membrane oxygenation (ECMO): a review of the pathophysiology. *Crit Care.* 2016;20(1):387.
29. Nalluri N, Patel N, Saouma S, et al. Utilization of the Impella for hemodynamic support during percutaneous intervention and cardiogenic shock: an insight. *Expert Rev Med Devices.* 2017;14(10):789-804.
30. O'Neill WW, Kleiman NS, Moses J, et al. A prospective, randomized clinical trial of hemodynamic support with Impella 2.5 versus intra-aortic balloon pump in patients undergoing high-risk percutaneous coronary intervention: the PROTECT II study. *Circulation.* 2012;126(14):1717-1727.

31. O'Neill W, Basir M, Dixon S, Patel K, Schreiber T, Almany S. Feasibility of early mechanical support during mechanical reperfusion of acute myocardial infarct cardiogenic shock. *JACC Cardiovasc Interv*. 2017;10(6):624-625.

32. Ouweneel DM, Eriksen E, Sjauw KD, et al. Percutaneous mechanical circulatory support versus intra-aortic balloon pump in cardiogenic shock after acute myocardial infarction. *J Am Coll Cardiol*. 2017;69(3):278-287.

33. Pappalardo F, Schulte C, Pieri M, et al. Concomitant implantation of Impella® on top of veno-arterial extracorporeal membrane oxygenation may improve survival of patients with cardiogenic shock. *Eur J Heart Fail*. 2017;19(3):404-412.

34. Pappalardo F, Scandroglio AM, Latib A. Full percutaneous biventricular support with two Impella pumps: the Bi-Pella approach. *ESC Heart Fail*. 2018;5(3):368-371.

35. Perera D, Stables R, Thomas M, et al. Elective intra-aortic balloon counterpulsation during high-risk percutaneous coronary intervention: a randomized controlled trial. *J Am Med Assoc*. 2010;304(8):867-874.

36. Pozzi M, Flagiello M, Armoiry X, et al. Extracorporeal life support in the multidisciplinary management of cardiogenic shock complicating acute myocardial infarction. *Catheter Cardiovasc Interv*. 2020;95(3):E71-E77.

37. Ravichandran AK, Baran DA, Stelling K, Cowger JA, Salerno CT. Outcomes with the tandem protek duo dual-lumen percutaneous right ventricular assist device. *ASAIO J*. 2018;64(4):570-572.

38. Rich JD, Burkhoff D. HVAD flow waveform Morphologies: theoretical foundation and implications for clinical practice. *ASAIO J*. 2017;63(5):526-535.

39. Schmack B, Weymann A, Popov AF, et al. Concurrent left ventricular assist device (LVAD) implantation and percutaneous temporary RVAD support via CardiacAssist protek-duo TandemHeart to Preempt Right Heart Failure. *Med Sci Monit Basic Res*. 2016;22:53-57.

40. Schmack B, Farag M, Kremer J, et al. Results of concomitant groin-free percutaneous temporary RVAD support using a centrifugal pump with a double-lumen jugular venous cannula in LVAD patients. *J Thorac Dis*. 2019;11(suppl 6):S913-S920.

41. Schrage B, Ibrahim K, Loehn T, et al. Impella support for acute myocardial infarction complicated by cardiogenic shock. *Circulation*. 2019;139(10):1249-1258.

42. Seyfarth M, Sibbing D, Bauer I, et al. A randomized clinical trial to evaluate the safety and efficacy of a percutaneous left ventricular assist device versus intra-aortic balloon pumping for treatment of cardiogenic shock caused by myocardial infarction. *J Am Coll Cardiol*. 2008;52(19):1584-1588.

43. Shah M, Patnaik S, Patel B, et al. Trends in mechanical circulatory support use and hospital mortality among patients with acute myocardial infarction and non-infarction related cardiogenic shock in the United States. *Clin Res Cardiol*. 2018;107(4):287-303.

44. Sjauw KD, Konorza T, Erbel R, et al. Supported high-risk percutaneous coronary intervention with the Impella 2.5 device the Europella registry. *J Am Coll Cardiol*. 2009;54:2430-2434.

45. Sklar MC, Sy E, Lequier L, Fan E, Kanji HD. Anticoagulation practices during venovenous extracorporeal membrane oxygenation for respiratory failure. A systematic review. *Ann Am Thorac Soc*. 2016;13(12):2242-2250.

46. Strom JB, Zhao Y, Shen C, et al. National trends, predictors of use, and in-hospital outcomes in mechanical circulatory support for cardiogenic shock. *EuroIntervention*. 2018;13(18):e2152-e2159.

47. Suga H. Ventricular energetics. *Physiol Rev*. 1990;70(2):247-277.

48. Sur JP, Pagani FD, Moscucci M. Percutaneous closure of an iatrogenic atrial septal defect. *Catheter Cardiovasc Interv*. 2009;73(2):267-271.

49. Thiele H, Sick P, Boudriot E, et al. Randomized comparison of intraaortic balloon support with a percutaneous left ventricular assist device in patients with revascularized acute myocardial infarction complicated by cardiogenic shock. *Eur Heart J*. 2005;26(13):1276-1283.

50. Thiele H, Zeymer U, Neumann FJ, et al. Intraaortic balloon support for myocardial infarction with cardiogenic shock. *N Engl J Med*. 2012;367(14):1287-1296.

51. Thiele H, Zeymer U, Thelemann N, et al. Intraaortic balloon pump in cardiogenic shock complicating acute myocardial infarction: long-term 6-year outcome of the randomized IABP-SHOCK II trial. *Circulation*. 2019;139(3):395-403.

52. Udesen NJ, Moller JE, Lindholm MG, et al. Rationale and design of DanGer shock: Danish-German cardiogenic shock trial. *Am Heart J*. 2019;214:60-68.

53. Vetrovec GW, Anderson M, Schreiber T, et al. The cVAD registry for percutaneous temporary hemodynamic support: a prospective registry of Impella mechanical circulatory support use in high-risk PCI, cardiogenic shock, and decompensated heart failure. *Am Heart J*. 2018;199:115-121.

25 Percutaneous Balloon Angioplasty and General Percutaneous Coronary Intervention[1]

Dotter and Judkins were the first to propose the concept of transluminal angioplasty—enlargement of the lumen of a stenotic vessel by a catheter—technique in 1964. The concept of "Dottering" vessels involved advancement of a series of progressively larger rigid dilators to dilate atherosclerotic peripheral arterial stenoses, and led to the development of balloons, which through sequential experiments and refinements culminated in the first percutaneous transluminal coronary angioplasty (PTCA) of a stenotic coronary artery performed by Andreas Gruentzig in a conscious human in 1977.

Balloon angioplasty remained the only coronary catheter-based revascularization technique in widespread use until the mid-1990s, when other modalities including atherectomy and stents were introduced, leading to the new concept of "percutaneous coronary intervention" (PCI). As the field has matured, an increasing number of patients undergo coronary intervention at the time of the initial angiogram. Several clinical situations have been responsible for this including the use of PCI for emergent/urgent care for patients presenting with ST-elevation myocardial infarction (STEMI) and non–ST-elevation acute coronary syndromes (NSTACS). The scientific underpinnings for this approach have been obtained in multiple randomized clinical trials (RCTs) and registries and now form the basis for a class 1 indication.

GENERAL PRINCIPLES OF PCI

Although PCI is often performed in an ad hoc fashion, consideration of staging is important in case of the following situations: (1) high anticipated procedural risk or technical complexity making surgical consultation or additional discussions with the patient and family desirable before proceeding with a nonemergency intervention; this is particularly true in patients with severe extensive multivessel disease and left ventricular dysfunction in whom coronary artery bypass graft (CABG) surgery is generally indicated as the treatment of choice; (2) the likelihood of the combined procedure leading to a large volume of contrast being used. Similar considerations apply to the decision to stage a complex multivessel procedure into 2 or more sessions (eg, patient tolerance, clinical stability, total contrast load, stability of the initial treatment results). This is of particular importance in patients with abnormal baseline renal function, or in patients who may have received preprocedural CT studies with contrast; (3) a consideration in staging for patients with multivessel disease who presented with either STEMI or non–ST-elevation myocardial infarction (NSTEMI). The timing of staged procedures in these patients has important clinical and reimbursement considerations; (4) counseling patients who are unwilling or unable to comply with the recommended duration of DAPT (dual antiplatelet therapy) following stent implantation, and especially drug-eluting stents (DESs), on the risks and benefits of DAPT and alternative therapies.

[1]We gratefully acknowledge the Grossman & Baim's *Cardiac Catheterization, Angiography, and Intervention*, 9th edition contributions of Drs Abhiram Prasad and David R. Holmes as portions of their chapter, "Percutaneous Balloon Angioplasty and General Coronary Intervention," were retained in this text.

Oral intake should be restricted after midnight on the evening prior to the procedure, and the patient should be pretreated with *aspirin* 325 mg/d and loaded with an adenosine diphosphate (ADP)-receptor antagonist unless there is clinical suspicion that the patient may require surgical intervention. In the aspirin-allergic patient requiring an elective PCI, a graded aspirin desensitization protocol may be considered prior to the procedure. An oral platelet ADP-receptor antagonist (such as clopidogrel, prasugrel, ticagrelor) should generally be administered prior to the procedure. This may require supplemental intravenous platelet glycoprotein IIb/IIIa receptor antagonists in patients with a large thrombus burden. Since aspirin reduces late cardiac mortality in patients with documented coronary disease, it is generally continued indefinitely after the procedure. Similar data now exist for longer-term clopidogrel treatment, and hence ADP-receptor antagonists may be used as an alternative to aspirin in patients with aspirin allergy. Statins appear to have some benefits when pretreatment is initiated from 7 days to just prior to PCI, especially in statin-naive patients. Hence, it is reasonable to administer a high dose of statin before PCI to reduce the risk of periprocedural myocardial infarction (MI).

Patients with a past history of a hypersensitivity reaction to contrast media should receive steroid and antihistamine prophylaxis; this prophylaxis is not beneficial in patients with a prior history of allergic reactions to shellfish or seafood. Finally, patients should be assessed for risk of contrast-induced acute kidney injury (nephropathy), and those identified at increased risk should be managed accordingly with preprocedure hydration and minimization of contrast dose (see Chapter 4).

Vascular access site complications have been found to result in increased morbidity and even mortality. The most important change has been the movement to use radial access. This has been studied in several randomized clinical trials and found to be associated with less vascular access bleeding, fewer transfusions, and a reduction in longer-term mortality. It is the access of choice for both diagnostic angiography and PCI. While both right and left radial arteries can be used, the right side is preferred. In patients who have previously undergone CABG with a left internal mammary artery (LIMA) graft, left radial access is preferred. For a detailed description of radial artery access, our readers are referred to Chapter 7.

There are clinical circumstances where femoral access is optimal including the use of larger sheaths for complex interventions. In these circumstances, micropuncture needle access and the use of fluoroscopic and/or preferably ultrasound guidance are essential to minimize complications such as femoral hematoma and pseudoaneurysm formation from a low puncture or retroperitoneal hemorrhage from a high puncture. A number of femoral vascular closure devices are available, each of which has its own specific potential complications and require specific expertise (Chapter 8).

After placement of the arterial sheath, intravenous antithrombin therapy is initiated. The most common agent is unfractionated heparin (70-100 U/kg), which may be reduced to 50 to 70 U/kg when there is concomitant administration of a platelet glycoprotein IIb/IIIa receptor antagonist. Alternatives include low-molecular-weight heparin (eg, enoxaparin) in patients who have been on such agents preprocedure or a direct thrombin antagonist (eg, bivalirudin [Angiomax], The Medicines Company). If unfractionated heparin is used, there is wide patient-to-patient variability in heparin binding and activity. So, ACT (activated clotting time) should be measured and additional heparin administered as needed to prolong the ACT to 250 to 300 seconds (reduced to 200 seconds if a platelet glycoprotein IIb/IIIa receptor blocker is to be given) before any angioplasty devices are introduced. Additional doses or an infusion of the antithrombotic agent may be required to maintain the ACT at this level throughout the case—ACTs <250 seconds are associated with an increase in the incidence of occlusive complications, whereas ACTs >300 to 350 seconds tend to increase the risk of bleeding. ACTs may also be used to monitor the effect of direct thrombin inhibitors such as bivalirudin. After an initial enthusiasm for the use of direct thrombin inhibitors, subsequent randomized controlled trials have not been overwhelmingly positive. In addition, a signal for early stent thrombosis has been reported. Low-molecular-weight heparin has relatively more activity against factor Xa than against thrombin; it causes less prolongation of the ACT so that specialized anti-Xa assays are required to monitor low-molecular-weight heparin effects.

EQUIPMENT

A PCI system consists of 3 basic components: (1) a guiding catheter, which provides access to the coronary ostium, a route for contrast administration, and a conduit for the advancement of the equipment; (2) a guidewire that can be passed through the guiding catheter, across the target lesion into the distal coronary vasculature to provide a rail over which devices can be advanced; and (3) the therapeutic devices (ie, balloon/stent/atherectomy catheter).

Guiding Catheters

To allow passage of therapeutic instruments, guiding catheters must have a lumen diameter at least twice that of a typical diagnostic catheter (eg, 0.076 in [2 mm] vs 0.038 in [1 mm]). To achieve this lumen in a catheter of outer diameter as small as 5F to 6F, the catheter walls must be very thin (<0.12 mm, or 0.005 in). Yet the catheter must still incorporate a Teflon liner to reduce friction, metal or plastic braid to transmit torque and provide sufficient stiffness to offer backup support during device advancement, and a smooth outer coating to resist thrombus formation. The complexity of this design requires use of special materials, the properties of which are typically varied along the length of the catheter to optimize the balance between support and flexibility at each point. Guiding catheters also include a very soft material in the most distal 2 mm of the catheter to reduce the risk of coronary dissection during engagement. They are available in virtually all of the conventional Judkins, multipurpose, and Amplatz curves, as well as a wide range of custom shapes (extra backup [XB, EBU], hockey stick, etc.) designed to ease engagement or provide better support during balloon advancement. Although most PCI procedures today are performed with 6F catheters, larger guiding catheters are sometimes still needed for rotational atherectomy, or treatment of bifurcation lesions (7F for kissing balloons and 8F for 2 stents) or chronic total occlusions (CTOs). 6F catheters can be readily used via radial access, although spasm may limit the ability to torque them. In that setting, 5F guiding catheters are available, though opacification is less optimal. From the radial approach, sheathless guides are available that have an outer diameter similar to a 6F sheath but an inner diameter comparable to a conventional 7F guide.

To function adequately, the guiding catheter must be able to selectively engage the ostium. This requires the selection of an appropriate catheter shape and the ability to manipulate the catheter under fluoroscopic guidance. Engagement of the desired vessel, however, should not interfere with arterial inflow. This is generally possible in the left coronary artery unless there is left main coronary disease, which may manifest itself as catheter damping. Identification of damping with engagement of the left main coronary artery mandates careful evaluation that includes reintubation, use of a different catheter to optimize coaxial placement, or intravascular ultrasound (IVUS) to document the underlying anatomy. Damping of the guiding catheter pressure is more common with engagement of the right coronary artery. This can be mitigated by changing the guiding catheter or changing its access plane. A second important function of the guiding catheter is to provide adequate support for advancement of interventional devices across the target stenosis. This support is derived from the intrinsic stiffness of the guiding catheter, the shape that allows it to buttress against the opposite aortic wall, and if needed, deep engagement of the guiding catheter into the coronary ostium (**Figure 25.1**).

While deep engagement of the guiding catheter is sometimes required in challenging cases, it is also well recognized as a potential cause of ostial or proximal coronary dissection. This complication has become less frequent with incorporation of an atraumatic tip on guiding catheters and by relying on coaxial advancement of the guiding catheter over the balloon catheter during deep engagement. After a deeply engaged guiding catheter has been used to position a dilatation balloon or other device across the lesion, it is important to then withdraw the guiding catheter back to avoid its migration into an even deeper position as the device is withdrawn. Development of guide extension devices (eg, GuideLiner [**Figure 25.2**] [Vascular Solutions Inc], TrapLiner [Vascular Solutions], Guidezilla [Boston Scientific], Guidion [IMDS]) has reduced the need for deep engagement. These devices are a major step forward in improving support in difficult lesion subsets (ie, tortuous and calcified).

Guidewires

The original dilatation balloon designed by Gruentzig had a short, fixed segment of guidewire (spring coil) attached to its tip to lead the balloon in the vessel lumen and help avoid subintimal passage as the catheter was advanced across the stenosis. However, neither the shape nor the orientation of the leading wire could be modified. In the early 1980s, Simpson designed a *movable* guidewire system in which a 0.018 in Teflon-coated wire extended and moved freely through a central lumen within a coaxial dilatation catheter. If this guidewire selected the desired vessel, it was advanced until it crossed the target lesion. If the guidewire instead selected a more proximal side branch, the balloon catheter was advanced to a point just before the side branch and the wire was withdrawn and reshaped in an effort to choose the desired path beyond.

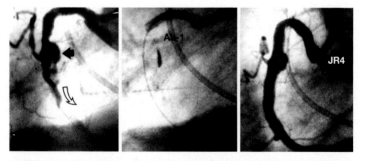

Figure 25.1 Use of deep guiding catheter engagement to facilitate coronary intervention. Left. Complex lesion in the right coronary artery including aneurysm (dark arrow) and diffuse distal disease (open curved arrow). Center. Left Amplatz guiding catheter (AL-1) is deeply engaged to provide optimal support for stent placement. Right. After stent placement, the vessel is widely patent, but replacement of the Amplatz catheter with a conventional right Judkins catheter (JR4) shows how effective the Amplatz has been in straightening out a severe upward bend (shepherd's hook) in the proximal right coronary artery. Deep seating of the guiding catheter needs to be done with great care and by coaxial advancement of the guiding catheter over a balloon catheter to avoid injuring the proximal coronary artery.

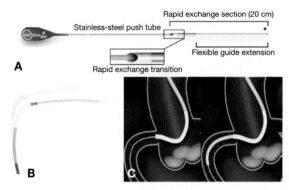

Figure 25.2 Schematic presentation of the GuideLiner catheter **(A)** and **(B)**. **C,** The GuideLiner has been advanced to the mid right coronary artery over a guidewire.
(Reproduced with permission from Burzotta F, Trani C, Mazzari MA, et al. Use of a second buddy wire during percutaneous coronary interventions: a simple solution for some challenging situations. *J Invasive Cardiol.* 2005;17:171-174.)

Modern guidewires (0.014 in diameter) are designed to combine tip softness, trackability around curves, radiographic visibility, and precise torque control. There is a distal tip taper helps retain torque control when the wire is steered around the series of bends located in the guiding catheter and proximal coronary anatomy and allows the stiffer proximal portions of the wire to follow the soft tip into side branches. This core is generally covered by a spring coil, and a coating (eg, Teflon, silicone) is applied to the body of the wire. Radiopaque platinum is often applied to the distal 3 to 25 cm. A family of hydrophilic polymer-covered tip guidewires is also available to aid in crossing vessels with extreme tortuosity, calcification, side branches through stent struts, and total occlusions. It must be remembered that hydrophilic wires allow reduced tactile feel and are more likely to cause dissections or perforations.

There is substantial choice of tip stiffness, driven by the way the tapered core wire is attached to the outer coil at the wire tip. In soft wires, the tapered core is generally welded to the coil via a flattened intermediary shaping ribbon that allows the operator to kink or bend the tip of the wire into a shape that is appropriate for navigating the vessel features. When larger probing force is required (eg, for crossing a CTO), stiffer tip designs are available. These "core-to-tip" guidewires are often graded by the force that the straight guidewire tip can apply to a strain gauge. Wires are available with force increments of 3, 4.5, 6, 9, and 12 g. The core-to-tip design also provides better torque control. Use of these stiff-tip guidewires requires a high degree of skill and feel to avoid unintentional vessel injury (dissection or perforation). Less stiff but more maneuverable CTO wires (Gaia, Asahi Intecc) have been developed using a composite-core, dual-coil construction, which enhances torque control and hence wiring of long tortuous occlusions.

Advancing certain devices around bends may require more shaft support from the guidewire. This is provided by extrasupport wires, which have a thicker and firmer inner core. Alternatively, some operators prefer to place a second guidewire across the lesion in parallel (a "buddy" wire) to straighten vessel bends and facilitate device passage. Some specialty CTO guidewires have a tapered tip (0.009-0.012) to help penetrate the plaque and find microchannels.

Standard coronary guidewires are approximately 190 cm long, approximately 50 cm longer than the average balloon catheter shaft. This allows the wire to be advanced across the lesion while the balloon catheter remains in the guiding catheter but does not offer sufficient length for exchange of one "over-the-wire" (OTW) device for another. Most guidewires are also available in a 300 cm exchange length. Such wires can be advanced across the target lesion and remain in place as a series of OTW devices (balloons, rotational atherectomy burrs, stents) are delivered or removed without the need for recrossing the lesion. OTW devices have largely been replaced by rapid-exchange (Rx) or monorail balloon catheters and stent delivery systems compatible with shorter guidewires.

Dilatation Catheters

An important characteristic of PTCA balloons is the diameter of the smallest opening through which the deflated balloon can be passed (its profile)—current balloons have profiles as small as 0.5 mm. To preserve the best balloon profile, a negative aspiration preparation should be performed in which a contrast-filled syringe is attached to the balloon inflation hub, the plunger is pulled back to apply a vacuum, and gently released to allow the balloon to draw in a small volume of 1:2 dilution saline-contrast. The crossing profile increases significantly after a balloon is used, as rewrapping of the balloon following deflation is suboptimal. This is particularly an issue with noncompliant high-pressure balloons.

PTCA balloons are available either as OTW catheters in which the guidewire runs through a central lumen in the shaft throughout its entire length or as monorail Rx catheters in which the wire is contained within the balloon shaft only over its distal 25 cm and then runs outside the balloon shaft more proximally. The latter type of catheters can be exchanged quickly by a single operator over a standard-length (190 cm) guidewire and generally have smaller shaft profiles, which allows better contrast injection and simultaneous placement of 2 balloons for the treatment of bifurcation lesions.

Although profile is important, the ability of the balloon to advance easily through tortuous vascular segments (trackability) and the presence of sufficient shaft stiffness (pushability) to force it through the stenosis are important. Delivery of the balloon is also aided by the incorporation of a friction-resistant coating to improve surface lubricity. Some special balloons exploit the concept of focused force angioplasty, in which a wire (AngioSculpt balloon, Philips), microblades (Cutting balloon, Boston Scientific, Natick, MA), or nitinol caging structure that creates pillows and grooves on the balloon surface (Chocolate XD Balloon [Teleflex]) concentrate the delivery of dilating force from the balloon to the lesion and reduce balloon slippage during inflation (the so-called watermelon seeding effect). These technologies have not, however, improved the long-term patency as compared with conventional PTCA.

An important characteristic of PTCA balloons is their ability to inflate to a precisely defined diameter despite application of pressures that average 10 to 16 atm. This can be readily achieved using balloons manufactured from high-density polyethylene, polyethylene terephthalate (PET), or nylon, despite balloon wall thicknesses as low as 7.6212.7 µm. Based on material and wall thickness, each balloon has a compliance characteristic reflecting the pressure at which the balloon reaches its specified (nominal) diameter and how much that diameter increases as the balloon is inflated to even higher pressures. More compliant balloon materials tend to reach their nominal diameter at 6 atm and then grow by <20% above their nominal size (ie, a 3.0 mm balloon growing to 3.5 mm) at 10 atm. Semicompliant balloon materials such as high-density polyethylene or nylon grow by <10% over this pressure range, whereas truly noncompliant balloon materials such as PET can retain their defined diameter up to 20 atm to allow dilatation of calcific stenoses or full expansion of coronary stents (**Figure 25.3**). Ultrahigh-pressure balloons are available for the treatment of severely calcified or fibrotic lesions (OPN NC [SIS Medical]). These PTCA balloons have a twin-layer construction with uniform expansion and a rated burst pressure up to 35 atm. They are bulky and suitable for expanding proximally located lesions or underexpanded stents.

Regardless of which balloon type is used, it is important to stay within the stated range of inflation pressures in order to avoid balloon rupture. This pressure range is specified in terms of the rated burst pressure (ie, an inflation pressure at which the probability of balloon rupture is <0.1%). Taking any balloon above its rated burst pressure (usually 16-20 atm) increases the risk of balloon rupture, with the potential for vessel rupture, local dissection, or difficulty in removing the balloon from an incompletely dilated lesion. Instead of relying solely on high balloon inflation pressures, we recommend the use of rotational atherectomy or electric lithotripsy for treating resistant lesions that are invariably associated with severe calcification.

PROCEDURE

Typically balloon dilation is not used as the definitive procedure, relying instead on stent placement. In the occasional patients in whom stand-alone angioplasty is selected, optimal results are obtained using a balloon with a diameter that closely approximates the diameter of a presumably nondiseased reference segment adjacent to the site being treated (balloon-artery ratio 0.9:1.1). Slightly larger balloons (approximately 1.1-1.2 times the size of the reference lumen) may be used if IVUS

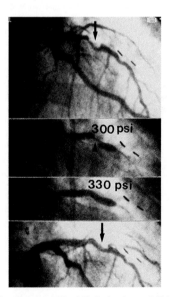

Figure 25.3 Successful dilatation of a rigid calcific lesion (arrows). This rigid lesion (top) in the mid left anterior descending coronary artery of a postbypass patient resisted dilatation at 300 lb/in (20 atm) (arrowhead), but yielded to an inflation pressure of 330 lb/in (22 atm; middle 2 views) with reduction in the stenosis (bottom). Such pressures are obtainable only with high-pressure noncompliant balloons.

shows that the vessel (external elastic membrane [EEM]) diameter in the reference segment is significantly larger than the reference lumen—positive remodeling. On the other hand, slightly smaller initial balloons are used when it is difficult to estimate the correct reference size, when difficulty is anticipated in crossing the lesion, or if the risk of complications must be minimized in a patient who cannot receive a stent. It is routine to predilate the target lesion with a balloon that is slightly undersized relative to the reference vessel and roughly the same length as the target lesion. While modern low-profile stents can often be delivered without predilation of the target lesion (direct stenting) provided that there is minimal calcification, predilation makes delivery and accurate placement of the stent within the lesion easier, facilitates the selection of the correct stent diameter and length, and ensures that lesion compliance is sufficient to allow full expansion of the stent without pretreatment by rotational atherectomy. Predilation is particularly important if a short stent is used, to avoid "geographic mismatch."

Once the dilatation catheter has been positioned within the target stenosis, the balloon is inflated progressively using a screw-powered handheld inflation device equipped with a pressure dial. At low pressures (ie, 2-4 atm), the balloon typically exhibits an hourglass appearance owing to central constriction by the coronary stenosis being treated. In soft lesions, this constriction (or "waist") may expand gradually as the inflation pressure is increased, allowing the balloon to assume its full cylindrical shape. In more rigid lesions, the constriction may remain prominent until the balloon expands abruptly at a stenosis resolution pressure that may be as high as 20 atm. If a calcified plaque resists balloon expansion at >16 atm, one may prefer to use rotational atherectomy or focused force cutting/scoring balloons rather than inflating the balloon to the very high pressures (>20 atm; **Figure 25.3**). Electric lithotripsy balloons (Shockwave Medical Inc.) have proven benefit at treating calcified lesions. They result in circumferential plaque modification by delivering acoustic pulses through a balloon inflated at low pressures.

The response of each lesion to balloon dilation must then be assessed individually. The most common way to assess lesion response to balloon dilation is repeat angiography. A typical result of even a successful angioplasty is approximately 30% residual diameter stenosis (ie, a 1.9 mm lumen in a 3 mm vessel) with some degree of intimal disruption (reflected as localized haziness, filling defect, or dissection). Although this once created a dilemma about whether to persist with additional balloon inflations (weighed against the risk of creating a vessel dissection), the need to obtain a perfect result with balloon angioplasty is now moot in the stent era—any lesion that can be stented is generally stented. In the current view, the best position for standalone balloon angioplasty is thus in lesions that are poorly suited to stenting owing to vessel size below 2 mm or branch ostial disease where bifurcation stenting is not contemplated. One exception is the development of drug-coated balloons to treat in-stent restenosis and small-caliber arteries. The balloons are semicompliant, coated with antiproliferative agents that are released locally into the intima during balloon inflation.

Given the importance of achieving the optimal acute angiographic result, if there is uncertainty based on angiographic assessment, a number of techniques are available to determine the quality of PCI result. Intravascular imaging is preferred with either IVUS or optical coherence tomography (OCT) because they can more accurately measure vessel/stent lumen diameter and cross-sectional area and detect vessel dissection or hematoma. Alternatively, 0.014 in pressure-measuring guidewires may be used to measure trans-stenotic gradient at baseline flow and during maximal hyperemia. The goal is to achieve a fractional flow reserve (FFR)—defined as the ratio of distal mean coronary pressure to aortic mean pressure during adenosine-induced hyperemia—of >0.95 in a successful PCI. Although IVUS/OCT/ FFR provide important mechanistic insights into balloon angioplasty, they are used in <10% of cases because of the added procedural time and expense. In most laboratories, the postdilation angiogram remains the gold standard to assess whether or not an adequate result has been obtained.

Once adequate dilatation is deemed to have been achieved, with PTCA alone, it is standard practice to withdraw the balloon completely from the guiding catheter, leaving the guidewire across the dilated segment to allow observation of the treated vessel for signs of angiographic deterioration for 10 minutes. With more predictable interventions such as stenting, however, a single set of postprocedure angiograms in orthogonal views with the guidewire removed is usually sufficient to document a suitable result.

POSTPROCEDURE MANAGEMENT

Postprocedural coronary complications are infrequent such that the sheath can be removed and manual compression applied when the ACT is <180 seconds in patients treated with unfractionated heparin. For bivalirudin, sheath removal and manual compression can occur at 2 hours post cessation of infusion in patients with normal renal function. In patients with a creatinine clearance <30 mL/min or those on dialysis, ACT should be checked and sheaths removed once the ACT is <180 seconds.

Ambulation is allowed 2 to 6 hours following manual compression hemostasis, depending on sheath size, and recurrent bleeding. In fact, with the wide adoption of radial access and femoral vascular closure devices it is common to remove the arterial sheath in the catheterization laboratory at the end of the interventional procedure, despite a fully anticoagulated state, allowing earlier ambulation 1 to 4 hours after removal. Increasingly, same-day discharge is being adopted in non–high-risk elective PCI, as it improves patient satisfaction and reduces costs.

Aspirin (81-325 mg/d) is continued indefinitely, and patients who have received a stent are given clopidogrel 600 mg (or prasugrel 60 mg, ticagrelor 180 mg) as a loading dose (300 mg with fibrinolytics) during or prior to the procedure. If ticagrelor is used, typically the dose of aspirin is reduced. The duration of DAPT varies depending on type of stent, technical factors (left main or bifurcation stenting), clinical factors (stable vs acute coronary syndrome), and the potential risk of bleeding. Patients should be counseled on the importance of compliance with DAPT and that therapy should not be discontinued without consultation with their cardiologist. Proton pump inhibitors should be used in patients with a history of prior gastrointestinal bleeding who require DAPT, and it is reasonable to prescribe those for patients at increased risk for bleeding. If the risk from bleeding outweighs the potential benefit of the recommended duration of DAPT, earlier discontinuation is reasonable.

MECHANISM OF PERCUTANEOUS TRANSLUMINAL CORONARY ANGIOPLASTY

Plaque compression accounts for a minority of the observed improvement in stenosis severity. Extrusion of liquid components from the plaque does permit some compression of soft plaques but contributes minimally to improvement in more fibrotic lesions. Most of the luminal improvement following PTCA seems to result from plaque redistribution—like footprints in wet sand. Some of this takes place by longitudinal displacement of plaque upstream and downstream from the lesion. The concept of geographic miss is important in this regard. While the position of the balloon can be captured radiographically, the stent may not cover the regions at the edges of the predilation balloon treatment site. Edge dissections and plaque shift may be mechanisms for restenosis. Maximum improvement in the lumen following balloon angioplasty or stenting results from stretching leading to fracture of the intimal plaque and partial disruption of the media and adventitia, with consequent enlargement of both the lumen and the overall outer diameter of the vessel (**Figure 25.4**).

Although use of a full-sized balloon (balloon-artery ratio of 1:1) should theoretically eliminate all narrowing at the treatment site, the overstretched vessel wall invariably exhibits elastic recoil following balloon deflation and some degree of local vasospasm. These processes typically leave the stretched vessel with a residual stenosis. A typical balloon angioplasty result also shows evidence of localized trauma to more superficial plaque components as an almost universal haziness of the lumen. Higher degrees of disruption are reflected by intimal filling defects (**Figure 25.5**), contrast caps outside the vessel lumen, or spiral dissections that may interfere with antegrade blood flow. Such local disruption has been seen on IVUS, angioscopy, and histologic examination of postmortem angioplasty specimens, and its extent correlates with the risk of an occlusive complication. In contrast, stenting or directional atherectomy reduces or even eliminates this elastic recoil, dissection, and vascular tone and thereby provides lower (0%-10% rather than 30%) postprocedural residual stenosis and a smooth and uniform lumen by angiography or IVUS, with less chance of acute closure.

There is good evidence that subclinical distal atheroembolization during balloon angioplasty and stent placement occurs frequently. This is most clearly established in patients undergoing dilatation of a saphenous vein bypass graft or patients with large thrombi adherent to the lesion. Distal embolization of large (>1 mm) plaque elements is usually manifest as an abrupt cutoff of flow in the embolized distal vessel. In contrast, microembolization of plaque debris or adherent thrombus may contribute to post-procedure chest pain, enzyme elevation, or the no-reflow phenomenon in which there is dramatic reduction in antegrade flow with manifestations of severe ischemia (chest pain and ST-segment elevation), in the absence of epicardial vessel stenosis, dissection, or macroembolic cutoff. No-reflow can usually be improved by distal intracoronary injection of an arterial vasodilator (adenosine 12-60 μg; nitroprusside 100 μg;

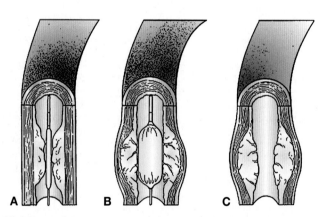

Figure 25.4 Proposed mechanism of angioplasty. **A,** Deflated balloon positioned across stenosis. **B,** Inflation of the balloon catheter within the stenotic segment causes cracking of the intimal plaque, stretching of the media and adventitia, and expansion of the outer diameter of the vessel. **C,** Following balloon deflation, there is partial elastic recoil of the vessel wall, leaving a residual stenosis and local plaque disruption that would be evident as haziness of the lumen contours on angiography.

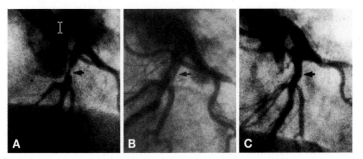

Figure 25.5 Normal healing of percutaneous transluminal coronary angioplasty (PTCA)-related coronary dissection. As compared with the baseline angiogram **(A)**, the immediate post-PTCA angiogram **(B)** shows enlargement of the left anterior descending (LAD) artery lumen with 2 small filling defects typical of an uncomplicated coronary dissection (arrows). Follow-up angiogram 3 mo later **(C)** shows preservation of luminal caliber with complete healing of the localized dissection (arrow). (Republished by permission of McGraw-Hill, from Baim DS. Percutaneous transluminal coronary angioplasty. In: Braunwald E, ed. *Harrison's Principles of Internal Medicine: Update VI.* McGraw-Hill; 1985.)

verapamil 100 µg; diltiazem 250 µg; nicardipine 200 µg—but not nitroglycerin, which has a greater effect on epicardial arteries). But such treatment does not prevent periprocedural MI. In contrast, the use of a distal embolic protection system in vein graft interventions recovers atheroembolic debris and reduces the incidence of these complications by nearly half. The SAFER trial of vein graft stenting thus showed that such enzyme elevations occurred in 17% of lesions, with evidence of no-reflow in 8% of lesions, which were reduced to 9.7% and 3.3%, respectively, through the use of distal embolic protection. Similar benefits have now been seen with distal embolic filter devices and in carotids. However, a recent meta-analysis has shown that the benefits of SVG distal protection are less in the current era, due to preloading of P2Y12 inhibitors and undersizing of stents, and the US guideline recommendation has been lowered from 1 to 2a. In addition, embolic protection devices have not been shown to improve outcomes in native coronary arteries but are selectively used by some interventionists in the presence of a large thrombus burden at the site of the culprit lesion.

COMPLICATIONS

The larger caliber guiding catheter used for angioplasty is more likely to result in damage to the proximal coronary artery and cause local bleeding complications at the catheter introduction site. Selective advancement of guidewires and balloons into diseased coronary arteries may lead to vessel injury if they are manipulated too aggressively.

The risk of in-hospital mortality is driven mostly by clinical factors such as age, cardiogenic shock, congestive heart failure, renal failure, and urgent or emergency PCI. An example of a contemporary risk model for the probability of cardiovascular complications from PCI using clinical variables is shown in **Figure 25.6**. Procedure success and overall complications, however, tend to be driven by lesion-related features. The original American Heart Association (AHA)/American College of Cardiology (ACC) type A, B, and C lesion categorization (**Table 25.1**) was modified by Ellis to discriminate between B1 and B2 lesions (ie, those with 1 or more than 1 B characteristic), but the continued validity of this classification scheme has come into question

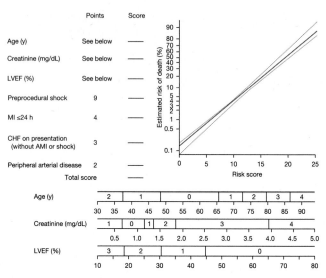

Figure 25.6 New Mayo Clinic risk model for prediction of in-hospital death. The coefficients for age, left ventricular ejection fraction (LVEF), and serum creatinine level can be determined from the nomograms at the bottom. Note that congestive heart failure (CHF) needs to be entered only for patients not presenting with myocardial infarction (MI) or shock. If LVEF is unavailable, enter 1 for the LVEF contribution if the patient presents with CHF; enter 0 otherwise. If serum creatinine level is unavailable, enter 1 for the creatinine contribution if the patient is a man presenting with CHF; enter 0 otherwise. (From Singh M, Rihal CS, Lennon RJ, Spertus J, Rumsfeld JS, Holmes DR Jr.. Bedside estimation of risk from percutaneous coronary intervention: the new Mayo Clinic risk scores. *Mayo Clin Proc.* 2007;82(6):701-708, with permission.)

in the stent era. The Society for Cardiovascular Angiography & Interventions has thus proposed a simplification into 4 risk categories (based on whether or not the lesion has a type C feature and whether it is patent or occluded). This offers a somewhat better predictive value for both procedural success and major complications (death, MI, emergency surgery, or emergency repeat angioplasty) and shows the potent effect of stenting in reducing those complications across the board (**Figure 25.7**).

Periprocedural Myocardial Infarction

The Fourth Universal Definition of Myocardial Infarction defines PCI-related injury (type 4a) as an elevation of cardiac troponin T (cTn) values more than 5 times the 99th percentile upper reference limit (URL) within 48 hours in patients with normal baseline values. In patients with elevated preprocedure cTn in whom the cTn level are stable (<20% variation) or falling, the postprocedure cTn must rise by >20% and >5 × 99th percentile URL. In addition, one of the following elements is required: (1) new ischemic ECG changes, (2) development of new pathological Q waves, (3) imaging evidence of new loss of viable myocardium or new regional wall motion abnormality in a pattern consistent with an ischemic etiology, and (4) angiographic or postmortem findings consistent with a procedural flow-limiting complication such as coronary dissection, occlusion of a major epicardial artery or a side branch occlusion/thrombus, disruption of collateral flow, or distal embolization. The definition is

Table 25.1 **Lesion Morphologic Predictors of Procedure Success and Complication Based on the AHA/ACC Lesion Classification System**

Characteristics of Type A, B1, B2, and C Lesions
Type A lesions (high success, >85%; low risk)
Discrete (<10 mm length)
Concentric
Readily accessible
Nonangulated segment <45°
Smooth contour
Little or no calcification
Less than totally occlusive
Not ostial in location
No major branch involvement
Absence of thrombus
Type B1 Lesions (Moderate Success, 60%-85%; Moderate Risk)
Tubular (10-20 mm length)
Eccentric
Moderate tortuosity of proximal segment
Moderately angulated segment, 45°-90°
Irregular contour
Moderate to heavy calcification
Ostial in location
Bifurcation lesions requiring double guidewires
Some thrombus present
Total occlusion <3 mo old
Type B2 Lesions (Ellis modification of AHA/ACC System)
Two or more type B characteristics
Type C Lesions (Low Success, <60%; High Risk)

(Continued)

Table 25.1	Lesion Morphologic Predictors of Procedure Success and Complication Based on the AHA/ACC Lesion Classification System (Continued)
Characteristics of Type A, B1, B2, and C Lesions	
Diffuse (>2 cm length)	
Excessive tortuosity of proximal segment	
Extremely angulated segment >90°	
Inability to protect major side branches	
Degenerated vein grafts with friable lesions	
Total occlusion >3 mo old	

ACC, American College of Cardiology; AHA, American Heart Association.

supported by studies correlating the magnitude of biomarker elevation to the extent of irreversible injury in the myocardium on magnetic resonance imaging and to worse in-hospital and long-term outcomes. However, there is considerable evidence to suggest that in the majority of cases, the periprocedural infarction is a reflection of increased preprocedural risk (atherosclerosis burden and disease acuity), and hence, the clinical significance of such periprocedural MI and its management remain a matter of considerable controversy and uncertainty.

Two measurements of post-PCI cTn level, starting 2 to 6 hours after PCI and separated by 2 to 6 hours, may be considered in patients with procedural complications (eg, large side-branch occlusion, flow-limiting dissection, no-reflow phenomenon, or coronary thrombosis), as well as in those who have symptoms, signs, or electrocardiographic evidence of myocardial ischemia, in order to quantify the extent of myocardial injury. The current PCI guidelines do not recommend routine measurement of periprocedural biomarkers in patients with uncomplicated successful PCI. It is unlikely that clinically relevant additional information can be gained in these patients, independent of preprocedural risk. Large periprocedural MI is likely at cTn levels 20 to 40× upper limit of normal, CK-MB (creatine kinase, myocardial band) elevation of >5× the upper reference limit and/or new Q-waves identify patients with extensive injury. These patients should be monitored in the hospital for an additional period of time because of an increased risk of arrhythmias, hemodynamic instability, heart failure, and death.

Coronary Artery Dissection

Although plaque disruption and dissection may be caused by the guiding catheter or overly vigorous attempts to pass the guidewire through a tortuous stenotic lumen, most dissections are actually the by-product of the "controlled injury" induced intentionally by inflation of the dilatation balloon. When these dissections are small and do not interfere with antegrade flow in the distal vessel, they have no clinical consequence. Follow-up angiography as soon as 3 weeks after the angioplasty procedure usually demonstrates complete healing of the dissected segment (see **Figure 25.5**), although occasional localized formation of aneurysms has been described at the site of dissection. Clinically significant dissections in contemporary stent-based PCI are generally seen at either the proximal or the distal stent edge. These can be managed

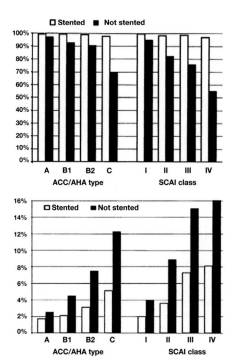

Figure 25.7 Lesion risk scores. Top. The probability of success by AHA type lesion (left) and the new SCAI class (right), treated with (open bars) and without (closed bars) coronary stenting. Bottom. The probability of a major complication based on AHA lesion type (left) and the new SCAI class (right), treated with (open bars) and without (closed bars) coronary stenting. The SCAI score, based simply on whether the vessel has 1 or more type C characteristics and is open or occluded, has a stronger predictive value for success and complications than that of the traditional AHA/ACC score. The beneficial effect of stenting on complications is evident (see also **Table 25.3**). ACC, American College of Cardiology; AHA, American Heart Association; SCAI, Society for Cardiovascular Angiography & Interventions. (From Krone RJ, Shaw RE, Klein LW, et al. Evaluation of the American College of Cardiology/American Heart Association and the Society for Coronary Angiography and Interventions lesion classification system in the current "stent era" of coronary interventions from the ACC- National Cardiovascular Data Registry. *Am J Cardiol.* 2003;92:389-394, with permission.)

conservatively if minor but may require treatment with a stent if abrupt closure is considered to be a possibility. Guide-induced dissections remain an infrequent but serious complication, generally occur in complex interventions, and invariably need to be treated with a stent.

Abrupt Closure

Prior to the widespread use of stents, large progressive dissections interfered with ante-grade flow and led to total occlusion of the dilated segment (known as abrupt closure). With balloon angioplasty alone, abrupt closure occurred in roughly 5% of patients as the result of compression of the true lumen by the dissection flap, with superimposed thrombus formation, platelet adhesion, or vessel spasm. Most abrupt closures after stand-alone balloon angioplasty developed within minutes of the final balloon inflation, so it became routine practice to observe the lesion for 10 minutes after the last balloon inflation, before leaving the catheterization laboratory.

Before 1985, most patients who experienced abrupt closure of a major epicardial coronary artery went directly to emergency surgery, in an effort to minimize the amount of consequent myocardial damage. The rate of emergency surgery was thus 5% to 6%, and even with emergency surgery within 90 minutes of the onset of vessel occlusion, up to 50% of patients sustained a Q-wave MI. The development of perfusion catheters—angioplasty balloons with multiple side holes along their distal shaft to allow 40 to 60 mL/min of blood to flow through the central lumen, and exit into the lumen distal to the point of occlusion—allowed patients to go to the operating room in a nonischemic state (**Figure 25.8**) and was shown to reduce the incidence of transmural infarction during emergency surgery to approximately 10%. Once it was realized that many abrupt closures can be reversed by simply readvancing the balloon dilatation catheter across the lesion to "tack up" the dissection via repeated balloon inflation, the emergency surgery rate fell in half to roughly 3%. Since 1993, the availability of coronary stents has made the certainty of reversing abrupt closure >90%, and with elective stenting, this problem has been largely eliminated.

It is clear that platelet-rich clots contribute significantly to abrupt closure. The role of thrombus in abrupt closure is further supported by an increased risk in patients with a subtherapeutic ACT and the reduction of ischemic end points seen in patients treated with glycoprotein IIb/IIIa inhibitors. Although platelets may adhere to a damaged vessel wall through a variety of receptors, activation of the glycoprotein IIb/IIIa receptors represents the final common pathway that allows them to bind avidly to fibrin to cause platelet aggregation and thrombosis. Vessels with moderate local dissection but preserved antegrade flow are thus more likely to stay patent in the presence of potent antiplatelet therapy (eg, glycoprotein IIb/IIIa antagonists and pretreatment with thienopyridines),

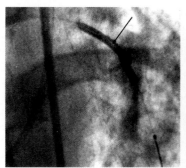 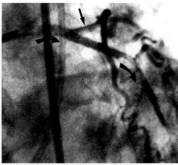

Figure 25.8 Use of a perfusion balloon catheter. left. The inflated perfusion balloon (arrow) is shown in the left anterior descending artery and can be recognized by the presence of the non–contrast-filled (white) perfusion lumen running through the center of the balloon. Bottom. Injection through the guiding catheter (left curved arrow) shows direct opacification of the circumflex (straight arrow) as well as contrast flow into the distal left anterior descending. This flow enters through proximal side holes, passes through the perfusion lumen within the balloon, and flows out into the distal vessel (right curved arrow). The 40- to 60-mL/min flow to the distal vessel through the perfusion lumen helps mitigate myocardial ischemia during prolonged balloon inflations. However, this device is no longer used in contemporary percutaneous coronary intervention (PCI) practice, since routine use of stents has made persistent abrupt closure a rare event.

thereby reducing the incidence of emergency surgery. These agents also significantly reduce the incidence of periprocedural MI, and particularly the incidence of biomarker elevations (non–Q-wave MI) that are seen in 20% to 30% of patients undergoing coronary intervention.

Branch Vessel Occlusion

Occlusion of a side branch originating from within the stenotic segment occurs in 14% of vessels at risk during angioplasty of the main vessel. This is generally owing to shifting of plaque which is sometimes referred to as the snowplow effect. If the branch vessel is small, this event usually has no significant clinical sequelae. On the other hand, if a large branch vessel originates from within the stenotic segment, simultaneous dilatation of the main vessel and the involved branch with 2 separate dilatation systems (the kissing balloon technique) may be required for preservation of both vessels. Current large-lumen guiding catheters and low-profile dilatation systems allow kissing balloon inflations through a 6F guiding catheter. The effective side-by-side balloon diameter in the proximal vessel can be estimated as the square root of the sum of the squares of the individual balloon diameters (two 3.0 mm balloons have an effective combined diameter of 4.25 mm [square root of 18 = 9 + 9]). Multiple studies have evaluated different bifurcation strategies and, in general, have concluded that provisional stenting is the best, with stent placement in the main branch and stenting of the side branch only if needed. The results of PCI for some true bifurcation lesions can be improved, however, by the use of various bifurcation stent strategies or atherectomy of both the parent and branch vessel.

Coronary Perforation

Guidewire-induced perforation occurs rarely; is typically seen with hydrophilic wires and in complex cases, especially during PCI for CTOs; and does not necessarily have dire consequences, unless a device is passed over the wire or the wire perforation takes place in a patient receiving a platelet IIb/IIIa receptor antagonist. Frank rupture of the coronary artery owing to the use of too large a dilatation balloon or the use of an atherectomy device can also cause vessel perforation that leads to rapid tamponade and hemodynamic collapse. For a detailed description of the management of coronary perforation, our readers are referred to Chapter 4.

Bleeding

The incidence of periprocedural bleeding ranges from 3% to 6% depending on the patient population and the definition used. Major periprocedural bleeding may be a risk factor for mortality. Several risk scores for periprocedural bleeding have been reported, but they are not typically used in clinical practice. Definitions for major bleeding, derived from clinical trials, are summarized in **Table 25.2**. The Bleeding Academic Research Consortium (BARC) has published a consensus classification that is likely to be helpful for standardizing definitions in clinical trials.

Risk factors for periprocedural bleeding include patient factors (eg, age >75 years, female gender, prior history of bleeding, low body mass index, preprocedural anemia, chronic kidney disease, acuity of presentation), potency of the anticoagulant and antiplatelet regimen used, vascular access site, and sheath size. Strategies to reduce the risks of bleeding include (1) the use of anticoagulation regimens associated with the optimal risk-benefit profile, (2) weight-based dosing of heparin and other agents, (3) use of activated clotting times to guide unfractionated heparin dosing, (4) dosing adjustments in patients with chronic kidney disease, and (5) use of radial artery access.

Table 25.2 Definitions of Major Bleeding

TIMI (1988)	GUSTO (1997)	ACUITY (2006)	REPLACE-2 (2007)	HORIZONS-AMI (2009)
Intracranial bleed	Intracranial bleed	Intracranial or intraocular	Intracranial, intraocular, or retroperitoneal	Intracranial or intraocular
Hgb > 5 g/dL or Hct > 15%		Hgb > 3 g/dL with overt bleeding Any Hgb > 4 g/dL	Hgb > 3 g/dL with overt bleeding Any Hgb > 4 g/dL	Hgb > 3 g/dL with overt bleeding Any Hgb > 4 g/dL
		Any transfusion	Transfusion > 2 units of red blood cells	Any transfusion
	Hemodynamic compromise requiring intervention	Access site bleeding requiring intervention Hematoma > 5 cm Reoperation for bleeding		Access site bleeding requiring intervention Hematoma > 5 cm Reoperation for bleeding

Hgb, hemoglobin.
TIMI and GUSTO trials were in patients receiving fibrinolytic therapy for acute myocardial infarction.
ACUITY, REPLACE-2, and HORIZONS-AMI trial recruited patients undergoing percutaneous coronary intervention.

Device Failures

Device failure can infrequently occur when any device is subjected to severe operating stresses (eg, when a guidewire is rotated repeatedly in a single direction while its tip is held fixed in a total occlusion or when a balloon catheter is inflated past its operating pressure range in an attempt to dilate a resistant stenosis). In a small percentage of cases, this may lead to detachment of a part of the wire with a fragment remaining in the coronary artery. In the stent era, this also includes dislodgment of the stent from its delivery balloon or failure of the stent delivery balloon to inflate or deflate properly. To avoid the need for surgical removal, the angioplasty operator should be familiar with various techniques (baskets, bioptomes, intertwined guidewires) for catheter retrieval.

THE HEALING RESPONSE TO CORONARY ANGIOPLASTY—RESTENOSIS

Following successful balloon angioplasty, there is a period of vascular repair. A layer of platelets and fibrin is deposited over minutes. Within hour to days, inflammatory cells infiltrate the site, cytokines are released, and vascular smooth muscle cells migrate from the media toward the lumen. These smooth muscle cells and fibroblasts transform into a synthetic phenotype and remain in this state as they undergo hypertrophy, proliferate, and begin to secrete extensive extracellular matrix (**Figure 25.9**). The luminal surface is simultaneously colonized by endothelial cells that slowly regain their normal barrier function and secretory functions (eg, tissue plasminogen activator and nitric oxide synthesis). Along with this proliferative neointimal response, there may also be further elastic

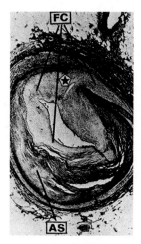

Figure 25.9 Mechanisms of restenosis: Cross section of a restenotic lesion in the left anterior descending artery 5 months after initial coronary angioplasty shows the original atherosclerotic (AS) plaque, the crack in the medial layer induced by the original procedure (star), and the proliferation of fibrocellular (FC) tissues that constitutes the restenotic lesion. In stent restenosis, the mechanism is purely proliferation, whereas in nonstent interventions such as balloon angioplasty, there is frequently an additional component owing to shrinkage of the overall vessel diameter (negative remodeling) at the treatment site. (From Serruys PW, Reiber JH, Wijns W, et al. Assessment of percutaneous transluminal coronary angioplasty by quantitative coronary angiography: diameter vs densitometric area measurements. *Am J Cardiol.* 1984;54:482-488.)

recoil and fibrotic contraction of the vessel wall (ie, negative vessel remodeling). The extent of proliferation and remodeling appears to vary according to the artery and type of intervention—for example, obstruction within stents is predominantly caused by neo-intimal hyperplasia, whereas significant amount of late narrowing following stand-alone angioplasty occurs owing to contraction of the vessel wall. Although vessel recoil is eliminated by coronary stenting, *incomplete stent expansion* at the time of implantation is an important mechanism for recurrent stenosis, especially in calcified and fibrotic lesions. *Stent fracture* owing to mechanical fatigue caused by repetitive cardiac contraction may also account for some cases of recurrent stenosis (at least 4%). Hypersensitivity to 1 or more components of the implanted stent has been proposed as a potential mechanism with systemic symptoms as well. There are also significant patient-to-patient variations in the late healing response after coronary intervention, reflected in variable amounts of late loss in lumen diameter between the completion of the intervention and the time when the repair process stabilizes (~6-12 months). Follow-up angiography shows continued maintenance of lumen diameter at the treated site beyond this period in the majority of patients.

If the healing response is excessive, however, most or all of the gain in lumen diameter produced by the initial intervention may be lost to the healing process. This causes the return of a severe stenosis and ischemic symptoms—a phenomenon known as *restenosis.* Initially, restenosis was considered a dichotomous outcome that either did or did not develop. More recently, restenosis has been considered as a continuous variable, and cumulative distribution curves have been used to show the population distribution of the late result for the whole treated population (**Figure 25.10**).

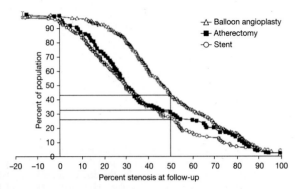

Figure 25.10 The view of restenosis as a continuous process that takes place to some degree in every treated segment favors displaying the late result (here, percent stenosis at follow-up) for the whole treated population. For patients treated by balloon angioplasty, directional atherectomy, or stenting, the *y* axis shows the percent of patients who have a stenosis larger than the stenosis value on the *x* axis. The ability of stenting and atherectomy to lower restenosis is shown by a shift of their cumulative distribution function curves to the left. If a dichotomous definition of restenosis is applied, the intersection of each curve with a late diameter stenosis of 50% (vertical axis) corresponds to a dichotomous restenosis rate of 43% for angioplasty, 31% for atherectomy, and 26% for stenting. (From Kuntz RE, Safian RD, Levine MJ, et al. Novel approach to the analysis of restenosis. *J Am Coll Cardiol.* 1992;19:1493-1499.)

On the diameter stenosis curve, the percentage of the population that has a late diameter stenosis of >50% (binary restenosis) serves as a useful benchmark for comparing the angiographic restenosis rates between different treatment groups.

Every treated lesion undergoes some degree of *late loss*, but fortunately late loss usually negates only part (roughly half) of the acute gain, so that a long-term net gain in lumen diameter results with alleviation of myocardial ischemia. In fact, there tends to be a roughly linear relationship between the acute gain in lumen diameter caused by the intervention and late loss in lumen diameter (caused by the proliferative and fibrotic reaction of the artery during the healing phase), with a slope (the *loss index*) of roughly 0.5 for most interventions. This means that larger lumen diameters immediately after intervention translate into larger lumen diameters at 6-month angiographic restudy (the "bigger is better" dictum). All new mechanical devices have been able to deliver a lower restenosis rate than that of balloon angioplasty by providing a larger acute lumen diameter (more acute gain), rather than by reducing the loss index. Angiographic restenosis following balloon angioplasty alone is common (up to 50%), is less frequent with bare-metal stents (20%-30%), and is least often seen with DESs (5%-10%).

Brachytherapy

Coronary brachytherapy was used in the past but is no longer performed given the superiority of DESs in preventing restenosis. The delivery of 2000 cGy of either beta or gamma radiation to the coronary arterial wall retards intimal proliferation within bare-metal coronary stents. Trials of primary radiation at the time of stenting for de novo lesions were less impressive. As with DESs, the inhibition of stent endothelialization by radiation treatment was associated with an increased risk of delayed stent thrombosis, which had to be mitigated by long-term DAPT.

Drug-Eluting Stents

The local release of antiproliferative drugs (eg, sirolimus, paclitaxel, zotarolimus, everolimus, Biolimus) from a polymer matrix over the first few months after stent implantation can substantially reduce inflammation and smooth muscle cell proliferation within a stent. For a detailed overview of coronary stenting, our readers are referred to Chapter 27.

CURRENT INDICATIONS

With the improvements in equipment and technique described above, PCI has become the dominant form of coronary revascularization compared to CABG. However, the previous trend of steady rise in PCI volumes in the United States has reversed; the numbers of diagnostic cardiac catheterization and PCI being performed have gradually decreased since the mid-2000s onward. Potential reasons for the decline include (1) reduction in smoking and improved treatment of cardiovascular risk factors, (2) use of DESs and the associated reduction in in-stent restenosis, and (3) impact of the COURAGE and ISCHEMIA trials demonstrating similar outcomes for both medical therapy and PCI in a select population with stable CAD.

Key issues that need to be addressed in patient selection for PCI include the following: (1) clinical justification for revascularization, (2) disease complexity which impacts the safety and efficacy of PCI, (3) potential advantages and disadvantages of PCI as compared to other therapeutic options such as medical therapy or bypass surgery, and (4) what combination of interventional devices would offer the best short- and long-term outcomes. This evaluation process thus involves integration of complex clinical, angiographic, pathophysiologic, and procedural knowledge and constitutes an important component of operator training.

The current guidelines recommend that this function be executed in stable patients with unprotected left main and complex multivessel disease (eg, SYNTAX score >22) via a multidisciplinary approach by establishing a *"Heart Team"* that is composed of an interventional cardiologist, a cardiac surgeon, and the patient's general cardiologist. Support for this strategy comes from studies showing that patients with complex CAD referred for revascularization in concurrent trial registries have lower mortality rates than those randomly assigned to PCI or CABG in the trials. Moreover, the guidelines state that it is reasonable to use the Society of Thoracic Surgeons (STS) and SYNTAX scores to assist making decisions regarding revascularization. The advantage of the SYNTAX score is that it is a unique tool that allows quantification of the angiographic complexity of CAD. However, it is complex to calculate and that introduces the potential for error. It may be calculated using an online calculator available at http://www.syntaxscore.com. The STS score is based on clinical characteristics and as such is easier to use and can also be derived from an online calculator at http://209.220.160.181/STSWebRiskCalc261/de.aspx.

With the rapid growth of PCI, there has been a series of guidelines and position papers published in Europe and the United States. The ACC/AHA first published Angioplasty Guidelines in 1988, updating them in 1993, 2001, 2005, and 2007. Comprehensive revisions were published in 2011 and 2021 with updates in 2015 and 2016. These statements are useful compilations that outline some well-accepted indications and contraindications for PCI and are available online at http://www.cardiosource.org/science-and-quality.aspx.

Percutaneous Coronary Intervention to Improve Survival in Stable Disease

The 2021 guidelines do not give a class I recommendation for patients with left main stenosis. They recommend that PCI for this purpose is *reasonable* (class IIa), as an alternative to CABG, in selected *stable* patients with significant (>50% diameter stenosis) unprotected left main disease with (1) anatomic conditions associated with a low risk of PCI procedural complications and a high likelihood of good long-term outcome (eg, a low SYNTAX score [<22], ostial or trunk left main stenosis) and (2) clinical characteristics that predict a significantly increased risk of adverse surgical outcomes (eg, STS-predicted risk of operative mortality >5%). In patients with unstable angina/NSTEMI, PCI is *reasonable* when an unprotected left main coronary artery is the culprit lesion and the patient is not a candidate for CABG. Finally, in patients with acute STEMI, PCI is reasonable for an unprotected left main coronary artery that hosts the culprit lesion causing decreased blood flow (Thrombolysis in Myocardial Infarction [TIMI] grade <3), and PCI can be performed more rapidly and safely than CABG.

The only recommendation for PCI to improve survival in patients without left main disease is for those who survive sudden cardiac death with presumed ischemia-mediated ventricular tachycardia caused by significant (>70% diameter) stenosis in a major coronary artery. This is a class I recommendation for which either PCI or CABG may be performed, as considered appropriate.

Percutaneous Coronary Intervention to Improve Symptoms in Stable Disease

PCI is more performed to relieve symptoms, not improve survival. For this purpose, the 2021 guidelines state that PCI (or CABG) is *beneficial* in patients with 1 or more significant (>70% diameter) coronary artery stenoses amenable to revascularization and unacceptable angina despite guideline-directed medical therapy. A lower level of indication (class IIa) is given by the guidelines for PCI (or CABG) to improve symptoms in patients with 1 or more significant (>70% diameter) coronary artery stenoses and unacceptable angina for whom guideline-directed medical therapy cannot be implemented because of medication contraindications, adverse effects, or patient preferences. Similarly, PCI is *reasonable* in patients with previous CABG, 1 or more significant (>70% diameter) coronary artery stenoses associated with ischemia, and unacceptable angina despite guideline-directed medical therapy.

Percutaneous Coronary Intervention in Acute Coronary Syndromes

The purpose of angiography and revascularization in NSTACS is to relieve ischemia and symptoms as well as reducing the risk of death and (recurrent) MI. Selection of patients for an early invasive strategy is based on risk stratification. Patients in whom this approach is indicated are individuals without serious comorbidities or contraindications to the procedures, who either have an elevated risk for clinical events or have refractory angina/hemodynamic compromise/electrical instability. The selection of PCI or CABG as the means of revascularization should generally be based on the same considerations as those for patients without ACS. The indications for angiography in STEMI are summarized in **Table 25.3**.

Complete Revascularization in Stable Disease

An important principle of myocardial revascularization is to minimize residual ischemia. Hence, completeness of revascularization has been proposed to be a determinant of prognosis and symptom relief. The extent to which initial incomplete revascularization influences outcomes is unclear, as there are no data from any randomized trial primarily comparing complete and incomplete revascularization.

However, as one would expect, the need for subsequent PCI/CABG is usually higher in those with initial incomplete revascularization with PCI.

Table 25.3 Recommendations for Revascularization of the Infarct Artery in Patients With STEMI

COR	LOE	Recommendations
1	A	In patients with STEMI and ischemic symptoms for <12 h, PCI should be performed to improve survival
1	B-R	In patients with STEMI and cardiogenic shock or hemodynamic instability. PCI or CABG (when PCI is not feasible) is indicated to improve survival, irrespective of the time delay from MI onset.
1	B-NR	In patients with STEMI who have mechanical complications (eg, ventricular septal rupture, mitral valve insufficiency because of papillary muscle infarction or rupture, or free wall rupture), CABG is recommended at the time of surgery, with the goal of improving survival.
1	C-LD	In patients with STEMI and evidence of failed reperfusion after fibrinolytic therapy, rescue PCI of the infarct artery should be performed to improve clinical outcomes.
2a	B-R	In patients with STEMI who are treated with fibrinolytic therapy, angiography within 3-24 h with the intent to perform PCI is reasonable to improve clinical outcomes.
2a	B-NR	In patients with STEMI who are stable and presenting 12-24 h after symptom onset, PCI is reasonable to improve clinical outcomes.
2a	B-NR	In patients with STEMI in whom PCI is not feasible or successful, with a large area of myocardium at risk, emergency or urgent CABG can be effective as a reperfusion modality to improve clinical outcomes.
2a	C-EO	In patients with STEMI complicated by ongoing ischemia, acute severe heart failure, or life-threatening arrhythmia, PCI can be beneficial to improve clinical outcomes, irrespective of time delay from MI onset.
3: no benefit	B-R	In asymptomatic stable patients with STEMI who have a totally occluded infarct artery >24 h after symptom onset and are without evidence of severe ischemia. PCI should not be performed).
3: Harm	C-EO	In patients with STEMI, emergency CABG should not be performed after failed primary PCI: • In the absence of ischemia or a large area of myocardium at risk, or • If surgical revascularization is not feasible because of a no-reflow state or poor distal targets.

CABG, coronary artery bypass graft; CAD, coronary artery disease; COR, class of recommendation; EO, expert opinion; LD, limited data; LOE, level of evidence; MI, myocardial infarction; NR, nonrandomized; PCI, percutaneous coronary intervention; R, randomized; SIHD, stable ischemic heart disease; STEMI, ST-elevation myocardial infarction.
Reprinted with permission from Lawton JS, Tamis-Holland JE, Bangalore S, et al. 2021 ACC/AHA/SCAI guideline for coronary artery revascularization: a report of the American College of Cardiology/American Heart Association Joint Committee on Clinical Practice Guidelines. *J Am Coll Cardiol*. 2022;79(2):e21-e129. ©2022 American Heart Association, Inc.

SUGGESTED READINGS

 1. Ahn JM, Park DW, Lee CW, et al. Comparison of stenting versus bypass surgery according to the completeness of revascularization in severe coronary artery disease: patient-level pooled analysis of the SYNTAX, PRECOMBAT, and BEST Trials. *JACC Cardiovasc Interv.* 2017;10(14):1415-1424.
 2. Baim DS, Wahr D, George B, et al. Randomized trial of a distal embolic protection device during percutaneous intervention of saphenous vein aorto-coronary bypass grafts. *Circulation.* 2002;105(11):1285-1290.
 3. Bech GJW, Pijls NHJ, DeBruyne B, et al. Usefulness of fractional flow reserve to predict clinical outcome after balloon angioplasty. *Circulation.* 1999;99(7):883-888.
 4. Blankenship JC, Krucoff MW, Werns SW, et al. Comparison of slow oscillating versus fast balloon inflation strategies for coronary angioplasty. *Am J Cardiol.* 1999;83(5):675-680.
 5. Boden W, O'Rourke R, Teo K, et al. Optimal medical therapy with or without PCI for stable coronary disease. *N Engl J Med.* 2007;356(15):1503-1516.
 6. Brinton TJ, Ali ZA, Hill JM, et al. Feasibility of shockwave coronary intravascular lithotripsy for the treatment of calcified coronary stenoses. *Circulation.* 2019;139(6):834-836.
 7. Chakravarty T, White AJ, Buch M, et al. Meta-analysis of incidence, clinical characteristics, and implications of stent fracture. *Am J Cardiol.* 2010;106(8):1075-1080.
 8. Dauerman HL, Higgins PJ, Sparano AM, et al. Mechanical debulking versus balloon angioplasty for the treatment of true bifurcation lesions. *J Am Coll Cardiol.* 1998;32(7):1845-1852.
 9. de Muinck ED, den Heijer P, van Dijk RB, et al. Autoperfusion balloon versus stent for acute or threatened closure during percutaneous transluminal coronary angioplasty. *Am J Cardiol.* 1994;74(10):1002-1005.
10. Dehmer GJ, Blankenship JC, Cilingiroglu M, et al. SCAI/ACC/AHA expert consensus document: 2014 update on percutaneous coronary intervention without on-site surgical backup. *Catheter Cardiovasc Interv.* 2014;84(2):169-187.
11. Dervan JP, McKay RG, Baim DS. The use of an exchange guide wire in coronary angioplasty. *Cathet Cardiovasc Diagn.* 1985;11(2):207-212.
12. Dotter CT, Judkins MP. Transluminal treatment of arteriosclerotic obstruction: description of a new technique and a preliminary report of its application. *Circulation.* 1964;30:654-670.
13. Ellis SG, Roubin GS, King SB III, et al. Angiographic and clinical predictors of acute closure after native vessel coronary angioplasty. *Circulation.* 1988;77(2):372-379.
14. Ellis SG, Vandormael MG, Cowley MJ, et al. Coronary morphologic and clinical determinates of procedural outcome with angioplasty for multivessel coronary disease: implications for patient selection. *Circulation.* 1990;82(4):1193-1202.
15. Ellis SG, Ajluni S, Arnold AZ, et al. Increased coronary perforation in the new device era: incidence, classification, management, and outcome. *Circulation.* 1994;90(6):2725-2730.
16. Fanaroff AC, Zakroysky P, Dai D, et al. Outcomes of PCI in relation to procedural characteristics and operator volumes in the United States. *J Am Coll Cardiol.* 2017;69(24):2913-2924.
17. Feit F, Brooks MM, Sopko G, et al. Long-term clinical outcome in the bypass angioplasty revascularization investigation registry: comparison with the randomized trial. BARI investigators. *Circulation.* 2000;101(24):2795-2802.
18. Feit F, Voeltz MD, Attubato MJ, et al. Predictors and impact of major hemorrhage on mortality following percutaneous coronary intervention from the REPLACE-2 Trial. *Am J Cardiol.* 2007;100(9):1364-1369.
19. George BS, Voorhees WD III, Roubin GS, et al. Multicenter investigation of coronary stenting to treat acute or threatened closure after percutaneous transluminal coronary angioplasty: clinical and angiographic outcomes. *J Am Coll Cardiol.* 1993;22(1):135-143.
20. Gruentzig AR, Senning A, Siegenthaler WE. Non-operative dilatation of coronary artery stenosis: percutaneous transluminal coronary angioplasty. *N Engl J Med.* 1979;301:61-68.
21. Grundy SM, Stone NJ, Bailey AL, et al. 2018 AHA/ACC/AACVPR/AAPA/ABC/ACPM/ADA/AGS/APhA/ASPC/NLA/PCNA Guideline on the management of blood cholesterol: executive summary—a Report of the American College of Cardiology/American Heart Association Task Force on Clinical Practice Guidelines. *J Am Coll Cardiol.* 2019;73(24):3168-3209.
22. Kuntz RE, Baim DS. Defining coronary restenosis: newer clinical and angiographic paradigms. *Circulation.* 1993;88(3):1310-1323.
23. Leon MB, Teirstein PS, Moses JW, et al. Localized intracoronary gamma-radiation therapy to inhibit the recurrence of restenosis after stenting. *N Engl J Med.* 2001;344(4):250-256.
24. Levine GN, Bates ER, Blankenship JC, et al. 2011 ACCF/AHA/SCAI guideline for percutaneous coronary intervention: a report of the American College of Cardiology Foundation/American Heart Association Task Force on Practice Guidelines and the Society for Cardiovascular Angiography and Interventions. *Circulation.* 2011;124(23):e574-e651.

25. Levine GN, Bates ER, Bittl JA, et al. 2016 ACC/AHA Guideline focused update on duration of dual antiplatelet therapy in patients with coronary artery disease: a Report of the American College of Cardiology/American Heart Association Task Force on Clinical Practice Guidelines. *J Am Coll Cardiol.* 2016;68(10):1082-1115.

26. Manoukian SV, Feit F, Mehran R, et al. Impact of major bleeding on 30-day mortality and clinical outcomes in patients with acute coronary syndromes: an analysis from the ACUITY Trial. *J Am Coll Cardiol.* 2007;49(12):1362-1368.

27. Mauri L, Bonan R, Weiner BH, et al. Cutting balloon angioplasty for the prevention of restenosis: results of the cutting balloon global randomized trial. *Am J Cardiol.* 2002;90(10):1079-1083.

28. Mehran R, Rao SV, Bhatt DL, et al. Standardized bleeding definitions for cardiovascular clinical trials: a consensus report from the Bleeding Academic Research Consortium. *Circulation.* 2011;123(23):2736-2747.

29. Mintz GS, Popma JJ, Pichard AD, et al. Arterial remodeling after coronary angioplasty—a serial intravascular ultrasound study. *Circulation.* 1996;94(1):35-43.

30. Morice MC, Serruys PW, Kappetein AP, et al. Outcomes in patients with de novo left main disease treated with either percutaneous coronary intervention using paclitaxel-eluting stents or coronary artery bypass graft treatment in the synergy between percutaneous coronary intervention with TAXUS and Cardiac Surgery (SYNTAX) trial. *Circulation.* 2010;121(24):2645-2653.

31. Moscucci M, Share D, Smith D, et al. Relationship between operator volume and adverse outcome in contemporary percutaneous coronary intervention practice: an analysis of a quality-controlled multicenter percutaneous coronary intervention clinical database. *J Am Coll Cardiol.* 2005;46(4):625-632.

32. Patel MR, Calhoon JH, Dehmer GJ, et al. ACC/AATS/AHA/ASE/ASNC/SCAI/SCCT/STS 2017 appropriate use criteria for coronary revascularization in patients with stable ischemic heart disease: a report of the American College of Cardiology Appropriate Use Criteria Task Force, American Association for Thoracic surgery, American Heart Association, American Society of Echocardiography, American Society of Nuclear Cardiology, Society for Cardiovascular Angiography and Interventions, Society of Cardiovascular Computed Tomography, and Society of Thoracic Surgeons. *J Am Coll Cardiol.* 2017;69(17):2212-2241.

33. Piana RN, Paik GY, Moscucci M, et al. Incidence and treatment of "no-reflow" after percutaneous coronary intervention. *Circulation.* 1994;89(6):2514-2518.

34. Popma JJ, Suntharalingam M, Lansky AJ, et al. Randomized trial of 90Sr/90Y beta-radiation versus placebo control for treatment of in-stent restenosis. *Circulation.* 2002;106(9):1090-1096.

35. Prasad A, Rihal CS, Lennon RJ, Singh M, Jaffe AS, Holmes DR Jr. Significance of periprocedural myonecrosis on outcomes after percutaneous coronary intervention: an analysis of preintervention and post intervention troponin T levels in 5487 patients. *Circ Cardiovasc Interv.* 2008;1:10-19.

36. Qureshi MA, Safian RD, Grines CL, et al. Simplified scoring system for predicting mortality after percutaneous coronary intervention. *J Am Coll Cardiol.* 2003;42(11):1890-1895.

37. Roubin GS, Douglas JS Jr, King SB III, et al. Influence of balloon size on initial success, acute complications, and restenosis after percutaneous transluminal coronary angioplasty. A prospective randomized study. *Circulation.* 1988;78(3):557-565.

38. Schulz-Schupke S, Helde S, Gewalt S, et al. Comparison of vascular closure devices vs manual compression after femoral artery puncture: the ISAR-CLOSURE randomized clinical trial. *J Am Med Assoc.* 2014;312(19):1981-1987.

39. Shaw LJ, Berman DS, Maron DJ, et al; COURAGE Investigators. Optimal medical therapy with or without percutaneous coronary intervention to reduce ischemic burden: results from the Clinical Outcomes Utilizing Revascularization and Aggressive Drug Evaluation (COURAGE) trial nuclear substudy. *Circulation.* 2008;117(10):1283-1291.

40. Simpson JB, Baim DS, Robert EW, Harrison DC. A new catheter system for coronary angioplasty. *Am J Cardiol.* 1982;49(5):1216-1222.

41. Singh M, Lennon RJ, Holmes DR Jr, Bell MR, Rihal CS. Correlates of procedural complications and a simple integer risk score for percutaneous coronary intervention. *J Am Coll Cardiol.* 2002;40(3):387-393.

42. Solensky R. Drug allergy: desensitization and treatment of reactions to antibiotics and aspirin. *Clin Allergy Immunol.* 2004;18:585-606.

43. Steinhubl SR, Berger PB, Mann JT III, for the CREDO Investigators. Early and sustained dual oral antiplatelet therapy following percutaneous coronary intervention: a randomized controlled trial. *J Am Med Assoc.* 2002;288(19):2411-2420.

44. Stone GW, Rogers C, Hermiller J, et al. Randomized comparison of distal protection with a filter-based catheter and a balloon occlusion and aspiration system during percutaneous intervention of diseased saphenous vein aortocoronary bypass grafts. *Circulation.* 2003;108(5):548-553.

45. Thygesen K, Alpert JS, Jaffe AS, et al. Fourth universal definition of myocardial infarction (2018). *Eur Heart J*. 2019;40(3):237-269.
46. Writing Committee Members; Lawton JS, Tamis-Holland JE, Bangalore S, et al. 2021 ACC/AHA/SCAI Guideline for Coronary Artery Revascularization: a Report of the American College of Cardiology/American Heart Association Joint Committee on Clinical Practice Guidelines. *J Am Coll Cardiol*. 2022;79(2):e21-e129. doi:10.1016/j.jacc.2021.09.006
47. Zhang F, Dong L, Ge J. Effect of statins pretreatment on periprocedural myocardial infarction in patients undergoing percutaneous coronary intervention: a meta-analysis. *Ann Med*. 2010;42(3):171-177.

ATHERECTOMY

The role of coronary atherectomy has evolved dramatically since its introduction as a method to improve the results of balloon angioplasty. Initially, it was hypothesized that plaque *removal* with atherectomy would achieve a larger postprocedural luminal diameter and yield reduced long-term restenosis rates. Despite great early enthusiasm for atherectomy as a definitive primary strategy, this technique now is utilized to modify calcified lesions to facilitate coronary stenting. Coronary atherectomy is performed using rotational and orbital techniques.

Rotational Atherectomy and Orbital Atherectomy

Mechanism of Rotational Atherectomy and Orbital Atherectomy

Percutaneous transluminal rotational atherectomy (PTRA) and orbital atherectomy (OA) operate on the principle of "differential cutting" in which hard, fibrocalcific plaque can be ablated by a rotating burr, while softer tissue in the treated coronary segment deflects away from the device. Plaque is pulverized into particles smaller than red blood cells (generally <10-15 μm in diameter) that can pass through the coronary microcirculation for uptake by the reticuloendothelial system.

Device Specifics

In rotational atherectomy (RA) systems, the burr spins *concentrically* on the guidewire. Two dominant RA systems are currently marketed: Rotablator and ROTAPRO (Boston Scientific, Boston, MA). The Rotablator 4-component system consists of a burr catheter, an advancer, a free-standing control console, and a foot pedal. The RotaLink burr consists of an elliptical, nickel-coated brass burr attached to a hollow flexible 4.3F drive shaft, which is encased in a Teflon sheath (**Figure 26.1**).

The sheath protects the artery proximal to the lesion from the rotating drive shaft and allows flush solution to lubricate the drive shaft and burr. The burr's ablative distal surface is embedded with 20 μm diamond chips, with 5 μm protruding from the surface. The proximal nonablative surface of the burr is smooth. Therefore, in contradistinction to OA crowns, the RA burr only ablates when advanced, not during retraction. The back end of the RotaLink burr catheter is connected to a RotaLink advancer, which allows the operator to extend and retract the burr within the vessel (**Figure 26.2**).

A control console delivers air or nitrogen to the turbine housed within the RotaLink advancer to pneumatically spin the drive shaft and the burr. The console is activated by a foot pedal; turbine pressure is adjusted by a control knob; and rotational speed is monitored by a fiberoptic tachometer. The RotaWire guidewires combine a 0.009-in diameter body with a 0.014-inch tip (**Figure 26.3**). These are supplied with a specific wire clip to facilitate wire manipulation. The burr can be advanced over the 0.009-in section, but its forward movement is limited by the wider wire tip. During turbine activation, a wire brake is engaged to prevent spinning of the guidewire,

[1]We gratefully acknowledge the *Grossman & Baim's Cardiac Catheterization, Angiography, and Intervention,* 9th edition contributions of Dr Robert N. Piana, as portions of his chapter, "Atherectomy, Thrombectomy, and Distal Protection Devices," were retained in this text.

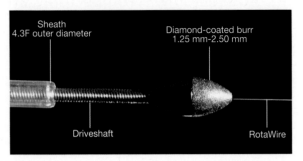

which could otherwise traumatize the distal vessel. The wire clip provides a secondary brake. The RotaWire guidewires have no lubricious coating, no shaping ribbon, and are easily kinked. Rotaglide, a lubricating solution, may be infused during RA to reduce friction.

The ROTAPRO system has been released to simplify the RA procedure without changing the underlying technology. The foot pedal is eliminated, a miniaturized console now mounts to an intravenous (IV) pole, and the controls are incorporated into the advancer.

Coronary orbital atherectomy is currently performed using the DIAMOND-BACK 360 Coronary Orbital Atherectomy System (Cardiovascular Systems, Inc, St. Paul, MN) (**Figure 26.4A**). The orbital atherectomy device (OAD) is composed of a sheath-covered drive shaft and an *eccentrically* mounted diamond-coated crown. A connected infusion pump lubricates and cools the system with ViperSlide, an emulsion composed of soybean oil, egg yolk phospholipids, glycerin, and water. The OAD is advanced over a 0.012″ Viper Wire Advance Coronary Guide Wire, which has an 0.014″ spring tip. A brake lever on the OAD is used to lock the wire to prevent it from spinning. A control button on the OAD *electronically* activates crown rotation with 2 optional speeds. As the eccentrically mounted crown spins, it begins to "orbit" and centrifugal force presses the crown into the calcified coronary plaque. The centrifugal force is directly proportional to the mass (M) of the crown and its rotational velocity (V) and inversely proportional to the radius (R) of rotation: $F_c = (MV^2)/R$. Due to its design, the OA crown ablates both on advancement and during retraction (**Figure 26.4B**).

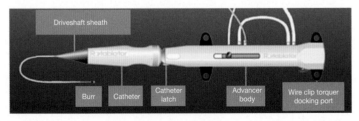

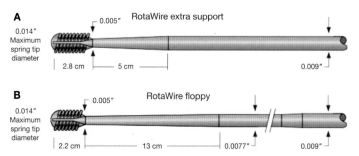

Figure 26.3 Rotablator wires. **A,** RotaWire extra support. **B,** RotaWire floppy. (© 2020 Boston Scientific Corporation or its affiliates. All rights reserved.)

Case Selection for Rotational Atherectomy and Orbital Atherectomy

Due to concerns for potential embolization, dissection, or no-reflow, these ablative atherectomy techniques are generally not applied in acute myocardial infarction, thrombotic lesions, coronary dissections, or saphenous vein grafts (SVGs) with poor distal runoff. Patients with severe left ventricular dysfunction are approached with extreme caution due to the risk of hemodynamic decompensation from ischemia or no-reflow during these complex procedures. Hemodynamic support may be required.

Adjunctive Therapies Patients are pretreated with aspirin and possibly a calcium channel blocker to counteract induced vasospasm. Glycoprotein (GP) IIb/IIIa receptor antagonists have shown benefit in limiting speed-dependent platelet activation with RA. Appropriate anticoagulation is unfractionated heparin over bivalirudin to facilitate reversal of anticoagulation in the event of vessel perforation.

Lipid emulsions (Rotaglide for RA, ViperSlide for OA) are utilized to reduce friction, limit heat generation, and facilitate device deliverability. Various combinations of vasodilators have often been added as well to counteract vasospasm and microvascular no-reflow. Typical "RotaFlush" solutions mix 4 mg of nitroglycerin and 5 mg of verapamil in 500 mL of saline. A temporary pacing wire or IV aminophylline have

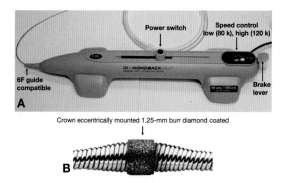

Figure 26.4 **A,** DIAMONDBACK 360″ coronary orbital atherectomy system. **B,** Orbital atherectomy diamond-coated crown. Note how the diamond-coated crown is eccentrically mounted. (A, Copyright ©2020 Cardiovascular Systems, Inc. Photo is used with permission from Cardiovascular Systems, Inc. CSI and Diamondback 360 are registered trademarks of Cardiovascular Systems, Inc.)

been utilized for RA of the right coronary or dominant circumflex owing to the risk of profound bradycardia, which is believed to result from adenosine release with red cell fragmentation. With current techniques of burr to artery ratios of 0.6 to 0.7 using RA and OA for plaque modification the complications of no-reflow and heart block are reduced.

Technique for Rotational Atherectomy A guiding catheter with a gentle curve with an inner diameter to accommodate the largest burr diameter is recommended. Complex lesions are often difficult to cross with RA wires owing to their poor torque. In such cases, a conventional exchange length coronary angioplasty wire is used to cross and then exchanged for the RA guidewire using a microcatheter. Typically, a RotaWire floppy is chosen in order to minimize guidewire bias—a phenomenon observed when a stiff guidewire straightens a curved vessel segment and causes deeper cuts or dissection as the burr is forced against the lesser curvature of the vessel. The floppy guidewire may fail to facilitate the burr's passage around tight bends. The RotaWire extra-support wire is generally utilized for distal or heavily calcified lesions. Burrs for coronary use are available in 1.25 to 2.5 mm diameters. The selection of burr size should not exceed a burr-to-artery ratio of 0.7 (eg, 2.15-mm burr in a 3.0-mm vessel). In treating long segments of disease, heavily calcified lesions, and subtotal de novo lesions, it is generally advisable to start with a smaller (1.25 or 1.5 mm) burr and step up to the final burr size in 0.5-mm increments.

Once the guidewire is placed across the lesion, the burr should be advanced to within a few centimeters of the rotating hemostatic valve. The compressed air or nitrogen source to the console is confirmed to have a pressure of at least 500 psi. A preprocedural checklist is then applied: (1) "Drip"—adequate flow of the pressurized heparinized flush through the Teflon sheath is visualized; (2) "Rotation"—while the operator holds the catheter so that the burr tip is not in contact with the sterile drapes, the system should be tested by depressing the foot pedal and having an assistant adjust the turbine pressure to achieve the desired burr speed; (3) "Advancer"—test whether the advancer moves the burr freely; (4) "Wire"—ensure that the wire clip is in place on the wire and test whether the brake locks the wire in place during rotation. Once these tests have been completed, the static burr can be advanced over the wire through the guiding catheter. The guiding catheter must remain well seated in the vessel ostium to prevent looping of the guidewire in the aortic root while the burr is advanced—such unrecognized loops can lead to its transection when the burr is activated at the ostium.

Once the burr has been advanced to 2 cm proximal to the target lesion, the advancer lever should be unlocked and pulled gently back as the entire catheter is withdrawn 2 mm. This relieves compression in the drive shaft that might cause the burr to lurch forward into the lesion on activation. Under fluoroscopy, the burr is then activated by the foot pedal and adjusted to the desired "platform" speed of 140,000 to 160,000. Advancement of the lever then brings the spinning burr slowly into contact with the lesion. It is important to be aware of the sound of the turbine, the rotational speed display, and tactile feedback during rotablation. When the burr face encounters excessive resistance to rotation, the speed will fall, but it is essential to avoid speed drops of >5000 rpm during advancement. Larger speed drops may result in the liberation of larger particles, frictional heating of the plaque, or dissection. We prefer advancing with a "pecking" motion in which brief (1-3 seconds) periods of plaque contact are alternated with longer (3-5 seconds) periods of reperfusion provided by pulling the burr back from the plaque.

After a brief run of <30 seconds, the device should be withdrawn into the proximal vessel and rotation suspended before advancing the burr again. During each pause, a small test injection should be performed to ensure antegrade flow. This sequence should be repeated until the device can be advanced through the full length of the lesion without any fluoroscopic or tactile resistance to burr advancement. The foot pedal is then used to activate the lower speed "Dynaglide" mode, and the burr is removed while depressing the brake-release button.

Technique for Orbital Atherectomy The DIAMONDBACK 360 OAD utilizes an eccentrically mounted, diamond-coated 1.25 mm crown. The ViperWire Advance (0.012″ diameter stainless steel wire with a silicone coating and a distal 0.014″ diameter spring tip) or ViperWire Advance Flex Tip (updated with a flexible nitinol core with a shapeable floppy tip to help navigate complex anatomy) is positioned well across the most distal aspect of the target lesion to maintain at least 5 mm distance between the spinning crown and the spring tip of the wire. The OAD is advanced to 1 cm proximal to the lesion, the wire brake is engaged, and the advancer knob is pulled back to its most proximal position to relieve any compression on the drive shaft. With constant infusion of ViperSlide, the device is activated. After a 2-second ramp, the rotational speed plateaus and the crown is advanced between 1 and 10 mm/s. It is recommended to limit runs to <30 seconds, followed by a rest period of equal time. As opposed to the pecking motion utilized with RA, in OA, it is recommended that crown movement be gradual and steady. In modeling tests, traversing the lesion slowly at lower speeds appears to achieve more effective ablation than more rapid advancement at higher speeds. The device ablates with both advancement and retraction.

Clinical Results

Rotational Atherectomy or Orbital Atherectomy as a Definitive Strategy Despite the intuitive appeal of plaque ablation, 3 randomized trials have failed to demonstrate the superiority of RA as a stand-alone procedure when compared to percutaneous transluminal coronary angioplasty (PTCA) for the treatment of native coronary lesions (**Table 26.1**).

Recognizing that debulking with RA is not superior to PTCA, current ACC/AHA/SCAI (American College of Cardiology/American Heart Association/Society for Cardiovascular Angiography & Interventions) guidelines do not support the use of RA for *routine coronary lesions* (class III recommendation). Orbital atherectomy has not been studied as a stand-alone strategy for percutaneous coronary interventions (PCIs), and its routine use is not addressed in current PCI guidelines.

Rotational Atherectomy or Orbital Atherectomy for In-Stent Restenosis Randomized trials have reported conflicting data regarding RA of in-stent restenosis (ISR). With randomized trials showing drug-eluting stenting (DES) to be superior for ISR, RA is generally no longer used for debulking of ISR. The 2011 guidelines for PCI provide a class III recommendation for RA of ISR, while the 2021 guidelines are mute.

Rotational Atherectomy or Orbital Atherectomy with Stenting for Calcified Lesions In several series, RA improved stent expansion even in calcified lesions. In a single-center series, RA followed by DES for calcified lesions was associated with reduced target lesion revascularization rates as compared to RA plus bare-metal stenting (BMS) (10.6% vs 25%, $P < .001$). Another single-center series has suggested that when RA is utilized to deliver and expand DES in heavily calcified lesions, clinical outcomes are similar to those of DES alone. However, no study has demonstrated the superiority of RA plus DES over DES alone, even in calcified lesions.

PCI guidelines provide a class IIa recommendation for RA in heavily calcified or fibrotic lesions that may not dilate with conventional techniques prior to stenting.

Table 26.1 Randomized Clinical Trials of Percutaneous Transluminal Rotational Atherectomy

Trial Focus	Design	Relevant End point[a]	Findings	Implication
Restenosis Trials				
ERBAC	RA vs PTCA in native vessels	TVR 6 mo	RA 42.4% PTCA 31.9% $P = .01$	Unfavorable effect of RA on TVR
COBRA	RA vs PTCA in native vessels	Binary restenosis 6 mo	RA 49% PTCA 51% $P = .33$	No reduction of restenosis with RA
DART	RA vs PTCA in small native vessels (2-3 mm)	TVF at 12 mo	RA 30.5% PTCA 31.2% $P = .98$	No reduction in TVF with RA
		Binary restenosis 8 mo	RA 50.5% PTCA 50.5% $P = 1.0$	No reduction in restenosis with RA
Aggressive Debulking				
STRATAS	RA (B/A <0.7) + standard PTCA vs RA (B/A 0.7-0.9) + minimal PTCA	Binary restenosis 6 mo	Standard 58% Aggressive 52% $P = NS$	No reduction in restenosis with aggressive debulking RA
CARAT	RA (B/A = 0.7) vs PTRA (B/A > 0.7)	MACE 6 mo	Standard 32.7% Aggressive 36.3% $P = NS$	No reduction in MACE with aggressive debulking RA
In-Stent Restenosis				
ROSTER	RA (B/A >0.7) vs PTCA for diffuse ISR. IVUS guided for all pts	TLR 9 mo	RA 32% PTCA 45% $P = .04$	Less repeat TLR with RA vs PTCA for diffuse ISR
ARTIST	RA (B/A >0.7) vs PTCA for diffuse ISR. IVUS guided in a subset.	MACE 6 mo	RA 80% PTCA 91% $P = .0052$	PTCA superior to RA for diffuse ISR
Optimization of Stenting				
ROTAXUS	DES vs RA plus DES alone for calcified complex native lesions	Late lumen loss in mm at 9 mo angiography	DES 0.44 ± 0.58 DES + RA 0.31 ± 0.52 $P = .04$	↑ Late lumen loss with routing RA prior to DES

B/A, balloon-to-artery ratio; DES, drug-eluting stent; ISR, in-stent restenosis; IVUS, intravascular ultrasound; MACE, major adverse cardiac events; PTCA, percutaneous transluminal coronary angioplasty; PTRA, percutaneous transluminal rotational atherectomy; RA, rotational atherectomy; TLR, target lesion revascularization; TVF, target vessel failure.
[a]Not necessarily the primary end point of the trial.

Lesion Selection for Rotational Atherectomy or Orbital Atherectomy

Based on the failure of atheroablation to improve clinical outcomes, current PCI guidelines do not recommend routine use of RA. With the superiority of DES firmly established, the primary role of RA is to facilitate delivery and expansion of DES. Heavily calcified lesions are the most common indication for RA. Rotablator should be avoided if there is angiographic evidence of dissection, thrombus, slow flow or no-reflow, or excessive vessel tortuosity. In patients with severe left ventricular dysfunction, hemodynamic support techniques may be considered. When aggressive balloon angioplasty has failed to dilate a lesion, balloon-generated dissection may be present, and RA in the same setting could compound the dissection or induce perforation.

Cutting balloon angioplasty (CBA) is designed to optimize acute luminal gain by creating controlled longitudinal incisions ("atherotomy") into coronary plaque with less barotrauma. CBA has been shown to increase luminal gains of RA followed by stenting compared to RA and POBA (plain old balloon angioplasty) followed by stenting.

Limitations and Complications of Rotational Atherectomy

Limitations of RA and OA include increased cost and lack of confirmed impact on restenosis. Procedural success is highly dependent on the operator's technique and experience. Particularly in longer lesions, RA and OA can be complicated by non–Q-wave myocardial infarction and no-reflow related to particle embolization and spasm. In addition, adenosine released secondary to microactivation and red cell hemolysis may lead to bradycardia and atrioventricular block. Therefore, temporary venous pacing may be required. Nevertheless, complication rates are low.

Cutting Balloon Angioplasty

Cutting balloons consist of a noncompliant balloon on which several longitudinal microtomes are mounted.

Mechanism of Cutting Balloon Angioplasty

CBA is designed to optimize acute luminal gain by creating controlled longitudinal incisions ("atherotomy") into coronary plaque with less barotrauma and with the goal of improving long-term outcomes.

Device Specifics

The Flextome and Wolverine Cutting Balloon dilation devices are available in 6, 10, and 15 mm lengths, and 2 to 4 mm in diameter. Based on the balloon diameter, 3 or 4 atherotomes are affixed longitudinally to the noncompliant nylon balloon. The 10- and 15-mm length devices integrate flex points into the atherotomes at 5-mm intervals to enhance deliverability (**Figures 26.5** and **26.6**).

Technique

The technique of CBA is similar to that of balloon angioplasty. However, slow inflation and deflation of the balloon and adherence to the maximal balloon inflation pressure are recommended in order to avoid disruption of the atherotomes.

Clinical Results

De Novo Lesions Large randomized trials have failed to demonstrate benefit of CBA over angioplasty (GRT and REDUCE trial; **Table 26.2**).

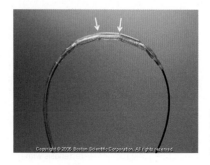

Figure 26.5 Cutting balloon. White arrows indicate flexion points on the atherotomes. (© 2020 Boston Scientific Corporation. All rights reserved.)

In-Stent Restenosis CBA has also not shown superiority over balloon angioplasty for the treatment of ISR. The Restenosis Cutting Balloon Evaluation Trial (RESCUT) randomized 428 ISR patients to CBA vs angioplasty; there was no difference in angiographic restenosis at 7 months (CBA 29.8%, PTCA 31.4%; $P = .82$). The REDUCE 2 trial from Japan also found no reduction in restenosis with CBA as compared to balloon angioplasty for ISR (**Table 26.2**).

Prestenting The REDUCE 3 trial randomized 521 patients to CBA vs angioplasty prior to BMS. In 453 patients with angiographic follow-up, restenosis at 6 months was reduced with CBA (11.8% vs 19.1%, $P = <.05$).

Lesion Selection for Cutting Balloon Angioplasty

Based on these findings, current guidelines do not recommend routine use of CBA for standard coronary lesions. The rigidity of CBA renders it less deliverable in tortuous or calcified vessels. Small vessels, bifurcations, and ostial lesions have all been proposed as appropriate targets, but the superiority of CBA over other techniques in these situations has not been proven. Reduced balloon slippage with CBA for ISR has led to a class IIb recommendation for CBA for this purpose. If predilation of ISR is required prior to repeat stenting of the lesion, reduced balloon slippage with CBA may minimize the trauma beyond the target lesion.

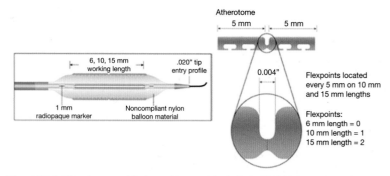

Figure 26.6 Atherotomes and flexion points on cutting balloon. (© 2020 Boston Scientific Corporation. All rights reserved.)

Table 26.2 Cutting Balloon Angioplasty Trials

Trial	Design	Relevant End point[a]	Findings	Implication
De Novo Lesions				
GRT	CBA vs PTCA in native vessels	Binary restenosis at 6 mo	CBA 31.4% PTCA 30.4% $P = .75$	No reduction of restenosis with CBA
REDUCE	CBA vs PTCA in native vessels	Binary restenosis at 6 mo	CBA 32.7% PTCA 25.5% $P = .75$	No reduction of restenosis with CBA
In-Stent Restenosis				
RESCUT	CBA vs PTCA for ISR	Binary restenosis at 7 mo	CBA 29.8% PTCA 31.4% $P = .82$	No reduction of repeat restenosis with CBA for ISR
REDUCE 2	CBA vs PTCA for ISR	Binary restenosis	CBA 24% PTCA 20%	No reduction of repeat restenosis with CBA for ISR
Korean Trial	CBA vs DES for focal ISR in DES	Binary restenosis at 9 mo	CBA 20.7% DES 3.1% $P = .06$	DES is superior to CBA for focal ISR in DES j

CBA, cutting balloon angioplasty; DES, drug-eluting stent; ISR, in-stent restenosis; PTCA, percutaneous transluminal coronary angioplasty.
[a]Not necessarily the primary end point of the trial.

Scoring Balloon Angioplasty

The AngioSculpt Scoring Balloon Catheter (AngioScore, Inc, Alameda, CA) utilizes a nitinol scoring element with 3 spiral struts that wrap around a semicompliant balloon (**Figure 26.7**). In one small, nonrandomized trial, predilation with AngioSculpt resulted in greater stent expansion by ultrasound criteria as compared to direct stenting or predilation with a standard semicompliant balloon. No randomized studies for coronary intervention have been performed with this device.

ABLATIVE LASER TECHNIQUES
Laser Angioplasty

LASER angioplasty was developed to achieve precise plaque removal and thereby lowering clinical restenosis and complication rates. Despite technological advancements, restenosis rates following laser angioplasty were not shown to be lower than with balloon angioplasty alone. Owing to the high cost of these systems and the lack of clinical benefit over other mechanical therapies, laser is now utilized infrequently, primarily as an adjunctive treatment to debulk lesions rather than as mainstream stand-alone therapy. Excimer Lasers used clinically vaporize water and clots, but were never designed to cut calcium. It is probably the residual blood and contrast in the laser field causing microcavitations which allows excimer lasers to have some success with calcium.

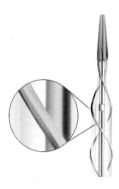

Figure 26.7 AngioSculpt scoring balloon catheter. (Illustration by courtesy of Koninklijke Philips N.V.)

Clinical Results

Randomized trials have not demonstrated an advantage of laser-assisted angioplasty as compared to balloon angioplasty (**Table 26.3**). In the Excimer Laser-Rotational Atherectomy Balloon Angioplasty Comparison (ERBAC) trial, 685 patients with a complex lesion were randomly assigned to balloon angioplasty ($n = 222$), ELCA ($n = 232$), or PTRA ($n = 231$). Despite higher procedural success with PTRA, target lesion revascularization at 6 months proved higher with both PTRA (42.4%) and ELCA (46.0%) than with angioplasty (31.9%; $P = .013$). The Laser Angioplasty vs Angioplasty (LAVA) trial randomized 215 patients with stable or unstable angina to holmium:YAG laser vs stand-alone angioplasty. Major in-hospital complications increased with laser (10.3% vs 4.1%; $P = .08$), with similar MACE-free survival rates at 6 months (71.1% vs 76.5%; $P = .55$). Finally, 308 patients with stable angina and lesions >10 mm long were randomized to ELCA vs balloon angioplasty in the Amsterdam-Rotterdam (AMRO) trial, which found no reduction in MACE (33.3% vs 29.9%) or angiographic restenosis (51.6% vs 41.3%) at 6 months.

Calcified/Undilatable Lesions The somewhat higher procedural failure rate of ELCA in the ERBAC trial was attributed to a significant proportion of heavily calcified lesions. In a prospective registry of undilatable lesions, procedural success with ELCA was significantly reduced in heavily calcified lesions as compared to other lesions (79% vs 96%; $P < .05$). Nevertheless, ELCA has a success rate similar to that of rotational atherectomy for the treatment of undilatable lesions. Despite its efficacy in undilatable lesions, laser angioplasty should not be attempted in cases where prior balloon dilation attempts have resulted in local vessel dissection. Use of excimer laser angioplasty in such substrates is invariably associated with worsened dissection or perforation.

In-Stent Restenosis Observational studies have shown no benefit of ELCA as compared to balloon angioplasty or PTRA for ISR. One important mechanism underlying ISR can be stent underexpansion. Lee et al. studied 81 patients (23 treated with ELCA, 58 without ELCA) who underwent OCT imaging both pre and post PCI for ISR with stent underexpansion. By OCT imaging, compared to high-pressure balloon dilation alone, ELCA was associated with more calcium fractures in the plaque surrounding the underexpanded stent, a larger final lumen diameter, and better stent expansion. This effect was more pronounced with the use of contrast flush, which is believed to result in greater photoacoustic modification of the plaque surrounding the underexpanded stent.

Table 26.3 Laser Angioplasty Trials

Trial	Design	Relevant End point[a]	Findings	Implication
Restenosis Trials				
ERBAC	ELCA vs PTCA in native vessels	TVR at 6 mo	ELCA 46.0% PTCA 31.9% $P = .01$	Unfavorable effect of ELCA on TVR
LAVA	ILCA vs PTCA in native vessels or SVG	MACE at 6 mo	ILCA 28.9% PTCA 23.5% $P = .55$	No reduction of MACE with ILCA
AMRO	ELCA vs PTCA in native vessels	MACE at 6 mo	ELCA 33.3% PTCA 29.9% $P = .55$	No reduction of MACE with ELCA
		Binary restenosis 6 mo	ELCA 51.6% PTCA 41.3% $P = .13$	No reduction of restenosis with ELCA

ELCA, excimer laser coronary angioplasty; ILCA, infrared laser coronary angioplasty; MACE, major adverse cardiac events; PTCA, percutaneous transluminal coronary angioplasty; SVG, saphenous vein graft; TVR, target lesion revascularization.
[a]Not necessarily the primary end point of the trial

MECHANICAL THROMBECTOMY

Acute myocardial ischemia is often precipitated by intracoronary thrombus formation. PCIs of these larger thrombi can lead to distal emboli, no-reflow, and abrupt closure. Mechanical devices that either disintegrate or aspirate and remove thrombus have therefore been developed as adjuncts in PCI for thrombotic lesions or in the setting of acute coronary syndromes.

Venturi/Bernoulli Suction

Use of a high-speed water jet to create suction via a Bernoulli/Venturi effect is the operating principle of the AngioJet (Boston Scientific) system (**Figure 26.8**).

Transient bradycardia is the most frequent complication during AngioJet rheolytic thrombectomy, particularly when utilized in the right coronary artery or a dominant circumflex system. This is probably owing to local adenosine release mediated by hemolysis. Temporary venous pacemaker placement is therefore recommended prior to AngioJet in these circumstances.

Clinical Results

AngioJet was approved for treatment of thrombus-containing native coronary arteries and SVGs based on the results of the second Vein Graft AngioJet Study (VeGAS-2). This study compared AngioJet vs intracoronary urokinase (6-30 hours) in thrombotic lesions prior to definitive revascularization. There was no difference in the primary composite clinical end point at 30 days (AngioJet, 29%; urokinase, 30%). However, the AngioJet strategy achieved higher procedural success (86% vs 72%, $P = .002$) with lower MACE at 30 days (16% vs 33%, $P < .001$) and fewer hemorrhagic and vascular complications.

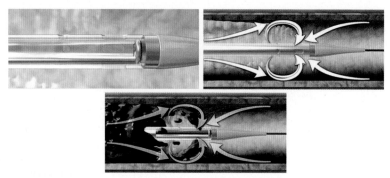

AngioJet was then applied in the setting of primary PCI for acute ST-elevation myocardial infarction (STEMI) where thrombus is prevalent (**Table 26.4**). In the AngioJet Rheolytic Thrombectomy in Patients Undergoing Primary Angioplasty for Acute Myocardial Infarction (AIMI) trial, compared to standard PCI, adjunctive AngioJet treatment was associated with larger infarct size, reduced TIMI flow grade, and higher 30-day MACE (6.7% vs 1.7%, $P = .01$), driven by an unexpectedly low mortality rate (0.8%) among control patients.

In the AngioJet Rheolytic Thrombectomy Before Direct Infarct Artery Stenting in Patients Undergoing Primary PCI for Acute Myocardial Infarction (JETSTENT), patients with visible thrombus were randomized to AngioJet plus stent vs direct stenting. AngioJet achieved disparate results with respect to the coprimary end points of ST-segment resolution at 30 minutes and scintigraphic infarct size, improving the former with no reduction in the latter. The 2011 and 2021 PCI guidelines conclude that rheolytic thrombectomy has demonstrated no clinical benefit in primary PCI.

Suction Thrombectomy

These devices generally have a double-lumen construction, allowing them to track over a guidewire passed through 1 lumen (generally a short monorail), while reserving the other full catheter length lumen for thrombus aspiration (TA). With most devices, suction is applied manually using a large syringe attached to the aspiration port.

Clinical Results

Acute Myocardial Infarction These aspiration systems have primarily been studied in primary PCI (**Table 26.4**). Early randomized trials comparing TA prior to PCI vs no TA prior to PCI suggested a significant benefit of TA. The strategy of routine TA prior to PCI appeared to improve indices of myocardial perfusion such as myocardial blush grade and resolution of ST elevation, and 1- to 2-year mortality was reduced in these trials. Based on these early data, the 2011 PCI guidelines assigned a class IIa recommendation to adjunctive aspiration thrombectomy during primary PCI, but mechanical thrombectomy and embolic protection were not recommended.

Table 26.4 Selected Major Prospective Randomized Trials of Embolic Protection Devices and Thrombus Removal Devices in Primary Percutaneous Coronary Intervention for Acute Myocardial Infarction

Trial Name	Trial Design	Device	Control	Primary End point	Results
Distal Protection					
EMERALD 2007	Prospective randomized multicenter (n = 501)	GuardWire	No distal protection	STR and infarct size at ^{99m}Tc Sestamibi Scan	No difference in STR at 30 min (63% vs 62%), MI size (12% vs 9.5%), or MACE at 6 mo (10% vs 11%)
PROMISE 2005	Prospective randomized (n = 200)	FilterWire (EZ)	No distal protection	Infarct related artery max flow velocity and infarct size at MRI	No difference in max flow velocity (34 vs 36 cm/s) or MI size (11.8% vs 10.4%)
DEDICATION 2008	Prospective randomized multicenter (n = 626)	FilterWire (EZ)	No distal protection	STR ≥70%	No difference in STR ≥70% (76% vs 72%)
PREMIAR 2007	Prospective randomized multicenter (n = 140)	Spider RX	No distal protection	STR ≥70%	No difference in STR ≥70% at 60 min (61% vs 60%)
PREPARE 2009	Prospective randomized multicenter (n = 284)	Proxis	No distal protection	STR ≥70%	No difference in STR ≥70% at 60 min (80% vs 72%). No difference in infarct size at 6 mo (6.1 vs 6.3 g/cm²)
Extraction/Aspiration					
AIMI 2006	Prospective randomized multicenter (n = 480)	AngioJet	No AngioJet	Infarct size by Tc Sestamibi perfusion scan	Final Infarct size higher in AngioJet group (12.5% vs 9.8%, P = .03)
X AMINE ST 2005	Prospective randomized multicenter (n = 201)	X-Sizer	No X-Sizer	STR	X-Sizer leads to better STR (7.5 vs 4.9 mm, P < .04)
JETSTENT 2010	Prospective randomized multicenter (n = 201)	AngioJet	No AngioJet	Coprimary: STR and ^{99m}Tc-Sestamibi infarct size	AngioJet achieved better STR (85.8% vs 78.8%, P = .043) with no improvement in infarct size (11.8% vs 12.7%, P = .4). One-year estimated freedom from MACE reduced with thrombectomy (85% vs 75%, P = .009)

(Continued)

Table 26.4 **Selected Major Prospective Randomized Trials of Embolic Protection Devices and Thrombus Removal Devices in Primary Percutaneous Coronary Intervention for Acute Myocardial Infarction (Continued)**

Trial Name	Trial Design	Device	Control	Primary End point	Results
TAPAS 2008	Prospective randomized multicenter (*n* = 1071)	Export	No aspiration	MBG ≤1	EXPORT reduced MBG ≤1 from 26.3%-17.1%, *P* < .001. One-year cardiac mortality reduced from 6.7%-3.6% (*P* = .02)
EXPIRA 2010	Prospective randomized (*n* = 175)	Export	No aspiration	MBG ≥2 and STR ≥70%	All patients received abciximab. EXPORT associated with improved MBG ≥2 (74% vs 60%, *P* < .001), reduced MACE at 24 mo (4.5% vs 13.7%, *P* = .038), and reduced cardiac death (0% vs 6.8%, *P* = .012)
TASTE 2013	Prospective randomized multicenter (*n* = 7244)	Multiple devices. 6F compatible, low profile	No Aspiration	30 d all-cause mortality	Death not reduced at 30 d (2.8% vs 3.0%, *P* = .06) or 1 y (5.3% vs 5.6%, *P* = .57). Stroke 0.5% in both groups (*P* = .87)
TOTAL	Prospective randomized multicenter (*n* = 10,732)	Export	No Aspiration	Composite of CV death, MI, cardiogenic shock, NYHA class IV CHF within 180 d	Composite end point not reduced at 180 d (6.9% vs 7.0%, *P* = .86) or at 1 y (8% vs 8%, *P* = .99). Stroke increased with aspiration at 30 d (0.7% vs 0.3%, *P* = .02) and at 1 y (1.2% vs 0.7%, *P* = .015)

CHF, congestive heart failure; CV, cardiovascular; MACE, major adverse cardiac events; MBG, myocardial blush grade; MI, myocardial infarction; MRI, magnetic resonance imaging; NYHA, New York Heart Association; STR, ST-segment resolution.

These favorable findings have now been refuted by several larger randomized trials comparing routine TA prior to primary PCI vs primary PCI alone for STEMI. The Thrombus Aspiration during ST-Segment Elevation Myocardial Infarction (TASTE) (*n* = 7244) and the ThrOmbecTomy with PCI vs PCI ALone in patients with STEMI (TOTAL) (*n* = 10,732) trials both demonstrated no clinical benefit of routine aspiration prior to primary PCI in early follow-up or at 1 year. In addition, the incidence of stroke was increased with routine TA in the TOTAL trial. Even when the analysis was restricted to patients in TOTAL with a high thrombus burden, there was still no improvement of clinical outcomes with routine TA.

In response to these data, the 2015 focused update of the 2011 PCI guidelines downgraded *routine* TA in primary PCI from a class IIa recommendation to a class III recommendation (no benefit). The usefulness of *selective* and *bailout* TA was considered not well established, a class IIb recommendation.

High-Risk Lesions The role of routine aspiration thrombectomy has also been assessed in high-risk lesions. In the recent INFUSE AMI study, 452 patients with high-risk lesions in the proximal or mid-LAD were treated with aspirin, clopidogrel, and bivalirudin, and randomized in a 2 × 2 factorial design to aspiration thrombectomy vs intracoronary abciximab. The primary end point of infarct size as assessed by cardiac MRI was reduced with abciximab (15.1% vs 17.9%, *P* = .03) but not with aspiration (17% vs 17.3%, *P* = .51). More recently, the CHEETAH study prospectively examined 400 patients with high thrombus burden resulting in coronary occlusion with the Penumbra Indigo Aspiration System with mechanical suction. TIMI-3 flow was obtained in 97.5% at final angiography. However, there was no control group enrolled. Thus, the role of clot aspiration systems in patients with high clot burden remains unresolved.

EMBOLIC PROTECTION DEVICES

Embolic protection devices (EPDs) were designed to minimize ischemic injury and no-reflow by trapping fragmented plaque and thrombus liberated during PCI. These devices can be divided into 3 types: (1) distal conduit occlusion, (2) proximal conduit occlusion, and (3) distal filtration (**Figure 26.9**). **Table 26.5** summarizes the technical aspects of many of the devices available currently or until recently.

Distal Occlusion Systems

These devices incorporate a balloon inflated distal to the target lesion during PCI to interrupt antegrade flow, trapping atherothrombotic debris and soluble vasoactive substances in the epicardial vessel. These components are then aspirated from the stagnant column prior to deflation of the occlusive balloon, thus avoiding embolization to the distal microvasculature when antegrade flow is restored. The theoretical advantage of distal occlusion is that debris of all sizes is captured and aspirated. This approach allows for the removal of soluble vasoactive or prothrombotic substances which would pass through alternative distal filtering devices. Distal occlusion has several important limitations, however. Ischemia during interruption of antegrade flow may not be tolerated in patients. With cessation of antegrade flow, angiography to guide the intervention is limited for the target lesion and impossible for the distal vasculature. The crossing profile of these devices is larger than those of low-profile coronary balloons, and the wires are less steerable than standard coronary guidewires. These factors lead to a risk of distal embolization before distal occlusion is established. PCI of a very proximal or ostial lesion without antegrade flow also risks debris embolization retrograde into the aorta with the potential for stroke.

The benefit of embolic protection for vein graft PCI was established in the SAFER (SVG Angioplasty Free of Emboli Randomized) trial, which assigned 801 patients to either a standard guidewire or the GuardWire distal occlusion system (**Figure 26.10**). Distal protection yielded a 42% relative risk reduction in MACE at 30 days (9.6% vs 16.5%; *P* = .004), driven by prevention of myocardial infarction (8.6% vs 14.7%; *P* = .008) and less coronary no-reflow (3% vs 9%; *P* = .02). These benefits were maintained even in the 61% of patients receiving GP IIb-IIIa inhibitors (10.7% vs 19.4%;

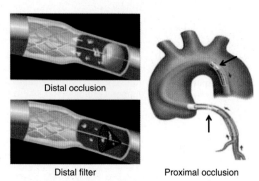

Distal occlusion

Distal filter   Proximal occlusion

Figure 26.9 Embolic protection devices. Top panel. Distal occlusion system such as GuardWire occludes antegrade flow during PCI. Liberated debris is then aspirated out from the stagnant column of blood above the balloon, followed by deflation of the balloon to restore antegrade coronary flow. Middle panel. Distal filter system is positioned beyond the target lesion in such a way that liberated debris during PCI is captured in the filter rather than embolizing to the distal vasculature. Bottom panel. Proximal occlusion system such as Proxis. Occlusion balloons on the device are inflated in the coronary segment above the target lesion and within the guide (black arrows), arresting antegrade flow. Once PCI is completed, aspiration of the stagnant column of blood is performed to remove liberated debris, followed by deflation of the occlusion balloons. PCI, percutaneous coronary intervention. (From MauriL, RogersC, BaimDS. Devices for distal protection during percutaneous coronary revascularization. *Circulation*. 2006;113:2651-2656.)

P = .008). Angiographic predictors of MACE in the SAFER trial included the degree of graft degeneration and estimated plaque volume in the lesion, but GuardWire demonstrated a significant benefit for all patients, not just high-risk patients.

Despite the benefits seen with distal occlusion devices in vein graft interventions, these devices have now been replaced by distal filter devices given the greater ease of use of the latter.

Distal Filters

Filtration devices utilize a nonocclusive basket deployed distal to the target lesion to capture embolic material larger than the interstices of the device mesh.

Advantages: Preserved antegrade coronary flow is a distinct advantage of the filter approach, minimizing ischemia and allowing angiographic visualization of the target lesion and distal vasculature during the period of embolic protection. The delivery and retrieval steps are intuitive to most interventionalists, often employing standard coronary guidewires to cross the lesion rather than a less responsive, bulkier occlusion balloon-wire apparatus.

Limitations: The need to traverse the target lesion incurs risk of device-induced distal embolization before protection is established. The completeness of distal protection may also be compromised when the filter is positioned in tortuous segments where apposition of the basket against the vessel wall is suboptimal. The pore size of the filter also determines the completeness of capture. Available devices have a pore size ranging from 80 to 150 μm to allow passage of red blood cells and leukocytes through the filter. Smaller particulate matter and soluble factors still traverse the filter and enter the microcirculation. A large burden of embolic material can occlude the filter and mimic no-reflow. This requires either prompt use of an aspiration catheter to clear the filter or filter retrieval to restore antegrade flow. In addition, filters require

Table 26.5 Coronary Embolic Protection Device Specifications

Device Type	FDA-Approved Devices	Manufacturer	Guide Compatibility	Guidewire Compatibility	Distal Landing Zone[a]	Advantages	Control
Distal filtration	SpiderFX	Medtronic Minneapolis, MN	6F	0.014″	20 mm	• Maintain antegrade flow • Allow angiography with device deployed • Rapid deployment and retrieval in most cases using techniques familiar to interventionalists	• Debris may embolize if smaller than filter pore size • Soluble factors not trapped • Filter crossing the lesion may cause distal embolization • Possibly difficult to place in the presence of tortuosity
Distal filtration	FilterWire EZ™	Boston Scientific Natick, MA	6F	0.014″	25 mm		

EPD, embolic protection device; FDA, U.S. Food and Drug Administration; PCI, percutaneous coronary intervention.
[a]Distal landing zone = disease-free segment distal to the lesion required to adequately deploy the device.

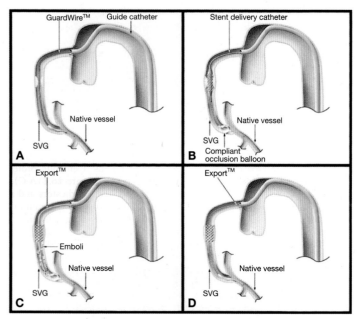

Figure 26.10 PercuSurge GuardWire (Medtronic) system. **A,** GuardWire is advanced across the lesion to the distal vessel. **B,** Stent is delivered, positioned, and deployed over the GuardWire and with distal balloon inflated to prevent embolization. **C,** Aspiration catheter is advanced into the vessel, and debris is aspirated with distal balloon inflated to prevent embolization. **D,** Distal balloon is deflated to restore antegrade flow. SVG, saphenous vein graft. (From BaimDS, WahrD, GeorgeB, et al. Randomized trial of a distal embolic protection device during percutaneous intervention of saphenous vein aorto-coronary bypass grafts. *Circulation.* 2002;105:1285-1290.)

a distal landing zone of approximately 18 to 30 mm from a graft anastomosis in order to accommodate the length of the device, thereby limiting use of distal filtration in the setting of very distal lesions.

FilterWire

FilterWire EX (Boston Scientific, Natick, MA) was the first filter approved by the U.S. Food and Drug Administration in 2003. It consists of a conventional guidewire to which an elliptical, radiopaque, nitinol loop is attached. A polyurethane filter bag with 110-pm pores is suspended from the nitinol loop. Intended for use in vessels 3.5 to 5.5 mm in diameter, FilterWire is delivered in its collapsed state within a 3.2F (6F guide-compatible) delivery sheath, which is withdrawn to allow the filter to expand and the procedure to be performed over the guidewire shaft. At the end of the intervention, a retrieval sheath is advanced over the wire to recollapse and withdraw the filter. A retrieval sheath with an angulated tip (EZ Bent Tip Retrieval Sheath) can be used to negotiate through the deployed stent if resistance is met with the standard sheath. The second-generation FilterWire EZ was designed to enhance filter centering even in curved segments and utilizes a lower-profile peel-away delivery sheath.

In the FilterWire EX Randomized Evaluation (FIRE) trial, the relative efficacy and safety of FilterWire were directly compared with those of distal occlusion using the

GuardWire in patients undergoing vein graft stenting (**Table 26.6**). A high 30-day MACE rate of 21.3% was observed with FilterWire in the early roll-in phase of FIRE, which was successfully reduced to 11.3% in the next phase by improvements in procedural technique including (1) ensuring >2.5 cm distance between lesion and distal anastomosis, (2) placement of the FilterWire in a straight landing zone segment (>2 cm), (3) use of orthogonal angiographic views to document circumferential filter apposition to the vessel wall prior to stenting, and (4) retracting only the proximal end of the debris-containing filter into the retrieval sheath. This favorable performance was continued in the randomized phase of the FIRE trial, which showed similar 30-day MACE rates with the FilterWire and the GuardWire (9.9% vs 11.6%, P = .0008 for noninferiority).

SpiderFX

The SpiderFX (ev3 Endovascular, Inc, Plymouth, MN) distal embolic protection system includes a capture wire and the SpiderFX catheter (**Figure 26.11A-C**). The capture wire has a nitinol mesh filter with proximal and distal indicators and a distal floppy tip, mounted on a 190-cm or convertible 320/190-cm polytetrafluoroethylene (PTFE)-coated 0.014-in stainless-steel wire. The filter has a heparin coating designed to maintain patency. The wire is designed to rotate and move longitudinally independent of the filter for enhanced stability during the procedure. The SpiderFX catheter has a 3.2F green delivery end and a 4.2F blue recovery end. The capture wire is provided preloaded into the SpiderFX catheter with the filter protruding from its distal tip. Submerged in saline to avoid air trapping, the wire is pulled into the tip of the catheter and back to a clear space in the catheter proximal to the coronary guidewire monorail exit. Any 0.014inch/0.018inch coronary wire is used to cross the target lesion. The SpiderFX catheter is advanced in a monorail fashion over the coronary guidewire and positioned so the proximal end of the filter can be deployed 2 cm beyond the target lesion (**Figures 26.12-26.16**). The coronary wire is then removed and the capture wire advanced out through the distal end of the SpiderFX catheter, allowing the nitinol filter to expand to provide distal protection. The catheter is removed, and PCI is performed over the capture wire. The capture wire has a score at the interface between its gold distal and black proximal ends. This can be used to break the wire if only a short wire is required for monorail systems. Once the PCI is completed, the recovery end of the SpiderFX catheter is advanced over the capture wire to retrieve the filter. At this point, wire positioning across the lesion is sacrificed.

In the SPIDER trial, 747 patients undergoing vein graft PCI were randomized to SpiderFX vs GuardWire with similar rates of MACE at 30 days (9.2% vs 8.7%, P = .012 for noninferiority). SpiderFX has subsequently been approved for both carotid and lower extremity intervention.

Embolic Protection During Acute Myocardial Infarction and Native Coronary Percutaneous Coronary Intervention

Randomized trials have failed to demonstrate significant benefit of routine embolic protection in primary PCI for STEMI (**Table 26.4**). In the EMERALD trial GuardWire, distal occlusion did not improve infarct size or ST-segment resolution as compared to a standard guidewire. Similarly, distal protection with the FilterWire in primary PCI did not improve maximal adenosine-induced flow velocity, infarct size, or 30-day mortality in the PROMISE trial, or complete (>70%) ST-segment resolution detected by continuous ST-segment monitoring in the DEDICATION trial.

Finally, proximal protection with PROXIS in the PREPARE trial did achieve more frequent immediate complete resolution of ST-segment elevation but did not improve the primary end point of ST-segment resolution at 60 minutes, and there was no reduction in infarct size or ventricular function at 6 months.

Table 26.6 Selected Major Trials of Embolic Protection Devices for SVG Intervention

Trial Name	Trial Design	Device	Control	Primary End point	Results
SAFER 2002	Prospective randomized SVG intervention ($n = 801$)	GuardWire (Occlusion Balloon)	No GuardWire	30-d MACE	MACE reduced with GuardWire (9.6% vs 16.5%, $P = .004$)
FIRE 2003	Prospective randomized SVG intervention ($n = 651$)	FilterWire EX	GuardWire (Occlusion Balloon)	30-d MACE	MACE similar for FilterWire and GuardWire (9.9% vs 11.6%; $P = .0008$ for *noninferiority*)
PRIDE 2005	Prospective randomized SVG intervention ($n = 631$)	TriActiv	GuardWire (Occlusion Balloon) or FilterWire EX	30-d MACE	MACE similar for TriActiv and control devices (11.2% vs 10.1%; $P = .02$ for *noninferiority*)
SPIDER 2006	Prospective randomized SVG intervention ($n = 732$)	SpiderFX	GuardWire (Occlusion Balloon) or FilterWire EX	30-d MACE	MACE similar for SpiderFX and control devices (9.2% vs 8.7%: $P = .012$ for *noninferiority*)
AMETHYST 2007	Prospective randomized SVG intervention ($n = 797$)	Interceptor PLUS	GuardWire or FilterWire	30-d MACE	MACE similar for Interceptor PLUS and control devices (8% vs 7.3%; $P = .025$ for *noninferiority*)
PROXIMAL 2007	Prospective randomized SVG intervention ($n = 594$)	Proxis	GuardWire or FilterWire	30-d MACE	MACE similar for Proxis and control devices (9.2% vs 10%; $P = .0061$ for *noninferiority*)

MACE, major adverse cardiac events; SVG, saphenous vein graft.

Embolic Protection Recommendations

The 2021 ACC/AHA/SCAI and 2018 ESC guidelines downgraded a class I recommendation for EPD use in SVG intervention based on the results of the SAFER and FIRE trials to a class IIa recommendation. This reduction from "should be used" to "reasonable to use" is based upon a recent large meta-analysis where the benefits of distal protection in contemporary practice were no longer demonstrated. As a result, an ACC National Cardiovascular Database Registry analysis revealed that EPDs were utilized in only 22% of SVG PCIs. Use of EPDs in STEMI has been disappointing with no significant benefit demonstrated. For this reason, no recommendations regarding EPD use in PCI for native coronary artery acute infarction have been offered.

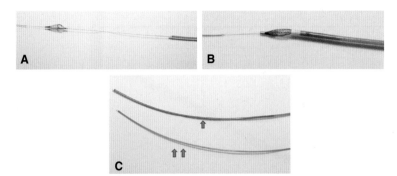

Figure 26.11 SpiderFX distal embolic protection system. **A,** Capture wire is seen extruded from the SpiderFX catheter. **B,** Capture wire is seen partially captured within the SpiderFX catheter. **C,** The filter is delivered through the green ("go") end of the SpiderFX catheter (double blue arrow). The filter is retrieved with the slightly larger blue ("back") end of the SpiderFX catheter (single blue arrow).

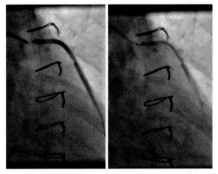

Figure 26.12 Severe ostial stenosis in vein graft to left anterior descending. Left panel shows coronary wire advanced across the lesion. Flow arrests due to guide occlusion of the ostium. Right panel shows SpiderFX catheter being advanced. It will not cross the critical ostial lesion.

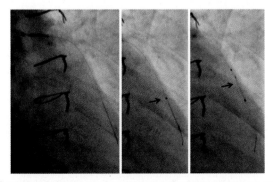

Figure 26.13 Predilation of the ostial lesion (left panel). SpiderFX catheter now successfully advanced beyond the lesion (middle panel, arrow). Coronary wire removed, and capture wire now advanced within the SpiderFX catheter (right panel, arrow). It is not yet extruded.

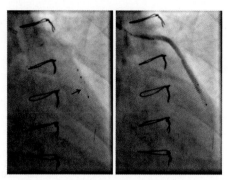

Figure 26.14 Capture wire desheathed from the SpiderFX catheter in the distal vein graft (left panel, arrow). Stent delivered to the ostial lesion (right panel).

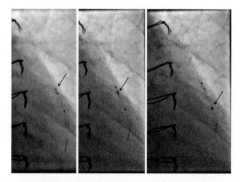

Figure 26.15 After successful stent deployment, blue retrieval end of the SpiderFX catheter is gradually advanced over the capture wire (black arrows show tip of the retrieval catheter as it is advanced). The capture wire and the SpiderFX catheter are then removed as a unit, leaving no wire in the graft.

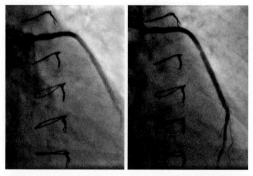

Figure 26.16 No-reflow occurs (left panel). After intragraft nitroprusside, there is return of brisk TIMI 3 flow (right panel).

SUGGESTED READINGS

1. Ahmed WH, al-Anazi MM, Bittl JA. Excimer laser-facilitated angioplasty for undilatable coronary narrowings. *Am J Cardiol.* 1996;78(9):1045-1046.
2. Albiero R, Silber S, Di Mario C, et al. Cutting balloon vs conventional balloon angioplasty for the treatment of in-stent restenosis: results of the restenosis cutting balloon evaluation trial (RESCUT). *J Am Coll Cardiol.* 2004;43(6):943-949.
3. Ali A, Cox D, Dib N, et al; AIMI Investigators. Rheolytic thrombectomy with percutaneous coronary intervention for infarct size reduction in acute myocardial infarction: 30-day results from a multicenter randomized study. *J Am Coll Cardiol.* 2006;48(2):244-252.
4. Appelman YE, Piek JJ, Strikwerda S, et al. Randomised trial of excimer laser angioplasty versus balloon angioplasty for treatment of obstructive coronary artery disease. *Lancet.* 1996;347(8994):79-84.
5. Baim DS, Wahr D, George B, et al. Randomized trial of a distal embolic protection device during percutaneous intervention of saphenous vein aorto-coronary bypass grafts. *Circulation.* 2002;105(11):1285-1290.
6. Burzotta F, De Vita M, Gu YL, et al. Clinical impact of thrombectomy in acute ST-elevation myocardial infarction: an individual patient-data pooled analysis of 11 trials. *Eur Heart J.* 2009;30(18):2193-2203.
7. Chambers JW, Feldman RL, Himmelstein SI, et al. Pivotal trial to evaluate the safety and efficacy of the orbital atherectomy system in treating de novo, severely calcified coronary lesions (ORBIT II). *JACC Cardiovasc Interv.* 2014;7(5):510-518.
8. Dauerman HL, Higgins PJ, Sparano AM, et al. Mechanical debulking versus balloon angioplasty for the treatment of true bifurcation lesions. *J Am Coll Cardiol.* 1998;32(7):1845-1852.
9. de Ribamar Costa J, Jr, Mintz GS, Carlier SG, et al. Nonrandomized comparison of coronary stenting under intravascular ultrasound guidance of direct stenting without predilation versus conventional predilation with a semi-compliant balloon versus predilation with a new scoring balloon. *Am J Cardiol.* 2007;100(5):812-817.
10. Deckelbaum LI, Natarajan MK, Bittl JA, et al. Effect of intracoronary saline infusion on dissection during excimer laser coronary angioplasty: a randomized trial. The Percutaneous Excimer Laser Coronary Angioplasty (PELCA) Investigators. *J Am Coll Cardiol.* 1995;26(5):1264-1269.
11. Dill T, Dietz U, Hamm CW, et al. A randomized comparison of balloon angioplasty versus rotational atherectomy in complex coronary lesions (COBRA study). *Eur Heart J.* 2000;21:1759-1766.
12. Dixon SR, Grines CL, O'Neill WW. The year in interventional cardiology. *J Am Coll Cardiol.* 2006;47(8):1689-1706.
13. Frobert O, Lagerqvist B, Olivecrona GK, et al. Thrombus aspiration during ST-segment elevation myocardial infarction. *N Engl J Med.* 2013;369(17):1587-1597.
14. Giugliano GR, Kuntz RE, Popma JJ, Cutlip DE, Baim DS; Saphenous Vein Graft Angioplasty Free of Emboli Randomized SAFER Trial Investigators. Determinants of 30-day adverse events following saphenous vein graft intervention with and without a distal occlusion embolic protection device. *Am J Cardiol.* 2005;95(2):173-177.
15. Halkin A, Masud AZ, Rogers C, et al. Six-month outcomes after percutaneous intervention for lesions in aortocoronary saphenous vein grafts using distal protection devices: results from the FIRE trial. *Am Heart J.* 2006;151(4):915.e1-915.e7.
16. Hamburger JN, Gijsbers GH, Ozaki Y, Ruygrok PN, de Feyter PJ, Serruys PW. Recanalization of chronic total coronary occlusions using a laser guide wire: a pilot study. *J Am Coll Cardiol.* 1997;30(3):649-656.
17. Hoffmann R, Mintz GS, Popma JJ, et al. Treatment of calcified coronary lesions with Palmaz-Schatz stents. An intravascular ultrasound study. *Eur Heart J.* 1998;19(8):1224-1231.
18. Isner JM, Rosenfield K, White CJ, et al. In vivo assessment of vascular pathology resulting from laser irradiation. Analysis of 23 patients studied by directional atherectomy immediately after laser angioplasty. *Circulation.* 1992;85(6):2185-2196.
19. Jolly SS, Cairns JA, Yusuf S, et al. Outcomes after thrombus aspiration for ST elevation myocardial infarction: 1-year follow-up of the prospective randomised TOTAL trial. *Lancet.* 2016;387(10014):127-135.
20. Jolly SS, James S, Džavík V, et al. Thrombus aspiration in ST-segment-elevation myocardial infarction. An individual patient meta-analysis: thrombectomy trialists collaboration. *Circulation.* 2017;135(2):143-152.
21. Kelbaek H, Terkelsen CJ, Helqvist S, et al. Randomized comparison of distal protection versus conventional treatment in primary percutaneous coronary intervention: the drug elution and distal protection in ST-elevation myocardial infarction (DEDICATION) trial. *J Am Coll Cardiol.* 2008;51(9):899-905.
22. Kini A, Reich D, Marmur JD, Mitre CA, Sharma SK. Reduction in periprocedural enzyme elevation by abciximab after rotational atherectomy of type B2 lesions: results of the Rota Reopro randomized trial. *Am Heart J.* 2001;142(6):965-969.

23. Koch KC, vom Dahl J, Kleinhans E, et al. Influence of a platelet GPIIb/IIIa receptor antagonist on myocardial hypoperfusion during rotational atherectomy as assessed by myocardial Tc-99m sestamibi scintigraphy. *J Am Coll Cardiol.* 1999;33(4):998-1004.

24. Koster R, Kahler J, Terres W, et al. Six-month clinical and angiographic outcome after successful excimer laser angioplasty for instent restenosis. *J Am Coll Cardiol.* 2000;36(1):69-74.

25. Kotani J, Nanto S, Mintz GS, et al. Plaque gruel of atheromatous coronary lesion may contribute to the no-reflow phenomenon in patients with acute coronary syndrome. *Circulation.* 2002;106(13):1672-1677.

26. Kuntz RE, Baim DS, Cohen DJ, et al. A trial comparing rheolytic thrombectomy with intracoronary urokinase for coronary and vein graft thrombus (the vein graft Angiojet study [VeGAS 2]). *Am J Cardiol.* 2002;89(3):326-330.

27. Levine GN, Bates ER, Blankenship JC, et al. 2011 ACCF/AHA/SCAI guideline for percutaneous coronary intervention. A report of the American College of Cardiology Foundation/American Heart Association Task Force on Practice Guidelines and the Society for Cardiovascular Angiography and Interventions. *J Am Coll Cardiol.* 2011;58(24):e44-e122.

28. Mauri L, Bonan R, Weiner BH, et al. Cutting balloon angioplasty for the prevention of restenosis: results of the cutting balloon global randomized trial. *Am J Cardiol.* 2002;90(10):1079-1083.

29. Mauri L, Reisman M, Buchbinder M, et al. Comparison of rotational atherectomy with conventional balloon angioplasty in the prevention of restenosis of small coronary arteries: results of the dilatation vs ablation revascularization trial targeting restenosis (DART). *Am Heart J.* 2003;145(5):847-854.

30. Mauri L, Cox D, Hermiller J, et al. The proximal trial: proximal protection during saphenous vein graft intervention using the proxis embolic protection system. A randomized, prospective, multicenter clinical trial. *J Am Coll Cardiol.* 2007;50(15):1442-1449.

31. Mehran R, Dangas G, Mintz GS, et al. Treatment of in-stent restenosis with excimer laser coronary angioplasty versus rotational atherectomy: comparative mechanisms and results. *Circulation.* 2000;101(21):2484-2489.

32. Mehta SK, Frutkin AD, Milford-Beland S, et al. Utilization of distal embolic protection in saphenous vein graft interventions (an analysis of 19,546 patients in the American College of Cardiology-National Cardiovascular Data Registry). *Am J Cardiol.* 2007;100(7):1114-1118.

33. Mintz GS, Kovach JA, Javier SP, et al. Mechanisms of lumen enlargement after excimer laser coronary angioplasty. An intravascular ultrasound study. *Circulation.* 1995;92(12):3408-3414.

34. Oesterle SN, Bittl JA, Leon MB, et al. Laser wire for crossing chronic total occlusions: "Learning phase" results from the US. Total trial. Total occlusion trial with angioplasty by using a laser wire. *Cathet Cardiovasc Diagn.* 1998;44(2):235-243.

35. Piana RN, Paik GY, Moscucci M, et al. Incidence and treatment of "no-reflow" after percutaneous coronary intervention. *Circulation.* 1994;89(6):2514-2518.

36. Rathore S, Matsuo H, Terashima M, et al. Rotational atherectomy for fibro-calcific coronary artery disease in drug eluting stent era: procedural outcomes and angiographic follow-up results. *Catheter Cardiovasc Interv.* 2010;75(6):919-927.

37. Reifart N, Vandormael M, Krajcar M, et al. Randomized comparison of angioplasty of complex coronary lesions at a single center. Excimer laser, rotational atherectomy, and balloon angioplasty comparison (ERBAC) study. *Circulation.* 1997;96(1):91-98.

38. Safian RD, Feldman T, Muller DW, et al. Coronary angioplasty and rotablator atherectomy trial (CARAT): immediate and late results of a prospective multicenter randomized trial. *Catheter Cardiovasc Interv.* 2001;53(2):213-220.

39. Sakakura K, Inohara T, Kohsaka S, et al. Incidence and determinants of complications in rotational atherectomy: insights from the national clinical data (J-PCI registry). *Circ Cardiovasc Interv.* 2016;9(11):e004278.

40. Sharma SK, Duvvuri S, Dangas G, et al. Rotational atherectomy for in-stent restenosis: acute and long-term results of the first 100 cases. *J Am Coll Cardiol.* 1998;32(5):1358-1365.

41. Song HG, Park DW, Kim YH, et al. Randomized comparison of optimal treatment strategies for in-stent restenosis after drug-eluting stent implantation. *J Am Coll Cardiol.* 2012;59(12):1093-1100.

42. Stone GW, de Marchena E, Dageforde D, et al. Prospective, randomized, multicenter comparison of laser-facilitated balloon angioplasty versus stand-alone balloon angioplasty in patients with obstructive coronary artery disease. The Laser Angioplasty versus Angioplasty (LAVA) Trial Investigators. *J Am Coll Cardiol.* 1997;30(7):1714-1721.

43. Stone GW, Cox DA, Babb J, et al. Prospective, randomized evaluation of thrombectomy prior to percutaneous intervention in diseased saphenous vein grafts and thrombus-containing coronary arteries. *J Am Coll Cardiol.* 2003;42(11):2007-2013.

44. Stone GW, Rogers C, Hermiller J, et al. Randomized comparison of distal protection with a filter-based catheter and a balloon occlusion and aspiration system during percutaneous intervention of diseased saphenous vein aorto-coronary bypass grafts. *Circulation.* 2003;108(5):548-553.
45. Stone GW, Webb J, Cox DA, et al. Distal microcirculatory protection during percutaneous coronary intervention in acute ST-segment elevation myocardial infarction: a randomized controlled trial. *J Am Med Assoc.* 2005;293(9):1063-1072.
46. Svilaas T, Vlaar PJ, van der Horst IC, et al. Thrombus aspiration during primary percutaneous coronary intervention. *N Engl J Med.* 2008;358(6):557-567.
47. Teirstein PS, Warth DC, Haq N, et al. High speed rotational coronary atherectomy for patients with diffuse coronary artery disease. *J Am Coll Cardiol.* 1991;18(7):1694-1701.
48. Vlaar PJ, Svilaas T, van der Horst IC, et al. Cardiac death and reinfarction after 1 year in the thrombus aspiration during percutaneous coronary intervention in acute myocardial infarction study (TAPAS): a 1-year follow-up study. *Lancet.* 2008;371(9628):1915-1920.
49. vom Dahl J, Dietz U, Haager PK, et al. Rotational atherectomy does not reduce recurrent in-stent restenosis: results of the angioplasty versus rotational atherectomy for treatment of diffuse in-stent restenosis trial (ARTIST). *Circulation.* 2002;105(5):583-588.
50. Whitlow PL, Bass TA, Kipperman RM, et al. Results of the study to determine rotablator and transluminal angioplasty strategy (STRATAS). *Am J Cardiol.* 2001;87(6):699-705.

27 Coronary Stenting[1]

The mechanism of balloon angioplasty involves plaque fracture (dissection) into the deep media, with expansion of the external elastic lamina, as well as partial axial plaque redistribution along the length of the treated vessel. The majority of vessels undergoing balloon angioplasty tolerate balloon dilatation and heal sufficiently to result in an adequate lumen. However, balloon-mediated injury to the vessel wall can be uncontrolled and excessive, resulting in balloon angioplasty's 2 major limitations: abrupt closure (occurring acutely) and restenosis (occurring later, within months after the procedure due to a combination of acute recoil and chronic constrictive remodeling). The coronary stent was thus devised as an endoluminal scaffold to create a larger initial lumen, to seal dissections, and to resist recoil.

Development of the Coronary Stent

Palmaz designed the first successful stent, a balloon-expandable slotted tube stainless steel stent in which rectangular slots were cut into thin-walled stainless steel tubing and deformed into diamond shaped windows during expansion by an underlying delivery balloon. However, its rigidity made delivery in the coronary vasculature difficult. In 1989, a design modification was made by Schatz, consisting of the placement of a 1-mm central articulating bridge connecting the 2 rigid 7-mm slotted segments, creating the 15-mm Palmaz-Schatz stent (**Figure 27.1**, right).

In 1989, enrollment commenced in 2 randomized multicenter studies (STRESS and BENESTENT) comparing balloon angioplasty alone with elective Palmaz-Schatz stenting. In these studies, the use of the Palmaz-Schatz stent was associated with markedly improved initial angiographic results, and with a 20% to 30% reduction in clinical and angiographic restenosis compared with conventional balloon angioplasty

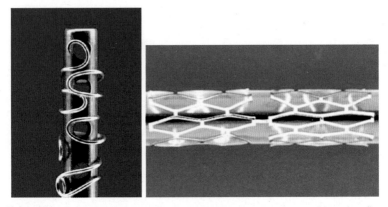

Figure 27.1 Left. The Gianturco-Roubin stent. Stainless steel sutures were wound around a cylindrical rod using pegs to shape the wire, resulting in a clamshell design. Right. The Palmaz-Schatz stent. Note the articulation between the 2 slotted tubes.

---

[1]We gratefully acknowledge the *Grossman & Baim's Cardiac Catheterization, Angiography, and Intervention*, 9th edition contributions of Drs David W. M. Muller and Ajay J. Kirtane as portions of their chapter, Coronary Stenting, were retained in this text.

(**Figure 27.2**). Long-term follow-up (to 15 years) subsequently demonstrated few late clinical or angiographic recurrences from years 1 to 5 after coronary stent implantation, with slight and progressive decrements in luminal size thereafter extending beyond 10 years. The mechanisms of this late progression of disease was related to the development of new atherosclerosis within the stented segment. Overall stent thrombosis rates remained low (1.5% at 15 years).

The anticoagulation regimen felt to be needed to prevent stent thrombosis included aspirin, dipyridamole, dextran, and warfarin. This profound degree of anticoagulation resulted in a marked increase in hemorrhagic and vascular complications. In 1994 to 1995, Dr. Antonio Colombo demonstrated reduced rates of stent thrombosis with intravascular ultrasound (IVUS)-guided deployment techniques including routine high-pressure dilatation (>14 atm), along with the combination of aspirin and a second antiplatelet agent (thienopyridine, ticlopidine) rather than prolonged warfarin therapy. These modifications reduced the incidence of stent thrombosis to ~1% to 2% and concomitantly reduced bleeding and vascular complications. The confirmation of Colombo's initial findings in several randomized clinical trials definitively established the superiority of dual-antiplatelet therapy (with aspirin and ticlopidine) over an anticoagulation-based approach for prevention of stent thrombosis.

Stent Design: Impact on Performance and Clinical Outcomes

Classification

Coronary stents may be classified based on their composition (eg, metallic or polymeric), configuration (eg, slotted tube, open cell, closed cell), bioabsorption (either inert [biostable or durable] or degradable [bioabsorbable]), coatings (none, passive [such as heparin or polytetrafluorethylene] or bioactive [such as those eluting rapamycin or paclitaxel]), and mode of implantation (eg, self-expanding or balloon-expandable). The ideal stent would be made of a nonthrombogenic radiopaque material to allow fluoroscopic visualization, have sufficient flexibility in its unexpanded state to permit passage through tortuous vessels, have an expanded configuration

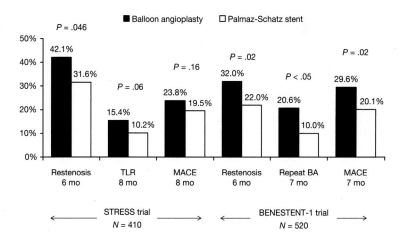

Figure 27.2 Results of STRESS and BENESTENT-1 landmark trials of the Palmaz-Schatz stent, which prevented restenosis in de novo lesions. BA, balloon angioplasty; MACEs, major adverse cardiac events; TLR, target lesion revascularization.

providing scaffolding with low recoil and maximal radial strength, and would allow access to side branches.

Stent Composition

Until recently, the most widely used stent material was 316L stainless steel. Cobalt chromium and platinum chromium alloys employed in more recent stent designs allow lower-profile thin stent struts (~75 μm, vs 100-150 μm in most stainless steel stents) that still maintain radial strength and visibility. Stent designs have also utilized Nitinol, a nickel/titanium alloy that has superelastic and thermal shape memory properties. Nitinol stents can be constrained on the delivery system and are able to return to the set shape when released.

Other than gold (which has been shown to increase restenosis), there is little evidence that thrombosis or restenosis rates vary with the specific stent metal. Biodegradable stents offer the advantages of increased longitudinal flexibility (though at the expense of radial force), and complete bioabsorption over a period of months to years, restoring underlying vascular reactivity. Bioabsorbable stents are either polymeric (eg, using proprietary biodegradable polymers or poly-L-lactic acid [PLLA], which is degraded to carbon dioxide and water) or nonpolymeric (eg, magnesium based).

Stent Configuration and Design

Stents can be assigned to 1 of 3 subgroups, based on construction: wire coils, slotted tubes/multicellular, and modular designs. Wire coil stents (eg, the Gianturco-Roubin stent, **Figure 27.1**) rapidly fell out of favor due to low axial and radial strength and recoil. Thus, the vast majority of stents in current use are either slotted tube/multicellular or modular in design. In an effort to preserve the radial strength and wall coverage of the original tubular designs (eg, the Palmaz stent) but improve flexibility in their collapsed states, several generations of slotted tube and multicellular stents were introduced by various manufacturers.

Multicellular stents can be broadly subclassified as either open cell or closed cell. Open-cell designs tend to have varying cell sizes and shapes along the stent and provide increased flexibility, deliverability, and side-branch access by staggering the cross-linking elements to provide radial strength. Open-cell designs tend to conform better on bends, although the cell area may open excessively on the outer curve of an angulated segment. Closed-cell designs typically incorporate a repeating unicellular element that provides more uniform wall coverage with less tendency for plaque prolapse, at the expense of reduced flexibility and side-branch access. Stents that possess better conformability, less rigidity, and greater circularity experimentally produce less vascular injury, thrombosis, and neointimal hyperplasia.

Ex vivo and clinical studies have suggested that thin stent struts may be associated with more rapid endothelial cell strut coverage, reduced neointimal hyperplasia, and lower rates of restenosis, in addition to inherently less thrombogenicity. While thin-strutted stents have obvious advantages, some of these stent platforms have been associated with a greater tendency for recoil (radial) or orthogonally, for axial (or "longitudinal") deformation and/or compression.

Balloon-Expandable vs Self-Expanding Stents

Balloon-expandable stents are mounted onto a delivery balloon and delivered into the coronary artery in their collapsed state. Once the stent is in the desired location, inflation of the delivery balloon expands the stent and embeds it into the arterial wall, following which the stent-delivery system is removed. Balloon-expandable stents are typically chosen to be 0.8 to 0.9 times the reference arterial luminal diameter, with the stent sized up to the closest 0.25 mm, and with a length several millimeters longer than the lesion. Almost all stents implanted in human coronary arteries are balloon expandable.

Self-expanding stents incorporate either specific geometric designs or nitinol shape-retaining metal to achieve a preset diameter. The stent is mounted onto the delivery system in its collapsed state and constrained by a restraining membrane or sheath. Retraction of the membrane allows the stent to reassume its unconstrained (expanded) geometry. While self-expanding stents are flexible and often easier to deliver compared with their balloon-expandable counterparts, restenosis has remained a concern, limiting their use in coronary arteries. Moreover, difficulties relating to accurate sizing and precise placement necessitate a longer operator learning curve and render these devices unsuitable for treating ostial lesions or stenoses adjacent to side branches.

DRUG-ELUTING STENT OVERVIEW
Limitations of Bare-Metal Stents

While coronary stents increase acute luminal diameters to a greater extent than balloon angioplasty, the vascular injury caused by stent implantation elicits an exaggerated degree of neointimal hyperplasia, resulting in greater decreases in luminal diameter (late lumen loss) compared with balloon angioplasty alone. However, the incremental gain in luminal dimensions with stenting compared with balloon angioplasty alone is typically greater than the incremental increase in late loss, resulting in a larger net gain in minimal luminal dimensions over the follow-up period. This observation was formulated as the "bigger is better" concept. Nonetheless, rates of clinical restenosis following bare-metal stent (BMS) implantation still approached 20% to 40% within 6 to 12 months. As such, coronary restenosis became known as the "Achilles heel" of coronary stenting. Drug-eluting stents (DESs), which maintain the mechanical advantages of BMS while delivering an antirestenotic pharmacologic therapy locally to the arterial wall, were shown to effectively and safely reduce the amount of in-stent tissue that accumulates after stent implantation, resulting in significantly reduced rates of clinical and angiographic restenosis.

Components of Drug-Eluting Stents

The 3 critical components of a DES include (1) the *stent* itself and its delivery system; (2) the *pharmacologic agent* being delivered; and (3) the *drug carrier*, which controls the drug dose and pharmacokinetic release rate (**Figure 27.3**, **Table 27.1**).

Stent Pharmacology

The antirestenotic properties of a wide range of pharmacologic agents have been tested in humans. The 2 most clinically effective classes of agents are the "rapamycin analogue" (or "-limus") family of drugs and paclitaxel (**Figure 27.4**). The principal mechanism of action of rapamycin (also known as sirolimus) and its analogues (including zotarolimus, everolimus, biolimus A9, novolimus, and amphilimus) is inhibition of the mammalian target of rapamycin (mTOR), which prevents cell cycle progression from the Go phase. The other agent that has been used effectively in coronary DES, drug-eluting balloons, and in peripheral DES applications is paclitaxel. By interfering with microtubule function, paclitaxel has multifunctional antiproliferative and anti-inflammatory properties, prevents smooth muscle migration, blocks cytokine and growth factor release and activity, interferes with secretory processes, is antiangiogenic, and impacts signal transduction. At low doses (similar to those in DES), paclitaxel affects the G0-G1 and G1-S phases (G1 arrest) resulting in cytostasis without cell death.

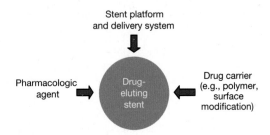

Figure 27.3 Components of drug-eluting stents.

Table 27.1 Generalized Classification of Drug-Eluting Stents

Generation	Drug	Polymer	Stent
First	*Sirolimus or Paclitaxel*	*Not specifically designed for biocompatibility*	*Early BMS platforms*
Cypher	Sirolimus	Biostable mix of poly-n-butyl methacrylate and polyethylene-vinyl acetate	Bx Velocity
TAXUS Express	Paclitaxel	Styrene-isobutylene-styrene (SIBS)	Express
TAXUS Liberté	Paclitaxel	Styrene-isobutylene-styrene (SIBS)	Liberté[a]
ION (TAXUS ELEMENT)	Paclitaxel	Styrene-isobutylene-styrene (SIBS)	Element (platinum-chromium)[a]
Second	*Limus analogues*	*Biocompatible polymers*	*More flexible, thinner-strut BMS*
Endeavor	Zotarolimus	Phosphorylcholine	Driver (cobalt alloy)
Xience V and Xience PRIME	Everolimus	Vinylidene fluoride and hexafluoropropylene	Multi-Link Vision and Multi-Link 8 (cobalt-chromium)
Xience Sierra	Everolimus	Vinylidene fluoride and hexafluoropropylene	Cobalt chromium
Promus Element Premier	Everolimus	Vinylidene fluoride and hexafluoropropylene	Element (platinum-chromium)
Synergy	Everolimus	Poly(lactide-co-glycolide) (PLGA)	Platinum chromium
Resolute	Zotarolimus	Biolinx polymer	Integrity, Onyx (cobalt alloy)

(Continued)

Table 27.1 **Generalized Classification of Drug-Eluting Stents (Continued)**

Generation	Drug	Polymer	Stent
BioMatrix	Biolimus A9	Abluminal poly-L-lactic acid (bioabsorbable)	Juno (stainless steel)
Nobori	Biolimus A9	Abluminal poly-L-lactic acid (bioabsorbable)	S-stent
Orsiro	Sirolimus	PLLA with silicon carbide layer	Cobalt chromium
Ultimaster	Sirolimus	Abluminal poly-D, L-lactic acid/polycaprolactone (PDLLA/PCL)	Cobalt chromium

[a]Liberte and, in particular, Element BMS platforms are newer BMS platforms but are included in the first-generation due to the presence of the original TAXUS polymer.

Polymers and Drug Delivery Systems

In order to more effectively regulate the dosing of antirestenotic agents, a *drug carrier* vehicle became necessary. Numerous polymer-based drug delivery systems have since been developed and are DES specific. While the polymer is instrumental in regulating the pharmacokinetics of drug delivery to the arterial wall, the polymer may also elicit deleterious vascular responses. Specifically, histopathologic studies have demonstrated hypersensitivity and eosinophilic inflammatory reactions and delayed endothelialization with first-generation DES that were not previously seen with BMS. It is believed that inflammation and delayed endothelialization play a role in the development of late stent malapposition, aneurysm formation, stent thrombosis, and restenosis.

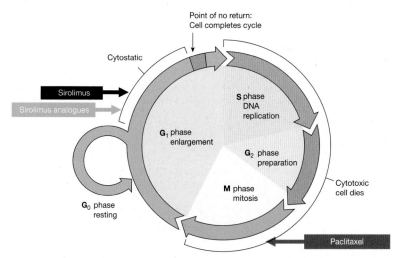

Figure 27.4 Diagram of the cell cycle showing the mechanisms of action of sirolimus and its analogues (phase G1) and paclitaxel (phase M). (Reproduced with permission from Seabra-Gomes R. Percutaneous coronary interventions with drug eluting stents for diabetic patients. *Heart*. 2006;92(3):410-419.)

GENERATIONS OF DRUG-ELUTING STENTS

DESs are often classified into several generations of development (**Table 27.1**). First-generation devices include the 2 DES that were initially approved for clinical use by most regulatory bodies, each of which utilized an early (currently outdated) BMS stent platform with early durable polymers (not specifically designed for biocompatibility) in order to deliver either sirolimus or paclitaxel. Second-generation devices (currently used in the vast majority of DES procedures) have incorporated more deliverable, thinner-strut stents with polymers that have been designed for biological compatibility.

Second-Generation Drug-Eluting Stents

Despite the demonstrated efficacy of first-generation sirolimus eluting stents (SES) and paclitaxel eluting stents (PES), concerns were raised about their late safety. Adverse reactions to first-generation DES polymers were described, with delayed endothelialization and late stent thrombosis. In order to mitigate some of the abnormal vessel responses associated with first-generation DES, several modifications of first-generation technology were implemented.

Everolimus-Eluting Stents (Xience V/Promus)

In the everolimus-eluting stents (EESs) (manufactured by Abbott Vascular [Santa Clara, California]; distributed as the Xience V, Xience PRIME, Xience Xpedition, Xience Alpine, and Xience Sierra stents, and by Boston Scientific as the Promus, Promus Element, and Synergy stents), everolimus (100 μg/cm^2) is released from a thin (7.8 μm), nonadhesive, durable, biocompatible, fluorocopolymer consisting of vinylidene fluoride and hexafluoropropylene monomers, coated onto a low-profile (81 μm strut thickness), flexible stent. The original cobalt chromium Xience V base stent platform has been progressively updated, most recently to the Xience Sierra platform, an 81-μm stent with a very low crossing profile (<100 μm). The release kinetics of EESs are similar to that seen with sirolimus from the SES (~80% of the drug released at 30 days, with none detectable after 120 days).

One intriguing attribute of EES that emerged was the low rate of stent thrombosis observed with this stent. First demonstrated in SPIRIT IV and COMPARE, these findings were also validated in several other studies, summarized in a meta-analysis of 13 randomized EES trials ($N = 17,101$) that demonstrated lower rates of ST with EES compared with non-EES DES.

Zotarolimus-Eluting Stents

Endeavor The zotarolimus-eluting Endeavor stent (ZES, Medtronic, Santa Rosa, California) was originally conceived as a second-generation DES, rapidly eluting zotarolimus (10 μg/1 mm stent length) from a thin layer (5.3 μm) of the biocompatible polymer phosphorylcholine from a flexible, low-profile (91 μm strut thickness) cobalt chromium stent. Phosphorylcholine is a naturally occurring phospholipid found in the membrane of red blood cells and is resistant to platelet adhesion. The potencies of zotarolimus, everolimus, and sirolimus are roughly comparable, and zotarolimus is somewhat more lipophilic. However, the release rate of zotarolimus from Endeavor (~90% within 7 days, 100% within 30 days) is significantly faster than the rate at which everolimus and sirolimus are released from EES and SES stents, respectively.

Resolute One potential explanation for the higher late lumen loss of the Endeavor platform was the fast rate of drug elution. The Resolute stent (Medtronic Inc) was designed to slow the release of zotarolimus. Like the Endeavor stent, zotarolimus is eluted from the thin-strut cobalt-alloy BMS platform. However, instead of the phosphorylcholine coating of the Endeavor stent, the Resolute stent employs the BioLinx tripolymer coating, consisting of a hydrophilic endoluminal component and a hydrophobic component adjacent to the metal stent surface. This polymer serves to slow the elution of zotarolimus, such that 60% of the drug is eluted by 30 days and 100% by 180 days, making this the slowest rapamycin analogue–eluting DES.

In summary, the ZES (Resolute platform) was the first stent to demonstrate comparable overall safety and efficacy to the EES platforms, with long-term follow-up suggesting durable safety and effectiveness of this stent.

CONCERNS REGARDING SAFETY OF DRUG-ELUTING STENTS AND POOLED COMPARISONS OF DRUG-ELUTING STENTS AND BARE-METAL STENTS

The evidence base for initial approvals by the US Food and Drug Administration (FDA) of DES consisted primarily of randomized controlled trials enrolling largely stable patients with relatively noncomplex, single, de novo coronary artery lesions. Data from these early studies demonstrated similar rates of death and myocardial infarction (MI) among DES- and BMS-treated patients. Yet, DES were quickly used "off label" (in higher-risk patients and in more complex lesions), which led to concerns about the safety and appropriateness of the routine use of DES in the "real world."

A number of analyses have amalgamated trial data across clinical studies to increase overall sample size. In the largest and most comprehensive meta-analysis of first-generation DES versus BMS studies (including 9470 patients from 22 randomized trials and 182,901 patients from 34 observational studies), the use of DES in randomized trials was associated with comparable rates of mortality and MI, with a 55% relative reduction in target vessel revascularization (TVR) (**Figure 27.5**). Another meta-analysis incorporated comparative data from SES versus BMS trials, PES versus BMS trials, and SES versus PES trials in a statistical "network" of trials to discern treatment effects across all included trials. In this analysis of 38 trials including data from 18,023 patients, target lesion revascularization (TLR) was lower with SES and PES compared with BMS, with similar mortality among patients treated with SES, PES, and BMS. A reduction in the hazard of MI was observed with SES compared with both BMS (hazard ratio [HR] 0.81, 95% credibility interval 0.66-0.97, $P = .030$) and PES (HR 0.83, 0.71-1.00, $P = .045$).

BIODEGRADABLE POLYMER DRUG-ELUTING METAL STENTS

Biolimus A9-Eluting Stents (BioMatrix, Nobori Stent)

Early data from clinical and histopathology studies raised concerns that durable polymer DES could lead to a foreign body–mediated chronic inflammation, poor arterial reendothelialization and healing and, subsequently, late stent thrombosis and neoatherosclerosis. As a consequence, platforms were developed with either a biodegradable polymer coating or a modified metallic surface that allows polymer-free drug delivery.

One of the first biodegradable polymer stent platforms was the BioMatrix stent (Biosensors International, Switzerland) (BES). The PLLA polymer on the abluminal surface of the BES elutes biolimus A9. The BioMatrix BES was first tested in the randomized STEALTH trial in which 120 patients with single de novo coronary lesions received either a BES or a BMS. Treatment with BES resulted in lower in-stent late loss at 6 months (0.26 vs 0.74 mm for BMS, $P < .001$). The largest trial examining the safety and efficacy of the BioMatrix stent was the LEADERS trial, which randomized 1707 "all-comer" patients (55% of whom had acute coronary syndromes) to BES or SES. Similar rates of all clinical endpoints were observed at 9 months with BES and SES, including the primary study endpoint, which was the composite of cardiac death, MI, or TVR (9.2% vs 10.5%, $P = .39$).

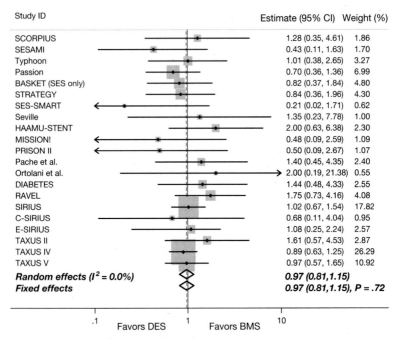

Study ID   Estimate (95% CI)   Weight (%)

Study ID	Estimate (95% CI)	Weight (%)
SCORPIUS	1.28 (0.35, 4.61)	1.86
SESAMI	0.43 (0.11, 1.63)	1.70
Typhoon	1.01 (0.38, 2.65)	3.27
Passion	0.70 (0.36, 1.36)	6.99
BASKET (SES only)	0.82 (0.37, 1.84)	4.80
STRATEGY	0.84 (0.36, 1.96)	4.30
SES-SMART	0.21 (0.02, 1.71)	0.62
Seville	1.35 (0.23, 7.78)	1.00
HAAMU-STENT	2.00 (0.63, 6.38)	2.30
MISSION!	0.48 (0.09, 2.59)	1.09
PRISON II	0.50 (0.09, 2.67)	1.07
Pache et al.	1.40 (0.45, 4.35)	2.40
Ortolani et al.	2.00 (0.19, 21.38)	0.55
DIABETES	1.44 (0.48, 4.33)	2.55
RAVEL	1.75 (0.73, 4.16)	4.08
SIRIUS	1.02 (0.67, 1.54)	17.82
C-SIRIUS	0.68 (0.11, 4.04)	0.95
E-SIRIUS	1.08 (0.25, 2.24)	2.57
TAXUS II	1.61 (0.57, 4.53)	2.87
TAXUS IV	0.89 (0.63, 1.25)	26.29
TAXUS V	0.97 (0.57, 1.65)	10.92
Random effects ($I^2 = 0.0\%$)	*0.97 (0.81, 1.15)*	
Fixed effects	*0.97 (0.81, 1.15), P = .72*	

.1   Favors DES   1   Favors BMS   10

Figure 27.5 Mortality in randomized trials comparing drug-eluting stents to bare-metal stents, demonstrating similar overall mortality of both stent types. DES, drug-eluting stent; BMS, bare-metal stent. (Reproduced with permission from Kirtane AJ, Gupta A, Iyengar S, et al. Safety and efficacy of drug-eluting and bare metal stents: comprehensive meta-analysis of randomized trials and observational studies. *Circulation.* 2009;119:3198-3206.)

Everolimus-Eluting Platinum-Chromium (SYNERGY) Stent

The SYNERGY stent (Boston Scientific Corporation, Natick, Massachusetts) is a thin strut (74 μm), platinum chromium, everolimus-eluting stent (PtCr-EES). The stents struts are covered on the abluminal surface by a thin coating of poly(D, L-lactic-co-glycolic acid) (PLGA) polymer, which is absorbed completely within 4 months. The stent platform was shown to be noninferior to a durable polymer EES (PROMUS Element, Boston Scientific) in the EVOLVE and EVOLVE II trials. In the EVOLVE study ($n = 291$), there was no difference at 5 years between the bioresorbable and durable platforms in incidence of TLF. Target-vessel revascularization was numerically lower in the SYNERGY arm (3.3% vs 10.2%, $P = .11$). In the larger EVOLVE II trial, the 5-year target lesion rates were 14.3% and 14.2%, respectively, with definite/probable stent thrombosis rates of 0.7% and 0.9% ($P = .75$).

POLYMER-FREE DRUG-ELUTING STENTS

In order to further reduce the potential for polymer-related inflammation and stent thrombosis, polymer-free drug eluting platforms have been developed. The successor to the BioMatrix stent platform is the BioFreedom stent (Biosensors Europe) (PF-BES), a stainless steel stent with a strut thickness of 112 μm. It has a modified abluminal surface that allows direct adhesion of biolimus to the stent without the need for a polymer coating. The majority (~90%) of the drug is released into the artery wall within 48 hours, with 100% of the drug released by 28 days. The platform was first evaluated in a patient population with a high bleeding risk. The LEADERS FREE trial randomly assigned 2466 patients with stable symptoms to receive a PF-BES or similar BMS. At 390 days, the primary safety endpoint (cardiac death, nonfatal MI, or stent thrombosis) occurred less frequently in the PF-BES-treated group (9.4% vs 12.9%, $P < .001$). The primary efficacy endpoint (clinically driven TLR) also occurred less frequently in the PF-BES group (5.1% vs 9.8%, $P < .001$). Subsequently, the PF-BES was compared with DP-EES in an all-comers population of 848 patients. At a median follow-up of 18.5 months, the incidence of major adverse events was 9.0% in the PF-BES compared with 4.5% in the DP-EES group ($P = .09$), with definite or probable stent thrombosis rates of 2.8% and 1.1%, respectively ($P = .123$). Restenosis occurred more commonly in the PF-BES group (2.3% vs 0.6%, $P = .041$).

The Cre8 stent (Alvimedica, Istanbul, Turkey) is a cobalt chromium stent with a strut thickness of 80 μm. Sirolimus, formulated with a nonpolymeric amphiphilic carrier mixture of long-chain fatty acids to form "amphilimus," is eluted from laser-drilled reservoirs on the abluminal surface of the stent. Approximately, 70% of the drug is released by 30 days and the remainder within 90 days. The Cre8 stent was shown to be noninferior to DP-EES in a small angiographic study (in-stent late loss 0.14 ± 0.24 mm vs 0.24 ± 0.57 mm, $P = .27$) and noninferior to ZES in a larger randomized trial of 1502 patients (TLF 5.6% vs 6.2%, P for noninferiority 0.0086).

Other similar approaches to polymer-free drug delivery have been reported. The Medtronic drug-filled stent (Medtronic) is a trilayered 86-μm wire stent that elutes sirolimus from laser-drilled holes that communicate with a central drug-filled lumen. The Medtronic Setagon stent consisted of a roughened metal surface that was "sponge-like" on electron microscopy and held drug within its metal recesses. However, drug release was unpredictable.

BIOABSORBABLE DRUG-ELUTING STENTS

The considerations that led to concerns about the potential for durable polymer DES resulted in a quest for completely resorbable drug-eluting polymers stents or scaffolds that had the following advantages over metallic stents: (1) complete resorption to allow restoration of physiological vasomotion, compensatory coronary dilatation, plaque reduction, and lumen enlargement; (2) improved endothelial coverage and reduced late stent thrombosis; (3) less interference with subsequent imaging by invasive or computed tomography angiography; and (4) less interference with coronary grafting in the event of subsequent coronary bypass surgery. The first drug-eluting bioresorbable stent was the Bioabsorbable Vascular Solutions EES (BVS-EES, Abbott Vascular). The BVS-EES (**Figure 27.6**) is a polymeric bioabsorbable scaffold constructed of PLLA with a thin mixture of poly-D, L-lactic acid (PDLLA) that serves as the drug-carrier vehicle for everolimus at a concentration of 8.2 μg/mm. The PDLLA enables controlled release of everolimus, with 80% elution by 30 days. The BVS-EES has an overall strut thickness of 150 μm in order to maintain structural integrity of the stent in coronary applications.

The BVS-EES platform was evaluated in a series of randomized controlled trials, each with the Xience EES as the comparator. These included ABSORB II, ABSORB III, ABSORB China, ABSORB Japan, AIDA, EVERBIO II, and TROFI II. Individually, several of these trials suggested an increased incidence of adverse events in the BVS-EES arm, a finding attributable to an increased incidence of scaffold thrombosis in the first 3 years of follow-up. As a consequence of the findings of these trials, the BVS-EES platform was withdrawn from commercial availability in the United States.

Although there appeared to be an early penalty for use of BVS, it was argued that the relatively short follow-up of the trials was insufficient to realize the potential

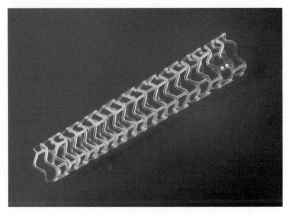

Figure 27.6 Bioabsorbable scaffold (BVS, Abbott Vascular).

advantages of BVS-EES once polymer degradation was complete. However, 5-year follow-up from the ABSORB III trial showed no difference in efficacy between BVS-EES and EES (TLF 17.5% vs 15.2%, P = .15; ischemia-driven TLR 9.5% vs 8.0%). There was a higher incidence of target-vessel MI (10.4% vs 7.5%, P = .04) and device thrombosis (2.5% vs 1.1%, P = .03). Currently, the European guidelines give the use of BVS a class IIIC indication for the treatment of coronary disease and do not recommend use of these devices outside clinical trials.

OTHER BIORESORBABLE SCAFFOLDS

An alternative to the fully reabsorbable polymer scaffolds is the magnesium alloy resorbable metallic scaffold (RMS). The second-generation RMS (Magmaris, Biotronik AG, Buelach, Switzerland) has a strut thickness of 150 μm with a PLLA coating that incorporates sirolimus at a dose of 1.4 μg/mm^2 (**Figure 27.7**). Degradation of the magnesium alloy occurs by conversion of the alloy to hydrated magnesium oxide and subsequent conversion to magnesium phosphate. Magnesium is eventually replaced by calcium, leaving an amorphous calcium phosphate as the only remaining element after 12 to 18 months. The Magmaris device has been evaluated in a series of clinical trials. The largest of these studies is the BIOSOLVE IV study, a single-arm study that plans to enroll 2054 patients. A prespecified interim analysis of the first 400 patients recently showed a device success rate of 96.1% and clinically driven TLR of 4.3%. There was 1 scaffold thrombosis.

Technical Aspects of Coronary Stent Implantation

Guide Catheter and Guidewire Selection Optimal guide catheter selection is critical for the successful completion of most stent procedures and requires the operator to consider *prior to the case* the amount of backup support required and the luminal dimensions of the guide to accommodate the devices likely to be used.

If the need of significant guide catheter backup support is anticipated (eg, fibrocalcific or tortuous vessels, distal lesions, or chronic total occlusions [CTOs]), or simultaneous delivery of multiple wires, stents, or use of atherectomy devices is planned, *larger-dimension guiding catheters* (eg, 7F) or those with specialized shapes (eg, Extra-Back Up or Voda shapes for the left coronary artery, and hockey stick or Amplatz shapes for the right coronary artery and saphenous vein grafts [SVGs]) should be chosen. Larger guiding catheters may also be required for stenting of bifurcation lesions when a 2-stent technique that requires contemporaneous delivery of both stents is required. An alternative to larger guide sizes to increase support is the use of a "mother-daughter" technique or coaxial deployment of a smaller catheter through an existing guide catheter system. Several guide extension catheters are now commercially available including the GuideLiner (Vascular Solutions, Maple Grove, Minnesota) and Guidezilla (Boston Scientific).

Stent Selection and Techniques to Optimize Acute and Long-Term Outcomes Optimal stent selection and implantation technique will minimize procedural complications, reduce the risk of stent thrombosis, and enhance long-term freedom from restenosis. Key issues include selection of the appropriate stent (including stent diameter and length), implantation pressure, the decision whether to predilate versus direct stent, and whether to postdilate or implant additional stents to achieve an optimal result (**Table 27.2**). Open-cell designs are generally more trackable than closed-cell stents and may be favored in tortuous vessels where conformability on bends is important or when stenting across bifurcation lesions (to reduce the risk of side-branch closure and preserve side-branch access). Closed-cell designs, in contrast, may be desirable when uniform or optimal scaffolding is required, such as in ostial lesions. If guide support is adequate and the stent does not easily pass across the lesion, it should be carefully withdrawn and the lesion should be aggressively predilated or modified (eg, by rotablation) before an attempt to readvance the stent is made.

High-pressure stent implantation with adjunctive IVUS has been shown to play an important role in achieving optimal stent expansion and apposition to the vessel wall. However, acceptable results have also been demonstrated with moderate-pressure implantation techniques without IVUS imaging. In a randomized trial of high (mean 16.9 atm) versus moderate (mean 11.1 atm) pressure for stent implantation in 934 patients, similar rates of stent thrombosis and restenosis were observed. In contrast, in a second randomized trial comparing routine high-pressure (17.0 atm) versus low-pressure (9.9 atm) stent implantation, high pressure resulted in greater initial and 6-month follow-up stent cross-sectional areas.

More important than the actual deployment pressure is the overall degree of expansion of the stent itself. Inadequate stent expansion has been linked to both stent thrombosis as well as restenosis. Complete lesion coverage without edge dissections is also important, as is the elimination of inflow and outflow stenoses that can compromise flow and lead to stent thrombosis. Implantation of additional short stents may be required to cover edge dissections and achieve optimal lumen dimensions. Although routine high-pressure stent implantation and high balloon-to-artery ratios result in greater stent expansion and optimize late outcomes, care must be taken to avoid edge dissections and perforation. The use of adjunctive imaging technologies including IVUS and OCT can be helpful to the operator.

Like adjunctive imaging technologies, physiologic lesion assessment (measurement of either coronary flow reserve or FFR) has utility during coronary stent implant procedures. FFR can be used to identify the hemodynamic significance of intermediate lesions, thereby providing direct physiologic evidence to the operator who can then address the suitability of the lesion for treatment.

Role of Plaque Modification Prior to Coronary Stent Implantation The amount of plaque present prior to and after stent implantation has been shown to be a strong determinant of subsequent restenosis, leading to the hypothesis that plaque debulking using either directional or rotational atherectomy devices prior to stenting would enhance event-free survival. However, randomized trials have been unable to demonstrate improved clinical or angiographic outcomes with atherectomy prior to stent implantation compared with stenting alone.

Table 27.2 Guidelines for Optimal Stent Selection and Implantation

1. **Choose the optimal stent length**
   a. Ensure adequate lesion coverage while avoiding excessively long stents, as stent length is a risk factor for periprocedural myonecrosis, stent thrombosis, and restenosis.
   b. Implant the stent from normal reference to normal reference if possible (starting 2 mm before and after the lesion shoulder), which will avoid edge dissections. An edge dissection, unless mild, often requires treatment with an additional short (8-10 mm) overlapping stent.
   c. In diffusely diseased vessels, a normal reference segment often cannot be identified. The most severe atherosclerotic segments should be stented, so there are no major inflow or outflow lesions proximal or distal to any stenosis. Spot stenting is likely preferable to the "full metal jacket." Avoid stenting over potential graft anastomosis site (eg, mid-distal left anterior descending).
   d. For long lesions, use 1 long stent if possible. If multiple stents are required, they should overlap by ~2 mm to ensure complete lesion coverage but minimizing the total length of overlap.
2. **Choose the optimal stent diameter**
   a. Size the stent diameter with a ratio of 1.0-1.1:1 to the *distal* reference vessel diameter. Be cognizant that the size of the distal vessel can be underestimated due to proximal severe disease or spasm (eg, in the setting of acute myocardial infarction).
   b. If the vessel is tapering, a larger noncompliant balloon can then be used to more fully expand the proximal stent segments.
   c. Be aware that within the same stent line, different-sized stents exist for different-diameter vessels. Oversizing stents designed for small vessels will lead to inadequate scaffolding and possibly strut fracture.
3. **Predilatation** versus **direct stenting**
   a. Direct stenting may be considered when guide catheter support is good to excellent. Lesions not generally amendable for direct stenting include those with excessive vessel or lesion tortuosity or calcification, diffuse disease or subtotal stenoses, bifurcations, acute myocardial infarction, or chronic total occlusions. While direct stenting is faster than predilatation prior to stenting, recognition of the potential for inadequate expansion is critical prior to deploying a stent that then cannot be expanded, which is a major risk factor for stent thrombosis and/or restenosis.
   b. If direct stenting is not feasible, predilatation should be performed with balloons undersized to the reference diameter by 0.5 mm and with length shorter than the lesion so as to not extend the length of stenosis requiring stenting. If this degree of predilatation does not allow stent passage, larger and/or higher pressure balloon inflations may be required.
4. **Implant and postdilate the stent at adequate pressure**
   a. Most stents (except those mounted on a very compliant delivery system) should be implanted using at least 12 atm of inflation pressure.
   b. Higher routine implantation pressures and/or requisite high pressure post dilation with a noncompliant balloon (16-18 atm or greater) are preferred by many to optimize stent expansion and are often required in fibrocalcific lesions.
   c. In diffusely diseased vessels, consider implanting the stent at 10-12 atm to avoid edge dissections, and then postdilate the stent at higher pressures using a short noncompliant balloon positioned within the stent margins.
5. **Strive for an optimal angiographic stent result, defined as**
   a. A residual stenosis <10%
   b. No edge dissection greater than national heart lung and blood institute type A
   c. Thrombolysis in myocardial infarction grade 3 flow
   d. Patency of all side branches >2.0 mm in diameter, absence of distal thromboemboli, perforation, or other angiographic complications with associated chest pain, electrocardiographic changes, or hemodynamic instability

At present, rotational atherectomy prior to stenting is used in "niche" indications, primarily to treat heavily calcified lesions or those resistant to balloon crossing or predilatation. In these cases, if rotational atherectomy is applied safely and with good operator technique, this technique can markedly improve the deliverability of coronary stents to the target lesion. Plaque modification of heavily fibrocalcific lesions can also be achieved using a cutting balloon or by delivering electric energy. The Coronary Lithoplasty System (Shockwave Medical, Fremont, California) has been evaluated in a multicenter registry. Plaque modification by fracturing of calcified lesions was evident by OCT.

COMPLICATIONS OF CORONARY STENTING
Stent Thrombosis

The most feared complication following stent placement is stent thrombosis, which, while fortunately rare (occurring in ~0.5% to 1% of patients within 1 year), in more than 80% of patients presents as acute MI. Treatment for stent thrombosis is almost always emergent repeat percutaneous coronary intervention (PCI), although optimal reperfusion is only achieved in two-thirds of patients. As a result, stent thrombosis has been associated with 30-day mortality rates of 10% to 25%. Moreover, approximately 20% of patients with a first stent thrombosis experience a recurrent stent thrombosis episode within 2 years.

The most widely used definition and timing classification of stent thrombosis was developed by the Academic Research Consortium, with definite or probable stent thrombosis considered the best trade-off between sensitivity and specificity. Stent thrombosis is also classified as primary if it is directly related to an implanted stent or secondary if it occurs at the stent site after an intervening TLR event. Primary stent thrombosis after BMS typically occurs within the first 30 days after implantation. In contrast, primary stent thrombosis after DES can occur years afterward, with an annual incidence of 0.2% to 0.3% in patients with noncomplex coronary artery disease and 0.4% to 0.6% in complex disease particularly with first-generation DES. Thus, primary stent thrombosis rates during long-term follow-up are higher with first-generation DES than with BMS, with the differences emerging predominately beyond the first year after implant. However, after taking into account secondary stent thrombotic events after TLR procedures for restenosis (which occur more commonly after BMS than DES), the overall incidence of stent thrombosis (primary plus secondary) does not seem to be increased with DES compared with BMS, and the overall late rates of death and MI have been similar with DES and BMS.

Patients who require oral anticoagulant therapy for atrial fibrillation and antiplatelet therapy for prevention of stent thrombosis remain a particularly difficult group. This challenge has been addressed by a number of trials. In the AUGUSTUS trial, 4616 patients who had an acute coronary syndrome and atrial fibrillation and underwent PCI or medical therapy with planned treatment with a P2Y12 inhibitor were randomly assigned in a 2 × 2 factorial design to apixaban or a vitamin K antagonist (VKA) and to aspirin or matching placebo. At 6-month follow-up, the incidence of major or clinically relevant nonmajor bleeding was lower for the apixaban group than the VKA group (10.5% vs 14.7%, $P < .001$) and for patients treated with placebo rather than aspirin (9.0% vs 16.1%, $P < .001$). Death or hospitalization was also lower in the apixaban group (23.5% vs 27.4%, $P = .002$) but was similar in the aspirin and placebo groups. In a recent network meta-analysis that included 11,542 patients undergoing PCI in 5 trials including AUGUSTUS, the optimal combination of antithrombotic and antiplatelet therapy was a direct oral anticoagulant and a P2Y12 antagonist.

The mechanisms underlying stent thrombosis are multifactorial and include patient-related factors, procedural factors (including stent choice), and postprocedural factors (including type and duration of antiplatelet therapy). Stent thrombosis occurs more frequently in complex patients and lesions, especially in patients with acute coronary syndromes and thrombotic lesions, diabetes, renal insufficiency, diffuse disease, small vessels, and bifurcation lesions requiring multiple stents. Variability in the antiplatelet response to clopidogrel (either identified through loss-of-function mutations to the enzyme responsible for conversion of clopidogrel to its active metabolite or through testing of platelet responsiveness) has been identified as an independent risk factor for early stent thrombosis. While more potent dual-antiplatelet therapies such as prasugrel or ticagrelor can reduce the incidence of stent thrombosis, these regimens are also associated with a greater risk of bleeding complications.

Procedural factors associated with stent thrombosis include the stent type selected and whether the stent is adequately expanded and apposed to the vessel wall and is placed in a vessel with sufficient "runoff" to support adequate flow through the stent. Hypersensitivity reactions to the DES polymer and vascular inflammation have been associated with stent thrombosis. Some DES polymers (particularly those not specifically designed for biocompatibility) may be inherently thrombogenic and prone to webbing and peeling, serving as a nidus for thrombosis. Strut fractures, which occur most commonly with stainless steel closed cell stent designs and especially with overlapping stents in the right coronary artery, have been pathologically and occasionally clinically linked to stent thrombosis. Whether late-acquired stent malapposition is a cause of late stent thrombosis or merely a reflection of underlying vascular toxicity to the drug or polymer with positive vessel remodeling is uncertain. It is also uncertain whether malapposition alone (in the absence of underexpansion) is a determinant of late stent thrombosis. The most commonly proposed explanation underlying the increased rate of very late primary stent thrombosis with DES compared with BMS is delayed or absent endothelialization of stent struts. In addition, some cases of very late stent thrombosis may be due to the development of neoatherosclerosis within stents with new plaque rupture.

The rates of stent thrombosis have clearly decreased with improvements in stent technology, imaging, adjunct pharmacology, and changes in deployment technique resulting from IVUS guidance. Less reactive and biocompatible polymers and improvements in stent design have significantly reduced the rates of early (EES) and late (EES, ZES(E), and BES) stent thrombosis. The role of potent antiplatelet therapy for the prevention of stent thrombosis, particularly in the early phase, is well established. While early observational studies uniformly documented that premature thienopyridine discontinuation within 6 months after DES placement was strongly associated with stent thrombosis, the role of prolonged dual-antiplatelet therapy is less clear with some studies in support of this hypothesis and others against.

Several trials have evaluated short-duration dual anti-platelet therapy (DAPT) and P2Y12 inhibitor monotherapy after second-generation DES. In Japan, Watanabe and colleagues compared 1-month DAPT followed by clopidogrel monotherapy with 1-year DAPT in 3045 patients. The composite primary endpoint, which included both ischemic and bleeding endpoints, occurred less frequently in the short-duration DAPT arm than in the 1-year DAPT arm (2.36% vs 3.70%, P for noninferiority <.001; P for superiority = .04). In Korea, 3-month DAPT followed by P2Y12 inhibitor monotherapy was compared with 1-year DAPT in 2993 patients. The short-duration DAPT regimen was noninferior to 1-year DAPT with respect to major adverse cardiac and cerebrovascular events, with less frequent bleeding (2.0% vs 3.4%, P = .02). Finally,

Mehran and colleagues compared ticagrelor monotherapy after 3 months' DAPT with 1-year ticagrelor and aspirin in 7119 patients undergoing complex PCI with at least 1 risk factor for ischemic or bleeding complications. The primary endpoint (Bleeding Research Academic Consortium type 2, 3, or 5 bleeding) was lower (4.0% vs 7.1%, $P < .001$) in the ticagrelor monotherapy arm, with no difference in the incidence of death, nonfatal MI, or nonfatal stroke (3.9% vs 3.9%, P for noninferiority <.001). Together, these trials suggest that short-duration DAPT (3-6 months), followed by P2Y12 inhibitor monotherapy, may provide optimal control of both ischemic and bleeding complications after PCI using second-generation DES.

Treatment of Stent Thrombosis

Prompt reperfusion is critical when treating stent thrombosis. Stent thrombosis may be treated with emergent thrombectomy (either aspiration or mechanical) or with balloon angioplasty alone, often in conjunction with administration of more potent antiplatelet regimens including glycoprotein IIb/IIIa inhibitors. The placement of additional stents should usually be avoided unless a mechanical reason for the initial thrombotic event is ascertained (eg, edge dissection or residual untreated disease). The use of adjunctive imaging such as IVUS or OCT will often reveal a possible cause of stent thrombosis, such as stent underexpansion or malapposition, residual dissection, or significant inflow or outflow stenosis, and is thus recommended following thrombectomy. Maintenance antiplatelet therapy is typically escalated in cases of stent thrombosis (eg, clopidogrel is switched to prasugrel or ticagrelor).

Restenosis

Restenosis is most commonly defined as renarrowing to a diameter stenosis >50%, either within the stent or within 5 mm proximal or distal to the stent margin. By increasing acute luminal gain and eliminating late recoil and negative vessel remodeling, stents reduce the rates of restenosis compared with balloon angioplasty. However, stents induce more arterial injury than stand-alone balloon angioplasty and therefore elicit a greater absolute amount of neointimal hyperplasia developing over the first 6 to 12 months after the procedure.

The causes of restenosis after stent implantation are multifactorial. In addition to excessive late neointimal hyperplasia, restenosis after BMS and DES has been associated with stent underexpansion, edge dissections, residual untreated disease, geographic miss, and strut fractures. Excessive inflammation from first-generation DES polymers (specifically eosinophilic reactions to PES and granulomatous reactions to SES) may provoke late restenosis.

Numerous studies have demonstrated that the most reproducible determinates of restenosis after BMS implantation are the presence of diabetes mellitus, small-vessel diameter, and long lesion length. Other factors associated with restenosis are treatment of ostial and/or calcified lesions, true bifurcation lesions requiring main vessel and side-branch stents, CTOs, and SVGs. The same factors are associated with higher rates of DES restenosis, although to a lesser degree because of the profound effects of DES in limiting the intimal hyperplastic response to stent implantation. Angiographic and clinical restenosis (as well as death, MI, and stent thrombosis) after DES occurs less frequently in FDA-approved "on-label" lesions than in more complex off-label lesions, although, in nearly all cases, DES have been shown to reduce TLR compared with BMS.

Patients who develop in-stent restenosis are at high risk for recurrence after percutaneous treatment, especially if the pattern of restenosis is diffuse. IVUS and/or OCT imaging is highly useful in patients with restenosis to differentiate neointimal hyperplasia from stent underexpansion, geographic miss, strut fracture, and other rare occurrences such as chronic recoil and stent embolization, which require directed approaches to successfully manage. Isolated restenosis at the stent edge can often be effectively treated with balloon angioplasty only or an additional short stent. Treatment options for diffuse BMS restenosis due to neointimal hyperplasia have been extensively studied. In the BMS era, cutting balloons, directional or rotational atherectomy, or repeat BMS did not prove better than balloon angioplasty for diffuse in-stent restenosis. Vascular brachytherapy with locally applied beta or gamma radiation was effective in reducing recurrent restenosis within 1 year but was logistically complex, and the resultant vascular toxicity from prolonged inflammation and obliteration of normal cell lines resulted in high rates of late stent thrombosis and restenosis. Following the introduction of DES, 2 multicenter randomized trials demonstrated that SES and PES significantly reduced angiographic restenosis and improved event-free survival compared with either beta or gamma vascular brachytherapy in patients with BMS restenosis. Treatment of in-stent restenosis with DES was shown to be superior to balloon angioplasty alone in the randomized ISAR-DESIRE trial. Angiographic follow-up at 6 months demonstrated recurrent restenosis after balloon angioplasty in 44.6% of patients treated versus 14.3% for SES ($P < .001$) and 21.7% for PES ($P = .001$). Based on the results of this and other trials, DES has become the standard of care for nearly all cases of BMS and DES restenosis due to intimal hyperplasia.

Compared with BMS restenosis, DES restenosis tends to be focal. If the stenosis is isolated to the margin of the stent, or is focal within the stent, balloon angioplasty is often selected. Management of diffuse DES restenosis has been less studied. Many operators consider diffuse in-stent restenosis after DES to represent "drug failure" and will treat with a different class of agent (eg, PES after SES failure). However, in the ISAR-DESIRE-2 trial, 450 patients with SES restenosis were randomized to SES versus PES. At 6- to 8-month follow-up, there were no differences between SES and PES in late loss (0.40 ± 0.65 mm vs 0.38 ± 0.59 mm; $P = .85$), binary restenosis (19.6% vs 20.6%; $P = .69$), or TLR (16.6% vs 14.6%; $P = .52$).

An alternative strategy for treating in-stent stenosis after either BMS or DES is the use of a drug-coated balloon (DCB). Paclitaxel-coated balloons, in particular, have been shown to be superior to plain balloon angioplasty, comparable with first-generation DES, and inferior or comparable with second-generation DES in preventing a further recurrent stenosis. The most recent European guidelines on myocardial revascularization recommend DCB use for treatment of in-stent restenosis after BMS or DES with a class IA indication.

Other Complications of Coronary Stent Implantation

Side-Branch Compromise/Occlusion

Side-branch compromise after stent implantation most commonly results from shifting of plaque during stent deployment. This has been termed the "snowplow" effect. Stent-induced occlusion of a large side branch may result in significant myocardial ischemia and infarction, although in most patients, the long-term prognosis is excellent and most initially occluded side branches are patent at late angiographic follow-up.

Side-branch compromise and/or occlusion should be anticipated whenever a stent is placed across a side branch. If the side branch is >2.5 mm in diameter and diseased at its ostium, it should be protected with a second guidewire prior to PCI. It is often beneficial to predilate the side branch prior to stent implantation in the main branch. Predilation of bifurcations is most commonly performed with conventional balloon angioplasty, but alternatives include use of debulking techniques such as atherectomy, although these approaches have not been clearly shown to preserve side-branch patency beyond that achieved by balloon angioplasty alone. Once the side branch is protected with a second wire and predilated if necessary, a stent may be placed in the main vessel across the branch origin, temporarily "jailing" the wire. This usually preserves patency of the side branch should occlusion otherwise occur and serves as a locator for the side-branch origin. If additional angioplasty is planned, a third wire should then be passed through the stent struts into the narrowed side branch, after which the jailed wire is removed. The likelihood of a jailed wire becoming "stuck" is rare if the parent vessel stent is implanted at ~12 atm of pressure, but jailing a long segment of wire in the parent vessel should be avoided, and hydrophilic wires should be used cautiously because of the risk of stripping the polymer coating on its withdrawal.

Stent Embolization

Embolization of the stent from the stent delivery system may occur during antegrade passage in a fibrocalcific or tortuous vessel or upon withdrawal of the device after failure to cross a lesion (often when the edge of the stent snags on the tip of the guide catheter or on another plaque proximal to the lesion itself). Risk factors for stent embolization include heavy vessel calcification, pronounced vessel tortuosity, diffuse disease, and attempting to deliver a stent to a distal lesion through a previously implanted proximal stent. Stent dislodgement within the coronary arterial tree is associated with significant rates of coronary thrombosis, coronary artery occlusion, and subsequent MI, with mortality rates as high as 17%. If the stent can be removed through percutaneous (nonsurgical) techniques, the majority of patients have a satisfactory outcome.

Success rates for percutaneous retrieval of lost stents from the coronary tree have ranged from 40% to 70% of patients. There are several basic strategies that can be employed to address stent embolization. If the coronary guidewire is still through the stent and has been maintained in the distal coronary artery, a low-profile balloon can sometimes be advanced through the stent, allowing the stent to be repositioned across the target lesion and expanded. If the stent cannot be repositioned, the balloon can be placed distal to the stent and inflated to trap the stent between the balloon and guiding catheter, and then all components can be withdrawn together into the femoral sheath. If guidewire position has been lost and the unexpanded stent is located in a proximal portion of the coronary artery or has embolized into a peripheral artery, it can sometimes be removed using snare devices or forceps. If the stent is displaced from the wire more distally within the artery, a snare or series of wires can be wrapped around it to attempt to ensnare it. Alternatively, a second stent may be expanded adjacent to the dislodged stent to trap and crush it against the vessel wall, effectively excluding it from the lumen.

Coronary Perforation

Although the routine use of high-pressure postdilatation improves stent expansion, the significant barotrauma imparted to the vessel may result in frank perforation, particularly if oversized or very compliant balloons are used either for deployment or post dilation. In a retrospective analysis, Ellis and colleagues documented a 0.5% incidence of perforation among 12,900 procedures. From most contemporary series with stents, perforation has been reported in 0.2% to 1.0% of patients, although mild perforations are likely underreported. Risk factors for perforation include female gender, advanced age, lesion calcification and angulation, CTOs, and adjunctive atherectomy use. Device oversizing is also a risk for perforation (balloon-to-artery ratio >1.2) and has a risk of perforation and vessel rupture ranging from 1.2% to 3.0%. Most small perforations can be sealed with prolonged balloon inflations and reversal of unfractionated heparin anticoagulation with protamine.

STENT USAGE IN SPECIFIC PATIENTS AND LESIONS

Acute ST-Segment Elevation Myocardial Infarction

Prompt reperfusion with either fibrinolytic therapy or PCI has been demonstrated to improve myocardial salvage and reduce mortality for patients with acute ST-segment elevation myocardial infarction (STEMI). Compared with fibrinolytic therapy, timely reperfusion with PCI results in improved myocardial salvage and reduced rates of recurrent ischemia, reinfarction, stroke, and death. Several studies have examined the use of stents compared with balloon angioplasty in patients with STEMI. In a meta-analysis of studies comparing the use of BMS with balloon angioplasty alone, implantation of BMS in STEMI was shown to result in similar rates of mortality and reinfarction but reduced rates of TVR.

Following the introduction of DES, several randomized trials compared the use of DES versus BMS in patients with STEMI. The largest trial was the HORIZONS-AMI trial, which randomized 3002 patients with evolving STEMI to PES versus BMS. At 12 months, PES compared with BMS reduced the rates of ischemia-driven TLR (4.5% vs 7.5%, HR [95% confidence interval (CI) = 0.59 (0.43, 0.83)], $P = .002$) with similar rates of major adverse cardiac events (MACE) (8.1% vs 8.0%, HR [95% CI] = 1.02 [0.76, 1.36], $P = .92$). Clinical follow-up from HORIZONS-AMI at 3 years demonstrated nonsignificantly different rates of death, reinfarction, stent thrombosis, and MACE with PES and BMS. TLR was reduced from 15.1% with BMS to 9.4% with PES (HR [95% CI] = 0.60 [0.48, 0.76], $P < .001$).

Multivessel and Left Main Disease

Although left main and multivessel disease are distinctly different conditions, revascularization decisions for these patients are often considered together because, historically, the default strategy for these lesion subtypes has been coronary artery bypass graft (CABG).

Among patients enrolled in trials using BMS, follow-up to 5 years demonstrated comparable rates of death, MI, or stroke between BMS and CABG (16.7% vs 16.9%, $P = .69$), with no heterogeneity noted in patients with diabetes versus those without diabetes or with double- versus triple-vessel disease. However, the 5-year rates of unplanned revascularization were significantly higher with BMS compared with CABG (29.0% vs 7.9%, $P < .001$).

The first sizable study to compare the relative safety and efficacy of DES versus CABG in multivessel and left main coronary artery (LMCA) disease was the SYNTAX trial, which randomized 1800 patients with triple-vessel disease ($N = 1095$) and/or left main disease ($N = 705$) to PES(E) versus CABG, with the primary aim of demonstrating noninferiority of PCI to CABG. However, the primary endpoint of SYNTAX, the 1-year composite rate of all-cause mortality, stroke, MI, or unplanned repeat revascularization occurred significantly less commonly with CABG than with PES and thus noninferiority could not be claimed. The major differences in the primary study endpoint were driven by greater rates of repeat revascularization with PCI compared with CABG. The composite endpoint of death, MI, or stroke was no different between the 2 study arms, and the rates of death or MI individually were similar between PCI and CABG. However, the 1-year rate of stroke was significantly lower with PCI than with CABG. At 5-year follow-up, the Kaplan-Meier estimates of major adverse cardiac or cerebrovascular event (MACCE) were lower in the CABG group (26.9% vs 37.3%, $P < .0001$). The estimates were lower for MI (3.8% vs 9.7%, $P < .0001$) and repeat revascularization (13.7% vs 25.9%, $P < .0001$) in the CABG group, but all-cause death and stroke were not statistically different. MACCE outcomes were similar in patients with left main coronary disease and in patients with a low SYNTAX score.

The SYNTAX score (www.syntaxscore.com) is an anatomy-based risk score that was prospectively defined prior to patient enrollment in the SYNTAX trial. Patients undergoing PCI had progressively higher MACCE rates with increasing SYNTAX scores, whereas MACCE outcomes after CABG were independent of SYNTAX score. MACCE outcomes were significantly lower for patients treated with CABG than for PCI in the intermediate SYNTAX score group (25.8% vs 36.0%, $P = .008$) and in the high SYNTAX score group (26.8% vs 44.0%, $P < .0001$). Ten-year follow-up data from the SYNTAX trial were recently published. All-cause mortality was similar in the 2 groups (PCI 28% vs CABG 24%, $P = .066$). However, there was a survival benefit for CABG in the 3-vessel disease group (CABG 21% vs PCI 28%, HR 1.42 [95% CI 1.11-1.81]) that was not seen in patients with left main coronary disease (CABG 28% vs PCI 27%). There was no apparent difference in outcomes for patients with diabetes or across the SYNTAX tertiles.

Nonetheless, on the basis of the SYNTAX trial and other first-generation DES trials, the US and EU guidelines elevated PCI of the left main to either a class IIb recommendation (US guidelines) or IIa or IIb (EU guidelines) depending on the relative risk and complexity for PCI versus CABG. However, the optimal treatment of unprotected LMCA disease has remained a subject of considerable debate. Two large trials have evaluated second-generation DES compared with CABG for LMCA disease. The EXCEL trial randomized 1905 patients with LMCA disease (>70% diameter stenosis) and a low to moderate SYNTAX score (0-32) to stenting (Xience EES) or CABG. The primary endpoint of all-cause death, stroke, or MI at 3 years was noninferior in the PCI group compared with CABG (15.4% vs 14.7%, P for noninferiority = 0.02). The secondary composite endpoint (death, stroke, MI, or ischemia-driven revascularization) was also noninferior (23.1% vs 19.1%, P for noninferiority = 0.01). At 5 years, the primary outcome of death, stroke, or MI occurred in 22.0% of the PCI cohort compared with 19.2% of the CABG cohort ($P = .13$).

In contrast, the NOBLE trial ($n = 1201$) reported a significant difference between the PCI group (BioMatrix BD-BES) and CABG at 5 years in favor of surgery. The composite primary endpoint (all-cause mortality, nonprocedural MI, or repeat revascularization) Kaplan-Meier estimate was 28% of the PCI group compared with 19% of the CABG group ($P = .0002$). Five-year estimates for all-cause mortality were 9% versus 9% ($P = .68$), for nonprocedural MI were 8% versus 3% ($P = .0002$), and for repeat revascularization were 17% versus 10% ($P = .0009$).

Current guidelines for myocardial revascularization remain supportive of PCI for LMCA disease. In Europe, CABG has a class 1, level A indication for LMCA disease, regardless of the SYNTAX score. In contrast, PCI is indicated for LMCA disease with a class 1, level A recommendation for patients with a low SYNTAX score (0-22), with a class IIa, level A recommendation for intermediate scores and class III, level B for high SYNTAX scores (>33).

Chronic Total Occlusions

Clinical and angiographic restenosis rates after both balloon angioplasty and stent implantation are increased following PCI of CTO lesions compared with nonoccluded stenoses, due principally to an increased incidence of diabetes, greater lesion length, plaque mass, and calcification. Stenting of CTO lesions has thus become the default strategy when PCI is planned and the use of DES is preferred.

Critical issues related to stenting of CTO lesions include selection of occlusions that are in viable and/or ischemic myocardial territories, minimizing stent overlap and overall stented length, avoidance of stent implantation in diffusely diseased distal territories, and optimization of lumen area in vessels that are chronically underfilled. It should be noted that, in spite of the technical improvements in achieving and maintain patency of chronically occluded coronary arteries, there are few randomized controlled trials documenting clinical benefit of the intervention. Some, but not all, trials have shown an improvement in angina frequency and quality of life, but no trial has demonstrated an improvement in hard endpoints such as left ventricular systolic function, ventricular arrhythmias, or survival when compared with optimal medical therapy.

Bifurcation Lesions

Bifurcation lesions represent 20% or more of stenoses undergoing angioplasty, and PCI of coronary bifurcation lesions is associated with increased procedural complications and worsened long-term outcomes. For true bifurcation lesions the major decision is whether to undertake a provisional or dual-stent strategy. With *provisional stenting*, the main vessel is stented (often after optimal predilatation of the side branch), and the side branch is dilated or stented only for a truly unacceptable result (typically a diameter stenosis >50% or severe dissection). A strategy of provisional stenting of the side branch is the generally accepted current approach to bifurcation disease unless there is significant high-grade and lengthy disease within the side branch. This approach is also usually preferred if the parent vessel is large and the side branch relatively small. Alternatively, when both the parent vessel and side branch are large (>2.5 mm), especially when the side branch arises at a shallow angle, planned stenting of both branches should be considered. Various approaches to dual stenting of bifurcation lesions have been developed and are briefly outlined in **Figure 27.7**.

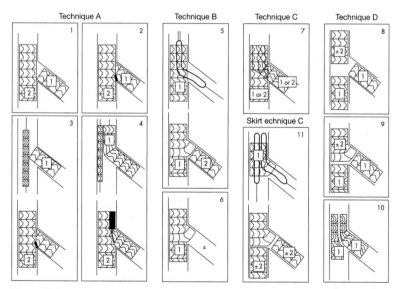

Figure 27.7 Strategies for the treatment of bifurcation disease. 1 and 2. Classic T-stenting beginning with side-branch stenting. 3. Modified T-stenting. 4. "Crush" technique. 5. Classic T-stenting beginning with main-branch stenting. 6. Provisional T-stenting. 7. "Culotte" or "trousers" technique. 8. Touching stents completed or not as Y technique. 9. "Trouser legs and seat" technique, a classic touching stents technique completed proximally by a "skirt" technique. 10. Kissing stents technique. 11. "Skirt" technique. (From Louvard Y, Lefevre T, Morice M-C. Percutaneous coronary intervention for bifurcation coronary disease. *Heart*. 2004;90:713-722.)

T-Stent Technique

A stent is deployed at the ostium of the side branch, followed by a second stent in the parent vessel. Unless the angle of origin of the side branch is 90°, however, the operator is faced with the dilemma of whether it is better to leave a portion of the ostial side-branch lesion unstented or risk having part of the stent protrude into the parent vessel. A modification of this technique to maximize ostial side-branch coverage is the T and protrusion technique, where the main-branch stent is deployed first, followed by stenting of the side branch with a balloon angioplasty catheter in the main vessel. The side-branch stent is brought back to protrude slightly into the main branch to maximize ostial coverage and is then deployed, impinging on the main-branch balloon, making a "T." A kissing balloon inflation (into the main branch and side branch simultaneously) is then performed to ensure adequate flow into both branches without compromise.

"Culotte" Stent Technique

A stent is deployed into the side branch with extension into the proximal aspect of the parent vessel. A wire is then passed through the side struts of this stent and into the distal parent vessel. After balloon dilatation, a second stent is passed through the side struts into the distal vessel, so that the proximal ends of the first and second stents overlap in the proximal vessel.

"Crush" Stent Techniques

After predilatation of both limbs, 2 stents are positioned simultaneously in the side branch and main branch. The side-branch stent extends into the proximal main vessel 2 to 3 mm (or less in the "mini-crush"); the parent branch stent extends at least several millimeters more proximally. The side-branch stent is inflated first, trapping the main-branch stent-delivery system. After confirmation of patency without dissection in the side branch, the side-branch guidewire and stent-delivery system are removed and the main-branch stent is implanted, "crushing" the side-branch stent. Following this, the side-branch stent is rewired and simultaneous kissing balloon inflations are performed (it is generally recommended that all bifurcation stent techniques be completed by kissing balloon technique). There have been many modifications of this technique, including modified sequences of stent implantation such as in the "reverse crush," which is applicable when side-branch stenting was not initially planned. In this case, after main-branch implantation, a second stent is placed in the side branch extending into the proximal parent vessel (within the previously placed stent) and a balloon is placed in the main vessel. The side-branch stent is then deployed, impinging on the balloon. After removal of the side-branch stent-delivery system and wire, the main-branch balloon is then inflated to crush the proximal portion of the side-branch stent and a final kissing balloon inflation is performed. Balloon crushing of the side-branch stent can also be used as the initial approach (prior to main-branch deployment) in the "step crush" technique, a technique that is useful when smaller guide and sheath sizes are used). Other modifications include performance of additional kissing balloon inflations prior to main-branch deployment (eg, "double-kissing crush" technique), which can improve procedural outcomes. Recrossing the crushed side-branch stent with a guidewire and balloon can be challenging and time consuming but is essential because late outcomes are significantly improved following a simultaneous kissing balloon inflation with this technique.

Simultaneous Kissing Stents/V-Stenting

Two stents are deployed simultaneously over separate guidewires: 1 in the parent vessel and 1 in the side branch. For simultaneous kissing stents, both stents extend side by side in the main vessel proximal to the bifurcation (for V-stenting, these stents are deployed at the ostia of both branches, minimizing the length of the "carina"). Although this technique offers the advantage of simplicity and control of both vessels, a new, more proximal carina is created in the center of the proximal parent vessel, which is unlikely to endothelialize fully and can be very difficult to wire if repeat PCI is required. Also, placement of an additional stent is problematic should a proximal dissection occur.

Saphenous Vein Grafts

The most common cause of recurrent ischemia following CABG surgery is atheromatous degeneration within the body of an SVG, and BMSs have been associated with improved outcomes compared with balloon angioplasty in SVG intervention. While DESs have the potential to further lower rates of restenosis of the target lesion within SVGs, disease progression at nontarget sites within SVGs are frequent, and additionally, due to the large caliber of most SVGs, the "tolerated late loss" within SVG lesions is typically greater than in native coronary vessels. With extended follow-up to a median of 32 months in one trial, the antirestenotic advantage of SES compared with BMS was lost and SES was associated with higher mortality. A more recent larger randomized trial, the ISAR-CABG trial, randomized 610 patients to BMS, SES, PES, or biodegradable polymer SES. At 1 year, the use of all DES versus BMS was associated with reductions in TLR (7% vs 13%, $P = .01$) as well as composite death, MI, and TLR (15% vs 22%, $P = .02$), with no differences observed in overall mortality or stent thrombosis. A meta-analysis of 1582 patients from 6 randomized controlled trials showed a lower short-term MACE rate for DES versus BMS (odds ratio: 0.56 [95% CI 0.35-0.91], $P = .02$) but no difference in MACE rate, mortality, TLR, or stent thrombosis with long-term follow-up.

SUGGESTED READINGS

1. Ali ZA, Serruys PW, Kimura T, et al. 2-year outcomes with the absorb bioresorbable scaffold for treatment of coronary artery disease: a systematic review and meta-analysis of seven randomised trials with an individual patient data substudy. *Lancet.* 2017;390(10096):760-772.
2. Baber U, Mehran R, Sharma SK, et al. Impact of the everolimus-eluting stent on stent thrombosis: a meta-analysis of 13 randomized trials. *J Am Coll Cardiol.* 2011;58(15):1569-1577.
3. Colombo A, Hall P, Nakamura S, et al. Intracoronary stenting without anticoagulation accomplished with intravascular ultrasound guidance. *Circulation.* 1995;91(6):1676-1688.
4. Colombo A, Drzewiecki J, Banning A, et al. Randomized study to assess the effectiveness of slow- and moderate-release polymer-based paclitaxel-eluting stents for coronary artery lesions. *Circulation.* 2003;108(7):788-794.
5. Cook S, Wenaweser P, Togni M, et al. Incomplete stent apposition and very late stent thrombosis after drug-eluting stent implantation. *Circulation.* 2007;115(18):2426-2434.
6. Cutlip DE, Windecker S, Mehran R, et al. Clinical end points in coronary stent trials: a case for standardized definitions. *Circulation.* 2007;115(17):2344-2351.
7. Daemen J, Boersma E, Flather M, et al. Long-term safety and efficacy of percutaneous coronary intervention with stenting and coronary artery bypass surgery for multivessel coronary artery disease: a meta-analysis with 5-year patient-level data from the ARTS, ERACI-II, MASS-II, and SoS trials. *Circulation.* 2008;118(11):1146-1154.
8. Dawkins KD, Grube E, Guagliumi G, et al. Clinical efficacy of polymer-based paclitaxel-eluting stents in the treatment of complex, long coronary artery lesions from a multicenter, randomized trial: support for the use of drug-eluting stents in contemporary clinical practice. *Circulation.* 2005;112(21):3306-3313.
9. Eisenstein EL, Wijns W, Fajadet J, et al. Long-term clinical and economic analysis of the endeavor drug-eluting stent versus the driver bare-metal stent: 4-year results from the ENDEAVOR II trial (randomized controlled trial to evaluate the safety and efficacy of the medtronic AVE ABT-578 eluting driver coronary stent in de novo native coronary artery lesions). *JACC Cardiovasc Interv.* 2009;2(12):1178-1187.
10. Farb A, Heller PF, Shroff S, et al. Pathological analysis of local delivery of paclitaxel via a polymer-coated stent. *Circulation.* 2001;104(4):473-479.

11. Finn AV, Joner M, Nakazawa G, et al. Pathological correlates of late drug-eluting stent thrombosis: strut coverage as a marker of endothelialization. *Circulation*. 2007;115(18):2435-2441.

12. Fischman DL, Leon MB, Baim DS, et al. A randomized comparison of coronary-stent placement and balloon angioplasty in the treatment of coronary artery disease. Stent restenosis study investigators. *N Engl J Med*. 1994;331(8):496-501.

13. Fujii K, Carlier SG, Mintz GS, et al. Stent underexpansion and residual reference segment stenosis are related to stent thrombosis after sirolimus-eluting stent implantation: an intravascular ultrasound study. *J Am Coll Cardiol*. 2005;45(7):995-998.

14. George BS, Voorhees WD III, Roubin GS, et al. Multicenter investigation of coronary stenting to treat acute or threatened closure after percutaneous transluminal coronary angioplasty: clinical and angiographic outcomes. *J Am Coll Cardiol*. 1993;22(1):135-143.

15. Grise MA, Massullo V, Jani S, et al. Five-year clinical follow-up after intracoronary radiation: results of a randomized clinical trial. *Circulation*. 2002;105(23):2737-2740.

16. Grube E, Silber S, Hauptmann KE, et al. Taxus I: six- and twelve-month results from a randomized, double-blind trial on a slow-release paclitaxel-eluting stent for de novo coronary lesions. *Circulation*. 2003;107(1):38-42.

17. Gwon HC, Hahn JY, Park KW, et al. Six-month versus 12-month dual antiplatelet therapy after implantation of drug-eluting stents: the efficacy of xience/promus versus cypher to reduce late loss after stenting (EXCELLENT) randomized, multi center study. *Circulation*. 2012;125(3):505-513.

18. Habara S, Iwabuchi M, Inoue N, et al. A multicenter randomized comparison of paclitaxel-coated balloon catheter with conventional balloon angioplasty in patients with bare-metal stent restenosis and drug-eluting stent restenosis. *Am Heart J*. 2013;166(3):527-533.

19. Jensen LO, Thayssen P, Hansen HS, et al. Randomized comparison of everolimus-eluting and sirolimus-eluting stents in patients treated with percutaneous coronary intervention: the Scandinavian organization for randomized trials with clinical outcome IV (SORT OUT IV). *Circulation*. 2012;125(10):1246-1255.

20. Joner M, Nakazawa G, Finn AV, et al. Endothelial cell recovery between comparator polymer-based drug-eluting stents. *J Am Coll Cardiol*. 2008;52(5):333-342.

21. Kaiser C, Galatius S, Erne P, et al. Drug-eluting versus bare-metal stents in large coronary arteries. *N Engl J Med*. 2010;363(24):2310-2319.

22. Kirtane AJ, Gupta A, Iyengar S, et al. Safety and efficacy of drugeluting and bare metal stents: comprehensive meta-analysis of randomized trials and observational studies. *Circulation*. 2009;119(25):3198-3206.

23. Kirtane AJ, Leon MB, Ball MW, et al. The "final" 5-year follow-up from the ENDEAVOR IV trial comparing a zotarolimus-eluting stent with a paclitaxel-eluting stent. *JACC Cardiovasc Interv*. 2013;6(4):325-333.

24. Kuntz RE, Safian RD, Carrozza JP, Fishman RF, Mansour M, Baim DS. The importance of acute luminal diameter in determining restenosis after coronary atherectomy or stenting. *Circulation*. 1992;86(6):1827-1835.

25. Leon MB, Baim DS, Popma JJ, et al. A clinical trial comparing three antithrombotic-drug regimens after coronary-artery stenting. Stent anticoagulation restenosis study investigators. *N Engl J Med*. 1998;339(23):1665-1671.

26. Leon MB, Teirstein PS, Moses JW, et al. Localized intracoronary gamma-radiation therapy to inhibit the recurrence of restenosis after stenting. *N Engl J Med*. 2001;344(4):250-256.

27. Leon MB, Mauri L, Popma JJ, et al. A randomized comparison of the Endeavor zotarolimus-eluting stent versus the TAXUS paclitaxel-eluting stent in de novo native coronary lesions 12-month outcomes from the ENDEAVOR IV trial. *J Am Coll Cardiol*. 2010;55(6):543-554.

28. Lopes RD, Hong H, Harskamp RE, et al. Optimal antithrombotic regimens for patients with atrial fibrillation undergoing percutaneous coronary intervention: an updated network meta-analysis. *JAMA Cardiol*. 2020;5:582-589. doi:10.1001/jamacardio. 2019.6175.

29. Lopes RD, Leonardi S, Wojdyla DM, et al. Stent thrombosis in patients with atrial fibrillation undergoing coronary stenting in the AUGUSTUS trial. *Circulation*. 2020;141(9):781-783.

30. Mauri L, Kereiakes DJ, Yeh RW, et al. Twelve or 30 months of dual antiplatelet therapy after drug-eluting stents. *N Engl J Med*. 2014;371(23):2155-2166.

31. Mehilli J, Byrne RA, Tiroch K, et al. Randomized trial of paclitaxel-versus sirolimus-eluting stents for treatment of coronary restenosis in sirolimus-eluting stents. The ISAR-DESIRE 2 (Intracoronary Stenting and Angiographic Results: Drug Eluting Stents for In-Stent Restenosis 2) study. *J Am Coll Cardiol*. 2010;55(24):2710-2716.

32. Mehran R, Baber U, Sharma SK, et al. Ticagrelor with or without aspirin in high-risk patients after PCI. *N Engl J Med*. 2019;381(21):2032-2042.

33. Morice MC, Serruys PW, Sousa JE, et al. A randomized comparison of a sirolimus-eluting stent with a standard stent for coronary revascularization. *N Engl J Med.* 2002;346(23):1773-1780.
34. Moses JW, Leon MB, Popma JJ, et al. Sirolimus-eluting stents versus standard stents in patients with stenosis in a native coronary artery. *N Engl J Med.* 2003;349(14):1315-1323.
35. Nakamura S, Colombo A, Gaglione A, et al. Intracoronary ultrasound observations during stent implantation. *Circulation.* 1994;89(5):2026-2034.
36. Nakazawa G, Otsuka F, Nakano M, et al. The pathology of neoatherosclerosis in human coronary implants bare-metal and drug-eluting stents. *J Am Coll Cardiol.* 2011;57(11):1314-1322.
37. Neumann FJ, Sousa-Uva M, Ahlsson A, et al. 2018 ESC/EACTS guidelines on myocardial revascularization. *Eur Heart J.* 2019;40(2):87-165.
38. Park SJ, Park DW, Kim YH, et al. Duration of dual antiplatelet therapy after implantation of drug-eluting stents. *N Engl J Med.* 2010;362(15):1374-1382.
39. Patel MR, Calhoon JH, Dehmer GJ, et al. ACC/AATS/AHA/ASE/ASNC/SCAI/SCCT/STS 2017 appropriate use criteria for coronary revascularization in patients with stable ischemic heart disease: a report of the American College of Cardiology Appropriate Use Criteria Task Force, American association for Thoracic Surgery, American Heart Association, American Society of Echocardiography, American Society of Nuclear Cardiology, Society for Cardiovascular Angiography and Interventions, Society of Cardiovascular Computed Tomography, and Society of Thoracic Surgeons. *J Am Coll Cardiol.* 2017;69(17):2212-2241.
40. Pinto DS, Stone GW, Ellis SG. Impact of routine angiographic follow-up on the clinical benefits of paclitaxel-eluting stents: results from the TAXUS-IV trial. *J Am Coll Cardiol.* 2006;48(1):32-36.
41. Rinfret S, Cutlip DE, Katsiyiannis PT, et al. Rheolytic thrombectomy and platelet glycoprotein IIb/IIIa blockade for stent thrombosis. *Cathet Cardiovasc Interv.* 2002;57(1):24-30.
42. Rittger H, Brachmann J, Sinha AM, et al. A randomized, multicenter, single-blinded trial comparing paclitaxel-coated balloon angioplasty with plain balloon angioplasty in drug-eluting stent restenosis: the PEPCAD-DES study. *J Am Coll Cardiol.* 2012;59(15):1377-1382.
43. Schatz RA, Baim DS, Leon M, et al. Clinical experience with the Palmaz-Schatz coronary stent. Initial results of a multicenter study. *Circulation.* 1991;83(1):148-161.
44. Serruys PW, Strauss BH, Beatt KJ, et al. Angiographic follow-up after placement of a self-expanding coronary-artery stent. *N Engl J Med.* 1991;324(1):13-17.
45. Sigwart U, Puel J, Mirkovitch V, Joffre F, Kappenberger L. Intravascular stents to prevent occlusion and restenosis after transluminal angioplasty. *N Engl J Med.* 1987;316(12):701-706.
46. Stettler C, Wandel S, Allemann S, et al. Outcomes associated with drug-eluting and bare-metal stents: a collaborative network metaanalysis. *Lancet.* 2007;370(9591):937-948.
47. Stone GW, Ellis SG, Cannon L, et al. Comparison of a polymer-based paclitaxel-eluting stent with a bare metal stent in patients with complex coronary artery disease: a randomized controlled trial. *J Am Med Assoc.* 2005;294(10):1215-1223.
48. Stone GW, Rizvi A, Newman W, et al. Everolimus-eluting versus paclitaxel-eluting stents in coronary artery disease. *N Engl J Med.* 2010;362(18):1663-1674.
49. Valgimigli M, Campo G, Monti M, et al. Short-versus long-term duration of dual-antiplatelet therapy after coronary stenting: a randomized multicenter trial. *Circulation.* 2012;125(16):2015-2026.
50. van der Giessen WJ, Lincoff AM, Schwartz RS, et al. Marked inflammatory sequelae to implantation of biodegradable and non-biodegradable polymers in porcine coronary arteries. *Circulation.* 1996;94(7):1690-1697.
51. Waksman R, Raizner AE, Yeung AC, Lansky AJ, Vandertie L. Use of localised intracoronary beta radiation in treatment of instent restenosis: the INHIBIT randomised controlled trial. *Lancet.* 2002;359(9306):551-557.
52. Wilson GJ, Marks A, Berg KJ, et al. The SYNERGY biodegradable polymer everolimus eluting coronary stent: porcine vascular compatibility and polymer safety study. *Cathet Cardiovasc Interv.* 2015;86(6):E247-E257.

28 General Overview of Interventions for Structural Heart Disease[1]

The introduction of valvuloplasty in the 1980s after the initial work in the 1950s by Rubio-Alvarez et al and the more recent development of new technology for closure of intracardiac shunts and for percutaneous valve repair and replacement have led to the new frontier of interventions for structural heart disease. This chapter provides a general overview of this developing field. The reader is referred to other sections of this book for more detailed information on techniques and indications of specific interventions.

CLASSIFICATION OF INTERVENTIONS FOR STRUCTURAL HEART DISEASE

Interventions for structural heart disease can be classified into 6 broad categories, as illustrated in **Table 28.1**.

Each intervention requires an in-depth knowledge of the pathophysiology and cardiac anatomy of the condition being treated, the acquisition of specific technical skills, and knowledge of indications for the procedure performed as well as of potential complications and bailout techniques.

Closure of Congenital and Acquired Cardiac Defects

This category includes closure of atrial and ventricular septal defects, closure of pervious ductus arteriosus, and closure of ventricular pseudoaneurysms (**Figure 28.1**). Beyond standard cardiac catheterization competency, additional knowledge base includes a full understanding of atrial and ventricular anatomy; understanding of indications and contraindications for closure; knowledge of occluder devices, specialized guidewires, and arterial sheath; and the development of technical skills needed for access to ventricular septal defects and ventricular pseudoaneurysm. Details on techniques and indications are listed in Chapter 36.

Percutaneous Valve Interventions

As of today mitral valvuloplasty is considered a valid alternative to surgical commissurotomy (see Chapter 33). In contrast, the initial enthusiasm for aortic valvuloplasty in the adult was met by disappointing intermediate and long-term results, leading to a class IIb indication for aortic valvuloplasty in the 2020 American College of Cardiology/American Heart Association guidelines for the management of patients with valvular heart disease: "Class IIb. In critically ill patients with severe AS, percutaneous aortic balloon dilation may be considered as a bridge to SAVR or TAVR. (Level of Evidence: C.)." The recent introduction of transcatheter aortic valve replacement (TAVR) has created a revolution in the management of patients with aortic stenosis, and it has resulted in a resurgence of aortic valvuloplasty as a component of TAVR (Chapter 34). Similar developments are occurring for the management of mitral and tricuspid valve disease through percutaneous mitral and tricuspid valve repair and replacement (see Chapter 33) and for the pulmonic valve (see Chapters 34 and 36). Thus, percutaneous valve interventions are emerging as an alternative to surgery in

---

[1]We gratefully acknowledge the Grossman & Baim's *Cardiac Catheterization, Angiography, and Intervention*, 9th edition contributions of Drs. Mauro Moscucci, John D. Carroll, and John G. Webb, as portions of their chapter, General Overview of Interventions for Structural Heart Disease, were retained in this text.

Table 28.1	General Classification of Interventions for Structural Heart Disease
Closure of congenital and acquired cardiac defects	• Atrial septal defect closure • Ventricular septal defect closure • Patent foramen ovale closure • Acquired post–myocardial infarction ventricular septal defects closure • Post–myocardial infarction pseudoaneurysm closure • Patent ductus arteriosus closure
Percutaneous valve interventions	• Pulmonic valvuloplasty • Transcatheter pulmonary valve replacement • Tricuspid valvuloplasty • Mitral valvuloplasty • Aortic valvuloplasty • Transcatheter mitral valve repair and replacement • Transcatheter tricuspid valve repair and replacement • Transcatheter aortic valve replacement • Closure of paravalvular leaks
Myocardial interventions	• Interventions with cell-based therapy • Alcohol septal ablation for hypertrophic cardiomyopathy
Intervention for the creation of intracardiac shunts	• Blade atrial septostomy • Balloon atrial septostomy • Balloon atrial septostomy for pulmonary hypertension • Balloon atrial septostomy to vent left ventricle in patients on percutaneous cardiopulmonary bypass
Pericardial interventions	• Pericardiocentesis • Balloon pericardiotomy • Epicardial access through the pericardial space
Miscellanea interventions	• Percutaneous cardiopulmonary bypass • Left atrial appendage occlusion • Transcatheter embolization of extracardiac shunts

high-, intermediate-, and low-surgical-risk patients and as a new option for patients who otherwise are not surgical candidates.

Myocardial Interventions

This group includes alcohol septal ablation as a treatment for obstructive hypertrophic cardiomyopathy (HCM) and the new field of interventions with cell therapies. Transcatheter ablation of the septum with ethanol was first reported by Sigwart in 1995. The procedure entails inducing a controlled myocardial infarction by injecting absolute ethanol in the septal perforator branch supplying the area of the septum participating in the creation of left ventricular outflow tract obstruction. Significant controversy still exists regarding the long-term risk of sudden death in patients undergoing alcohol septal ablation, although a recent metanalysis has suggested that the benefits of alcohol septal ablation are similar to the benefits of surgical myectomy. Given the complexity of HCM and the fact that alcohol ablation has a steep learning curve and unusual complications (see Chapter 30), it has been recommended that alcohol ablation should be performed only by experienced operators within a multidisciplinary program and in centers offering comprehensive care for patients with HCM.

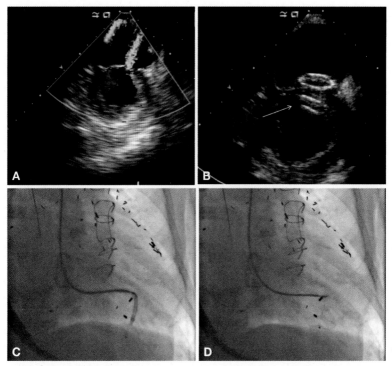

Figure 28.1 Closure of ventricular pseudoaneurysm. **A,** Transesophageal image showing the communication between the left ventricular cavity and the pseudoaneurysm. **B,** Transesophageal image showing exclusion of the pseudoaneurysm following deployment of an Amplatzer atrial septal occluder (arrow). **C and D,** Deployment of the Amplatzer atrial septal occluder. (Courtesy of Alan W. Heldman, MD.)

Cardiac cell–based therapy has emerged as a new exciting field that hopefully will provide novel therapeutic options for patients with dilated or ischemic cardiomyopathies.

Interventions for the Creation of Intracardiac Shunts

The development of the Fontan procedure was a major breakthrough in the management of patients with single ventricles, tricuspid atresia, and pulmonary atresia. It involves redirecting venous blood to the pulmonary arteries through an intracardiac or extracardiac cavopulmonary connection, or via an atriopulmonary connection, thus bypassing the ventricle. Pulmonary blood flow will be driven by a pressure gradient between the venous circulation and the pulmonary circulation. Any alteration in pulmonary vascular resistance will result in an increase in venous pressure leading to right-sided heart failure and in some patients to protein-losing enteropathy secondary to the high venous pressure and bowel edema. In these patients, the creation of a small right-to-left shunt through a fenestration can be beneficial in reducing venous pressure and increasing cardiac output. The fenestration can be performed at the time of surgery or later percutaneously using balloon septostomy.

Balloon atrial septostomy has also been used in patients with pulmonary hypertension to increase left ventricular filling at the expense of mild systemic desaturation (**Figure 28.2**) and to vent the left ventricle in patients with cardiogenic shock on percutaneous extracorporeal membrane oxygenator (ECMO) circulatory support. In patients on ECMO support, the creation of a left-to-right shunt through a balloon atrial septostomy can decompress the left atrium and prevent or reverse pulmonary hemorrhages.

Pericardial Interventions

Pericardiocentesis, balloon pericardiotomy, and pericardial access to the epicardium are described in Chapter 38. Interventions for structural heart disease might be rarely complicated by the development of cardiac perforation. Thus, proficiency in pericardiocentesis should be part of the skill set of contemporary interventional cardiologists.

Miscellanea Intervention

This last group includes percutaneous cardiopulmonary bypass (see Chapter 24), left atrial appendage exclusion, and transcatheter embolization of extracardiac shunts (see Chapters 32 and 36).

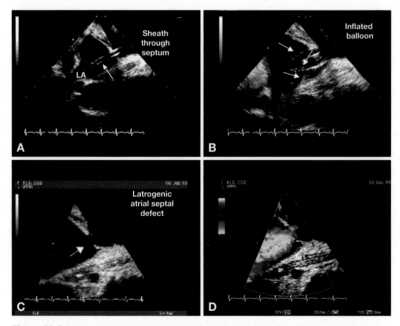

Figure 28.2 Intracardiac, 2D-Doppler echocardiography-guided balloon atrial septostomy in a patient with pulmonary hypertension. **A,** The Mullins sheath has been advanced through the septum (white arrow). **B,** Inflation of the balloon (white arrows). **C,** Iatrogenic atrial septal defect (ASD) (white arrow). **D,** Color Doppler flow through a moderate-size ASD with continuous right-to-left flow. (Reproduced with permission from Moscucci M, Dairywala IT, Chetcuti S, et al. Balloon atrial septostomy in end-stage pulmonary hypertension guided by a novel intracardiac echocardiographic transducer. *Catheter Cardiovasc Interv.* 2001;52(4):530-534.)

Table 28.2	Interventions for Structural Heart Disease: Knowledge Base and Interventional Skills
Knowledge base	• Natural history • Cardiac anatomy • Pathophysiology • Alternative treatment strategies to the interventional strategy • Practice guidelines from professional societies • Assessment of patient preferences and individualized patient-centric decision making
Interventional skills	• Baseline cardiac catheterization skills • Hemodynamics • Transseptal catheterization • Direct left ventricular apical puncture • Transhepatic access • Intravascular ultrasound imaging and integration of multiple imaging modalities for navigation in cardiac chambers • Knowledge of available devices • Additional technical skills related to the specific procedure • Procedural complications and bailout techniques

TRAINING AND CREDENTIALING CRITERIA

Several consensus statements and position papers have provided recommendations on training and credentialing criteria (**Table 28.2**). For a detailed list of knowledge base elements and interventional skills related to each procedure, the reader is referred to an excellent expert consensus statement from the Society for Cardiovascular Angiography and Interventions endorsed by the American College of Cardiology Foundation. The consensus recommendation is that training in structural heart disease interventions or in interventions for adult with congenital heart disease should include at least 1 year of additional dedicated time, recognizing that learning in structural heart disease is a lifelong endeavor. It should be noted that third-party payers, at least in the United States, have been developing criteria for reimbursement and that those criteria can have an effect on credentialing (**Table 28.3**). Most institutions have incorporated these criteria in the credentialing process for operators performing TAVR. As the field of structural heart disease interventions continues to evolve, new criteria are being developed (**Table 28.4**).

INFORMED CONSENT AND THE USE OF APPROVED DEVICES FOR NONAPPROVED INDICATIONS

Interventions for structural heart disease might require the use of approved devices for a nonapproved indication (off-label use). For example, specific devices for the closure of paravalvular leaks have not yet been developed and a combination of coils, septal occluders, and ductal occluders has been used by several operators. In the United States, the Food and Drug Administration (FDA) does not regulate the practice of medicine, and in particular, the Federal Food Drug and Cosmetic Act specifically states that "nothing in this Act shall be construed to limit or interfere with the authority of a health care practitioner to prescribe or administer any legally marketed device to a patient for any condition or disease within a legitimate health care practitioner-patient relationship." Thus, the off-label use of approved devices is implicitly allowed, as long as the general requirements for good medical practice as listed in the following statement are followed: "Good medical practice and the best

Table 28.3	**Qualification for Transcatheter Aortic Valve Replacement Programs Required by the Center for Medicare and Medicaid Services Within the National Coverage Determination**

Qualifications to begin a TAVR program for heart teams *without* TAVR experience	A. Cardiovascular surgeon with:
	  i. ≥ 100 Career open heart surgeries of which ≥25 are aortic valve related.
	B. Interventional cardiologist with:
	  i. Professional experience *of* ≥100 *career* structural heart disease procedures; or, ≥30 left-sided structural procedures per year; and
	  ii. Device-specific training as required by the manufacturer.
	
	The hospital program must have the following:
	
	A. ≥50 Open heart surgeries in the previous year prior to TAVR program initiation;
	B. ≥20 Aortic valve–related procedures in the 2 y prior to TAVR program initiation;
	C. ≥2 Physicians with cardiac surgery privileges;
	D. ≥1 Physician with interventional cardiology privileges; and
	E. ≥300 Percutaneous coronary interventions (PCIs) per year.

Qualifications for hospital programs *with* TAVR experience	**The hospital program must maintain the following:** a. ≥50 AVRs (TAVR or SAVR) per year including ≥20 TAVR procedures in the prior year; b. ≥100 AVRs (TAVR or SAVR) every 2 y, including ≥40 TAVR procedures in the prior 2 y; c. ≥2 Physicians with cardiac surgery privileges; d. ≥1 Physician with interventional cardiology privileges; and e. ≥300 Percutaneous coronary interventions (PCIs) per year. The heart team and hospital are participating in a prospective, national, audited registry that: 1. Consecutively enrolls TAVR patients; 2. Accepts all manufactured devices; 3. Follows the patient for at least 1 y; and 4. Complies with relevant regulations relating to protecting human research subjects, including 45 CFR Part 46 and 21 CFR Parts 50 and 56.

CMS, Center for Medicare and Medicaid Services; TAVR, transcatheter aortic valve replacement.

interests of the patient require that physicians use legally available drugs, biologics, and devices according to their best knowledge and judgment". If physicians use a product for an indication not in the approved labeling, they have the responsibility to be well informed about the product, to base its use on firm scientific rationale and on sound medical evidence, and to maintain records of the product's use and effects.

Use of a marketed product in this manner when the intent is the "practice of medicine" does not require the submission of an Investigational New Drug Application, Investigational Device Exemption, or review by an Institutional Review Board (IRB). However, the institution at which the product will be used may, under its own authority, require IRB review or other institutional oversight, and while the off-label use of approved device does not violate FDA or other regulatory bodies' rules, the decision to reimburse is often independently made by insurance companies and government agencies such as the Center for Medicare and Medicaid Services (CMS). Disclosure of the off-label use is highly recommended, and a well-executed and documented informed consent process is paramount. In addition, the FDA also

Table 28.4	Qualification for Transcatheter Mitral Valve Repair (TMVR) Programs Required by the Center for Medicare and Medicaid Services Within the National Coverage Determination
Institutional and operator requirements for performing TMVR	**The hospital must have the following:** 1. A surgical program that performs ≥25 total mitral valve surgical procedures for severe mitral regurgitation (MR) per year of which at least 10 must be mitral valve repairs; 2. An interventional cardiology program that performs ≥1000 catheterizations per year, including ≥400 percutaneous coronary interventions (PCIs) per year, with acceptable outcomes for conventional procedures compared with National Cardiovascular Data Registry (NCDR) benchmarks; 3. Each interventional cardiologist performs ≥50 structural procedures per year including atrial septal defects (ASDs), patent foramen ovale (PFO), and transseptal punctures; 4. Additional members of the heart team including echocardiographers, cardiac imaging specialists, heart valve and heart failure specialists, electrophysiologists, cardiac anesthesiologists, intensivists, nurses, nurse practitioners, physician assistants, data/research coordinators, and a dedicated administrator; 5. Interventional cardiologist(s) must receive prior suitable training on the devices to be used; 6. All cases must be submitted to a single national database; 7. Ongoing continuing medical education (or the nursing/technologist equivalent) of 10 h/y of relevant material; 8. The interventional cardiologist(s) must be board-certified in interventional cardiology or board-certified/eligible in pediatric cardiology or similar boards from outside the United States; 9. The cardiothoracic surgeon(s) must be board-certified in thoracic surgery or similar foreign equivalent; and 10. Participation to a national audited registry.

specifies that the investigational use of an approved device, when the intent is to develop information about the safety of efficacy of the device in treating a specific condition, may require submission of an Investigational Device Exemption. For detailed information, the reader is referred to the FDA website listed in the recommended readings.

MULTIDISCIPLINARY PROGRAMS AND THE CARDIAC TEAM

The evolution of interventions for structural heart disease has introduced the new concept of the cardiac team, with inclusion of interventional cardiologists, vascular surgeons, cardiac surgeons, imaging specialists, heart failure specialists, noninvasive cardiologists, intensivists, nurses, and cardiovascular technologists. The complexity of the procedure performed, the different types of vascular access that can be used, the need of the input from different subspecialists in the evaluation of best treatment options, and the integration of multiple imaging modalities within the hybrid cardiac catheterization suite make this multidisciplinary approach a critical component of interventions for structural heart disease. This new paradigm, which promotes appropriate and optimal patient care, is emphasized in several chapters in this textbook.

CLINICAL REGISTRIES

Quality assurance has become an integral component of interventional cardiology programs, and it has led to the development of clinical registries that provide the opportunity to benchmark individual operators and hospital data with national data.

Most importantly, the Center for Medicare and Medicaid Services NCD requires as a condition for reimbursement of TAVR and TMVR (transcatheter mitral valve repair) participation to a prospective, national, audited registry that meets the following requirements: (1) consecutively enrolls TAVR and TMVR patients; (2) accepts all manufactured devices; (3) follows the patient for at least 1 year; and (4) complies with relevant regulations relating to protecting human research subjects, including 45 CFR Part 46 and 21 CFR Parts 50 and 56.

The STS/ACC TVT (transcatheter valve therapy) registry was originally created as a collaboration between the Society of Thoracic Surgeon and the American College of Cardiology to track real-world procedure and outcome data of TAVR. Recently, it has been expanded with the inclusion of TMVR, and it will be further expanded with the inclusion of tricuspid valve transcatheter interventions. The registry has been approved by CMS as meeting the requirements for reimbursement. The data collected in the registry have been used in postapproval studies, in safety surveillance, and for expansion and approval of new indications such as alternative access for TAVR and valve-in-valve procedures for failing aortic and mitral bioprosthetic valves in patients at high risk for surgery.

The Left Atrial Appendage Occlusion Registry is similar to the TVT registry, and it was developed to track real-world outcomes of left atrial appendage occlusion procedures. Like the TVT registry, this registry is approved by CMS to meet the NCD requirements for left atrial appendage occlusion.

ACADEMIC RESEARCH CONSORTIUM

The growth of interventional cardiology, the expansion of clinical trials, and a quest to standardize definitions of safety and effectiveness endpoints led in 2006 to the development of the Academic Research Consortium as a collaboration between 4 academic research organizations, with input from the US Food Administration and participation of industry stakeholders as nonvoting members. Endpoints definitions have been developed for coronary interventions, transcatheter aortic valve and mitral valve trials, and bleeding complications. These definitions provide a level framework for the assessment of safety and effectiveness, and they are currently used in ongoing clinical trials of cardiovascular devices.

SUGGESTED READINGS

1. Alvarez VR, Lason RL. Tricuspid commissurotomy by means of a modified catheter. *Arch Inst Cardiol Mex.* 1955;25(1):57-69.
2. Bavaria JE, Tommaso CL, Brindis RG, et al. 2018 AATS/ACC/SCAI/STS expert consensus systems of care document: operator and institutional recommendations and requirements for transcatheter aortic valve replacement. A joint report of the American Association for Thoracic Surgery, American College of Cardiology, Society for Cardiovascular Angiography and Interventions, and Society of Thoracic Surgeons. *J Am Coll Cardiol.* 2019;73(3):340-374.
3. Centres for Medicare and Medicaid Services. *National Coverage Determination (NCD) for Transcatheter Aortic Valve Replacement (TAVR) (20.32).* Accessed August 3, 2020. https://www.cms.gov/medicare-coverage-database/details/ncd-details.aspx?NCDid=355
4. Freeman JV, Varosy P, Price MJ, et al. The NCDR left atrial appendage occlusion registry. *J Am Coll Cardiol.* 2020;75(13):1503-1518. doi:10.1016/j.jacc.2019.12.040
5. Garcia-Garcia HM, McFadden EP, Farb A, et al. Standardized end point definitions for coronary intervention trials: the academic research consortium-2 consensus document. *Eur Heart J.* 2018;39(23):2192-2207.
6. Genereux P, Head SJ, Hahn R, et al. Paravalvular leak after transcatheter aortic valve replacement: the new Achilles' heel? A comprehensive review of the literature. *J Am Coll Cardiol.* 2013;61(11):1125-1136.
7. Gersh BJ, Maron BJ, Bonow RO, et al. 2011 ACCF/AHA guideline for the diagnosis and treatment of hypertrophic cardiomyopathy: a report of the American College of Cardiology Foundation/American Heart Association Task Force on practice guidelines. *Circulation.* 2011;124(24):e783-e831.

8. Harold JG, Bass TA, Bashore TM, et al. ACCF/AHA/SCAI 2013 update of the clinical competence statement on coronary artery interventional procedures: a report of the American College of Cardiology Foundation/American Heart Association/American College of Physicians Task Force on Clinical Competence and Training (writing committee to revise the 2007 clinical competence statement on cardiac interventional procedures). *Circulation.* 2013;128(4):436-472. doi:10.1161/CIR.0b013e318299cd8a

9. Holzer R, Hijazi Z. The off-versus on-label use of medical devices in interventional cardiovascular medicine? Clarifying the ambiguity between regulatory labeling and clinical decision making, part III: structural heart disease interventions. *Catheter Cardiovasc Interv.* 2008;72(6):848-852.

10. Johnston TA, Jaggers J, McGovern JJ, O'Laughlin MP. Bedside transseptal balloon dilation atrial septostomy for decompression of the left heart during extracorporeal membrane oxygenation. *Catheter Cardiovasc Interv.* 1999;46(2):197-199.

11. Kappetein AP, Head SJ, Genereux P, et al. Updated standardized endpoint definitions for transcatheter aortic valve implantation: the Valve Academic Research Consortium-2 consensus document (VARC-2). *Eur J Cardio Thorac Surg.* 2012;42(5):S45-S60. doi:10.1093/ejcts/ezs533

12. Krucoff MW, Mehran R, van Es GA, Boam AB, Cutlip DE. The academic research Consortium governance charter. *JACC Cardiovasc Interv.* 2011;4(5):595-596.

13. Lakkis NM, Nagueh SF, Kleiman NS, et al. Echocardiography-guided ethanol septal reduction for hypertrophic obstructive cardiomyopathy. *Circulation.* 1998;98(17):1750-1755.

14. Leon MB, Smith CR, Mack M, et al. Transcatheter aortic-valve implantation for aortic stenosis in patients who cannot undergo surgery. *N Engl J Med.* 2010;363(17):1597-1607.

15. Mehran R, Rao SV, Bhatt DL, et al. Standardized bleeding definitions for cardiovascular clinical trials: a consensus report from the Bleeding Academic Research Consortium. *Circulation.* 2011;123(23):2736-2747.

16. Moscucci M, Dairywala IT, Chetcuti S, et al. Balloon atrial septostomy in end-stage pulmonary hypertension guided by a novel intracardiac echocardiographic transducer. *Catheter Cardiovasc Interv.* 2001;52(4):530-534.

17. Rich S, Dodin E, McLaughlin VV. Usefulness of atrial septostomy as a treatment for primary pulmonary hypertension and guidelines for its application. *Am J Cardiol.* 1997;80(3):369-371.

18. Rubio-Alvarez V, Limon R, Soni J. Intracardiac valvulotomy by means of a catheter. *Arch Inst Cardiol Mex.* 1953;23(2):183-192.

19. Ruiz CE, Feldman TE, Hijazi ZM, et al. Interventional fellowship in structural and congenital heart disease for adults. *JACC Cardiovasc Interv.* 2010;3(9):e1-e15.

20. Sandoval J, Gaspar J, Pena H, et al. Effect of atrial septostomy on the survival of patients with severe pulmonary arterial hypertension. *Eur Respir J.* 2011;38(6):1343-1348.

21. Sigwart U. Non-surgical myocardial reduction for hypertrophic obstructive cardiomyopathy. *Lancet.* 1995;346(8969):211-214.

22. Stone GW, Adams DH, Abraham WT, et al. Clinical trial design principles and endpoint definitions for transcatheter mitral valve repair and replacement: part 2. Endpoint definitions. A consensus document from the Mitral Valve Academic Research Consortium. *Eur Heart J.* 2015;66(3):308-321.

23. Urban P, Mehran R, Colleran R, et al. Defining high bleeding risk in patients undergoing percutaneous coronary intervention: a consensus document from the Academic Research Consortium for High Bleeding Risk. *Eur Heart J.* 2019;40(31):2632-2653.

24. US Food and Drug Administration. *"Off-Label" and investigational use of marketed drugs, biologics, and medical devices.* Accessed August 6, 2020. https://www.fda.gov/regulatory-information/search-fda-guidance-documents/label-and-investigational-use-marketed-drugs-biologics-and-medical-devices

25. Warnes CA, Williams RG, Bashore TM, et al. ACC/AHA 2008 guidelines for the management of adults with Congenital Heart Disease. Executive summary: a report of the American College of Cardiology/American Heart Association Task Force on practice guidelines (writing committee to develop guidelines for the management of adults with congenital heart disease). *Circulation.* 2008;118(23):2395-2451.

26. Webb JG, Pate GE, Munt BI. Percutaneous closure of an aortic prosthetic paravalvular leak with an Amplatzer duct occluder. *Catheter Cardiovasc Interv.* 2005;65(1):69-72.

29 Patent Foramen Ovale, Atrial Septal Defect, and Ventricular Septal Defect Closure[1]

Clinically important left-to-right as well as right-to-left shunts can result from congenital defects of the cardiac septa or anomalous venous connections to the heart. The degree of shunting and the patient's tolerance of that shunt depend on the defect size, the resistance of each of the alternate paths of flow, and to a large degree on ventricular compliance. Since left ventricular compliance diminishes as part of the normal aging process, many shunt lesions that have been well tolerated through childhood can become hemodynamically burdensome for patients later in life, similar to chronic aortic or mitral regurgitation.

ATRIAL-LEVEL COMMUNICATIONS: ANATOMY OF THE ATRIAL SEPTUM

The formation of the atrial septum involves a complex embryologic process whereby 2 independent crescent-shaped tissue membranes (septum primum and septum secundum) form the elements of the septum and grow to overlap one another centrally. The compliant septum primum is situated to the left of the more rigid septum secundum and acts as a 1-way flap valve, a patent foramen ovale (PFO) that allows ongoing right-to-left flow during fetal life. After birth, left atrial pressure rises, the flap valve of the foramen ovale closes, and the septum primum and secundum fuse to one another (in 75%-80% of the population) to complete septation of the atrial chambers. The remaining 20% to 25%, however, have a persistent flap valve, a PFO, with the potential for continuous or intermittent right-to-left flow.

Other failures in the normal development of the septum primum and septum secundum can result in true holes in the septal wall, known as atrial septal defects (ASDs). These defects are named for their normal embryologic counterparts and include septum primum ASDs at the crux of the heart, adjacent to the semilunar valves (an actual defect of the endocardial cushion); secundum ASDs located centrally in the fossa ovale (a defect of the septum primum); and sinus venosus ASDs, most commonly at the superior margin of the septum between the superior vena cava (SVC) and right pulmonary venous return (improper incorporation of the sinus venosus portion of the fetal heart into the right atrium [RA]). Shunting defects of the atrial septum are by far the most common congenital heart disease discovered de novo in adults.

PATHOPHYSIOLOGY OF ATRIAL-LEVEL SHUNTS

Shunt direction and magnitude across an ASD depends primarily on the differences between left and right ventricular compliance (diastolic filling properties). In most patients with an ASD, there is left-to-right flow across the defect throughout the cardiac cycle. In diastole, the more compliant right ventricle (RV) fills more easily than the stiffer left ventricle (LV) and blood flows from the left atrium (LA) to the RV preferentially than to the LV. This increased RV volume traverses the lungs, overloading the LA, and is the driving force of left-to-right shunting when the atrioventricular

---

[1]We gratefully acknowledge the Grossman & Baim's *Cardiac Catheterization, Angiography, and Intervention*, 9th edition contributions of Drs. Alejandro J. Torres and Robert J. Sommer as portions of their chapter, Interventions for Pediatric and Adult Congenital Heart Disease, were retained in this text.

valves are closed in systole. The RV will dilate to accommodate the increased volume and is the best indicator of a hemodynamically important left-to-right shunt.

Because of the ability of the RV to maintain its systolic performance in a dilated state, children are virtually never symptomatic with ASDs. But physiologic parameters change with maturation. The LV walls begin to hypertrophy as afterload increases (part of the normal aging process), resulting in a stiffer chamber that is harder to fill. This leads to increasing left-to-right shunt across the ASD as patients age. It is for this reason that patients with ASD typically only become symptomatic in the third to fifth decades of life. Symptoms are most often new-onset, progressive exercise intolerance and atrial arrhythmia secondary to volume overload and stretching of the right-sided chambers and the conduction system.

Rarely pulmonary vascular disease (Eisenmenger syndrome) can be associated with ASD. When the RV hypertrophies to compensate for its increased afterload, its compliance changes as well. If RV compliance is nearly equal, or becomes worse than LV compliance, right-to-left shunting can occur across the defect. Other factors such as tricuspid valve (TV) disease, congenital right ventricular hypoplasia, or right ventricular myocardial infarction can also change physiologic conditions and augment the potential for right to left flow. With sufficient right-to-left flow, the patient may present with chronic hypoxemia, positional hypoxemia, or transient changes in saturation with exercise that presents as exertional breathlessness.

Even in patients with normal right-sided mechanics, following Valsalva/strain, there is a momentary augmentation of systemic venous return and a transient elevation of RA volume and pressure. With any defect of the atrial septum, including the 1-way "valve" of the PFO, this can result in transient right-to-left flow of varying magnitude across the defect. Right-to-left shunts have been associated with a number of other clinical symptoms including thromboembolic stroke, paradoxical thromboembolization to the systemic circulation, hypoxemia, migraine headache (particularly with aura), decompression illness in divers, and obstructive sleep apnea.

Since September 2017, the role of the PFO in thromboembolic stroke has been redefined. Four randomized trials (RESPECT, REDUCE, CLOSE, and DEFENSE-PFO) demonstrated a substantial reduction in stroke risk with transcatheter PFO closure and chronic blood thinner therapy, when compared with patients who received blood thinners alone. These statistically significant reductions ranged from 45% to 100% in the 4 trials, in populations of young patients with cryptogenic stroke. After more than 2 decades of debate, these trials have led to the US Food and Drug Administration (FDA) approval of 2 PFO closure devices in 2016 and in 2017 (the Amplatzer PFO Occluder, Abbott Medical, and the GORE Cardioform Septal Occluder, WL Gore & Associates).

TRANSCATHETER CLOSURE OF AN ATRIAL SEPTAL DEFECT

Only the secundum-type ASD is currently amenable to transcatheter repair. Both the primum-type and the sinus venosus-type defects lack sufficient surrounding septal rims for a device to be stable, and the device may impede upon surrounding venous and valvar structures. Closure of sinus venosus ASD with covered stents has been reported. Closure of large ASDs, either by surgery or by a transcatheter approach, has been shown to significantly increase exercise capacity. Right ventricular volume usually returns to normal or near-normal levels, but the RA may remain enlarged even after device closure. This may account for the early observation that closing an ASD in adults may not eliminate the increased long-term risk of developing atrial fibrillation seen with ASDs. Closure eliminates the risk of paradoxical embolization. Severe pulmonary hypertension, with persistent right-to-left shunt at the defect resulting in systemic desaturation, is a contraindication to defect closure.

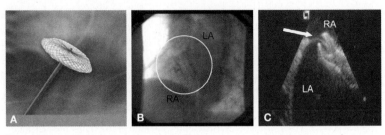

Figure 29.1 **A,** Amplatzer Septal Occluder (Abbott, Santa Clara, USA). **B,** Postimplant fluorosco-py. **C,** Postimplant intracardiac echo image, showing device entrapping the thin septum primum (white arrow). LA, left atrium; RA, right atrium.

In the last decade, transcatheter closure of ASD has become a routine clinical procedure. Currently, the Amplatzer Septal Occluder (ASO) (**Figure 29.1**), the Amplatzer Cribriform Device (ACO) (**Figure 29.2**), the GORE Cardioform Septal Occluder (GSO) (**Figure 29.3**), and the GORE Cardioform ASD Occluder (**Figure 29.4**) are approved for use in the United States. A number of other devices are in use outside of the United States.

The ASO (**Figure 29.1**) is a self-centering device, with 2 nitinol mesh discs that act to secure the device to the surrounding tissue rims and cover the defect on each septal surface, with a smaller central "waist" that actually fills the defect. The center waist of the device is chosen to be equal to or minimally larger than the balloon stop-flow diameter of the defect (the balloon size at which all flow across the defect is stopped by echo imaging). This design produces a rigid implant, providing stability to close ASDs up to 36 mm in diameter. However, when used for ASDs positioned anteriorly/superiorly in the septum with deficiency of the "retroaortic rim" (<5 mm), the ASO has been associated with rare but potentially catastrophic device erosions.

The ACO (**Figure 29.2**) has 2 connected nitinol mesh discs, similar to the ASO, but without the central waist portion of the device. This device was designed and subsequently approved for the closure of the multiply fenestrated atrial septum, in which a series of small defects are located within a small area, allowing the device to span and cover the entire field of defects with a single device.

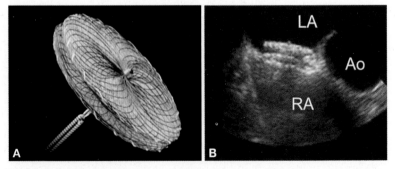

Figure 29.2 **A,** Amplatzer Cribriform Occluder (Abbott, Santa Clara, USA) differs from the Am-platzer Septal Occluder (ASO) in that the discs are the same size, and there is no central "waist" (non-self-centering device). **B,** Amplatzer Cribriform Occluder successfully deployed. Ao, aorta; LA, left atrium; RA, right atrium.

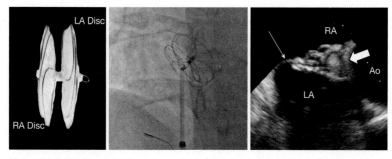

Figure 29.3 GORE cardioform septal occluder (WL Gore & Associates, Flagstaff, Arizona). Left: Non-self-centering device, approved for both ASD and PFO closure, with 2 discs that cover the defect on both septal surfaces. Center: Postimplant fluoroscopy demonstrates the wire frame of the device. Right: Postimplant intracardiac echocardiography demonstrates device entrapping septal rims in good position. The thin septum primum (thin arrow) is seen caught between the device discs. The "retroaortic rim" is much thicker (thick arrow) and causes the 2 discs to splay apart from one another. Ao, aorta; ASD, atrial septal defect; LA, left atrium; PFO, patent foramen ovale; RA, right atrium.

The GSO (**Figure 29.3**), similarly, is made of 2 connected discs that cover the ASD on each septal surface. The frame is made of platinum-filled nitinol wires, covered on each side by expanded polytetrafluoroethylene. There is no central waist portion to fill the defect, limiting this device to closure of small to moderate-sized ASDs (<18 mm in diameter) (GORE Cardioform Septal Occluder IFU, March 2018).

The device is soft and compliant with no reported device erosions with this, or with any prior GORE device, even when used in patients with deficient retroaortic rim. In the Gore Septal Occluder pivotal study, wire frame fractures were observed in 9.3% (4/43) of subjects who underwent fluoroscopic evaluation at 6 months. The fractures were not associated with device instability or clinical sequelae (GORE Cardioform Septal Occluder IFU, March 2018).

The technique for implanting any of the double-disc occluders is similar, regardless of the specific device chosen. The device implant is performed in the catheterization laboratory under transesophageal (TEE) or intracardiac echocardiography (ICE). Femoral venous access is obtained. After a hemodynamic assessment including shunt calculation, a 6F or 7F multipurpose catheter with an A-2 curve is passed to the SVC. The catheter is then withdrawn slowly, aiming the tip toward the patient's left shoulder, until it "jumps" into the defect. A guidewire can then be advanced through the septum to the left upper pulmonary vein, the most stable wire position. Echocardiographic confirmation of the wire position crossing the ASD is confirmed prior to proceeding to the next steps of the procedure.

Alternatively, with the catheter placed in the inferior vena cava (IVC), angled toward the patient's left shoulder, a J-wire can be passed through the defect to the left side of the heart. This technique is particularly useful in cases where additional smaller fenestrations may surround the larger defect and best assures that the largest defect is crossed. The wire is exchanged for a stiffer, more supportive exchange length wire. A sizing balloon is then passed over the wire to straddle the defect. With gentle inflation, the balloon will expand at each end, where it is unconstrained, and will remain narrowed centrally at the site of the ASD. With echo imaging, the balloon is inflated slowly until all shunt flow is eliminated. The size of the balloon can then be measured, and an appropriately sized device can be selected. After careful deairing of the delivery sheath, the device is advanced to the LA. The left atrial occluder is opened and pulled back against the septum, ensuring that no portion of the device prolapses back through the defect into the RA. The right atrial occluder is then opened. The device position is carefully evaluated with echo imaging, reassessing the entrapment of all septal rims, and the elimination of shunting by color flow mapping. Agitated saline injections can also be used to rule out significant residual right-to-left shunting. If the device position is suboptimal, the device can be recaptured and redeployed. Once in good position, the device stability can be tested with a push-pull test on the connecting catheter. The device is then released and the procedure is completed.

The GORE Cardioform ASD Occluder (**Figure 29.4**) is designed to leverage the structural advantages of both the ASO and the GSO in order to be able to close ASDs that might previously have required surgical intervention. The soft, conformable nitinol wire frame of the GSO was retained, while an "anatomically adaptable" central waist portion was added to allow for self-centering and the closure of larger defects. The pivotal cohort of the ASSURED Trial demonstrated a 96% technical success rate for implantation and shunt elimination comparable with the pivotal trials of both ASO and HELEX.

TRANSCATHETER CLOSURE OF PATENT FORAMEN OVALE

The techniques for PFO closure are generally the same as for ASD closure. For an inexperienced operator, the biggest challenge can be finding and crossing the defect. Using the techniques as outlined above, the catheter or wire will naturally

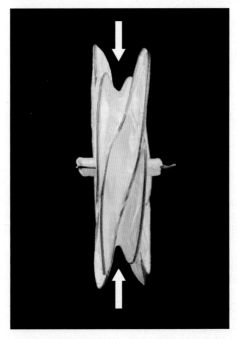

Figure 29.4 GORE cardioform ASD occluder (WL Gore & Associates, Flagstaff, Arizona). In profile, the "anatomically adaptable" center waist of the device is demonstrated (white arrows). This device, like the ASO is self-centering. ASD, atrial septal defect; ASO, Amplatzer Septal Occluder.

be directed into the fossa ovale. Echo imaging can be quite helpful as an adjunct. Balloon sizing is less helpful in determining device size with the PFO, as the flap can be opened to very large sizes with sufficient balloon pressure. However, balloon occlusion and agitated saline injection can help to identify the patient with an alternative source of right-to-left shunt prior to the implant and may give important anatomic information about the length and compliance of the PFO tunnel.

SPECIAL TECHNIQUES

1. Additional fenestrations: In some patients, there will be additional fenestrations of the septum primum. If these defects are clustered in the fossa ovale as is usually the case, a single, larger, non-self-centering device (ACO or GSO) can be used. Occasionally, the distance between these defects is too great for closure with a single device, and additional devices can be placed during the same procedure. To ensure that the first device does not partially cover the distal defects and make subsequent crossing more difficult, we will often obtain an additional femoral venous access and cross both the main ASD/PFO as well as the additional defect with separate catheters and wires. With the wire in place through the second defect, the first ASD/PFO is closed using the usual technique. A second sheath is then advanced over the wire through the additional fenestration, and a second device is placed. Occasionally, when the defects are close enough together that significant device interaction is anticipated, simultaneous deployment of the 2 LA discs to settle them into place can be useful.

2. Long, rigid PFO tunnel: Rarely, if the septum primum is relatively inflexible and the overlap of septum primum and septum secundum is long (>1 cm), it may be difficult to withdraw the closure device back far enough into the tunnel to successfully open the right atrial occluder. This may leave a partially opened RA occluder or extra traction on the LA occluder that may back it into the tunnel in a partially collapsed position. This is less of an issue when using the Amplatzer PFO Occluder (**Figure 29.5**), as it is more rigid and tends to adapt the septal anatomy to the native configuration of the device, rather than the softer devices that tend to conform more to the anatomy of the tunnel. There are 2 techniques for dealing with this unusual situation:

    a. Transseptal puncture technique: Instead of crossing the septum through the PFO, a standard Brockenbrough transseptal puncture can be performed under echo guidance. The septum primum is punctured just at the over-

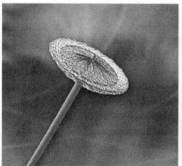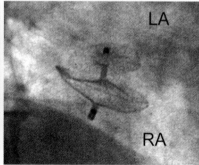

Figure 29.5 Left. Amplatzer PFO occluder. Right. Postimplant fluoroscopy of PFO device, note different-sized discs with RA disc larger than then LA disc. LA, left atrium; PFO, patent foramen ovale; RA, right atrium.

lap site of the septum secundum (**Figure 29.6**). Once across the septum, the wires are exchanged to place the super stiff guidewire in the left upper pulmonary vein as above. Echo guidance is critical here, as it is imperative that the puncture be performed as close to the overlap as possible and that the puncture position be checked from orthogonal angles prior to device placement.

b. Balloon detunnelization: Once the wire is through the PFO to the pulmonary vein, a sizing balloon can be advanced over the wire to the LA. The balloon when initially inflated will demonstrate a sizable distance between the indentation at the entrance to the PFO tunnel and the indentation at the exit on the LA side. With increasing balloon pressure, the indentations on the balloon move toward one another as the balloon straightens. With sufficient force, some of the LA attachments of septum primum can be disrupted, leaving a more compliant tunnel. There are some risks of tearing the septum if sufficient force is employed.

3. Rarely, femoral venous access to the heart will be unavailable, owing to previous instrumentation, venous thrombosis, or an IVC filter that will not allow passage of the necessary catheters. In these cases, a right internal jugular approach or right subclavian approach is possible. However, because of the orientation of the PFO's flap valve, the catheter from the SVC impacts the septum on the wrong angle to cross the defect. This has become more straightforward with the introduction of deflectable sheaths from a number of manufacturers, now available in sizes large enough to deliver the septal occluder. The delivery angle from above usually makes it difficult to maintain a support wire in the left upper pulmonary vein. From the superior approach, the most stable wire position is usually in the LV apex, where a stiff wire with a ventricular loop can help the delivery system to

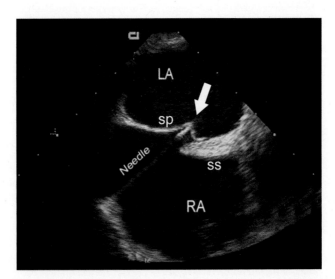

Figure 29.6 Transseptal puncture under transesophageal echo guidance, target site just below the overlap of septum primum and septum secundum. Septum primum "tents" as needle pushes it toward the left atrium (arrow). LA, left atrium; RA, right atrium; sp, septum primum; ss, septum secundum.

cross the septum. Care must be taken to avoid injuring the mitral valve on device deployment with this approach. A separate access will still be required if intracardiac echocardiography is used to guide the procedure. Transhepatic access can also be used, for those experienced with the technique. Once access is obtained, the procedure is no different from the traditional femoral approach, because the catheter course from the IVC to the fossa ovale is maintained.

RESULTS—ATRIAL SEPTAL DEFECT/PATENT FORAMEN OVALE CLOSURE

In a wide array of reviews and collected cohorts, transcatheter closure of an ASD or a PFO is a safe and effective procedure with closure rates >95%. Minor procedural complications, including femoral venous access complications, transient atrial arrhythmia during the procedure, and impingement of the device on surrounding valvar and venous structures occurred in about 5%. More serious complications, such as pericardial effusions/perforations, valve injury, air embolization, device embolization and retrieval, and retroperitoneal bleeding occur in ~2% of patients. Post implant, the incidence of new-onset atrial arrhythmia, including simple premature atrial contractions, supraventricular tachycardia, and other atrial tachyarrhythmias, wase not significantly different from that of surgical series.

Atrial fibrillation has been cited as a reason NOT to close a PFO or an ASD with a transcatheter approach. In the randomized trials, this incidence ranged from 1.5% to 6%, was seen more frequently in an older population, and was transient in all patients who did not previously have atrial fibrillation. Ultimately, the patients receiving the closure device had a lower stroke rate than those treated with medical therapy alone, despite the incidence of atrial fibrillation.

Following successful closure, the dilated RV normalized in dimensions in over 75% of patients, with a significant relationship between older age and failure to return to normal. Transcatheter closure is now the procedure of choice for secundum ASD repair, as it offers significant advantages in terms of pain, length of hospital stay, cosmesis, and recovery time with comparable closure rates in all but the largest defects.

PFO closure rates, whether for stroke prevention, migraines, and other symptoms, are comparable with that seen with ASD closure. In all of the recently published randomized PFO-stroke trials, >90% of patients with PFO implants had no or minimal residual shunting at 12-month follow-up. However, the residual shunts in patients with PFO are held to a different level of scrutiny than in patients with ASDs. In the latter, a reduction in RV volume overload, regardless of the appearance of the residual shunt, typically by color flow Doppler, is the standard definition of a successful closure. In the PFO population, particularly those with prior paradoxical embolic stroke, agitated saline injections are the standard by which closure is judged, a far higher bar.

Several other important issues remain with the currently approved devices for atrial septal repair. Based on reporting to the US FDA's Medical Device Complication website, the former CardioSEAL device (NMT Medical, Boston, Massachusetts) was afflicted with thrombus formation on the device in the first few months after implantation. This issue is still seen occasionally but is far less common in the GORE and Amplatzer devices. Device erosion (cardiac perforation) is the most commonly reported serious long-term complication with the Amplatzer devices. In a recent postapproval, multicenter study, the rate of erosion was 0.3% occurring 12 to 171 days from implant.

Thrombus formation has been reported with the Amplatzer device as well. The Cardioform Septal Occluder has a reported 9% rate of wire-frame fracture, an issue not seen in the Amplatzer devices. An FDA panel review of this issue in 2012 found no significant complications associated with the wire fractures in the GORE HELEX device. There is no indication that either thrombosis or erosion is a significant issue, to date, with the GORE devices.

There is no consensus yet on the appropriate degree of antithrombotic therapy after device implantation. Aspirin alone has been used in many centers, with a combination of aspirin, clopidogrel, and warfarin being used by others. In children, only aspirin (5 mg/kg/d, maximum dose 325 mg) for 6 months is recommended. Adolescents and adults are most often treated with aspirin 325 mg daily for 6 months and clopidogrel 75 mg for 3 months.

The incidence of infective endocarditis of the device is also unknown. Most centers recommend antibiotic prophylaxis for dental work or other minor surgical procedures for a period of 6 to 12 months from the time of device implantation.

VENTRICULAR SEPTAL DEFECTS

Like ASDs, congenital deficiencies in the ventricular septum are varied in anatomy. The most common ventricular septal defects (VSDs) occur in the membranous septum. Endocardial cushion defects affecting the ventricular septum, malalignment defects of the outflow septum, and defects of the muscular portion of the septum are less common. Left-to-right shunts at the ventricular level result in pulmonary overcirculation, but with a concomitant LV volume overload. With a large enough defect, the pressure head of LV contraction is transmitted to the PA in systole. This makes VSDs physiologically different from ASDs in which there is simply volume loading of the right side of the heart. The resistance to flow at the defect itself is the primary determinant of shunt volume in children. As a direct sequela of the magnitude of the LV volume load, patients with small defects may be symptom free, without significant LV enlargement by imaging. With larger defects, the patient will present with the classic symptoms of congestive heart failure (CHF) early in infancy. With a moderate-sized defect, the patient may be asymptomatic in childhood, despite a significantly dilated LV. These patients may present in adulthood with new symptoms of CHF as with expected aging changes in the LV myocardium, the chamber compliance decreases. The volume load associated with the VSD will then no longer be handled at low diastolic pressures, as when the patient was younger. LA pressures rise, and pulmonary venous congestion may ensue, particularly with exertion, when blood flow through the left heart increases further. Patients with unrestrictive defects, who do not undergo repair in the first 2 to 3 years of life, risk the development of irreversible pulmonary vascular disease (Eisenmenger syndrome).

TRANSCATHETER CLOSURE OF VENTRICULAR SEPTAL DEFECTS

Transcatheter closure of inlet (endocardial cushion-type) VSDs is not yet possible based both on the embryologic and anatomic relationship of these defects to abnormalities of the atrioventricular valves and to the lack of surrounding support structures to stabilize such a device. Similarly, the design of devices to close *membranous* VSDs was quite challenging, as the aortic valve, the TV, and the conduction system all abut this portion of the septum. The Amplatzer Membranous VSD was the first device specifically designed for closure of membranous VSD. Despite high closure rates, it was associated with unacceptable high rates of complete AV block of 3.6%, which increased to almost 5% on follow-up since 25% of the cases of AV block occurred as a late event. (This is in contradistinction to 1% incidence of heart block following surgical closure.) A second version of the same device has undergone evaluation with improved outcomes in a small number of patients. Currently, there are no approved devices for closure of membranous VSD in the United States.

Although much less common than membranous VSDs, large *muscular* VSDs, which may occur anywhere in the muscular portion of the septum, present a difficult challenge for the surgeon. Apical and anterior defects may be impossible to visualize and repair through the TV. Right ventricular septal trabeculations make identification from the RV septal surface difficult. The original surgical approach was through a left ventriculotomy. However, long-term follow-up of these patients revealed a high rate of LV aneurysm formation and an equally disturbing number of patients with global LV dysfunction.

The need for successful transcatheter therapy has therefore been more pressing in patients with muscular rather than with the membranous defects. At the same time, the anatomy is more favorable to a transcatheter approach as most have good surrounding tissue rims to support the device, without concerns of valvar or electrophysiologic compromise. Reports of successful transcatheter muscular VSD closures have appeared since the early 1990s. Percutaneous VSD closure is indicated in infants >5 kg with hemodynamically significant defects (left ventricular or left atrial volume overload or pulmonary-to-systemic blood flow ratio >2:1). In babies with Down syndrome, closure should be undertaken prior to 6 months of age, since these patients tend to develop irreversible pulmonary vascular disease sooner than non-Down babies.

The procedure remains technically challenging in small children, and a number of strategies have evolved to incorporate transcatheter management in infants with CHF due to a large muscular VSD. Initially, a staged approach was used. PA banding was performed in the infant (a closed heart procedure) to limit pulmonary flow and eliminate symptoms of CHF. With subsequent growth of the child, transcatheter defect closure would become technically easier and could be followed with surgical band removal (also a closed heart procedure). More recently, periventricular "hybrid" surgical approaches have been described, in which a surgical incision exposes the RV free wall. This approach is recommended in infants <5 kg. A needle can be used to puncture the RV free wall (under echocardiographic guidance), and a wire advanced through the needle to the defect and into the LV. A sheath is advanced over the wire into the LV, and the closure device is deployed in the usual fashion. The puncture site in the RV free wall can be closed with a purse-string suture. Numerous devices have been used for closing muscular VSDs in the past. These were primarily devices designed for closure of ASDs that were used off-label in the ventricular septum. The Amplatzer Muscular VSD Occluder (**Figure 29.7**) is designed specifically for closure of congenital muscular VSDs. The device is similar in design and concept to the ASD devices, but both discs are the same diameter and the center waist of the Muscular VSD Occluder is longer than that of the ASD devices to account for the increased thickness of the ventricular septum.

TECHNIQUE OF MUSCULAR VENTRICULAR SEPTAL DEFECT CLOSURE

After a complete left- and right-sided heart hemodynamic assessment and an echocardiographic assessment of the defect and the surrounding anatomy by TEE or ICE, an LV angiogram is performed to best profile the defect. The defect is then crossed from the left ventricular septal surface, either with a torquable coronary catheter or with a balloon-tipped catheter (balloon wedge catheter) introduced retrograde via the femoral artery or antegrade via a transvenous transseptal approach. The defect is typically easier to cross from the LV side, as it is a smooth, less heavily trabeculated surface, and the catheter crosses in the direction of the high-velocity flow.

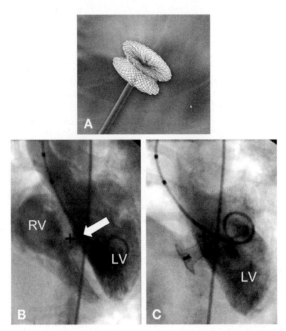

Figure 29.7 A, Amplatzer Muscular VSD Occluder. **B,** Left ventricle (LV) angiogram showing left-to-right shunt across a midmuscular VSD (arrow), filling the right ventricle (RV). **C,** Defect closed with Amplatzer Muscular VSD Occluder. VSD, ventricular septal defect. (Images courtesy of Z. Hijazi.)

A soft extension-length guidewire (ie, Benson wire) is passed through the defect to the RV and advanced to the PA. From a transvenous approach (femoral for anterior muscular defects and jugular for midmuscular and apical defects produce the straightest course for device delivery), a balloon wedge catheter is advanced through the right side of the heart to the PA and exchanged for a snare catheter, which is used to capture and exteriorize the wire. This creates a reliable "rail" over which the device delivery sheath can be advanced. Using the balloon catheter to cross through the TV and capturing the wire in the PA minimizes the risk of having the wire become entangled in the TV and disrupting chordal attachments. The largest dimension of the defect may then be confirmed with balloon sizing (the balloon introduced over wire to straddle the defect—see ASD closure earlier), but unlike an ASD, the VSD dimensions as measured on echo do not stretch as they do with ASD balloon sizing. The device is then chosen to exceed the defect size by 1.6 to 2.0 times when a double-umbrella device is used or by 2 to 3 mm when an Amplatzer Muscular VSD Occluder is selected.

Next, the appropriate size delivery system is advanced from the venous access, over the exteriorized wire to the RA, RV, and through the defect to the LV. Echocardiography and hand injections through the sheath will confirm its position. The wire is then removed from the arterial side, and the device is delivered through the long sheath in the usual fashion. The LV occluder is opened and pulled back against the septum. Resistance will be felt as the device is pulled into the defect. Echo and angiographic injections will confirm LV septal position, and the RV septal occluder is then delivered. When angiographic and/or echo images confirm the position of the device on both sides of the septum, the device is released.

RESULTS—VENTRICULAR SEPTAL DEFECT CLOSURE

Twenty-three European centers collaborated to report the largest experience so far with transcatheter closure of congenital VSDs. Of the 430 cases that underwent attempted closure of a congenital VSD, 119 were muscular defects, 250 were perimembranous, 45 were residual defects post surgery, and 16 had multiple defects. The procedure was technically successful in 95% of the cases. The procedures were done primarily with the Amplatzer group of devices. Failures were primarily related to complications or device malposition requiring immediate surgical intervention.

Complications occurred in 12.7% (6.5% were serious) and included device embolization (1.3%), creation of aortic regurgitation (3.4%), creation of tricuspid regurgitation (6.6%), minor rhythm disturbances (2.5%), and complete heart block (4%, the majority of whom required pacemaker implantation). Only 0.8% of patients with defects in the muscular septum developed rhythm disturbances. There was 1 death. In the multivariate analysis, the only definitive risks for procedural complication were patient age ($P = .012$) and patient weight ($P = .0035$). A US registry had very similar results.

VSD closure has been described with other devices on an off-label basis including free and detachable Gianturco coils, the Nit-Occlud device, the Amplatzer Duct Occluder I, and the Amplatzer Duct Occluder II.

While transcatheter closure of the VSD is technically feasible, careful patient and defect selection remains the most important aspect of the procedure. For asymptomatic patients with small defects, the closure may not be clinically indicated. For patients with membranous-type defects sufficiently large to cause clinical symptoms, the surgical option remains an excellent alternative.

POST MYOCARDIAL INFARCTION
Ventricular Septal Rupture

One additional area of interest for adult interventionalists is postinfarction ventricular septal rupture. These defects are always muscular in location and occur in the distribution of the distal left anterior descending artery (LAD), yielding mid and apical muscular VSDs, or in the right coronary artery (RCA) producing inferior (inlet) VSDs. These VSDs classically present in a bimodal fashion with a higher incidence in the first 24 hours and then again 3 to 5 days after myocardial infarction. In an era of aggressive angioplasty at the first signs of ischemia, this complication of myocardial infarction is far less common than in previous generations.

Untreated, large defects are nearly always fatal, as a large left-to-right shunt, pulmonary overcirculation, pulmonary hypertension, and LV volume overload are superimposed on to a severely compromised/ischemic pump. Acute surgical intervention with patch closure has been difficult, because the surgeon has little reliable tissue in the margins of the defect in which to place sutures. Exclusion strategies similar to those used for apical aneurysms are now being more commonly employed. Similarly, following transcatheter closure of these defects, ongoing necrosis of surrounding tissue can lead to important residual shunts and device instability after early implantation. Small defects are interesting from a diagnostic perspective but do not impose a significant hemodynamic burden. However, with ongoing tissue necrosis, the defect can become more hemodynamically important over the first few weeks.

Once identified as hemodynamically important, these defects should be closed as soon as possible, whether by a surgical or transcatheter approach. Waiting to stabilize the patient medically is an unreliable approach, as the shunt may only increase with time and the onset of multisystem organ failure over several days of poor cardiac output makes the patient less likely to recover from either intervention.

The transcatheter device implantation technique is identical to the treatment of congenital muscular VSDs (as above). Transcatheter intervention is an excellent approach for patients with infarcts in the LAD distribution, while surgical intervention is probably more likely to succeed when the defect arises from an RCA infarct. Catheter repair of these posterior defects is complicated by the proximity to the atrioventricular valves and their support structures. A hybrid approach technique for closure of postinfarct ventricular septal rupture has also been described.

SUGGESTED READINGS

1. Bridges ND, Perry SB, Keane JF, et al. Preoperative transcatheter closure of congenital muscular ventricular septal defects. *N Engl J Med.* 1991;324(19):1312-1317.
2. Carminati M, Butera G, Chessa M, et al. Transcatheter closure of congenital ventricular septal defects: results of the European Registry. *Eur Heart J.* 2007;28(19):2361-2368.
3. Crystal MA, Vincent JA, Gray WA. The wedding cake solution: a percutaneous correction of a form fruste superior sinus venosus atrial septal defect. *Catheter Cardiovasc Interv.* 2015;86(7):1204-1210.
4. Duong P, Ferguson LP, Lord S, et al. Atrial arrhythmia after transcatheter closure of secundum atrial septal defects in patients >40 years of age. *Europace.* 2017;19(8):1322-1326.
5. El-Said H, Hegde S, Foerster S, et al. Device therapy for atrial septal defects in a multicenter cohort: acute outcomes and adverse events. *Catheter Cardiovasc Interv.* 2015;85(2):227-233.
6. Jones TK, Latson LA, Zahn E, et al. Results of the U.S. multicenter pivotal study of the HELEX septal occluder for percutaneous closure of secundum atrial septal defects. *J Am Coll Cardiol.* 2007;49(22):2215-2221.
7. King TD, Mills NL. Historical perspective on ASD device closure. In: Hijazi ZM, Feldman T, Abdullah Al-Qbandi MH, Sievert H, eds. *Transcatheter Closure of ASDs and PFOs.* Cardiotext; 2010:37-64.
8. Lee PH, Song JK, Kim JS, et al. Cryptogenic stroke and high-risk patent foramen ovale: the DEFENSE-PFO trial. *J Am Coll Cardiol.* 2018;71(20):2335-2342.
9. Mas JL, Derumeaux G, Guillon B, et al; CLOSE Investigators. Patent foramen ovale closure or anticoagulation vs. antiplatelets after stroke. *N Engl J Med.* 2017;377(11):1011-1021.
10. Saver JL, Carroll JD, Thaler DE, et al. Long-term outcomes of patent foramen ovale closure or medical therapy after stroke. *N Engl J Med.* 2017;377(11):1022-1032.
11. Sondergaard L, Kasner SE, Rhodes JF, et al; Gore REDUCE Clinical Study Investigators. Patent foramen ovale closure or antiplatelet therapy for cryptogenic stroke. *N Engl J Med.* 2017;377(11):1033-1042.
12. Tobis JM, Narasimha D, Abudayyeh I. Patent foramen ovale closure for hypoxemia. *Interv Cardiol Clin.* 2017;6(4):547-554.
13. Turner DR, Owada CY, Sang CJ, Khan M, Lim DS. Closure of secundum atrial septal defects with the AmplatzerTM Septal Occluder: a prospective, multicenter, post-approval study. *Circ Cardiovasc Interv.* 2017;10:e004212.
14. Tzikas A, Ibrahim R, Velasco-Sanchez D, et al. Transcatheter closure of perimembranous ventricular septal defect with the Amplatzer® membranous VSD occluder 2: initial world experience and one-year follow-up. *Catheter Cardiovasc Interv.* 2014;83(4):571-580.

30 Alcohol Septal Ablation[1]

Hypertrophic cardiomyopathy (HCM) is the most common genetic cardiovascular disease, with an estimated prevalence in the general population of 0.2%. It is transmitted as a Mendelian autosomal-dominant trait, and some if not all the sporadic forms are due to spontaneous mutations. At least 15 different genes and over 1500 mutations have been identified (**Figure 30.1**). HCM can present with different phenotypes, the most common of which is a hypertrophied, nondilated, hyperdynamic, left ventricle (LV). The hypertrophy can vary from focal (<3 segments) to multisegmental, and in 5% to 25% of cases, it can have a predominantly apical distribution. Left ventricular outflow tract obstruction (LVOTO) is usually associated with multisegmental hypertrophy, and it is the result of the combination of asymmetric septal hypertrophy and systolic anterior motion (SAM) of the mitral valve (**Figure 30.2**). While medical therapy is effective in relieving symptoms in a majority of patients, some patients remain severely symptomatic or might be intolerant of medical therapy. Surgical myectomy involving the resection of the hypertrophied septal muscle from the outflow tract was first performed by Cleland in 1958 and described in 1960. The procedure was later modified by Morrow, and since Morrow's initial publication in 1975, different surgical techniques have been proposed. Surgical results in experienced tertiary centers have been excellent, but broad expertise is currently lacking.

Transcatheter ablation of the septum with ethanol emerged as an alternative to surgical myectomy in selected symptomatic patients with LVOTO in 1994. The concept

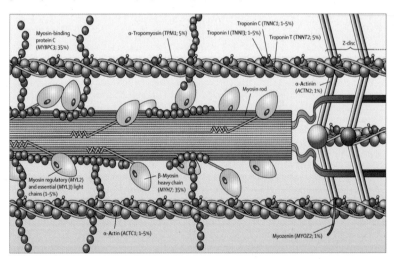

Figure 30.1 Locations of genes within the cardiac sarcomere known to cause hypertrophic cardiomyopathy. Prevalence of every gene (derived from data of unrelated hypertrophic cardiomyopathy probands with positive genotyping) is shown in parentheses. (Reproduced with permission from Maron BJ, Maron MS. Hypertrophic cardiomyopathy. *Lancet*. 2013;381(9862):242-255.)

---

[1]We gratefully acknowledge the *Grossman & Baim's Cardiac Catheterization, Angiography, and Intervention*, 9th edition contributions of Drs. Mauro Moscucci and Stanley Chetcuti, as portions of their chapter, "Nonvalvular Interventions: Left Atrial Appendage Closure and Alcohol Septal Ablation," were retained in this text.

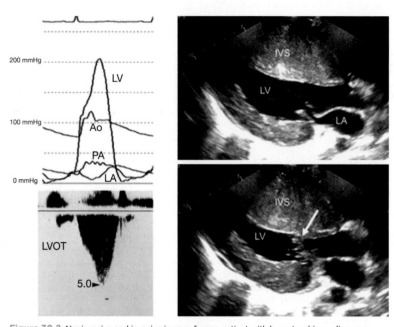

Figure 30.2 Noninvasive and invasive images from a patient with hypertrophic cardiomyopathy. **Top left**, Pressure tracings obtained at cardiac catheterization demonstrating a severe left ventricular (LV) outflow tract obstruction. The LV shows a late peaking systolic pressure exceeding 200 mmHg. There is a spike and dome pattern in the ascending aorta (Ao) pressure, with a gradient of 95 mmHg between the LV and Ao. There are slight elevations of the left atrial (LA) and LV end-diastolic pressures. **Bottom left**, Continuous-wave Doppler echocardiogram across the left ventricular outflow tract (LVOT). There is a dagger-shaped late peaking systolic velocity of 5 m/s correlating with a peak gradient of 100 mmHg. **Top right**, Parasternal long-axis view showing severe increase in thickness of the interventricular septum (IVS) of 3.5 cm, resulting in asymmetrical septal hypertrophy. There is a normal left ventricular (LV) cavity and a normal left atrial (LA) volume. The images are taken during the onset of systole, in which there is the start of mild anterior motion of the mitral valve leaflets. **Bottom right**, The 2-dimensional echocardiogram is now shown during late systole, in which there is severe systolic anterior motion of the mitral valve (arrow). PA, pulmonary artery. (Reproduced with permission from Nishimura RA, Seggewiss H, Schaff HV. Hypertrophic obstructive cardiomyopathy. *Circ Res.* 2017;121(7):771-783.)

behind the development of the procedure was based on the observation that inflating a balloon in a septal perforator artery would result in akinesia or hypokinesia of the corresponding septal myocardial segment and a reduction of the gradient, and on prior experience related to alcohol injection for the management of ventricular arrhythmias.

Patient Selection for Alcohol Septal Ablation

Septal reduction therapy with surgical myectomy or alcohol septal ablation (ASA) is appropriate for patients with hypertrophic obstructive cardiomyopathy (HOCM) who have symptoms that interfere with their lifestyle and are refractory to optimal medical therapy. The choice of alcohol ablation versus surgical myectomy depends on anatomical factors. Abnormalities of the mitral valve and papillary muscle that would require a surgical approach and underlying coronary artery disease with an indication for coronary artery bypass surgery should be ruled out. The most recent recommendation is also to avoid ASA when the intraventricular septum is felt to be inadequate to perform the procedure safely in the judgment of the operator, given the high risk of ventricular septal defect (VSD) in the setting of mild hypertrophy. Recommendation according to the 2020 American College of Cardiology (ACC)/American Heart Association (AHA) guidelines for the management of HCM are shown in **Table 30.1**. The 2014 European Society of Cardiology guidelines for the management of HCM provide more general recommendations regarding septal reduction therapies including septal myectomy or septal alcohol ablation (SAA), as follows (class 1 indications):

1. "Septal reduction therapies be performed by experienced operators, working as part of a multidisciplinary team expert in the management of HCM."
2. "Septal reduction therapy to improve symptoms is recommended in patients with a resting or maximum provoked LVOT gradient of >50 mmHg, who are in NYHA functional class III-IV, despite maximum tolerated medical therapy."
3. "Septal myectomy, rather than SAA, is recommended in patients with an indication for septal reduction therapy and other lesions requiring surgical intervention (eg, mitral valve repair/replacement, papillary muscle intervention)."

The relief of LVOTO with ASA is associated with significant regression of LV hypertrophy (**Figure 30.3**). However, concerns have been expressed that, when compared with surgical myectomy, the septal scar resulting from ASA would generate a milieu for malignant ventricular arrhythmias. While as of today it remains unclear whether ASA might have a proarrhythmogenic effect, several reported case series and a systematic review have failed to show worse survival in patients treated with ASA when compared with patients treated with surgical myectomy.

Procedure

Transthoracic echocardiographic guidance is routinely (and should be) used to guide the procedure. The procedural steps commonly used are as follows:

1. A dual-lumen catheter (Langston Catheter, Teleflex) is inserted into the LV to measure intraventricular pressure and simultaneous systemic arterial pressure.

Table 30.1	ACC/AHA Guidelines Recommendation for Alcohol Septal Ablation	
Class of Recommendation	**Level of Evidence**	**Recommendations**
1	C-Limited Data	In adult patients with obstructive HCM who remain severely symptomatic, despite GDMT and in whom surgery is contraindicated or the risk is considered unacceptable because of serious comorbidities or advanced age, alcohol septal ablation in eligible patients,[a] performed at experienced centers,[b] is recommended.

GDMT, guideline directed medical therapy.
[a]General eligibility criteria for septal reduction therapy: (a) Clinical: Severe dyspnea or chest pain (usually New York Heart Association functional class III or class IV), or occasionally other exertional symptoms (eg, syncope, near syncope), when attributable to LVOTO, that interfere with everyday activity or quality of life despite optimal medical therapy. (b) Hemodynamic: Dynamic LVOT gradient at rest or with physiologic provocation with approximate peak gradient of ≥50 mmHg, associated with septal hypertrophy and SAM of the mitral valve. (c) Anatomic: Targeted anterior septal thickness sufficient to perform the procedure safely and effectively in the judgment of the individual operator.
[b]Comprehensive or primary HCM centers with demonstrated excellence in clinical outcomes for these procedures.
Reprinted with permission from Ommen SR, Mital S, Burke MA, et al. 2020 AHA/ACC guideline for the diagnosis and treatment of patients with hypertrophic cardiomyopathy: a report of the American College of Cardiology/American Heart Association Joint Committee on Clinical Practice Guidelines. *Circulation*. 2020;142(25):e558-e631. ©2020 American Heart Association, Inc.

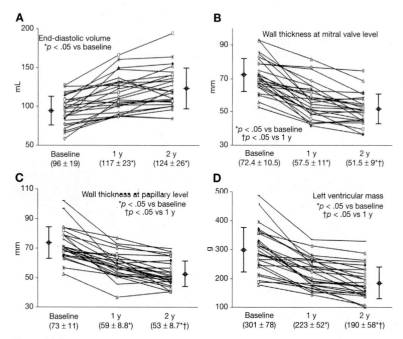

Figure 30.3 Individual data points of left ventricular end-diastolic volume **(A)**, wall thickness score at mitral valve level **(B)**, wall thickness score at papillary muscle level **(C)**, and mass **(D)** at baseline and 1 and 2 y after nonsurgical septal reduction therapy. (Reproduced with permission from Mazoor W, Nagueh SF, Lakkis NM, et al, Regression of left ventricular hypertrophy after nonsurgical septal reduction therapy for hypertrophic obstructive cardiomyopathy. *Circulation.* 2001;103:1492-1496.)

    A resting or provoked (Valsalva) left ventricular outflow tract (LVOT) gradient is demonstrated before proceeding with ASA.

2. The coronary and septal anatomy is evaluated with coronary angiography to assess whether the anatomy is suitable for ASA. We recommend angiography also of the right coronary artery (RCA) to rule out the possibility of anomalous RCA to septal collaterals.

3. A transvenous pacemaker is inserted in patients who do not have a preexisting permanent pacemaker or implantable cardioverter-defibrillator (ICD).

4. Therapeutic anticoagulation is administered.

5. A 0.014-in guidewire is inserted into the first septal artery of the left anterior descending (LAD) artery, and a short other-the-wire balloon is advanced into the septal artery.

6. The balloon is inflated to occlude the septal artery. Confirmation that the inflated balloon is not obstructing flow in the LAD artery is obtained by contrast injection in the LAD through the guiding catheter (**Figure 30.4**).

7. The septal guidewire is removed, and the position of the inflated balloon is confirmed again by angiography.

8. The septal anatomy is defined by angiographic contrast injection through the balloon lumen, making sure that there is no leakage of contrast into the LAD (**Figure 30.5**).

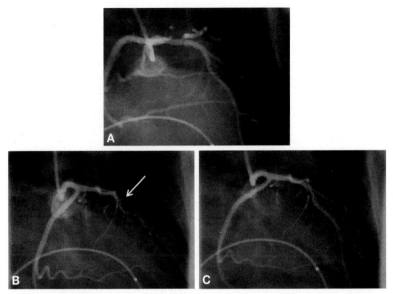

Figure 30.4 **Panel A,** Baseline coronary angiogram—left anterior descending (LAD) artery. **Panel B,** Coronary angiogram after inflation of the balloon in the septal perforator artery. The balloon is clearly obstructing flow in the LAD (arrow). **Panel C,** Repeat coronary angiogram after repositioning of the balloon. (Reproduced with permission from Fernades V, Moscucci M, Spencer WH. Complications of alcohol septal ablation for hypertrophic obstructive cardiomyopathy. In: Moscucci M, ed. *Complications of Cardiovascular Procedures. Risk Factors, Management, and Bailout Techniques.* Wolters Kluwer; 2011.)

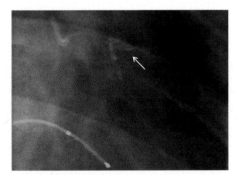

Figure 30.5 Contrast injection through the inflated balloon. There is extravasation of contrast in the left anterior descending (arrow). Injection of alcohol in this case would lead to catastrophic consequences. (Reproduced with permission from Fernades V, Moscucci M, Spencer WH. Complications of alcohol septal ablation for hypertrophic obstructive cardiomyopathy. In: Moscucci M, ed. *Complications of Cardiovascular Procedures. Risk Factors, Management, and Bailout Techniques.* Wolters Kluwer; 2011.)

9. Agitated angiographic contrast or echo contrast is injected into the occluded septal artery via the balloon lumen, and the location of the intended infarct at the mitral-septal contact site is correctly identified by transthoracic echocardiography.

10. Additional analgesia is administered.

11. Finally, 1 to 3 mL absolute alcohol is injected slowly (over 2-5 min) into the septal artery via the balloon lumen. Arteriovenous (AV) conduction is closely monitored during the alcohol injection. The rate of injection may need to be slowed significantly or stopped altogether if significant AV block occurs. Our practice is to perform the alcohol injection under continuous fluoroscopic visualization to ensure that, during injection, the balloon does not slip back in the LAD and thus to avoid potentially catastrophic consequences of alcohol injection in the native LAD.

12. The balloon is left inflated for an additional 5 min after the alcohol administration.

13. The balloon central lumen is then continually aspirated while the balloon is deflated and withdrawn. Continual aspiration through the lumen of the balloon prevents any alcohol seepage into the LAD or guiding catheter. Care must be taken during balloon withdrawal to limit the guiding catheter's tendency to telescope further into the left main and LAD and cause dissections.

14. Confirmation by hemodynamic measurements and by Doppler echocardiography that the LVOT gradient is successfully reduced is obtained.

15. A final coronary angiogram is performed to demonstrate the septal occlusion and absence of coronary complications.

16. If inadequate gradient reduction is achieved, then another septal artery may be injected with alcohol to reduce the gradient. However, alcohol injection in multiple septal perforator branches has been found to be associated with increased risk of complications, and therefore it is not generally recommended.

17. Our practice is to keep the transvenous pacemaker for 48 to 72 hours, as we have observed occasionally the development of third-degree AV block >24 hours after the procedure.

Complications of ASA

It cannot be overemphasized that the procedure should be performed only in experienced centers with a dedicated program in HCM and by experienced operators. ASA involves occluding a coronary artery branch and inducing a therapeutic infarction in a targeted area of myocardium; its complexity and the type of complications require a critical skill set.

In general, complications of ASA can be divided into 2 main groups—early complications and late complications. An alternative classification includes 3 secondary groups. The first group includes complications related to cardiac catheterization, the second group includes complications related to percutaneous coronary intervention (PCI), and the third group includes complications specific to ASA (**Table 30.2**). Further discussion in this chapter will focus on the complications specific to ASA.

Early Periprocedural Death

In a case series including 850 patients who underwent ASA, there were 9 procedure-related deaths (1.05%). The causes of periprocedural deaths are shown in **Table 30.3**.

Nontargeted Remote Myocardial Infarction

Remote infarction following ASA can be due to extravasation of ethanol or the presence of collateral circulation. The common areas of nontargeted infarct are the anterior wall and apex from the extravasation of alcohol from the septal artery (**Figure 30.6**) or the distal LAD and RCA territory from egress of alcohol through septal collaterals (**Figures 30.7** and **30.8**). ASA can also result in undesirable infarction in the

Table 30.2 **Complications of Alcohol Septal Ablation (ASA)**

Related to Cardiac Catheterization	Related to PCI	Related to ASA		
		Periprocedural		Late
Death	Contrast nephropathy	Dissection	Death	V tachycardia	V tachycardia
MI	Atheroembolism	Perforation	Remote MI	Mitral regurgitation	Mitral regurgitation
Stroke	Local complications	Distal embolization	High-grade block	VSD	VSD
TIA	Hematoma	MI	Hypotension	Septal hematoma	CHF
Embolic events	Pseudoaneurysm	Death	Dissection	Delayed infarction	Death
Arrhythmia	Bleeding	Stroke	Tamponade	Takotsubo cardiomyopathy	
Perforation	AV fistula		Alcohol leak into LAD		
Tamponade	Distal emboli				
Allergic reactions	Arterial thrombosis				
	Infection				

AV, arteriovenous; CHF, congestive heart failure; LAD, left anterior descending; MI, myocardial infarction; PCI, percutaneous coronary intervention; TIA, transient ischemic attack; VSD, ventricular septal defect. Reproduced with permission from Fernades V, Moscucci M, Spencer WH. Complications of alcohol septal ablation for hypertrophic obstructive cardiomyopathy. In: Moscucci M, ed. *Complications of Cardiovascular Procedures. Risk Factors, Management, and Bailout Techniques*. Wolters Kluwer; 2011.

location of the right ventricular (RV) free wall, LV free wall, or the papillary muscles. Echocardiographic guidance with the use of agitated X-ray contrast or echo contrast agents will identify inappropriate sites for alcohol injection. With contrast echocardiography, we have observed 1 case in which the septal branch provided blood supply to the anterior papillary muscle, 1 case in which it provided blood supply to the RV papillary muscles, and a third case in which the septal branch drained into the RV. In all these cases, the procedure was aborted.

Electrocardiogram Changes and High-Grade AV Block

Electrocardiogram (ECG) changes are frequent during ASA and include QT prolongation, Q-waves, right bundle branch block (72% of cases), left bundle branch block (LBBB, 6%), first-degree heart block (53%), and complete heart block (CHB).

The incidence of CHB requiring a pacemaker has been reported to be up to 40% in early series. The incidence of AV block has decreased significantly after modification of the procedure with slower injection of smaller amounts of ethanol per septal

Table 30.3	**Procedure-related Deaths (of 850 Patients Series BAYLOR/MUSC)**
1. LAD dissection and ventricular fibrillation during ASA	
2. Retroperitoneal bleed	
3. Acute septal perforation (VSD) with pulmonary edema	
4. Left main dissection	
5. Sudden death 10 d after ASA	
6. Late inferior MI with RV infarct and cardiogenic shock (10 d post ASA)	
7. RV perforation and tamponade from temporary pacemaker lead	
8. Cardiogenic shock	
9. Stress cardiomyopathy	

ASA, alcohol septal ablation; LAD, left anterior descending; MI, myocardial infarction; RV, right ventricular; VSD, ventricular septal defect.
Reproduced with permission from: Fernades V, Moscucci M, Spencer WH. Complications of alcohol septal ablation for hypertrophic obstructive cardiomyopathy. In: Moscucci M, ed. *Complications of Cardiovascular Procedures. Risk Factors, Management, and Bailout Techniques.* Wolters Kluwer; 2011.

perforator artery, the use of myocardial contrast echocardiography (MCE), and avoidance of injecting multiple septal perforator branches. The rate of new pacemaker implantation in high-volume centers is currently <10%.

It is important to note that patients referred for ASA might have previously undergone implantation of a permanent pacemaker or an ICD. Therefore, the reported case series might underestimate the actual pacemaker requirement following ASA.

Significant predictors of new pacemaker implantation are preexisting LBBB or first-degree heart block, injection of ethanol by bolus rather than slow infusion, lack of use of MCE, injection of more than 1 septal artery, and female sex.

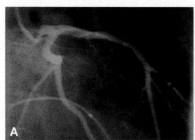 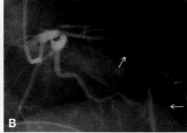

Figure 30.6 Leakage of alcohol in the left anterior descending. **Panel A,** Baseline coronary angiogram. **Panel B,** Coronary angiogram obtained after injection of alcohol (arrows). (Reproduced with permission from: Fernades V, Moscucci M, Spencer WH. Complications of alcohol septal ablation for hypertrophic obstructive cardiomyopathy. In: Moscucci M, ed. *Complications of Cardiovascular Procedures. Risk Factors, Management, and Bailout Techniques.* Wolters Kluwer; 2011.)

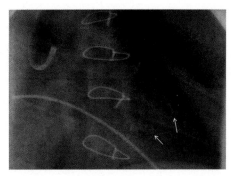

Figure 30.7 Injection of contrast through the inflated balloon in the septal perforator branch. There is filling of the distal left anterior descending (LAD) via septal to LAD collaterals (arrows).

Hypotension

Mild hypotension can be seen in up to 25% of patients after ASA. The etiology of hypotension includes hypovolemia, the effect of medications, cardiogenic shock due to coronary artery dissection or alcohol extravasation, remote infarct, stress cardiomyopathy, pericardial tamponade, bleeding, mitral regurgitation, and the development of a VSD. The differential diagnosis is critical because treatment options can be quite different.

Perforation and Tamponade

Perforation and tamponade, while rare, are usually due to temporary pacemaker leads perforating through the RV free wall. Anticoagulation should be held or reversed with protamine, and immediate pericardiocentesis should be done with echocardiographic guidance when appropriate.

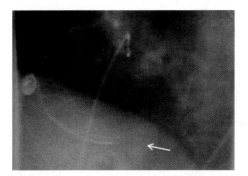

Figure 30.8 Coronary angiogram of the right coronary artery (RCA) after injection of alcohol in a septal perforator branch of the left anterior descending. There is no flow in the distal RCA, likely due to extravasation of alcohol in the RCA territory through collateral flow (arrow). (Reproduced with permission from Fernades V, Moscucci M, Spencer WH. Complications of alcohol septal ablation for hypertrophic obstructive cardiomyopathy. In: Moscucci M, ed. *Complications of Cardiovascular Procedures. Risk Factors, Management, and Bailout Techniques.* Wolters Kluwer; 2011.)

Alcohol Extravasation into the LAD

Alcohol extravasation is a potentially disastrous complication of ASA. Alcohol can leak back into the LAD either during the injection of alcohol into the septal artery or when the balloon is withdrawn from the septal artery. Extravasation of alcohol causes no-reflow or complete occlusion of the LAD, and it can manifest with antero-lateral ST elevation, severe chest pain, hemodynamic or electrical instability, and cardiac arrest.

This complication can be avoided by meticulous technique, the use of a slightly oversized balloon (1.2:1 balloon:septal diameter ratio), confirmation that the inflated balloon is occlusive, and with slow injection of alcohol under continuous fluoroscopic and ECG monitoring to ensure that the balloon has not migrated from its position. After alcohol injection is completed, the inflated balloon can be flushed with a saline solution and left in the septal artery for ~5 min. Negative aspiration on the balloon lumen should be maintained when the balloon is withdrawn into the guiding catheter and out of the guide. After withdrawal of the balloon from the guide catheter, we recommend aspirating and discarding blood from the guide, followed by flushing the guide before any contrast injection.

If the LAD flow is compromised, the differential diagnosis includes dissection, spasm, or LAD alcohol leak. A guidewire should be placed into the LAD, and intracoronary nitroglycerine should be administered. Intravascular ultrasound may be helpful to rule out dissection. Intracoronary agents that help no-reflow like adenosine, nitroprusside, nicardipine, or verapamil may help restore or improve flow. An intra-aortic balloon pump (IABP) can be used to improve coronary perfusion. There is no role for coronary artery bypass graft surgery or PCI in this situation, and the treatment is mostly supportive.

Ventricular Arrhythmia

Ventricular arrhythmia can occur in 5% of patients during and after ASA. Most episodes of ventricular tachycardia are transient and are due to catheter irritation or to the septal infarction itself. However, they can also be secondary to other acute complications of the procedure and can occur after the procedure has been completed.

Mitral Regurgitation

Acute mitral regurgitation can result from inadvertent injection of alcohol into the papillary muscle. It is poorly tolerated, and it can be associated with hemodynamic instability or acute pulmonary edema. Treatment includes intravenous nitroprusside and IABP support as a bridge to surgery.

Ventricular Septal Defect

It has been recommended that, to prevent the occurrence of VSDs, the anterior septal wall thickness should be >1.6 cm if ASA is to be considered and aortic stenosis must be excluded. In the setting of acute VSD, patients can be hemodynamically supported by intravenous nitroprusside and IABP as a bridge to surgery. Successful percutaneous closure with VSD closure devices has also been reported.

Septal Dissection and Hematoma

Septal dissection and hematoma with extravasations of contrast into the septal myocardium have also been described. These complications can occur during guidewire manipulation in the septal branch, and they are usually benign. However, in these cases, abortion of the procedure might be advisable.

Delayed Infarction

Delayed myocardial infarction has also been described. **Figure 30.**7 illustrates a case of collateral flow from the septal branches to the distal LAD artery. This anatomy is an absolute contraindication to ASA.

Late Complications

Complications observed >30 days after ASA are classified as late complications and include ventricular arrhythmias, mitral regurgitation, the late development of VSD, congestive heart failure, and the need for repeat procedures.

Conclusion

Short-term, mid-term, and long-term results have demonstrated the effectiveness of ASA in relieving LVOTO and improving symptoms in patients with HCM. Appropriate patient selection, the steep learning curve, and the unique complications make it best suited for dedicated interventional cardiologists in centers offering comprehensive care for patients with HOCM.

SUGGESTED READINGS

1. Alam M, Dokainish H, Lakkis N. Alcohol septal ablation for hypertrophic obstructive cardiomyopathy: a systematic review of published studies. *J Interv Cardiol*. 2006;19(4):319-327.
2. Aroney CN, Goh TH, Hourigan LA, Dyer W. Ventricular septal rupture following non-surgical septal reduction for hypertrophic cardiomyopathy: treatment with percutaneous closure. *Catheter Cardiovasc Interv*. 2004;61(3):411-414.
3. Authors/Task Force members; Elliott PM, Anastasakis A, et al. 2014 ESC guidelines on diagnosis and management of hypertrophic cardiomyopathy: the Task Force for the Diagnosis and Management of Hypertrophic Cardiomyopathy of the European Society of Cardiology (ESC). *Eur Heart J*. 2014;35(39):2733-2779.
4. Chang SM, Nagueh SF, Spencer WH III, Lakkis NM. Complete heart block: determinants and clinical impact in patients with hypertrophic cardiomyopathy undergoing non-surgical septal reduction therapy. *J Am Coll Cardiol*. 2003;42(2):296-300.
5. Faber L, Welge D, Fassbender D, Schmidt HK, Horstkotte D, Seggewiss H. Percutaneous septal ablation for symptomatic hypertrophic obstructive cardiomyopathy: managing the risk of procedure-related AV conduction disturbances. *Int J Cardiol*. 2007;119(2):163-167.
6. Fernades V, Moscucci M, Spencer WH. Complications of alcohol septal ablation for hypertrophic obstructive cardiomyopathy. In: Moscucci M, ed. *Complications of Cardiovascular Procedures. Risk Factors, Management, and Bailout Techniques*. Wolters Kluwer; 2011.
7. Fernandes VL, Nielsen C, Nagueh SF, et al. Follow-up of alcohol septal ablation for symptomatic hypertrophic obstructive cardiomyopathy the Baylor and Medical University of South Carolina experience 1996 to 2007. *JACC Cardiovasc Interv*. 2008;1(5):561-570.
8. Gietzen F, Leuner C, Gerenkamp T, Kuhn H. Abnahme der Obstruktion bei hypertrophischer Kardiomyopathie wahrend pas-sagerer Okklusion des ersten Septalastes der linken Koronararterie. *Z Kardiol*. 1994;83:146.
9. Goodwin JF, Hollman A, Cleland WP, Teare D. Obstructive cardiomyopathy simulating aortic stenosis. *Br Heart J*. 1960;22(3):403-414.
10. Ingles J, Burns C, Barratt A, Semsarian C. Application of genetic testing in hypertrophic cardiomyopathy for preclinical disease detection. *Circ Cardiovasc Genet*. 2015;8(6):852-859.
11. Lakkis NM, Nagueh SF, Kleiman NS, et al. Echocardiography-guided ethanol septal reduction for hypertrophic obstructive cardiomyopathy. *Circulation*. 1998;98(17):1750-1755.
12. Liebregts M, Vriesendorp PA, Mahmoodi BK, Schinkel AF, Michels M, ten Berg JM. A systematic review and meta-analysis of long-term outcomes after septal reduction therapy in patients with hypertrophic cardiomyopathy. *JACC Heart Fail*. 2015;3(11):896-905.
13. Maron BJ, McKenna WJ, Danielson GK, et al. American College of Cardiology/European Society of Cardiology clinical expert consensus document on hypertrophic cardiomyopathy. A report of the American College of Cardiology Foundation Task Force on clinical expert Consensus Documents and the European Society of Cardiology Committee for practice guidelines. *Eur Heart J*. 2003;24(21):1965-1991.
14. Maron MS, Olivotto I, Betocchi S, et al. Effect of left ventricular outflow tract obstruction on clinical outcome in hypertrophic cardiomyopathy. *N Engl J Med*. 2003;348(4):295-303.

15. Maron MS, Olivotto I, Zenovich AG, et al. Hypertrophic cardiomyopathy is predominantly a disease of left ventricular outflow tract obstruction. *Circulation.* 2006;114(21):2232-2239.

16. Maron BJ, Rastegar H, Udelson JE, Dearani JA, Maron MS. Contemporary surgical management of hypertrophic cardiomyopathy, the need for more myectomy surgeons and disease-specific centers, and the Tufts initiative. *Am J Cardiol.* 2013;112(9):1512-1515.

17. Maron BJ, Dearani JA, Ommen SR, et al. Low operative mortality achieved with surgical septal myectomy: role of dedicated hypertrophic cardiomyopathy centers in the management of dynamic subaortic obstruction. *J Am Coll Cardiol.* 2015;66(11):1307-1308.

18. Mazur W, Nagueh SF, Lakkis NM, et al. Regression of left ventricular hypertrophy after non-surgical septal reduction therapy for hypertrophic obstructive cardiomyopathy. *Circulation.* 2001;103(11):1492-1496.

19. McCully RB, Nishimura RA, Tajik AJ, Schaff HV, Danielson GK. Extent of clinical improvement after surgical treatment of hypertrophic obstructive cardiomyopathy. *Circulation.* 1996;94(3):467-471.

20. Ommen SR, Maron BJ, Olivotto I, et al. Long-term effects of surgical septal myectomy on survival in patients with obstructive hypertrophic cardiomyopathy. *J Am Coll Cardiol.* 2005;46(3):470-476.

21. Ommen SR, Mital S, Burke MA, et al. 2020 AHA/ACC guideline for the diagnosis and treatment of patients with hypertrophic cardiomyopathy: a report of the American College of Cardiology/American Heart Association Joint Committee on clinical practice guidelines. *Circulation.* 2020;142(25):e558-e631.

22. Runquist LH, Nielsen CD, Killip D, Gazes P, Spencer WH III. Electrocardiographic findings after alcohol septal ablation therapy for obstructive hypertrophic cardiomyopathy. *Am J Cardiol.* 2002;90(9):1020-1022.

23. Samardhi H, Walters DL, Raffel C, et al. The long-term outcomes of transcoronary ablation of septal hypertrophy compared to surgical myectomy in patients with symptomatic hypertrophic obstructive cardiomyopathy. *Catheter Cardiovasc Interv.* 2014;83(2):270-277.

24. Sedehi D, Finocchiaro G, Tibayan Y, et al. Long-term outcomes of septal reduction for obstructive hypertrophic cardiomyopathy. *J Cardiol.* 2015;66(1):57-62.

25. Sigwart U. Non-surgical myocardial reduction for hypertrophic obstructive cardiomyopathy. *Lancet.* 1995;346(8969):211-214.

26. Sorajja P, Ommen SR, Holmes DR Jr, et al. Survival after alcohol septal ablation for obstructive hypertrophic cardiomyopathy. *Circulation.* 2012;126(20):2374-2380.

27. ten Cate FJ, Soliman OI, Michels M, et al. Long-term outcome of alcohol septal ablation in patients with obstructive hypertrophic cardiomyopathy: a word of caution. *Circ Heart Fail.* 2010;3(3):362-369.

28. Vriesendorp PA, Liebregts M, Steggerda RC, et al. Long-term outcomes after medical and invasive treatment in patients with hypertrophic cardiomyopathy. *JACC Heart Fail.* 2014;2(6):630-636.

31 Closure of Paravalvular Leaks[1]

The growth of percutaneous valve interventions has been paralleled by a growth in interventions for the management of paravalvular leaks (PVLs). It has been estimated that PVLs can occur in 5% to 17% of patients following surgical valve replacement. In addition, PVLs are a recognized occurrence following transcatheter aortic valve and mitral valve replacement. The clinical spectrum varies from asymptomatic status to heart failure and/or severe hemolysis. Moderate to severe PVLs are associated with an increased risk of mortality, and reoperation in these patients is also associated with high morbidity and mortality. Thus, there has been a large body of work attempting to address this problem with transcatheter techniques (**Figures 31.1 and 31.2**).

While several case reports and case series have been published using a variety of devices, from vascular coils to vascular plugs (**Figure 31.1**), currently, there are no devices that have been approved by the U.S. Food and Drug Administration specifically for the management of PVLs. Among the devices that have been used, the Amplatzer Vascular Plug III is currently undergoing evaluation in a "prospective, international, multi-center, single-arm study to demonstrate its safety and effectiveness for percutaneous, transcatheter closure of PVL occurring after aortic or mitral valve replacement with a surgically-implanted mechanical or bioprosthetic valve" (ClinicalTrials.gov: NCT04489823).

Interventional skills required for the management of PVLs include proficiency in transseptal catheterization, access to the left ventricle through direct apical puncture (**Figure 31.3**), the ability to evaluate 3D echocardiographic and computed tomography reconstructions of the defect (**Figure 31.4**), and familiarity with guidewire snaring and exteriorization techniques (**Figure 31.5**). Most importantly, 3D echo-

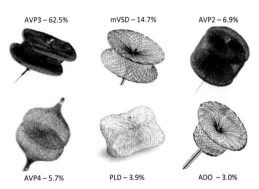

Figure 31.1 Devices frequently used for paravalvular leak closure in a large case series (380 PVL closures), with frequencies. AVP3 (Amplatzer Vascular Plug 3, Abbott Vascular [AV]), ADO (Amplatzer Duct Occluder, AV), mVSD (muscular Ventricular Septal Defect Occluder, AV), PLD (Paravalvular Leak Device, Occlutech). (Reproduced with permission from Calvert PA, Northridge DB, Malik IS, et al. Percutaneous device closure of paravalvular leak: combined experience from the United Kingdom and Ireland. *Circulation*. 2016;134(13):934-944. Fig. 3.)

---

[1]We gratefully acknowledge the *Grossman & Baim's Cardiac Catheterization, Angiography, and Intervention*, 9th edition contributions of Drs. Mauro Moscucci, John D. Carroll, John G. Webb as portions of their chapter, General Overview of Interventions for Structural Heart Disease, were retained in this text.

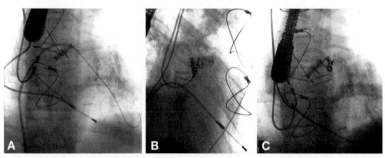

Figure 31.2 Paravalvular leak closure with coils in a patient with severe hemolytic anemia. **A,** Right anterior oblique view of a prosthetic mitral valve. A hydrophilic wire has been advanced into the left ventricle through a paravalvular mitral defect. The transesophageal echocardiogram probe can be seen in the top portion of the figure. **B and C,** Radiographic images after deploying the coils are shown. Both coils have been symmetrically deployed across the mitral valve ring. (Reproduced with permission from Moscucci M, Deeb GM, Bach D, Eagle KA, Williams DM. Coil embolization of a periprosthetic mitral valve leak associated with severe hemolytic anemia. *Circulation.* 2001;104(16):E85-E86.)

cardiography has a critical role in defining the anatomic characteristics of the leak, including location within the valve annulus, size, and orientation with respect to other cardiac structures. Identification of the precise location of the leak has an essential role in procedure planning. For example, mitral valve PVL are generally closed through an antegrade transseptal approach. However, a retrograde approach either via transapical access or through the aortic valve via femoral artery access can also be used and might be preferred when the leak is in the proximity of the interatrial septum. Hydrophilic guidewires and delivery sheaths, as well as steerable transseptal sheaths, are commonly used.

Current recommendations for PVL closure according to the 2020 guidelines for the management of valvular heart disease are listed in **Table 31.1.** As the field evolves, it can be expected that the growing experience will lead to the development of dedicated devices and further expansion of the use of percutaneous approaches.

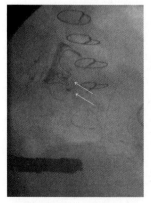

Figure 31.3 Paravalvular leak closure in a bioprosthetic mitral valve. In this case, given the size of the defect, 2 Amplatzer ventricular septal defect occluders were implanted (arrows). As shown by the position of the devices (arrows), the deployment was performed in a retrograde fashion using a transapical approach. (Courtesy of Claudia C. Martinez, MD.)

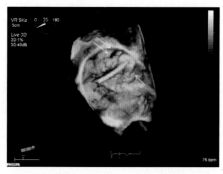

Figure 31.4 Online 3D echocardiographic reconstruction during closure of a paravalvular mitral valve leak. An Amplatzer septal occluder is being deployed (*single arrow*). There is still a residual defect as shown by the *double arrow*. In cases like this, 2 devices can be used to achieve complete closure of the leak.

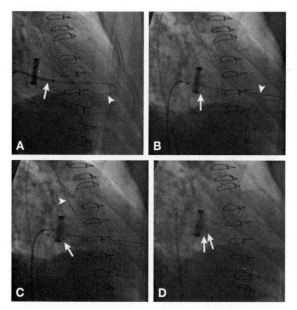

Figure 31.5 Closure of paravalvular leak with the anchor wire technique. Sequential device deployment **(A)**: an extra support guidewire (arrowhead) is passed across the paravalvular defect, through the aortic valve, and is exteriorized through a femoral arterial sheath, creating an arteriovenous rail. An 8F Flexor Shuttle sheath (Cook Medical) is advanced across the paravalvular defect (arrow). **B,** A vascular plug (arrowhead) is deployed in the defect while the arteriovenous wire loop is maintained through the defect (arrow). **C,** A second vascular plug is deployed (arrow) alongside the first device, leaving the arteriovenous loop in position (arrowhead). **D,** Final position with 2 devices released (arrows) and the arteriovenous loop wire removed. (Reproduced with permission from Rihal CS, Sorajja P, Booker JD, Hagler DJ, Cabalka AK. Principles of percutaneous paravalvular leak closure. *JACC CardiovascInterv*. 2012;5(2):121-130.)

Table 31.1 Recommendations for Intervention for Transvalvular or Paravalvular leak

COR	LOE	Recommendations
1	B-NR	1. In patients with intractable hemolysis or HF attributable to prosthetic transvalvular or paravalvular leak, surgery is recommended unless surgical risk is high or prohibitive.
2a	B-NR	2. In asymptomatic patients with severe prosthetic regurgitation and low operative risk, surgery is reasonable.
2a	B-NR	3. In patients with prosthetic paravalvular regurgitation with the following: (1) either intractable hemolysis or NYHA class III or IV symptoms and (2) who are at high or prohibitive surgical risk and (3) have anatomic features suitable for catheter-based therapy, percutaneous repair of paravalvular leak is reasonable when performed at a Comprehensive Valve Center.
2a	B-NR	4. For patients with severe HF symptoms caused by bioprosthetic valve regurgitation who are at high to prohibitive surgical risk, a transcatheter ViV procedure is reasonable when performed at a Comprehensive Valve Center.

COR, class of recommendation; HF, heart failure; LOE, level of evidence; NR, nonrandomized; NYHA, New York Heart Association.
Reprinted with permission from Otto CM, Nishimura RA, Bonow RO, et al. 2020 ACC/AHA guideline for the management of patients with valvular heart disease: executive summary: a report of the American College of Cardiology/American Heart Association Joint Committee on Clinical Practice Guidelines. *Circulation*. 2021;143:e72-e227. ©2020 American Heart Association, Inc.

SUGGESTED READINGS

1. Binder RK, Webb JG. Percutaneous mitral and aortic paravalvular leak repair: indications, current application, and future directions. *Curr Cardiol Rep*. 2013;15(3):342.
2. Calvert PA, Northridge DB, Malik IS, et al. Percutaneous device closure of paravalvular leak: combined experience from the United Kingdom and Ireland. *Circulation*. 2016;134(13):934-944.
3. Cruz-Gonzalez I, Rama-Merchan JC, Calvert PA, et al. Percutaneous closure of paravalvular leaks: a systematic review. *J Interv Cardiol*. 2016;29(4):382-392.
4. Genereux P, Head SJ, Hahn R, et al. Paravalvular leak after transcatheter aortic valve replacement: the new Achilles' heel? A comprehensive review of the literature. *J Am Coll Cardiol*. 2013;61(11):1125-1136.
5. Giblett JP, Williams LK, Moorjani N, Calvert PA. Percutaneous management of paravalvular leaks. *Heart*. 2022;108(13):1005-1011.
6. Janmohamed IK, Mishra V, Geragotellis A, Sherif M, Harky A. Mitral valve paravalvular leaks: comprehensive review of literature. *J Card Surg*. 2022;37(2):418-430.
7. Martinez CA, Cohen H, Ruiz CE. Simultaneous aortic and mitral metallic paravalvular leaks repaired through one delivery sheath. *J Invasive Cardiol*. 2011;23(2):E19-E21.
8. Moscucci M, Deeb GM, Bach D, Eagle KA, Williams DM. Coil embolization of a periprosthetic mitral valve leak associated with severe hemolytic anemia. *Circulation*. 2001;104(16):E85-E86.
9. Pate G, Webb J, Thompson C, et al. Percutaneous closure of a complex prosthetic mitral paravalvular leak using transesophageal echocardiographic guidance. *Can J Cardiol*. 2004;20(4):452-455.
10. Pate GE, Al Zubaidi A, Chandavimol M, Thompson CR, Munt BI, Webb JG. Percutaneous closure of prosthetic paravalvular leaks: case series and review. *Catheter Cardiovasc Interv*. 2006;68(4):528-533.
11. Pate GE, Thompson CR, Munt BI, Webb JG. Techniques for percutaneous closure of prosthetic paravalvular leaks. *Catheter Cardiovasc Interv*. 2006;67(1):158-166.
12. Rihal CS, Sorajja P, Booker JD, Hagler DJ, Cabalka AK. Principles of percutaneous paravalvular leak closure. *JACC Cardiovasc Interv*. 2012;5(2):121-130.
13. Ruiz CE, Jelnin V, Kronzon I, et al. Clinical outcomes in patients undergoing percutaneous closure of periprosthetic paravalvular leaks. *J Am Coll Cardiol*. 2011;58(21):2210-2217.
14. Webb JG, Pate GE, Munt BI. Percutaneous closure of an aortic prosthetic paravalvular leak with an Amplatzer duct occluder. *Catheter Cardiovasc Interv*. 2005;65(1):69-72.

32 Left Atrial Appendage Closure[1]

Atrial fibrillation (AF) is the most common arrhythmia, with an estimated global prevalence of 1368/100,000 males and 856/100,000 females >35 years of age in 2010. In the United States alone, it has been estimated that 2.7 to 6.1 million people have AF and that by the year 2050, the number of people affected by AF will double. Several studies have evaluated the morbidity and mortality associated with AF. In the Framingham study, AF was associated with a 5-fold increased risk of stroke and the mortality rate of AF-related stroke was twice as high as that of stroke unrelated to AF. The observation that >80% of AF-related strokes are thromboembolic and that approximately 90% of thrombi are believed to originate in the left atrial appendage (LAA) has led to the emergence of left atrial appendage closure (LAAC) as a new modality to reduce the risk of thromboembolic stroke in patients with AF.

WATCHMAN Device

The WATCHMAN device (Boston Scientific, Natick, Massachusetts) comprises a 10-struts nitinol frame with 10 active fixation anchors in 1 row designed to engage the LAA tissue for stability and a 160-PM membrane polyethylene terephthalate cap designed to block emboli and to promote endothelialization (**Figure 32.1**).

The device is available in 21, 24, 27, 30, and 33 mm sizes, and it is delivered with a 12F delivery system advanced through a 75-cm-long, 14F access system. The access system is currently available as a single curve, double curve, and anterior curve, which should be selected depending on the anatomic characteristics of the LAA.

The WATCHMAN-Flex is the newest-generation WATCHMAN device. It comprises a nitinol frame with 12 anchors in 2 rows. It differs from the original WATCHMAN device by having an atraumatic closed distal end with a fluoroscopy marker, a flat and recessed screw hub, 12 anchors in 2 rows and 18 struts in the frame. In addition, it allows redeployment after full or partial recapture.

LAAC with the WATCHMAN Left Atrial Appendage System was evaluated in 2 randomized clinical trials (RCTs), the PROTECT-AF trial (Embolic Protection in Patients with Atrial Fibrillation) and the PREVAIL trial (Prospective Randomized Evaluation of the WATCHMAN LAA Closure Device in Patients With Atrial Fibrillation Versus Long-Term Warfarin Therapy), and in 2 single-arm continuous access registries, CAP1 (Continued Access to PROTECT-AF) and CAP2 (Continued Access to PREVAIL). In the PROTECT-AF trial, the primary safety endpoint included major bleeding, pericardial effusion, and device embolization. At a mean follow-up of 18 months (1065 patient-years), the primary efficacy rate was 3.0 per 100 patient-years in the intervention group and 4.9 per 100 patient-years in the control group (device/warfarin rate ratio [RR] 0.62%, 95% credible interval [CrI] 0.35-1.25) (**Figure 32.2**). The probability of noninferiority of the intervention was more than 99% to 9%. The primary safety event rate was 7.4 per 100 patient-years in the intervention group (95% CrI 5.5-9.7) and 4.4 per 100 patient-years in the control group (RR 1.69%, 96% CrI 1.01-3.1). The higher event rate in the device group was due to procedural complications. The most frequent safety adverse event in the device group was serious pericardial effusion requiring percutaneous or surgical drainage, which occurred in 22 (4.8%) of patients. The rate of pericardial effusion declined with increasing operator experience. The clinical trial design included additional follow-up through 5 years. At a

[1]We gratefully acknowledge the *Grossman & Baim's Cardiac Catheterization, Angiography, and Intervention*, 9th edition contributions of Drs. Mauro Moscucci and Stanley Chetcuti, as portions of their chapter, Nonvalvular Interventions: Left Atrial Appendage Closure and Alcohol Septal Ablation, were retained in this text.

627

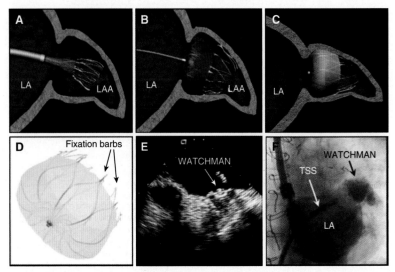

Figure 32.1 The top 3 panels illustrate a cartoon showing delivery **(Panel A)**, deployment **(Panel B)**, and release **(Panel C)** of a WATCHMAN left atrial appendage (LAA) device, through a transseptal delivery system (Altritech Inc., Plymouth, Minnesota). **Panel D,** shows a close-up view of the WATCHMAN device consisting of a self-expanding nitinol frame structure with fixation barbs designed to engage the LAA wall. **Panel E,** shows a transesophageal echocardiography image of an occluded LAA following deployment of a WATCHMAN LAA device (white arrow). **Panel F,** shows a cine image of a left atrial (LA) angiogram demonstrating a WATCHMAN device properly deployed inside the LAA (black arrow). TSS, transseptal sheath. (Reproduced with permission from Aryana A, Saad EB, d'Avila A. Left atrial appendage occlusion and ligation devices: what is available, how to implement them, and how to manage and avoid complications. *Curr Treat Options Cardiovasc Med.* 2012;14:503-519.)

mean follow-up of 3.8 years (2621 patient-years), the primary endpoint event rate was 8.4% in the device group compared with an event rate of 13.9% in the control group (2.3 events per 100 patients years in the device group and 3.8 events per 100 patient-years in the control group, RR, 0.60%; 95% CrI, 0.41-1.05), meeting prespecified criteria for both noninferiority (posterior probability, >99.9%) and superiority(posterior probability, 96.0%). Patients in the device group had lower rates of cardiovascular mortality (3.7% vs 9.0%; hazard ratio [HR], 0.40; 95% confidence interval [CI], 0.21-0.75; P = .005) and all-cause mortality (12.3% vs 18.0%; HR, 0.66; 95% CI, 0.45-0.98; P = .04). In the PREVAIL trial, patients with non valvular atrial fibrillation (NVAF) who had a $CHADS_2$ score >2 or 1 and another risk factor were randomized in a 2:1 ratio to undergo LAA occlusion and subsequent discontinuation of warfarin (intervention group, n = 269) or receive chronic warfarin therapy (control group, n = 138). Two efficacy coprimary endpoints and 1 primary safety endpoint were assessed. The first efficacy coprimary endpoint was a composite of stroke, systemic embolism, and cardiovascular/unexplained death, while the second coprimary endpoint was stroke or systemic embolism >7 days from the index procedure. The primary safety endpoint was a composite of all-cause death, ischemic stroke, systemic embolism (SE), or device-/procedure-related events requiring open cardiovascular surgery or major endovascular intervention between randomization and within 7 days of the procedure or during the index hospitalization. At 18 months, the rate of the coprimary efficacy endpoint was surprisingly low at 0.064 in the device group and 0.063 in the control group (RR 1.07, 95% CrI 0.57-1.89) and did not reach the prespecified noninferiority criteria (upper boundary for noninferiority 95% CrI > 1.75). The rate for the

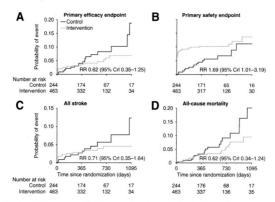

Figure 32.2 Kaplan-Meier curves of incidence of study endpoints in intervention and control groups, RR = rate ratio. Incidence probabilities for the intention-to-treat analysis are shown with time calculated as the days since randomization for the primary efficacy endpoint **(A)**, the primary safety endpoint **(B)**, all stroke **(C)**, and all-cause mortality **(D)**. (Reproduced with permission from Holmes DR, Reddy VY, Turi ZG, et al. Percutaneous closure of the left atrial appendage vs warfarin therapy for prevention of stroke in patients with atrial fibrillation: a randomised noninferiority trial. *Lancet*. 2009;374(9689):534-542.)

second coprimary efficacy endpoint (stroke or SE > 7 days from the index procedure) was 0.0253 in the device group versus 0.0200 in the control group, and it achieved noninferiority. Early safety events were significantly lower than in the PROTECT-AF trial (2.2% rate in the WATCHMAN group) and met a prespecified safety performance goal. The 5-year results from the 2 RCTs and their respective continued access studies were further evaluated in 2 separate patient-level meta-analysis. The first meta-analysis included data from the 2 randomized clinical trials, and the second meta-analysis included data from the 2 randomized clinical trials and the 2 continuous access registries. Both meta-analyses have shown that LAAC with the WATCHMAN device is comparable with warfarin in preventing stroke in patients with NVAF, with a reduction in major bleeding, hemorrhagic stroke, and mortality. Based on the results of the 2 randomized clinical trials and the 2 continuous access registries, the WATCHMAN device in 2015 received US Food and Drug Administration (FDA) approval as the first-of-a-kind device intended for transcatheter nonsurgical closure of the LAA.

Patient Selection

In the United States, the WATCHMAN device currently "is indicated to reduce the risk of thromboembolism from the left atrial appendage (LAA) in patients with nonvalvular atrial fibrillation who: are at increased risk for stroke and systemic embolism based on $CHADS_2$ or CHA_2DS_2-VASc scores and are recommended for anticoagulation therapy; are deemed by their physicians to be suitable for warfarin; and have an appropriate rationale to seek a nonpharmacologic alternative to warfarin, taking into account the safety and effectiveness of the device compared to warfarin."[2] As for other recently approved devices for the management of structural heart disease, the Center for Medicare and Medicaid Services (CMS) National Coverage Determination (NCD) follows the FDA indication (**Table 32.1**). Most importantly, a "formal shared decision-making interaction with an independent noninterventional physician using an evidence-based decision tool on oral anticoagulation in patients with NVAF prior to LAAC," is included in the CMS NCD.

---

[2]Accessed April 29, 2022. https://www.accessdata.fda.gov/scripts/cdrh/cfdocs/cfpma/pma.cfm?id=P130013

Table 32.1 Center for Medicare and Medicaid Services National Coverage Determination for LAAC

LAAC devices are covered when the device has received Food and Drug Administration (FDA) Premarket Approval (PMA) for that device's FDA-approved indication and meets all the conditions specified below

The patient must have:	• A CHADS$_2$ score ≥2 or CHA$_2$DS$_2$-VASc score ≥3. • A formal shared decision-making interaction with an independent noninterventional physician using an evidence-based decision tool on oral anticoagulation in patients with NVAF prior to left atrial appendage closure (LAAC). In addition, the shared decision-making interaction must be documented in the medical record. • A suitability for short-term warfarin but deemed unable to take long-term oral anticoagulation following the conclusion of shared decision-making, as LAAC is only covered as a second-line therapy to oral anticoagulants. • The patient (preoperatively and postoperatively) is under the care of a cohesive, multidisciplinary team (MDT) of medical professionals. The procedure must be furnished in a hospital with an established structural heart disease and/or electrophysiology program.
The procedure must be performed by an interventional cardiologist(s), electrophysiologist(s), or cardiovascular surgeon(s) who meet the following criteria:	• Has received training prescribed by the manufacturer on the safe and effective use of the device prior to performing LAAC; • Has performed ≥25 interventional cardiac procedures that involve transseptal puncture through an intact septum; • Continues to perform ≥25 interventional cardiac procedures that involve transseptal puncture through an intact septum, of which at least 12 are LAAC, over a 2-year period.

The patient is enrolled in, and the MDT and hospital must participate in, a prospective, national, audited registry that:

1. Consecutively enrolls patients with LAAC	
2. Tracks the following annual outcomes for each patient for a period of at least 4 y from the time of the LAAC:	• Operator-specific complications • Device-specific complications including device thrombosis • Stroke, adjudicated, by type • Transient ischemic attack • Systemic embolism • Death • Major bleeding, by site and severity

The registry must be designed to permit identification and analysis of patient-, practitioner-, and facility-level factors that predict patient risk for these outcomes. The registry must collect all data necessary to conduct analyses adjusted for relevant confounders and have a written executable analysis plan in place to address the following questions:

• How do the outcomes listed above compare with outcomes in the pivotal clinical trials in the short term (≤12 mo) and in the long term (≥4 y)?
• What is the long-term (≥4 y) durability of the device?
• What are the short-term (≤12 mo) and the long-term (≥4 y) device-specific complications including device thromboses?

Adapted from Centers for Medicare and Medicaid Services. Accessed April 29, 2022. https://www.cms.gov/medicare-coverage-database/details/ncd-details.aspx?NCDId=367

Preprocedural and procedural assessment, as well as postprocedural management, are summarized in **Tables 32.2 to 32.5**. Preprocedural assessment must include a thorough evaluation through transesophageal echocardiography of the suitability of the LAA for device implantation (**Figures 32.3 and 32.4; Tables 32.2 and 32.3**). As previously mentioned, device embolization at the time of implant or post implant is a possibility, and its occurrence can be minimized by the prerelease checklist illustrated in **Table 32.4**.

Complications of LAAC with the WATCHMAN device include pericardial effusion/tamponade secondary to cardiac perforation during the transseptal puncture or advancement of the delivery system in the LAA, ischemic stroke due to air embolism or related to the procedure, device embolization, suboptimal deployment (**Figure 32.5**), and vascular complications. Both the PROTECT-AF and the PREVAIL trials have shown the importance of the learning curve in the occurrence of these complications. In a post hoc analysis Device Release Criteria: PASS of the PROTECT-AF and PREVAIL trials and their respective continuous access registry, device-related

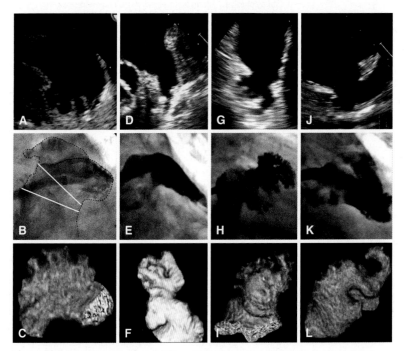

Figure 32.3 Left atrial appendage (LAA): morphologies and modalities. The 4 different LAA morphologies as shown by transesophageal echocardiography (top), cine angiography (middle), and 3D computed tomography (bottom). Cauliflower **(A-C)**, windsock **(D-F)**, cactus **(G-I)**, and chicken wing **(J-L)**. (Reproduced with permission from Beigel R, Wunderlich NC, Ho SY, Arsanjani R, Siegel RJ. The left atrial appendage: anatomy, function, and noninvasive evaluation. *JACC Cardiovasc Imaging*. 2014;7(12):1251-1265.)

---

[3]For a further and detailed review of each procedure step, our readers are referred to the excellent Instruction for Use document available at https://www.accessdata.fda.gov/cdrh_docs/pdf13/P130013D.pdf

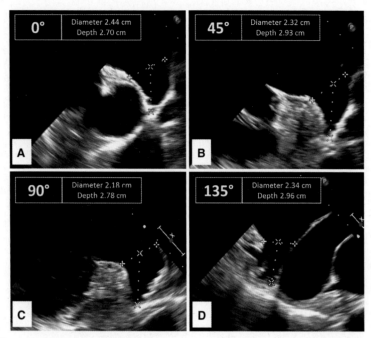

Figure 32.4 Left atrial appendage (LAA) sizing for WATCHMAN device on 2D transesophageal echocardiography (TEE). Two-dimensional TEE demonstrates sizing for the WATCHMAN device. The LAA orifice diameter and depth are measured at 0° **(A)**, 45° **(B)**, 90° **(C)**, and 135° **(D)**. (Reproduced with permission from Vainrib AF, Harb SC, Jaber W, et al. Left atrial appendage occlusion/exclusion: procedural image guidance with transesophageal echocardiography. *J Am Soc Echocardiogr.* 2018;31(4):454-474.)

Table 32.2	**Baseline Transesophageal Echocardiographic Assessment of LAA Anatomy for Suitability of WATCHMAN Device Implant**

1. **Assess the following parameters through multiple imaging planes (0°, 45°, 90°, and 135° sweep)**:
   - Left atrial appendage (LAA) size/shape, number of lobes in LAA, and location of lobes relative to the ostium.
   - Confirm the absence of thrombus (use color Doppler and echo contrast as necessary).
2. **Record LAA ostium and LAA length measurements (0°, 45°, 90°, and 135° sweep). Measure the LAA ostium at approximately these angles**:
   - at 0° measure from coronary artery marker to a point 2 cm from tip of the "limbus"
   - at 45° measure from top of the mitral valve annulus to point 2 cm from tip of the limbus
   - at 90° measure from top of the mitral valve annulus to a point 2 cm from tip of the limbus
   - at 135° measure from top of the mitral valve annulus to a point 2 cm from tip of the limbus

Measured maximum LAA ostium width must be ≥17 mm or ≤31 mm to accommodate available device size.

Data from WATCHMAN Left Atrial Appendage Closure Device with Delivery System, https://www.access-data.fda.gov/cdrh_docs/pdf13/P130013D.pdf.

Table 32.3 WATCHMAN Device Selection

Max LAA Ostium (mm)	Device Size (mm)
17-19	21
20-22	24
23-25	27
26-28	30
29-31	33

Data from WATCHMAN Left Atrial Appendage Closure Device with Delivery System, https://www.access-data.fda.gov/cdrh_docs/pdf13/P130013D.pdf.

thrombus (DRT) associated with an increased risk of stroke has also been described in 3.7% of cases. However, further analysis of the outcomes of patients with DRT in the context of the expected rate of stroke without treatment still showed a predicted 28% relative reduction in the rate of ischemic stroke.

AMPLATZER AMULET DEVICE

The AMPLATZER AMULET LAAC device (Abbott Vascular, Santa Clara, California) can be considered an evolution of the Amplatzer cardiac plug device. The Amulet device is constructed from a nitinol mesh and a polyester patch, and it comprises

Table 32.4 Device Release Criteria: PASS (All the Criteria Must Be Met Prior to Device Release)

A. **P**osition: Plane of maximum diameter is at or just distal to and spans the entire left atrial appendage (LAA) ostium.
B. **A**nchor: Fixation anchors engaged/device is stable. Gently pull back, then release deployment knob to visualize movement of device and LAA together.
C. **S**ize (compression): Measure plane of maximum diameter of the device. The device is compressed 8%-20% of original size according to the following table as a guide.

Original Diameter (mm)	Deployed Diameter (80%-92% of original, or 8%-20% compression)
21	16.8-19.3
24	19.2-22.1
27	21.6-24.8
30	24.0-27.6
33	26.4-30.4

D. **S**eal: Device spans ostium. Ensure all lobes are distal to device and sealed, ie, ≤5 mm jet.

Data from WATCHMAN Left Atrial Appendage Closure Device with Delivery System, https://www.access-data.fda.gov/cdrh_docs/pdf13/P130013D.pdf.

Table 32.5 Antithrombotic Regimen

A. Aspirin should be started 1 d prior to the procedure.

B. Patients should be fully heparinized during the procedure with recommended activated clotting time of 200-300 s recorded after transseptal puncture.

C. Postprocedural warfarin therapy is required in ALL patients receiving a WATCHMAN device.

D. Patients should remain on 81-100 mg of aspirin, and warfarin should be taken post implant (INR 2.0-3.0)

E. At 45 d (±15 d) post implant, perform WATCHMAN device assessment with TEE.

F. Cessation of warfarin is at physician discretion provided that any peridevice flow demonstrated by TEE is ≤ 5 mm.

G. If adequate seal is not demonstrated, subsequent warfarin cessation decisions are contingent on demonstrating flow ≤5 mm.

H. At the time the patient ceases warfarin, the patient should begin clopidogrel 75 mg daily and increase aspirin dosage to 300-325 mg daily. This regimen should continue until 6 mo have elapsed after implantation. Patients should then remain on aspirin 300-325 mg indefinitely.

I. If a patient remains on warfarin and aspirin 81-100 mg for at least 6 mo after implantation, and then ceases warfarin, the patient should not require clopidogrel but should increase aspirin dosage to 300-325 mg daily, which should be taken indefinitely.

Data from WATCHMAN Left Atrial Appendage Closure Device with Delivery System, https://www.accessdata.fda.gov/cdrh_docs/pdf13/P130013D.pdf.
INR, international normalized ratio; TEE, transesophageal echocardiography.

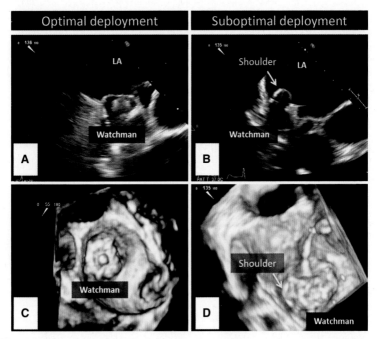

Figure 32.5 Suboptimal WATCHMAN device deployment. Two-dimensional transesophageal echocardiography (TEE) at 135° view and 3D TEE demonstrating optimal and suboptimal WATCHMAN device deployment. The device should optimally be deployed parallel to the left atrial appendage orifice **(A and B)**. If the device is excessively tilted, a device "shoulder" will be visualized **(C and D)**. To ensure an adequate seal, the extent of the shoulder cannot be >40% to 50% of the device height. (Reproduced with permission from Vainrib AF, Harb SC, Jaber W, et al. Left atrial appendage occlusion/exclusion: procedural image guidance with transesophageal echocardiography. *J Am Soc Echocardiogr.* 2018;31(4):454-474.)

a lobe and a disc connected by a flexible waist (**Figure 32.6**). The function of the lobe is to anchor the device within the neck of the LAA, while the disc seals the LAA orifice. The Amulet device is available in 8 different sizes that can be divided into 2 groups: devices 16 to 22 mm that have a shorter (7.5 mm) lobe length and a disc diameter 6 mm larger than the base device diameter, and devices 25 to 34 mm that have a longer (10 mm) lobe length and disc diameter 7 mm larger than the lobe diameter. It received CE Mark in 2008 and FDA approval in 2021. The device underwent evaluation in the AMPLATZER AMULET LAA Occluder IDE Trial. The trial was a prospective, randomized, multicenter worldwide trial, designed to evaluate the safety and effectiveness of the AMPLATZER Amulet Left Atrial Appendage Occluder when compared with the WATCHMAN LAAC device (control) (ClinicalTrials.gov Identifier: NCT02879448). The primary safety endpoint was a composite of procedure-related complications, all-cause death, or major bleeding at 12 months, and the primary effectiveness endpoint was a composite of ischemic stroke or systemic embolism at 18 months and the rate of LAA occlusion at 45 days. The trial enrolled a total of 1878 patients. The AMULET device was found to be noninferior to the WATCHMAN device both for the primary safety endpoint (14.5% vs 14.7%; difference = −0.14 [95% CI, −3.42 to 3.13]; $P < .001$ for noninferiority) and for the primary effectiveness endpoint (2.8% vs 2.8%; difference = 0.00 [95% CI, −1.55 to 1.55]; $P < .001$ for noninferiority).

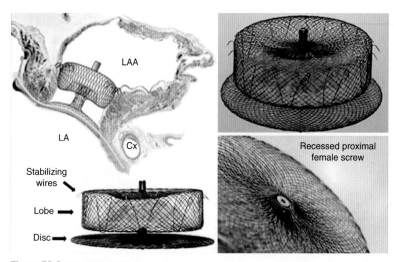

Figure 32.6 The AMPLATZER Amulet device: main components and mechanism of action. The main components of the AMPLATZER Amulet device are the lobe and the disc. The lobe is implanted into the LAA neck, 12 to 15 mm from the LAA ostium, and its role is to anchor the device and close the LAA neck. It is self-expanding, so in order to sit tight, it needs to be slightly compressed. In addition, the lobe has 6 to 10 pairs of stabilizing wires around its distal perimeter. The disc covers the LAA ostium at the atrial side. Proper apposition of the disc and creation of continuity (yellow line) with the atrial walls allow faster endocardialization and complete LAA closure at a second, more proximal level. Cx, left circumflex coronary artery; LA, left atrium; LAA, left atrial appendage. (Reproduced with permission from Tzikas A, Gafoor S, Meerkin D, et al. Left atrial appendage occlusion with the AMPLATZER Amulet device: an expert consensus step-by-step approach. *EuroIntervention.* 2016;11(13):1512-1521.)

LARIAT DEVICE

The LARIAT device (SentreHEART, Redwood City, California) provides a percutaneous "ligation" approach to LAAC. The device consists of a 15-mm compliant balloon catheter, a 0.025-in endocardial magnet-tipped guidewire, a 0.035-in magnet-tipped epicardial guidewire, and a 12F snare/suture delivery device (**Figure 32.7**). The procedure requires a combined transseptal and epicardial approach. Following transseptal access and epicardial access (as described in Chapters 6 and 40), the 0.025 endocardial magnet-tipped guidewire is backloaded in the 15-mm balloon and advanced through the transseptal sheath to the apex of the LAA. The origin of the LAA is identified by inflation of the compliant balloon. Through the epicardial access, the 0.035-in opposite-polarity magnet-tipped guidewire is advanced in the epicardial space and connected end to end with the endocardial magnet-tipped guidewire advanced to the apex of the LAA. The 2 attached guidewires function as an over-the-wire system over which the LARIAT snare is advanced to the base of the LAA. After confirmation of the position of the balloon at the os of the LAA, the suture is released from the snare, tightened to exclude the LAA, and then cut (**Figure 32.8**). Single-arm, nonrandomized trials have shown the feasibility of LAAC with the LARIAT device. In the United States, the LARIAT has FDA approval for the following intended use: "The LARIAT Loop Applicator facilitates suture placement and knot tying for use in surgical applications where soft tissue are being approximated and/or ligated with a pre-tied polyester suture soft tissue closure."[4]

It does not have specific approval for LAAC and the prevention of thromboembolism in patients with AF, and its use for LAAC is (at the time of this writing, April 29, 2022) undergoing evaluation in the aMAZE Study: LAA Ligation Adjunctive to PVI for Persistent or Longstanding Persistent Atrial Fibrillation (aMAZE). The study is a prospective, multicenter, randomized (2:1) controlled study to evaluate the safety and effectiveness of the LARIAT system to isolate and ligate the LAA as an adjunct to pulmonary vein isolation catheter ablation in subjects with symptomatic persistent or longstanding persistent AF (ClinicalTrials.gov Identifier: NCT02513797).

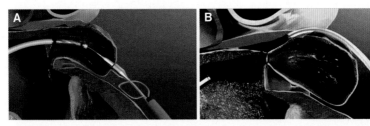

Figure 32.7 A, Lariat guidewires (SentreHEART, Redwood City, California) coupled to control left atrial appendage. **B,** Left atrial appendage closed by suture using Lariat. (Reproduced with permission from Khawar W, Smith N, Masroor S. Managing the left atrial appendage in atrial fibrillation: current state of the art. *Ann Thorac Surg.* 2017;104(6):2111-2119.)

---

[4]https://www.accessdata.fda.gov/cdrh_docs/pdf6/k060721.pdf

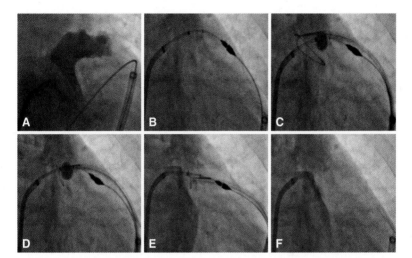

Figure 32.8 Fluoroscopic guidance to assist in the closure of the left atrial appendage (LAA). All images are in the right anterior oblique projection. Left atrial (LA) angiography identifies the ostium and body of the LAA **(A)**. Attachment of the magnet-tipped endocardial and epicardial guidewires **(B)** allows for the LARIAT suture delivery device to be guided over the LAA by the magnet-tipped epicardial guidewire using an over-the-wire approach **(C)**. After verification of the correct position of the snare with the balloon catheter **(D)**, an LA angiogram is performed prior to the release of the pretied suture to exclude the existence of a remnant trabeculated LAA lobe **(E)**. A final LA angiogram is performed to verify LAA exclusion **(F)**. (Reproduced with permission from Bartus K, Han FT, Bednarek J, et al. Percutaneous left atrial appendage suture ligation using the LARIAT device in patients with atrial fibrillation: initial clinical experience. *J Am Coll Cardiol.* 2013;62(2):108-118.)

SUGGESTED READINGS

1. https://www.cdc.gov/dhdsp/data_statistics/fact_sheets/fs_atrial_fibrillation.htm
2. Bartus K, Han FT, Bednarek J, et al. Percutaneous left atrial appendage suture ligation using the LARIAT device in patients with atrial fibrillation: initial clinical experience. *J Am Coll Cardiol.* 2013;62(2):108-118.
3. Bartus K, Gafoor S, Tschopp D, et al. Left atrial appendage ligation with the next generation LARIAT(+) suture delivery device: early clinical experience. *Int J Cardiol.* 2016;215:244-247.
4. Beigel R, Wunderlich NC, Ho SY, Arsanjani R, Siegel RJ. The left atrial appendage: anatomy, function, and noninvasive evaluation. *JACC Cardiovasc Imaging.* 2014;7(12):1251-1265.
5. Benjamin EJ, Wolf PA, D'Agostino RB, Silbershatz H, Kannel WB, Levy D. Impact of atrial fibrillation on the risk of death: the Framingham Heart study. *Circulation.* 1998;98(10):946-952.
6. Blackshear JL, Odell JA. Appendage obliteration to reduce stroke in cardiac surgical patients with atrial fibrillation. *Ann Thorac Surg.* 1996;61(2):755-759.
7. Block PC, Burstein S, Casale PN, et al. Percutaneous left atrial appendage occlusion for patients in atrial fibrillation suboptimal for warfarin therapy: 5-year results of the PLAATO (Percutaneous Left Atrial Appendage Transcatheter Occlusion) Study. *JACC Cardiovasc Interv.* 2009;2(7):594-600.
8. Chugh SS, Havmoeller R, Narayanan K, et al. Worldwide epidemiology of atrial fibrillation: a global burden of disease 2010 study. *Circulation.* 2014;129(8):837-847.
9. De Backer O, Arnous S, Ihlemann N, et al. Percutaneous left atrial appendage occlusion for stroke prevention in atrial fibrillation: an update. *Open Heart.* 2014;1(1):e000020.
10. Dukkipati SR, Kar S, Holmes DR, et al. Device-related thrombus after left atrial appendage closure: incidence, predictors, and outcomes. *Circulation.* 2018;138(9):874-885.

11. El-Chami MF, Grow P, Eilen D, Lerakis S, Block PC. Clinical outcomes three years after PLAATO implantation. *Catheter Cardiovasc Interv.* 2007;69(5):704-707.
12. Holmes DR, Reddy VY, Turi ZG, et al. Percutaneous closure of the left atrial appendage versus warfarin therapy for prevention of stroke in patients with atrial fibrillation: a randomised noninferiority trial. *Lancet.* 2009;374(9689):534-542.
13. Holmes DR Jr, Alkhouli M. The history of the left atrial appendage occlusion. *Card Electrophysiol Clin.* 2020;12(1):1-11.
14. Holmes DR Jr, Kar S, Price MJ, et al. Prospective randomized evaluation of the Watchman Left Atrial Appendage Closure device in patients with atrial fibrillation versus long-term warfarin therapy: the PREVAIL trial. *J Am Coll Cardiol.* 2014;64(1):1-12.
15. Holmes DR Jr, Doshi SK, Kar S, et al. Left atrial appendage closure as an alternative to warfarin for stroke prevention in atrial fibrillation: a patient-level meta-analysis. *J Am Coll Cardiol.* 2015;65(24):2614-2623.
16. Lakkireddy D, Thaler D, Ellis CR, et al. Amplatzer Amulet left atrial appendage occluder versus Watchman device for stroke prophylaxis (Amulet IDE): a randomized, controlled trial. *Circulation.* 2021;144(19):1543-1552.
17. Nakai T, Lesh MD, Gerstenfeld EP, Virmani R, Jones R, Lee RJ. Percutaneous left atrial appendage occlusion (PLAATO) for preventing cardioembolism: first experience in canine model. *Circulation.* 2002;105(18):2217-2222.
18. Omran H, Tzikas A, Sievert H, Stock F. A history of percutaneous left atrial appendage occlusion with the PLAATO device. *Interv Cardiol Clin.* 2018;7(2):137-142.
19. Ostermayer SH, Reisman M, Kramer PH, et al. Percutaneous left atrial appendage transcatheter occlusion (PLAATO system) to prevent stroke in high-risk patients with non-rheumatic atrial fibrillation: results from the international multicenter feasibility trials. *J Am Coll Cardiol.* 2005;46(1):9-14.
20. Parashar A, Tuzcu EM, Kapadia SR. Cardiac plug I and Amulet devices: left atrial appendage closure for stroke prophylaxis in atrial fibrillation. *J Atr Fibrillation.* 2015;7(6):1236.
21. Reddy VY, Sievert H, Halperin J, et al. Percutaneous left atrial appendage closure vs warfarin for atrial fibrillation: a randomized clinical trial. *J Am Med Assoc.* 2014;312(19):1988-1998.
22. Reddy VY, Doshi SK, Kar S, et al. Percutaneous left atrial appendage closure: from the PREVAIL and PROTECT AF trials. *J Am Coll Cardiol.* 2017;70(24):2964-2975.
23. Sievert H, Lesh MD, Trepels T, et al. Percutaneous left atrial appendage transcatheter occlusion to prevent stroke in high-risk patients with atrial fibrillation: early clinical experience. *Circulation.* 2002;105(16):1887-1889.
24. Tzikas A, Gafoor S, Meerkin D, et al. Left atrial appendage occlusion with the AMPLATZER Amulet device: an expert consensus step-by- step approach. *EuroIntervention.* 2016;11(13):1512-1521.
25. Vainrib AF, Harb SC, Jaber W, et al. Left atrial appendage occlusion/exclusion: procedural image guidance with transesophageal echocardiography. *J Am Soc Echocardiogr.* 2018;31(4):454-474.

33 Percutaneous Therapies for Mitral and Tricuspid Valve Disease[1]

Building upon long-standing experience derived from mitral valvuloplasty and transcatheter aortic valve intervention, technologies aimed at leaflet repair, annular reduction, and even complete valve replacement are now under development or in clinical use for the treatment of mitral and tricuspid valve (TV) disease.

PERCUTANEOUS BALLOON MITRAL VALVULOPLASTY

Percutaneous mitral valvuloplasty (PMV) is an important therapeutic tool in treating rheumatic mitral stenosis. Although the prevalence of rheumatic heart disease has declined significantly in the United States, this procedure remains an important therapeutic option for the symptomatic patient with mitral stenosis. In the developing countries where rheumatic heart disease remains prevalent, percutaneous mitral valvuloplasty is the treatment of choice. Percutaneous mitral valvuloplasty is more appropriately called percutaneous mitral *commissurotomy* because the balloon dilatation improves the valve orifice by separating the fused mitral commissures. As shown by echocardiographic, fluoroscopic, and anatomic studies, the expanding balloon splits fused commissures in the same manner as surgical commissurotomy does.

Patient Selection for Mitral Valvuloplasty

Patients should be selected for percutaneous mitral valvuloplasty based on both clinical and anatomic factors. In general, they should be symptomatic, and mitral valve area, as measured by echocardiography and hemodynamics, should be <1.5 cm². Unlike for valve surgery, the presence of pulmonary hypertension or abnormal left ventricular function is not a contraindication. Patients with anatomically suitable valves who have developed restenosis (commissural refusion) after prior surgical or balloon commissurotomy can also undergo percutaneous mitral valvuloplasty with results almost as good as those for previously untreated patients. Although the procedure can be performed in patients of almost any age, the best clinical results are observed in younger patients, with less predictable long-term results occurring in patients older than 70 years, who are more likely to have deformed and calcified valves. Percutaneous mitral valvuloplasty is a particularly valuable tool in treating the symptomatic pregnant woman with critical mitral stenosis. It can also be a lifesaving emergency procedure in the patient with mitral stenosis and refractory pulmonary edema or cardiogenic shock.

Asymptomatic patients should be considered for percutaneous mitral commissurotomy when they develop pulmonary hypertension or new-onset atrial fibrillation.

Contraindications

Thrombus within the left atrium or on the interatrial septum is a contraindication to this procedure. Moderate or severe (>2+ on a scale of 0-4, determined angiographically) mitral regurgitation is also a contraindication to percutaneous mitral valvuloplasty. Patients with mitral stenosis and aortic or TV lesions that require cardiac surgery should be referred for surgery. Concomitant coronary disease can be treated

We gratefully acknowledge the Grossman & Baim's *Cardiac Catheterization, Angiography, and Intervention*, 9th edition contributions of Drs Azeem Latib And Duane S. Pinto as portions of their chapter, "Percutaneous Therapies for Mitral and Tricuspid Valve Disease," were retained in this text.

with percutaneous coronary intervention in conjunction with valvuloplasty when the coronary anatomy is suitable.

Anatomic Factors in Patient Selection for Mitral Valvuloplasty

Echocardiography provides valuable information that helps the interventional cardiologist select patients and predict results. The ideal patient has pliable, noncalcified mitral leaflets and mild subvalvular disease. As the degree of subvalvular disease increases, the quality of the result with percutaneous mitral valvuloplasty decreases. Similarly, increasing degrees of calcification of the mitral valve diminish the effectiveness of mitral valve dilatation and increase the complication rate. Dilating mitral valves with commissural calcification may lead to leaflet tearing along noncommissural lines and is associated with a higher incidence of procedure-related mitral regurgitation. Heavy calcification of the valve and bicommissural calcification are also associated with poorer outcomes. When commissural fusion is symmetric, even in the presence of calcification, bicommissural splitting is more likely than when commissural fusion is asymmetric.

Many find the echocardiographic scoring system of Wilkins et al. useful in assessing patients for percutaneous mitral valvuloplasty. This echocardiographic classification system is shown in **Table 33.1**. Points are given for leaflet mobility, valve thickening, subvalvular thickening, and valvular calcification. The final score is determined by adding up the points from each category. Higher scores indicate more severe anatomic disease and less likelihood of a successful procedure. The maximum score is 16, and percutaneous mitral commissurotomy results are generally excellent in patients with an echo score of <8, indicating favorable anatomy, for example, pliable leaflets, mild or moderate subvalvular disease, and mild or absent valve calcification.

Table 33.1 **Echocardiographic Scoring System[a] for Assessing Patients for Percutaneous Mitral Valvuloplasty**

Leaflet mobility
1. Highly mobile valve with restriction of only the leaflet tips
2. Midportion and base of leaflets have reduced mobility
3. Valve leaflets move forward in diastole mainly at the base
4. No or minimal forward movement of the leaflets in diastole

Valvular thickening
1. Leaflets near normal (4-5 mm)
2. Midleaflet thickening, marked thickening of the margins
3. Thickening extends through the entire leaflets (5-8 mm)
4. Marked thickening of all leaflet tissue (>8-10 mm)

Subvalvular thickening
1. Minimal thickening of chordal structures just below the valve
2. Thickening of chordae extending up to one-third of chordal length
3. Thickening extending to the distal third of the chordae
4. Extensive thickening and shortening of all chordae extending down to the papillary muscle

Valvular calcification
1. A single area of increased echo brightness
2. Scattered areas of brightness confined to leaflet margins
3. Brightness extending into the midportion of leaflets
4. Extensive brightness through most of the leaflet tissue

[a]Adding each of the components determines the final score (maximum 16 points).
From Wilkins GT, Weyman AE, Abascal VM, et al. Percutaneous balloon dilatation of the mitral valve: an analysis of echocardiographic variables related to outcome and the mechanism of dilatation. *Br Heart J.* 1988;60:299.

Technique

The most commonly used approaches for percutaneous mitral valvuloplasty are transvenous antegrade (ie, transseptal) techniques, using either a double balloon or the Inoue balloon system. The Inoue balloon is the only device approved specifically for percutaneous mitral valvuloplasty in the United States and is the most commonly used device worldwide. Alternatively, a double-balloon technique can be used with 2 balloons advanced over separate guidewires from the femoral vein to the left atrium, across the mitral valve into the left ventricle. The 2 balloons are then inflated simultaneously across the mitral valve. **Figure 33.1** illustrates the 2-balloon technique. In this patient, the mitral valve was first dilated with a single balloon, after which double balloons were used to achieve the desired hemodynamic result. When properly performed, the double-balloon technique results in an excellent improvement in mitral valve area. Multiple studies have shown no significant difference in hemodynamic results (mitral valve gradient or mitral valve area) post procedure between the double-balloon technique and the Inoue balloon system.

However, the Inoue balloon technique is faster and less cumbersome, and generally requires less fluoroscopy time than these other approaches. The Inoue balloon allows simple progressive upsizing of the balloon without withdrawing the balloon from the left atrium—an important advantage if larger balloon sizes are needed. The Inoue balloon system may, however, result in a slightly higher incidence of mitral regurgitation.

Inoue Balloon Technique

All antegrade approaches begin with the crucial first step of successful transseptal catheterization. This technique not only requires successful access to the left atrium but must also be performed through the posterior and superior part of the atrial septum to allow easy access to the mitral valve. After successful placement of a Mullins-type dilator and sheath into the left atrium and confirmation of its position by hand injection of contrast, the patient is anticoagulated with heparin. Baseline hemodynamic measurements are then recorded, confirming the appropriateness of the degree of mitral stenosis for PMV. Subsequently, a special solid-core coiled 0.025-in guidewire is introduced into the left atrium, and the Mullins sheath dilator system is removed. The femoral vein

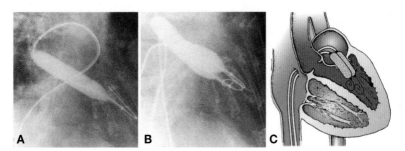

Figure 33.1 Mitral balloon valvuloplasty in a 72-year-old woman who presented with progressive dyspnea on exertion. Her hemodynamic evaluation showed a mean mitral valve gradient of 22 mmHg. This was reduced to 10 mmHg after single-balloon valvuloplasty **(A)** and 4 mmHg after double-balloon dilatation **(B)**. **C,** A schematic drawing showing the anatomic path and catheter positions for double-balloon mitral valvuloplasty.

and interatrial septum are then dilated with a long 14F dilator over the coiled guidewire within the left atrium. The previously prepared, tested, and now slenderized Inoue balloon is then introduced over the guidewire into the left atrium. The Inoue balloon (**Figure 33.2**) is made of nylon and rubber micromesh. Owing to the variable elasticity along its length, the balloon inflates in distinct stages as illustrated in **Figure 33.3**. This allows for stable positioning of the balloon catheter across the mitral valve.

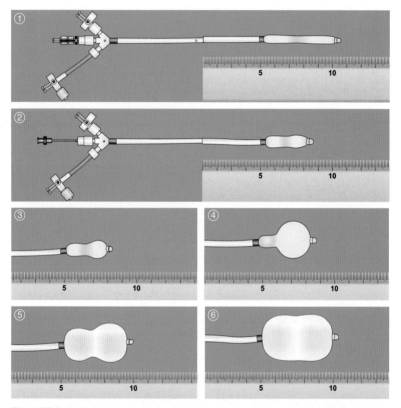

Figure 33.2 The Inoue balloon catheter. The **top panel** shows the length of the catheter. On the far left, at the hub, the stretching metal tube has been fully advanced, resulting in stretching and elongation of the balloon catheter, seen on the right side of the figure. This results in a minimized profile to facilitate passage through a femoral venous sheath or directly through the skin. In the **second panel**, the stretching metal tube on the far left has been pulled back, allowing the balloon to shorten and fatten. The stretching tube is pulled back in this manner after the balloon is passed across the atrial septal puncture. This is seen on the right side of the second panel. **Panels 3-6** show the stepwise inflation characteristics of the balloon. In **panel 3**, the balloon is uninflated. In **panel 4**, the distal portion has been inflated. This portion of the balloon can be "floated" or manipulated across the mitral valve from the left atrium to the left ventricle in a manner analogous to crossing the tricuspid valve with a right heart balloon floatation catheter. In **panel 5**, the balloon is further inflated to create a "dog bone" configuration. This allows the balloon to self-position within the mitral valve. Upon final inflation, as seen in **panel 6**, the waist of the balloon is fully expanded, ultimately resulting in commissural splitting.

After the slenderized balloon has been positioned within the left atrium, the stretching tube is removed, and a preshaped "J" stylet is introduced into the Inoue balloon. The distal portion of the balloon is inflated slightly to aid in crossing the valve and to prevent intrachordal passage. By maneuvering the balloon catheter while rotating and withdrawing the stylet, the balloon tip can be moved anteriorly and inferiorly toward the mitral orifice. Once the balloon catheter is placed across the mitral orifice, the distal portion of the balloon is inflated more fully and the catheter is pulled back gently to confirm that the inflated distal portion of the balloon is secure across the mitral valve. As further volume is added to the balloon, the proximal end inflates to lock the valve between the proximal and distal ends of the balloon. Inflation to precalibrated volume then dilates the valve orifice to the corresponding preset size. **Figure 33.3** illustrates the sequential filling and positioning of the Inoue balloon. It is then allowed to deflate passively before it is withdrawn into the left atrium.

The pressure gradient across the mitral valve is measured after each balloon dilatation, and echocardiography may be used to assess the mitral valve area, leaflet mobility, and the degree of mitral regurgitation. If the first inflation has not resulted in a satisfactory increase in the mitral valve area, and the degree of mitral regurgitation has not increased, the balloon is then readvanced across the mitral valve and inflation repeated with the balloon diameter increased by 1 or 2 mm by delivery of slightly more of the precalibrated syringe volume in a stepwise dilatation process, which is repeated until the desired result is achieved.

The Inoue balloon comes in 4 sizes—24, 26, 28, and 30 mm, referring to the fully inflated maximal balloon diameter. However, since actual balloon size is dependent on the volume used for inflation, the actual diameter can be varied over a range from 6 mm less than nominal up to the full rated diameter, as required. We generally estimate the expected maximal inflated balloon diameter using an empirical formula based on the height of the patient (one-tenth the height in centimeter plus 10 mm). It is important to start with a smaller balloon diameter, especially for valves that are very much thickened or rigid or have moderate amounts of subvalvular disease, to minimize the development of mitral regurgitation, which can develop suddenly with as little as a 1- to 2-mm increase in inflation diameter of the balloon.

The Inoue balloon is fundamentally different from conventional balloons, being volume-driven. The balloon is precalibrated so that inflation with volumes labeled on the inflation syringe results in corresponding inflated diameters of the balloon. The pressure that the balloon is inflated to is thus different for different inflation volumes. A smaller maximal-size balloon, such as a 26-mm balloon, when inflated to its maximal size, will be at a higher pressure than a balloon that has a larger capacity, such as a 30-mm balloon, inflated to the same diameter of 26 mm. The Inoue balloon has a low-pressure zone encompassing the first two-thirds of its range of inflation. The balloon pressure in this zone typically is approximately 2 or 3 atm. As the balloon is inflated to its last couple of millimeters of diameter with increasing inflation volumes, the balloon pressure rises toward 4 atm. Randomized trials have examined the effects of using balloons in the low-pressure zone as compared with using them in the high-pressure zone. With similar maximal inflated diameters, inflations in the low-pressure zone resulted in less mitral regurgitation than did inflations in the high-pressure zone. Thus, using a 30-mm balloon inflated to a maximum diameter of 28 mm will overall result in causing less mitral regurgitation than will using a maximal nominal 28-mm balloon inflated to 28 mm (in the high-pressure zone).

It is important to assess for increases in mitral regurgitation after each inflation before proceeding to the next inflation diameter. Changes in the V wave must be assessed carefully during percutaneous commissurotomy procedures, but additional information obtained using techniques such as Doppler echocardiography or repeat left

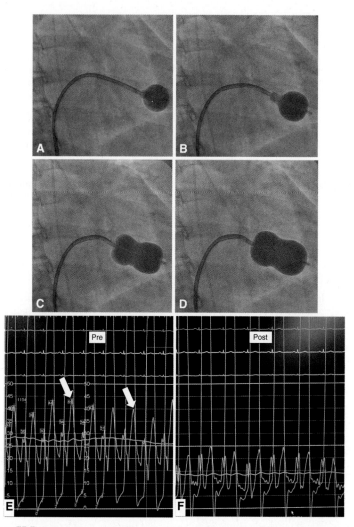

Figure 33.3 Balloon mitral valvuloplasty in a 42-year-old man who presented with dyspnea on exertion. **A,** Distal tip of the Inoue balloon has crossed the mitral valve. **B,** With the distal tip of the balloon filled, the catheter was withdrawn to straddle the mitral valve. **C,** Partial filling of the balloon. **D,** Complete filling of the Inoue balloon across the mitral valve. Following this dilation, the mitral valve gradient was reduced from 18 to 2 mmHg. **E,** A large V wave is seen prior to percutaneous mitral valvuloplasty. There is a large diastolic transmitral valve gradient. The white arrows denote the peak of the V waves. No mitral regurgitation was noted at this point by either echocardiography or left ventriculography. **F,** Post mitral valvuloplasty, the transmitral gradient has been dramatically reduced, as has the V wave. Ventriculography and Doppler echocardiography at this point show no mitral regurgitation.

ventriculography is necessary to interpret these findings fully. After each balloon inflation, the mean left atrial pressure should be expected to decrease in conjunction with a decrease in the transmitral pressure gradient. When the left atrial pressure remains unchanged both in magnitude and in the morphology of the waveform after balloon inflation, it is likely that no progress has been made. If a persistent gradient is present, an additional inflation is warranted.

Following successful mitral valve dilatation, the Inoue balloon is reslenderized by reintroducing first the guidewire and then the stretching tube. The slenderized balloon is subsequently withdrawn from the body over the guidewire. If no sheath has been used, a 10F sheath is inserted into the femoral vein over the guidewire before removal of the wire.

Immediate Results

Figure 33.4 illustrates a typical reduction in left atrial pressure and transmitral gradient immediately after balloon mitral valvuloplasty. The mitral valve orifice area will generally be increased to >1 cm²/m² body surface area. By echocardiographic assessment in the laboratory, particularly by planimetry of the mitral valve orifice image in the 2-dimensional echocardiogram short-axis view, another confirmation of improvement of mitral valve orifice area can be obtained. The accuracy of Doppler measurements during valvuloplasty can be variable, but color Doppler assessment is the method of choice for sequential evaluation of the degree of mitral regurgitation. When Doppler echocardiography is not available in the catheterization lab, serial left ventriculograms can be done to evaluate the degree of mitral regurgitation. The appearance of new mitral regurgitation or an increase of greater than one grade on the 0 to 4 classification of preexisting mitral regurgitation in general signals an end point of the procedure. In addition, if the mitral valve area has increased to >2 cm², or if the mean gradient has been reduced to <5 mmHg without a decrease in cardiac output, the procedure has been completed successfully.

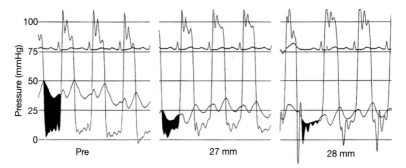

Figure 33.4 Before valvuloplasty, there is a large transmitral valve pressure gradient, filled in black in the first diastolic period in the prevalvuloplasty tracing. After a 27-mm balloon inflation, the transmitral valve pressure gradient is significantly reduced, and following a 28-mm diameter balloon inflation, the gradient is nearly resolved. (Effect of balloon size and stepwise inflation technique on the results of Inoue mitral commissurotomy. Reproduced from Feldman T, Carroll JD, Herrmann HC, et al. Effect of balloon size and stepwise inflation technique on the acute results of Inoue mitral commissurotomy. *Cathet Cardiovasc Diagn.* 1993;28:199-205.)

Long-Term Hemodynamic and Clinical Results

Numerous studies have demonstrated the effectiveness of balloon valvuloplasty in increasing mitral valve area. There is a consistent increase in mitral valve area to >1.5 cm^2, a decrease in left atrial pressure, and usually a slight increase in cardiac output. Over time, there is a gradual decrease in pulmonary artery pressure and pulmonary vascular resistance. In a multicenter series, the National Heart, Lung, and Blood Institute Balloon Valvuloplasty Registry reported results in 736 patients older than 18 years who were followed up for 4 years. The actuarial survival rates at 1, 2, 3, and 4 years were 93%, 90%, 87%, and 84%, respectively. The event-free survival (freedom from death, mitral valve surgery, or repeat balloon valvuloplasty) at 1, 2, 3, and 4 years was 80%, 71%, 66%, and 62%, respectively. Multivariate predictors of mortality were New York Heart Association (NYHA) functional class IV, echocardiographic mitral valve score of >12, systolic pulmonary artery pressure of >40 mmHg post procedure, and left ventricular end-diastolic pressure of >15 mmHg. More recently, Bouleti et al reported long-term follow-up data for up to 20 years in 912 patients who had had successful mitral valvuloplasty, defined by a valve area of >1.5 cm^2 with mitral regurgitation of <2. During a median follow-up of 12 years, 561 patients (62%) were free of reintervention. In the 351 patients (38%) who underwent a reintervention, surgery was performed in 266 patients and repeat balloon valvuloplasty in 85 patients. Importantly, cardiovascular survival without surgery was 60 ± 7% at 10 years in the 85 patients who underwent repeat valvuloplasty. These data support the concept that percutaneous mitral balloon valvuloplasty is an effective therapy for mitral stenosis and that a repeat valvuloplasty can allow further postponement of surgery in a significant number of patients.

Complications

In skilled hands, the failure rate of the procedure should be <5%. Failure usually results from the inability to safely puncture the interatrial septum because of anatomic difficulties or, in some cases, to position the balloon catheter successfully across the mitral valve. Procedural mortality rate varies from 0% to 3% in most series. Hemopericardium related to transseptal catheterization, atrial puncture, or, rarely, left ventricular apical perforation by the balloon or wires varies in incidence from 0.5% to 10%. Systemic embolization has been encountered in 0.5% to 5% of cases. These complications diminish with increasing operator experience.

Severe mitral regurgitation is fortunately uncommon, ranging in incidence from 2% to 9%, and is related to noncommissural leaflet tearing or chordal rupture. Leaflet tears are largely unpredictable and unpreventable, but chordal rupture can be minimized by careful application of the technique. Usually, in these circumstances one or both of the mitral commissures might have been too tightly fused to be split successfully by the balloon, and the leaflets might have torn along noncommissural lines. Most cases of severe mitral regurgitation occur in patients with unfavorable mitral valve anatomy. Same-day surgical mitral valve replacement is necessary in 2% to 3% of patients. Usually, even severe mitral regurgitation is well tolerated for a time by the patient, and in the acute setting, it is usually responsive to intravenous nitroglycerin or nitroprusside. In general, elective surgical replacement rather than repair of the valve will be necessary when severe mitral regurgitation occurs because of the severity of the underlying valvular and subvalvular disease.

PERCUTANEOUS MITRAL VALVE REPAIR AND REPLACEMENT

Mitral regurgitation previously has been treatable only by surgical methods (placement of an annuloplasty ring, leaflet resection, chordal replacement, or the edge-to-edge Alfieri stitch repair). Percutaneous approaches to mitral valve repair have now been successful, and both annuloplasty and edge-to-edge repair approaches are in use. Understanding the mechanism of mitral regurgitation is important for treatment and procedure planning. Conventionally, the etiology of mitral regurgitation is classified based on leaflet motion and anatomic lesions. Carpentier classification stratifies mitral regurgitation into type I (normal leaflet motion with organic leaflet pathology including perforation or cleft), type II (leaflet prolapse due to chordal rupture or leaflet elongation, papillary muscle dysfunction/rupture), type IIIa (restricted leaflet motion in systole and diastole due to chordal and/or leaflet thickening and calcification), and type IIIb (restricted leaflet motion in systole only).

Complementary to the Carpentier classification, there are 2 pathophysiologic categories of mitral regurgitation. Primary (or degenerative) mitral regurgitation is due to primary pathology of the mitral valve; secondary (or functional) mitral regurgitation is due to primary pathology and remodeling of the left ventricle (**Figure 33.5**). While there may be changes in the valve as a consequence of this remodeling, the primary disorder relates to remodeling and geometric changes occurring in the left ventricle. Degenerative disorders account for the majority of cases compared with functional mitral regurgitation.

Percutaneous Annular Modification

Indirect annuloplasty may be accomplished via the coronary sinus, the course of which parallels that of the mitral annulus, by stretching or reshaping the coronary sinus to cause

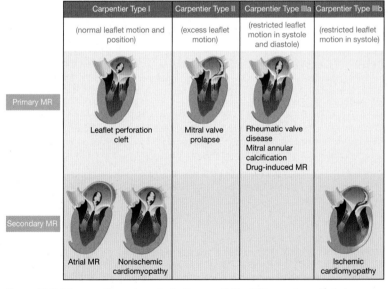

Figure 33.5 Primary and secondary mitral valve regurgitation (MR) groupings with their respective Carpentier functional classification. Carpentier type I represents normal leaflet motion and position. Carpentier type II represents excess leaflet motion. Carpentier type IIIa represents restricted leaflet motion in systole and diastole. Carpentier type IIIb represents restricted leaflet motion in systole. (Reproduced with permission from El Sabbagh A, Reddy YNV, Nishimura RA. Mitral valve regurgitation in the contemporary era: insights into diagnosis, management, and future directions. *JACC Cardiovasc Imaging.* 2018;11(4):628-643.)

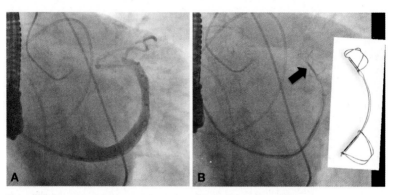

Figure 33.6 Coronary sinus annuloplasty with Cardiac Dimensions' CARILLON device. **A,** A measuring catheter is placed in the coronary sinus. **B,** The distal anchor of the device has been released (arrow). The inset shows the device in a similar orientation to that in the right-hand side panel.

contraction of the mitral annulus, with displacement of the posterior mitral annulus toward the septum. Several devices have shown efficacy in preclinical experience and are now entering clinical trials. Some of the challenges involved with this approach include the variability of the coronary sinus in its anatomic relation to the mitral valve annulus, the course of the circumflex coronary artery and its branches over or under the coronary sinus, and the potential for injury to the thin-walled sinus. The Carillon Mitral Contour System (Cardiac Dimensions, Inc.) has proximal and distal nitinol anchors connected by a nitinol wire, which is inserted after appropriate sizing with a catheter. The device applies direct tension, thus reducing the anterior-medial diameter of the mitral valve annulus (**Figure 33.6**).

Direct annuloplasty systems are also in development (**Figure 33.7**). The Cardioband Mitral Reconstruction System (Edwards Lifesciences Corp, Irvine, CA, United States) is designed to reduce MR through annular reduction. The device is delivered transseptally and consists of a fabric covered band that is deployed along the anterior and posterior regions of the annulus on the atrial side and is affixed using a series of anchors in a stepwise manner under echocardiographic and fluoroscopic guidance for optimal placement. Once the implant is affixed to the annulus, the size-adjustment tool is introduced over a

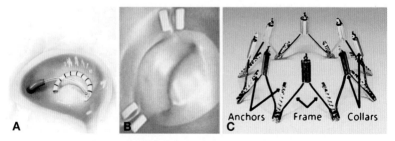

Figure 33.7 Transcatheter direct annuloplasty systems. **(A)** Cardioband (Edwards Lifesciences); **(B)** Mitralign (Mitralign Inc.); **(C)** Millipede (Boston Scientific Corporation). (Reproduced with permission from Testa L, Latib A, Montone RA, Bedogni F. Transcatheter mitral valve regurgitation treatment: state of the art and a glimpse to the future. *J Thorac Cardovasc Surg.* 2016;152:319-327.

wire to contract the Cardioband implant. The first anchor is deployed in the lateral commissure, and additional anchors are deployed at short intervals until the last anchor is implanted in the medial commissure. The band is then contracted, reducing the annular size. A randomized controlled trial comparing the Cardioband Mitral System treatment with medical therapy versus medical therapy alone is active in the United States (Annular Reduction for Transcatheter Treatment of Insufficient Mitral Valve; NCT03016975).

Leaflet Repair or Plication

Another surgical approach for mitral valve repair involves the plication of the free edges of the 2 mitral leaflets using a suture or pledget, with a resultant bow tie or double-orifice mitral valve. This edge-to-edge repair technique was pioneered by Alfieri in the early 1990s. A percutaneous method to deliver a clip (MitraClip Abbott Vascular, Santa Clara, CA) is currently in widespread use with over 150,000 procedures having been performed worldwide. Using this device, the resultant double-orifice repair is similar to surgical repair, ultimately maintained by fibrosis of the clip with a tissue bridge.

Candidates for the MitraClip procedure are symptomatic patients with moderate to severe mitral regurgitation, left ventricular ejection fraction (LVEF) >30%, left ventricular end-diastolic diameter (LVEDD) <40 mm, or asymptomatic patients with one or more of the following: LVEF between 25% and 60%, LVEDD >45 mm, new-onset atrial fibrillation, and pulmonary hypertension defined as sPAP (systolic pulmonary artery pressure) >50 mmHg at rest or >60 mmHg on effort. Patients should be high-risk candidates for mitral valve surgery based on a consensus between a local cardiologist and cardiac surgeon.

The randomized EVEREST II trial comparing percutaneous edge-to-edge mitral repair to surgical mitral repair showed that surgery is more effective in reducing mitral regurgitation, but that percutaneous repair is safer and achieves both reductions in left ventricular chamber volumes and symptoms and improvements in quality of life that are similar to those achieved with surgery. Subgroup analysis from this trial showed that the best results for percutaneous repair were achieved in older patients with poor left ventricular function and functional mitral regurgitation. The reductions in NYHA classification, mitral regurgitation, and end-diastolic volumes have been durable in reports out to 5 years among surviving patients.

Two studies have evaluated the MitraClip system in functional mitral regurgitation and achieved discordant findings: the Multicentre Study of Percutaneous Mitral Valve Repair MitraClip Device in Patients with Severe Secondary Mitral Regurgitation (MITRA-FR), and the Cardiovascular Outcomes Assessment of the MitraClip Percutaneous Therapy for Heart Failure Patients with Functional Mitral Regurgitation (COAPT). COAPT showed that in 614 patients with heart failure and severe functional mitral regurgitation, transcatheter percutaneous mitral valve repair using the MitraClip device in conjunction with guidelines-directed medical therapy (GDMT) when compared with GDMT alone not only significantly reduced the primary end point of heart failure rehospitalizations (hazard ratio, 0.53; 95% confidence interval [CI], 0.40-0.70; $P < .001$) but also reduced mortality at 2 years (hazard ratio, 0.62; 95% CI, 0.46-0.82; $P < .001$). Conversely, MITRA-FR primary outcome results in 304 patients at 12 months showed no significant difference in the rate of death or unplanned heart failure hospitalizations in the intervention and control groups (54.6% vs 51.3%; OR 1.16; 95% CI 0.73-1.84; $P = .53$).

Potential explanations for the discordant results include differences in patient selection and in the severity of mitral regurgitation graded according to several criteria: Using the effective regurgitant orifice area (EROA), the MITRA-FR trial had only 16% of patients with severe mitral regurgitation as defined by EROA >40 mm^2 versus

41% of COAPT patients. In the COAPT trial, the EROA was ~30% higher and LV volumes were ~30% smaller than in the MITRA-FR trial. The patients in MITRA-FR had more profound LV damage with larger LV end-diastolic volumes (MITRA-FR: 135 ± 35 mL/m^2 vs COAPT: 101 ± 34 mL/m^2).

One possible explanation of the observed difference in outcomes among the 2 trials is that the COAPT trial enrolled patients with more severe mitral regurgitation, but with less severe underlying cardiomyopathy. The only COAPT subgroup that did not benefit from MitraClip with GDMT was the group of patients who had an EROA <30 mm^2 in the setting of a dilated LV (>96 mL/m^2). Furthermore, there were differences in procedural outcomes; residual mitral regurgitation class >3+ was higher post clip in the MITRA-FR trial compared with COAPT, both acutely (9% vs 5%) and at 12 months (17% vs 5%).

Anatomic Considerations

Favorable anatomy with high likelihood of successful percutaneous repair includes the presence of A2/P2 noncalcified mitral valve leaflet prolapse, mitral valve area >4 cm^2, and mean gradient <4 mmHg, with a flail width (length of leaflet along the coaptation line that has flail segment on echocardiographic short-axis view) <15 mm and flail gap (the greatest distance between the edges of the flail leaflet and opposing leaflet on echocardiographic 4- or 5-chamber view) <10 mm. A new version of the MitraClip system, the XTr system, was introduced in 2018. Compared with the first generation and NT system, MitraClip XTr has arms that are 3 mm longer and grippers that are designed to facilitate leaflet grasping. Further enhancements introduced with the MitraClip G4 include an expanded range of clip sizes, as well facilitation of leaflet grasping and of real time procedure assessment, aimed at facilitating its use in less favorable anatomies.

MitraClip Procedure

The procedure (**Figure 33.8**) is divided into 5 parts: (1) transseptal puncture and catheter insertion, (2) steering of the clip, (3) alignment with the valve and commissure, (4) grasping of the leaflets, and (5) standardized imaging and hemodynamic evaluation. The transseptal puncture is often guided by echocardiography. The optimal position in the posterior and superior portion of the fossa is approximately 40 mm above the plane of the mitral valve. The location of the puncture may be modified according to the type and location of the disease. A puncture higher (50 mm) from the plane of the mitral valve may be beneficial in degenerative disease, and lower (35 mm) for functional disease since tethering results in coaptation below the mitral annular plane. This general approach allows for sufficient space to maneuver the delivery system and for the system to reach the leaflets. If the lesion is lateral, a lower puncture can be selected, while if the lesion is medial, the puncture should be higher.

The left superior pulmonary vein is cannulated and a stiff exchange length 0.035″ wire is left in place. Dilation of the interatrial septum can be performed with a 10 mm balloon. The 24F catheter is advanced through the interatrial septum, and then the dilator is removed avoiding entraining air. The catheter is steerable and can be adjusted in the anteroposterior and mediolateral planes using transesophageal echocardiographic guidance so that it is perpendicular and central to the valve orifice. Typically, this requires posteromedial rotation. The clip is then advanced in the open position to the left ventricle. With echocardiographic guidance, the clip is closed to 120° and pulled back until the leaflets are captured. The clip is then progressively closed and the leaflets are grasped. The clip can be readjusted depending upon the imaging and hemodynamic findings. In some cases, multiple clips can be placed to control the mitral regurgitation but creation of mitral stenosis is a concern. Once a suitable position is selected, the arms are closed, locked, and released.

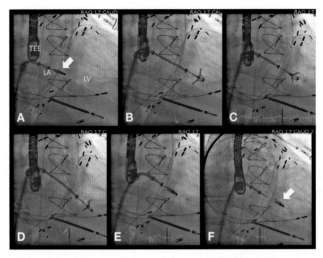

Figure 33.8 Fluoroscopic images of the steps of the MitraClip procedure. **A,** The arrow shows the clip in the left atrium (LA). **B,** The open clip has been advanced into the left ventricle. **C,** The clip arms are everted to allow withdrawal back into the left atrium without chordal entanglement. **D,** The open clip has been readvanced into the left ventricle to attempt a better grasp of the leaflet edges. **E,** The clip has been closed to grasp the mitral leaflet free edges. **F,** The arrow shows the clip after release from the delivery system. LV, left ventricle; TEE, transesophageal echo probe.

The PASCAL Transcatheter Valve Repair System (Edwards Lifesciences, Irvine, CA) system is a leaflet repair technology designed to reduce mitral regurgitation and minimize the coaptation gap. Larger implant size and broader paddles enhance the ability to grasp individual leaflets independently and maximize leaflet coaptation, while a central spacer within the device fills the central regurgitant orifice area.

Transcatheter Mitral Valve Replacement

Transcatheter mitral valve replacement (TMVR) has the potential to reduce mitral regurgitation to a similar extent as surgery and has the potential for application in a broader array of patients and mitral valve anatomies. Percutaneous mitral valve replacement in deteriorated bioprosthetic valves, annuloplasty rings, and annular calcification has been performed using the SAPIEN 3 29 mm balloon-expandable aortic-designed transcatheter valves delivered through transseptal (**Figure 33.9,** panels A and B), transatrial, or transapical approach.

Numerous dedicated mitral valve devices are in development but face several design challenges. The mitral valve annulus is elliptical and saddle-shaped (**Figure 33.10**) with a complex and interconnected subvalvular apparatus making entanglement and paravalvular leaks possible. The mitral valve itself is dynamic with reductions in the area of approximately 30% and circumference of 15%, which can result in valve dislodgement. Because the anterior leaflet is contiguous with the left ventricular outflow tract (LVOT), and as TMVR devices consist of circumferentially covered stent frames, significant protrusion into the LV cavity can occur or the anterior mitral leaflet can be displaced. Thus, the device anterior leaflet and septum create a "neo-LVOT," which may not be of sufficient size and can lead to obstruction. The consequences of this complication are dire, with procedural mortality exceeding

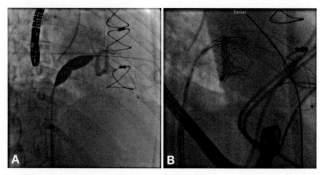

Figure 33.9 Fluoroscopic image of Edwards SAPIEN 3 valve implanted via a transseptal approach. The interatrial septum has been punctured in **A** and a 10 mm balloon has been advanced and inflated to facilitate delivery of the device. **B** shows the valve at deployment. A preshaped wire has been placed on the left ventricle.

30%. Predictors of this complication have been identified, and CT imaging is performed to identify suitability. Alcohol septal ablation and percutaneous laceration of the anterior leaflet (LAMPOON) and septum (SESAME) have been performed in some cases to allow for valve implantation.

PERCUTANEOUS APPROACHES TO TRICUSPID VALVE DISORDERS

The prevalence of tricuspid regurgitation (TR) is underestimated, and there is a mistaken belief that moderate to severe TR has minimal prognostic impact. While patients with TR may have a long asymptomatic latent period, they eventually present with symptoms. TR is often not considered for treatment within a multitude of medical problems as it is mistakenly not considered important. The available infor-

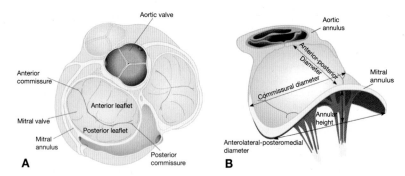

Figure 33.10 Three-dimensional anatomic relationships of mitral and aortic valves. **A,** Mitral and aortic valves viewed from above. **B,** Three-dimensional shape of the mitral valve, with relation to the aortic valve. (Reproduced with permission from Three-dimensional mitral valve morphology and age-related trends in children and young adults with structurally normal hearts using transthoracic echocardiography. *J Am Soc Echocardiography*. 2017;6:561-571).

mation evaluating the pathophysiology, natural history, and novel therapeutic agents for TR is small compared to the data for aortic and mitral valve disease. There is a mistaken belief that diuretics or treating left-sided disease is sufficient to treat severe TR with annular dilatation and that cardiac surgery is the only intervention for severe TR. As a result, even though there are more than 1.6 million cases of moderate to severe TR in the United States, only 8000 surgical procedures are performed annually with the majority of patients presenting late and not being offered any intervention.

TR is characterized by a pathological amount of blood regurgitating from the right ventricle (RV) into the right atrium (RA) during systole. Secondary or functional tricuspid regurgitation (FTR) accounts for over 90% of the causes of TR and occurs predominantly as a result of left-sided heart disease increasing left atrial pressure (valvular in 49.5% and myocardial in 12.9%), or pulmonary hypertension from pulmonary disease or idiopathic causes in 23%. Functional, "atrial" TR associated with atrial fibrillation has been recently identified as an important subset of TR. It tends to be associated with better long term outcomes when compared with functional "ventricular" TR. There is a significant interdependence between the TV and RV, left heart, and pulmonary vasculature. TR is associated with a subsequent rise in RA-RV pressures as well as progressive dysfunction and dilatation. The result is (1) annular dilatation due to the eccentric forces applied by the dilating RV free wall that makes the valve more planar, less mobile, and (2) leaflet tethering as a result of papillary muscle displacement in lateral and apical directions that causes reduced leaflet coaptation and an increase in tenting volume. As FTR worsens, it results in a vicious cycle with a negative impact on both the left and right side of the heart as well as the pulmonary vasculature.

There are now numerous studies showing that not only severe TR but also moderate TR is associated with a worse prognosis and poor quality of life, independent of the severity of pulmonary hypertension, RV dysfunction or dilatation, and LV dysfunction. This has been shown in various heart failure populations, post mitral valve surgery, after transcatheter procedures such as transcatheter aortic valve replacement (TAVR) and MitraClip, in patients with isolated TR. The cause of FTR has also been shown to have an impact on prognosis with severe TR associated with left-sided valvular disease and LV systolic dysfunction having a worse prognosis.

Until recently, surgery has been the only treatment option for patients with severe TR who remain symptomatic despite diuretic therapy. However, current guidelines recommend surgery for functional TR only in patients undergoing left-sided valve surgery. Indeed, corrective surgery for isolated TR is not commonly done and when performed it is associated with significantly high in-hospital mortality, even in highly selected patients. Two recent analyses evaluating outcomes over a 10-year period from the National Inpatient Database showed that although the absolute number of TV surgeries has increased, the majority (85%) is performed in conjunction with other cardiac surgery and only 15% is performed as isolated TV surgery; in-hospital mortality ranges from 8.1% to 10.9% and has remained constant over the past 10-year period.

When performed in isolation, the majority of TV is replaced (60%) rather than repaired, and the in-hospital mortality is higher for replacement probably because these patients have more advanced RV remodeling. The morbidity and mortality of isolated TV surgery are high because these patients are older with more comorbidities and more severe end-organ disease. A recent analysis by Curio et al provides insights into why so few patients with severe TR undergo surgery other than the higher in-hospital mortality. The analysis showed that patients with severe TR present late to tertiary centers in advanced stages of TR with multiple comorbidities, and as a result, the majority are not good surgical candidates.

Anatomy of the TV and Relevance for Transcatheter Procedures

The TV is crescent-shaped (**Figure 33.11A**), consisting of 3 very thin and translucent leaflets of unequal size: anterior (generally the largest and longest), posterior (shortest circumferentially), and septal (shortest radially and least mobile). The TV is the most anatomically variable cardiac valve and can have 4, 5, or 6 leaflets, which can be sometimes visualized as distinct leaflets or as having prominent folds and deep clefts. These anatomical characteristics could explain some of the challenges of leaflet based devices to capture the leaflets, especially the difficulty in capturing the septal leaflet, the lack of reproducibility, and the increased risk of clip detachment. The TV has a rich and dense subannular structure with multiple chordae that may interact and entrap catheters and devices. It is also important to evaluate whether there is a prominent moderator band when performing valve replacement procedures that could impede the advancement of the valve delivery system. The tricuspid annulus (TA) is D-shaped composed of a relatively straight and flat septal region and a larger C-shaped curved anterior and posterior region corresponding to the free wall of the RV.

There are a number of structures in close proximity to the TV that are important not only as anatomical landmarks but also due to the risk of injury from transcatheter devices. The noncoronary sinus of Valsalva is adjacent to the anteroseptal commissure and there is a risk of aortic perforation with annuloplasty devices that require fixation in this region (**Figure 33.11A**). The atrioventricular (AV) node and the bundle of His cross the septal leaflet attachment 3 to 5 mm posterior (more septal) to the anteroseptal commissure and can be injured by annular devices or catheter manipulation resulting in transient or permanent AV block. The right coronary artery (RCA) originates from the right coronary sinus, and courses in the AV groove along the anterior and posterior parts of the annulus, with its bifurcation occurring after the anteroposterior commissure (**Figure 33.11A and B**). The RCA on angiography or with the aid of a coronary wire is an excellent marker of the approximate location of the annulus such that when manipulating annular devices, navigation is aided by following the RCA and being above or below the RCA is a useful fluoroscopic marker of being too atrial or too ventricular, respectively. Furthermore, the distance of the RCA from the annulus is variable with a larger distance in the proximal RCA (anterior

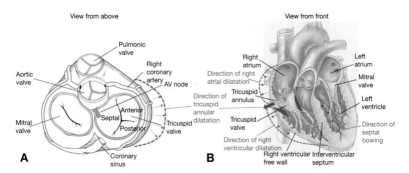

Figure 33.11 Anatomy of the tricuspid valve and associated structures. **Panels A** and **B** show the proximity of the anterior (ant) and septal (sept) leaflets to the aorta (Ao) and conduction system as well as the relation of the right coronary artery (RCA) to the anterior and posterior (post) leaflets. (Reproduced with permission from Dahou A, Levin D, Reisman M, Hahn R. Anatomy and physiology of the tricuspid valve. *JACC Cardiovasc Imaging.* 2019;12:458-468.)

annulus) and a much shorter distance near the mid-RCA, which corresponds to the inferior part of the anterior annulus and the posterior annulus. Thus, there is a higher risk of injury to the RCA in the regions on either side of the anteroseptal commissure. The RCA can be damaged directly from penetration by an anchor or due to spasm or kinking from the torsion of tissue from the insertion of screw-type anchors or during cinching of annular devices. Finally, the coronary sinus is a good landmark to identify the posteroseptal commissure.

In FTR, the free wall dilates resulting in dilation of lateral and posterior aspects of the annulus. Thus, all annular reshaping devices are designed to pull the anterior and/or posterior segments of the annulus toward the relatively fixed septal part. Also, there is significant heterogeneity in muscle and fatty tissue in the TA with discontinuous fibrous support that may explain the increased risk of dehiscence seen with all of the transcatheter annular devices.

Percutaneous Treatment of Functional Tricuspid Regurgitation

The recognition that there are numerous patients with symptomatic FTR without treatment options has sparked the development of numerous transcatheter devices that are currently undergoing preclinical or clinical testing. Currently, there are no U.S. Food and Drug Administration (FDA)-approved devices, and there are 2 devices approved in Europe. In general, the majority of the tricuspid devices have been developed to reproduce surgical techniques and can be broadly divided into the following categories:

1. Annuloplasty
2. Leaflet approximation/coaptation enhancement
3. Valve replacement
4. Caval valve implantation (CAVI)

Annuloplasty Devices

Trialign

The Trialign device (Mitralign, Tewksbury, United States) uses transcatheter suture annuloplasty to reproduce the surgical Kay bicuspidization. Through jugular vein access, an insulated radiofrequency wire is advanced into the RV to then retrogradely cross the TA tissue. In this way, 2 pledgets are placed at the posteroseptal as well as the anteroposterior commissures that are then cinched to obliterate the posterior tricuspid leaflet, creating a bicuspid valve and thus reducing TR. The small footprint of the device, leaving a significant amount of native anatomy undisturbed for subsequent procedures, was an important advantage of this device. In the early feasibility SCOUT I trial (NCT02574650), implantation success was achieved in all 15 patients. However, 1 patient required right coronary artery stenting because of extrinsic compression. At 30-day follow-up, the technical success rate was 80% because of 3 patients developing single-pledget TA detachment. Reintervention was not required in these patients.

In the remaining patients, significant reductions of TA areas and EROA were observed while left ventricular stroke volume improved. In addition, NYHA class, 6-minute walk distance, and quality of life (QoL) were significantly improved. After 12 months, improvements in NYHA class and QoL were sustained at follow-up. Although enrollment had started on a larger 60-patient study, the device is no longer available due to a lack of funding.

Nevertheless, as the first transcatheter device to be implanted in a large group of patients, the experience provided the basis for standardization and improvement in TEE guidance of tricuspid procedures, recognition of the fragility of TA tissue as compared to the mitral, and the increased risk of dehiscence and the heterogeneity of the patients with severe TR including those who may require treatment with multiple devices (ie, annuloplasty plus edge-to-edge) or TV replacement. It was also noted that the improvement in symptoms was disproportionately larger than the reduction in TR.

Cardioband Tricuspid Valve Reconstruction System

The Cardioband Tricuspid Valve Reconstruction System (Edwards Lifesciences, Irvine, United States) is the first transcatheter device that received CE mark approval for TR treatment. Similar to the Cardioband Mitral System, it consists of a fabric covered band that is deployed along the anterior and posterior regions of the annulus and the size adjustment tool contracts the Cardioband implant. The reduction in annular diameters and TR are assessed by real-time echocardiography while the heart is beating and adjusted as appropriate to minimize TR.

The Cardioband Tricuspid System evaluated in the European TRI-REPAIR CE mark trial (NCT02981953), and a US-based study evaluating early feasibility is underway (NCT03382457). Six-month results of the TRI-REPAIR trial showed technical success (including access, deployment, and positioning) was achieved in 100% of the 30 enrolled patients. At 30-day follow-up, 1 device-related death was observed. Significant reductions of TA diameter, EROA, and vena contracta (VC) were sustained at 6-month follow-up. Furthermore, there was a significant increase in 6-minute walk distance and Kansas City Cardiomyopathy Questionnaire scores and reduction in NYHA class at 6-month follow-up.

Leaflet Approximation/Coaptation Devices

Extensive operator experience, as well as the availability of MitraClip, led to its use in the tricuspid position in over 2000 cases of severe TR. Thus, the TriValve registry that evaluated 304 transcatheter tricuspid procedures performed around the world showed that MitraClip was used in 69% of patients. The MitraClip device has several limitations when utilized on the TV because (1) the clip delivery system has to be miskeyed in order to have more ability to navigate and orientate the clip, (2) it is more difficult to be coaxial to the coaptation line, (3) navigation is often limited by a lack of height above the TV and/or the delivery system hugging the atrial septum, (4) there are larger coaptation gaps and a wide TR jet, (5) the presence of 3 commissures necessitates multiple clips for TR reduction, (6) the septal leaflet is often more tethered and immobile making grasping more challenging, and (7) there can be interference by a pacing lead.

The technique involves implanting multiple clips on the anteroseptal leaflets and/ or posteroseptal leaflets, often starting at the commissures before moving more centrally. This results in bicuspidization of the valve by approximating the anterior and septal leaflets. A clover technique can be mimicked by connecting the septal with the anterior and posterior leaflets, resulting in a triple orifice. Clipping the anteroposterior leaflets is generally avoided in functional TR, as it may distort the valve and worsen TR.

A multicenter European registry showed reduction of TR by at least 1 grade in 91% of patients, accompanied by a significant reduction in EROA, VC width, and regurgitant volume, as well as an improvement in NYHA class and 6-minute walk distance. Of note, predominantly central and anteroseptal jets have been identified as predictors of procedural success. In many cases, procedures were successfully performed in combination with repair of the mitral valve, and procedural success is associated with a reduction in mortality. A modified version of the MitraClip device, called TriClip, uses the same clip but a dedicated guiding catheter and clip delivery system specifically designed for the TV that overcomes many of the limitations of using the mitral system. This device was evaluated in the prospective, multicenter, single-arm TRILUMINATE study (NCT03227757) in 21 sites in Europe and the United States. Implantation was successful in all 85 patients enrolled with implantation of >2 clips in 80% (average of 2.2 clips/patient), resulting in a reduction of TR grade severity by at least 1 grade in 30 days in 71 (86%) of 83 patients who had available echocardiogram data and imaging. Clinical outcomes at 6 months were as follows: major adverse events in 4% (3/84), single leaflet attachment in 7% (5/72), and all-cause mortality in 5% (4/84). The TriClip has been further evaluated in a large FDA-approved TRILUMINATE Pivotal Trial (NCT03904147) randomizing symptomatic patients with severe TR to TriClip or medical therapy. In that study, 175 patients were assigned to TriClip, and 175 patients were assigned to medical therapy. The primary endpoint was a hierarchical composite that included death from any cause, tricuspid valve surgery, hospitalization for heart failure, and an improvement of at least 15 points in quality of life measured with the Kansas City Cardiomyopathy Questionnaire. At 1-year follow-up, there were no significant differences in the incidence of death, tricuspid valve surgery, or heart failure hospitalization among the two groups. There was, however, a significant improvement in quality of life scores in the TriClip group when compared with the medical therapy group (12.3 ± 1.8 points vs 0.6 ± 1.8 points, respectively, $P < 0.001$).

PASCAL TRANSCATHETER VALVE REPAIR SYSTEM

The repositionable and recapturable PASCAL Repair System (Edwards Lifesciences, Irvine, United States) was initially designed for the treatment of mitral regurgitation. However, the same system was successfully evaluated in the repair of a regurgitant TV with few limitations to the deliverability of the implant. The first case of the PASCAL Repair System in the tricuspid position was reported in early 2018, and recently the compassionate use experience in 28 patients treated at 6 sites was published. Procedural success was 86%, there were no intraprocedural complications and 1.4 + 0.6 devices were implanted. At 30-day follow-up there was a reduction of TR to grade <2 in 85% and no intraprocedural complications. Additionally, mortality was 7.1%, 88% of patients with NYHA I-II, improvement in 6-Minute Walk Test from 240 to 335 m, with 2 single-leaflet device attachments. The PASCAL Repair System is currently undergoing further evaluation in the PASCAL Tricuspid Pivotal Trial (CLASP II TR) that randomizes symptomatic patients with severe TR to PASCAL or medical therapy (NCT04097145).

VALVE REPLACEMENT SYSTEMS

The distinctive characteristics of the tricuspid valve have precluded the widespread use of available transcatheter valves in the tricuspid position and have led to the development of dedicated tricuspid valve replacement systems. There are several devices in different stages of clinical development. At the time of this writing, a search on ClinicalTrial.gov using the search terms (1) "Tricupid valve regurgitation" and (2) "Transcatheter valve replacement" has led to the identification of 22 ongoing clinical trials. Our readers are encouraged to go through the list for additional details that are beyond the scope of this handbook (https://www.clinicaltrials.gov/search?cond=Tricuspid%20Valve%20Regurgitation&term=Transcatheter%20Valve%20Replacement. Access date:07/06/2023).

CAVAL IMPLANTATION SYSTEMS

Caval valve implantation (CAVI) has recently emerged as an alternative therapy for patients with tricuspid regurgitation. The concept is based on implanting transcatheter valves in the IVC and SVC to prevent backflow, reduce venous congestion and improve the associated symptoms. Also for CAVI, several devices are in different stages of clinical evaluation.

SUGGESTED READINGS

1. Asmarats L, Puri R, Latib A, Navia JL, Rodes-Cabau J. Transcatheter tricuspid valve interventions: landscape, challenges, and future directions. *J Am Coll Cardiol.* 2018;71(25):2935-2956.

2. Babaliaros VC, Greenbaum AB, Khan JM, et al. Intentional percutaneous laceration of the anterior mitral leaflet to prevent outflow obstruction during transcatheter mitral valve replacement: first-inHuman experience. *JACC Cardiovasc Interv.* 2017;10(8):798-809.

3. Besler C, Meduri CU, Lurz P. Transcatheter treatment of functional tricuspid regurgitation using the Trialign device. *Interv Cardiol.* 2018;13(1):8-13.

4. Blanke P, Naoum C, Dvir D, et al. Predicting LVOT obstruction in transcatheter mitral valve implantation: concept of the neo-LVOT. *JACC Cardiovasc Imaging.* 2017;10(4):482-485.

5. Bouleti C, Iung B, Himbert D, et al. Reinterventions after percutaneous mitral commissurotomy during long-term follow-up, up to 20 years: the role of repeat percutaneous mitral commissurotomy. *Eur Heart J.* 2013;34(25):1923-1930.

6. Braun D, Orban M, Orban M, et al. Transcatheter edge-to-edge repair for severe tricuspid regurgitation using the triple-orifice technique versus the bicuspidalization technique. *JACC Cardiovasc Interv.* 2018;11(17):1790-1792.

7. Carpentier A. Cardiac valve surgery—the "French correction." *J Thorac Cardiovasc Surg.* 1983;86(3):323-337.

8. Carroll JD, Feldman T. Percutaneous mitral balloon valvotomy and the new demographics of mitral stenosis. *J Am Med Assoc.* 1993;270(14):1731-1736.

9. Cohen DJ, Kuntz RE, Gordon SP, et al. Predictors of long-term outcome after percutaneous balloon mitral valvuloplasty. *N Engl J Med.* 1992;327(19):1329-1335.

10. Complications and mortality of percutaneous balloon mitral commissurotomy. A report from the National Heart, Lung, and Blood Institute Balloon Valvuloplasty Registry. *Circulation.* 1992;85:2014-2024.

11. Cribier A, Rath PC, Letac B. Percutaneous mitral valvotomy with a metal dilatator. *Lancet.* 1997;349(9066):1667.

12. Dahou A, Levin D, Reisman M, Hahn RT. Anatomy and Physiology of the tricuspid valve. *JACC Cardiovasc Imaging.* 2019;12(3):458-468.

13. Dean LS, Mickel M, Bonan R, et al. Four-year follow-up of patients undergoing percutaneous balloon mitral commissurotomy. A report from the National Heart, Lung, and Blood Institute Balloon Valvuloplasty Registry. *J Am Coll Cardiol.* 1996;28(6):1452-1457.

14. Fam NP, Braun D, von Bardeleben RS, et al. Compassionate use of the PASCAL transcatheter valve repair system for severe tricuspid regurgitation: a multicenter, observational, first-in-Human experience. *JACC Cardiovasc Interv.* 2019;12(24):2488-2495.

15. Feldman T, Herrmann HC, Inoue K. Technique of percutaneous transvenous mitral commissurotomy using the Inoue balloon catheter. *Cathet Cardiovasc Diagn.* 1994(suppl 2):26-34.

16. Feldman T, Foster E, Glower DD, et al. Percutaneous repair or surgery for mitral regurgitation. *N Engl J Med.* 2011;364(15):1395-1406.

17. Grayburn PA, Sannino A, Packer M. Proportionate and disproportionate functional mitral regurgitation: a new Conceptual Framework that reconciles the results of the MITRA-FR and COAPT trials. *JACC Cardiovasc Imaging.* 2019;12(2):353-362.

18. Hahn RT, Meduri CU, Davidson CJ, et al. Early feasibility study of a transcatheter tricuspid valve annuloplasty: SCOUT trial 30-day results. *J Am Coll Cardiol.* 2017;69(14):1795-1806.

19. Inoue K, Owaki T, Nakamura T, Kitamura F, Miyamoto N. Clinical application of transvenous mitral commissurotomy by a new balloon catheter. *J Thorac Cardiovasc Surg.* 1984;87(3):394-402.

20. Kuwata S, Taramasso M, Nietlispach F, Maisano F. Transcatheter tricuspid valve repair toward a surgical standard: first-in-man report of direct annuloplasty with a cardioband device to treat severe functional tricuspid regurgitation. *Eur Heart J.* 2017;38(16):1261.

21. Latib A, Grigioni F, Hahn RT. Tricuspid regurgitation: what is the real clinical impact and how often should it be treated? *EuroIntervention.* 2018;14(AB):AB101-AB111.

22. Levin TN, Feldman T, Bednarz J, Carroll JD, Lang RM. Transesophageal echocardiographic evaluation of mitral valve morphology to predict outcome after balloon mitral valvotomy. *Am J Cardiol.* 1994;73(9):707-710.

23. Lurz P, Besler C, Noack T, et al. Transcatheter treatment of tricuspid regurgitation using edge-to-edge repair: procedural results, clinical implications and predictors of success. *EuroIntervention.* 2018;14(3):e290-e297.

24. Maisano F, Taramasso M, Nickenig G, et al. Cardioband, a transcatheter surgical-like direct mitral valve annuloplasty system: early results of the feasibility trial. *Eur Heart J.* 2016;37(10):817-825.

25. McElhinney DB, Aboulhosn JA, Dvir D, et al. Mid-term valve-related outcomes after transcatheter tricuspid valve-in-valve or valve-in- ring replacement. *J Am Coll Cardiol.* 2019;73(2):148-157.

26. McKay RG, Lock JE, Safian RD, et al. Balloon dilation of mitral stenosis in adult patients: postmortem and percutaneous mitral valvuloplasty studies. *J Am Coll Cardiol*. 1987;9(4):723-731.

27. Nickenig G, Kowalski M, Hausleiter J, et al. Transcatheter treatment of severe tricuspid regurgitation with the edge-to-edge MitraClip technique. *Circulation*. 2017;135(19):1802-1814.

28. Nickenig G, Weber M, Lurz P, et al. Transcatheter edge-to-edge repair for reduction of tricuspid regurgitation: 6-month outcomes of the TRILUMINATE single-arm study. *Lancet*. 2019;394(10213):2002-2011.

29. Nishimura RA, Otto CM, Bonow RO, et al. 2014 AHA/ACC guideline for the management of patients with valvular heart disease: a report of the American College of Cardiology/American Heart Association Task Force on Practice Guidelines. *J Am Coll Cardiol*. 2014;63(22):e57-e185.

30. Obadia JF, Messika-Zeitoun D, Leurent G, et al. Percutaneous repair or medical treatment for secondary mitral regurgitation. *N Engl J Med*. 2018;379(24):2297-2306.

31. Otto CM, Davis KB, Holmes DR Jr., et al. Methodologic issues in clinical evaluation of stenosis severity in adults undergoing aortic or mitral balloon valvuloplasty. The NHLBI Balloon Valvuloplasty Registry. *Am J Cardiol*. 1992;69(19):1607-1616.

32. Patel JJ, Shama D, Mitha AS, et al. Balloon valvuloplasty versus closed commissurotomy for pliable mitral stenosis: a prospective hemodynamic study. *J Am Coll Cardiol*. 1991;18(5):1318-1322.

33. Reyes VP, Raju BS, Wynne J, et al. Percutaneous balloon valvuloplasty compared with open surgical commissurotomy for mitral stenosis. *N Engl J Med*. 1994;331(15):961-967.

34. Rodes-Cabau J, Hahn RT, Latib A, et al. Transcatheter therapies for treating tricuspid regurgitation. *J Am Coll Cardiol*. 2016;67(15):1829-1845.

35. Sanon S, Cabalka AK, Babaliaros V, et al. Transcatheter tricuspid valve-in-valve and valve-in-ring implantation for degenerated surgical prosthesis. *JACC Cardiovasc Interv*. 2019;12(15):1403-1412.

36. Schofer J, Siminiak T, Haude M, et al. Percutaneous mitral annuloplasty for functional mitral regurgitation: results of the CARILLON Mitral Annuloplasty Device European Union Study. *Circulation*. 2009;120(4):326-333.

37. Stone GW, Lindenfeld J, Abraham WT, et al. Transcatheter mitral-valve repair in patients with heart failure. *N Engl J Med*. 2018;379(24):2307-2318.

38. Taramasso M, Alessandrini H, Latib A, et al. Outcomes after current transcatheter tricuspid valve intervention: mid-term results from the International TriValve registry. *JACC Cardiovasc Interv*. 2019;12(2):155-165.

39. Turi ZG, Reyes VP, Raju BS, et al. Percutaneous balloon versus surgical closed commissurotomy for mitral stenosis. A prospective, randomized trial. *Circulation*. 1991;83(4):1179-1185.

40. Wang DD, Guerrero M, Eng MH, et al. Alcohol septal ablation to prevent left ventricular outflow tract obstruction during transcatheter mitral valve replacement: first-in-Man Study. *JACC Cardiovasc Interv*. 2019;12(13):1268-1279.

41. Williams AM, Bolling SF, Latib A. The five Ws of transcatheter tricuspid valve repair: who, what, when, where, and why. *EuroIntervention*. 2019;15(10):841-845.

34 Percutaneous Therapies for Aortic and Pulmonary Valvular Heart Disease[1]

PERCUTANEOUS AORTIC VALVE THERAPIES

After the initial introduction in 1960, and following improvements in device and surgical techniques, surgical aortic valve replacement (SAVR) became the cornerstone of therapy for both severe aortic valve regurgitation and stenosis. While SAVR is remarkably effective in ideal candidates, the surgery is still associated with a relatively high morbidity and mortality in older patients with geriatric syndromes like frailty, multimorbidity, and physical and cognitive dysfunction. The high morbidity and mortality associated with SAVR in high-risk patients led to the development of aortic valvuloplasty as a less invasive approach and more recently to the development of transcatheter aortic valve replacement (TAVR).

BALLOON AORTIC VALVULOPLASTY

Dilatation of the stenotic aortic valve, whether by surgical technique or by percutaneous balloon, has not enjoyed the same level of success as has balloon therapy for the pulmonic and mitral valves. Surgical mechanical dilatation of the stenotic adult aortic valve has been attempted since the 1950s, but the various valvulotomy approaches have failed to provide a significant solution for the problem of calcific aortic stenosis, and they have largely been abandoned in favor of AVR in eligible surgical or transcatheter candidates.

Noncalcific Aortic Stenosis

Considerable experience exists of using balloon aortic valvuloplasty (BAV) in children and adolescents with noncalcified congenital stenotic aortic valves, with excellent short-term and satisfactory long-term results. The predominantly fibrotic nature of these congenitally stenotic valves makes them well suited for balloon valvuloplasty (**Figure 34.1**). The procedure is effective 80% to 90% of the time, with a mortality rate of approximately 0.7%. Survival at 8 years has been reported as 95% with a need for repeat intervention of 25% at 4 years and 50% at 8 years. There may be a role for balloon valvuloplasty in the treatment of young adult patients without significant valve calcification. One study of young adults aged 17 to 40 years (mean age 23 years) with congenital aortic stenosis showed that balloon aortic valvuloplasty produced a significant reduction in the gradient across the aortic valve and an increase in the aortic valve area. In this series, there were no deaths or embolic cerebrovascular events. Intermediate follow-up at 38 months showed that 50% of patients required no further intervention. The absence of significant valve calcification is an important predictor of a good short- and long-term result.

Calcific Aortic Stenosis

The more typical patient encountered by the adult cardiologist is the older patient with acquired calcific aortic stenosis. Although experience with balloon valvuloplasty for this condition dates back to 1986, the procedure has a limited role at present

[1]We gratefully acknowledge the Grossman & Baim's *Cardiac Catheterization, Angiography, and Intervention*, 9th edition contributions of Drs. Abdulla A. Damluji, Wayne B. Batchelor, and Jon R. Resar as portions of their chapter, Percutaneous Therapies for Aortic and Pulmonary Valvular Heart Disease, were retained in this text.

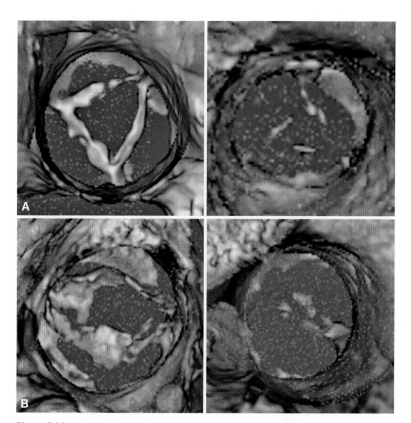

Figure 34.1 3D volume-rendering view of thickened leaflets in tricuspid and bicuspid aortic valve with normal controls. **A,** Noncalcific aortic leaflet thickening in a tricuspid patient **(on the left)** with a normal control **(on the right)**. **B,** Noncalcific aortic leaflet thickening in a bicuspid patient **(on the left)** with a normal control **(on the right)**. (Used with permission from Xiong TY, Feng Y, Liao YB, et al. Transcatheter aortic valve replacement in patients with non-calcific aortic stenosis. *EuroIntervention.* 2018;13(15):e1756-e1763.)

because of limited durability owing to the high rate of recurrence or restenosis. Virtually, all symptomatic patients with calcific aortic stenosis should undergo AVR as the treatment of choice. There are, however, specific settings where balloon valvuloplasty may play an important palliative role in patients who are poor candidates for immediate valve replacement. Balloon aortic valvuloplasty is useful in patients presenting with cardiogenic shock owing to aortic stenosis and can serve as a successful bridge to definitive valve replacement (surgical or transcatheter) in these hemodynamically unstable patients. It may also be used for palliation in patients with severe comorbid conditions or end-stage disease processes. While most patients with severe aortic stenosis in a compensated state can safely undergo noncardiac surgery, aortic balloon valvuloplasty can be used in selected patients if it is felt that more conservative medical therapy presents an excessive risk. Last, valvuloplasty may be useful as a diagnostic tool. Patients with low gradient, low cardiac output, and markedly depressed ejection fraction have poor outcomes with surgical valve replacement. Balloon valvuloplasty may be used to assess the potential for improvement in left ventricular function: those patients who do not improve represent a group that has underlying cardiomyopathy, while those who do improve after balloon dilatation generally have a good outcome with subsequent AVR. More recently, the indication for aortic balloon valvuloplasty has expanded with the introduction of TAVR; valvuloplasty predilatation before transcatheter aortic valve implantation in patients with *critical* aortic stenosis can be used as a bridge to TAVR. Also, predilatation of the aortic valve with aortic balloon valvuloplasty can be utilized as a component of the standard TAVR protocol (see below).

Mechanism of Improved Aortic Orifice Area

Postmortem and intraoperative dilatations have demonstrated how balloon aortic valvuloplasty improves the adult aortic valve with calcific degenerative aortic stenosis. Balloon dilatation increases the mobility of leaflets, thus enlarging the aortic valve orifice. The mechanism of dilatation appears predominantly to be fracturing of the calcific aortic valve nodules. In addition, in patients who have rheumatic disease with superimposed calcification, separation of postinflammatory fused commissures might contribute to the results of dilatation. The likely mechanism of restenosis is fusion of the cracks or crevices in calcific nodules on the aortic leaflets. The fractured calcific nodules may heal with fibrosis, which is probably the most common occurrence.

Technique

The retrograde aortic technique for balloon aortic valvuloplasty is the one most commonly used. One or both femoral arteries may be used. A 5F pigtail catheter is inserted from the left femoral artery and positioned in the ascending aorta for pressure monitoring and gradient determination. Right-sided heart catheterization is done from the left femoral vein. A balloon flotation thermodilution catheter is placed in the pulmonary artery, which remains there throughout the procedure to allow determination of the cardiac output. A second venous puncture may be "stacked" under the first for a 5F sheath for insertion of a temporary pacemaker, which is utilized for rapid right ventricular pacing during balloon inflation. Using the right femoral artery, a 6F sheath is introduced to allow left-sided heart catheterization to be performed. A 0.035 straight-tipped guidewire is used to cross the aortic valve, which is advanced through an angled pigtail catheter, a left Amplatz catheter, a Judkins right 4 catheter, or a specialized catheter designed to cross the aortic valve. The aortic valve gradient is measured, and the aortic valve area is determined using the Gorlin formula. Patients may be heparinized prior to any attempt to cross the aortic valve.

Following these prevalvuloplasty baseline measurements, an extra-stiff 0.035-in exchange-length (260-300 cm) guidewire, shaped with a pigtail or ram's horn curve at its tip, is inserted into the left ventricle. The wire tip can be shaped by pulling the wire between a finger and the edge of a hemostat, which helps it lie benignly in the left ventricular apex (without causing perforation or undue ventricular arrhythmia). However, this technique can potentially result in unraveling the distal ribbon of the guidewire. Precurved wires like the Safari (Boston Scientific, Marlborough, Massachusetts) and Confida (Medtronic, Minneapolis, Minnesota), are used frequently during routine structural heart procedures, including aortic balloon valvuloplasty. The previously placed left ventricular catheter is removed, and a 10F to 14F sheath is placed over this wire into the femoral artery, depending on the size and type of balloon that has been selected. Through the sheath, the previously prepared dilatation balloon is advanced over the guidewire. Under fluoroscopy and using 2 operators, the extra-stiff guidewire is kept in the left ventricle as the balloon valvuloplasty catheter is advanced and positioned to straddle the aortic valve. Using the proximal and distal markers of the balloon, the operator attempts to place the middle of the balloon at the level of the calcific aortic valve. **Figure 34.2** illustrates the unfilled balloon straddling the aortic valve.

In most normal-sized adult patients with an adequate aortic valve annulus, we begin with a 20- or 22-mm-diameter, 4- to 6-cm-long balloon. Measurement of the aortic annulus diameter from echocardiography, usually in a long-axis view, improves balloon size selection. A balloon-to-annulus ratio of about 1:1 based on 2-dimensional transthoracic echocardiographic or computed tomography (CT) measurements is desirable. In small or frail patients, the operator can start with an 18-mm balloon or (very rarely) a 15-mm balloon. The balloon is filled with a contrast medium diluted 9 to 1 using either a large syringe or an angioplasty end-deflator-type device. Care must be taken to maintain balloon position within the valve orifice to achieve an effective dilatation. The balloon catheter tends to jump either forward or backward with the force of ventricular systole. Therefore, the procedure is performed with rapid ventricular pacing. A pacing catheter is advanced into the right ventricle. Immediately before balloon inflation, rapid pacing at a rate between 180 and 220 beats/min is instituted. The rapid pacing results in a marked reduction in left ventricular ejection and prevents ejection of the balloon during inflation.

When the systemic pressure falls below 60 mmHg, the balloon can be inflated and will usually remain in a stable position within the annulus. Pacing should be used only for a minimum amount of time to avoid causing myocardial ischemia. Achievement of optimal balloon positioning, pacing, and balloon inflation requires significant coordination among the operators and the person running the pacemaker. The electrocardiogram (ECG) and the aortic pressure should be constantly monitored. If tolerated clinically, the balloon can be left inflated for 5 to 10 seconds. It is then withdrawn into the aorta as it begins to deflate, maintaining guidewire position in the left ventricle. Pulling the balloon back immediately after full infla-

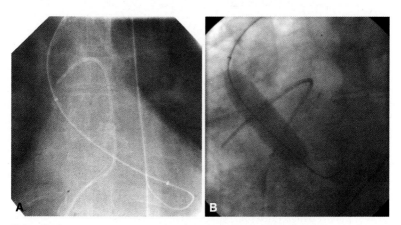

Figure 34.2 **A,** Anteroposterior projection shows passage of the deflated aortic valvuloplasty balloon across a stenotic aortic valve. Balloon markers are positioned in such a way that the balloon straddles the calcified aortic valve. **B,** Anteroposterior projection showing an inflated aortic valvuloplasty balloon across the stenotic aortic valve. The tip of the guidewire has been formed into a concentric curve to minimize the potential for left ventricular apical trauma.

tion is reached minimizes the duration of hypotension caused by obstruction of the aortic valve. A period of stabilization for blood pressure and ECG changes to return to baseline should be allowed before further dilatations.

It is often necessary to exert considerable force on these balloons to expand them fully and relieve the "waist" caused by the stenotic aortic valve, and it might be difficult to achieve full inflation of these large balloons using a 50-mL syringe. With the balloon connected to the 50-mL syringe with a short pressure tubing and a high-pressure stopcock, the sidearm of the stopcock can be attached to a 10-mL syringe filled with diluted contrast to boost the inflation after the larger syringe has been used to its maximal volume. After several dilatations with a single balloon, the balloon is withdrawn through the sheath, leaving the exchange-length, heavy-duty wire in place. It is frequently necessary to remove the arterial sheath along with the deflated valvuloplasty balloon, since valvuloplasty balloons do not always rewrap adequately to allow removal through the sheath.

A pigtail catheter is then reintroduced over the exchange-length guidewire back into the left ventricle, and measurements of the pressure gradient and cardiac output are repeated. The aortic valve area is calculated. Our usual goal is to achieve a valve area of at least 1 cm². If a desirable result has not been achieved, we may then change to a larger-diameter balloon and repeat the procedure (a 14F sheath may be necessary to accommodate a 23- to 26-mm balloon). If an adequate result is still not achieved, a dual-balloon technique (using a pair of 15- or 18-mm balloons if aortic annulus size permits) could be attempted, although this requires accessing the contralateral femoral artery for introduction of the second balloon. Of course, the potential for aortic insufficiency increases with larger balloon sizes. Pressure is monitored through the side arm of the large arterial sheath during the procedure. **Figure 34.3** illustrates the dual-balloon technique, and **Figure 34.4** shows the progressive reduction in gradient with single-balloon, followed by dual-balloon, valvuloplasty.

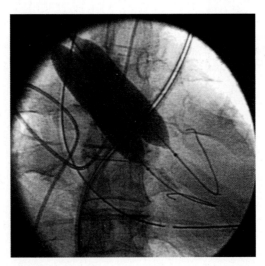

Figure 34.3 Balloon aortic valvuloplasty using the double-balloon technique in a 94-year-old woman who presented with syncope and heart failure. Full inflation of two 18-mm-diameter, 5.5-cm-long Scimed balloons across the stenotic aortic valve.

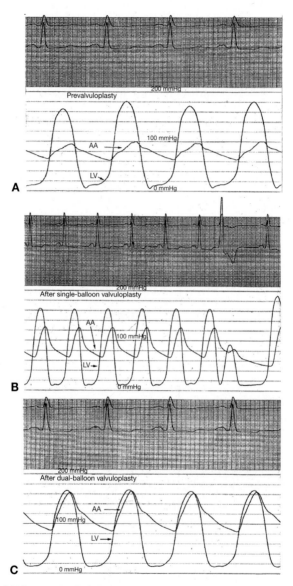

Figure 34.4 Balloon aortic valvuloplasty in an elderly patient with severe calcific aortic stenosis. **A,** Baseline pressure gradient across the stenotic aortic valve measured with one catheter in the left ventricle (LV) and a separate pigtail catheter in the ascending aorta (AA). There is a 58-mmHg mean gradient and an 80-mmHg peak-to-peak gradient across the valve. **B,** A reduction in the aortic valve gradient after a series of progressive single-balloon dilatations of the aortic valve. **C,** A marked reduction in aortic valve gradient after dual-balloon valvuloplasty.

Clinical Results and Complications

In the large Mansfield Scientific balloon aortic valvuloplasty registry, data were collected from 27 clinical centers across the United States and Europe from 6742 patients with calcific aortic stenosis undergoing balloon aortic valvuloplasty between 1986 and 1987. Balloon aortic valvuloplasty resulted in an increase in aortic valve area from 0.5 ± 0.18 to 0.81 ± 0.18 cm^2 and a decrease in mean aortic valve pressure gradient from 60 ± 24 to 30 ± 14 mmHg. There was also an accompanying increase in cardiac output from 3.86 ± 0.55 to 4.01 ± 0.51 L/min. Complications were experienced in 22.6% of patients, which included a procedural death rate of 4.9%, death within 7 days of 2.6%, emboli 2.2%, ventricular perforation 1.4%, and emergency AVR 1.2%. The NHLBI balloon valvuloplasty registry enrolled patients from 1987 to 1989 at 24 clinical centers. Similar results were obtained, with balloon aortic valvuloplasty increasing aortic valve area from 0.5 ± 2 to 0.8 ± 0.5 cm^2, decreasing aortic valve pressure gradient from 57 ± 30 to 29 ± 13 mmHg, and increasing cardiac output from 3.9 ± 1.2 to 4.1 ± 1.2 L/min. These results were reproduced in more contemporary data. In a study population of 262 patients with severe symptomatic aortic stenosis from January 2000 to December 2009, 301 balloon aortic valvuloplasty procedures were performed. The indication for BAV was mostly symptom relief, but 14% were performed for patients with cardiogenic shock or as a bridge to TAVR. The mean aortic valve area increased from 0.58 ± 0.3 to 0.96 ± 0.4 cm^2, decreasing the mean aortic valve pressure gradient from 46.3 ± 19.7 to 21.4 ± 12.4 mmHg and increasing cardiac output from 3.8 ± 1.1 to 4.1 ± 1.2 L/min. Despite the improved hemodynamic results, the mortality rate for patients who received aortic balloon valvuloplasty remains dismal (mortality rate 30%-50%) at a median follow-up period of 6 months.

The most common complication associated with aortic balloon valvuloplasty was local vascular injury, requiring surgical repair in 5.7% to 9.8% of patients. The requirement for transfusions has been significantly diminished by the use of percutaneous suture closure for the management of the large-caliber arterial puncture necessary for retrograde aortic valvuloplasty. Perclose (Abbott Cardiovascular, North Plymouth, MN) devices must be preplaced after arterial access is obtained. After placing a 6F or 8F sheath in the femoral artery, the sheath is exchanged for a Perclose device, the sutures of which are deployed but not tied. A wire is replaced in the Perclose device, and an exchange is made for a 12F or 14F sheath for valvuloplasty. At the conclusion of the procedure, a wire is replaced in the sheath so that vascular access can be protected while the Perclose knots are tied. If hemostasis is secure, the wire is removed and the knots are tightened. If hemostasis with Perclose fails, Angioseal can be deployed. In one report, this approach decreased the need for transfusions after aortic valvuloplasty from 23% to 0% of patients. Preclosure techniques may be used in the same manner for large-bore venous punctures for antegrade aortic valvuloplasty, mitral valvuloplasty, or pulmonic valvuloplasty. In addition, a figure-of-8 suture can also be used effectively to achieve hemostasis in large-bore venous punctures.

Long-Term Results

Restenosis with recurrent symptoms is common in the first year following balloon aortic valvuloplasty in an adult with calcific aortic stenosis. The mean duration of relief of symptoms is about 1 year. The 1-year survival rate in the Mansfield registry of 492 patients was 64%, with an event-free survival rate of 43%. Therefore, it must be emphasized that, when at all feasible, definitive AVR is the technique of choice for managing the adult patient with severe calcific aortic stenosis.

Short-term clinical improvements associated with balloon aortic valvuloplasty may be accompanied by improvement in systolic and diastolic left ventricular function in some patients. Patients with significantly depressed left ventricular function undergoing this procedure have a very poor long-term prognosis. In a cohort of patients with severe symptomatic aortic stenosis (New York Heart Association class IV and/or Canadian Cardiovascular Society functional class IV) and impaired left ventricular function (left ventricular ejection fraction of <40%) who underwent a total of 114 aortic balloon valvuloplasty from October 2012 to July 2015, a significant improvement of left ventricular ejection fraction was observed at 1-month follow-up (median +16%). The effect on improved left ventricular function was sustained up to 6 months of follow-up. In patients with cardiogenic shock who have been stabilized with successful balloon aortic valvuloplasty, cardiac surgery with definitive AVR or TAVR should be undertaken soon after stabilization. Patients with a good acute clinical response are most likely to benefit from TAVR.

PERCUTANEOUS VALVE REPLACEMENT AND REPAIR

Surgical valve replacement and repair has been the gold standard for valve disease for several decades. Recently, however, great progress has been made in adapting these surgical approaches to the percutaneous arena, and percutaneous valve replacement and repair today is one of the therapeutic options available for some patients with valvular heart disease.

PERCUTANEOUS PULMONIC VALVE REPLACEMENT

Percutaneous prosthetic treatment for pulmonic stenosis has been pioneered in children with congenital heart disease who have been previously treated with Fontan conduits in the pulmonary circulation. These conduits contain a porcine prosthetic valve that degenerates as the children age. Reoperation for degeneration of the pulmonic prosthetic valve is frequently necessary in patients who have already undergone 2 or 3 prior surgical procedures for their congenital heart disease. As a nonsurgical alternative, Bonhoeffer et al. pioneered the use of a bovine jugular venous valve prosthesis for stent delivery, which led to the development of implantable pulmonary valves. The Melody valve (Medtronic) has been approved in the United States for pediatric patients with dysfunctional right ventricular outflow tract (RVOT) conduits and with a clinical indication for intervention represented by either moderate/severe regurgitation or stenosis with a mean RVOT gradient of >35 mmHg. The valve is made from a cow's jugular vein valve sewn onto a metal stent. The Edwards Sapien valve is currently undergoing evaluation in clinical trials for intermediate-risk patients and for re-replacement in patients with degenerated tissue valves.

PERCUTANEOUS AORTIC VALVE REPLACEMENT

Although the results of aortic valvuloplasty as a standalone therapy have been disappointing, the results of percutaneous AVR have been outstanding. Cribier et al. in 2002 became the first to use equine pericardial leaflets placed on a balloon-expandable stent to treat aortic stenosis in older patients deemed nonsurgical or poor surgical candidates. Since then, the positive results of randomized clinical trials and registry analyses have led to the introduction in clinical practice of different types of valve prosthesis. In 2023, a variety of percutaneous devices are available in clinical practice: (1) balloon-expandable devices (Sapien XT and Sapien 3, Sapien 3 Ultra), and (2) self-expanding devices (CoreValve Evolut R, CoreValve Evolut PRO, Acurate Neo, Portico, Allegra) (**Figure 34.5**).

Valve Construction

The Edwards Sapien valve is made with bovine pericardial leaflets mounted on a balloon-expandable cobalt-chromium stent. It is currently available in 4 sizes in the

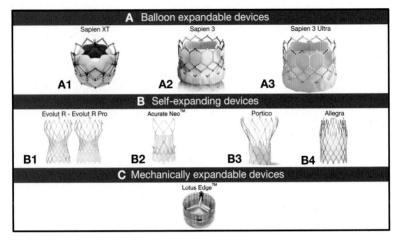

Figure 34.5 Percutaneous transcatheter aortic valve replacement devices approved in the United States and Europe. **A,** Balloon expandable devices: Sapien XT (A1), Sapien 3 (A2), Sapien 3 Ultra (A3). **B,** Self-expanding devices: Evolut R-Evolut R Pro (B1), Acurate Neo (B2), Portico (B3), Allegra (B4). **C,** Mechanically expandable devices: Lotus Edge.

United States: 20 mm for annulus size (CT) of 273 to 345 mm², 23 mm for annulus size (CT) ranging between 338 and 430 mm², 26 mm for annulus size (CT) ranging between 430 and 546 mm², and 29 mm for annulus size (CT) ranging between 540 and 683 mm². The Edwards Sapien valve has been approved for clinical use. A lower-profile delivery system (Sapien XT) was evaluated in the PARTNER II clinical trial, and it became available for clinical use in the United States (**Figure 34.6**). In June 2015, the FDA approved the Edwards Sapien 3 transcatheter heart valve, 20, 23, 26, and 29 mm, and associated delivery system (Edwards Commander delivery system) for high-surgical-risk patients. The indication was expanded to include patients at intermediate or greater risk for open surgery therapy (ie, predicted risk of surgical mortality >3% at 30 days) in 2016. Most recently, the indication was further expanded to include patients at low risk for SAVR in 2019, utilizing Edwards Sapien 3 or its design iteration Edwards Sapien 3 Ultra transcatheter heart valve system.

The Medtronic CoreValve is also made of porcine pericardial leaflets, although mounted on a self-expanding nitinol stent. The valve is approved for clinical use in several countries, including the United States. It is available in 23 mm size for annular perimeter (CT) ranging from 56.5 to 62.8, 26 mm size for annular perimeter (CT) ranging from 62.8 to 72.3, 29 mm size for annular perimeter (CT) ranging from 72.3 to 81.7, and 34 mm size for annular size ranging from 81.7 to 94.2 mm. Given their rather different characteristics and shapes, each valve has specific positioning within the aortic annulus. The Medtronic valve results in a supra-annular position of the neovalve leaflets.

The Abbott Portico valve is a self-expanding nitinol valve. The valve includes a cuff made from porcine pericardium sutured to the stent frame, which provides a sealing area for implantation, and 3 valve leaflets. The cuff and leaflet pericardial tissue is preserved and cross-linked in glutaraldehyde. In the United States, at the time of this writing, the Portico valve is indicated for transcatheter delivery in patients with symptomatic severe native aortic stenosis who are considered high surgical risk.

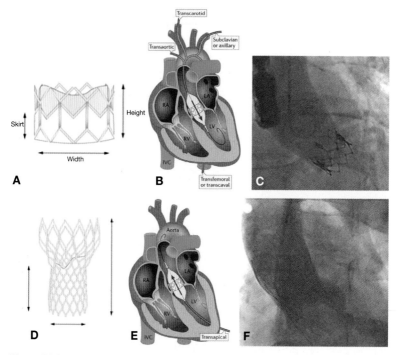

Figure 34.6 **A and D,** Edwards Sapien valve **(A)** and CoreValve **(D)**. **B and E,** Drawing showing the positioning within the aortic annulus of the Edward Sapien valve from the transfemoral retrograde approach **(B)** and the transapical antegrade approach **(E)**. **C and F,** Images of Edwards Sapien valve **(C)** and CoreValve **(F)** in actual use. IVC, inferior vena cava; LA, left atrium; LV, left ventricle; RA, right atrium; RV, right ventricle. (Reproduced with permission from van der Boon RM, Nuis RJ, van Mieghem NM, et al.
New conduction abnormalities after TAVI - frequency and causes. *Nat Rev Cardiol.* 2012;9:454-463.)

Patient Selection, Preparation, and Valve Delivery

TAVR presents a significant degree of complexity in terms of appropriate patient selection, identification of the optimal vascular access site for valve delivery, and accurate measurement of the aortic annulus for selection of the valve of appropriate size, in addition to the complexities related to aortic valvuloplasty and valve implantation.

Patient Selection

When compared with mechanical or bioprosthetic aortic valves approved for surgical implantation, data on percutaneous aortic valve durability are still limited. Therefore, current indications for TAVR include patients with severe symptomatic aortic stenosis at low, intermediate, or high risk for standard SAVR. Several risk calculators have been developed for the assessment of surgical risk in patients undergoing coronary artery bypass surgery and valve replacement (**Figure 34.7**). As of today, the Society of Thoracic Surgeons (STS) score and the EuroScore are the most widely used risk calculators. High risk is defined as a EuroScore of >20% or an STS score of >8%, or

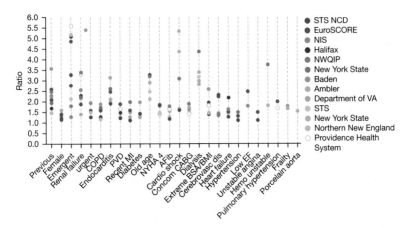

Figure 34.7 Odds ratio of the variables included in different surgical risk models. (Reproduced with permission from van Mieghem NM, Head SJ, van der Boon RMA, et al. The SURTAVI model: proposal for a pragmatic risk stratification for patients with severe aortic stenosis. *EuroIntervention*. 2012;8:258-266.)

presence of additional risk factors that might not be included in the EuroScore or STS score such as chest radiation therapy, porcelain aorta, hepatic cirrhosis, prior cardiac surgery, and any other major contraindication to open chest surgery. The STS score defines as intermediate risk patients with a predicted surgical mortality of 3% to 8% and as low risk those with a risk of <3%.

Choice of Delivery Approach

Both antegrade and retrograde techniques have been utilized for the delivery of the aortic valve prosthesis. The antegrade techniques include the transapical approach and the transvenous/transseptal approach. The retrograde techniques include the transfemoral, transsubclavian, transcarotid, transcaval, and direct transaortic approaches (**Figure 34.6**). Each approach has benefits and limitations. The profile of the aortic valve prosthesis was 24F in its initial iteration, which made the use of the antegrade transvenous approach attractive, although the delivery of a large prosthesis through the turns involved in traversing the left atrium and left ventricular apex en route to the aortic valve was difficult. The retrograde approach through the femoral artery was limited by the size of the femoral artery (minimum 7-8 mm) and by the presence of aortoiliac tortuosity and peripheral vascular disease. The introduction of second- and third-generation delivery systems has expanded the use of the retrograde approach by allowing the performance of retrograde femoral access in vessels of 5 mm minimal lumen diameter. The transcarotid, transcaval, transapical, and transaortic approaches have the advantage of overcoming remaining limitations, thus allowing treatment of patients who otherwise might not be suitable candidates for percutaneous valve replacement because of peripheral vascular disease or a small femoral artery. In addition, the antegrade transvenous or transapical approaches can be used successfully in patients with heavily calcified or "porcelain" aorta. However, when feasible, the transfemoral approach is preferred over a nontransfemoral approach due to observational studies suggesting lower vascular complications, major bleeding, and 30-day mortality. During TAVR planning, it is routine to obtain a

CT with inclusion of the distal aorta, iliac arteries, and femoral artery for assessment of minimum vessel diameter (from the femoral artery entry site to the aorta) as well as the presence of calcification and tortuosity.

Prosthesis Size Selection

Sizing of the aortic annulus and assessment of the aortic root are critical components in preparation for the procedure. They can be performed using transthoracic echocardiography and transesophageal echocardiography but mainly involve assessment by pre-TAVR CT. It should be noted that the aortic annulus has an oval shape, and therefore measurements should be obtained for the 2 perpendicular diameters. Once the measurements are obtained, a valve that is generally 10% to 20% larger than the measured diameter should be selected.

Deployment of the Valve

TAVR includes all the steps of aortic valvuloplasty described above, with the addition of insertion of a larger arterial sheath, insertion of another contralateral femoral (or radial) arterial sheath (5F or 6F) for placement of a pigtail catheter for thoracic aortography, and delivery of the valve itself.

Aortic valvuloplasty is occasionally performed in preparation for deployment of the valve. After removal of the valvuloplasty balloon, the valve delivery system is advanced over the guidewire and positioned across the aortic valve annulus. Thoracic aortography is generally performed to identify a coplanar view that lines up the leaflets and facilitates accurate valve placement. Appropriate positioning of the valve is critical, as a position of the valve either too high or too low can result in valve embolization, paravalvular leaks, an increased risk of heart block, or obstruction of the origin of a coronary artery. The optimal view is the view that places the aortic valve annulus on edge and that results in alignment of the coronary and noncoronary cusps on a single line. In the past, multiple views used to be obtained with aortography. The introduction of multimodality imaging and the ability to import CT images in the cardiac catheterization suite have markedly improved the ability to identify the ideal view for valve deployment (**Figure 34.8**). More

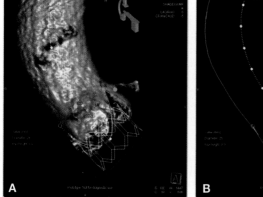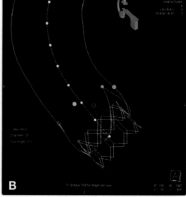

Figure 34.8 **A,** CT 3D reconstruction of the aortic arch and aortic annulus in preparation for transcatheter aortic valve replacement. The coronary and noncoronary cusps are aligned on a single line. **B,** Automatic segmentation and contouring of leaflet. (Courtesy of Mauricio Cohen, University of Miami.)

recently, 3-dimensional angiographic reconstruction of rotational aortic root angiography has emerged as a new modality for the identification of the optimal view for valve positioning in the cardiac catheterization laboratory.

Clinical Results

Patients at Extreme Surgical Risk The Placement of Aortic Transcatheter Valves (PARTNER) trial has provided landmark data on the effectiveness of TAVR. In the first cohort reported (PARTNER Cohort B), 358 patients with aortic stenosis who were not considered to be candidates for surgery (defined as >50% risk of death or other major adverse events at 30 days based on STS score) were randomized to medical therapy versus transcatheter aortic valve implantation with the Edwards Sapien valve. At 1-year follow-up, the mortality rate was 30.7% in the TAVR group when compared with 50.7% in the standard medical therapy group (hazard ratio [HR] with TAVR, 0.55; 95% confidence interval [CI], 0.40-0.74; P < .001). The benefit of TAVR was also observed when a combined endpoint including death from any cause or repeat hospitalization was analyzed (42.5% with TAVR vs 71.6% with standard therapy, P < .001) and when New York Heart Association functional class was evaluated.

Patients at High Surgical Risk In the PARTNER trial Cohort A, 699 patients with severe, symptomatic aortic stenosis and at high risk for traditional AVR (STS score >10%) were randomized to either the Edwards Sapien valve implantation via transfemoral or transapical delivery or the standard SAVR. The mortality rate was 3.4% in the transcatheter group and 6.5% in the surgical group (P = .07) at 30 days, and 24.2% and 26.8%, respectively, at 1 year (P = .44). A trend toward a higher rate of major stroke was observed in the TAVR group when compared with the surgical group at 30 days (3.8% vs 2.1%, P = .20) and 1 year (5.1% and 2.4%, respectively, P = .07). Major vascular complications were significantly more frequent with TAVR, while the incidence of major bleeding and atrial fibrillation was significantly higher in the surgical group. At 2-year follow-up, the noninferiority of TAVR when compared with conventional AVR was maintained.

The efficacy of TAVR utilizing the first-generation self-expanding CoreValve was demonstrated in the CoreValve Extreme Risk Pivotal Trial. Among the 795 randomized patients with increased surgical risk (ie, risk of death with 30 days after surgery was 15% as assessed by the Heart Team), 394 patients were assigned to the TAVR group and 401 were assigned to the conventional SAVR. The rate of death in the as-treated analysis was significantly better in the TAVR group than in the surgical group (14.2% vs 19.1%) with an absolute risk reduction of 4.9% (95% CI interval −0.4, P < 0.001 for noninferiority; P = 0.04 for superiority). There was a nonsignificant trend toward a lower incidence of stroke in the TAVR group when compared with the surgical group both at 30 days (4.9% vs 6.2%, respectively, P = .46) and at 1 year (8.8% and 12.6%, respectively, P = .10). These results were sustained at 2 and 5 years, respectively.

Patients at Intermediate Surgical Risk Following the evaluation of TAVR in high- and extreme-risk cohorts, TAVR was evaluated in intermediate-surgical-risk populations (STS predicted mortality of 3%-8%). The PARTNER 2A trial enrolled 2032 intermediate-risk patients (mean STS score 5.8%) with severe symptomatic aortic stenosis and randomized them to TAVR or surgical therapy. At 2-year follow-up, TAVR was noninferior to surgery with respect to the composite outcome of death from any cause or disability from stroke (HR 0.87, 95% CI 0.71, 1.09, P = .05). When the individual components of these composite outcomes were evaluated separately, the TAVR and surgical groups were similar with respect to death or stroke at 2 years. The SURTAVI trial enrolled 1746 patients with intermediate risk (mean STS score 4.5%) and randomized them to TAVR with a self-expanding bioprosthesis versus conventional SAVR. Similar to results obtained from PARTNER 2A trial, TAVR with self-expanding prosthesis (Medtronic CoreValve Systems) was noninferior to conventional surgery with similar rates of a composite endpoint of death or disabling stroke at 2 years (TAVR: 12.5% vs surgery: 14%, 95% CI for difference: −5.2 to 2.3). Analysis limited to individual outcomes showed that the rate of death (TAVR: 11.4% vs SAVR: 11.6%) and disability stroke (TAVR: 2.6% vs SAVR: 4.5%) were also similar at 2-year follow-up. Based on these results, the FDA granted commercial approval for the use of Sapien XT, Sapien 3, Sapien 3 Ultra, CoreValve Evolut R, and CoreValve Evolut Pro for intermediate-risk patients.

Patients at Low Surgical Risk Building on the results from the intermediate-risk cohort, TAVR has now extended to the low-risk patients. The PARTNER 3 trial enrolled 1000 patients at low surgical risk (mean STS score 1.9%) and randomized them to transfemoral TAVR with a balloon-expandable valve versus conventional surgery. At 1 year, TAVR showed a remarkable superiority over surgery regarding the primary composite outcome of death, stroke, or rehospitalizations (HR 0.54, 95% CI 0.37, 0.79, P = .001). Examination of each individual endpoint was mostly favorable toward TAVR, as compared with conventional SAVR. The overall death from any cause at 1 year was 1.0% for TAVR versus 2.5% for surgery (HR 0.41, 95% CI 0.14, 1.17). The self-expanding valve (Medtronic CoreValve Evolut R and Evolut Pro) was tested in a multinational, randomized, noninferiority clinical trial and compared with conventional surgery. Among the 1468 patients randomized in a 1:1 ratio, the mean STS score was 1.9%. At 2-year follow-up, the primary endpoint of death from any cause or disability stroke was similar between TAVR and surgery (TAVR 5.3% vs surgery 6.7%, 95% CI 4.4-9.6) rendering TAVR as a noninferior therapy to surgery (posterior probability of noninferiority >0.999). Similar to results obtained from PARTNER 3 trials, death from any cause was the same between TAVR and surgery (TAVR: 4.5% vs surgery: 4.5%), but the rate of stroke was significantly lower with TAVR (TAVR: 1.1% vs surgery: 3.5%, differences = 2.4% points, 95% CI −4.8 to 0.4). Based on these results, the FDA expanded the indication for TAVR to include patients at low risk for death or major complications associated with conventional surgery. The approval included both the balloon-expandable Sapien 3 and Sapien 3 Ultra and the self-expanding CoreValve Evolut R and Evolut PRO.

Additional Indications SAVR using bioprosthetic surgical devices remains the most utilized form of AVR procedures. Bioprosthetic valve failure is not uncommon and in severe forms of structural valve dysfunction may lead to valve reintervention. In one study, the rate of redo-valve intervention was 7.3% at 10 years. The advent of TAVR technology has introduced an additional line of therapy for those with degenerated heart valves. In a multinational valve-in-valve registry that included 459 patients with degenerated bioprosthetic valves who underwent valve-in-valve procedures using self-expandable CoreValve (Medtronic) and balloon-expandable Edwards Sapien devices (Edwards LifeSciences), the mechanism of failure was stenosis in 39% of cases, regurgitation in 30% of cases, and mixed disease accounted for 30% of cases. The overall survival rate at 1 year was 83.2%, and predictors of mortality were small surgical bioprosthesis (<21 mm) and baseline stenosis. Risks associated with valve-in-valve TAVR procedures include coronary obstruction, a rare event that is associated with increased risk of mortality.

Predictors of coronary obstructions include the distance between the virtual ring and the coronary ostia (VTC—valve to coronary ring ostia <4 mm), externally mounted bioprosthetic valve leaflets, stentless bioprosthetic valves, bioprosthetic valve fracture, and absent coronary filling on balloon aortic valvuloplasty angiography. Bioprosthetic or native aortic scallop intentional laceration to prevent iatrogenic coronary artery obstruction during TAVR (BASILICA), which is a novel transcatheter technique, was shown to be feasible and effective in preventing coronary artery obstruction in high-risk patients. Other valve-in-valve procedural complications include valve thrombosis, high residual gradients, and paravalvular leak. While valve-in-valve is a promising therapy for failed surgical and transcatheter heart valve, it is only approved in high- or extreme-risk patients. Longer-term outcomes for valve-in-valve patients are yet to be determined, and while uncommon, complications of this form of transcatheter therapy represent a significant challenge in clinical practice.

Guideline Recommendations

In 2017, the American Heart Association and the American College of Cardiology published a focused update on the clinical guidelines for patients with valvular heart disease. In that document, TAVR is considered class IA as a treatment for symptomatic patients with severe aortic stenosis (stage D) and prohibitive or high-risk for SAVR. The most recent guideline recommendations have changed, and they now reflect the clinical trial evidence for patients at low to intermediate risk (**Figure 34.9**).

Special Clinical Scenarios

As TAVR extends to the low-surgical-risk populations, many unique or challenging clinical scenarios have emerged. For example, in cases of poor expected survival due to other concomitant medical conditions or the presence of severe forms of geriatric impairment (frailty or physical dysfunction), the utilization of TAVR to prolong life and relieve symptoms becomes more challenging. The presence of concomitant valvular heart disease, like severe mitral or tricuspid valve regurgitation, seems to impair the efficacy of TAVR to improve health outcomes and health-related quality of life. In these cases, percutaneous therapies for mitral or tricuspid valve disease may be an option, but these therapies were not evaluated in randomized trials. The presence of concomitant coronary artery disease is a frequent encounter in patients with severe symptomatic aortic stenosis, but most patients with noncritical disease are managed medically.

It is only in patients with severe impairments to the coronary circulations (eg, left main or 3-vessel disease with proximal left anterior descending artery involvement) percutaneous revascularizations could be considered. Other special situations related to the size of the annulus and coronary height are more frequently encountered now with the extended indication of TAVR to the low-risk group by the FDA. Very small or very large annulus or the presence of low coronary ostium may impair the utilization of TAVR, and surgery could be considered instead when such challenging clinical scenarios arise in clinical practice.

Complications

The complications of TAVR include complications related to the aortic valvuloplasty and those related to the valve implantation. Vascular complications are the most common. Additional complications include stroke, valve embolization (extremely rare), aortic annulus rupture, obstruction of the origin of a coronary artery (very rare), development of paravalvular leaks, and development of complete heart block, requiring permanent pacemaker placement. Permanent pacing may be needed in up to 20% of patients receiving the self-expanding CoreValve device and 10% in patients receiving the Sapien S3 device (**Table 34.1**).

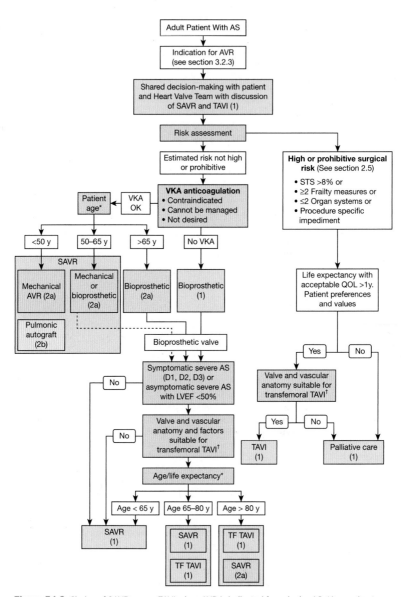

Figure 34.9 Choice of SAVR versus TAVI when AVR is indicated for valvular AS. *Approximate ages, based on US Actuarial Life Expectancy tables, are provided for guidance. The balance between expected patient longevity and valve durability varies continuously across the age range, with more durable valves preferred for patients with a longer life expectancy. Bioprosthetic valve durability is finite (with shorter durability for younger patients), whereas mechanical valves are very durable but require lifelong anticoagulation. Long-term (20-y) data on outcomes with surgical bioprosthetic valves are available; robust data on transcatheter bioprosthetic valves

Figure 34.9 Continued

extend to only 5 y, leading to uncertainty about longer-term outcomes. The decision about valve type should be individualized on the basis of patient-specific factors that might affect expected longevity. †Placement of a transcatheter valve requires vascular anatomy that allows transfemoral delivery and the absence of aortic root dilation that would require surgical replacement. Valvular anatomy must be suitable for placement of the specific prosthetic valve, including annular size and shape, leaflet number and calcification, and coronary ostial height. AS, aortic stenosis; AVR, aortic valve replacement; LVEF, left ventricular ejection fraction; QOL, quality of life; SAVR, surgical aortic valve replacement; STS, Society of Thoracic Surgeons; TAVI, transcatheter aortic valve implantation; TF, transfemoral; VKA, vitamin K antagonist. (Reprinted with permission from: Otto CM, Nishimura RA, Bonow RO, Carabello BA, Erwin JP, Gentile F, et al. 2020 ACC/AHA guideline for the management of patients with valvular heart disease: a report of the American College of Cardiology/American Heart Association Joint Committee on Clinical Practice Guidelines. *Circulation*. 2021;143(5):e72-e227. ©2020 American Heart Association, Inc.).

Follow-Up

Structural Valve Degeneration While structural valve degeneration is an important risk for transcatheter heart valves, the durability of these valves were bench tested, and the tests found excellent nominal and nonnominal valve deployments to 1 billion and 200 million cycles. Sathananthan et al. tested the 20-, 23-, 26-, and 29-mm-sized balloon-expandable Sapien S3 using nominal and nonnominal deployment. Although the number of cycles represents 25 years of valve wear with excellent durability, concerns regarding long-term (ie, >10-year follow-up) valve degeneration exist. In the intermediate term, data from the PARTNER I trial showed no structural valve deterioration requiring surgery at 5 years. In the Medtronic CoreValve device trials, the incidence of midterm prosthesis failure at 5 years was 1.4%.

Anticoagulation and Subclinical Leaflet Thrombosis Valve leaflet thickening and reduced leaflet motions are occasionally observed after TAVR or conventional SAVR. These structural changes can occur without hemodynamic effects. These structural phenomena are called hypoattenuating leaflet thickening and hypoattenuation affecting motion on CT. In one pooled analysis, the incidence of hypoattenuating leaflet thickening was noted in up to 38% of patients and the incidence of the more severe hypoattenuation affecting motion in up to 20% of cases. Anticoagulation does not appear to have a beneficial effect against these structural valve changes. The Galileo trial (ClinicalTrials.gov Identifier: NCT02556203) aimed to evaluate the efficacy of rivaroxaban (10 mg once a day) and aspirin (75-100 mg once daily) versus the conventional antiplatelet therapy of clopidogrel (75 mg once daily) and aspirin (75-100 mg once daily) within the first 90 days after randomization. The primary outcome was death or first thromboembolic event through study completion. The study cohort consisted of 1644 patients who received TAVR and were free of atrial fibrillation at baseline. After 17 months, the incidence rate of death or a first thromboembolic event was higher in the rivaroxaban group versus the antiplatelet group (9.8 vs 7.2 per 100 person-years, HR 1.45: 95% CI 1.01-1.81, $P = .04$). In addition, major, disabling, or life-threatening bleeding occurred more in the rivaroxaban group. Given this increased risk, the trial was stopped prematurely and new anticoagulation therapy after TAVR is not recommended for bioprosthetic transcatheter valves. In clinical practice, the use of dual-antiplatelet therapy was derived from the protocols of the original PARTNER trials.

Until more evidence regarding the best anticoagulation strategy is devised, the current recommendation is to use dual-antiplatelet therapy (aspirin plus clopidogrel) for 3 to 6 months for patients who do not have other indications for oral anticoagulation.

Table 34.1 Rates of Major Complications in Pivotal Clinical Trials Comparing TAVI and SAVR

Trial (Population)	N	All Stroke (%)	Disabling Stroke (%)	TIA (%)	Major Vascular Complications (%)	Life-Threatening/ Disabling Bleeding (%)	AKI (%)	New AF (%)	Pacemaker Implantation (%)
PARTNER 1A (TAVI Population)[44]	348	5.5	3.8	0.9	11.0	9.3	2.9	8.6	3.8
PARTNER 1A (SAVR Population)[44]	351	2.4	2.1	0.3	3.2	19.5	3.0	16.0	3.6
CoreValve High-Risk (TAVI Population)[54]	390	4.9	3.9	0.8	5.9	13.6	6.0	11.7	19.8
CoreValve High-Risk (SAVR Population)[54]	357	6.2	3.1	0.3	1.7	35.0	15.1	30.5	7.1
PARTNER IIA (TAVI Population)[57]	994	5.5	3.2	0.9	7.9	10.4	1.3	9.1	8.5
PARTNER IIA (SAVR Population)[57]	1021	6.1	4.3	0.4	5.0	43.4	3.1	26.4	6.9

(Continued)

Table 34.1 Rates of Major Complications in Pivotal Clinical Trials Comparing TAVI and SAVR (Continued)

Trial (Population)	N	All Stroke (%)	Disabling Stroke (%)	TIA (%)	Major Vascular Complications (%)	Life-Threatening/ Disabling Bleeding (%)	AKI (%)	New AF (%)	Pacemaker Implantation (%)
PARTNER S3I Intermediate-Risk (TAVI Population)[75]	1077	2.7	1.0	NA	5.6	5.4	0.5	5.0	10.2
SURTAVI (TAVI Population)[58]	864	3.4	1.2	1.5	6.0	12.2	1.7	12.9	25.9
SURVATI (SAVR Population)[58]	794	5.6	2.5	1.1	1.1	9.3	4.4	43.4	6.6
NOTION (TAVI Population)[76]	145	2.8	1.4	1.4	5.6	11.3	0.7	16.9	34.1
NOTION (SAVR Population)[76]	135	3.0	3.0	0	1.5	20.9	5.7	57.8	1.6

AF, atrial fibrillation; AKI, acute kidney injury; SAVR, surgical aortic valve replacement; TAVI, transcatheter aortic valve implantation; TIA, transient ischemic attack.
Adapted with permission from Jones BM, Krishnaswamy A, Tuzcu EM, et al. Matching patients with the ever-expanding range of TAVI devices. *Nat Rev Cardiol.* 2017;14(10): 615-626. doi:10.1038/nrcardio.2017.82.

SUGGESTED READINGS

1. Adams DH, Popma JJ, Reardon MJ. Transcatheter aortic-valve replacement with a self-expanding prosthesis. *N Engl J Med.* 2014;371(10):967-968.

2. Bagur R, Rodes-Cabau J, Gurvitch R, et al. Need for permanent pacemaker as a complication of transcatheter aortic valve implantation and surgical aortic valve replacement in elderly patients with severe aortic stenosis and similar baseline electrocardiographic findings. *JACC Cardiovasc Interv.* 2012;5:540-551.

3. Barbanti M, Petronio AS, Ettori F, et al. 5-year outcomes after transcatheter aortic valve implantation with CoreValve prosthesis. *JACC Cardiovasc Interv.* 2015;8:1084-1091.

4. Batchelor W, Patel K, Hurt J, et al. Incidence, prognosis and predictors of major vascular complications and percutaneous closure device failure following contemporary percutaneous transfemoral transcatheter aortic valve replacement. *Cardiovasc Revasc Med.* 2020;21(9):1065-1073, S1553-8389(20)30016-6. doi:10.1016/j.carrev.2020.01.007

5. Ben-Dor I, Pichard AD, Satler LF, et al. Complications and outcome of balloon aortic valvuloplasty in high-risk or inoperable patients. *JACC Cardiovasc Interv.* 2010;3(11):1150-1156.

6. Bleiziffer S, Ruge H, Horer J, et al. Predictors for new-onset complete heart block after transcatheter aortic valve implantation. *JACC Cardiovasc Interv.* 2010;3(5):524-530.

7. Bonhoeffer P, Boudjemline Y, Saliba Z, et al. Percutaneous replacement of pulmonary valve in a right-ventricle to pulmonary-artery prosthetic conduit with valve dysfunction. *Lancet.* 2000;356(9239):1403-1405.

8. Bonhoeffer P, Boudjemline Y, Qureshi SA, et al. Percutaneous insertion of the pulmonary valve. *J Am Coll Cardiol.* 2002;39(10):1664-1669.

9. Bonow RO, Carabello BA, Chatterjee K, et al; American College of Cardiology/American Heart Association Task Force on Practice Guidelines. 2008 focused update incorporated into the ACC/AHA 2006 guidelines for the management of patients with valvular heart disease: a report of the American College of Cardiology/American Heart Association Task Force on Practice Guidelines (writing committee to revise the 1998 guidelines for the management of patients with valvular heart disease). Endorsed by the Society of Cardiovascular Anesthesiologists, Society for Cardiovascular Angiography and Interventions, and Society of Thoracic Surgeons. *J Am Coll Cardiol.* 2008;52(13):e1-e142.

10. Brown JM, O'Brien SM, Wu C, Sikora JA, Griffith BP, Gammie JS. Isolated aortic valve replacement in North America comprising 108,687 patients in 10 years: changes in risks, valve types, and outcomes in the Society of Thoracic Surgeons National Database. *J Thorac Cardiovasc Surg.* 2009;137(1):82-90.

11. Chieffo A, Buchanan GL, van Mieghem NM, et al. Transcatheter aortic valve implantation with the Edwards SAPIEN versus the medtronic CoreValve revalving system devices: a multicenter collaborative study. The PRAGMATIC plus initiative (Pooled- RotterdAm-Milano-Toulouse in Collaboration). *J Am Coll Cardiol.* 2013;61(8):830-836.

12. Cribier A, Savin T, Saoudi N, Rocha P, Berland J, Letac B. Percutaneous transluminal valvuloplasty of acquired aortic stenosis in elderly patients: an alternative to valve replacement? *Lancet.* 1986;1(8472):63-67.

13. Dangas GD, Tijssen JGP, Wohrle J, et al; GALILEO Investigators. A controlled trial of rivaroxaban after transcatheter aortic-valve replacement. *N Engl J Med.* 2020;382(2):120-129.

14. Daniec M, Nawrotek B, Sorysz D, et al. Acute and long-term outcomes of percutaneous balloon aortic valvuloplasty for the treatment of severe aortic stenosis. *Catheter Cardiovasc Interv.* 2017;90(2):303-310.

15. Dvir D, Webb JG, Bleiziffer S, et al. Transcatheter aortic valve implantation in failed bioprosthetic surgical valves. *J Am Med Assoc.* 2014;312(2):162-170.

16. Edelman JJ, Khan JM, Rogers T, et al. Valve-in-valve TAVR: state-of- the-art review. *Innovations.* 2019;14(4):299-310.

17. Feldman T, Carroll JD, Chiu YC. An improved catheter design for crossing stenosed aortic valves. *Cathet Cardiovasc Diagn.* 1989;16(4):279-283.

18. Genereux P, Head SJ, Wood DA, et al. Transcatheter aortic valve implantation: 10-year anniversary part II. Clinical implications. *Eur Heart J.* 2012;33(19):2399-2402.

19. Genereux P, Webb JG, Svensson LG, et al; PARTNER Trial Investigators. Vascular complications after transcatheter aortic valve replacement: insights from the PARTNER (Placement of AoRTic TraNscathetER Valve) trial. *J Am Coll Cardiol.* 2012;60(12):1043-1052.

20. Gleason TG, Reardon MJ, Popma JJ, et al; CoreValve U.S. Pivotal High Risk Trial Clinical Investigators. 5-year outcomes of self-expanding transcatheter versus surgical aortic valve replacement in high-risk patients. *J Am Coll Cardiol.* 2018;72(22):2687-2696.

21. Holmes DR Jr., Nishimura RA, Reeder GS. In-hospital mortality after balloon aortic valvuloplasty: frequency and associated factors. *J Am Coll Cardiol.* 1991;17(1):189-192.

22. Koziarz A, Makhdoum A, Butany J, Ouzounian M, Chung J. Modes of bioprosthetic valve failure: a narrative review. *Curr Opin Cardiol.* 2020;35(2):123-132.

23. Leon MB, Smith CR, Mack M, et al; PARTNER Trial Investigators. Transcatheter aortic-valve implantation for aortic stenosis in patients who cannot undergo surgery. *N Engl J Med.* 2010;363(17):1597-1607.

24. Leon MB, Smith CR, Mack MJ, et al; PARTNER 2 Investigators. Transcatheter or surgical aortic-valve replacement in intermediaterisk patients. *N Engl J Med.* 2016;374(17):1609-1620.
25. Mack MJ, Leon MB, Smith CR, et al; PARTNER 1 trial investigators. 5-year outcomes of transcatheter aortic valve replacement or surgical aortic valve replacement for high surgical risk patients with aortic stenosis (PARTNER 1): a randomised controlled trial. *Lancet.* 2015;385(9986):2477-2484.
26. Mack MJ, Leon MB, Thourani VH, et al; PARTNER 3 Investigators. Transcatheter aortic-valve replacement with a balloon-expandable valve in low-risk patients. *N Engl J Med.* 2019;380(18):1695-1705.
27. Malkin CJ, Judd J, Chew DP, Sinhal A. Balloon aortic valvuloplasty to bridge and triage patients in the era of trans-catheter aortic valve implantation. *Catheter Cardiovasc Interv.* 2013;81(2):358-363.
28. Moreno PR, Jang IK, Newell JB, Block PC, Palacios IF. The role of percutaneous aortic balloon valvuloplasty in patients with cardiogenic shock and critical aortic stenosis. *J Am Coll Cardiol.* 1994;23(5):1071-1075.
29. Moretti C, Chandran S, Vervueren PL, et al. Outcomes of patients undergoing balloon aortic valvuloplasty in the TAVI Era: a multicenter registry. *J Invasive Cardiol.* 2015;27(12):547-553.
30. Nishimura RA, Otto CM, Bonow RO, et al. 2017 AHA/ACC focused update of the 2014 AHA/ACC guideline for the management of patients with valvular heart disease: a report of the American College of Cardiology/American Heart Association task force on clinical practice guidelines. *J Am Coll Cardiol.* 2017;70(2):252-289.
31. O'Neill WW. Predictors of long-term survival after percutaneous aortic valvuloplasty: report of the mansfield scientific balloon aortic valvuloplasty registry. *J Am Coll Cardiol.* 1991;17(1):193-198.
32. Otto CM, Nishimura RA, Bonow RO, et al. 2020 ACC/AHA guideline for the management of patients with valvular heart disease: a report of the American College of Cardiology/American Heart Association Joint Committee on clinical practice guidelines. *Circulation.* 2021;143(5):e72-e227.
33. Percutaneous balloon aortic valvuloplasty. Acute and 30-day follow-up results in 674 patients from the NHLBI Balloon Valvuloplasty Registry. *Circulation.* 1991;84:2383-2397.
34. Petronio AS, De Carlo M, Bedogni F, et al. 2-year results of CoreValve implantation through the subclavian access: a propensity-matched comparison with the femoral access. *J Am Coll Cardiol.* 2012;60(6):502-507.
35. Piazza N, Grube E, Gerckens U, et al. Procedural and 30-day outcomes following transcatheter aortic valve implantation using the third generation (18 Fr) corevalve revalving system: results from the multicentre, expanded evaluation registry 1-year following CE mark approval. *EuroIntervention.* 2008;4(2):242-249.
36. Popma JJ, Deeb GM, Yakubov SJ, et al; Evolut Low Risk Trial Investigators. Transcatheter aortic-valve replacement with a self-expanding valve in low-risk patients. *N Engl J Med.* 2019;380(18):1706-1715.
37. Reardon MJ, Adams DH, Kleiman NS, et al. 2-year outcomes in patients undergoing surgical or self-expanding transcatheter aortic valve replacement. *J Am Coll Cardiol.* 2015;66(2):113-121.
38. Reardon MJ, Van Mieghem NM, Popma JJ, et al; SURTAVI Investigators. Surgical or transcatheter aortic-valve replacement in intermediate-risk patients. *N Engl J Med.* 2017;376(14):1321-1331.
39. Rodriguez-Gabella T, Voisine P, Puri R, Pibarot P, Rodes-Cabau J. Aortic bioprosthetic valve durability: incidence, mechanisms, predictors, and management of surgical and transcatheter valve degeneration. *J Am Coll Cardiol.* 2017;70(8):1013-1028.
40. Rosenfeld HM, Landzberg MJ, Perry SB, Colan SD, Keane JF, Lock JE. Balloon aortic valvuloplasty in the young adult with congenital aortic stenosis. *Am J Cardiol.* 1994;73(15):1112-1117.
41. Safian RD, Mandell VS, Thurer RE, et al. Postmortem and intraoperative balloon valvuloplasty of calcific aortic stenosis in elderly patients: mechanisms of successful dilation. *J Am Coll Cardiol.* 1987;9(3):655-660.
42. Sager SJ, Damluji AA, Cohen JA, et al. Transient and persistent conduction abnormalities following transcatheter aortic valve replacement with the Edwards-Sapien prosthesis: a comparison between antegrade vs. retrograde approaches. *J Interv Card Electrophysiol.* 2016;47(2):143-151.
43. Sathananthan J, Hensey M, Landes U, et al. Long-term durability of transcatheter heart valves: insights from bench testing to 25 years. *JACC Cardiovasc Interv.* 2020;13(2):235-249.
44. Smith CR, Leon MB, Mack MJ, et al; PARTNER Trial Investigators. Transcatheter versus surgical aortic-valve replacement in high-risk patients. *N Engl J Med.* 2011;364(23):2187-2198.
45. Sondergaard L, De Backer O, Kofoed KF, et al. Natural history of subclinical leaflet thrombosis affecting motion in bioprosthetic aortic valves. *Eur Heart J.* 2017;38(28):2201-2207.
46. Thourani VH, Kodali S, Makkar RR, et al. Transcatheter aortic valve replacement versus surgical valve replacement in intermediate-risk patients: a propensity score analysis. *Lancet.* 2016;387(10034):2218-2225.
47. Thyregod HG, Steinbruchel DA, Ihlemann N, et al. Transcatheter versus surgical aortic valve replacement in patients with severe aortic valve stenosis: 1-year results from the All-Comers NOTION Randomized Clinical Trial. *J Am Coll Cardiol.* 2015;65(20):2184-2194.
48. van der Boon RM, Nuis RJ, Van Mieghem NM, et al. New conduction abnormalities after TAVI—frequency and causes. *Nat Rev Cardiol.* 2012;9(8):454-463.

35 Peripheral Intervention[1]

Management of patients with carotid, renal, or peripheral arterial disease (PAD) is complex. It requires not only excellent technical skills but also a full understanding of the natural history of the disease, of therapeutic options, and of the risk and benefit associated with any procedure.

CAROTID ARTERIES

Carotid endarterectomy (CEA) has long been considered the gold standard for carotid artery intervention. In the last 50 years since CEA was initially reported, significant technical advancements have improved morbidity, mortality, cost, and patient comfort. It was only after 40 years of widespread application of CEA, however, that definitive proof of its benefit was obtained. The landmark North American Symptomatic Carotid Endarterectomy Trial (NASCET) and Asymptomatic Carotid Atherosclerosis Study (ACAS) investigations demonstrated that surgical endarterectomy, when performed for carotid bifurcation disease by experienced vascular surgeons on appropriately selected patients, effectively reduced the likelihood of ipsilateral stroke compared with standard medical therapy in both symptomatic and asymptomatic patients, respectively.

Clinical trials have provided level I evidence for CEA for both symptomatic and asymptomatic patients with severe carotid disease. However, these studies have been limited by a number of factors. First, the patients selected for these trials were low to moderate risk. For example, the presence of severe coronary artery disease or heart failure was an exclusion for many of these trials. Furthermore, medical therapy in that era was limited to aspirin and occasional lipid-lowering agents. Therefore, contemporary data for CEA versus medical therapy are currently not available pending completion of the CREST-2 trial. Lastly, myocardial infarction (MI), a well-known complication of CEA, has not been included in the composite endpoints in any of these trials.

Because of the limitations and the need for general anesthesia in many cases, a less invasive approach was developed. In 2001, Roubin published a 5-year single-center follow-up of 528 consecutive patients undergoing carotid stenting, with a 98% success rate, 1.6% mortality, and a combined endpoint of death and stroke of 7.4% at 30-day follow-up. Of note, the rate of stroke decreased significantly over the 5-year study period, from 7.1% within the first year to 3.1% in the fifth year. This was felt to reflect improvements in technique, interventional devices, and pharmacotherapy. The seminal work of Roubin and colleagues highlighted the need for randomized controlled studies to determine the optimal treatment strategy.

The first such randomized controlled trial was the Carotid and Vertebral Artery Transluminal Angioplasty Study (CAVATAS) trial. In this study, the procedure included stent insertion in only 26% of cases with the remainder of patients being treated with balloon angioplasty alone. Distal protection was not available. Despite these limitations, the immediate and long-term results of angioplasty and endarterectomy were equivalent. Subsequently, smaller studies confirmed the benefits of carotid stenting, although the potential for distal embolization and consequent stroke

[1]We gratefully acknowledge the *Grossman & Baim's Cardiac Catheterization, Angiography, and Intervention,* 9th edition contributions of Drs Joseph D. Campbell, Samir R. Kapadia, and Mehdi H. Shishehbor, as portions of their chapter, Peripheral Intervention, were retained in this text.

remained a limiting factor (**Table 35.1**). To address this concern, distal protection devices were developed to minimize or prevent distal embolization.

The first randomized trial comparing carotid stenting with embolic protection to CEA was the Stenting and Angioplasty with Protection in Patients at High Risk for Endarterectomy (SAPPHIRE) trial. The SAPPHIRE study randomized 307 patients from 29 centers to either carotid artery stenting (CAS) with distal protection or CEA. Entry criteria included asymptomatic carotid stenosis (>80% by ultrasound) or symptomatic stenosis (>50%), plus at least 1 feature placing the patient at higher risk for surgical endarterectomy. These features included age older than 80 years, the presence of congestive heart failure, severe chronic obstructive pulmonary disease, previous endarterectomy with restenosis, previous radiation therapy or radical neck surgery, or lesions distal or proximal to the usual cervical location. At 30 days, the major adverse clinical events were reduced by more than 50% with CAS as compared with surgery (5.8% for CAS, 12.6% for CEA, $P = .047$). Interestingly, 408 patients in the SAPPHIRE study were deemed inappropriate for CEA and were therefore enrolled in the stent arm. Only 7 patients were deemed inappropriate for CAS.

More recently, 5 additional randomized trials have evaluated the role of CEA versus CAS (**Table 35.2**). These trials collectively failed to show equivalency between CAS and CEA, instead reported a significantly higher 30-day stroke risk with CAS as compared with CEA. Unfortunately, these data resulted in the Center for Medicare and Medicaid Services (CMS) limiting the use of CAS for asymptomatic high-risk individuals only, despite widespread criticism of the results being heavily biased by lack of operator experience and suboptimal embolic protection device (EPD) use. On the contrary to the above European trials, the National Institutes of Health (NIH)-sponsored Carotid Revascularization Endarterectomy versus Stenting Trial (CREST), which had strict criteria regarding operator experience and EPD use, showed equivalent 30-day outcome between CEA and CAS for the composite endpoint of death, stroke, and MI. In this trial, CEA was associated with higher rates of periprocedural

Table 35.1 **Comparison of Periprocedural and 30-d Risk Associated With Carotid Endarterectomy and Stenting**[a]

Characteristics	Carotid Endarterectomy	Carotid Artery Stenting
Periprocedural myocardial infarction	↑↑	↓
Periprocedural minor stroke	↓	↑
Periprocedural major stroke	=	=
Cranial nerve damage	↑↑	↓
Wound complications	↑	↓
Requirement for general anesthesia	↑↑	↓
Longer recovery	↑	↓

[a]Arrow indicates increased or decreased incidence when comparing carotid endarterectomy with stenting.

Table 35.2 Outcomes (30 d) of Selected Contemporary Randomized Trials of Carotid Endarterectomy vs Stenting

Trial[a]	n	Year	EPD (%)	Symptomatic (%)	Death		Stroke		Myocardial Infarction	
					CEA (%)	CAS (%)	CEA (%)	CAS (%)	CEA (%)	CAS (%)
SAPPHIRE	334	2004	96	29	2.5	1.2	3.1	3.6	6.1	2.4
EVA-3S	527	2008	92	100	0.1	0.1	3.5	9.2	0.8	0.4
SPACE	1200	2008	27	100	0.9	0.7	6.2	7.5	NR	NR
ICSS	1713	2010	72	100	0.8	2.3	4.1	7.7	0.4	0.6
CREST	2502	2010	96	53	0.3	0.7	2.3	4.1	2.3	1.1
ACT 1	1453	2016	98	0	0.3	0.1	1.4	2.8	0.9	0.5

[a]CAS, carotid artery stenting; CEA, carotid endarterectomy; CREST, Carotid Revascularization Endarterectomy Versus Stenting Trial; EPD, embolic protection device; EVA-3S, Endarterectomy Versus Stenting in Patients with Symptomatic Severe Carotid Stenosis; ICSS, International Carotid Stenting Study; NR, not reported; SAPPHIRE, Stenting and Angioplasty with Protection in Patients at High Risk for Endarterectomy; SPACE, Stent-Protected Angioplasty Versus Carotid Endarterectomy.

MI and cranial nerve damage, whereas CAS had a higher incidence of minor stroke. The 10-year follow-up data for CREST demonstrated no difference between the CAS of CEA groups with regard to the primary outcome or with regard to postprocedural ipsilateral stroke rates. Similar to CREST, the Randomized Trial of Stent versus Surgery for Asymptomatic Carotid Stenosis (ACT 1) demonstrated noninferiority between CEA and CAS with regard to the composite primary outcome of death, stroke, or MI within 30 days of the index procedure or ipsilateral stroke within 1 year in asymptomatic patients not deemed high risk for surgical complications.

Collectively, the data from randomized clinical trials to date support that clinical and anatomic features in addition to operator experience should guide the best revascularization strategy in patients with severe carotid disease (**Table 35.3**). How modern-day optimal medical therapy will influence the incremental benefit of surgical or endovascular carotid revascularization is the subject of the ongoing CREST-2 trial.

Treatment Considerations and Technique

Preprocedural Evaluation

A thorough history should be obtained to elucidate symptom status, relevant cardiovascular risk factors, and other comorbid conditions that might influence treatment decisions. This is done in conjunction with a full neurologic examination performed by an individual certified in the NIH stroke scale. A baseline carotid duplex is done, and if intervention is being considered, cross-sectional imaging with either a computed tomography angiogram (CTA) or magnetic resonance angiogram (MRA) should be obtained. Once revascularization is deemed necessary, clinical and anatomical features need to be considered and a decision regarding the best approach should be made in conjunction with the patient and family. In patients scheduled for CAS, premedication with aspirin and clopidogrel (at least 300 mg prior to intervention with sufficient time to achieve efficacy) in addition to consideration of prehydration to minimize hypotension has been advocated.

Angiographic Evaluation

Arch aortography is performed under digital subtraction in the left anterior oblique (LAO) 30° to 40° projection. In this image, the patient's head should be turned toward the right and tilted upward. Arch aortography is important in identifying the aortic arch anatomy (whether it is type I, II, or III), which will impact the endovascular approach and the selection of appropriate catheters in order to engage the carotid arteries (**Figure 35.1**). In addition, the takeoff of carotid and vertebral arteries should be examined. Other factors, such as degree of calcification, tortuosity, presence of ostial common carotid or innominate artery disease, and involvement of the external carotid artery may affect the procedural approach and success (**Figure 35.2**). Subsequently, using appropriate diagnostic catheters such as 5F angled glide, Vertebral, JR4 for type I arch and Vitek, Simmons, or JB2 for more challenging anatomy, selective 2-vessel (or 4-vessel if indicated) cerebral angiography is performed after the patient is fully anticoagulated. When performing selective angiography, the patient's head should be secured to the table using carotid head gear. Images in the ipsilateral 30° to 40° and lateral projections should be obtained. Formal measurements must be made of the target lesion using NASCET criteria where distal reference is used beyond the carotid bulb. Intracranial cerebral angiography should be routinely performed at baseline in the anteroposterior cranial and lateral projections to rule out intracerebral arterial abnormalities and to establish the baseline arterial anatomy (**Figure 35.3**). Of particular importance in baseline diagnostic angiography are the lesion morphology, degree of distal vessel tortuosity, presence of collateral flow, patency of the circle of Willis, and dominance of the intracerebral arterial supply.

Table 35.3 Clinical and Anatomical Characteristics that May Favor Carotid Endarterectomy or Stenting

Characteristics	Endarterectomy	Stenting
Clinical		
Age ≥ 70 y		++
Age < 70 y	++	
Congestive heart failure (class III/IV)		++
Ejection fraction < 35%		++
Planned open heart surgery		++
Recent myocardial infarction (<4-6 wk)		++
Unstable angina		++
Severe pulmonary disease		++
Contralateral cranial nerve injury		++
Symptomatic carotid disease	++	
Intolerance to antiplatelet therapy	++	
Inability to tolerate conscious sedation	++	
Low carotid volume operator/center	++	
Anatomical		
High-cervical lesion (≥C2)		++
Restenosis after previous endarterectomy		++
Ostial/below clavicle lesions		++
Contralateral carotid occlusion		++
Post neck radiation		++
Prior radical neck surgery		++
Severe tandem lesions		++
Spinal immobility of the neck		++
Type III aortic arch	++	
Heavily calcified lesion	++	
Significant thrombus burden	++	
Redundant internal carotid artery	++	
Significant common carotid artery disease	++	

++ refers to generally preferred revascularization strategy based upon given clinical or anatomical variable.

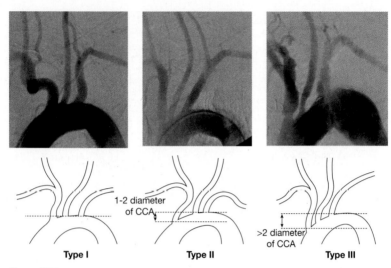

Figure 35.1 Aortic arch and the takeoff of great vessels are important aspects of carotid and cerebral intervention. Shown here are the 3 arch types. Note, in addition to arch type, careful attention should be given to the presence of severe ostial common carotid and innominate disease. CCA, common carotid artery.

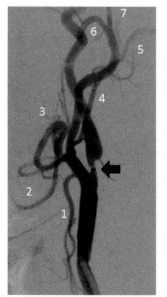

Figure 35.2 Note the presence of severe internal carotid artery disease (*black arrow*). Branches of external carotid artery are outlined. (1) Superior thyroid artery, (2) lingual artery, (3) facial artery, (4) ascending pharyngeal artery, (5) occipital artery, (6) internal maxillary artery, and (7) superficial temporal artery. (Adapted from Krishnaswamy A, Klein JP, Kapadia SR. Clinical cerebrovascular anatomy. *Catheter Cardiovasc Interv*. 2010;75(4):530-539.)

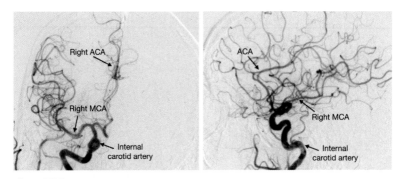

Figure 35.3 Right internal carotid artery cerebral angiogram showing middle and anterior cerebral arteries. ACA, anterior cerebral artery; MCA, middle cerebral artery. (Adapted from Krishnaswamy A, Klein JP, Kapadia SR. Clinical cerebrovascular anatomy. *Catheter Cardiovasc Interv*. 2010;75(4):530-539.)

Carotid Angioplasty and Stenting Procedure

A list of available equipment for carotid angioplasty and stenting is provided in **Tables 35.4** and **35.5**. The femoral approach is typically used, although the radial approach in selected cases is possible and may be preferred (ie, right internal carotid artery [ICA] lesion with bovine arch). Almost all devices are 6F compatible, allowing the use of an 80-cm-long nonkinkable sheath (ie, Cook Shuttle, Destination, Pinnacle, or ArrowFlex sheaths). Unlike a 90-cm sheath, the 80-cm sheaths are compatible with standard bailout equipment that are typically 100 cm long. A telescoping system for carotid artery intervention is typically used. A 5F-long diagnostic catheter is placed inside a sheath once the sheath has already been advanced to the mid descending aorta. Once the patient is fully anticoagulated, the carotid artery of interest is engaged using the diagnostic catheter. Subsequently, the glidewire is carefully advanced into the external carotid artery. Occasionally, the wire is left in distal common carotid artery under close watch not to accidently touch the lesion with sheath manipulation. The sheath is advanced up to the ostium of the innominate or left common carotid artery. The 5F diagnostic catheter is then advanced to the distal common or external carotid artery holding the wire and sheath in place.

The sheath is then advanced over the diagnostic catheter. The process may require several iterations of advancing catheters and removing slack from the system to achieve final positioning. Once a desired location is reached, the glidewire and catheter are slowly removed to prevent air trapping. One should never cross the carotid lesion with a 0.035-in wire or diagnostic catheters.

Certain safety precautions are necessary for CAS procedures: (1) Catheters should always be bled back to avoid any air or cholesterol embolization. (2) Anticoagulation and antiplatelet therapy should commence prior to advancing any catheters into the carotid system. (3) Less time in the carotid system is better. Although one should be cautious and deliberate in the performance of these procedures, the number of complications increases with additional intra-arterial time. (4) Catheter advancement should always be over a wire, and larger catheters should be transitioned in a stepwise, coaxial fashion over smaller catheters. (5) CAS procedures should not be done if proximal or distal protection is not possible. In select cases, it is appropriate to predilate an ICA lesion with a 2.0-mm balloon in order to facilitate the passage of an EPD. (6) Only

Table 35.4 Currently Available Distal and Proximal Cerebral Protection Devices

Distal Protection

Device	Diameter (mm)	Pore Size (μm)	Manufacturer
Guardwire	Balloon occlusion	–	Medtronic
FiberNet	3.5-5, 5-6, 6-7	40	Medtronic
Accunet OTW Accunet RX	4.5, 5.5, 6.5, 7.5	120	Abbott Laboratories
Emboshield NAV[6]	2.5-4.8, 4-7	140	Abbott Laboratories
Angioguard XP Angioguard Rx	4, 5, 6, 7, 8	100	Cordis
FilterWire EZ	4.5, 5.5, 6.5	100	Boston Scientific
Spider	3, 4, 5, 6, 7	50-200	Covidien
Gore Embolic Filter	5, 7	100	Gore

Proximal Protection

Gore Flow Reversal	Reversal of flow	–	Gore
Mo.Ma	Flow clamping	–	Medtronic

Table 35.5 Currently Available Self-Expanding Carotid Stents

Stent	Metal Composition	Design	Tapered	Manufacturer
AccuLink[a]	Nitinol	Open cell	Yes	Abbott Laboratories
X-Act[a]	Nitinol	Closed cell	Yes	Abbott Laboratories
Cristallo Ideale	Nitinol	Hybrid	Yes	Medtronic
Zilver	Nitinol	Open cell	No	Cook
Protégé[a]	Nitinol	Open cell	No	Covidien
Precise[a]	Nitinol	Open cell	No	Cordis
Exponent[a]	Nitinol	Open cell	No	Medtronic
WALLSTENT[a]	Cobalt chromium	Closed cell	No	Boston Scientific

[a]US Food and Drug Administration–approved carotid stents.

atraumatic guidewires should be advanced into the ICA to minimize the risk of spasm or dissection. (7) Predilation is recommended to confirm the ability to adequately dilate the stenosis. (8) The use of self-expanding (SE) stents is preferred for the carotid bifurcation and other compressible sites. Balloon-expandable (BE) stents should be used only for aorto-ostial carotid lesions and distal (eg, intracranial) ICA lesions. (9) When encountering resistance during advancement of balloons or stent delivery systems, removal and redilation with lower-profile devices is appropriate.

If an SE stent will not easily cross a predilated lesion, it should not be forced. (10) Careful periprocedural hemodynamic monitoring is essential. Manipulation within the area of the carotid sinus can cause both acute and prolonged hypotension and bradycardia, requiring fluid resuscitation, atropine, or adrenergic agents. Pacing is rarely needed but should be readily available. In most cases, atropine should be administered prophylactically to mitigate this. Postprocedural hypertension must also be avoided, so as to minimize the chances of hyperperfusion syndrome, a potentially devastating entity that is occasionally seen following revascularization, particularly in elderly patients with previous near-occlusion and underperfused cerebral circulation. (11) Postdilation should be performed to relatively low or nominal pressure using no more than a 5-mm noncompliant balloon. It is not necessary to completely eliminate the stenosis to achieve an excellent result. Indeed, attempts to reduce the stenosis to 0% relative to the reference segment significantly increase the risk of distal embolization, dissection, or resistant hypotension relating to carotid body stimulation or compression. (12) When retrieving a distal EPD, care must be taken not to force the retrieval catheter through the proximal stent edge or ICA. If there is difficulty with passage, often gentle neck rotation will solve the problem. In select cases, alternate catheters may be required. Note that there is occasionally mild spasm at the site of the EPD deployment, and this does not require further treatment. (13) If a proximal protection device is being used, the interventional team should be mindful of the stump pressure and carefully monitor neurologic status, especially in patients with compromised collateral reserve. Often, early signs of impending neurologic compromise may be as simple as the patient yawning, and these must be promptly recognized as such. In the setting of clinically evident cerebral ischemia (ie, new deficit or seizure), it is critical that the team remain calm. If needed, the patient's head and neck should be supported. The timing of this relative to the procedural sequence will dictate whether the procedure should be efficiently completed or if temporary cessation of proximal protection is needed to allow for recovery (after appropriate aspiration of debris from the carotid according to standard technique) prior to completing the case.

Stent Selection

If not all, the majority of stents used for carotid disease are nitinol SE stents. Whether open- or closed-cell design will have an important clinical significance is not well known. Newer hybrid stents, where the middle of the stent is closed cell but ends are open, are being developed. In general, the closed cell design stents are more rigid (**Table 35.5**), which is relevant in tortuous vessel segments as these rigid stents can result in kinking of the vessel.

Distal Protection

The combination of carotid stenting with distal protection has revolutionized carotid intervention (**Table 35.4**). The first randomized trial demonstrating outstanding results of carotid stenting with distal protection was the SAPPHIRE trial, and this was quickly followed by several registries like ARCHeR and SECuRITY. In general, cerebral protection devices function either by filtering atheromatous debris out of the flowing blood distal to the lesion or by occluding antegrade flow proximal or distal to the lesion to allow removal of atheromatous debris. Each design has relative merits and potential disadvantages. The filtering devices allow for continuous visualization for precise stent placement and allow cerebral perfusion as antegrade blood flow is unobstructed. The current filter pore size ranges from 80 to 150 μm, raising the question of what diameter of atheromatous debris is required to cause neurologic sequelae. The occluding devices, by design, limit visualization and, in the absence of adequate collateral circulation, may result in prolonged cerebral ischemia. Retrograde embolization to the aortic arch may occur if aggressive injection is performed. However, occluding devices offer the theoretical advantage of protecting against a wider range of particulate sizes. The optimal protection device or combination of protection device and stent remains unclear and is a source of intense clinical investigation.

Complications

The most feared complication of carotid stenting is stroke at the time of the procedure. This complication most frequently happens from distal embolization prior to placement of the EPDs or potential overload of the filters. Manipulation of the catheters and wires to place the sheath in the common carotid artery should be done in a deliberate but delicate manner. Proper selection of patients and equipment is critical to prevent such complications. If the filter is filled and there is slow flow in the carotid, aspiration of the proximal column of blood is necessary prior to filter retrieval. Cerebral angiogram has to be carefully assessed for vessel cutoff. Depending on the size and location of the cutoff, wiring of the lesions or other techniques can be used to minimize the size of infarction. Sometimes glycoprotein IIb/IIIa inhibitors can be useful in this situation. Intracranial hemorrhage is another complication that can be devastating. One cause of this is cerebral hyperperfusion, which may be prevented by careful blood pressure monitoring in most cases. Wire-related hemorrhage should be preventable by proper techniques.

Aside from access site–related complications, the most common carotid stenting complications are bradycardia and hypotension. The primary operator should be extremely careful during the procedure as cerebral hypoperfusion due to bradycardia and hypotension may result in seizure activity and sudden movement by the patient. Securing the devices during predilation, stenting, and postdilation is therefore important. In general, bradycardia is transient and improves on its own. Occasionally, atropine or adrenergic drugs might be required for the management of bradycardia and hypotension.

VESSELS OF THE AORTIC ARCH
Subclavian, Common Carotid, and Innominate Arteries

Atherosclerosis is commonly the cause of stenosis in the subclavian and great vessels. However, other conditions such as giant cell arteritis, Takayasu arteritis, and fibromuscular dysplasia (FMD) should be considered. Disease of the subclavian and innominate arteries is frequently asymptomatic. However, patients may occasionally present with subclavian steal or upper limb ischemia (**Figure 35.4**). Less frequently, patients with prior coronary bypass surgery with in situ internal mammary artery (IMA) grafts may experience angina due to severe subclavian disease. In patients with bilateral subclavian disease in whom accurate blood pressure measurement is important, intervention to one side may also be appropriate (**Table 35.6**).

In general, angioplasty and stenting of the great vessels are the preferred primary approaches; however, when there is total occlusion with extensive ostial calcification, surgery (carotid-subclavian, aortosubclavian, or axilloaxillary bypass or endarterectomy) may be the best option. Stent fracture in patients with severe calcification and

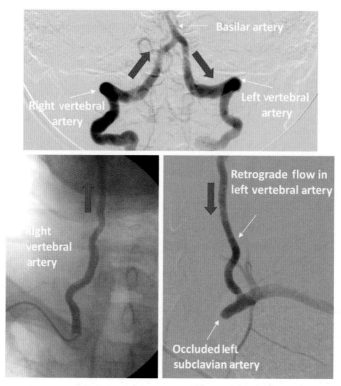

Figure 35.4 Left subclavian steal syndrome. Red arrows show direction of flow. Flow is antero-grade in the right vertebral artery and retrograde in the left vertebral artery. Note, totally occluded left subclavian artery.

ostial disease can occur, and it is usually not associated with significant clinical man-ifestations, but it may increase the likelihood of restenosis. In general, intervention to the great vessels has a success rate of greater than 90% with a low complication rate. Primary stenting may further improve these results; however, it may not be possible in heavily calcified total or subtotal occlusions. No randomized comparison between surgery and stenting for great vessels is available; however, observational studies directly comparing surgery to an endovascular approach showed a stroke risk of 3%, mortality of 2%, and an overall complication rate of 13% with surgery; the stent series had 0% stroke, 0% death, and 6% overall complications rates. The recurrence rate was 12% for the surgical series and 3% for the stent series.

Treatment Considerations and Technique

Understanding the patient's symptoms and whether they relate to great vessel disease is essential to prevent inappropriate intervention. Bilateral blood pressures should be obtained, and palpation of upper extremity pulses should be performed. Auscul-tation for bruits is important, but their absence does not negate the presence of great vessel disease. In our clinic, the first test to confirm great vessel stenosis or occlusion is a noninvasive duplex ultrasound evaluation. In this examination, the presence of

Table 35.6	Indication for Subclavian, Common Carotid, and Innominate Artery Revascularization
Vertebrobasilar insufficiency	
Bilateral vertebral artery stenosis	
Subclavian steal syndrome	
Before and after coronary bypass surgery to improve blood flow into left or right internal mammary artery	
Disabling upper extremity claudication	
Inability to obtain accurate blood pressure	
Preservation of inflow to axillary graft or dialysis conduit	
Blue digit syndrome (embolization to fingers)	
Asymptomatic severe stenosis (peak systolic velocity >275 cm/s) of the innominate or left common carotid artery	

elevated velocities, flow turbulence, and bidirectional or retrograde ipsilateral verte-bral artery flow may indicate a subclavian or innominate artery stenosis. If there is a clinical suggestion of vasculitis, an erythrocyte sedimentation rate or C-reactive pro-tein should be measured. Frequently, CTA of the arch and great vessels is performed to help with the interventional approach. Once a decision regarding intervention has been made, premedication with aspirin is standard, with addition of clopidogrel.

The choice of access site is dependent on location of the lesion, involvement of the ostium, stenosis versus occlusion, and visualization of great vessels. In most cases, either a radial artery approach or a femoral artery approach will be sufficient. However, dual access may be beneficial in the setting of total occlusions to facilitate lesion crossing or in cases where precise stent positioning relative to branch vessels is needed. In the latter case, the radial access will help with dye injection and stent positioning, which will allow precise stent placement without jailing the vertebral, right common carotid, or internal mammary artery. When starting the intervention, the first step is to perform an arch aortogram in the LAO projection at 30° to 40°. This will provide a "road map" prior to gaining selective access into the subclavian or innominate artery. If needed, a selective RAO caudal angiogram can be helpful to separate the right common carotid and right subclavian bifurcation. For subclavian intervention via a femoral approach, a telescoping technique with a 5F diagnostic catheter inside a 6F sheath is typically used. After the lesion is crossed, the diagnostic catheter and the sheath are then advanced over the wire. From the radial approach, a 6F hydrophilic 55-cm sheath can be placed proximal to the lesion, which can facil-itate contrast injection and support for lesion crossing. Either a 0.014- or 0.018-in workhorse peripheral wire or a 0.035-in angled 90-cm braided microcatheter for additional support can be used to start. If needed, stiffer 0.018-in chronic total occlu-sion (CTO) wires, a nested 0.018-in braided microcatheter, or 0.035-in wires, such as stiff-angled glide or glide advantage wires, may be necessary to cross difficult lesions. After crossing, intervention may be pursued via a radial approach, or if needed, the wire can be externalized via a femoral sheath and intervention can be then pursued via that approach. Once the lesion is crossed and adequately predilated, an appropriate stent is then chosen. SE stents are reserved for distal locations. Balloon-expanding stents are better for lesions extending from the ostium to the origin of the vertebral artery. Inflation of the balloon for about a minute will reverse the flow in the vertebral artery, and this technique can be used to minimize embolization to the brain. Embolic prevention devices are typically not used in subclavian interventions. Occasionally, covered stents are chosen for highly calcified lesions or in the setting of in-stent restenosis (ISR).

For innominate and common carotid artery interventions an 8F guide catheter is used. In most laboratories, these interventions are almost always performed with carotid distal embolic protection.

Before stenting the great vessels, predilation using a 4- to 6-mm balloon is advisable. This will help to ensure that the stent will fully expand and also may help with stent size selection. Intravascular ultrasound (IVUS) may also be selectively used if needed for stent sizing. Some operators suggest crossing the lesion with the sheath and then unsheathing the stent in order to prevent stent dislodgment and embolization. However, with the newer stents, this may not be necessary, and it may actually be less traumatic to cross the lesion with the stent than with the guide or sheath. When using covered stents, it is also notable to recognize that aggressive postdilation may result in foreshortening, so ensuring adequate margins for lesion coverage is crucial to achieving optimal results. For lesions located beyond the internal mammary artery, SE stents should probably be used to avoid dissection and possibly late stent compression by extravascular structures. Stents should be postdilated to match the size of the subclavian artery (generally between 5 and 8 mm). Overdilation should be avoided to minimize the risk of dissection that might extend into the vertebral or internal mammary artery or rupture with intrathoracic bleeding. If such dissections do occur, they can often be salvaged by placement of a stent within the origin of the affected branch vessel, although distal extension of the dissection within the branch vessel may render attempts at salvage futile. Following postdilatation, pressure gradients may be repeated to demonstrate complete elimination of the gradient.

In general, a postprocedural duplex ultrasound is obtained. Resolution of symptoms is the best marker to monitor; bilateral arm blood pressure measurements are also usually recommended and are a simple bedside test to assess patency. Restenosis within subclavian arteries occurs in 10% to 20% of patients and may be treated by stenting (if not stented initially), drug-coated balloon angioplasty (for ISR), or covered stent placement. Stent compression or fracture may occur. If clinically relevant, these can be treated by balloon reexpansion, angioplasty with a drug-coated balloon, restenting, and even placement of an SE stent within the old BE stent; however, data regarding these approaches are limited.

Complications

Complications associated with great vessel intervention may include problems at the access site, as well as inadvertent "jailing," dissection, or embolization of the vertebral or left internal mammary arteries, which may require balloon angioplasty.

RENAL ARTERIES

Renal artery stenosis (RAS) is a common manifestation of generalized atherosclerosis; however, its treatment has been extremely controversial. In general, RAS can lead to resistant hypertension via the renin-angiotensin-aldosterone system or lead to ischemic nephropathy. While theoretically RAS should be treated to prevent renal ischemia, randomized trials to date have not shown a significant benefit from renal artery intervention to prevent progression of renal failure. However, the trials conducted to date have been criticized for including patients with stenosis of less than 70% and for including individuals not at risk of renal ischemia or resistant hypertension (**Table 35.7**).

The current gold standard for renal artery intervention is endovascular therapy with balloon angioplasty and stenting.

Fibromuscular Dysplasia

FMD is a nonatherosclerotic, noninflammatory disorder of unknown etiology that constitutes the second most common cause of RAS after atherosclerosis. It typically affects women from 15 to 50 years of age and is more common in first-degree relatives and in the presence of the ACE-I allele. FMD can also involve carotid and peripheral arteries, although renal artery involvement is seen in 60% of cases of FMD, with frequent bilateral involvement. Progressive renal stenosis is seen in 37% of cases and loss of renal mass in 63%. FMD has a distinctive angiographic appearance, with a beaded, aneurysmal pattern (**Figure 35.5**). Medical management of hypertension is frequently successful; however, due to high rates of procedural success, elimination of hypertension, and low recurrence rate (10%),

Table 35.7 Randomized Trials of Renal Artery Stenting for Renal Artery Revascularization vs Medical Therapy[a]

Study	n	Year	Indication	Angioplasty Alone (%)	Blood Pressure Outcome	Renal Function Outcome
EMMA	59	1998	HTN with unilateral RAS	91	NS	–
SNRASCG	55	1998	Resistant HTN	80	–	NS
DRASTIC	106	2000	Resistant HTN	96	NS	–
ASTRAL	803	2009	Resistant HTN unexplained CRI	7.0	NS	NS
STAR	138	2009	CRI	1.6	NS	NS
NITER	52	2009	Resistant HTN with CRI	0	NS	NS
RASCAD	84		Ischemic heart disease + RAS	0	NS	NS
CORAL	947	2014	Resistant HTN or CRI	5	$P = .03^b$	NS

[a]ASTRAL, Revascularization Versus Medical Therapy for Renal Artery Stenosis; CORAL, Stenting and Medical Therapy for Atherosclerotic Renal Artery Stenosis; CRI, chronic renal insufficiency; EMMA, Essai Multicentrique Medicaments Versus Angioplastie; HTN, hypertension; NS, none significant; RAS, renal artery stenosis; STAR, Atherosclerotic Ostial Stenosis of the Renal Artery.
[b]SBP modestly lower on longitudinal analysis in stent group (−2.3 mmHg; 95% CI, −4.4 to −0.2 mmHg; $P = .03$) with no change in number of BP medications.

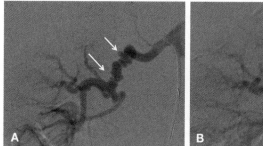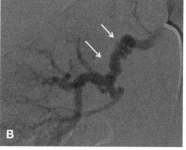

Figure 35.5 Fibromuscular dysplasia involving the right renal artery in a female with resistant hypertension (see arrows) **(A)**. The same patient after serial dilatation with 4.0- and 5.0-mm balloons **(B)**.

percutaneous intervention with balloon angioplasty is usually recommended. FMD localized within the main renal artery or its primary branches can be treated quite effectively with balloon angioplasty alone, with stenting reserved for failure or complications of balloon angioplasty (**Figure 35.5**).

Atherosclerotic Renal Artery Stenosis

A number of observational studies have shown benefit with renal artery intervention to treat atherosclerotic RAS. However, a meta-analysis of the 8 randomized trials conducted to date failed to show preservation or reversal of renal function (**Table 35.7**). The only clear advantage was the use of less antihypertensive medications for blood pressure control. For this reason, the current guidelines have given a class IIa indication for renal artery intervention for resistant hypertension or for preservation of renal function. Resistant hypertension is defined as a blood pressure of over 150 mmHg while on maximum dose of 3 antihypertensive medications including a diuretic. There are other conditions where renal artery intervention may also have a role, including recurrent flash pulmonary edema or congestive heart failure. A number of factors may predict blood pressure response after renal artery intervention. These include (1) rapid acceleration of hypertension over the prior weeks or months, (2) presence of "malignant" hypertension (eg, end-organ effect), (3) hypertension in association with flash pulmonary edema, (4) contemporaneous rise in serum creatinine, and (5) development of azotemia in response to angiotensin-converting enzyme (ACE) inhibitors administered for control of hypertension. Predictors of successful salvage or preservation of renal function are similar and include (1) recent rapid rise in creatinine, unexplained by other factors; (2) azotemia resulting from ACE inhibitors; (3) absence of diabetes or other cause of intrinsic kidney disease; and (4) the presence of global renal ischemia, wherein the entire functioning renal mass is subtended by bilateral critically narrowed renal arteries or a vessel supplying a solitary kidney. Conversely, predictors of poor functional renal recovery following renal artery stenting include (1) renal atrophy demonstrated by kidney length less than 7.5 cm on ultrasound, (2) high (>0.8) renal resistance index (RRI) measured from the peak systolic velocity (V_{max}) and the end-diastolic velocity (V_{min}) using the formula $RRI = 1 - (V_{max} - V_{min}/V_{max})$, (3) proteinuria greater than 1 g/L, (4) hyperuricemia, and finally (5) creatinine clearance less than 40 mL/min. None of these, however, constitutes an absolute contraindication, as individual patient responses are unpredictable.

It is important to note that the clinical spectrum of RAS is wide and not every patient with RAS needs to be stented. Determining the optimum timing for intervention is complex, often requiring close interaction between a nephrologist and an interventionalist. Although the approach of delayed intervention allows instigation of comprehensive antihypertensive therapy and risk factor modification, there is mounting evidence that earlier RAS intervention yields greater preservation of renal function, better control of renovascular hypertension, and reduced cardiovascular morbidity.

Treatment Considerations and Technique

Renal artery intervention can be performed via the femoral, brachial, or radial approach. For downward takeoffs, usually a brachial or radial approach is preferred. However, most other angulations can be treated via the femoral approach. In general, the radial approach is preferred over the brachial approach.

Diagnostic Angiography

Nonselective arteriography is recommended prior to selective cannulation to identify the location of the renal ostia and the configuration of the aorta and to minimize the need for catheter manipulation in a diseased aorta. However, when renal artery stenting is performed to preserve kidney function in patients with renal insufficiency, every measure should be taken to decrease contrast use. In these cases, abdominal aortography is usually not performed. The "no-touch" technique is used to wire the renal artery, and then 1 picture in shallow LAO projection can be taken (**Figure 35.6**). A 3-mL contrast mixed with 3 to 4 mL of saline will be enough to outline the renal arteries and parenchymal flow. This injection is usually enough to also identify accessory renal arteries, which are present in roughly 25% of patients. This approach can be supplemented with IVUS to better assess lesion severity and to have a better understanding of lumen size and plaque burden. Diagnostic renal angiography can be performed using a variety of catheters. Catheter selection should depend on angle

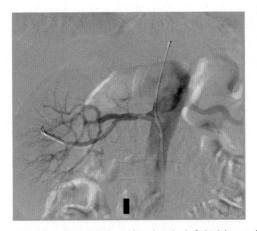

Figure 35.6 The "no-touch" technique is the preferred method of obtaining renal angiography. With this technique, a 0.035-in wire is placed above the renal artery in the aorta. This prevents scrapping of the aortic wall with the catheter. Subsequently, using a 0.014-in wire, the renal artery is engaged.

of renal artery takeoff. Most renal arteries can be cannulated using an IMA, Judkins right, hockey stick, renal double curve, or SOS Omni. Hemodynamic assessment of a renal artery lesion is recommended if severity is ever a question. This should only be performed via the fractional flow reserve (FFR) 0.014-in wire. Traditional advancement of a diagnostic catheter through the lesion to assess hemodynamic significance should be avoided due to associated trauma, risk of embolization, and false gradients created by the occlusion of the vessel lumen by the diagnostic catheter. Although the data in general are sparse, a significant pressure gradient can be considered to be greater than 10 mmHg mean and/or 20 mmHg peak to peak. A resting FFR value of 0.9 is also considered significant. Additional information can be obtained from hyperemia using dopamine or papaverine.

In a study by Lesser et al., a hyperemic systolic gradient of >21 mmHg was the strongest predictor of blood pressure response to renal artery stenting.

Renal Artery Intervention

Once the severity of RAS is confirmed and a decision is made to intervene, angioplasty and stenting can be performed. It is not necessary to perform angioplasty prior to every stenting; however, if there is any doubt as to whether the lesion is expandable or not, angioplasty should be undertaken.

The location of the ostial renal artery can be identified with IVUS (**Figure 35.7**). Fluoroscopic picture of the IVUS catheter is taken when the ostium is visualized on IVUS imaging. The position of the IVUS catheter is then used to place a stent in order to cover the ostium. In addition, IVUS is used not only to select appropriate stent size but also to evaluate stent apposition and edge dissection.

Complications

Complications associated with renal artery intervention are infrequent, but they could be catastrophic. Death has been reported, and renal and aortic dissection can occur. Furthermore, embolization and perforation are other known complications.

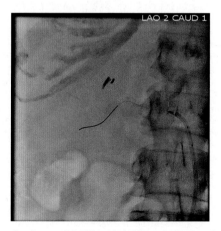

Figure 35.7 Intravascular ultrasound (IVUS)-guided placement of the renal artery stent. Using IVUS, the renal artery ostium is identified. Subsequently, using bony landmarks on the vertebral bodies (*dashed lines*), the appropriate stent position is marked. This technique can be used to minimize contrast use.

Some of these complications can be prevented by proper technique and potential use of IVUS for stent selection and procedural guidance. Atheroembolization has been reported, and in general, it is associated with aggressive guide manipulation. Distal protection devices have been studied in renal arteries; however, currently there is no conclusive evidence that their use is associated with better outcomes in all patients.

LOWER EXTREMITY

PAD represents a spectrum of disease predominantly due to atherosclerotic narrowing of the lower extremity vasculature. An estimated 8 to 12 million Americans carry a diagnosis of PAD, but owing to a high burden of asymptomatic disease (approximately 50% of patients with only a small percentage presenting with typical symptoms) and lack of awareness among both patients and providers, large numbers of patients are undiagnosed.

Critical limb ischemia (CLI) represents the most advanced stage of lower extremity occlusive disease with severe impairment of tissue perfusion resulting in ischemic rest pain, ischemic ulcers, or gangrene (see **Table 35.8**). Although 5% to 10% of patients with PAD will progress to a CLI diagnosis, this is often the index presentation at which time a patient is found to have PAD. Although cardiovascular risk reduction remains critical, outcomes with patients with CLI are predominantly driven by limb-related events with the subsequent sequelae that result from them. At 1 year, 25% of patients with CLI will be dead, 30% will require a major amputation, and 20% will have ongoing CLI. Alarmingly, in a study of 72,199 Medicare beneficiaries published in 2018, 4-year mortality was 54% (median survival 3.5 years), which portends a worse prognosis than most malignancies. Although survival is known to be lower in patients undergoing major amputation (21% at 4 years), surprisingly more than 50% of patients receive a primary amputation without a prior attempt at revascularization.

Clinical Presentation

The classic presentation is that of pain, tightness, aching, soreness, hardness, or heaviness that occur in the calf, buttock, hip, or arch of the foot during ambulation and resolves with rest (intermittent claudication). In more severe cases (CLI), patients present with rest pain, ulcer, or even gangrene (**Table 35.9**). CLI, usually a chronic progressive process, should be differentiated from acute limb ischemia, a medical emergency. Acute limb ischemia typically occurs suddenly and is associated with the classic 5 "'P's." These include sudden pain, pulselessness, pallor, paresthesias, and paralysis. Acute limb ischemia typically requires an endovascular or an open surgical intervention and has been described as the ST elevation MI equivalent of the legs.

Diagnosis

History and physical examination are the foundation for correct diagnosis and subsequent timely treatment of PAD. Attention to the timing of symptoms, location, duration, and risk factors related to atherosclerosis is critical. Any history of back surgery, trauma, arthritis, or neuropathy should be ascertained. Furthermore, the severity of symptoms including its impact on the patient's quality of life and ability to perform physical activity should be obtained. This will guide the level of treatment including whether or not an endovascular or surgical intervention is necessary. Subsequently, a full physical examination that includes a close inspection of skin for breakdowns, pulses, bruits, and temperature should be performed. Once PAD is suspected, confirmatory noninvasive tests should be obtained. If patients can tolerate it, a segmental pulse volume recording (PVR) with exercise is used as a start. Segmental PVRs are useful since they may help localize diseased segments within the lower extremities. In patients with CLI, the presence of noncompressible vessels can render the ankle brachial index

Table 35.8 Clinical (Rutherford) Categories of Chronic Limb Ischemia

Grade	Category	Clinical Description	Objective Criteria
0	0	Asymptomatic	Normal treadmill/stress test
	1	Mild claudication	Completes treadmill exercise,[a] ankle pressure after exercise <50 mmHg but >25 mmHg less than brachial
I	2	Moderate claudication	Between categories 1 and 3
	3	Severe claudication	Cannot complete treadmill exercise and ankle pressure after exercise <50 mmHg
II	4	Ischemic rest pain	Resting ankle pressure < 60 mmHg, ankle or metatarsal pulse volume recording flat or barely pulsatile; toe pressure < 40 mmHg
	5	Minor tissue loss—no healing ulcer, focal gangrene with diffuse pedal ischemia	Resting ankle pressure < 40 mmHg, flat or barely pulsatile ankle or metatarsal pulse volume recording; toe pressure < 30 mmHg
III	6	Major tissue loss—extending above transmetatarsal level, functional foot no longer salvageable	Same as for category 5

[a]Five minutes at 2 mph on a 12% incline.
Adapted from Rutherford RB, Flanigan DP, Gupta SK. Suggested standards for reports dealing with lower extremity ischemia. *J Vasc Surg.* 1986;4:80.

Table 35.9 Clinical Categories of Acute Limb Ischemia

Category	Description	Capillary Return	Muscle Weakness	Sensory Loss	Doppler Signals	
					Arterial	Venous
Viable	Not immediately threatened	Intact	None	None	Audible (ankle pressure > 30 mmHg)	Audible
Threatened	Salvageable if promptly treated	Intact, slow	Mild, partial	Mild, incomplete	Inaudible	Audible
Irreversible	Major tissue loss, amputation regardless of treatment	Absent (marbling)	Profound, paralysis	Profound, anesthetic	Inaudible	Inaudible

Adapted from Rutherford RB, Flanigan DP, Gupta SK. Suggested standards for reports with lower extremity ischemia. *J Vasc Surg.* 1986;4:80.

near-normal or normal in approximately 30% of cases, in which case evaluation of segmental pressure waveforms or alternate measurements such as toe pressure or toe brachial index can be instrumental in making a PAD/CLI diagnosis. Occasionally, additional anatomic data are required in which case a duplex ultrasound, CTA, or MRA may be obtained depending on the desired information and specific clinical scenario.

AORTOILIAC OBSTRUCTIVE DISEASE

Obstructive disease involving the distal abdominal aorta and the iliac vessels may present as buttock or hip claudication, erectile dysfunction in men, lower extremity claudication, or even CLI. Given the size of the aorta and the iliac vessels, endovascular therapy should be the first line of therapy. The current indication for aortoiliac revascularization is listed in **Table 35.10**.

Surgical revascularization for aortoiliac disease includes aortofemoral or aortoiliac bypass, which has a long-term patency of 90% at 1 year, 75% to 80% at 5 years, and 60% to 70% at 10 years but carries a mortality between 2% and 3%. More importantly, it is associated with significant morbidity. Despite these limitations, surgical revascularization remains the best option for selected groups of patients where endovascular treatment would not be ideal. In general, endovascular repair of the abdominal aorta requires a relatively normal landing zone below the renal arteries for stent deployment. In cases where the renal arteries or suprarenal aorta are involved, endovascular repair would not be recommended. Occasionally a hybrid technique might be the ideal approach. The current guidelines also recommend surgery for TASC D (TransAtlantic InterSociety Consensus D) lesions; however, many operators would consider endovascular repair, and if this fails, then the patients are referred to surgery (**Figure 35.8**).

Stents for Aortoiliac Disease

In 1993, the US Food and Drug Administration approved the use of Palmaz BE stents (P-308 series, 30 mm long and 8 mm in diameter) for iliac arteries. The SE Wall-stent prosthesis was approved for similar indications in 1996. Initially, stents were primarily employed following failed percutaneous transluminal angioplasty (PTA), which was defined as a residual mean gradient of >5 mm, residual stenosis of >30%, or presence of a flow-limiting dissection. However, with time, the favorable acute results, relative ease of use, and paucity of complications encountered during aortoiliac stenting led to expanded use of stents to reduce recoil and improve on the immediate hemodynamic and angiographic result of PTA. With the use of stents,

---

Table 35.10 Aortoiliac Revascularization Is Currently Recommended for the Following Indications

Relief of symptomatic lower extremity ischemia, including claudication, rest pain, ulceration or gangrene, or embolization causing blue digit syndrome

Restoration and preservation of inflow to the lower extremity in the setting of preexisting or anticipated distal bypass

Procurement of access to more proximal vascular beds for anticipated invasive procedures (ie, cardiac catheterization)

Improvement of blood flow in patients with buttock claudication and vasculogenic erectile dysfunction

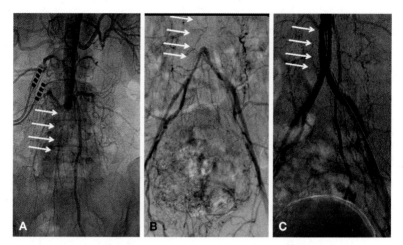

Figure 35.8 Totally occluded infrarenal abdominal aorta (**A**, *arrows*) with reconstitution right above the iliac bifurcation (**B**, *arrows*). Total reconstruction of the aorta and the aortoiliac vessels (**C**, *arrows*).

acute technical success ranged from 90% to 100%, with average 1-year patency of 90% and average 3-year patency of 75%.

Because of these superior acute and long-term results, a strategy of primary stent deployment for aortoiliac vessels has become standard of care within the field.

Treatment Considerations and Technique

The 2 most important aspects of aortoiliac artery endovascular intervention are degree of disease (occlusion vs stenosis) and location. In general, if the *stenotic* lesion involves the distal common iliac and proximal external iliac artery, but distal external and common femoral artery are patent, a retrograde approach via the ipsilateral common femoral artery is appropriate. The ipsilateral retrograde approach also works well for stenotic lesions involving the ostium or proximal common iliac artery; however, in these situations, a 6F access in the contralateral common femoral artery or left radial artery can be very helpful (**Figure 35.9**). This will allow placement of a diagnostic catheter right above the aortoiliac bifurcation. Injection via this catheter will then allow accurate placement of the stent at the common iliac artery ostium and it provides direct access to the aorta in case of inadvertent jailing of the contralateral iliac or plaque shifting. A general approach for *occlusive* lesions in the distal aorta, bifurcation, and iliac systems is the antegrade approach along with retrograde access. This is typically achieved via the left brachial or radial approach, or via contralateral crossover technique (**Figure 35.10**). When the brachial or radial approach is used, an ipsilateral 5F common femoral sheath is also placed. This will allow externalization of the wire once the occlusive lesion has been crossed. When attempting recanalization of totally occluded lesions, it is extremely important to ensure true final luminal position (**Figure 35.11**). This can be achieved by injecting dye.

A straight or an angled glidewire supported by a 4F or 5F glide catheter can be used when traversing stenotic or occlusive lesions. Although one aim, when crossing these lesions, is to remain intraluminal, this may be difficult. The subintimal approach is appropriate, but it should be performed very carefully, and luminal entry should be gained as

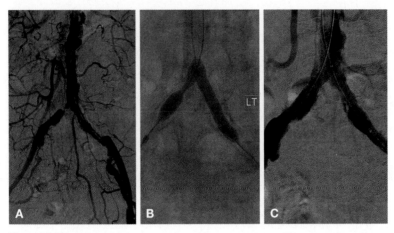

Figure 35.9 Treatment of complex aortoiliac diseased segment **(A)**. Balloon angioplasty **(B)** followed by stenting and final angiographic result **(C)**.

soon as the lesion has been traversed. Reentry into true lumen should always be above the common femoral artery. This will prevent jailing of the profunda femoris or the requirement for common femoral artery stenting.

Both SE and BE stents have been used when performing aortoiliac interventions. BE stents are generally preferred for aorta, aortoiliac bifurcation, and ostial and proximal common iliac arteries. SE stents are typically used from distal common and external iliac arteries. BE stents have higher radial strength and allow more precise placement; therefore, they are the preferred stents for bifurcation lesions in our laboratory. Covered stents have also been used to treat aortoiliac lesions. In the COBEST trial, which randomized 125 patients (168 iliac arteries) to treatment with a

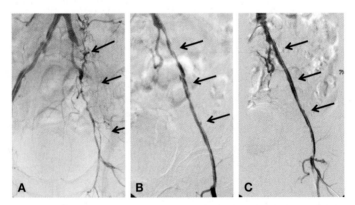

Figure 35.10 Contralateral crossover technique to treat a totally occluded external iliac artery **(A)**. Using angle glidewire and 5F angle glide catheter, the external iliac artery was crossed and dilated using 5-mm balloons **(B)**. The external iliac artery was subsequently stented using self-expanding nitinol stents **(C)**. Arrows refer to site of intervention.

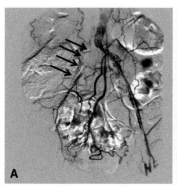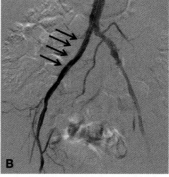

Figure 35.11 Complex TASC D lesion with a total occlusion of the common and external iliac artery **(A)**. A brachial approach was used to cross and externalize the wire from the right common femoral artery. Subsequently, angioplasty and stenting of the common and external iliac arteries were performed with good result **(B)**. Arrows refer to site of intervention.

standard BMS or covered stents, both devices were safe and effective in TASC B lesions, whereas covered stents performed better in TASC C and D lesions. This benefit was sustained out to 5-year follow-up, which translated into less need for target limb revascularization in patients treated with covered stents.

On occasion, other modalities can be used to guide endovascular repair of the aortoiliac system. IVUS and pressure assessment can facilitate endovascular repair. By convention, a 10-mmHg mean resting pressure gradient is taken as indicative of a significant residual stenosis. IVUS is also very helpful in defining the anatomy and in guiding stent diameter.

In summary, percutaneous therapy has now become the first line of therapy for aortoiliac obstructive disease. With the exception of patients with very extensive disease, PTA with stent deployment is associated with a highly successful acute and long-term outcome. If this strategy fails, subsequent surgical intervention remains feasible. While the current guidelines continue to recommend surgical revascularization for TASC C and D lesions, most experienced operators prefer endovascular therapy over open surgery, even for complex totally occlusive aortoiliac lesions.

Complications

Complications are relatively infrequent with aortoiliac angioplasty (<6% based on multiple series). Arterial rupture must be recognized promptly and controlled by inflation of a balloon within the lesion (balloon tamponade), reversal of anticoagulation, and volume resuscitation. Surgery may be required, but stent grafts are increasingly being used to treat this complication. Other complications include distal embolization, which was encountered in alarming frequency in early studies of recanalized total iliac occlusion. More recent studies indicate an incidence of <5%. An aortic occlusive balloon (CODA, Cook Medical) with a 10F to 14F sheath should always be available in the laboratory, and all personnel should be aware of its location.

COMMON FEMORAL ARTERY

The common femoral artery, the so-called left main of the leg, has previously been considered the exclusive purview of the vascular surgeon, whose approach through a local incision (often under local anesthesia) allows endarterectomy and patch angioplasty with good results. Owing to concerns regarding stent fracture and compression, elastic recoil, or compromise of the profunda femoral artery, most experts continue to avoid endovascular therapy for this artery. However, recent series from Europe and other centers have shown good results in highly selected patients. In general, younger patients and those with heavy calcification should be considered for surgery. For older patients with significant cardiac disease, those with poorly controlled diabetes mellitus, obese patients, and individuals who are at increased risk of wound infection, an endovascular approach may be better. However, all efforts should be to minimize the use of stents in this location. Our current approach is atherectomy followed by drug-coated balloon angioplasty.

PROFUNDA FEMORAL ARTERY

The deep femoral artery is the main source of collaterals to the lower extremity. In the face of occlusion of the superficial femoral artery (SFA) or a fem-pop bypass graft, the profunda alone becomes responsible for maintaining viability of the lower extremity. Surgery for disease involving the ostia of the SFA and profunda involves endarterectomy and patch angioplasty. Balloon angioplasty has been reserved for situations in which severe ischemia is present (Rutherford category 4, 5, or 6) and surgery is absolutely contraindicated, or when critical lesions involve the mid or distal portions of the descending branch of the profunda that are less accessible to the surgeon. Because of the potential for producing limb-threatening ischemia or limb loss if the vessel occludes, treatment of this site should generally be reserved for patients with rest pain or CLI in whom no good surgical options are available.

SUPERFICIAL FEMORAL AND POPLITEAL ARTERIES

This vessel, the longest nonbranching artery in the body, continues to present a challenge for both endovascular and surgical approaches. Despite a mean vessel diameter between 5 and 6 mm, restenosis is nearly twice that of coronary interventions. Furthermore, due to the presence of significant collaterals from profunda femoris to the popliteal and lower leg, most patients do not become symptomatic until the artery has totally occluded. Unfortunately, once the occlusion occurs, it is typically long and over 20 cm making endovascular intervention more challenging. Occasionally, patients modify their activity level to prevent claudication; therefore, they frequently present with critical limb or rarely acute limb ischemia. In general, there is direct correlation between lesion length and presence of occlusion and long-term patency. Moreover, the SFA undergoes significant mechanical stress such as torsion, compression, expansion, and rotation, and these forces can create fractures and restenosis. Because of these limitations, revascularization for SFA disease in non-CLI settings has been reserved for lifestyle-limiting claudication only after risk factor modification and a supervised exercise program.

Considerable controversy remains as to the relative role of percutaneous therapy versus surgery. The results of balloon angioplasty in the SFA have improved over time. Similarly, the success rate in crossing occluded segments of the SFA and popliteal arteries has improved dramatically as a consequence of technical advances. These include improvement in guidewire and microcatheter technology in addition to utilization of alternative access. Among 8 large series of patients undergoing PTA of femoral-popliteal stenoses and occlusions, most of whom were claudicants, the acute technical success ranged between 82% and 96%. Primary patency rates at 1, 3, and 5 years averaged 60%, 50%, and 45%. Several factors influence long-term outcome following SFA-POP angioplasty. Patients with intermittent claudication (vs tissue loss), a more severe lesion at baseline, and lower posttreatment residual stenosis tend to have a better outcome at 1 year, whereas those with diabetes, threatened limb loss, or diffuse atherosclerotic vascular disease with 0- to 1-vessel runoff have a worse outcome. The excellent acute results that can be obtained from percutaneous techniques in the current era, and the fact that subsequent surgical bypass is still possible if needed, have led most to support a strategy of initial endovascular therapy, including for the treatment of CLI.

Adjunct Therapies

Traditionally, the approach to SFA and popliteal intervention relied on the utilization of angioplasty, and although acute results were often acceptable, this strategy was plagued by high rates of restenosis, with primary patency rates often <50% at 1-year follow-up. Understanding this limitation led to the development of drug-eluting technology and atherectomy devices. With regard to stents, initially, several studies of nitinol bare-metal SE stents demonstrated improved patency rates compared with that of standard balloon angioplasty, although with variable rates of stent fracture. To better address the complex mechanical forces present in the SFA and popliteal space, a wire interwoven nitinol stent was developed, and in the SUPERB trial, high primary patency rates with only 1 stent fracture at 3-year follow-up time point were demonstrated.

Another concern that arose from the initial stent experience was poor primary patency rates in long lesions. A strategy aimed at addressing the issue of restenosis was the use of drug-coated technology. Given that the primary mechanism of stent failure tends to be neointimal hyperplasia leading to ISR, the utilization of drug-coated technology has recently increased. Several studies of drug-coated balloons and drug-eluting stents in the peripheral space have demonstrated improved primary patency rates when compared with standard balloon angioplasty.

Despite superior patency rates, there have been 2 critical challenges with regard to drug-eluting technology in PAD. First, the CMS made a decision to remove the transitional pass-through payment for drug coated balloon (DCB) reimbursement, which significantly affected reimbursement with DCB use. Second, in 2018, Katsanos published a meta-analysis suggesting increased mortality with the use of paclitaxel drug-coated technology in the femoropopliteal space. In 2 separate analyses of DCBs and drug-eluting stents among Medicare beneficiaries, this finding was unable to be reproduced.

Recognizing the concern regarding long-term patency of stents, especially in complex lesion types, many operators have advocated for adjunctive use of atherectomy devices in an attempt to modify plaque and thereby improve outcomes with subsequent angioplasty. Currently, there are several devices on the market indicated in the femoropopliteal space, each of which mechanistically is uniquely suited for the various plaque morphologies encountered in this vascular territory (**Figure 35.12**). Numerous trials regarding atherectomy devices have demonstrated this strategy to be safe and effective with low bailout stent use when used in appropriately selected patients in de novo SFA and popliteal lesions. EXCITE-ISR specifically evaluated the utility of laser atherectomy in ISR and found this strategy to be superior to balloon angioplasty alone with lower TLR rates and major adverse events in the laser atherectomy group. Furthermore, the use of atherectomy in CLI revascularization was shown to be cost-effective, primarily due to reduction in revascularization rates, amputation rates, and end-of-life care over a 6- to 12-month period following intervention. Although concern exists regarding up-front cost, risk of distal embolization, and long-term efficacy, atherectomy devices remain a valuable tool within the armamentarium of the endovascular specialist.

Treatment Considerations and Technique

Access

The most important aspect of SFA intervention is access. Before approaching a case, all noninvasive and invasive tests including prior angiograms should

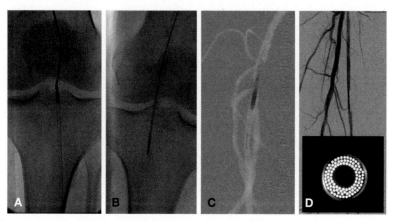

Figure 35.12 Currently available atherectomy devices for treatment of infrainguinal vessels. Silverhawk **(A)**. Pathway **(B)**. Diamondback **(C)**. Laser **(D)**.

be reviewed. This will guide the best access site selection. The most common approach for SFA disease is contralateral crossover technique. However, radial, brachial, ipsilateral antegrade, popliteal, and pedal access may also be needed (**Figure 35.13**).

Adapting from experience in the coronary CTO space, several recent treatment algorithms have been developed, including CTOP and P-CTO, in order to help guide choice of access site. Familiarity with the local anatomy at the level of the common femoral artery is essential. The use of a kink-resistant sheath is critical to maintaining access around the bifurcation of the aorta, especially in the case of the acutely angulated bifurcation. Any number of curved (Cobra, IMA, RIM) or retroflexed (Omni,

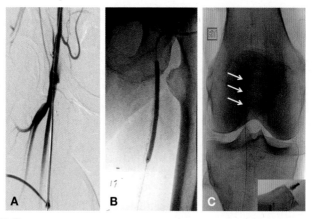

Figure 35.13 Various access sites are required when performing infrainguinal intervention. Retrograde common femoral artery **(A)**. Antegrade ipsilateral common femoral artery **(B)**. Pedal access with retrograde wire *(arrows)* at the level of popliteal artery above the knee (P2 segment) **(C)**.

SOS, Simmons) catheters may be used to obtain access to the contralateral common iliac artery. The advantages to this approach include the ability to image the common femoral and its bifurcation and the ability to treat iliac and infrainguinal disease in the same setting.

In general, all stenoses are crossed through the lumen; however, total occlusions typically require a subintimal pass. A number of chronic total occlusion devices have become available. These include the Crosser device (BARD), Frontrunner (Cordis), and even laser atherectomy; however, to date, little data exist regarding the efficacy of these devices. Knowledge about each device is important.

Occasionally, reentry to true lumen can be very difficult when a subintimal technique has been selected. Many experts use 0.014- or 0.018-in stiff chronic total occlusion wires. This approach works around 30% to 40% of the time. Alternatively, an Outback or a Pioneer reentry device can be used. The Outback device uses fluoroscopy to direct a needle toward the true lumen. The Pioneer device uses IVUS to detect the lumen. Subsequently, similar to the Outback device, a needle is pushed toward the true lumen and reentry is obtained.

INFRAPOPLITEAL ARTERIES

Although traditionally alternative access options were only considered after failure of a conventional "up and over" approach, most experienced operators have now adopted up-front use of alternative access when indicated, given its favorable safety profile combined with high procedural success rates. While isolated below-knee disease is generally not responsible for claudication symptoms, most patients (between 70% and 80%) with CLI have below-knee disease. Of these, 30% to 40% have isolated below-knee disease only.

In a large series reported by Dorros success was achieved in 406 of 417 patients (96%); the success rate in stenoses (98%) was superior to that in occlusions (76%). In-hospital complications were extremely low. The vast majority of patients with CLI (95%) improved following revascularization. Such improvement does not necessarily imply ongoing patency. Restoration of flow through only 1 of the 3 major vessels to the foot may be sufficient to heal a distal ischemic lesion. Once healed, most patients will do well even in the face of documented reocclusion or restenosis. However, recent data indicate that improving blood flow to the area that is responsible for tissue loss (known as the angiosome concept) is most likely the best option for patients with Rutherford class V and VI. There are also data that achieving pedal arch patency may be more important than angiosome-guided revascularization with regard to wound healing and limb salvage. In the RENDEVOUS registry, patients who underwent successful pedal arch angioplasty had higher limb salvage rates and a shorter time to wound healing.

Many of the patients treated with infrapopliteal angioplasty to date have been those who were too high risk or otherwise not candidates for bypass surgery. The BASIL trial is the first randomized clinical trial to compare angioplasty with open surgical revascularization in patients with CLI. In this trial, both surgery and angioplasty resulted in similar amputation-free survival; however, in the short term, surgery was more expensive. In general, surgery was associated with a higher incidence of bleeding and wound infection, while angioplasty was associated with a higher revascularization rate.

Techniques

Similar to iliac and SFA disease, appropriate preparation including a full review of prior noninvasive and invasive tests is critical. The diagnostic portion of the angiogram will need to focus on the foot and distal pedal vessels. Selective injection using digital subtraction angiography via the catheter placed at the level of the knee is recommended. This will allow identification of pedal and tibial vessels in case retrograde pedal or tibial access is necessary. Of note, poor opacification of tibial vessels often results from low pressure distal to an occlusion with consequent underfilling of these vessels. Also, many tibial CTOs comprise long segments of hibernating lumen and can be safely accessed and traversed using ultrasound guidance and standard CTO equipment. Not infrequently, anatomic variants will be present, such as the anterior tibial arising above the knee joint or a dominant peroneal artery directly supplying the medial and lateral plantar branches. In addition, it is not unusual to mistake one of the small side branches or collaterals for the main arterial trunk. Adequate anticoagulation is critical, and administration of vasodilator therapy (nitroglycerin or papaverine) may be useful. Initial attempts to cross tibial lesions should use standard 0.014-in coronary guidewires in stenotic lesions or workhorse CTO wires (ie, Command or Gladius) in the case of an occlusion. If unsuccessful, escalation to 0.014-in wires with higher penetrating force (ie, Halberd, Astato) or, in some cases, 0.018- and 0.035-in platforms may be needed. If available, real-time extravascular ultrasound guidance can help traversing complex occlusions. Confirmation of a luminal position in the distal vessel should always be obtained prior to dilating, by removing the wire from the catheter and injecting a small amount of diluted contrast through the guide or the support catheter into the distal vessel. IVUS is also valuable to confirm wire position throughout a lesion, obtain accurate vessel size, and help define plaque morphology to guide treatment strategy.

Orbital atherectomy, directional atherectomy, excimer laser angioplasty, and intravascular lithotripsy can be useful as adjunctive therapy. Specifically, lesions that have unfavorable morphology, such as total occlusions, heavy calcification, and ostial disease, may benefit from these niche devices. Given the risk of distal embolization, distal protection devices should be used when possible. Alternately, inflation of a blood pressure cuff on the calf followed by mechanical thrombectomy using a standard coronary aspiration device can be helpful. When neither option is possible, limiting run time to less than 30 seconds, liberal use of vasodilators (usually intra-arterial nitroglycerin every other run), and, when a pedal sheath is present, opening the sidearm during device use can help minimize the risk of distal embolization and poor outflow. The use of stents, including drug-eluting stents, has been advocated and evaluated in a number of small studies.

VENOUS DISEASE AND INTERVENTION

An estimated 100 persons per 100,000 each year are newly diagnosed with venous thromboembolism in the United States. Of these, about two-thirds have acute deep venous thrombosis (DVT), while one-third have pulmonary embolism. Over 30% to 40% of patients with DVT may suffer from postthrombotic syndrome (PTS) after lower extremity DVT. Similarly, with the rising prevalence of malignancy, the incidence of upper extremity DVT has also been on the rise. While typically more benign, it has been associated with superior vena cava syndrome and upper extremity discomfort.

Chronic DVT has also been a target of intervention in patients with venous claudication or in those with venous ulcers. Unfortunately, currently tools to treat chronic venous disease are limited in the United States. Recently, the ATTRACT trial demonstrated a lack of efficacy with regard to PTS incidence at 24 months in addition to increased bleeding risk with a pharmacomechanical approach versus anticoagulation alone. Although this trial has been widely criticized for several reasons, including the inclusion of patients without iliofemoral DVT, the volume of DVT interventions has since declined following its publication.

Techniques

Popliteal vein access is obtained with ultrasound guidance and patient in a prone position. The lesion is crossed using a 0.035-in stiff-angled glidewire over a 4F angled glide catheter. Care is taken to avoid inadvertent wiring of the lumbar branches. Once the lesion is crossed, a contrast injection is used to confirm wire position in the inferior vena cava. For acute (within 2-4 weeks) lower extremity DVT, pulse spray lytic therapy followed by mechanical thrombectomy using one of the available devices, such as Angiojet Zelante catheter, is typically used. An alternate approach, which is gaining traction given the ability to avoid thrombolysis, is manual aspiration thrombectomy using the INARI ClotTriever system. Regardless of which option is chosen, the utilization of IVUS following thrombectomy can be used to further evaluate for extrinsic compression, especially in left iliofemoral DVTs. When needed, adjunctive angioplasty and/or stenting can then be pursued using IVUS for appropriate sizing. For subacute or chronic DVT, lytic therapy infusion over 24 to 72 hours may be required. These individuals require close monitoring in the intensive care unit. When placing patients on a lytic infusion, low-dose heparin (600-800 U/h) should also be administered simultaneously with a partial thromboplastin time goal of 40 to 60. These individuals should be monitored for signs of intracranial bleeding. Furthermore, complete blood counts and fibrinogen levels should be monitored. Following thrombolysis, adjunctive thrombectomy, angioplasty, and/or stenting is pursued in a manner similar to above.

TRAINING AND CREDENTIALING

Percutaneous intervention for the treatment of PVD has been adopted by multiple specialties, including interventional cardiology, vascular surgery, and interventional radiology. Such widespread application necessitates the development of standardized guidelines for training and credentialing to ensure that patients will receive optimal care. Current guidelines regarding the minimal requirements necessary to care for patients with PAD and perform peripheral vascular procedures have been described in the multidisciplinary Clinical Competence Statement on vascular medicine and catheter-based peripheral vascular interventions. More specific recommendations apply to carotid interventions and have recently been ratified by the cardiology, vascular surgery, and vascular medicine communities, with a view to establishing a common set of criteria for training and credentialing to facilitate safe and orderly dissemination of this new therapy into clinical practice.

SUGGESTED READINGS

1. Abou-Chebl A, Yadav JS, Reginelli JP, Bajzer C, Bhatt D, Krieger DW. Intracranial hemorrhage and hyperperfusion syndrome following carotid artery stenting: risk factors, prevention, and treatment. *J Am Coll Cardiol.* 2004;43(9):1596-1601.
2. Adam DJ, Beard JD, Cleveland T, et al. Bypass versus angioplasty in severe ischaemia of the leg (BASIL): multicentre, randomised controlled trial. *Lancet.* 2005;366(9501):1925-1934.
3. Banerjee S, Shishehbor MH, Mustapha JA, et al. A percutaneous crossing algorithm for femoropopliteal and tibial artery chronic total occlusions (PCTO algorithm). *J Invasive Cardiol.* 2019;31(4):111-119.
4. North American Symptomatic Carotid Endarterectomy Trial Collaborators; Barnett HJM, Taylor DW, Haynes RB, et al. Beneficial effect of carotid endarterectomy in symptomatic patients with high-grade carotid stenosis. *N Engl J Med.* 1991;325(7):445-453.
5. Bonvini RF, Rastan A, Sixt S, et al. Endovascular treatment of common femoral artery disease: medium-term outcomes of 360 consecutive procedures. *J Am Coll Cardiol.* 2011;58(8):792-798.
6. Brott T, Howard G, Roubin G, et al. Long-term results of stenting versus endarterectomy for carotid-artery stenosis. *N Engl J Med.* 2016;374(11):1021-1031.
7. Cooper CJ, Murphy TP, Cutlip DE, et al. Stenting and medical therapy for atherosclerotic renal-artery stenosis. *N Engl J Med.* 2014;370(1):13-22.

8. Dake MD, Ansel GM, Jaff MR, et al. Durable Clinical effectiveness with paclitaxel-eluting stents in the femoropopliteal artery: 5-year results of the Zilver PTX randomized trial. *Circulation.* 2016;133(15):1472-1483; discussion 1483.

9. Dattilo R, Himmelstein SI, Cuff RF. The COMPLIANCE 360° Trial: a randomized, prospective, multicenter, pilot study comparing acute and long-term results of orbital atherectomy to balloon angioplasty for calcified femoropopliteal disease. *J Invasive Cardiol.* 2014;26(8): 355-360.

10. Dormandy JA, Rutherford RB. Management of peripheral arterial disease (PAD). TASC working group: TransAtlantic Inter-Society Consensus (TASC). *J Vasc Surg.* 2000;31(1 pt. 2):S1-S296.

11. Dotter CT, Judkins MP. Transluminal treatment of arteriosclerotic obstruction. Description of a new technic and a preliminary report of its application. *Circulation.* 1964;30:654-670.

12. Dworkin LD, Cooper CJ. Clinical practice. Renal-artery stenosis. *N Engl J Med.* 2009;361(20):1972-1978.

13. Feiring AJ, Krahn M, Nelson L, Wesolowski A, Eastwood D, Szabo A. Preventing leg amputations in critical limb ischemia with below-the-knee drug-eluting stents: the PaRADISE (PReventing Amputations using Drug eluting StEnts) trial. *J Am Coll Cardiol.* 2010;55(15):1580-1589.

14. Garcia L, Jaff MR, Metzger C, et al. Wire-interwoven nitinol stent outcome in the superficial femoral and proximal popliteal arteries: twelve-month results of the SUPERB trial. *Circ Cardiovasc Interv.* 2015;8(5):e000937.

15. Hadjipetrou P, Cox S, Piemonte T, Eisenhauer A. Percutaneous revascularization of atherosclerotic obstruction of aortic arch vessels. *J Am Coll Cardiol.* 1999;33(5):1238-1245.

16. Hirsch AT, Haskal ZJ, Hertzer NR, et al. ACC/AHA 2005 practice guidelines for the management of patients with peripheral arterial disease (lower extremity, renal, mesenteric, and abdominal aortic). A collaborative report from the American Association for Vascular Surgery/Society for Vascular Surgery, Society for Cardiovascular Angiography and Interventions, Society for Vascular Medicine and Biology, Society of Interventional Radiology, and the ACC/AHA task force on practice guidelines (writing committee to develop guidelines for the management of patients with peripheral arterial disease): endorsed by the American Association of Cardiovascular and Pulmonary Rehabilitation; National Heart, Lung, and Blood Institute; Society for Vascular Nursing; TransAtlantic InterSociety Consensus; and Vascular Disease Foundation. *Circulation.* 2006;113(11):e463-e654.

17. Iida O, Soga Y, Hirano K, et al. Long-term results of direct and indirect endovascular revascularization based on the angiosome concept in patients with critical limb ischemia presenting with isolated below-the-knee lesions. *J Vasc Surg.* 2012;55(2):363-370.e5.

18. Inzitari D, Eliasziw M, Gates P, et al. The causes and risk of stroke in patients with asymptomatic internal-carotid-artery stenosis. North American Symptomatic Carotid Endarterectomy Trial Collaborators. *N Engl J Med.* 2000;342(23):1693-1700.

19. Johnston KW. Femoral and popliteal arteries: reanalysis of results of balloon angioplasty. *Radiology.* 1992;183(3):767-771.

20. Kahn SR, Ginsberg JS. Relationship between deep venous thrombosis and the postthrombotic syndrome. *Arch Intern Med.* 2004;164(1):17-26.

21. Katsanos K, Spiliopoulos S, Kitrou P, Krokidis M, Karnabatidis D. Risk of death following application of paclitaxel-coated balloons and stents in the femoropopliteal artery of the leg: a systematic review and meta-analysis of randomized controlled trials. *J Am Heart Assoc.* 2018;7(24):e011245.

22. Laird JR, Jain A, Zeller T, et al. Nitinol stent implantation in the superficial femoral artery and proximal popliteal artery: twelve month results from the complete SE multicenter trial. *J Endovasc Ther.* 2014;21(2):202-212.

23. Leesar MA, Varma J, Shapira A, et al. Prediction of hypertension improvement after stenting of renal artery stenosis: comparative accuracy of translesional pressure gradients, intravascular ultrasound, and angiography. *J Am Coll Cardiol.* 2009;53(25):2363-2371.

24. Leriche R. Des obliterations arterielles hautes comme cause des insuffisances circulatoires des membres inferieurs. *Bull Mem Soc Chir.* 1923:1404-1406.

25. Marmagkiolis K, Sardar P, Mustapha JA, et al. Transpedal access for the management of complex peripheral artery disease. *J Invasive Cardiol.* 2017;29(12):425-429.

26. Mathur A, Dorros G, Iyer SS, Vitek JJ, Yadav SS, Roubin GS. Palmaz stent compression in patients following carotid artery stenting. *Cathet Cardiovasc Diagn.* 1997;41(2):137-140.

27. McKinsey JF, Zeller T, Rocha-Singh KJ, Jaff MR, Garcia LA; DEFINITIVE LE Investigators. Lower extremity revascularization using directional atherectomy: 12-month prospective results of the DEFINITIVE LE study. *JACC Cardiovasc Interv.* 2014;7(8):923-933.

28. Mendelsohn FO, Weissman NJ, Lederman RJ, et al. Acute hemodynamic changes during carotid artery stenting. *Am J Cardiol.* 1998;82(9):1077-1081.

29. Rosenfield K, Jaff MR, White CJ, et al. Trial of a paclitaxel-coated balloon for femoropopliteal artery disease. *N Engl J Med*. 2015;373(2):145-153.
30. Rosenfield K, Matsumura J, Chaturvedi S, et al. Randomized trial of stent versus surgery for asymptomatic carotid stenosis. *N Engl J Med*. 2016;374(11):1011-1020.
31. Rothwell PM, Eliasziw M, Gutnikov SA, et al. Analysis of pooled data from the randomised controlled trials of endarterectomy for symptomatic carotid stenosis. *Lancet*. 2003;361(9352):107-116.
32. Roubin GS, Yadav S, Iyer SS, Vitek J. Carotid stent-supported angioplasty: a neurovascular intervention to prevent stroke. *Am J Cardiol*. 1996;78(3A):8-12.
33. Roubin GS, New G, Iyer SS, et al. Immediate and late clinical outcomes of carotid artery stenting in patients with symptomatic and asymptomatic carotid artery stenosis: a 5-year prospective analysis. *Circulation*. 2001;103(4):532-537.
34. Saab F, Jaff MR, Diaz-Sandoval LJ, et al. Chronic total occlusion crossing approach based on plaque cap morphology: the CTOP classification. *J Endovasc Ther*. 2018;25(3):284-291.
35. Safian RD, Textor SC. Renal-artery stenosis. *N Engl J Med*. 2001;344(6):431-442.
36. Scheinert D, Scheinert S, Sax J, et al. Prevalence and clinical impact of stent fractures after femoropopliteal stenting. *J Am Coll Cardiol*. 2005;45(2):312-315.
37. Shishehbor MH, White CJ, Gray BH, et al. Critical limb ischemia: an expert statement. *J Am Coll Cardiol*. 2016;68(18):2002-2015.
38. Slovut DP, Olin JW. Fibromuscular dysplasia. *N Engl J Med*. 2004;350(18):1862-1871.
39. Tepe G, Laird J, Schneider P, et al. Drug-coated balloon versus standard percutaneous transluminal angioplasty for the treatment of superficial femoral and popliteal peripheral artery disease: 12month results from the IN.PACT SFA randomized trial. *Circulation*. 2015;131(5):495-502.
40. Troisi N, Turini F, Chisci E, et al. Pedal arch patency and not direct-angiosome revascularization predicts outcomes of endovascular interventions in diabetic patients with critical limb ischemia. *Int Angiol*. 2017;36(5):438-444.
41. White RH. The epidemiology of venous thromboembolism. *Circulation*. 2003;107(23 suppl 1): I4-I8.
42. White CJ. Chronic mesenteric ischemia: diagnosis and management. *Prog Cardiovasc Dis*. 2011;54(1):36-40.
43. Wholey M. The role of embolic protection in peripheral arterial atherectomy. *Tech Vasc Interv Radiol*. 2011;14(2):65-74.
44. Yadav JS, Roubin GS, King P, Iyer S, Vitek J. Angioplasty and stenting for restenosis after carotid endarterectomy. Initial experience. *Stroke*. 1996;27(11):2075-2079.
45. Yadav JS, Wholey MH, Kuntz RE, et al. Protected carotid-artery stenting versus endarterectomy in high-risk patients. *N Engl J Med*. 2004;351(15):1493-1501.

36 Interventions for Pediatric and Adult Congenital Heart Disease[1]

The successes of both pediatric cardiac medicine and pediatric cardiac surgery over the past 40 years have resulted in a rapidly growing population of adults with corrected and palliated congenital cardiac lesions that few adult cardiologists have experience in managing. This chapter focuses on a series of interventions for congenital heart disease (CHD) that apply to *both* the pediatric and the adult population, noting procedural modifications that are required to accommodate a neonate or an adult patient. Since knowledge of the physiologic and hemodynamic consequences of these lesions is at least as critical as knowing the steps of the procedures, a brief review of the underlying pathophysiology is also included in each section.

CONGENITAL OBSTRUCTIVE LESIONS

Obstructive Lesions of the Right Ventricular Outflow Tract

Congenital obstruction of the right ventricular outflow tract (RVOT) can occur in the muscular RVOT (subvalvular obstruction), at the valvular level, in the main pulmonary artery (MPA) (supravalvular obstruction), or at the level of the branch pulmonary arteries. Although the level of obstruction can usually be determined noninvasively, each lesion has a unique hemodynamic pattern and angiographic appearance. The clinical symptoms associated with these lesions depend on the degree of obstruction and the age of the patient.

Subvalvular Pulmonary Stenosis

Subvalvular obstruction is usually muscular in nature and is not generally amenable to catheter intervention (**Figure 36.1A**). Residual or recurrent "infundibular" obstruction is most commonly found in patients who have undergone repair of tetralogy of Fallot. Double-chambered right ventricle (DCRV) also features hypertrophy of the infundibular muscle, causing it to closely appose the free wall of the RV in systole and narrow the outflow tract below the pulmonary valve. In children, this lesion may be associated with small membranous ventricular septal defects (VSDs) or membranous subaortic obstruction. Over time, the membranous VSD may close spontaneously as the infundibular obstruction progresses, so that DCRV may present in the adult as an apparently isolated subvalvular obstruction.

Pulmonary valve annular hypoplasia may also present in the setting of significant RVOT obstruction and can be found in patients as residua of surgically corrected CHD. This lesion is not generally amenable to transcatheter intervention owing to the fibrous ring of the hypoplastic annulus that resists balloon dilation.

Supravalvular Pulmonary Stenosis

Supravalvular obstruction generally occurs at the sinotubular junction and is congenital. It is commonly seen in a variety of different congenital diseases including congenital rubella, tetralogy of Fallot, and Alagille and Williams syndromes. Scarring from previous surgical interventions can also produce narrowing of the MPA (ie, following arterial reconstruction in neonatal transposition of the great arteries, or tetralogy of Fallot). Sinotubular junction stenosis can be confused echocardiographically

[1]We gratefully acknowledge the Grossman & Baim's *Cardiac Catheterization, Angiography, and Intervention*, 9th edition contributions of Drs. Alejandro J. Torres and Robert J. Sommer, as portions of their chapter, Intervention for Pediatric and Adult Congenital Heart Disease, were retained in this text.

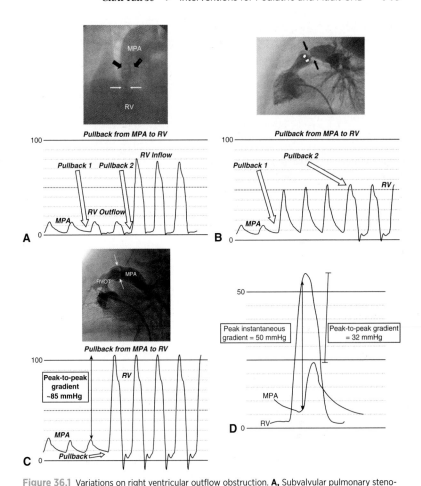

Figure 36.1 Variations on right ventricular outflow obstruction. **A,** Subvalvular pulmonary steno-sis (PS) in an adult patient with double-chambered right ventricle (RV). Severe muscular narrow-ing of the RV outflow tract (white arrow), well below the level of the valve leaflets (black arrows). Bottom. Systolic pressure remains unchanged (Pullback 1) as diastolic pressure falls, indicating transition into the RV outflow tract. On further withdrawal of the catheter (Pullback 2), there is a large systolic gradient with no change in diastole, consistent with an intraventricular obstruction. **B,** Supravalvular PS in a patient with Noonan syndrome. The thickened pulmonary valve leaflets (white arrows) abut the supravalvular muscular ridge at the sinotubular junction (black arrows), not allowing full leaflet excursion. **C,** Top. Valvular PS. Doming valve leaflets (white arrows) are fused and cannot open fully. Jet of contrast through valve orifice is well profiled. Bottom. Systolic pressure gradient occurs at same site/time where diastolic pressure falls, indicating transition through the valve from artery to ventricle. **D,** Simultaneous RV and main pulmonary artery (MPA) tracings in a patient with valvular PS. The bracket demonstrates the peak-to-peak gradient as measured in the cath lab. The arrow shows the peak instantaneous pressure difference, which corresponds to the peak velocity as measured by Doppler echocardiography. In general, the echo overestimates the degree of obstruction found in the cath lab.

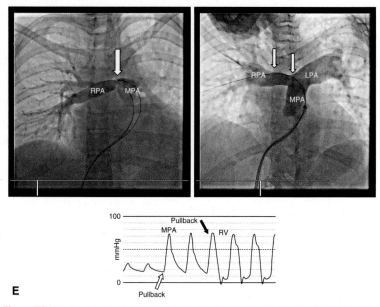

E

Figure 36.1 Continued **E,** Top left. Right pulmonary artery (RPA) stenosis at the takeoff of the RPA from the MPA. Bottom. Normal PA pressure in the RPA. Pullback into the MPA (white arrow) shows a systolic pressure gradient, with no change in the diastolic pressure. On further pullback (black arrow) into the RV, the fall in diastolic pressure indicates that the catheter has crossed the pulmonary valve. The lack of change in systolic pressure from MPA to RV indicates an unobstructed RV outflow tract. Top right. RPA takeoff after stent angioplasty.

with valvular disease, because the normal leaflets are limited in their forward motion by the distal ridge of muscular tissue (**Figure 36.1B**), appear to dome, and exhibit turbulent flow at the leaflet tips on Doppler, just as seen in valvular pulmonary stenosis (PS). Balloon dilation of supravalvular obstructions is largely unsuccessful owing to the muscular/elastic nature of the arterial wall in the MPA, and has been associated with MPA rupture. Stents have been placed successfully to relieve obstruction in the supravalvular region, but carry the risk of stenting open the pulmonary valve and causing severe insufficiency, most often a poor trade-off for moderate PS.

Valvular Pulmonary Stenosis

Valvular stenosis is the most common form of PS, accounting for 80% to 90% of cases of RVOT) obstruction. There are 3 subtypes of valvular morphology with different clinical presentations: (1) Dome-shaped valves account for 40% to 60% of valvular PS. It is typically caused by commissural fusion that precludes full separation of the leaflets (**Figure 36.1C**). Poststenotic dilation of the MPA is frequently present, and balloon valvuloplasty is highly successful in this group. (2) Dysplastic pulmonary valves are present in 20% of patients with valvular PS and are commonly associated with Noonan syndrome. PV leaflets are usually thickened with little commissural fusion but with limited mobility. It is commonly associated with different degrees of stenosis at different levels of the RVOT. Usually, there is no poststenotic dilation of the pulmonary artery (PA). Balloon valvuloplasty may relieve some of the obstruction, but it is not effective in most cases. (3) Bicuspid PV is often seen in patients with other congenital heart anomalies such as tetralogy of Fallot. Quadricuspid valves are rare and present with pulmonary insufficiency rather than stenosis.

The natural history studies of isolated valvular PS in children indicate that a pressure gradient >50 mmHg is associated with poor long-term outcomes, including RV myocardial dysfunction, ventricular arrhythmia, and sudden death, whereas pressure gradients <30 mmHg are not associated with symptoms, changes in lifestyle, or decreased life expectancy.

Balloon valvuloplasty is currently recommended in symptomatic patients with moderate obstruction (peak Doppler gradient of 36-64 mmHg) or asymptomatic patients with severe obstruction (peak/mean Doppler gradient >64 and >35 mmHg, respectively).

Neonatal Critical Pulmonary Stenosis

Neonates with critical valvular PS present with cyanosis. Desaturated blood returning to the right atrium (RA) can either enter the severely hypertrophied, sometimes diminutive RV chamber or flow right to left across the patent foramen ovale (PFO), as it did throughout fetal life. This shunt adds desaturated blood to the pulmonary venous return on the left side of the heart, accounting for the systemic hypoxemia. If the atrial level shunt is large enough, and resulting antegrade pulmonary flow is limited, the patient will be dependent on the coexistence of a patent ductus arteriosus (PDA) to provide pulmonary blood flow. As the PDA begins to close within hours after birth, the child becomes progressively hypoxemic, requiring prostaglandin E1 (PGE1) to reopen and maintain ductal patency until an appropriate intervention is performed.

Even after successful balloon intervention in the neonate (see below), the hypertrophied RV continues to present a diastolic impediment to forward flow, fostering a continued right-to-left shunt at the PFO, and ongoing systemic desaturation. When PGE1 is discontinued, and the PDA begins to close, pulmonary blood flow will be reduced, and systemic oxygen saturations will fall. As long as the infant maintains oxygen saturations greater than 70% and does not develop a systemic metabolic acidosis, PGE1 does not need to be restarted. Over a course of days to weeks, after elimination of the elevated RV afterload, the myocardium thins out and becomes more compliant. It becomes easier to fill the RV, right-to-left shunting diminishes across the PFO, and the patient's oxygen saturation normalizes. Rarely, ongoing RV noncompliance, often in combination with right ventricular and tricuspid valve (TV) hypoplasia, can result in persistent desaturation in the absence of significant residual PS. In these cases, stent implantation in the PDA or surgical placement of an aortopulmonary shunt may be indicated in order to secure an additional source of pulmonary flow and be able to discontinue PGE1. If the RV and TV have poor growth and remain small, the RV can be partially "unloaded" by performing a bidirectional superior cavopulmonary shunt (Glenn shunt) once the pulmonary vascular resistance has normalized at 4 to 8 months of life.

Pulmonary Stenosis After the Neonatal Period

In most children, PS presents as an asymptomatic heart murmur. Gradients are followed noninvasively with Doppler echocardiography. It is important to note that the peak instantaneous echo gradient usually overestimates the peak-to-peak gradient measured in the cath lab (**Figure 36.1D**). when considering the timing of the intervention in a child. Severe obstruction is associated with surprisingly few symptoms in young children. Rarely, children with severe PS may maintain patency of the PFO allowing right-to-left shunt at times of peak exercise (exercise-induced cyanosis). In patients who are cyanotic at rest, it is important to recognize that neither the echo nor catheter estimates of valve gradient accurately reflect the degree of obstruction, since only part of the cardiac output is traversing the valve.

Adolescent/Adult Patients

Valvular PS rarely presents de novo in the adolescent and adult population. The harsh systolic murmur invariably brings these patients to attention early in childhood. However, the lack of symptoms, and lesser gradients, in the pediatric age group, may delay early intervention. Mild degrees of obstruction are tolerated without issues for many decades but can occasionally be associated with new onset symptoms of exercise intolerance, breathlessness, and fatigue in the older adult. Classic signs of right heart failure—peripheral edema, jugular venous distension, and ascites—are rare. However, the excessive afterload limits RV systolic performance, thereby diminishing left ventricle (LV) preload and cardiac output during exertion.

Valvular PS in the adult may also be acquired as part of carcinoid heart disease. These valves become thickened and dense and more closely resemble dysplastic neonatal valves, where resistance to flow is not related to valve leaflet fusion, but rather to the force required to push open the thickened leaflets. As is the case in the newborn disease, these thickened valves are generally not responsive to balloon valvuloplasty.

Branch Pulmonary Artery Stenosis

Branch PA stenosis (**Figure 36.1E**) or hypoplasia may be acquired (eg, either at sites of prior surgery, or from extrinsic compression) or congenital (ie, tetralogy of Fallot). Numerous congenital syndromes are also associated with branch PA stenosis/hypoplasia (Williams syndrome, congenital rubella, Alagille syndrome, and others). Branch PA stenosis is typically a hemodynamic burden that must be dealt with in children but can be seen in adults as residue of earlier congenital heart surgery or rarely as an isolated congenital lesion. Anatomy ranges from single stenotic areas, to multiple stenoses, to diffuse hypoplasia of the vessel. In contrast with other right-sided obstructive lesions, the branch PA stenosis not only increases RV afterload but also results in maldistribution of the pulmonary blood flow with hypoperfusion of selected lung segments or of an entire lung causing overcirculation and hypertension of others because of the parallel pathways available to the pulmonary blood flow. Quantitative lung perfusion scans, and more recently MRI/MRA, have been extremely useful in the ongoing assessment of these patients. Flow to each individual lobe can be quantified, yielding information about relative severity of individual stenotic lesions. This can help direct therapy prior to arrival in the cath lab and avoid unnecessary catheter/wire manipulation during often lengthy procedures. Indications for angioplasty include significant obstruction with gradients of 20 to 30 mmHg across the stenotic area, elevation of the RV or proximal MPA pressure to greater than one-half to two-thirds of systemic pressure, or when there is relative flow discrepancy between the 2 lungs of 35%/65% or worse. In children, growth of the distal vessels depends on the blood flow to those segments. Segmental hypoperfusion in childhood is associated with poor growth of the affected PA and is itself an indication for intervention.

Percutaneous Balloon Pulmonary Valvuloplasty

The current static balloon technique for pulmonary valvuloplasty was, reported by Kan et al in 1982. Results have demonstrated the safety and effectiveness of this technique and have established it as the treatment of choice for children and adults with isolated pulmonary valve stenosis.

Pediatric Technique

Echocardiographic evaluation is critical to successful outcome prior to intervention. It defines both the degree of obstruction as well as the valve morphology, allows accurate measurement of the pulmonary valve annulus, and can rule out any associated defects. Balloon dilation catheters are now available on catheter shafts as small as 3F, allowing pulmonary balloon valvuloplasty even in premature infants less than 2 kg.

After administration of appropriate anesthesia, femoral venous access is obtained. In most cases, femoral arterial access is not required, as complications from arterial access probably far outweigh the complications of the valvuloplasty especially in children less than 5 kg. The need for heparin administration (50-100 U/kg), in a purely right-sided catheter procedure is unclear. A balloon-tipped angiography or end-hole catheter is used to perform the right heart catheterization. In the absence of associated defects, the PA saturation is used to estimate predilation cardiac index (Fick calculation). The catheter is advanced across the valve to a branch PA, and a pressure pullback is performed. The peak-to-peak and mean gradients across the pulmonary outflow are measured. Right ventricular angiography is then performed using both lateral and cranial-angled AP projections to localize the valve and confirm the echocardiographic annulus size by measuring the valve diameter at the level of the valve hinge points. A balloon diameter 1.2 to 1.4 times that of the annulus is selected, since the use of oversized balloons in pulmonary valvuloplasty has been shown to produce optimal results in children. In larger patients, with an annulus size >20 mm, modifications in technique are required (see "Adult Patients" section). A balloon length of 2 to 3 cm, depending on patient size, is adequate in most children and avoids some of the potential complications of RVOT trauma or injury to the TV.

A balloon end-hole catheter can be floated to the distal right or left PA (angled, torquable catheters may also be used), and a stiff exchange-length guidewire is placed in the branch PA, taking care not to injure the small distal branches of the PA. The catheter is removed, and the desired valvuloplasty balloon is introduced over the guidewire. Once the balloon catheter is centered on the pulmonary valve, the position can be adjusted quickly using a series of very-low-pressure partial inflations to look for the valve "waist." When in the appropriate position, the balloon is inflated rapidly, with mild traction to prevent forward motion, until the waist disappears, most often with a "popping" sensation. The balloon is then immediately deflated. The pop of the valve corresponds to the tearing of the stenotic valve commissures.

After successful opening of the valve, the balloon will usually jump forward with forward flow, which must be distinguished from the forward "squirting" of a balloon that has been positioned too far into the PA, since the latter indicates that the valve has not been effectively dilated. In patients with dysplastic or thickened pulmonary valves, there will be no pop as the balloon is inflated to full pressure but only a gradual resolution of the waist with increasing balloon pressure and a return of the waist as balloon pressures fall. As mentioned, these valves are rarely amenable to balloon valvuloplasty.

A monorail-type angiographic catheter can be advanced over the wire to assess the residual gradient, without removing the guidewire. Alternatively, a larger-lumen end-hole catheter (ie, a guide catheter) with a Y-adapter (Tuohy-Borst valve) can be advanced over the wire to perform a pullback, measuring pressure from the side port of the Tuohy-Borst as the catheter is withdrawn across the valve. In this way, residual pressure gradients can be measured and accurately localized to either the valvular or infundibular level (see "Complications" section). Residual valvular gradients of more than 20 to 30 mmHg are unusual and suggest suboptimal balloon size or position and warrant repeat dilation with use of a larger balloon over the guidewire that is still in place in the distal PA.

Age-Related Modifications of the Procedure

In neonates, access for the procedure is usually obtained in the femoral vein. Maneuvering catheters through the RV and pulmonary valve from umbilical vein access is technically difficult and should only be used if no other access is available. In older patients, internal jugular and subclavian approaches are also acceptable for the procedure. Percutaneous transhepatic access has also been used.

With severe PS and a closed PDA, the catheter across the tiny valve lumen may completely or virtually completely obstruct flow. In this setting, the RV angiogram is performed prior to crossing the valve to minimize the potential for hemodynamic compromise. Once the valve is crossed, the catheter is removed quickly, leaving only the guidewire (to minimize obstruction to flow). In neonates, it is almost never possible to pass a balloon-tipped catheter through the valve, making our catheter of choice a torquable 4F or 5F end-hole catheter with a Judkins right coronary or Berenstein curve. This catheter is manipulated through the TV and flipped up into the RV outflow tract, and either a 0.014-in torque-control guidewire or a small hydrophilic guidewire can be used to probe for the valve orifice. Once the valve is crossed, the wire is positioned either in a branch PA or through the ductus arteriosus into the descending aorta where it could be snared from the descending aorta to stabilize the position further, if needed. Most often, in this setting, a smaller balloon on a smaller catheter shaft is used to predilate the valve, followed by an oversized balloon to finish the procedure.

Valvular pulmonary atresia also presents with cyanosis in the neonate. In these neonates, patency of the ductus arteriosus is required to provide pulmonary blood flow. In some cases, the size of the pulmonary valve annulus, the RV chamber volume, and the TV annulus may be sufficient to allow handling of the normal pulmonary blood flow. In these patients, several techniques have been used to perforate the atretic valve, including stiff guidewires, transseptal needles, or radiofrequency ablation—the most common choice today. Once the valve is perforated and a wire advanced into one of the branches or down the descending aorta (through the PDA), balloon dilation proceeds as if for critical neonatal PS. In some cases, ductal stenting can also be performed to maintain adequate pulmonary flow, while the RV becomes more compliant over time.

Adolescent/Adult Technique

Percutaneous balloon valvuloplasty in adults is similar to what is described above for younger children. The principal difference is that the valve annulus is larger, and owing to the need for balloon diameter oversizing to 120% to 140% of the valve annulus, balloons of 25 mm or larger are often required. There are 3 solutions to this size issue:

Custom balloons are available in sizes greater than 30 mm. With a balloon of this size, there is no difference in the technique, but the balloons have longer inflation and deflation times, lower burst pressures, and require larger sheath sizes.

Double-balloon technique. A second venous access is obtained and a balloon-tipped end-hole catheter is passed to the distal PA. A second stiff exchange-length guidewire is placed across the valve. The perimeter of the combined balloons is selected to be 20% to 40% larger than the measured annulus and the balloons are inflated simultaneously. The double balloon technique allows the use of 2 smaller sheaths but requires additional venous access and additional personnel; it is also more technically challenging, requiring accurate positioning of 2 balloons during simultaneous inflation.

In these cases, an Inoue balloon can be used for adolescent/adult pulmonary valvuloplasty. After hemodynamic evaluation and RV angiography, a 14F sheath is exchanged over a wire and a 0.032-in stiff exchange guidewire is positioned in the branch PA. An Inoue balloon is selected with a diameter 1.2 times the valve annulus. The balloon is stretched/slenderized and passed over the wire to the RA. At that point, the balloon is softened by retraction of the metal support rod, and the distal portion of the balloon is inflated slightly to help float the catheter through the valve. If there is difficulty in manipulating the Inoue balloon through the RV to the PA, a long 14F Mullins sheath can be passed over a wire into the PA, and the Inoue can be advanced through the long sheath (the sheath may need to be cut shorter to accommodate the Inoue length). Once positioned in the main PA, the valvuloplasty is performed exactly as a mitral valvuloplasty.

Procedural Complications

Acute Subvalvular (Infundibular) Obstruction With severe valvular PS, particularly in older children and adults, concentric RV hypertrophy is present universally. When the afterload at the valve is acutely removed, a hypercontractile RV outflow tract may create a dynamic subvalvular muscular obstruction, which has been termed the "suicide RV." The total gradient across the outflow tract may actually be higher after dilation than it was prior to the balloon dilation. It is critical to recognize the difference between residual valvular obstruction and subvalvular reactive obstruction, so as not to perform unnecessary additional valve dilations. A careful pullback pressure recording performed over a wire (as outlined earlier) is the best way to determine the level of residual obstruction. The subvalvular area can also be visualized with an RV angiogram. With an intact atrial septum, if the subvalvular obstruction is severe enough, cardiac output may fall acutely. In patients with the potential for right-to-left shunt at the atrial level, hypoxemia will ensue. Acute treatment of these patients is much like that with left-sided hypertrophic obstructive cardiomyopathy. Volume loading should be combined with beta and/or calcium channel blockers. Over the course of several weeks to months, as the hypertrophy of the outflow tract muscle recedes after reduction of the RV afterload, subvalvular obstruction will resolve.

Other complications are rare and include TV injury, as a result of wire tension on the TV leaflet during inflation or in pulling the partially deflated balloon back through the TV. Pulmonary insufficiency after dilation is common, occurring in 10% to 40% of patients, but is usually well tolerated acutely. Long-standing valvular regurgitation, however, may lead to RV dilation and dysfunction in adults. In neonates and small children, long balloons may rarely injure/rupture the curved RV outflow tract as the balloon straightens, and a long balloon advanced or propelled too far into one of the branch PAs may cause injury at that site. Finally, the wire tracking through the TV can pinch or damage the atrioventricular node, resulting in high-degree atrioventricular block. In our experience, however, more than 94% of pulmonary valve procedures in all age groups were uncomplicated, with most complications clustered in the smaller infants.

Balloon Angioplasty for Branch Pulmonary Artery Stenosis

Balloon angioplasty for hemodynamically important branch PA lesions can be accomplished with small peripheral vascular balloon catheters. Placement of intravascular stents has become the treatment of choice in older children and adults who have completed or nearly completed their growth. Particularly in the proximal, more muscular branches of the pulmonary tree, stents reliably improve vessel size, overcoming the recoil of these elastic vessels, and reduce the need for oversized balloons.

Technique Branch PAs may be dilated from any venous access, depending on the catheter course required. Often, access to the left PA can best be achieved from the femoral approach, while a superior approach may be the easiest to get to the right PA. Following a Glenn shunt, the only access to the branch PAs would be from above. In the case of an aortic to PA shunt, the PAs would need to be accessed from the femoral artery.

After heparinization and the placement of a small arterial catheter for blood pressure monitoring, right heart hemodynamics are measured, and the magnitude and location of gradients in the PAs are determined. In patients with severely hypertensive and dysfunctional RV, advancing large sheaths into the pulmonary arteries across the TV may not be tolerated. Creation of an atrial septal defect (to maintain cardiac output by allowing right-to-left shunting) prior to the PA intervention may decrease morbidity and mortality, by maintaining LV preload even with the balloon inflated in the lungs. Pulmonary angiograms should include selective biplane injections in each lung and in affected lobes or segments.

Selective catheterization of the lung segments is best accomplished using a torquable end-hole catheter and a floppy-tipped torque wire. Once satisfactory wire position is attained, an angiographic monorail catheter is the tool of choice to image and to assess the severity of the stenosis. Alternatively, a larger-lumen angiographic catheter may be passed over the wire, with a Y-adaptor at its end, to allow angiography and pressure measurement from the side-port. Either technique allows pressure measurements, angiograms, and dilations to be performed without losing wire position. Lower-volume, selective injections in the affected lobes almost always yield superior images compared to injections in the central PA. Prior to dilation, a stiffer exchange-length wire should be passed to the largest vessel distal to the stenosis to support balloon positioning. Use of the largest vessel also minimizes the risk of rupture/vessel injury of small distal vessels with balloon inflation.

The balloon diameter is chosen to be 2 to 4 times the diameter of the lesion but not more than 2 times the diameter of the normal vessel on either side. The balloon is inflated until the waist disappears or until maximum inflation pressure is reached. Inflation times range from 10 to 60 seconds, depending on the response of the waist and how well the cardiac output is maintained. Like with coronary angioplasty, successful dilation generally results in tearing of the intima and media.

Following dilation, the balloon catheter is exchanged again over the guidewire for a monorail catheter, and hemodynamics are repeated. Angiograms are performed to measure the diameter of the stenosis and to look carefully for tears and aneurysms that may preclude further balloon dilation. For this reason, distal lesions are generally dilated prior to proximal lesions, and more severe stenoses are dilated prior to milder ones.

Results The criteria for successful dilation have been arbitrarily defined as an increase in diameter of >50%, an increase in flow in the affected segment of >20%, and/or a decrease of >20% in the systolic right ventricular-to-aortic pressure ratio. Using these criteria, the early success rate using low-pressure balloons with inflation pressures up to 10 atmospheres was approximately 50% of the vessels treated. The use of high-pressure balloons with inflation pressures greater than 20 atmospheres increased success rates to 70%. The success rate for postoperative stenosis is higher than for congenital, unrepaired stenosis which tends to be much more resistant to dilation. The incidence of subsequent restenosis following balloon angioplasty is approximately 10%. Adverse events are more common when interventions are performed on distal vessels compared with proximal vessels. In patients undergoing any type of PA intervention (balloon and/or stent), life-threatening complications as a direct result of the procedure occur in 2.8% and death in approximately 0.15%. Aneurysms occur in 3% of dilations and are most common in small vessels distal to the stenosis. Although the success rate using low-pressure balloons has changed little over the years, the complication rate has decreased owing primarily to improved technique. The use of high-pressure balloons does not seem to have significantly altered the complication rate. Balloon angioplasty at surgical sites should be used with caution in patients less than 4 to 6 weeks after surgery to minimize the risk of vessel rupture.

Use of Bladed Cutting Balloons

Later experience with bladed cutting balloon catheters has shown improved outcomes for the treatment of what were previously considered nondilatable lesions. Small studies, under compassionate use protocols, have shown significant improvement in vessel size using oversized cutting balloons that cut through intimal and medial layers. Cutting balloons have been demonstrated to be more effective than high-pressure balloons following failed low-pressure balloon dilation. Furthermore, after high-pressure balloons, subsequent use of cutting-balloon inflation, has improved outcomes with increase in lumen diameter of >90% than initial diameter.

Use of Intravascular Stents

Branch PA placement of stents was first reported in humans in 1991, with excellent short-term and midterm results and they are now the most commonly used in patients with CHD. Although balloon angioplasty remains the treatment of choice in peripheral lesions and in infants/small children, stent implantation in the PA bed has become first-line therapy for proximal obstructions, lesions due to surgical distortion, external compression, inadequate results of balloon angioplasty, and obstructive intimal flaps following balloon angioplasty. Infants who undergo surgical repairs such as the arterial switch for transposition of the great arteries, repair of tetralogy of Fallot with branch PA plasty, and palliations such as shunts or PA banding may have acute postoperative obstructions that create hemodynamic instability or place the obstructed lung at risk for long-term hypoperfusion. Stent usage in the immediate postoperative period, as an alternative to repeat surgical intervention, can be lifesaving and is more reliable than balloon angioplasty alone. Since early stent use in the branch PAs, technology has improved both in the stents themselves and in the delivery balloons. The use of stents has improved the success rate of branch PA interventions to >90%.

Current stents are available in a combination of different formats: open and closed cell designs, bare-metal and covered stents, and premounted and unmounted, each offering advantages and disadvantages. Because of their lower profile and greater stability on the balloon than manually crimped stents, premounted stents are preferred in infants and children. Current premounted stents can be dilated to medium (up to 12 mm) and large diameters (up to 20 mm) which allows subsequent balloon redilation to accommodate somatic growth even up to adult size vessel diameters. In patients whose stents cannot be dilated to an adult size diameter, surgery is required unless the stent can be "unzipped" with high-pressure angioplasty.

Unmounted stents have a greater radial force than premounted stents and are more commonly used in bigger patients with larger diameter proximal PAs. Innovations in balloon design include a marked reduction in catheter shaft diameter and slip-/scratch-resistant balloon surfaces (to reduce the incidence of the stent slipping off or puncturing the balloon). The BIB (balloon-in-balloon) balloon dilation catheter system (Nu-Med, Hopkinton, NY) is being used for many indications and helps minimize the risks of stent malposition.

Stent and balloon sizes are selected for the individual lesion. For premounted stents, the use of a long sheath is optional depending on the anatomy, need of angiography prior and during implantation and operator preference. If an unmounted stent is used, the stent is crimped onto the balloon and can be delivered using 1 of 2 techniques. With a standard approach, an oversized long sheath or guiding catheter is passed over a stiff exchange-length guidewire (with a short floppy tip) such that the sheath tip is distal to the lesion to be stented. The balloon-stent combination is then advanced over the guidewire through the sheath to the implantation site. Alternatively, the front-loading technique involves passing the balloon catheter fully through the sheath outside the body, crimping the stent onto the balloon, and pulling it back into the front of the sheath before introducing this assembly over the wire. Combined techniques are also used in which the long sheath is advanced over the wire to the inferior vena cava (IVC), the stent then mounted on the balloon, and advanced over the wire to the tip of the sheath *prior* to advancing the entire system over the wire to the target lesion. The front-loading approach decreases the risk of the stent slipping from the balloon as the entire system is advanced through tight intracardiac curves. Antiplatelet therapy is the norm, for a period of 3 to 6 months to prevent in-stent thrombosis. For patients with normal pulsatile flow in the PAs, aspirin alone should be sufficient. For patients with nonpulsatile flow (bidirectional Glenn shunt or Fontan), dual antiplatelet therapy or warfarin is recommended, though there are little data available on which to base such a decision. In-stent stenosis, angiographically defined as a 25% narrowing of the lumen relative to the stent diameter, is diagnosed in ~24% of patients following stent implantation and is a common source of recurrent stent obstruction. Heparinization and prophylactic antibiotic use are recommended in these typically long procedures.

Stents in Extracardiac Conduits

Stents may also be used to extend the life of surgical conduits inserted between the heart and the branch PAs. With rapid growth of the infant, such conduits may kink and/or develop intraluminal obstruction. Balloon angioplasty alone in this setting has been largely unsuccessful because the conduit will reassume its kinked course on balloon deflation. In several patients, it is possible to hold off conduit replacement for several years using this approach, removing the stent with the explanted conduit at later surgery. This may allow for placement of an adult-sized conduit at the next surgery, and future placement of transcatheter valve implants (see above). For patients with obstructions in full-sized conduits, stenting of the conduit followed by pulmonary valve implantation would be the current procedure of choice.

Pulmonary Valve Stenosis With Significant Regurgitation

When pulmonary valve stenosis or obstruction within a surgically placed RV to PA conduit or bioprosthetic valve coexists with significant pulmonary regurgitation, the result is both a volume overload and afterload increase on the RV. In this setting, relief of the obstruction alone may not alleviate the most severe hemodynamic derangement, the regurgitant flow, and may actually make it worse. Until recently, surgical intervention with valve or conduit replacement was the only alternative available to the patient.

Over the past decades, however, beginning with the work of Bonhoeffer's group in Europe, the development and subsequent clinical use of transcatheter implantable pulmonary valves has revolutionized the management of patients with residual post-surgical pulmonary valve disease. Since so many complex congenital malformations, including pulmonary valve atresia, tetralogy of Fallot, double-outlet RV, and some of the aortic valve malformations require placement of prosthetic RV to PA connection in the form of a conduit or bioprosthetic valve, the need for later valve replacement is growing due to the limited life span of these prostheses. This is particularly true in light of the growing recognition of the deleterious long-term effect of pulmonary valve insufficiency on the RV myocardium. Currently approved transcatheter pulmonary valves in the United States are the Melody Valve (Medtronic Inc, Dublin, Ireland) and the Edwards SAPIEN XT (Edwards Lifesciences, Irvine, CA). The Melody Valve is derived from a bovine jugular vein valve, sewn into a platinum iridium stent. It comes in one size that can be expanded up to 22 mm. The Edwards SAPIEN XT is produced from 3 equal-sized bovine pericardial leaflets that are sewn to a cobalt-chromium frame balloon-expandable stent, in 3 sizes: 23, 26, and 29 mm in diameter. Patients with tetralogy of Fallot who have had valved conduits or prosthetic valves placed, and patients who underwent the Ross procedure, where the pulmonary valve is autotransplanted to replace the diseased aortic valve and a valved conduit is used between the RV and the branch pulmonary arteries, represent the 2 largest patient populations who are receiving these valves.

Careful evaluation of the underlying coronary anatomy is critical in determining the appropriateness of the intervention (**Figure 36.2**). When the conduit is placed on the anterior surface of the heart, coronary branches may pass directly beneath it and may be potentially compressed by placement of the stented valve and distension of the conduit. Evaluation and pretreatment of the valve landing site is critical for optimal valve longevity. Because the conduits sit directly beneath the sternum, there is often an element of compression of the conduit which is dynamic and can lead to stent fracture. Prestenting the landing site of the new valve, potentially with several stents layered inside each other, has significantly improved the survival of the implant, minimizing stent fracture, which affected 23% of the initially reported series. Placement of transcatheter pulmonary valve within an existing bioprosthetic valve (valve-in-valve procedure) is

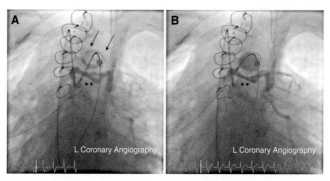

Figure 36.2 A, In this patient with a conduit repair of tetralogy of Fallot, imaged from a steep caudal angulation, the calcified, oval-shaped conduit (black arrows) passes over the left coronary system (black asterisks) which are being selectively injected. **B,** Balloon dilation within the conduit expands the conduit posteriorly, producing coronary compression in both the LAD and circumflex (black asterisks).

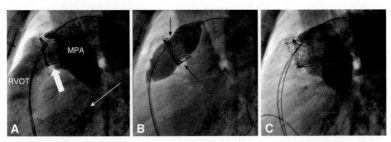

Figure 36.3 **A,** PA angiogram in a patient with a severely insufficient bioprosthetic pulmonary valve (thick white arrow). An atrial septal defect had been previously closed with an Amplatzer Septal Occluder Device (thin white arrow). **B,** Balloon sizing of the bioprosthetic valve. The waist on the balloon (black arrows) indicates the true inner diameter of the valve. **C,** Follow-up PA angiogram after placement of an Edwards SAPIEN valve (valve-in-valve) inside the ring of the existing bioprosthetic valve, showing no significant residual pulmonary insufficiency. MPA, main pulmonary artery; PA, pulmonary artery; RVOT, right ventricular outflow tract.

not associated with stent fracture as the valve framework is protected by the existing valve ring (**Figure 36.3**).

OBSTRUCTION OF THE LEFT VENTRICULAR OUTFLOW TRACT
Anatomy/Physiology

Similar to obstructions of the RVOT, congenital obstruction of the left ventricular outflow tract can occur at the subvalvular level, at the valvular level, at the supravalvular level, or in the aortic arch itself (coarctation of the aorta). The increased afterload on the LV myocardium results in concentric hypertrophy and reduced diastolic compliance of the ventricle as a receiving chamber with a corresponding increase in left atrial and pulmonary venous pressures.

Patients may present with angina, syncope, dyspnea on exertion, and/or orthopnea. Most children tolerate significant LV outflow tract obstruction without symptoms, presenting with a murmur alone, but symptoms become more common in the older child and adult.

Transcatheter Therapy for Left-Sided Obstruction

Subaortic stenosis encompasses a spectrum of disorders ranging from simple membranous obstruction of the subaortic area, to fibromuscular tunnel obstructions, to the more familiar hypertrophic cardiomyopathy. Like subvalvular lesions of the right side, subaortic obstruction is primarily a surgical issue. Membranous obstructions of the left ventricular outflow were treated with balloon angioplasty early in the interventional era with limited success and with routine recurrence of obstruction. Fibromuscular tunnel obstructions are generally not amenable to catheter intervention. Stents have been used in a few patients with critical postoperative obstructions, with very limited success, high morbidity, and a significant incidence of stent failure.

In hypertrophic cardiomyopathy with muscular subaortic obstruction, septal myectomy can be used in symptomatic children and adolescents with severe degrees of obstruction. Although alcohol ablation of septal tissue has been widely adopted in adults as an alternative to surgical muscle resection, there is no significant experience with this technique in children and adolescents. As for dual-chamber pacing that was initially reported to alleviate obstruction in younger patients, outcomes in later studies have been controversial. This therapy should only be considered as an alternative to surgical or transcatheter septal reduction in symptomatic patients with severe obstruction despite maximal medical therapy who are poor candidates for other interventions.

Supravalvular aortic stenosis (AS) typically occurs at the sinotubular junction, as a congenital lesion. This is the pathognomonic lesion for Williams syndrome, a genetic deletion syndrome associated with developmental delay, abnormalities of calcium metabolism, and diffuse arteriopathy including peripheral PA stenosis. Patients with Williams syndrome can experience significant hemodynamic lability; thus, any invasive procedure is associated with high mortality rates. This lesion should be treated surgically as the stenotic segment often is in close relationship to and can compromise the ostium of the coronary arteries.

Valvular Aortic Stenosis

Balloon aortic valvuloplasty for congenital AS in a child was first reported in 1983. It has been performed subsequently in large numbers of patients with both congenital and acquired valvular stenosis. In children, adolescents, and young adults with congenital valvular AS, balloon valvuloplasty is an excellent alternative to surgical valvulotomy or to valve replacement, since the pathology involves more commissural fusion and less leaflet rigidity than that seen in adult patients with senescent and densely calcified aortic valves.

Acquired calcific valve stenosis is almost exclusively seen in adults. Acute relief of gradient with balloon valvuloplasty is possible in these patients. However, the rapid rate of restenosis, the risk of cerebral calcium embolization, and the risk of disrupting the valve leaflets and causing severe valvular insufficiency, along with unpredictable and suboptimal degrees of obstruction relief have left balloon valvuloplasty for calcified valves as an emergency option only, when surgical valve replacement is not an option. The recent successes of transcatheter aortic valve replacement are changing the paradigms for treatment of older adults with severe aortic valve disease.

Neonatal Critical Aortic Stenosis

Physiologically, critical AS is a different entity from severe AS in older children, since the valve may be virtually atretic and the left ventricular cavity may be moderately to severely hypoplastic. The term "critical," in the neonate, implies that the infant's ability to maintain an adequate systemic cardiac output is dependent on flow reaching the aorta from the right ventricle via the PDA.

The clinical presentation of neonates with critical AS is variable and depends primarily on the proportion of cardiac output supplied by the LV, but also may be affected by restriction of the PFO, and ductus arteriosus patency. With severe not critical AS, the LV will fill adequately and pump enough blood through the aortic valve to maintain cardiac output when the ductus closes. With even more severe AS, forward flow through the valve is diminished either by LV hypoplasia, by LV hypocontractility (from excessive afterload), by left-to-right shunting at the atrial communication, or by any combination of the 3. With some forward flow through the valve, the arms and head receive primarily pulmonary venous blood and will have normal saturations by pulse oximetry, while the lower half of the body receives flow augmented by systemic venous return through the ductus arteriosus and will be desaturated. With no flow (or nearly no flow) through the aortic valve, all 4 extremities will be desaturated due to the mixing of the systemic and pulmonary venous returns in the right heart.

Newborns may be relatively asymptomatic immediately after birth because of the normal remnants of the fetal circulation. Pulmonary venous return to the left atrium can cross the PFO to the RA, rather than entering the LV and in the presence of limited antegrade flow across the aortic valve, the mixture of systemic and pulmonary venous return from the RV is pumped to the MPA, where flow is distributed between the lungs and the systemic circulation via the ductus arteriosus, based on the relative resistance of each pathway. If pulmonary resistance remains high enough, a normal blood volume reaches the aorta and cardiac output is maintained. But retrograde flow in the transverse arch and even ascending aorta may be evident on echocardiography. As pulmonary resistance falls and as the ductus arteriosus starts to close, RV output preferentially flows to the lungs. A corresponding fall in systemic blood flow results in diminished tissue oxygen delivery, profound metabolic acidosis, and circulatory collapse. Reestablishing and maximizing systemic flow is the key to resuscitating the acidotic newborn. Prostaglandin is required to reopen the ductus, while raising pulmonary vascular resistance is the primary goal of resuscitative therapy (minimizing FiO_2, allowing pCO_2 to rise).

None of these hemodynamic scenarios is sustainable over long periods of time. Thus, neonates with AS and evidence of hemodynamic compromise should be urgently intervened upon. In the newborn, when most of the systemic flow arises from the ductus arteriosus, rather than the LV, the measured valvular pressure gradient across the stenotic valve is not a meaningful number, as antegrade flow across the aortic valve is very limited. In the most severe cases, when systemic cardiac output is exclusively maintained by flow across the PDA, there will be no aortic valve gradient.

Unlike hypoplasia of the right ventricle in critical PS (in which right atrial blood may cross the PFO to maintain LV preload and cardiac output), the size of the LV has a direct impact on survival. If LV hypoplasia is a concern, the alternative is to assign these patients to a stage I palliation for hypoplastic left heart syndrome. A retrospective analysis of a group of patients with critical AS undergoing surgical valvulotomy or balloon dilation at Boston Children's Hospital led to a scoring system (based on echocardiographic measurement of left-sided structures) that can be used to triage such patients.

Fetal aortic valvuloplasty for severe AS with evolving hypoplastic left heart syndrome has been reported and associated with high technical success rates. Overall outcomes for patients who achieve a biventricular circulation after fetal balloon valvuloplasty are encouraging. However, results of attempts to recruit borderline-sized LVs in order to achieve biventricular circulation in patients who initially underwent single ventricle palliation have been suboptimal.

Technique for Critical Neonatal Aortic Stenosis

The techniques for performing balloon aortic valvuloplasty in neonates are similar to those in older children (see below). However, some adaptations are required for the neonate. Before the catheterization begins, the neonate's hemodynamic status must be optimized. This procedure is performed with the baby intubated and paralyzed and receiving a prostaglandin infusion. The FiO_2 is turned down to 21%, and pCO_2 is allowed to rise to the mid-40s to increase pulmonary vascular resistance and maximize systemic flow across the PDA. Body temperature is carefully monitored.

The umbilical artery can usually be used in the first week of life. Catheter manipulation is more difficult from the umbilical artery owing to the inferoposterior loop in its course before it enters the descending aorta, but its use avoids damage to the femoral artery in these very small infants. Surgical cutdown or percutaneous access at the carotid artery for catheter access has also been employed. This approach simplifies crossing the valve because of the straight path to the valve from the neck. As with older patients, a transseptal approach can be used from either the femoral or umbilical vein, with no arterial puncture required since all neonates have a PFO. But this approach is rarely used since it carries a much higher risk of mitral valve injury than in the older population. However, a balloon-tipped angiographic catheter placed in the LV during the procedure facilitates measuring gradients before and after balloon valvuloplasty.

Pediatric Technique

Indications for intervention in children and adolescents include a peak-to-peak systolic ejection gradient (PSEG) (by catheter) of >50 mmHg in the absence of symptoms or >40 mmHg in the presence of symptoms or new ST-T wave changes at rest or during exercise. A >40 mmHg gradient is also used as an indication for intervention in asymptomatic women willing to become pregnant. As most pediatric procedures are performed under sedation or general anesthesia, PSEG found during the procedure may be an underestimation of the actual gradient. Mean Doppler gradient correlates well with PSEG in aortic valve stenosis; thus, a mean Doppler gradient of ~50 mmHg in a nonsedated patient should serve as indicator of the need of intervention.

Using routine sedation, a femoral vein and artery are entered percutaneously and the patient is heparinized. The venous catheter is used to measure right heart pressures and cardiac output (when no shunts are present) before and after dilation. An ascending aortogram is performed to define the anatomic landmarks. The aortic annulus is measured at the hinge points of the valve and the orientation of the jet of unopacified blood arising from the ventricle is visualized which may help to aim the catheter/wire in order to cross the valve. The typical method for crossing the stenotic aortic valve from the aorta is to advance the soft end of a straight wire out of a steerable catheter (multipurpose or Judkins Right curve) and use it to probe for the valve orifice. A hydrophilic guidewire can be used, as the reduced friction of its surface allows for more rapid in and out movements, but probing must be done gently to avoid perforating a cusp or damaging the coronary arteries. When the LV is entered, a transvalvular gradient is measured by simultaneously recording pressure from the catheter and from the femoral sheath (1F size larger than the catheter). A pigtail catheter is exchanged over a wire, a left ventriculogram may be performed and the aortic annulus is measured again.

In contrast to the pulmonary valvuloplasty, the balloon diameter is chosen to be only 75% to 90% of the annulus diameter. Animal and clinical studies demonstrate that aortic valvuloplasty with a balloon-annulus ratio greater than 1.0 is more likely to be associated with occurrence of aortic regurgitation. A double-balloon technique was used in the past to allow for the use of smaller sheaths, when the annulus was larger, and there was concern for femoral artery injury in small children. However, with balloons on shafts as small as 3F and 4F today, there is little indication for such an approach. The pigtail catheter is exchanged for the balloon dilation catheter, which is centered across the valve, inflated and deflated rapidly, and pulled back to the descending aorta. The gradient and the cardiac output are remeasured following dilation, and an aortogram is performed to look for aortic regurgitation. If the residual gradient is >35 mmHg and an aortogram shows no or only mild regurgitation, a larger balloon may be used. It is far better, however, to leave a residual gradient than to cause significant aortic insufficiency (AI) in the small child, as surgical backout options are limited (Ross procedure).

In bigger patients who require large, slow inflating balloons, it can be difficult to keep the balloon positioned in the valve during inflation, against the force of left ventricular ejection. A stiff catheter shaft, long balloon, and extra stiff exchange wire will help stabilize the position, or the balloon can be advanced so that it lies along the top of the aortic arch rather than around the underside of the arch. Rapid RV pacing (rate is dependent on the age of the patient) during balloon inflation to reduce ventricular ejection is now the most commonly used and the most effective technique for balloon stabilization as has been demonstrated in transcatheter aortic valve replacement procedure in adults. However, this is rarely needed in neonates or infants since it carries a higher risk of RV perforation.

Results/Complications

Balloon valvuloplasty for congenital AS has been an effective palliation in the pediatric population with excellent gradient reduction and increase in valve area. Classification of procedural success has been defined as it follows: (1) Optimal outcome, PSEG < 35 mmHg and no AI; (2) adequate outcome, PSEG < 35 mmHg + mild AI or no worsening of baseline AI; and (3) inadequate outcome, PSEG > 35 mmHg or AI > mild or worsening AI in those with AI at baseline.

A recent study with the outcomes of 1020 patients from the IMPACT registry (Improving Pediatric and Adult Congenital Treatments) reported procedural success rates (optimal + adequate) of ~70% for noncritical and 62.5% for critical AS. New moderate or severe AI develops in 12% to 18% of patients. Although there were no intraprocedural deaths, hospital mortality was 1.5% in noncritical AS and 10% in critical AS patients. Severe adverse events were also more common in critical AS patients (27%) compared with noncritical AS (9.6%). Vascular complications occurred in 9.1% of critical AS neonates.

COARCTATION OF THE AORTA

The location of the obstruction in a patient with coarctation of the aorta (typically just distal to the takeoff of the left subclavian artery—**Figure 36.4A** and **B**) creates not only an increase in left ventricular afterload but also differential hypertension, with high pressures proximal to the obstruction and low to normal pressures distal (**Figure 36.4C** and **D**).

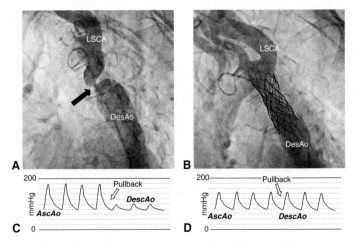

Figure 36.4 Coarctation of the aorta. **A,** Prior to stent implant. Discreet, severe coarctation site distal to left subclavian artery (black arrow). **B,** Post stent implant, the luminal diameter of the aorta is normalized. **C,** Pullback tracings from ascending to descending aorta prior to stent implant with a large systolic gradient indicating obstruction. **D,** Post stent implantation, there is no remaining pressure gradient through the aorta. Systolic pressure in the ascending aorta has fallen, and the descending aorta systolic pressure has normalized.

High pressure in the ascending aorta and its branches predisposes these patients to many of the usual risks associated with hypertension. Intracranial aneurysms may be present in as many as 10% of patients with coarctation. As a result, the natural history of untreated coarctation includes risks of developing premature coronary artery disease and cerebral aneurysm rupture. Because of the presence of a fixed obstruction, hypertension may be difficult to control with standard pharmacologic therapy. Unlike patients with essential systemic hypertension, pharmacologic reduction of upper extremity (cerebral and coronary) pressures will proportionally decrease descending aortic pressure and can produce iatrogenic claudication with exercise, abdominal cramping with splanchnic hypoperfusion, and significant renal dysfunction (prerenal azotemia).

Multiple levels of obstruction are possible—a bicuspid aortic valve is associated with coarctation of the aorta in >70% of patients and echocardiographic screening is recommended in all patients. Turner syndrome is associated with coarctation of the aorta.

Although any patient with coarctation of the aorta has a lifetime higher risk of developing hypertension or remaining hypertensive following transcatheter or surgical repair, the risk is even higher in patients undergoing treatment in adulthood compared with those treated as neonates or at a young age.

In neonatal coarctation of the aorta, the transverse and isthmic portions of the aortic arch may be hypoplastic and also in need of repair. The newborn with critical coarctation will be asymptomatic initially as the carotids and subclavian arteries are supplied adequately by the ascending aorta, while right-to-left shunting at the ductus arteriosus supplies flow to the lower part of the body (as discussed earlier). At this time, there may be differential cyanosis, with significantly lower arterial saturations in the legs than in the arms. The pulse and blood pressure in the lower extremities may not be substantially different from those in the arms. With the onset of ductal closure, the critical obstruction of the aorta precludes adequate flow to the lower portion of the body. Pulses vanish in the lower extremities only, and a severe metabolic acidosis ensues. Left ventricular dysfunction is common. Prostaglandin is required to reestablish flow to the lower portion of the body.

In older children and adults, the most common form of presentation is systemic hypertension. Less common are a history of headaches, an abnormal electrocardiogram with left ventricular hypertrophy, or the presence of a murmur of related to the bicuspid aortic valve. Indications for intervention beyond neonatal age include a transcatheter systolic gradient >20 mmHg across the coarctation or a gradient of <20 mmHg in the presence of significant collaterals, decreased left ventricular function or in patients with single ventricle palliation. Surgical arch repair remains the standard of care for neonatal coarctation of the aorta in most centers, reserving transcatheter intervention for older patients and those with recurrent postoperative obstruction.

Percutaneous balloon angioplasty of coarctation was first described in 1982 as an alternative to surgery and has been used since in pediatric patients for both native (unoperated) coarctation as well as with recurrent (postoperative) coarctation. However, due to the elastic nature of the aorta, balloon oversizing beyond the diameter of the normal segments of the aorta is often needed. As a result, balloon dilation of native coarctation of the aorta has been associated with higher rates of recurrence and higher risk of aneurysm formation in patients of any age. Thus, balloon angioplasty as a primary therapy for native coarctation remains controversial and is generally reserved for postoperative, recurrent coarctation or for temporary palliation in neonates presenting with significant hemodynamic compromise and a prohibitive surgical risk. Stent implantation has become the procedure of choice in older children, adolescents, and adults in whom the stent can be expanded to a full, or nearly full, adult aortic diameter so as to avoid the need for later redilation of the stent.

Pediatric Balloon Angioplasty Technique

Under routine sedation, femoral venous and arterial access is obtained percutaneously. The patient is heparinized to an activated clotting time (ACT) > 200 seconds. Coarctation is almost always best approached from a retrograde femoral arterial approach, though transvenous, transseptal, and antegrade approaches have been reported (when residual aortic arch obstruction must be addressed following stage I surgical palliation of single ventricles, a venous approach is commonly used). Right and left heart hemodynamics are measured (including cardiac output), and pullbacks are performed with an end-hole catheter from the LV back through the aortic valve and through the area of the coarctation. Biplane aortography is best performed with left anterior oblique (LAO) and straight lateral projections. The diameters of the narrowest area of coarctation and of the normal proximal and distal aorta are measured. For postoperative recurrent coarctation, the balloon is chosen to be 2.5 to 3.0 times the narrowest area but not greater than 1.5 times the normal proximal or distal aorta. For native obstructions, the balloon is commonly chosen to be equal to the diameter of the aorta at the isthmus or at the diaphragm. The balloon dilation catheter is centered across the coarctation, inflated until the waist disappears, and deflated. The balloon catheter is exchanged for a smaller pigtail catheter to allow simultaneous measurement of the ascending aortic pressure with the pigtail in comparison with the distal pressure from the side arm of the existing sheath.

A repeat aortogram should be performed following dilation to determine the angiographic effect of the inflation and to detect tears, ruptures, or dissections. If significant obstruction remains despite disappearance of the balloon waist during inflation, a larger balloon can be used. Although chest discomfort may be quite significant during balloon inflation, persistent pain after balloon deflation suggests aortic rupture or dissection.

Results

Procedural success for the treatment of coarctation of the aorta has been historically defined as a residual upper to lower extremity blood pressure gradient of <20 mmHg. Current studies have demonstrated that the procedure is safe with reasonable acute outcomes. Neonatal coarctation is, however, less responsive to balloon dilation, likely due to the presence of ductal tissue and only indicated as a salvage procedure. A recent prospective multicenter study in 130 patients >10 kg comparing outcomes of balloon angioplasty in native and recurrent coarctation of the aorta showed an acute residual gradient <15 mmHg in 73% to 80% and <10 mmHg in 54% to 68% of patients, respectively. The rate of angiographically identifiable acute aortic wall injury was similar in both groups at approximately 10%. At intermediate follow-up, native coarctation patients had a higher incidence of recurrent obstruction and aneurysm formation compared with the other group. Other studies have also demonstrated recurrent coarctation rates of up to 50% in native coarctation patients. Balloon angioplasty of native coarctation has also been shown to have an increased risk of aneurysm formation in 8% to 20% of patients on follow-up. Another multicenter study also found superior hemodynamic results with stent placement and surgery compared to balloon angioplasty in native coarctation. Furthermore, complication rate was lower among stent patients compared with the balloon angioplasty group. Single-ventricle patients often develop recurrent coarctation following surgical palliation. Residual coarctation needs to be treated aggressively in these patients. A fairly large study showed that balloon angioplasty is effective in this group. In the current era, most centers favor primary stent placement in older children and adults while surgery remains the preferred approach in young children for the management of native coarctation. Balloon angioplasty remains the best therapeutic option for recurrent obstruction following surgical repair and occasionally as a temporizing alternative to surgery in young children who are too small (<25-30 kg) to initially accommodate a stent that can be serially dilated to adult size.

A common complication in children is loss of the arterial pulse secondary to large catheter/artery size ratio. Iliac artery rupture and a retroperitoneal hemorrhage resulting in death have been reported in infants. The incidence of femoral artery injury has decreased with the availability of lower-profile balloons.

Coarctation of the Aorta in the Adult

The technique as outlined above is also applicable to adult patients, and several series have reported excellent outcomes in adult patients with low incidences of rupture, dissection, aneurysm formation, or restenosis.

Stent implantation is now the procedure of choice in most laboratories for either native or recurrent coarctation in older children, adolescents, and adult patients (see **Figure 36.4B**). Stent implantation has advantages over balloon angioplasty in terms of lower residual gradients and reduced rates of restenosis and is markedly more effective than balloon angioplasty alone in the patient with mild coarctation. Implantation of a stent eliminates the elastic recoil of the aortic tissue and allows the use of substantially smaller balloons which may result in a smaller number of aortic wall injuries, such as acute dissections and aneurysm formation. To reduce the incidence of these complications, the use of the covered Cheatham-platinum (CP) stents (NuMED, Inc., Hopkinton, New York) has become popular. In 2016, the U.S. Food and Drug Administration approved the CP-covered stents for the prevention and/or treatment of aortic wall injury in patients with coarctation of the aorta. CP stents are composed of a bare platinum/iridium stent with a polytetrafluoroethylene sleeve that can exclude aneurysms from the circulation. The stents are available in 8 zig and 10 zig designs, range in length from 16 to 60 mm and can be dilated up to a diameter of 24 to 30 mm. The choice of stent ultimately will be tailored to the needs of the patient. For stenting within the more proximal aortic arch, for example, bare-metal stents will remain the treatment of choice to minimize the risk of occluding carotid or subclavian arteries. In contrast, for patients with a tight coarctation remote to the aortic branches or with aneurysm formation at the site of a native or previously repaired coarctation, a covered stent is the clear choice.

Stent Angioplasty Procedure

The procedure is generally performed from a femoral arterial access with deep sedation or general anesthesia. Radial access is also obtained by some operators to maintain continuous monitoring of the arterial pressure and to facilitate management of the blood pressure after the procedure. Hemodynamics and angiography are performed as above. Over a stiff guidewire, often placed into the subclavian artery, a long sheath is advanced through the coarctation. The sheath size will generally need to be at least 2F sizes larger than the sheath size needed for introducing the dilation catheter to allow for the thickness of the stent. For premounted covered CP stents, the size of the sheath recommended is indicated in the package and ranges between 12F and 14F. Once the long sheath is passed through the coarctation, the stent is crimped onto the balloon (unless preloaded) and passed through the sheath to the delivery site. Rapid right ventricular pacing is employed; pressure measurements are performed, and redilation can be performed with a larger or higher-pressure balloon if needed. The goal is to eliminate the obstruction, not necessarily to create a pristine aortic profile angiographically. It is acceptable to leave a mild waist, if there is no further gradient at the site. There is certainly more leeway to aggressively reinflate the stent when a covered stent is implanted, as the risk of dissection or tears is reduced.

Stent malposition may occur as the balloon-stent assembly is pushed distally by the systolic force of the forward aortic flow, particularly with milder coarctation. In cases with bare-metal stents, the stent can be safely reexpanded lower in the aorta, avoiding coverage of side branches. However, with the use of covered stents, redeployment in the abdominal aorta may be problematic. The use of BIB balloons and rapid ventricular pacing during balloon inflation minimize these issues. Balloon puncture by the partially inflated stent is also possible as the stent needs to conform to the curved structure that is the distal aortic arch. This is also less of an issue using BIB balloons and stiffer wires than it had been in the past. Stent fracture is an unusual but potentially late complication of the procedure. The loss of structural integrity and radial strength may lead to recurrent obstruction at the site, to thrombus formation, or to injury of the aorta at the site of fracture.

Results

Numerous clinical studies have documented the effectiveness and safety of stent placement for treatment of both native and recurrent postoperative coarctation of the aorta. Forbes et al. reported procedural success (defined as gradient <20 mmHg and coarctation of the aorta to descending aorta ratio of >0.8) in ~98% of almost 600 procedures performed in patients older than 4 years treated predominantly with bare-metal stents. Procedural complications occurred in 14% of patients including 2 procedure-related deaths. Acute aortic wall rupture/dissection occurred in 1.6% of the procedures. On follow-up, abnormalities of the aortic wall were found in ~25% of the patients who underwent imaging, including aneurysm formation in 9% and intimal proliferation in 16%. Intimal proliferation was more common in children and those with a smaller poststent diameter. Aortic wall complications were associated with prestent angioplasty, balloon diameter–coarctation diameter ratio >3.5, abdominal coarctation, and age >40 years. At intermediate-term follow-up, no significant differences in resting hypertension have been found between stent versus surgically treated patients. Among stented patients, most common indications for reintervention include severe intimal stenosis, stent fracture, stent recoil, and adjustment for somatic growth and have been reported in 2.7% to 4% of the patients. Several studies have reported success using covered stents as a primary therapy for native or recurrent coarctation of the aorta and others have reported the utility of covered stents for managing acute aortic wall injury with or without coarctation. Covered stent outcomes are similar to bare-metal stents with the added advantage of the covering which adds a margin of safety particularly in patients with known high risk for aortic wall injury including those with Turner syndrome and older adults. Covered CP stents should be immediately available any time an intervention is planned in the aorta in the catheterization laboratory.

Management of antihypertensive medications following stent placement is based on individual response with most patients being able to decrease the dose and/or the number of medications over time. Patients are usually restricted from contact sports for at least 1 month after the procedure. They are also placed on daily antiplatelet medication and recommended endocarditis antibiotic prophylaxis for 6 months after stent placement. Even if the coarctation repair appears satisfactory, thoracic aortic imaging should be performed within 12 months after the procedure and every 5 years thereafter to assess for aortic dilatation or aneurysm formation. Imaging strategies for surveillance after stenting remain controversial. MRI is feasible but may be hindered by metallic artifact, particularly with stainless steel stents. Computed tomography

(CT) scan is the best imaging modality for the assessment of stent integrity and post-procedural aneurysm formation. However, its use is associated with cumulative doses of radiation, which is particularly concerning in young patients.

Congenital Mitral Stenosis

Congenital mitral stenosis usually involves abnormalities of the chordae tendineae, with either shortened or abnormal chordal attachments, such as in the "parachute" mitral valve. Unlike patients with acquired rheumatic mitral valve stenosis, congenital mitral stenosis is generally not suited for balloon valvuloplasty. In young children, the morbidity and mortality rate make this a treatment of last resort.

CONGENITAL LESIONS ASSOCIATED WITH EXTRACARDIAC SHUNTS

Systemic Arteriovenous Fistulas

Fistulous connections between a systemic artery and a systemic vein may create a sizable left-to-right shunt, with symptoms of exercise intolerance or frank congestive heart failure. The vein provides a lower-resistance runoff for the blood in the involved arterial branch. Unlike other left-to-right shunt lesions, systemic arteriovenous fistulas create a volume load for both ventricles. These fistulas may be congenital but may be acquired through trauma or complications from surgery or catheterization.

Coronary Fistulas

Coronary fistulas are hemodynamically similar to other systemic fistulas. Drainage is most commonly to the coronary sinus or directly to the RA, RV, or PA. In addition to the usual symptoms of exercise intolerance and shortness of breath secondary to the magnitude of the left-to-right shunt, these patients may present with a coronary steal, in which the low-resistance runoff to the fistula will reverse diastolic flow in the normal coronary artery branches. With diminished forward flow, ischemia may occur with exertion.

Aortopulmonary (Bronchial) Collaterals

Aortopulmonary collaterals may be congenital or may develop in children who undergo single ventricle repairs involving venous supply of pulmonary blood flow (Glenn shunt, Fontan operation) or in patients with pulmonary hypertension. These vessels most often arise from the thoracic aorta, the internal mammary arteries, and other branches of the subclavian. The left-to-right shunt creates a volume load on the LV, similar to a PDA. Patients with aortopulmonary collaterals can present with hemoptysis which can be life-threatening and require emergent heart catheterization for embolization of the culprit collateral. Bronchoscopy is useful to identify the area of the bleeding.

Old Surgical Shunts

In patients who have undergone previous congenital surgical palliations, an old Blalock-Taussig or other surgical shunt that either recanalized or was never taken down at later surgical stages may present as an ongoing left-to-right shunt. When this connection is no longer needed, it also creates a left ventricular volume load.

Pulmonary Fistulas

These unusual defects connect pulmonary arterioles, proximal to the air-containing spaces to pulmonary venules, resulting in the return of unoxygenated blood to the LA. If a defect is large enough or if there are multiple defects present (most often in hereditary hemorrhagic telangiectasia, formerly Osler-Weber-Rendu syndrome) or some patients with Fontan physiology, patients may be quite cyanotic. These defects have been a source of paradoxical thromboembolism in some patients who were erroneously diagnosed with PFO.

Venovenous Collaterals

In patients with single ventricle repairs where the systemic veins bypass the right heart and connect directly to the PAs, a pressure difference exists between those veins that lead to the lungs and those that return to the heart. This differential will result in rerouting of blood flow away from the lungs to return via the lower-resistance pathway back to the atrium. In the patient dependent on venous flow to the lungs, these venous connections result in diminished pulmonary flow and cyanosis.

Techniques of Device Embolization

All types of extracardiac vascular anomalies can be treated with catheter-based embolization techniques. These techniques are largely the same, regardless of the vessel designated for closure or the device chosen for the task. Coils are often the simplest and least expensive devices in part because of the variety of delivery catheters that can be used. Special considerations must be taken for large fistulae, which are discussed below. The vessel to be embolized is identified angiographically. Regional as well as selective injection in the vessel is essential, as some defects have multiple feeding sources (ie, pulmonary fistula, see **Figure 36.5A-C**), all of which must be occluded for a successful intervention, and some target vessels supply normal structures as well as the fistulous connection (ie, coronary fistula), making the positioning of the occlusion device more critical.

A multipurpose catheter with distal side holes can be used for the selective injections. Once the vessel has been acceptably imaged, a site for placement of the embolic device should be selected. Optimal locations include native narrowing, turns in the vessel course, bifurcation points, or long, straight, tubular segments. The target vessel is measured at the desired embolization site. For coil embolization, a device diameter 1 to 2 mm larger than the site diameter is selected. The delivery catheter is an end-hole catheter of a shape that approximates the wire course for stability of the catheter position.

The delivery catheter is exchanged over a wire and advanced past the desired site of implantation. The coil is then introduced to the catheter and pushed to the tip of the catheter (with a guidewire of a diameter approximating the catheter's inner lumen

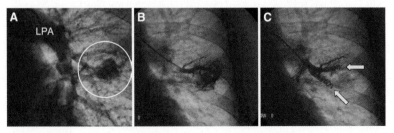

Figure 36.5 **A,** Large isolated pulmonary arteriovenous malformation (AVM) in left lower lobe (circle) in a patient with Osler-Weber-Rendu syndrome. **B,** Selective injection in 1 of 2 arterial feeding vessels filling the AVM. **C,** Following coil embolization of the 2 feeding vessels (arrows), there is no further filling of the AVM, with a concurrent increase in systemic saturation from 89% to 94% on room air. LPA, left pulmonary artery.

dimension), just distal to the site of implantation. The first loop of coil is delivered just distal to the optimal site by advancing the guidewire as the delivery catheter is withdrawn slightly. The remainder of the coil can be delivered in 1 of 2 ways: by fixing the delivery catheter and advancing the guidewire into the catheter to push out the coil; or by fixing the guidewire in place, and withdrawing the catheter over the wire, exposing the coil. A repeat angiogram is performed, and additional coils may be placed to complete the occlusion. Antibiotic prophylaxis is recommended for a period of 3 to 6 months to allow for complete endothelialization. MRI scanning will put significant stress on the original Gianturco coils (steel), can heat the coils significantly, and can create tremendous local reverberation artifacts. Newer, MRI-compatible coils have largely replaced the use of steel devices.

The use of coils has limitations, particularly for larger vessels with high-flow states. A series of Amplatzer Vascular Plugs (VP) are the current standards for embolization, when coils are not appropriate. These devices range from the cylindrical VP1, to the multilobed VP2, and to the more rectangular VP3. The VP4 is a dual-lobed device, designed to be delivered through a 4F catheter, similar to a coil. All but the VP3 are available in the United States. All are attached to a delivery cable with a screw mechanism, making it completely retrievable, until the operator wishes to release it. To a varying degree, the devices will conform to the size/shape of the target vessel.

Results/Complications

Embolization techniques are straightforward and are limited only by the operator's ability to achieve a stable catheter position in the vessel to be occluded. Once such a position is achieved, the procedure should be successful in 100% of cases. Complications include device embolization and potential obstruction of nearby side branches. Embolization occurs most frequently in arterial structures with high flow states when the device selected is not large enough or when a selected coil is too large, does not coil appropriately in the target vessel, and pushes the delivery catheter back out of the target vessel. Embolized coils can usually be retrieved with a snare technique. Hemolysis has been seen with incomplete closure of high flow defects.

CARDIAC CATHETERIZATION IN ADULT PATIENTS WITH FONTAN PHYSIOLOGY

Perhaps the greatest accomplishment in congenital heart disease in the last generation has been the combined surgical/interventional management of patients with functional single ventricles. In these patients, the systemic venous return is surgically rerouted directly to the PAs, no longer returning to the heart, leaving only the pulmonary venous return filling the single ventricle and being pumped to the aorta. Since Fontan described this approach to bypass the right side of the heart over 40 years ago, the concept has been applied to all congenital lesions in which the heart cannot be fully septated. Currently, the Fontan is performed between 2 and 4 years of age as the final step in a staged surgical approach. Over the last decade, a growing number of patients are reaching adulthood with Fontan physiology, presenting difficulties for adult cath labs that are not comfortable in dealing with this physiology on a regular basis. In a 2-ventricle circulation, pulmonary venous return is pumped by the LV to the systemic circulation with sufficient energy to traverse the systemic vascular bed (overcoming systemic vascular resistance). The blood then returns through the systemic veins to the RV, which adds enough additional energy to the blood to traverse the pulmonary vascular bed (overcoming pulmonary resistance). In a Fontan circulation, the 1 functional ventricle must generate enough energy to traverse both systemic and pulmonary vascular beds in series. Since there is no additional energy added after crossing through the systemic vascular bed, flow to the lungs is a passive flow system, where the blood from the SVC and IVC flows "downhill" through the PA, pulmonary veins, LA, and then into the single ventricle. It is clear, therefore, that any derangements of pulmonary vasculature, including elevated pulmonary vascular resistance, competitive flow (aortopulmonary collaterals), atrioventricular valve stenosis or regurgitation, elevation of (left) ventricular end-diastolic pressure, or even rhythm disturbances with loss of atrioventricular synchrony, will impede forward flow in this circulation and create higher systemic venous pressures. When systemic venous pressures begin to exceed 18 to 20 mmHg, venous stasis/pooling will occur. The result is diminished pulmonary flow, diminished left atrial return, and inadequate left ventricular preload, resulting in low cardiac output. Patients with failing Fontan physiology typically present with classic right heart failure: fluid retention, peripheral edema, ascites, and low output. In some children, a small Fontan "fenestration" may be created at the time of surgery. This communication between the systemic venous Fontan pathway and the pulmonary venous atrium allows a limited right-to-left shunt at the atrial level. This technique has been shown to improve outcomes of the surgery by better maintaining cardiac output in the perioperative period, at the expense of mild cyanosis. Secondary Fontan fenestration creation may be helpful later in the patient with a failing Fontan circulation and has been performed both in the operating room and in the cath lab as an interventional procedure.

Other issues that are common in a failing Fontan patient are as follows:

Protein-losing enteropathy is a syndrome seen in Fontan patients, in which there is enteral loss of serum proteins. The exact mechanism for these losses is unknown, but in some cases, it may be related to bowel edema as a result of high venous pressures. These protein losses include albumin, resulting in lower serum oncotic pressure, worsening the patient's fluid retention. Antithrombotic factors, such as antithrombin III, may also be lost, promoting hypercoagulable states.

Atrial arrhythmias, due to stretching of the atria or to extensive atrial surgery, may be the chief presentation of a failing Fontan or may be one of the underlying causes of the physiologic derangement.

Ventricular dysfunction is a common endpoint for Fontan patients. The mechanism of ventricular failure is unknown, but may be related to the amount of time prior to the Fontan, when the ventricular myocardium withstood multiple cardiopulmonary bypass runs in addition to the chronic oxygen deficiency. Stretching of the myocardium due to the volume overload associated with the first stage of the Fontan palliation is another contributing factor. Interestingly, Fontan patients cannot develop pulmonary venous congestion like other patients with poor left ventricular function. Mean left atrial/PA pressures cannot get high enough to cause pulmonary edema before systemic venous stasis occurs. These patients will present with "right heart failure" long before they develop typical symptoms of left heart failure. Because Fontan patients have begun to reach adult age in significant numbers, careful invasive assessment of the Fontan physiology will be required in the adult cath lab.

Hemodynamic Evaluation

Right and left heart hemodynamics should be obtained with particular focus on mechanical obstructions in the Fontan pathway. Ventricular end-diastolic pressure and PA wedge pressures should be compared to rule out pulmonary vein or atrioventricular valve obstruction. Pullbacks through both branch PAs should be done, looking for pressure gradients. Surgical anastomoses are a site of particular attention. Cardiac output should be assessed using the Fick calculation. Saturations must be obtained in the central and distal PAs to rule out competitive aortopulmonary collateral flow. Angiographically, all of the limbs of the Fontan pathway should be imaged, particularly because of the difficulties in imaging these using echocardiography. Venous collaterals draining to the heart or via a pulmonary vein directly to the atrium and via the coronary sinus should be ruled out, particularly in a patient presenting with systemic desaturation. An aortogram should be performed at the distal arch to rule out aortopulmonary collaterals providing competitive flow and to exclude aortic arch obstructions that may be affecting ventricular afterload. Atrial pacing can be performed to assess its effect on cardiac output and on atrial filling pressures for patients who are not in sinus rhythm. The interventions that may be required to improve Fontan physiology include a virtual manual of the procedures outlined in this chapter. Branch PA stenosis should be ballooned or stented to relieve any pathway obstruction. Venous pathways and surgical anastomoses may also require enlargement/angioplasty. Aortopulmonary collaterals should be aggressively embolized. Fontan fenestrations may need to be occluded in a patient who is excessively cyanotic. The devices for atrial septal closure can be used for this purpose. Pulmonary arteriovenous malformations may be present in patients who previously underwent a Glenn shunt and may need to be embolized.

Most long-term complications in Fontan patients, including protein losing enteropathy and chronic hepatic dysfunction, are related to long-standing elevated venous pressures and/or venous congestion. Thus, careful hemodynamic evaluation is recommended in patients with patent fenestrations or venovenous collaterals as closure of any right-to-left shunting invariably will result in further Fontan pressure elevation, which may not be well tolerated. In patients with failing Fontan physiology, creation of a Fontan fenestration has been shown to improve the symptoms of protein-losing enteropathy in some and to improve cardiac output in all.

SUGGESTED READINGS

1. Boe BA, Zampi JD, Kennedy KF, et al. Acute success of balloon aortic valvuloplasty in the current era: a National Cardiovascular Data Registry Study. *JACC Cardiovasc Interv.* 2017;10(17):1717-1726.
2. Bridges ND, Mayer JE Jr, Lock JE, et al. Effect of baffle fenestration on outcome of the modified Fontan operation. *Circulation.* 1992;86(6):1762-1769.
3. Butera G, Giugno L, Basile D, Piazza L, Chessa M, Carminati M. The Edwards Valeo lifestents in the treatment and palliation of congenital heart disease in infants and small children. *Catheter Cardiovasc Interv.* 2015;86(3):432-437.
4. Cabalka AK, Hellenbrand WE, Eicken A, et al. Relationships among conduit type, pre-stenting, and outcomes in patients undergoing transcatheter pulmonary valve replacement in the prospective North American and European Melody valve trials. *JACC Cardiovasc Interv.* 2017;10(17):1746-1759.
5. Cohen MS. Assessing the borderline ventricle in a term infant: combining imaging and physiology to establish the right course. *Curr Opin Cardiol.* 2018;33(1):95-100.
6. Devanagondi R, Peck D, Sagi J, et al. Long-term outcomes of balloon valvuloplasty for isolated pulmonary valve stenosis. *Pediatr Cardiol.* 2017;38(2):247-254.
7. Dijkema EJ, Sieswerda G-JT, Takken T, et al. Long-term results of balloon angioplasty for native coarctation of the aorta in childhood in comparison with surgery. *Eur J Cardiothorac Surg.* 2018;53(1):262-268.
8. Feltes TF, Bacha E, Beekman RH III, et al. Indications for cardiac catheterization and intervention in pediatric cardiac disease: a scientific statement from the American Heart Association. *Circulation.* 2011;123(22):2607-2652.
9. Fontan F, Baudet E. Surgical repair of tricuspid atresia. *Thorax.* 1971;26(3):240-248.
10. Forbes TJ, Kim DW, Du W, et al. Comparison of surgical, stent, and balloon angioplasty treatment of native coarctation of the aorta: an observational study by the CCISC (Congenital Cardiovascular Interventional Study Consortium). *J Am Coll Cardiol.* 2011;58(25):2664-2674.
11. Freud LR, McElhinney DB, Marshall AC, et al. Fetal aortic valvuloplasty for evolving hypoplastic left heart syndrome: postnatal outcomes of the first 100 patients. *Circulation.* 2014;130(8):638-645.
12. Gersony WM, Hayes CJ, Driscoll DJ, et al. Second natural history study of congenital heart defects. Quality of life of patients with aortic stenosis, pulmonary stenosis, or ventricular septal defect. *Circulation.* 1993;87(2 suppl I):I52-I65.

13. Golden AB, Hellenbrand WE. Coarctation of the aorta: stenting in children and adults. *Cathet Cardiovasc Interv.* 2007;69(2):289-299.
14. Harris KC, Du W, Cowley CG, Forbes TJ, Kim DW, Congenital Cardiac Intervention Study Consortium CCISC. A prospective observational multicenter study of balloon angioplasty for the treatment of native and recurrent coarctation of the aorta. *Catheter Cardiovasc Interv.* 2014;83(7):1116-1123.
15. Holzer R, Qureshi S, Ghasemi A, et al. Stenting of aortic coarctation: acute, intermediate, and long-term results of a prospective multi-institutional registry—Congenital Cardiovascular Interventional Study Consortium (CCISC). *Catheter Cardiovasc Interv.* 2010;76(4):553-563.
16. Holzer RJ, Gauvreau K, Kreutzer J, et al. Safety and efficacy of balloon pulmonary valvuloplasty: a multicenter experience. *Catheter Cardiovasc Interv.* 2012;80(4):663-672.
17. Justino H, Petit CJ. Percutaneous common carotid artery access for pediatric interventional cardiac catheterization. *Circ Cardiovasc Interv.* 2016;9(4):e003003.
18. Law MA, Shamszad P, Nugent AW, et al. Pulmonary artery stents: long-term follow-up. *Catheter Cardiovasc Interv.* 2010;75(5):757-764.
19. Maskatia SA, Ing FF, Justino H, et al. Twenty-five year experience with balloon aortic valvuloplasty for congenital aortic stenosis. *Am J Cardiol.* 2011;108(7):1024-1028.
20. Morray BH, McElhinney DB, Cheatham JP, et al. Risk of coronary artery compression among patients referred for transcatheter pulmonary valve implantation: a multicenter experience. *Circ Cardiovasc Interv.* 2013;6(5):535-542.
21. Ohye RG, Sleeper LA, Mahony L, et al. Comparison of shunt types in the Norwood procedure for single-ventricle lesions. *N Engl J Med.* 2010;362(21):1980-1992.
22. Pham PP, Moller JH, Hills C, Larson V, Pyles L. Cardiac catheterization and operative outcomes from a multicenter consortium for children with Williams syndrome. *Pediatr Cardiol.* 2009;30(1):9-14.
23. Rhodes LA, Colan SD, Perry SB, Jonas RA, Sanders SP. Predictors of survival in neonates with critical aortic stenosis. *Circulation.* 1991;84(6):2325-2335.
24. Schwartz MC, Glatz AC, Dori Y, Rome JJ, Gillespie MJ. Outcomes and predictors of reintervention in patients with pulmonary atresia and intact ventricular septum treated with radiofrequency perforation and balloon pulmonary valvuloplasty. *Pediatr Cardiol.* 2014;35(1):22-29.
25. Slesnick TC, Schreier J, Soriano BD, et al. Safety of magnetic resonance imaging after implantation of stainless steel embolization coils. *Pediatr Cardiol.* 2016;37(1):62-67.
26. Sohrabi B, Jamshidi P, Yaghoubi A, et al. Comparison between covered and bare Cheatham-Platinum stents for endovascular treatment of patients with native post-ductal aortic coarctation: immediate and intermediate-term results. *JACC Cardiovasc Interv.* 2014;7(4):416-423.
27. Stout KK, Daniels CJ, Aboulhosn JA, et al. 2018 AHA/ACC guideline for the management of adults with congenital heart disease: executive summary—a report of the American College of Cardiology/American Heart Association task force on clinical practice guidelines. *J Am Coll Cardiol.* 2019;73(12):1494-1563.
28. Taggart NW, Minahan M, Cabalka AK, et al. Immediate outcomes of covered stent placement for treatment or prevention of aortic wall injury associated with coarctation of the aorta (COAST II). *JACC Cardiovasc Interv.* 2016;9(5):484-493.

37 Endovascular Aortic Repair[1]

While endovascular aortic repair (EVAR) is most frequently performed in patients with degenerative infrarenal abdominal aortic aneurysms (AAAs), this chapter will also discuss its application for diseases of the thoracic aorta. Thoracic endovascular aortic repair (TEVAR) has been broadly utilized not only for degenerative pathology such as fusiform or saccular aneurysm (thoracic aortic aneurysm [TAA]) but also for aortic dissection (AD), blunt thoracic aortic injury, congenital aortic pathology (coarctation, Kommerell diverticulum), and infectious complications. This chapter will focus on the 2 most common pathologies of degenerative fusiform aneurysms and AD to highlight the procedure.

INDICATIONS FOR REPAIR

EVAR is indicated for the treatment of degenerative AAA over 5.5 cm or for AAAs that grow more than 0.5 cm/y. Multiple recent trials have suggested that while crossover does occur, surveillance of smaller aneurysms is associated with similar late survival and reduced cost when compared to earlier elective repair. In addition, the strategy of open surgical repair (OAR) vs EVAR for AAA has been studied in 2 randomized trials. These have suggested that late survival is similar between treatment strategies, but cost and reinterventions are higher after EVAR.

TEVAR is indicated for the treatment of degenerative TAA over 5.5 cm or a saccular aneurysm of any size. For patients with AD, TEVAR has become the first-line therapy for acute type B dissection with malperfusion or rupture and is also indicated when dissection-associated aneurysm size exceeds 5.5 cm or grows by more than 0.5 cm/y. For the chronic phase of dissection, however, it is unclear whether open repair is better in the long run.

ENDOGRAFT DESIGN

Endografts have evolved but essentially consist of a stent frame of either nitinol or stainless steel and fabric of either polyester or expanded polytetrafluoroethylene. For AAA, there are either unibody endografts (main body with 2 limbs with proximal extension) or bifurcated modular endografts (built "bottom down"). Recently, an endograft became available for juxtarenal aneurysms and has a fenestrated proximal component for renal artery branch stents. For TAA, stent grafts essentially are single components that can be "shingled" to extend the length of treatment. For both TEVAR and EVAR, each subsequent iterative product addresses anatomic limitations and these changes include improved conformability for curved aortas, profile reductions to allow for passage through smaller diameter access vessels, and changes in deployment to allow for a more controlled release in difficult anatomy.

PREOPERATIVE EVALUATION

For this anatomically limited treatment, preoperative imaging is key. EVAR works best when landing zones are of adequate length (1.5 cm for EVAR to 2 cm for TEVAR) free of thrombus or calcium, uniform in diameter, in straight segments, and within size

[1]We gratefully acknowledge the *Grossman & Baim's Cardiac Catheterization, Angiography, and Intervention*, 9th edition contributions of Dr. Himanshu J Patel, as portions of his chapter, "Endovascular Aortic Repair," were retained in this text.

windows of available devices. Therefore, 3-dimensional evaluation is critical in assessing the suitability for treatment (**Figure 37.1**). Armed with this information, one must evaluate the degree of deviation from this stated ideal anatomy and with experience can decide whether the extent of deviation will still allow successful treatment.

Device size selection is determined based upon underlying anatomy. Typically, oversizing by 10% to 20% is adequate to ensure seal and exclusion of pathology. In acute type B dissection, however, to reduce the risk of inducing stent graft–induced new entry tears, the selected device is oversized by 5% to 10% of the proximal nondissected aorta. The distal landing zone size is selected to total aortic diameter in acute dissection to account for the immediate increase in aortic diameter that occurs during the dissection event. There is, however, no consensus on how to select the distal diameter for the stent graft for chronic AD. Different devices require sizing based upon luminal diameter with or without including the thickness of the aortic wall.

For TEVAR, two unique questions arise. Since a large proportion of pathology requires coverage of the left subclavian artery to extend the proximal landing zone, one must decide whether subclavian revascularization is necessary. The absolute indications include the presence of patent left internal thoracic artery to left anterior descending coronary artery bypass and dominant left vertebral artery. In other instances, the indication to proceed with subclavian artery revascularization is at the

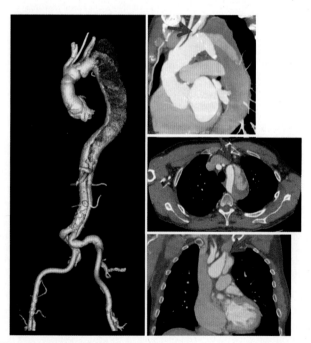

Figure 37.1 Three-dimensional (3D) analysis of this thoracic aneurysm suggests proximity of the thoracic aortic aneurysm to the left subclavian artery, and the curvature of the neck suggests better apposition may occur if the left subclavian artery is excluded. This 3D analysis is much more instructive in visualizing the surgical plan than its isolated cross-sectional imaging may provide alone. The associated arrow depicts the location of the left subclavian artery.

discretion of the physician and can be done to potentially reduce risks of spinal cord ischemia (SCI) and stroke.

The second question in TEVAR is the decision to utilize spinal canal drains to reduce the risks of SCI. While no randomized trial exists, and practice is variable, factors increasing the risk for paraplegia include extensive (>20 cm) aortic coverage, distal thoracic aortic coverage, prior AAA repair, and occluded spinal collateral circulation (hypogastric or vertebral arteries). The decision to use lumbar drains should also reflect expertise in their placement, as complications are not infrequent following their use.

A unique option includes the endoconduit approach (**Figure 37.2**) to stay transfemoral, but this often requires femoral artery patch repair. In this strategy, the diminutive iliac artery is lined with a stent graft and then overexpanded to prerupture the vessel to the intended diameter. The endograft is then advanced through this "endoconduit."

The access vessel is then cannulated with a stiff wire. The endograft is advanced over this wire to the intended target zone. The contralateral femoral artery is then used to deliver catheters for intravascular ultrasound (IVUS) or angiograms. IVUS is mandatory in the setting of AD to ensure the stent graft is deployed in the true lumen completely. Critical adjacent branch vessels are identified and marked prior to stent graft deployment. The correct orientation for image acquisition during angiography is aided by evaluation of the preoperative imaging study. The stent grafts are then deployed in the target landing zones. Completion angiography is performed to verify exclusion of pathology and patency of adjacent critical branches. The access vessels are then controlled by direct repair or manual hemostasis.

In acute AD, if TEVAR was performed for malperfusion, an assessment of ongoing branch vessel obstruction with either direct cannulation and pressure gradient assessment (>20 mmHg) or imaging evaluation. If ongoing obstruction exists, branch vessel stenting may be necessary to relieve malperfusion (**Figure 37.3**). Finally, in the setting of rupture of AD, the entire descending aorta is covered to ensure exclusion of the site of rupture.

NOTABLE EARLY COMPLICATIONS

Acute limb ischemia remains a rare early complication. Etiologies for this complication include thromboembolism or atheroembolism during the procedure, dissection of the access vessel, or occasionally in the setting of EVAR, graft limb thrombosis. Limb thrombosis is more frequent if iliac and femoral outflows were compromised at the outset or by embolism.

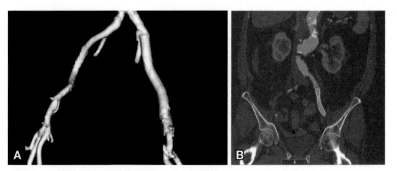

Figure 37.2 Three-dimensional **(A)** and coronal **(B)** reconstructions demonstrate a left external iliac artery stent graft.

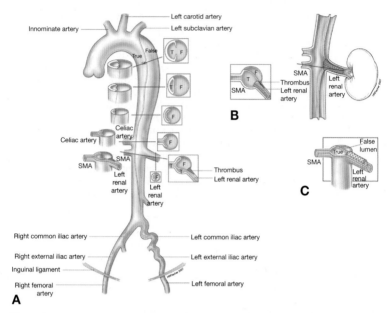

Figure 37.3 This schematic **(A)** demonstrates that the acute type B dissection has a compressed true lumen in the visceral segment. This is the source of dynamic obstruction, and the entry tear sits within the proximal descending aorta. After the primary entry tear is covered with the thoracic endograft **(B and C)**, persistent static obstruction exists in the left renal artery. This responds well to placement of a branch vessel bare metal self-expanding stent. SMA, superior mesenteric artery. (Reprinted with permission from Patel HJ, Williams DM. Endovascular therapy for malperfusion in acute type B aortic dissection. *Oper Tech Thorac Cardiovasc Surg.* 2009;14(1):2-11.)

Ischemic colitis is a rare event after EVAR and usually occurs in the sigmoid colon. While the inferior mesenteric artery is covered in EVAR, the mechanism of ischemia is multifactorial. Symptoms of ischemic colitis include left lower quadrant pain and tenderness, diarrhea, or hematochezia. The diagnostic test of choice is sigmoidoscopy, and the treatment often involves bowel resection.

SCI is seen more frequently after TEVAR than EVAR. Management includes the use of spinal canal drains, and permissive hypertension with mean blood pressures kept over 90 mmHg. Patients can get either temporary or permanent SCI, and it can occur immediately or in a delayed fashion. Understanding the collateral network concept of spinal cord perfusion, permissive hypertension is maintained for at least 2 weeks to allow robust formation of collaterals and prevent delayed paraplegia.

UNIQUE LATE COMPLICATIONS

The Achilles heel for endovascular aortic repair in the long term is the endoleak, defined as persistent blood flow into the aneurysm sac. Postoperative imaging surveillance is mandatory and typically occurs within the first month, at 6 months, and annually thereafter to ensure the diagnosis of aneurysm exclusion. There are 5 types of endoleaks. Type I is related to the failure of proximal (IA) or distal (IB) landing zone. This requires treatment with endograft extension to avoid aortic rupture. Type II occurs due to back bleeding from covered branch vessels. Type II endoleaks require treatment if the aneurysm sac is expanding or if it is secondary to left subclavian artery coverage in TEVAR. Otherwise, these are relatively benign and will likely thrombose in the first 6 to 12 months. Type III endoleaks occur due to fabric tears or from ineffective seal between 2 modular components. A flush aortogram with the catheter in the endograft is diagnostic, and treatment is mandatory with placement of another endograft at the offending site. Type IV endoleaks are related to graft porosity and require reversal of procedural anticoagulation. Finally, type V endoleaks describe a scenario where sac expansion occurs despite lack of flow within it. The treatment is often via open surgical repair and stent graft removal.

Stent graft–induced new entry tears are a unique complication occasionally seen after TEVAR for AD. If this occurs proximally, a retrograde type A dissection can occur and requires emergent proximal aortic repair. The frequency of this complication is highest after treatment for acute dissection and decreases the farther one gets from the initial time of dissection.

Finally, another unique complication appears to be emerging particularly following TEVAR. The elimination of the Windkessel function of the aorta with stiff endograft placement has led to a concern of increased impedance for left ventricular ejection. The long-term consequences are yet unknown but may include left ventricular hypertrophy or reduction in ejection fraction.

SUGGESTED READINGS

1. Dong Z, Fu W, Wang Y, et al. Stent graft induced new entry after endovascular repair for Stanford type B aortic dissection. *J Vasc Surg.* 2010;52(6):1450-1457.
2. Estrera AL, Sheinbaum R, Miller CC, et al. Cerebrospinal fluid drainage during thoracic aortic repair: safety and current management. *Ann Thorac Surg.* 2009;88(1):9-15.
3. Griepp RB, Griepp EB. Spinal cord protection in surgical and endovascular repair of thoracoabdominal aortic disease. *J Thorac Cardiovasc Surg.* 2015;149(2 suppl l):S86-S90.
4. Hiratzka LF, Bakris GL, Beckman JA, et al. ACCF/AHA/AATS/ACR/SCA/SCAI/SIR/STS/SVM guidelines for diagnosis and management of patients with thoracic aortic disease: executive summary. *J Am Coll Cardiol.* 2010;55(14):e27-e129.
5. Kreibich M, Morlock J, Beyersdorf F, et al. Decreased biventricular function following thoracic endovascular aortic repair. *Interact Cardiovasc Thorac Surg.* 2020;30(4):600-604.
6. Lederle FA, Wilson SE, Johnson GR, et al. Immediate repair compared with surveillance of small abdominal aortic aneurysms. *N Engl J Med.* 2002;346(19):1437-1444.
7. Ouriel K, Clair DG, Kent KC, Zarins CK; Positive Impact of Endovascular Options for Treating Aneurysms Early PIVOTAL Investigators. Endovascular repair compared with surveillance for patients with small abdominal aortic aneurysms. *J Vasc Surg.* 2010;51(5):1081-1087.
8. Parodi JC, Palmaz JC, Barone HD. Transfemoral intraluminal graft implantation for abdominal aortic aneurysms. *Ann Vasc Surg.* 1991;5(6):491-499.
9. Powell JT, Brown LC, Forbes JF, et al. Final 12-year follow-up of surgery versus surveillance in the UK small aneurysm trial. *Br J Surg.* 2007;94(6):702-708.
10. Rylski B, Blanke P, Beyersdorf F, et al. How does the ascending aorta geometry change when it dissects? *J Am Coll Cardiol.* 2014;63(13):1311-1319.
11. Van Bakel TMJ, Arthurs CJ, Nauta FJH, et al. Cardiac remodelling following thoracic endovascular aortic repair for descending aortic aneurysms. *Eur J Cardio Thorac Surg.* 2019;55(6):1061-1070.
12. Van Bogerijen GH, Williams DM, Eliason JL, Dasika NL, Deeb GM, Patel HJ. Alternative access techniques with thoracic endovascular aortic repair: open iliac conduit versus endoconduit technique. *J Vasc Surg.* 2014;60(5):1168-1176.
13. Van Bogerijen GH, Patel HJ, Williams DM, et al. Propensity adjusted analysis of open and endovascular thoracic aortic repair for chronic type B dissection: a twenty-year evaluation. *Ann Thorac Surg.* 2015;99(4):1260-1266.

38

Pericardial Interventions: Pericardiocentesis, Balloon Pericardiotomy, and Epicardial Approach to Cardiac Procedures[1]

INTRODUCTION

The pericardium consists of both a visceral and a parietal component, each composed of an inner layer of mesothelial cells covering an underlying fibrosa. The visceral pericardium is attached to the heart by loose connective tissue and surrounds the epicardial fat pads and coronary arteries. At the pericardial reflections, it extends onto the pulmonary veins (PVs), superior and inferior vena cavae, and several centimeters of proximal pulmonary artery and aorta, before folding around to continue as the parietal (or free) pericardium. The parietal pericardial then envelops the heart and visceral pericardium as a separate 1- to 2-mm-thick layer (**Figure 38.1**). As described in Chapter 20, pericardial disease can manifest with a variety of presentations, of which acute fluid accumulation leading to tamponade physiology and chronic fluid accumulation is relatively common. In addition, the growth in the performance of complex coronary interventions and catheter-based procedures for ablation of arrhythmias and for structural heart disease has been associated with an increase in coronary artery and cardiac perforation and pericardial tamponade as a complication of these procedures. Thus, familiarity with elective or emergency management of pericardial effusion and tamponade continues to be an important component of contemporary interventional cardiology.

PERICARDIOCENTESIS

The etiology of pericardial effusion varies, and the role of pericardiocentesis in its management depends on the presence of tamponade physiology, the size of the effusion, and the ability to obtain the appropriate diagnosis on the basis of clinical history and other noninvasive diagnostic tests. **Figure 38.2** depicts a proposed algorithm for the management of pericardial effusion. Pericardial tamponade is a class I indication for pericardiocentesis. Pericardiocentesis can also be considered for effusions >20 mm in size on echocardiography and for the diagnosis of smaller effusions when obtaining pericardial fluid is felt to aid in the diagnosis (**Table 38.1**).

Fluoroscopy-Guided Pericardiocentesis

At most centers, pericardiocentesis is performed in the cardiac catheterization laboratory using a combination of echocardiographic and fluoroscopic guidance. It is recommended that a 2-dimensional echocardiogram be obtained just prior to the procedure to document the presence, location, and size of the effusion; to determine the presence of loculation or significant stranding; and to determine the location on the body surface where the effusion lies closest to the surface and at which the fluid depth overlying the heart is maximal. Once an entry location is selected, the echo can indicate the optimal direction for needle passage and the approximate depth of needle insertion that will be required.

---

[1]We gratefully acknowledge the *Grossman & Baim's Cardiac Catheterization, Angiography, and Intervention*, 9th edition contributions of Drs. Juan Viles-Gonzalez, Andre D'Avila, and Mauro Moscucci, as portions of their chapter, Pericardial Interventions: Pericardiocentesis, Balloon Pericardiotomy, and Epicardial Approach to Cardiac Procedures, were retained in this text.

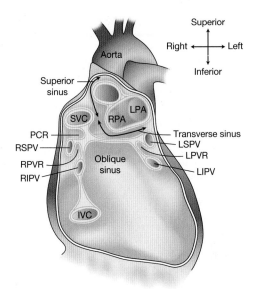

Figure 38.1 The anatomy of the pericardium space and its reflections along the great vessels, sinuses, and recesses is shown in an anterior view after removal of the heart. The transverse sinus is limited by a pericardial reflection between the superior pulmonary veins. The oblique sinus is confined by the pericardial reflections around the pulmonary veins and the inferior vena cava. IVC, inferior vena cava; LIPV, left inferior pulmonary vein; LPA, left pulmonary artery; LPVR, left pulmonary vein recess; LSPV, left superior pulmonary vein; PCR, postcaval recess; RIPV, right inferior pulmonary vein; RPA, right pulmonary artery; RPVR, right pulmonary vein recess; RSPV, right superior pulmonary vein; SVC, superior vena cava.

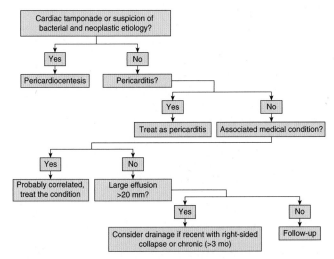

Figure 38.2 Management of pericardial effusion. (Reproduced with permission from Imazio M, Spodick DH, Brucato A, et al. Controversial issues in the management of pericardial disease. *Circulation.* 2010;121:916-928.)

Table 38.1 Utility of Diagnostic Tests for the Etiologic Diagnosis of Pericarditis According to Targeted Causes

Test	General	Tuberculous	Systemic Disease	Neoplastic	Purulent
Auscultation	+++	+/–	+/–	+/–	+/–
ECG	+++	+/–	+/–	+/–	+/–
Echocardiography	+++	+++	++	+++	+++
Markers of inflammation	+++	+++	+++	+++	+++
Markers of myocardial lesion	+++	+/–	+	+/–	+/–
Tumor markers	–	–	+/–	+	–
Tuberculin skin test	–	+/–	+/–	–	–
QuantiFERON-TB	–	+	+/–	–	–
ANA, ENA (anti-SSA)	–	–	+	–	–
HIV testing	–	+	+	–	+
Viral serology	–	–	–	–	–
Blood culture	–	–	–	–	+
Chest x-ray	++	+++	+++	+++	++
CT	–	+++	+++	+++	+++
CMR	–	++	++	+++	+++
Mammography	–	–	–	+++	–
Pericardiocentesis	–	+++	+/–	+++	+++
Pericardial biopsy	–	+++	+/–	+++	+

ANA, antinuclear antibody; CMR, cardiac magnetic resonance; CT, computed tomography; ECG, electrocardiography; ENA, extractable nuclear antigen; HIV, human immunodeficiency virus; SSA, Sjogren syndrome type A; +++, very high; ++, high/good; +, discrete; +/–, low/insufficient; –, not useful. QuantiFERON-TB is an interferon-release assay used in tuberculosis diagnosis.

Reproduced with permission from Imazio M, Spodick DH, Brucato A, et al. Controversial issues in the management of pericardial disease. *Circulation*. 2010;121:916-928.

We believe that in the cardiac catheterization laboratory, access to pressure measurement, continuous electrocardiography (ECG) and vital sign monitoring, and fluoroscopy with the ability to inject radiographic contrast are highly preferable, particularly in difficult or challenging cases, in patients with small or localized effusions, or when complications ensue. It is important to have access to adequate ancillary support and other technologies in hemodynamically unstable patients, unless an emergency requires a bedside procedure. Performing the procedure in the catheterization laboratory in conjunction with right heart pressure measurement is also required if the diagnosis of effusive-constrictive pericarditis is suspected, if the effusion is small or loculated, or if the patient is hemodynamically unstable.

The patient's torso is propped up to a level of about 45° using a wedge, and the transducers are zeroed to the level of the heart in this position. The subxiphoid approach is classic: a skin nick is made 1 to 2 cm below the costal margin just to the left of the xiphoid process, to allow the needle to "hug" the ribs. The desired needle path is generally toward the posterior aspect of the left shoulder, passing anterior to the anterior capsule of the liver, and entering the pericardial space overlying the right ventricle (**Figure 38.3**). Echocardiography from the subxiphoid window is thus very useful to confirm the optimal direction toward the pericardial entry point and the approximate depth below the skin. When this geometry is unfavorable—as in posterior effusions or patients with large body habitus—a low parasternal intercostal puncture site is a potential alternative. Care should be taken in the parasternal approach to avoid the internal mammary artery that runs 3 to 5 cm from the parasternal border, and also the neurovascular bundle at the lower margin of each rib (puncture above the rib).

After a sterile prep and draping, the skin and subcutaneous tissues are infiltrated with lidocaine with a small-gauge needle along the proposed path of entry. We use a 5- to 8-cm, 18-gauge needle attached to a 10-mL syringe filled with saline or lidocaine, which is inserted following the echo-determined trajectory. As the needle is advanced, the syringe is alternately aspirated to determine pericardial space entry and injected to deliver more local anesthesia along the route. If a 3-way stopcock is interposed between the syringe and the needle, it can be used to connect to a pressure manifold via a fluid-filled extension tube. Classically, electrocardiographic

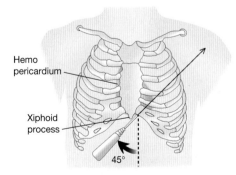

Hemo
pericardium

Xiphoid
process

45°

Figure 38.3 Schematic representation of the standard subxiphoid approach for pericardiocentesis. The procedure is usually performed by inserting a thin-walled 18-gauge or a 20-gauge spinal needle below the xiphoid process at a 45° angle toward the left shoulder. (From Fleisher GR, Ludwig S, Baskin MN. *Atlas of Pediatric Emergency Medicine.* Lippincott Williams & Wilkins; 2004.)

monitoring of the needle (by attaching its shaft to the V lead of the ECG system using a sterile alligator clip) can be used to provide an additional measure of safety (**Figure 38.4**): the ST segment recorded from the needle should be isoelectric during advancement, but dramatic elevation of the ST segment appears if the needle contacts the right ventricular epicardium. The needle must be withdrawn slightly until ST elevation resolves, to minimize the chance of right ventricular puncture or laceration. Use of a properly grounded ECG system is imperative to avoid introducing leakage currents through the needle. With the use of fluoroscopy and the ability to inject radiographic contrast and monitor pressure to confirm entry into the pericardial space, most operators no longer use ST segment monitoring during fluoroscopy-guided pericardiocentesis. Importantly, it should be emphasized that ST segment monitoring alone is inadequate as a safeguard from complications. A blunt-tip epicardial needle (Tuohy-17) can also be used to minimize risk of right ventricular puncture. This technique may be modified to enable access to the normal pericardium for drug delivery and epicardial mapping (see below).

When the needle enters the pericardial space, a distinct pop is usually felt and it is possible to aspirate fluid. If there is an interposed stopcock connected to a pressure transducer, turning the stopcock will allow display of intrapericardial pressure, which should be superimposable on the simultaneously displayed right atrial pressure from the right heart catheter. The waveform should not resemble that of right ventricular pressure. If the pericardial needle tip displays a right ventricular waveform, the tip is

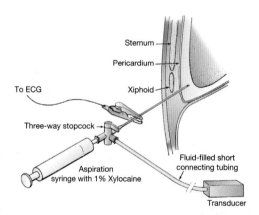

Figure 38.4 Diagram showing the subxiphoid approach to pericardiocentesis with pressure and ST segment monitoring. A hollow, thin-walled, 18-gauge needle is connected via a 3-way stopcock to an aspiration syringe filled with 1% Xylocaine and to a short length of fluid-filled tubing connected to a pressure transducer. A sterile V lead of an electrocardiographic recorder may be attached to the metal needle hub. The needle is advanced until pericardial fluid is aspirated or an injury current appears on the V-lead electrocardiographic recording. Once fluid is aspirated, the stopcock is turned so that needle-tip pressure is displayed against simultaneously measured right atrial pressure from a right heart catheter. When needle-tip position within the pericardial space is confirmed, a J-tipped guidewire is passed through the needle into the pericardial space, the needle is removed, and a catheter with end and side holes is advanced over the guidewire and subsequently connected via the 3-way stopcock to both the transducer and the syringe. This permits, first, thorough drainage of the pericardial effusion using a catheter rather than a sharp needle and, second, documentation that tamponade physiology is relieved when right atrial pressure falls and intrapericardial pressure is restored to a level at or below zero. ECG, electrocardiography.

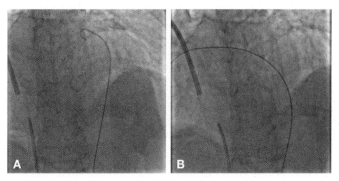

Figure 38.5 **A and B,** Guidewire advanced in the pericardial space with its characteristic path wrapping around the heart.

quickly but smoothly withdrawn slightly under continuous hemodynamic monitoring until the overlying pericardial space is entered.

Entry into the pericardial space can be confirmed by injection of radiographic contrast or agitated saline echo contrast, or the advancement of a 0.035-in J wire in the characteristic path wrapping around the heart (**Figure 38.5A and B**). A 6F to 8F dilator is then introduced over the guidewire, followed by a drainage catheter (straight or pigtail shaped, with multiple side holes) (**Figure 38.6**). If difficulty is encountered in advancing the drainage catheter, the dilator can be reintroduced and used to substitute an extra-stiff J wire for better support. We usually attach a 50-mL syringe and a 3-way stopcock to the drainage catheter, connecting an extension tube from the other port of the 3-way stopcock to a drainage bag or vacuum bottle. This allows fluid to be aspirated into the syringe and transferred to the bottle. Removal of as little as 50 mL of fluid is often sufficient to relieve frank tamponade and improve hemodynamics. After removal of 100 to 200 mL of fluid, it is informative to remeasure the pericardial and right atrial pressures before resuming aspiration. Resolution of tamponade physiology usually occurs after aspiration of 50 to 200 mL of fluid. It is recommended that pericardial fluid be removed slowly, as rapid removal can precipitate the development of acute postprocedure ventricular dysfunction (see

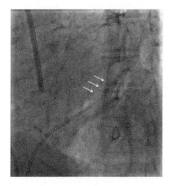

Figure 38.6 Pericardial drain in the pericardial space. The cardiac silhouette and its relation with the catheter are shown by the arrows.

"Complications of Pericardiocentesis" section). Occasionally, patients will experience pericardial pain when the effusion is tapped dry. In this case, parenteral narcotic analgesics and benzodiazepines can be administered, and if the pain is severe, 50 mL of pericardial fluid, sterile saline, or 10 to 20 mL of 1% Xylocaine can be reintroduced to help ease the pain. The patient should be laid flat and a final set of pericardial and right heart pressures measured. A fall in pericardial pressure to a level <0 mmHg and separation from the right atrial pressure, with a return of the normal diastolic y descent, indicate relief of tamponade physiology. These changes will be accompanied by a resolution of pulsus paradoxus. In previously hypotensive patients, systemic arterial pressure usually rises in association with an increase in mixed venous oxygen content, indicative of an increase in cardiac output. Failure of pericardial pressure to fall close to 0 mmHg indicates that the reference height of the transducers is incorrect or that free or loculated pericardial fluid is still under pressure. If the pericardial pressure falls appropriately but the right atrial pressures remain elevated with prominent x and y descents, the diagnosis of effusive-constrictive pericarditis must be entertained, with an ongoing element of constriction after the tamponade physiology has been relieved.

The drainage catheter is then sewn in place and attached to a sterile fluid path (stopcock, syringe, and drainage bag) to allow the postprocedure nursing staff to periodically attempt additional aspiration. Sterility must be strictly maintained with this technique because regularly interrupting the integrity of the drainage circuit may introduce infectious agents. Some institutions rely on continuous or intermittent suction applied via a water-seal device. The pericardial catheter is removed when the drainage has decreased to <25 to 50 mL/24 h, and there is no echocardiographic evidence of reaccumulation of fluid. Subsequently, periodic echo reassessment for fluid reaccumulation should be performed. Larger effusions may benefit from slightly more prolonged drainage, but >48-hour dwell time should be avoided to reduce the risk of infection. Analysis of pericardial fluid can aid in the diagnosis of infectious pericarditis (fungal, bacterial, viral, and tuberculous), as well as in the diagnosis of malignant and cholesterol effusions. **Table 38.2** summarizes recommended diagnostic tests to be performed on pericardial fluid, as indicated.

Echocardiography-Guided Pericardiocentesis

When performing pericardiocentesis, the ideal entry site would be the point at which the distance from skin to maximal fluid accumulation is minimal, with no intervening vital organs. Echocardiographic guidance has emerged as a technique to identify the ideal entry site and to perform pericardiocentesis safely without fluoroscopy (**Figure 38.7**).

Complications of Pericardiocentesis

The safety and success of percutaneous pericardiocentesis are related to the choice of entry site as well as to the size of the effusion. Pericardiocentesis is most likely to be uncomplicated if both anterior and posterior echo-free spaces are at least 10 mm. In smaller effusions, there is an increased risk of cardiac injury, so pericardiocentesis should usually be avoided in minimally symptomatic patients with small incidental effusions, unless there is clear echocardiographic evidence of hemodynamic compromise. The risk is also higher in patients who are anticoagulated with warfarin, so pericardiocentesis should be deferred if possible until the international normalized ratio (INR) is within normal range. If hemodynamic status demands urgent

Table 38.2 Diagnostic Tests of Pericardial Fluid

Suspected malignant effusion	Cytology and tumor markers (carcinoembryonic antigen—CEA), alpha-fetoprotein (AFP), carbohydrate antigens (CA 125, CA 72-4, CA 15-3, CA 19-9, CD-30, CD-25, etc.). Differentiation of tuberculous and neoplastic effusion is virtually absolute with low levels of adenosine deaminase (ADA) and high levels of CEA.
Suspected tuberculosis	Acid-fast bacilli staining; mycobacterium culture or radiometric growth detection (eg, BACTEC 460); adenosine deaminase (ADA), interferon (IFN)-gamma, pericardial lysozyme, and Polymerase chain reaction (PCR) analyses for tuberculosis (level of evidence B, indication I). Very high ADA levels have prognostic value for pericardial constriction. PCR analysis is as sensitive (75% vs 83%), but more specific (100% vs 78%) than ADA estimation for tuberculous pericarditis.
Suspected bacterial infection	At least 3 cultures of pericardial fluid for aerobes and anaerobes as well as blood cultures are mandatory (level of evidence B, indication I). Gram stains in pericardial fluid have a specificity of 99%, but a sensitivity of only 38% for exclusion of infection.
Viral infections	PCR analyses for cardiotropic viruses discriminate viral from autoreactive pericarditis (indication IIa, level of evidence B).
Nonspecific tests	Specific gravity (>1015), protein level (>3.0 g/dL; fluid/serum ratio >0.5), lactate dehydrogenase (LDH) (>200 mg/dL; serum/fluid ratio >0.6), and glucose (exudates vs transudates: 77.9 ± 41.9 vs 96.1 ± 50.7 mg/dL) can separate exudates from transudates but are not directly diagnostic (class IIb). However, purulent effusions with positive cultures have significantly lower fluid glucose levels (47.3 ± 25.3 vs 102.5 ± 35.6 mg/dL) and fluid-to-serum ratios (0.28 ± 0.14 vs 0.84 ± 0.23) than those of noninfectious effusions.
Cell counts	White blood cell (WBC) count is highest in inflammatory diseases, particularly of bacterial and rheumatologic origin. Very low WBC count found in myxedema. Monocyte count is highest in malignant effusions and hypothyroidisms (79% ± 27% and 74% ± 26%), while rheumatoid and bacterial effusions have the highest proportions of neutrophils (78% ± 20% and 69% ± 23%).
Cholesterol levels	As compared with controls, both bacterial and malignant pericardial fluids have higher cholesterol levels (49 ± 18 vs 121 ± 20 and 117 ± 33 mg/dL).
Epithelial membrane antigen, CEA, vimentin	Combination of epithelial membrane antigen, CEA, and vimentin immunocytochemical staining can be useful to distinguish reactive mesothelial and adenocarcinoma cells.

Adapted from Maisch B, Seferovic PM, Ristic AD, et al. Guidelines on the diagnosis and management of pericardial diseases: executive summary; the task force on the diagnosis and management of pericardial diseases of the European Society of Cardiology. *Eur Heart J.* 2004;25:587-610.

pericardiocentesis in the patient with elevated INR, fresh frozen plasma should be administered in the catheterization suite immediately after catheter access to the pericardium is achieved by an expert operator and drainage is initiated (to avoid conversion of a free hemorrhagic effusion into a mixture of fluid and gelatinous clot). Major and minor complications of pericardiocentesis are summarized in **Table 38.3**.

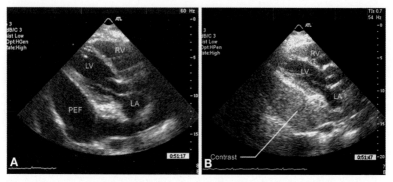

Figure 38.7 Parasternal long-axis echocardiogram recorded in a patient with a large posterior pericardial effusion (PEF). Pericardiocentesis is being undertaken with echocardiographic guidance. **A,** There is a large posterior pericardial fluid collection. **B,** Agitated saline has been injected via the pericardiocentesis needle. There is now echo contrast in the previously clear pericardial space confirming that the pericardiocentesis needle is in the pericardium. LA, left atrium; LV, left ventricle; RV, right ventricle.

PERCUTANEOUS BALLOON PERICARDIOTOMY

Percutaneous balloon pericardiotomy is an alternative approach to the treatment of cardiac tamponade in patients with large recurrent malignant effusions or idiopathic effusions that have recurred or not abated after prolonged catheter drainage (eg, catheter drainage of >100 mL/d for 3 days). Of the patients who undergo pericardiocentesis for malignant effusion, 66% have recurrence after simple drainage by pericardiocentesis. In comparison, in most series of cardiac tamponade not related to malignant effusion, pericardiocentesis with prolonged catheter drainage was effective without further intervention in >80% of patients. An analysis has suggested that balloon pericardiotomy, surgical pericardiectomy, pleuropericardial window, and subxiphoid window are all superior in terms of freedom from recurrence to repeat simple pericardiocentesis, instillation of sclerosing agents, radiation, or prolonged catheter drainage.

Patients with recurrent tamponade from malignant effusions often are poor surgical candidates. Hence in this patient population, percutaneous balloon pericardiotomy has emerged as an alternative to a subxiphoid window. The technique begins with pericardiocentesis via the subxiphoid approach. After pericardiocentesis, approximately 20 mL of contrast is injected to aid visualization of the pericardial space. A 0.035-in J-tip guidewire is then introduced and looped in the pericardium. The pericardiocentesis catheter is withdrawn, the tract is dilated with a 10F dilator, and a 10F to 12F sheath is inserted under fluoroscopy. A 20-mm-diameter by 3- to 4-cm-long dilating balloon (eg, Mansfield, Z-Med) is advanced over the guidewire. The balloon is positioned to straddle the pericardial border, and the sheath is withdrawn to uncover the balloon. The balloon is slightly inflated to define a waist at the parietal pericardial border as illustrated in **Figure 38.8**, and then fully expanded to create a rent in the pericardium. Depending on the stiffness of the pericardium, the balloon may "watermelon seed" into the pericardium and requires strong countertraction. In thin patients, the skin and subcutaneous tissues may need to be retracted inferiorly to avoid dilating through the skin. If the 20-mm balloon cannot

Table 38.3 Major and Minor Complications Following Echocardiography-Guided Pericardiocentesis in 1127 Procedures

Major complications	14 (1.2%)
Death	1 (0.09%)
Chamber laceration requiring surgery	5 (0.44%)
Injury to intercostal vessels requiring surgery	1 (0.09%)
Pneumothorax requiring chest tube	5 (0.44%)
Ventricular tachycardia	1 (0.09%)
Bacteremia	1 (0.09%)
Minor complications	40 (3.5%)
Chamber entry	11 (0.97%)
Small pneumothorax	8 (0.71%)
Pleuropericardial fistula	9 (0.8%)
Vasovagal reaction	2 (0.18%)
Nonsustained ventricular tachycardia	2 (0.18%)
Catheter occlusion	8 (0.71%)

Complications were deemed major if intervention was required. Minor complications were those that did not require intervention.
From Tsang TS, Enriquez-Sarano M, Freeman WK, et al. Consecutive 1127 therapeutic echocardiographically guided pericardiocenteses: clinical profile, practice patterns, and outcomes spanning 21 years. *Mayo Clin Proc.* 2002;77:429-436.

be successfully inflated, we have found that moving to a 12- or 18-mm balloon may allow dilation, with subsequent upsizing of the balloon to 20 to 22 mm in diameter. Balloon dilatation across the pericardium tends to cause severe pain, and adequate prophylactic narcotic analgesics should be administered prior to inflation to minimize discomfort.

The balloon is removed, the pericardial catheter is reintroduced, and about 10 mL of contrast may be injected to confirm free exit of fluid through the rent in the pericardium. Any remaining fluid is evacuated, and the catheter is left in place for drainage for 24 hours or until the catheter drainage is <50 mL/24 h. Sometimes more than 1 site must be dilated to ensure rapid emptying of the pericardial space, or balloon pericardiotomy may need to be repeated for recurrent tamponade. Chest roentgenography must be performed within 24 hours to evaluate for left pleural effusion, which is common, or pneumothorax, which is uncommon. Echocardiography should be performed 48 hours after catheter removal to confirm resolution of the pericardial effusion.

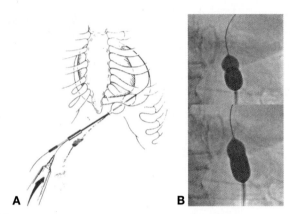

Figure 38.8 A, Illustration of the percutaneous balloon pericardiotomy technique. After partial drainage of the pericardium using a pericardial catheter, a 0.038-in stiff J-tip wire is introduced into the pericardial space. A 3-cm-long dilating balloon is then advanced over the guidewire to straddle the parietal pericardial membrane and is manually inflated to create a rent in the pericardium. **B,** Still frames from a percutaneous balloon pericardiotomy. (From Ziskind AA, Pearce AC, Lemmon CC, et al. Percutaneous balloon pericardiotomy for the treatment of cardiac tamponade and large pericardial effusions: description of technique and report of the first 50 cases. *J Am Coll Cardiol.* 1993;21:1-5.)

Modifications of the procedure include the use of a double-balloon technique and the use of the Inoue balloon catheter. With the double-balloon technique, 2 J-tip guidewires are advanced into the pericardial space through the same sheath after initial drainage of fluid. An 8- to 12-mm-diameter by 2-cm-long balloon and a second 8- to 12-mm-diameter by 4-cm-long balloon are advanced over the guidewires. The advantage of using 2 guidewires relates to the fact that the pericardial border can be identified as the point of separation of the 2 guidewires as they enter the pericardial space, thus facilitating positioning of the 2 balloons (**Figure 38.9**).

The Inoue balloon catheter is unique in that its inflation is sequential, that is, inflation of the distal portion is followed by inflation of the proximal portion. This sequential inflation dynamics can allow optimal positioning of the balloon across the pericardium. The technique requires inflating the distal portion of the balloon, pulling the balloon back against the parietal pericardium, and then full inflation, thus locking the pericardium in the middle of the balloon (**Figure 38.10**). In 11 patients who underwent Inoue balloon pericardiotomy for treatment of recurrent large effusion, the procedure was successful in 10 patients (91%), who remained free of recurrent effusion for a follow-up period of 4 months.

It has been established that balloon pericardiotomy causes drainage and absorption of fluid within the peritoneal cavity and the pleura. Given the experience with subxiphoid surgical pericardial window, it is unlikely that the communication between the pericardium and pleura or peritoneum produced by balloon pericardiotomy stays open for the long term as inflammatory fusion of the opposed parietal and visceral pericardium occurs over time and obliterates the potential space.

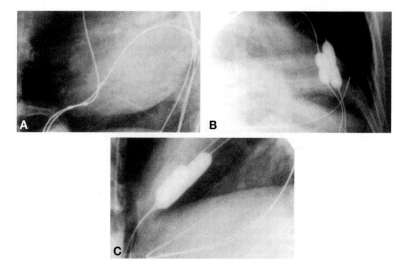

Figure 38.9 Double-balloon technique for balloon pericardiotomy. **A,** The pericardial border can be defined clearly as the 2 guidewires in the same tract separate from each other after entering the pericardial space. **B,** Double balloons are straddled over the pericardium and partially inflated, showing a central waist appearance. **C,** Fully expanded double balloons creating a pericardial window. (Reproduced with permission from Iaffaldano BA, Jones P, Lewis BE, et al. Percutaneous balloon pericardiotomy: a double balloon technique. *Cathet Cardiovasc Diagn.* 1995;36:79-81.)

THERAPEUTIC INTRAPERICARDIAL INTERVENTION AND EPICARDIAL ACCESS

There has been a significant development of the use of epicardial access for mapping and ablation of cardiac arrhythmias. Arrhythmogenic substrates have traditionally been approached endocardially with radiofrequency (RF) ablation procedures. Percutaneous epicardial access for the purpose of mapping and ablation of cardiac arrhythmias has now become an established and important adjunct and at times the

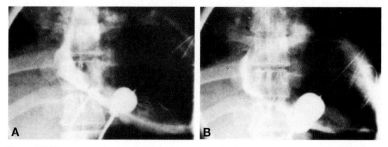

Figure 38.10 Anteroposterior projection showing Inoue balloon across the parietal pericardium during partial (A) and full (B) inflation over the coiled steel guidewire. Contrast medium has been instilled into the pericardial space. (Reproduced with permission from Bahl VK, Chandra S, Goel A, Goswami KC, Wasir HS. Versatility of Inoue balloon catheter. *Int J Cardiol.* 1997;59:75-83.)

preferred approach to eliminate certain cardiac arrhythmias. The prevalence of epicardial substrates responsible for tachyarrhythmias such as supraventricular tachycardia, atrial fibrillation, idiopathic ventricular tachycardia (VT), and scar-related VT has been confirmed. In addition, this approach is currently being considered for other cardiovascular applications such as left atrial appendage (LAA) occlusion.

Technical Aspects

Conceptually, entering the pericardial space is as simple as draining pericardial effusions. However, in the absence of an effusion, epicardial access can be intimidating since there is little room for error. The normal pericardial cavity contains only 15 to 35 mL of physiologic fluid. Thus, there is an increased risk of perforating the right ventricular (RV) wall and/or of damaging epicardial vessels when attempts are made to access the space percutaneously with a regular pericardiocentesis needle. In a series of 200 patients, a bleeding rate of 10% and "dry" RV puncture rate of 4.5% was reported. A step-by-step approach is illustrated in **Figure 38.11**.

After a 3-mm incision is made on the skin of the subxiphoid area using an 11-blade, a blunt-tipped epidural needle (Tuohy) designed to enter virtual spaces is routinely employed. The skin incision is often made to allow easy entry of the needle into the deeper tissues, and this also helps in transmitting the tactile sensation of various structures encountered on the way, especially the contracting walls of the heart. The needle is then advanced gently at an angle (depending on whether an anterior or inferior approach is required) aiming for the left scapula with the patient in the supine position. The preferred entry point is 2 to 3 cm below a line that joins the xiphoid process and the costal margin, left of the midline. Under fluoroscopic guidance, the needle is continually advanced until the operator can feel cardiac motion. X-ray can be deceiving, especially in single view. As the border of the heart is approached, small injections of contrast are made to delineate proximity to the pericardium.

It is preferable to perform percutaneous access after induction of general anesthesia as this allows to puncture during apnea, allowing for a more controlled puncture. Some operators prefer the use of conscious sedation to maximize the chance of

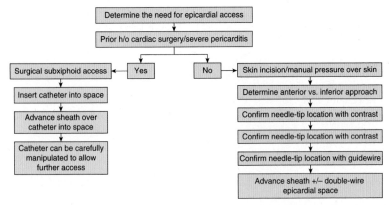

Figure 38.11 Percutaneous epicardial access: a step-by-step approach. As the needle is advanced toward the heart border, location of its tip is confirmed with small injections of contrast. h/o, history of.

arrhythmia induction. A small amount of contrast may then be injected to demonstrate entry of the needle into the pericardial space. Occasionally, the parietal pericardium can be stained and tenting of the pericardium can be seen before the needle suddenly enters the space. The appearance of layering of the contrast medium within the pericardial space indicates that the needle is correctly positioned within the pericardial cavity. This transition into the virtual space is usually accompanied by a sensation of "give," which is noted with experience.

Once within the pericardial space, a guidewire is passed through the needle. This step again allows confirmation of entry in the pericardial space. Occasionally, in some patients, cardiac motion and/or the sensation of "give" is difficult to perceive and direct entry into the RV cavity may occur inadvertently. In such cases, aspiration of blood or passage of the guidewire into the right ventricular outflow tract (RVOT) accompanied by salvoes of premature ventricular contractions indicates entry into the RV cavity. If this occurs, the needle should be slowly withdrawn a few millimeters and the guidewire pulled back into the needle tip and readvanced. This can be repeated until one gains entry into the pericardial space as opposed to withdrawing the needle entirely.

As a general rule, when the guidewire is advanced, it should slide unrestricted over the epicardial surface until it outlines the fluoroscopic entire heart border. This is usually achieved and confirmed in the left anterior oblique (LAO) view by advancing the guidewire, forcing it into a loop and observing the loop glide across the various chambers until it outlines the cardiac silhouette. Once the wire position within the pericardial space is confirmed beyond any doubt, the introducer and sheath are advanced over the wire under fluoroscopy maintaining adequate length of guidewire distal to the sheath tip. The introducer/guidewire is then removed and a standard ablation/pigtail catheter is advanced through the sheath and manipulated into the pericardial space. Double wiring of the epicardial space to avoid inadvertent loss of pericardial access during sheath manipulation is often helpful. The pigtail catheter is particularly useful to accurately assess the presence of hemopericardium as it has implications for subsequent anticoagulation with heparin.

The guidewire is always advanced under fluoroscopy typically in the anteroposterior (AP)/LAO projection (**Figure 38.12**). When the AP projection is chosen, it is difficult to discriminate whether the guidewire is actually in the pericardium along the lateral surface of the left ventricle or is instead being advanced into a dilated right ventricle and pulmonary artery. The operator can be sure that the guidewire is

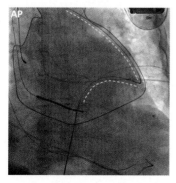

Figure 38.12 Anteroposterior (AP) view of guidewire through the epicardial needle during an anterior approach forming a large loop (white dashed line) that lies along the cardiac silhouette suggesting pericardial location.

wrapping around the heart only in the LAO projection. When it does occur, inadvertent RV puncture with the epidural needle or the guidewire does not cause severe complications. However, if the sheath is inadvertently advanced into the RV, surgical repair may be required to control the resulting hemopericardium. Thus, until the location of the guidewire is confirmed by fluoroscopic visualization in an LAO projection, the sheath should not be placed.

Special care should be taken when contrast is injected as it can obscure relevant fluoroscopic details if too much contrast is used. In this situation, the operator should consider waiting until the contrast dissipates allowing for clear visualization of the cardiac silhouette before attempting another puncture. Some operators try not to use contrast since if no contrast is used, the views are preserved. However, it can be difficult to confirm the correct access without contrast, using the current tools.

Contact forces on the epicardial surface can be suboptimal leading to ineffective RF lesion generation. Although soft-tip long vascular sheaths (eg, BRITE TIP, Johnson & Johnson) are often adequate in most situations, deflectable sheaths (Agilis EPI steerable sheath, St Jude Medical) can be used to enhance contact. An important measure when using sheaths is to ensure that the lumen of the sheath is always occupied either with an ablation catheter or a pigtail catheter so as to prevent the distal edge of the sheath from causing local trauma.

Anterior and Posterior Approach

Depending on the indication and/or the location of the potential ablation target, either an inferior or an anterior approach to pericardial puncture may be chosen. Typically, an inferior puncture allows for better mapping and ablation of the inferolateral wall of the ventricles and the posterior wall of the left atrium (LA) and for epicardial left ventricular lead placement. Conversely, an anterior puncture may be preferable when the anterior walls of the heart, such as the anterior RV or the left and right atrial appendages, are the target regions. When needle access is attempted in patients with history of prior cardiac surgery, posterior access may be chosen. In order to enter at the inferior surface of the pericardium, the puncture can be performed in LAO projection because it gives the operator a better view of the inferior wall of the heart. When an anterior puncture is chosen, the entry point should be 3 to 4 cm below the junction of the xiphoid appendage and the costal bone, and the needle should be advanced in a slightly shallow approach angle, often with gentle downward pressure to keep the left lobe of the liver away from the needle path. In this situation, the AP projection may facilitate visualization of the free wall of the right ventricle. When performing an epicardial LAA closure procedure, the anterior approach is mandatory and a more lateral angulation is preferred so as to approach the LAA with the catheters from a more favorable and stable position.

Fluoroscopic Navigation of the Epicardial Space

The right anterior oblique (RAO) and LAO positions project the heart in its anatomic sagittal and coronal planes such that, in RAO, the left and right sides are superimposed, but there is good atrioventricular differentiation, whereas in LAO, there is left-right differentiation, but the atria and ventricles are superimposed. A catheter placed in the coronary sinus marks the mitral valve annulus from the interatrial septum medially. These landmarks can be used to determine the position of the epicardial catheter as it is navigated within the pericardial space. Once a catheter is inserted into the pericardial space, it can be moved freely laterally, anteriorly, and inferiorly over various parts of the ventricle ranging from the RVOT to the posterior crux.

Damage to the coronary arteries during ablation is a major concern, particularly when it becomes necessary to ablate at the base of the heart or septum, for example, the case of accessory pathways that cannot otherwise be ablated with an endocardial or intravenous approach. Fluoroscopic identification of anatomic landmarks, supplemented by intracardiac catheters, including retrograde placement at the aortic root, will help avoid this.

The mitral and tricuspid annuli are intimately related to the major arteries and veins of the heart. The mitral annulus is outlined by the coronary sinus catheter, and the tricuspid annulus is identified by the endoluminal diagnostic quadripolar RV catheter, while the septum is defined fluoroscopically by the diagnostic catheter placed in the His-bundle area. Any remaining doubt regarding proximity to a coronary artery should prompt performing coronary angiography. Also it is important to appreciate the close relation of the RVOT to the proximal coronary arteries and distal coronary veins. The LAA is easily reachable and is the first atrial structure to be encountered when a catheter is advanced laterally and cranially; it is identifiable by the characteristic change in intracardiac electrograms. Understanding its fluoroscopic anatomy is important because of its proximity to the RVOT and the proximal coronary arterial system. It should be noted that the left ventricular outflow tract (LVOT) cannot be reached using this approach because it is covered by the RVOT anteriorly and the mitral valve or the LA posteriorly.

The blind-ending oblique sinus, its opening being bounded by the 2 inferior PVs, can be reached by passing the catheter superiorly behind the heart. Its importance in the contemporary practice of atrial arrhythmias ablation is related to its unique anatomic location behind the pulmonary venous atrium and the posterior left atrial wall. Within it rests the vein of Marshall, which can itself be a source of arrhythmia amenable to ablation. The esophagus is directly behind the LA and is vulnerable to thermal injury.

The transverse sinus lies superior to the oblique sinus and can be reached by passing the catheter around the lateral wall of the left ventricle and LA and then under the pulmonary arteries. It is of functional importance because a catheter placed at this site may ablate the roof of the LA or Bachmann bundle, both of which are important sites for certain atrial arrhythmias. It is intimately related to the aorta, which arches around it; the pulmonary arteries; and the LA. The floor of the transverse sinus is formed by the pericardial reflection between the right and left superior PVs, which separates it from the oblique sinus and the roof of the LA, which is the location of Bachmann's bundle. It allows access to the anterior LVOT as it communicates with the epicardial aspect of the noncoronary and right coronary aortic cusps via the inferior aortic recess. It also communicates with the SVC by way of the aortocaval sinus, a small virtual space between the SVC and the ascending aorta, which in some individuals is large enough to bypass with a catheter and reach the right heart border.

Complications of Epicardial Access

Pericarditis is the most common adverse event of epicardial procedures such as ablation or LAA closure. Adequate pain control immediately post procedure is required to minimize patient discomfort. Intrapericardial steroid injection at the end of the case can minimize the severity of pericarditis and either triamcinolone or methylprednisolone can be utilized.

Hemopericardium is a common adverse event seen with pericardial access, ranging from 5% up to 30% when accessing normal pericardial space. Pericardial bleeding can be categorized into early bleeding, bleeding during mapping, and bleeding at the end of the procedure. Right ventricular puncture/laceration, coronary vessel puncture/laceration, and/or adhesion disruption are common reasons for early hemopericardium. Bleb rupture, multiple punctures especially in the setting of anticoagulation, and steam pops with RF ablation can cause bleeding during mapping and ablation. Double right ventricular perforation could lead to extensive bleeding when the sheath is removed at the end of the case.

Prompt diagnosis, assessment of the extent of bleeding, and strategy for containing or fixing the cause are critical and can be lifesaving. As such, intracardiac echocardiography (ICE) plays a crucial role for identifying and managing this complication. ICE can identify the location of guidewire when gaining initial access. Inadvertent puncture of the right ventricle is easily diagnosed when the guidewire is seen in RV with ICE. Most bleeding with RV punctures from the access needle stop bleeding without any intervention as long as the sheath is not advanced over the guidewire into the RV. Lacerations are more likely to continue to bleed and require surgical intervention. Similarly, most small vessel punctures or adhesion disruptions also stop bleeding without major intervention other than aspiration of the blood from the pericardial space. Major vessel puncture or chamber laceration requires cardiac surgery or interventional cardiology. For these reasons, we recommend epicardial procedures to be done only when surgical backup is available. Each cardiac catheterization and electrophysiology laboratory needs to have rapid anticoagulation reversal and blood transfusion protocols in anticipation of potential major bleeding.

Conclusion

The percutaneous epicardial puncture technique is now well established and has been embraced by electrophysiologists owing to the importance of epicardial substrate for arrhythmia ablation and other interventional procedures such as percutaneous LAA occlusion. In experienced hands, it has a low complication rate. It is important to note that this safety profile reflects practices at centers that specialize in arrhythmia management and may not be applicable to less experienced operators or centers. With up to a 20% risk for ventricular perforation, careful patient selection is important, and the procedure should be performed solely by experienced operators with surgical backup.

SUGGESTED READINGS

1. Bernal JM, Pradhan J, Li T, Tchokonte R, Afonso L. Acute pulmonary edema following pericardiocentesis for cardiac tamponade. *Can J Cardiol.* 2007;23(14):1155-1156.
2. Bruce CJ, Stanton CM, Asirvatham SJ, et al. Percutaneous epicardial left atrial appendage closure: intermediate-term results. *J Cardiovasc Electrophysiol.* 2011;22(1):64-70.
3. Chow WH, Chow TC, Cheung KL. Nonsurgical creation of a pericardial window using the Inoue balloon catheter. *Am Heart J.* 1992;124(4):1100-1102.
4. Fujita M, Ikemoto M, Kishishita M, et al. Elevated basic fibroblast growth factor in pericardial fluid of patients with unstable angina. *Circulation.* 1996;94(4):610-613.
5. Hammond HK, White FC, Bhargava V, Shabetai R. Heart size and maximal cardiac output are limited by the pericardium. *Am J Physiol.* 1992;263(6 Pt 2):H1675-H1681.
6. Horkay F, Szokodi I, Selmeci L, et al. Presence of immunoreactive endothelin-1 and atrial natriuretic peptide in human pericardial fluid. *Life Sci.* 1998;62(3):267-274.
7. Iaffaldano RA, Jones P, Lewis BE, Eleftheriades EG, Johnson SA, McKiernan TL. Percutaneous balloon pericardiotomy: a double balloon technique. *Cathet Cardiovasc Diagn.* 1995;36(1):79-81.
8. Imazio M, Spodick DH, Brucato A, Trinchero R, Adler Y. Controversial issues in the management of pericardial diseases. *Circulation.* 2010;121(7):916-928.

9. Isselbacher EM, Cigarroa JE, Eagle KA. Cardiac tamponade complicating aortic dissection: is pericardiocentesis harmful?. *Circulation.* 1994;90(5):2375-2378.

10. Laham R, Simons M, Hung D. Subxyphoid access of the normal pericardium: a novel drug delivery technique. *Cathet Cardiovasc Diagn.* 1999;47(1):109-111.

11. Landau C, Jacobs AK, Haudenschild CC. Intrapericardial basic fibroblast growth factor induces myocardial angiogenesis in a rabbit model of chronic ischemia. *Am Heart J.* 1993;129:924-931.

12. Mannam AP, Ho KK, Cultip DE, et al. Safety of subxyphoid pericardial access using a blunt-tip needle. *Am J Cardiol.* 2002;89(7):891-893.

13. Reddy VY, Neuzil P, Ruskin JN. Extra-ostial pulmonary venous isolation: use of epicardial ablation to eliminate a point of conduction breakthrough. *J Cardiovasc Electrophysiol.* 2003;14(6):663-666.

14. Sacher F, Roberts-Thomson K, Maury P, et al. Epicardial ventricular tachycardia ablation: a multicenter safety study. *J Am Coll Cardiol.* 2010;55(21):2366-2372.

15. Soejima K, Couper G, Cooper JM, Sapp JL, Epstein LM, Stevenson WG. Subxiphoid surgical approach for epicardial catheter-based mapping and ablation in patients with prior cardiac surgery or difficult pericardial access. *Circulation.* 2004;110(10):1197-1201.

16. Sosa E, Scanavacca M, d'Avila A, et al. Endocardial and epicardial ablation guided by nonsurgical transthoracic epicardial mapping to treat recurrent ventricular tachycardia. *J Cardiovasc Electrophysiol.* 1998;9(3):229-239.

17. Sosa E, Scanavacca M, d'Avila A, Oliveira F, Ramires JA. Nonsurgical transthoracic epicardial catheter ablation to treat recurrent ventricular tachycardia occurring late after myocardial infarction. *J Am Coll Cardiol.* 2000;35(6):1442-1449.

18. Spodick DH. *The Pericardium, a Comprehensive Textbook.* Marcel Dekker; 1997.

19. Syed F, Lachman N, Christensen K, et al. The pericardial space: obtaining access and an approach to fluoroscopic anatomy. *Card Electrophysiol Clin.* 2010;2(1):9-23.

20. Tsang TSM, Freeman WK, Sinak LJ, Seward JB. Echocardiographically guided pericardiocentesis: evolution and state of the art technique. *Mayo Clin Proc.* 1998;73(7):647-652.

21. Tsang TS, Enriquez-Sarano M, Freeman WK, et al. Consecutive 1127 therapeutic echocardiographically guided pericardiocenteses: clinical profile, practice patterns, and outcomes spanning 21 years. *Mayo Clin Proc.* 2002;77(5):429-436.

22. Tsang SM, Barnes ME, Gersh BJ, Bailey KR, Seward JB. Outcomes of clinically significant idiopathic pericardial effusion requiring intervention. *Am J Cardiol.* 2003;91(6):704-707.

23. Tyberg JV, Smith ER. Ventricular diastole and the role of the pericardium. *Hertz.* 1999;15:354-361.

24. Uemura S, Kagoshima T, Hashimoto T, et al. Acute left ventricular failure with pulmonary edema following pericardiocentesis for cardiac tamponade—a case report. *Jpn Circ J.* 1995;59(1):55-59.

25. Vaitkus PT, Herrmann HC, LeWinter MM. Treatment of malignant pericardial effusion. *J Am Med Assoc.* 1994;272(1):59-64.

26. Wolfe MW, Edelman ER. Transient systolic dysfunction after relief of cardiac tamponade. *Ann Intern Med.* 1993;119(1):42-44.

27. Ziskind AA, Pearce AC, Lemmon CC, et al. Percutaneous balloon pericardiotomy for the treatment of cardiac tamponade and large pericardial effusions: description of technique and report of the first 50 cases. *J Am Coll Cardiol.* 1993;21:1-5.

28. Ziskind AA, Lemmon CC, Rodriguez S, et al. Final report of the percutaneous balloon pericardiotomy registry for the treatment for effusive pericardial disease. *Circulation.* 1994;90(suppl I):1-21.

Note: Pages followed by b, t, or f refer to boxes, tables, or figures, respectively.